W9-BOM-964

http://connection.LWW.com

Get Connected!

Connect to a one-of-a-kind educational resource!

connection

Register in 3 easy steps...

1. Visit the connection website and click log- on...
2. Set up a new user profile
3. Enter your name and e-mail address, and create a user name and password.

With registration you'll receive email notification whenever this site is updated.

Resource Centers include

for Faculty...

• Guidelines for teaching research

for Students....

• Guidelines for critiquing research
• Quick Review Charts

Connect today.
http://connection.LWW.com/go/polit

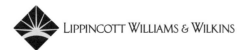
LIPPINCOTT WILLIAMS & WILKINS

G452-01   N1NXG452

Nursing Research: Principles and Methods

Seventh Edition

Denise F. Polit, PhD
President
Humanalysis, Inc
Saratoga Springs, New York

Adjunct Professor
Research Centre for Clinical Practice Innovation
Griffith University School of Nursing
Gold Coast, Queensland, Australia

Cheryl Tatano Beck, DNSc, CNM, FAAN
Professor
School of Nursing
University of Connecticut
Storrs, Connecticut

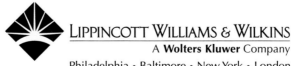

LIPPINCOTT WILLIAMS & WILKINS
A **Wolters Kluwer** Company
Philadelphia • Baltimore • New York • London
Buenos Aires • Hong Kong • Sydney • Tokyo

Acquisitions Editor: Margaret Zuccarini
Managing Editor: Barclay Cunningham
Editorial Assistant: Helen Kogut
Senior Production Manager: Helen Ewan
Managing Editor/ Production: Erika Kors
Design Coordinator: Brett MacNaughton
Cover Designer: Armen Kojoyian
Interior Designer: B. J. Crim
Manufacturing Manager: William Alberti
Compositor: TechBooks
Printer: R. R. Donnelly/Willard

7th Edition

Library of Congress Cataloging-in-Publication Data

Polit, Denise F.
   Nursing research: principles and methods / Denise F. Polit, Cheryl Tatano Beck.—7th ed.
      p.; cm.
   Includes bibliographical references and index.
   ISBN 0-7817-3733-8 (alk. paper)
      1. Nursing—Research—Methodology.   I. Beck, Cheryl Tatano.   II. Title.
   [DNLM: 1. Nursing Research—methods. WY 20.5 P769n 2003]
RT81.5.P64 2003
610.73'072—dc21

                                                        2002043422

Care has been taken to confirm the accuracy of the information presented and to describe generally accepted practices. However, the authors, editors, and publisher are not responsible for errors or omissions or for any consequences from application of the information in this book and make no warranty, express or implied, with respect to the content of the publication.

The authors, editors, and publisher have exerted every effort to ensure that drug selection and dosage set forth in this text are in accordance with the current recommendations and practice at the time of publication. However, in view of ongoing research, changes in government regulations, and the constant flow of information relating to drug therapy and drug reactions, the reader is urged to check the package insert for each drug for any change in indications and dosage and for added warnings and precautions. This is particularly important when the recommended agent is a new or infrequently employed drug.

Some drugs and medical devices presented in this publication have Food and Drug Administration (FDA) clearance for limited use in restricted research settings. It is the responsibility of the health care provider to ascertain the FDA status of each drug or device planned for use in his or her clinical practice.

TO DOROTHY

IN LOVING MEMORY OF DOROTHY
her charm, her extraordinary wit,
her strength, and her love
were inspirational.

PREFACE

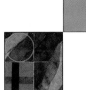

This seventh edition of *Nursing Research: Principles and Methods* presents many important changes to this textbook. This edition retains the features that have made this an award-winning textbook, while introducing revisions that will make it more relevant in an environment that is increasingly focused on evidence-based nursing practice.

New to This Edition

- **Emphasis on producing and evaluating research evidence.** This edition focuses more squarely on the fact that research is an evidence-building enterprise. We stress throughout that the decisions researchers make in designing and implementing a study have implications for the quality of evidence the study yields—and that the quality of evidence affects the utility of study findings for nursing practice. We have also expanded the final chapter on using research in an evidence-based nursing practice.

- **Expanded coverage of qualitative research methods.** As in the sixth edition, this textbook discusses the methods associated with naturalistic inquiries (qualitative studies) in a manner roughly parallel to the description of methods more typically used in traditional scientific research (quantitative studies). This edition, which is coauthored by a prominent qualitative nurse researcher, goes even further than previous ones in offering assistance to those embarking on a qualitative research project. For example,

differences in the approaches used by grounded theory researchers, phenomenologists, and ethnographers are noted throughout.

- **Better "how to" assistance.** There are even more "how to" tips in this edition than in previous ones, with many new ones aimed at qualitative researchers. Moreover, these tips are interspersed throughout the text rather than clustered at the end, which not only places them in more relevant locations, but also makes for a livelier presentation.

- **Improved readability.** This textbook has been widely hailed for its clear, concise, and "user-friendly" presentation. In this edition, however, we have gone to great lengths to write in an even simpler, more straightforward fashion, in recognition of the fact that research methods are an inherently complex topic. Additionally, the readability of the text is enhanced by several visual features, such as the use of a new, full-color design.

- **Greater acknowledgment of international efforts.** This edition gives better recognition to the contributions of nurse researchers from around the globe.

Organization of the Text

The content of this edition is organized into seven main parts.

- **Part I—Foundations of Nursing Research** introduces fundamental concepts in nursing research. Chapter 1 summarizes the history and future of nursing research, introduces the topic of using research evidence for nursing practice, discusses the philosophical underpinnings of qualitative research versus quantitative research, and describes the major purposes of nursing research. Chapter 2 introduces readers to key terms, with new emphasis on terms related to the quality of research evidence. Chapter 3 presents an overview of steps in the research process for both qualitative and quantitative studies.

- **Part II—Conceptualizing a Research Study** further sets the stage for learning about the research process by discussing issues relating to a study's conceptualization: the formulation of research questions and hypotheses (Chapter 4); the review of relevant research (Chapter 5); and the development of theoretical and conceptual contexts (Chapter 6).
- **Part III—Designs for Nursing Research** presents material on the design of qualitative and quantitative nursing research studies. Chapter 7 discusses issues important to the design of research that is ethically sound. Chapter 8 describes fundamental principles and applications of quantitative research design, while Chapter 9 describes mechanisms of research control for quantitative studies. Chapter 10 examines quantitative research with different purposes. Chapter 11 is devoted to research designs for qualitative studies, with new material added on critical theory, feminist, and participatory action research. Chapter 12 discusses mixed method research designs in which methods for qualitative and quantitative inquiry are blended. Chapter 13 presents designs and strategies for selecting samples of study participants.
- **Part IV—Measurement and Data Collection** deals with the gathering of information in a study. Chapter 14 discusses the overall data collection plan, and the subsequent three chapters present materials on specific data collection methods such as self-reports (Chapter 15), observation (Chapter 16), and biophysiologic and other methods (Chapter 17). Chapter 18 discusses the concept of measurement, and then focuses on methods of assessing data quality.

- **Part V—The Analysis of Research Data** discusses methods of analyzing qualitative and quantitative data. Chapters 19, 20, and 21 present an overview of univariate, inferential, and multivariate statistical analyses, respectively. Chapter 22 describes the development of an overall analytic strategy for quantitative studies. Chapter 23 discusses methods of doing qualitative analyses, with specific information about grounded theory, phenomenologic, and ethnographic analyses.
- **Part VI—Communicating Research** focuses on two types of research communication. Chapter 24 discusses how to write about research and, greatly expanded in this edition, how to publish a research report and prepare a thesis or dissertation. Chapter 25 offers suggestions and guidelines on preparing research proposals.
- **Part VII—Using Research Results** is intended to sharpen the critical awareness of nurses with regard to the use of research findings by practicing nurses. Chapter 26 discusses the interpretation and appraisal of research reports. The concluding chapter (Chapter 27) offers suggestions on utilizing research to build an evidence-based practice, and includes guidance on performing integrative reviews.

Key Features

This textbook was designed to be helpful to those who are learning how to do research, as well as to the growing number of nurses who are learning to appraise research reports critically and to use research findings in practice. Many of the features successfully used in previous editions have been retained in this seventh edition. Among the basic principles that helped to shape this and earlier editions of this book are (1) an unswerving conviction that the development of research skills is critical to the nursing profession; (2) a fundamental belief that research is an intellectually and professionally rewarding enterprise; and (3) a judgment that learning about research methods need be neither intimidating nor dull. Consistent with these principles, we have tried to present the fundamentals of research methods in a way that both facilitates understanding and arouses curiosity and interest. Key features of our approach include the following:

- **Research Examples.** Each chapter concludes with one or two actual research examples (usually one quantitative and one qualitative study) designed to highlight critical points made in the chapter and to sharpen the reader's critical thinking skills. In addition, many research examples are used to illustrate key points in the text and to stimulate students' thinking about a research project.
- **Clear, "user friendly" style.** Our writing style is designed to be easily digestible and nonintimidating. Concepts are introduced carefully and systematically, difficult ideas are presented clearly and from several vantage points, and readers are assumed to have no prior exposure to technical terms.
- **Specific practical tips on doing research.** The textbook is filled with practical guidance on how to translate the abstract notions of research methods into realistic strategies for conducting research. Every chapter includes several tips for applying the chapter's lessons to real-life situations. The inclusion of these suggestions acknowledges the fact that there is often a large gap between what gets taught in research methods textbooks and what a researcher needs to know in conducting a study.
- **Aids to student learning.** Several features are used to enhance and reinforce learning and to help focus the student's attention on specific areas of text content, including the following: succinct, bulleted summaries at the end of each chapter; tables and figures that provide examples and graphic materials in support of the text discussion; study suggestions at the end of each chapter; and suggested methodologic and substantive readings for each chapter.

Teaching-Learning Package

Nursing Research: Principles and Methods, seventh edition, has an ancillary package designed with both students and instructors in mind.

- **The Study Guide** augments the textbook and provides students with exercises that correspond to each text chapter. Answers to selected exercises are included at the end of the Study Guide. The Study Guide also includes two actual research reports that students can read, analyze, and critique.
- Free CD-ROM: The Study Guide also includes a CD-ROM providing hundreds of review questions to assist students in self-testing. This review program provides a rationale for both correct and incorrect answers, helping students to identify areas of strength and areas needing further study.
- **The Instructor's Resource CD-ROM** includes a chapter corresponding to every chapter in the textbook. Each chapter of the Instructor's Manual contains a statement of intent, student objectives, new terms in the chapter, comments on selected research examples in the textbook, answers to certain Study Guide exercises, and test questions (true/false and multiple choice) and answers. New to this edition are PowerPoint slides summarizing key points in each chapter, and test questions have been placed into a program that allows instructors to automatically generate a test complete with instructions and an answer key. A gradebook is also included in this program.

It is our hope that the content, style, and organization of this book continue to meet the needs of a broad spectrum of nursing students and nurse researchers. We also hope that the book will help to foster enthusiasm for the kinds of discoveries that research can produce, and for the knowledge that will help support an evidence-based nursing practice.

DENISE F. POLIT, PHD

CHERYL TATANO BECK, DNSC, CNM, FAAN

ACKNOWLEDGMENTS

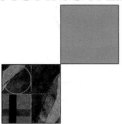

This seventh edition, like the previous six editions, depended on the contribution of many individuals. We are deeply appreciative of those who made all seven editions possible. In addition to all those who assisted us with the earlier editions, the following individuals deserve special mention.

Many faculty and students who used the text during the past 25 years have made invaluable suggestions for its improvement, and to all of you we are very grateful. In particular, we would like to acknowledge the comments of ten reviewers of the previous edition, whose feedback guided our revisions. We would also like to acknowledge the valuable contributions of David Garnes and Jill Livingston, reference librarians at the University of Connecticut, to Chapter 5. Mary Ann Cordeau's thoughtful review of Chapter 11 strengthened our historical research section. Finally, we are grateful for the insights of Dr. Robert Gable regarding instrument development in Chapter 18.

We also extend our warmest thanks to those who helped to turn the manuscript into a finished product. The staff at Lippincott Williams & Wilkins has been of tremendous assistance in the support they have given us over the years. We are indebted to Margaret Zuccarini, Barclay Cunningham, Helen Kogut, Erika Kors, and all the others behind the scenes for their fine contributions.

Finally, we thank our family, our loved ones, and our friends, who provided ongoing support and encouragement throughout this endeavor.

REVIEWERS

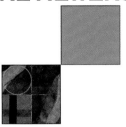

Eileen Chasens, DSN, RN
Assistant Professor
Wayne State University
Detroit, Michigan

Celia R. Colon-Rivera, RN, PhD
Professor
University of Puerto Rico-Mayaguez Campus
Mayaguez, Puerto Rico

Carol Cornwell, PhD, MS, CS
Director of Nursing Research and
Assistant Professor of Nursing
Georgia Southern University School of Nursing
Statesboro, Georgia

Linda Goodfellow, RN, MNEd
Assistant Professor of Nursing
Duquesne University
Pittsburgh, Pennsylvania

Janice S. Hayes, PhD, RN
Associate Professor
Florida Atlantic University College of Nursing
Davie, Florida

Joan R. S. McDowell, MN
Lecturer
University of Glaston
Nursing & Midwifery School
Glasgow, Scotland

Virginia Nehring, PhD, RN
Associate Professor
Wright State University
Dayton, Ohio

Marlene Reimer, RN, PhD, CNN(C)
Associate Professor
Faculty of Nursing
University of Calgary
Calgary, Alberta, Canada

Beth L. Rodgers, PhD, RN
Professor and Chair, Foundations of
Nursing Department
University of Wisconsin-Milwaukee
School of Nursing
Milwaukee, Wisconsin

Janet S. Secrest, PhD, RN
Assistant Professor
University of Tennessee at Chattanooga
School of Nursing
Chattanooga, Tennessee

Gloria Weber, PhD, RN, CNAA
Associate Professor
The University of Texas at Tyler
College of Nursing
Tyler, Texas

CONTENTS

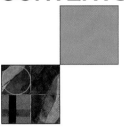

PART 3
Designs for
Nursing Research   139

PART

1

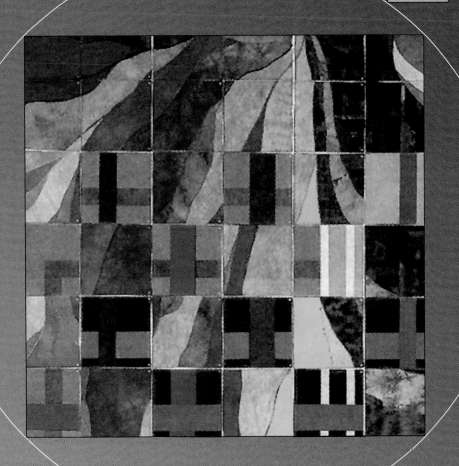

Foundations
of Nursing
Research

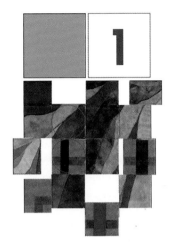

Introduction to Nursing Research

NURSING RESEARCH IN PERSPECTIVE

It is an exciting—and challenging—time to be a nurse. Nurses are managing their clinical responsibilities at a time when the nursing profession and the larger health care system require an extraordinary range of skills and talents of them. Nurses are expected to deliver the highest possible quality of care in a compassionate manner, while also being mindful of costs. To accomplish these diverse (and sometimes conflicting) goals, nurses must access and evaluate extensive clinical information, and incorporate it into their clinical decision-making. In today's world, *nurses must become lifelong learners,* capable of reflecting on, evaluating, and modifying their clinical practice based on new knowledge. And, nurses are increasingly expected to become producers of new knowledge through nursing research.

What Is Nursing Research?

Research is systematic inquiry that uses disciplined methods to answer questions or solve problems. The ultimate goal of research is to develop, refine, and expand a body of knowledge.

Nurses are increasingly engaged in disciplined studies that benefit the profession and its patients, and that contribute to improvements in the entire health care system. **Nursing research** is systematic inquiry designed to develop knowledge about issues of importance to the nursing profession, including nursing practice, education, administration, and informatics. In this book, we emphasize **clinical nursing research**, that is, research designed to generate knowledge to guide nursing practice and to improve the health and quality of life of nurses' clients.

Nursing research has experienced remarkable growth in the past three decades, providing nurses with an increasingly sound base of knowledge from which to practice. Yet as we proceed into the 21st century, many questions endure and much remains to be done to incorporate research-based knowledge into nursing practice.

 Examples of nursing research questions:

- What are the factors that determine the length of stay of patients in the intensive care unit undergoing coronary artery bypass graft surgery (Doering, Esmailian, Imperial-Perez, & Monsein, 2001)?
- How do adults with acquired brain injury perceive their social interactions and relationships (Paterson & Stewart, 2002)?

The Importance of Research in Nursing

Nurses increasingly are expected to adopt an **evidence-based practice (EBP)**, which is broadly defined as the use of the best clinical evidence in making patient care decisions. Although there is not a consensus about what types of "evidence" are appropriate for EBP (Goode, 2000), there is general agreement that research findings from rigorous studies constitute the best type of evidence for informing nurses' decisions, actions, and interactions with clients. Nurses are accepting the need to base specific nursing actions and decisions on evidence indicating that the actions are clinically appropriate, cost-effective, and result in positive outcomes for clients. Nurses who incorporate high-quality research evidence into their clinical decisions and advice are being professionally accountable to their clients. They are also reinforcing the identity of nursing as a profession.

Another reason for nurses to engage in and use research involves the spiraling costs of health care and the cost-containment practices being instituted in health care facilities. Now, more than ever, nurses need to document the social relevance and effectiveness of their practice, not only to the profession but to nursing care consumers, health care administrators, third-party payers (e.g., insurance companies), and government agencies. Some research findings will help eliminate nursing actions that do not achieve desired outcomes. Other findings will help nurses identify practices that improve health care outcomes and contain costs as well.

Nursing research is essential if nurses are to understand the varied dimensions of their profession. Research enables nurses to describe the characteristics of a particular nursing situation about which little is known; to explain phenomena that must be considered in planning nursing care; to predict the probable outcomes of certain nursing decisions; to control the occurrence of undesired outcomes; and to initiate activities to promote desired client behavior.

 Example of an EBP project:

• The Association of Women's Health, Obstetric, and Neonatal Nurses (AWHONN) is one nursing organization that has demonstrated a strong commitment to evidence-based nursing practice. For example, AWHONN undertook a project that developed and tested an evidence-based protocol for urinary incontinence in women, and then designed procedures to facilitate the protocol's implementation into clinical practice (Samselle et al., 2000a, 2000b). More recently, AWHONN and the National Association of Neonatal Nurses designed and tested an evidence-based protocol for neonatal skin care, and also instituted procedures for implementing it (Lund, Kuller, Lane, Lott, Raines, & Thomas, 2001; Lund, Osborne, Kuller, Lane, Lott, & Raines, 2001).

The Consumer–Producer Continuum in Nursing Research

With the current emphasis on EBP, it has become *every* nurse's responsibility to engage in one or more roles along a continuum of research participation. At one end of the continuum are those nurses whose involvement in research is indirect. **Consumers of nursing research** read research reports to develop new skills and to keep up to date on relevant findings that may affect their practice. Nurses increasingly are expected to maintain this level of involvement with research, at a minimum. **Research utilization**—the use of research findings in a practice setting—depends on intelligent nursing research consumers.

At the other end of the continuum are the **producers of nursing research:** nurses who actively participate in designing and implementing research studies. At one time, most nurse researchers were academics who taught in schools of nursing, but research is increasingly being conducted by practicing nurses who want to find what works best for their patients.

Between these two end points on the continuum lie a rich variety of research activities in which nurses engage as a way of improving their effectiveness and enhancing their professional lives. These activities include the following:

- Participating in a **journal club** in a practice setting, which involves regular meetings among nurses to discuss and critique research articles
- Attending research presentations at professional conferences
- Discussing the implications and relevance of research findings with clients
- Giving clients information and advice about participation in studies
- Assisting in the collection of research information (e.g., distributing questionnaires to patients)
- Reviewing a proposed research plan with respect to its feasibility in a clinical setting and offering clinical expertise to improve the plan
- Collaborating in the development of an idea for a clinical research project
- Participating on an institutional committee that reviews the ethical aspects of proposed research before it is undertaken
- Evaluating completed research for its possible use in practice, and using it when appropriate

In all these activities, nurses with some research skills are in a better position than those without them to make a contribution to nursing knowledge. An understanding of nursing research can improve the depth and breadth of *every* nurse's professional practice.

NURSING RESEARCH: PAST, PRESENT, AND FUTURE

Although nursing research has not always had the prominence and importance it enjoys today, its long and interesting history portends a distinguished future. Table 1-1 summarizes some of the key events in the historical evolution of nursing research.

The Early Years: From Nightingale to the 1950s

Most people would agree that research in nursing began with Florence Nightingale. Her landmark publication, *Notes on Nursing* (1859), describes her early interest in environmental factors that promote physical and emotional well-being—an interest that continues among nurses nearly 150 years later. Nightingale's most widely known research contribution involved her data collection and analysis relating to factors affecting soldier mortality and morbidity during the Crimean War. Based on her skillful analyses and presentations, she was successful in effecting some changes in nursing care—and, more generally, in public health.

For many years after Nightingale's work, the nursing literature contained little research. Some attribute this absence to the apprenticeship nature of nursing. The pattern of nursing research that eventually emerged at the turn of the century was closely aligned to the problems confronting nurses. Most studies conducted between 1900 and 1940 concerned nurses' education. For example, in 1923, a group called the Committee for the Study of Nursing Education studied the educational preparation of nurse teachers, administrators, and public health nurses and the clinical experiences of nursing students. The committee issued what has become known as the Goldmark Report, which identified many inadequacies in the educational backgrounds of the groups studied and concluded that advanced educational preparation was essential. As more nurses received university-based education, studies concerning nursing students—their differential characteristics, problems, and satisfactions—became more numerous.

During the 1940s, studies concerning nursing education continued, spurred on by the unprecedented demand for nursing personnel that resulted from World War II. For example, Brown (1948) reassessed nursing education in a study initiated at the request of the National Nursing Council for War Service. The findings from the study, like those of the Goldmark Report, revealed numerous inadequacies in nursing education. Brown recommended that the education of nurses occur in collegiate settings. Many subsequent research investigations concerning the functions performed by nurses, nurses' roles and attitudes, hospital environments, and nurse—patient interactions stemmed from the Brown report.

TABLE 1.1 Historical Landmarks Affecting Nursing Research

YEAR	EVENT
1859	Nightingale's *Notes on Nursing* published
1900	*American Nursing Journal* begins publication
1923	Columbia University establishes first doctoral program for nurses Goldmark Report with recommendations for nursing education published
1930s	*American Journal of Nursing* publishes clinical cases studies
1948	Brown publishes report on inadequacies of nursing education
1952	The journal *Nursing Research* begins publication
1955	Inception of the American Nurses' Foundation to sponsor nursing research
1957	Establishment of nursing research center at Walter Reed Army Institute of Research
1963	*International Journal of Nursing Studies* begins publication
1965	American Nurses' Association (ANA) begins sponsoring nursing research conferences
1966	Nursing history archive established at Mugar Library, Boston University
1968	*Canadian Journal of Nursing Research* begins publication
1971	ANA establishes a Commission on Research
1972	ANA establishes its Council of Nurse Researchers
1976	Stetler and Marram publish guidelines on assessing research for use in practice
1978	The journals *Research in Nursing & Health* and *Advances in Nursing Science* begin publication
1979	*Western Journal of Nursing Research* begins publication
1982	The Conduct and Utilization of Research in Nursing (CURN) project publishes report
1983	*Annual Review of Nursing Research* begins publication
1985	ANA Cabinet on Nursing Research establishes research priorities
1986	National Center for Nursing Research (NCNR) established within U.S. National Institutes of Health
1987	The journal *Scholarly Inquiry for Nursing Practice* begins publication
1988	The journals *Applied Nursing Research* and *Nursing Science Quarterly* begin publication Conference on Research Priorities (CORP #1) in convened by NCNR
1989	U.S. Agency for Health Care Policy and Research (AHCPR) is established
1992	The journal *Clinical Nursing Research* begins publication
1993	NCNR becomes a full institute, the National Institute of Nursing Research (NINR) CORP #2 is convened to establish priorities for 1995–1999 The Cochrane Collaboration is established The journal *Journal of Nursing Measurement* begins publication
1994	The journal *Qualitative Health Research* begins publication
1997	Canadian Health Services Research Foundation is established with federal funding
1999	AHCPR is renamed Agency for Healthcare Research and Quality (AHRQ)
2000	NINR issues funding priorities for 2000–2004; annual funding exceeds $100 million The Canadian Institute of Health Research is launched The journal *Biological Research for Nursing* begins publication

A number of forces combined during the 1950s to put nursing research on a rapidly accelerating upswing. An increase in the number of nurses with advanced educational degrees, the establishment of a nursing research center at the Walter Reed Army Institute of Research, an increase in the availability of funds from the government and private foundations, and the inception of the American Nurses' Foundation—which is devoted exclusively to the promotion of nursing research—were forces providing impetus to nursing research during this period.

Until the 1950s, nurse researchers had few outlets for reporting their studies to the nursing community. The *American Journal of Nursing*, first published in 1900, began on a limited basis to publish some studies in the 1930s. The increasing number of studies being conducted during the 1950s, however, created the need for a journal in which findings could be published; thus, *Nursing Research* came into being in 1952.

Nursing research took a twist in the 1950s not experienced by research in other professions, at least not to the same extent as in nursing. Nurses studied themselves: Who is the nurse? What does the nurse do? Why do individuals choose to enter nursing? What are the characteristics of the ideal nurse? How do other groups perceive the nurse?

Nursing Research in the 1960s

Knowledge development through research in nursing began in earnest only about 40 years ago, in the 1960s. Nursing leaders began to express concern about the lack of research in nursing practice. Several professional nursing organizations, such as the Western Interstate Council for Higher Education in Nursing, established priorities for research investigations during this period. Practice-oriented research on various clinical topics began to emerge in the literature.

The 1960s was the period during which terms such as *conceptual framework, conceptual model, nursing process,* and *theoretical base of nursing practice* began to appear in the literature and to influence views about the role of theory in nursing research. Funding continued to be available both for the educational preparation of nurses and, increasingly, for nursing research.

Nursing research began to advance worldwide in the 1960s. The *International Journal of Nursing Studies* began publication in 1963, and the *Canadian Journal of Nursing Research* was first published in 1968.

 Example of nursing research breakthroughs in the 1960s:

- Jeanne Quint Benoliel began a program of research that had a major impact on medicine, medical sociology, and nursing. Quint explored the subjective experiences of patients after diagnosis with a life-threatening illness (1967). Of particular note, physicians in the early 1960s usually did not advise women that they had breast cancer, even after a mastectomy. Quint's (1962, 1963) seminal study of the personal experiences of women after radical mastectomy contributed to changes in communication and information control by physicians and nurses.

Nursing Research in the 1970s

By the 1970s, the growing number of nurses conducting research studies and the discussions of theoretical and contextual issues surrounding nursing research created the need for additional communication outlets. Several additional journals that focus on nursing research were established in the 1970s, including *Advances in Nursing Science, Research in Nursing & Health*, the *Western Journal of Nursing Research*, and the *Journal of Advanced Nursing*.

In the 1970s, there was a decided change in emphasis in nursing research from areas such as teaching, curriculum, and nurses themselves to the improvement of client care—signifying a growing awareness by nurses of the need for a scientific base from which to practice. Nursing leaders strongly endorsed this direction for nursing studies. Lindeman (1975), for example, conducted a study to ascertain the views of nursing leaders concerning the focus of nursing studies; clinical problems were identified as the highest priorities. Nurses also began to pay attention to the utilization of research findings in nursing practice. A seminal article by Stetler and Marram (1976) offered guidance on assessing research for application in practice settings.

In the United States, research skills among nurses continued to improve in the 1970s. The cadre of nurses with earned doctorates steadily increased, especially during the later 1970s. The availability of both predoctoral and postdoctoral research fellowships facilitated the development of advanced research skills.

 Example of nursing research breakthroughs in the 1970s:

• Kathryn Barnard's research led to breakthroughs in the area of neonatal and young child development. Her research program focused on the identification and assessment of children at risk of developmental and health problems, such as abused and neglected children and failure-to-thrive children (Barnard, 1973, 1976; Barnard & Collar, 1973; Barnard, Wenner, Weber, Gray, & Peterson, 1977). Her research contributed to work on early interventions for children with disabilities, and also to the field of developmental psychology.

Nursing Research in the 1980s

The 1980s brought nursing research to a new level of development. An increase in the number of qualified nurse researchers, the widespread availability of computers for the collection and analysis of information, and an ever-growing recognition that research is an integral part of professional nursing led nursing leaders to raise new issues and concerns. More attention was paid to the types of questions being asked, the methods of collecting and analyzing information being used, the linking of research to theory, and the utilization of research findings in practice.

Several events provided impetus for nursing research in this decade. For example, the first volume of the *Annual Review of Nursing Research* was published in 1983. These annual reviews include summaries of current research knowledge on selected areas of research practice and encourage utilization of research findings.

Of particular importance in the United States was the establishment in 1986 of the National Center for Nursing Research (NCNR) at the National Institutes of Health (NIH) by congressional mandate, despite a presidential veto that was overridden largely as a result of nurse-scientists' successful lobbying efforts. The purpose of NCNR was to promote—and financially support—research training and research projects relating to patient care. In addition, the Center for Research for Nursing was created in 1983 by the American Nurses' Association. The Center's mission is to develop and coordinate a research program to serve as the source of national information for the profession. Meanwhile, funding for nursing research became available in Canada in the 1980s through the National Health Research Development Program (NHRDP).

Several nursing groups developed priorities for nursing research during the 1980s. For example, in 1985, the American Nurses' Association Cabinet on Nursing Research established priorities that helped focus research more precisely on aspects of nursing practice. Also in the 1980s, nurses began to conduct formal projects designed to increase research utilization. Finally, specialty journals such as *Heart & Lung* and *Cancer Nursing* began to expand their coverage of research reports, and several new research-related journals were established: *Applied Nursing Research*, *Scholarly Inquiry for Nursing Practice*, and *Nursing Science Quarterly*. The journal *Applied Nursing Research* is notable for its intended audience: it includes research reports on studies of special relevance to practicing nurses.

Several forces outside of the nursing profession in the late 1980s helped to shape today's nursing research landscape. A group from the McMaster Medical School in Canada designed a clinical learning strategy that was called evidence-based medicine (EBM). EBM, which promulgated the view that scientific research findings were far superior to the opinions of authorities as a basis for clinical decisions, constituted a profound shift for medical education and practice, and has had a major effect on all health care professions.

In 1989, the U.S. government established the Agency for Health Care Policy and Research (AHCPR). AHCPR (which was renamed the Agency for Healthcare Research and Quality, or AHRQ, in 1999) is the federal agency that has been charged with supporting research specifically designed to improve the quality of health care, reduce health costs, and enhance patient safety, and thus plays a pivotal role in the promulgation of EBP.

 Example of nursing research break-throughs in the 1980s:

• A team of researchers headed by Dorothy Brooten engaged in studies that led to the development and testing of a model of site transitional care. Brooten and her colleagues (1986, 1988, 1989), for example, conducted studies of nurse specialist–managed home follow-up services for very-low-birth-weight infants who were discharged early from the hospital, and later expanded to other high-risk patients (1994). The site transitional care model, which was developed in anticipation of government cost-cutting measures of the 1980s, has been used as a framework for patients who are at health risk as a result of early discharge from hospitals, and has been recognized by numerous health care disciplines.

Nursing Research in the 1990s

Nursing science came into its maturity during the 1990s. As but one example, nursing research was strengthened and given more national visibility in the United States when NCNR was promoted to full institute status within the NIH: in 1993, the **National Institute of Nursing Research (NINR)** was born. The birth of NINR helps put nursing research more into the mainstream of research activities enjoyed by other health disciplines. Funding for nursing research has also grown. In 1986, the NCNR had a budget of $16.2 million, whereas 16 years later in fiscal year 2002, the budget for NINR was over $120 million. Funding opportunities for nursing research expanded in other countries as well during the 1990s. For example,

the Canadian Health Services Research Foundation was established in 1997 with an endowment from federal funds, and plans for the Canadian Institute for Health Research were underway.

Several research journals were established during the 1990s, including *Qualitative Health Research*, *Clinical Nursing Research*, *Clinical Effectiveness*, and *Outcomes Management for Nursing Practice*. These journals emerged in response to the growth in clinically oriented and in-depth research among nurses, and interest in EBP. Another major contribution to EBP was inaugurated in 1993: the Cochrane Collaboration, an international network of institutions and individuals, maintains and updates systematic reviews of hundreds of clinical interventions to facilitate EBP.

Some current nursing research is guided by priorities established by prominent nurse researchers in the 1990s, who were brought together by NCNR for two Conferences on Research Priorities (CORP). The priorities established by the first CORP for research through 1994 included low birth weight, human immunodeficiency virus (HIV) infection, long-term care, symptom management, nursing informatics, health promotion, and technology dependence.

In 1993, the second CORP established the following research emphases for a portion of NINR's funding from 1995 through 1999: developing and testing community-based nursing models; assessing the effectiveness of nursing interventions in HIV/AIDS; developing and testing approaches to remediating cognitive impairment; testing interventions for coping with chronic illness; and identifying biobehavioral factors and testing interventions to promote immunocompetence.

 Example of nursing research break-throughs in the 1990s:

• Many studies that Donaldson (2000) identified as *breakthroughs* in nursing research were conducted in the 1990s. This reflects, in part, the growth of **research programs** in which teams of researchers engage in a series of related research on important topics, rather than discrete and unconnected studies. As but one example, several nurse researchers had breakthroughs during the 1990s in the area of psychoneuroimmunology, which has been adopted as the model of mind—body interactions. Barbara Swanson and Janice Zeller, for example, conducted several studies relating to HIV infection and neuropsychological function (Swanson, Cronin Stubbs, Zeller, Kessler, & Bielauskas, 1993; Swanson, Zeller, & Spear, 1998) that have led to discoveries in environmental management as a means of improving immune system status.

Future Directions for Nursing Research

Nursing research continues to develop at a rapid pace and will undoubtedly flourish in the 21st century. Broadly speaking, the priority for nursing research in the future will be the promotion of excellence in nursing science. Toward this end, nurse researchers and practicing nurses will be sharpening their research skills, and using those skills to address emerging issues of importance to the profession and its clientele.

Certain trends for the beginning of the 21st century are evident from developments taking shape in the 1990s:

- *Increased focus on outcomes research.* **Outcomes research** is designed to assess and document the effectiveness of health care services. The increasing number of studies that can be characterized as outcomes research has been stimulated by the need for cost-effective care that achieves positive outcomes without compromising quality. Nurses are increasingly engaging in outcomes research focused both on patients and on the overall delivery system.
- *Increased focus on biophysiologic research.* Nurse researchers have begun increasingly to study biologic and physiologic phenomena as part of the effort to develop better clinical evidence. Consistent with this trend, a new journal called *Biological Research for Nursing* was launched in 2000.
- *Promotion of evidence-based practice.* Concerted efforts to translate research findings

into practice will continue and nurses at all levels will be encouraged to engage in evidence-based patient care. In turn, improvements will be needed both in the quality of nursing studies and in nurses' skills in understanding, critiquing, and using study results.

- *Development of a stronger knowledge base through multiple, confirmatory strategies.* Practicing nurses cannot be expected to change a procedure or adopt an innovation on the basis of a single, isolated study. Confirmation is usually needed through the deliberate **replication** (i.e., the repeating) of studies with different clients, in different clinical settings, and at different times to ensure that the findings are robust. Replication in different settings is especially important now because the primary setting for health care delivery is shifting from inpatient hospitals to ambulatory settings, the community, and homes. Another confirmatory strategy is the conduct of multiple-site investigations by researchers in several locations.
- *Strengthening of multidisciplinary collaboration.* Interdisciplinary collaboration of nurses with researchers in related fields (as well as intradisciplinary collaboration among nurse researchers) is likely to continue to expand in the 21st century as researchers address fundamental problems at the biobehavioral and psychobiologic interface. As one example, there are likely to be vast opportunities for nurses and other health care researchers to integrate breakthroughs in human genetics into lifestyle and health care interventions. In turn, such collaborative efforts could lead to nurse researchers playing a more prominent role in national and international health care policies.
- *Expanded dissemination of research findings.* The Internet and other electronic communication have a big impact on the dissemination of research information, which in turn may help to promote EBP. Through such technological advances as on-line publishing (e.g., the *Online Journal of Knowledge Synthesis for Nursing*, the *Online Journal of Clinical Innovation*); on-line resources such as Lippincott's NursingCenter.com; elec-

tronic document retrieval and delivery; e-mail; and electronic mailing lists, information about innovations can be communicated more widely and more quickly than ever before.

- *Increasing the visibility of nursing research.* The 21st century is likely to witness efforts to increase the visibility of nursing research, the onus for which will fall on the shoulders of nurse researchers themselves. Most people are unaware that nurses are scholars and researchers. Nurse researchers must market themselves and their research to professional organizations, consumer organizations, and the corporate world to increase support for their research. They also need to educate upper-level managers and corporate executives about the importance of clinical outcomes research. As Baldwin and Nail (2000) have noted, nurse researchers are one of the best-qualified groups to meet the need in today's world for clinical outcomes research, but they are not recognized for their expertise.

Priorities and goals for the future are also under discussion. NINR has established scientific goals and objectives for the 5-year period of 2000 to 2004. The four broad goals are: (1) to identify and support research opportunities that will achieve scientific distinction and produce significant contributions to health; (2) to identify and support future areas of opportunity to advance research on high quality, cost-effective care and to contribute to the scientific base for nursing practice; (3) to communicate and disseminate research findings resulting from NINR-funded research; and (4) to enhance the development of nurse researchers through training and career development opportunities. For the years 2000, 2001, and 2002, topics identified by NINR as special areas of research opportunity included:

- Chronic illnesses or conditions (e.g., management of chronic pain; care of children with asthma; adherence to diabetes self-management)
- Behavioral changes and interventions (e.g., research in informal caregiving; disparities of infant mortality; effective sleep in health and illness)

- Responding to compelling public health concerns (e.g., reducing health disparities in cancer screening; end-of-life/palliative care)

SOURCES OF EVIDENCE FOR NURSING PRACTICE

Nursing students are taught how best to practice nursing, and best-practice learning continues throughout nurses' careers. Some of what students and nurses learn is based on systematic research, but much of it is not. In fact, Millenson (1997) estimated that 85% of health care practice has not been scientifically validated.

Clinical nursing practice relies on a collage of information sources that vary in dependability and validity. Increasingly there are discussions of **evidence hierarchies** that acknowledge that certain types of evidence and knowledge are superior to others. A brief discussion of some alternative sources of evidence shows how research-based information is different.

Tradition

Many questions are answered and problems solved based on inherited customs or tradition. Within each culture, certain "truths" are accepted as given. For example, as citizens of democratic societies, most of us accept, without *proof*, that democracy is the highest form of government. This type of knowledge often is so much a part of our heritage that few of us seek verification.

Tradition offers some advantages. It is efficient as an information source: each individual is not required to begin anew in an attempt to understand the world or certain aspects of it. Tradition or custom also facilitates communication by providing a common foundation of accepted truth. Nevertheless, tradition poses some problems because many traditions have never been evaluated for their validity. Indeed, by their nature, traditions may interfere with the ability to perceive alternatives. Walker's (1967) research on ritualistic practices in nursing suggests that some traditional nursing practices, such as the routine taking of a patient's temperature, pulse, and respirations, may be dysfunctional. The Walker study illustrates the potential value of critical appraisal of custom and tradition before accepting them as truth. There is growing concern that many nursing interventions are based on tradition, customs, and "unit culture" rather than on sound evidence (e.g., French, 1999).

Authority

In our complex society, there are authorities—people with specialized expertise—in every field. We are constantly faced with making decisions about matters with which we have had no direct experience; therefore, it seems natural to place our trust in the judgment of people who are authoritative on an issue by virtue of specialized training or experience. As a source of understanding, however, authority has shortcomings. Authorities are not infallible, particularly if their expertise is based primarily on personal experience; yet, like tradition, their knowledge often goes unchallenged. Although nursing practice would flounder if every piece of advice from nursing educators were challenged by students, nursing education would be incomplete if students never had occasion to pose such questions as: How does the authority (the instructor) *know*? What evidence is there that what I am learning is valid?

Clinical Experience, Trial and Error, and Intuition

Our own clinical experiences represent a familiar and functional source of knowledge. The ability to generalize, to recognize regularities, and to make predictions based on observations is an important characteristic of the human mind. Despite the obvious value of clinical expertise, it has limitations as a type of evidence. First, each individual's experience is fairly restricted. A nurse may notice, for example, that two or three cardiac patients follow similar postoperative sleep patterns. This observation may lead to some interesting discoveries with implications for nursing interventions, but does one nurse's observations justify broad changes in nursing care? A second limitation of experience is

that the same objective event is usually experienced or perceived differently by two individuals.

Related to clinical experience is the method of trial and error. In this approach, alternatives are tried successively until a solution to a problem is found. We likely have all used trial and error in our lives, including in our professional work. For example, many patients dislike the taste of potassium chloride solution. Nurses try to disguise the taste of the medication in various ways until one method meets with the approval of the patient. Trial and error may offer a practical means of securing knowledge, but it is fallible. This method is haphazard, and the knowledge obtained is often unrecorded and, hence, inaccessible in subsequent clinical situations.

Finally, intuition is a type of knowledge that cannot be explained on the basis of reasoning or prior instruction. Although intuition and hunches undoubtedly play a role in nursing practice—as they do in the conduct of research—it is difficult to develop policies and practices for nurses on the basis of intuition.

Logical Reasoning

Solutions to many perplexing problems are developed by logical thought processes. Logical reasoning as a method of knowing combines experience, intellectual faculties, and formal systems of thought. **Inductive reasoning** is the process of developing generalizations from specific observations. For example, a nurse may observe the anxious behavior of (specific) hospitalized children and conclude that (in general) children's separation from their parents is stressful. **Deductive reasoning** is the process of developing specific predictions from general principles. For example, if we assume that separation anxiety occurs in hospitalized children (in general), then we might predict that (specific) children in Memorial Hospital whose parents do not room-in will manifest symptoms of stress.

Both systems of reasoning are useful as a means of understanding and organizing phenomena, and both play a role in nursing research. However, reasoning in and of itself is limited because the validity of reasoning depends on the accuracy of the information (or premises) with which one starts, and reasoning may be an insufficient basis for evaluating accuracy.

Assembled Information

In making clinical decisions, health care professionals also rely on information that has been assembled for a variety of purposes. For example, local, national, and international **bench-marking data** provide information on such issues as the rates of using various procedures (e.g., rates of cesarean deliveries) or rates of infection (e.g., nosocomial pneumonia rates), and can serve as a guide in evaluating clinical practices. **Cost data**—that is, information on the costs associated with certain procedures, policies, or practices—are sometimes used as a factor in clinical decision-making. **Quality improvement and risk data**, such as medication error reports and evidence on the incidence and prevalence of skin breakdown, can be used to assess practices and determine the need for practice changes.

Such sources, although offering some information that can be used in practice, provide no mechanism for determining whether improvements in patient outcomes result from their use.

Disciplined Research

Research conducted within a disciplined format is the most sophisticated method of acquiring evidence that humans have developed. Nursing research combines aspects of logical reasoning with other features to create evidence that, although fallible, tends to be more reliable than other methods of knowledge acquisition.

The current emphasis on evidence-based health care requires nurses to base their clinical practice to the greatest extent possible on research-based findings rather than on tradition, authority, intuition, or personal experience. Findings from rigorous research investigations are considered to be at the pinnacle of the evidence hierarchy for establishing an EBP. As we discuss next, disciplined research in nursing is richly diverse with regard to questions asked and methods used.

PARADIGMS FOR NURSING RESEARCH

A **paradigm** is a world view, a general perspective on the complexities of the real world. Paradigms for human inquiry are often characterized in terms of the ways in which they respond to basic philosophical questions:

- *Ontologic*: What is the nature of reality?
- *Epistemologic*: What is the relationship between the inquirer and that being studied?
- *Axiologic*: What is the role of values in the inquiry?
- *Methodologic*: How should the inquirer obtain knowledge?

Disciplined inquiry in the field of nursing is being conducted mainly within two broad paradigms, both of which have legitimacy for nursing research. This section describes the two alternative paradigms and outlines their associated methodologies.

The Positivist Paradigm

One paradigm for nursing research is known as **positivism**. Positivism is rooted in 19th century thought, guided by such philosophers as Comte, Mill, Newton, and Locke. Positivism is a reflection of a broader cultural phenomenon that, in the humanities, is referred to as **modernism**, which emphasizes the rational and the scientific. Although strict positivist thinking—sometimes referred to as **logical positivism**—has been challenged and undermined, a modified positivist position remains a dominant force in scientific research.

The fundamental ontologic assumption of positivists is that there is a reality *out there* that can be studied and known (an **assumption** refers to a basic principle that is believed to be true without proof or verification). Adherents of the positivist approach assume that nature is basically ordered and regular and that an objective reality exists independent of human observation. In other words, the world is assumed not to be merely a creation of the human mind. The related assumption of **determinism** refers to the belief that phenomena are not haphazard or random events but rather have antecedent causes. If a person has a cerebrovascular accident, the scientist in a positivist tradition assumes that there must be one or more reasons that can be potentially identified and understood. Much of the activity in which a researcher in a positivist paradigm is engaged is directed at understanding the underlying causes of natural phenomena.

Because of their fundamental belief in an objective reality, positivists seek to be as objective as possible in their pursuit of knowledge. Positivists attempt to hold their personal beliefs and biases in check insofar as possible during their research to avoid contaminating the phenomena under investigation. The positivists' scientific approach involves the use of orderly, disciplined procedures that are designed to test researchers' hunches about the nature of phenomena being studied and relationships among them.

The Naturalistic Paradigm

The **naturalistic** paradigm began as a countermovement to positivism with writers such as Weber and Kant. Just as positivism reflects the cultural phenomenon of modernism that burgeoned in the wake of the industrial revolution, naturalism is an outgrowth of the pervasive cultural transformation that is usually referred to as **postmodernism**. Postmodern thinking emphasizes the value of **deconstruction**—that is, of taking apart old ideas and structures—and **reconstruction**—that is, putting ideas and structures together in new ways. The naturalistic paradigm represents a major alternative system for conducting disciplined research in nursing. Table 1-2 compares the major assumptions of the positivist and naturalistic paradigms.

TABLE 1.2 Major Assumptions of the Positivist and Naturalistic Paradigms

ASSUMPTION	POSITIVIST PARADIGM	NATURALISTIC PARADIGM
Ontologic (What is the nature of reality?)	Reality exists; there is a real world driven by real natural causes.	Reality is multiple and subjective, mentally constructed by individuals.
Epistemologic (How is the inquirer related to those being researched?)	The inquirer is independent from those being researched; findings are not influenced by the researcher.	The inquirer interacts with those being researched; findings are the creation of the interactive process.
Axiologic (What is the role of values in the inquiry?)	Values and biases are to be held in check; objectivity is sought.	Subjectivity and values are inevitable and desirable.
Methodologic (How is knowledge obtained?)	Deductive processes Emphasis on discrete, specific concepts Verification of researchers' hunches Fixed design Tight controls over context Emphasis on measured, quantitative information; statistical analysis Seeks generalizations	Inductive processes Emphasis on entirety of some phenomenon, holistic Emerging interpretations grounded in participants' experiences Flexible design Context-bound Emphasis on narrative information; qualitative analysis Seeks patterns

For the naturalistic inquirer, reality is not a fixed entity but rather a construction of the individuals participating in the research; reality exists within a context, and many constructions are possible. Naturalists thus take the position of relativism: if there are always multiple interpretations of reality that exist in people's minds, then there is no process by which the ultimate truth or falsity of the constructions can be determined.

Epistemologically, the naturalistic paradigm assumes that knowledge is maximized when the distance between the inquirer and the participants in the study is minimized. The voices and interpretations of those under study are crucial to understanding the phenomenon of interest, and subjective interactions are the primary way to access them. The findings from a naturalistic inquiry are the product of the interaction between the inquirer and the participants.

Paradigms and Methods: Quantitative and Qualitative Research

Broadly speaking, **research methods** are the techniques used by researchers to structure a study and to gather and analyze information relevant to the research question. The two alternative paradigms have strong implications for the research methods to be used. The methodologic distinction typically focuses on differences between **quantitative research**, which is most closely allied with the positivist tradition, and **qualitative research**, which is most often associated with naturalistic inquiry—although positivists sometimes engage in qualitative studies, and naturalistic researchers sometimes collect quantitative information. This section provides an overview of the methods associated with the two alternative paradigms. Note that this discussion accentuates differences in methods as a heuristic device; in reality, there is often greater overlap of methods than this introductory discussion implies.

The "Scientific Method" and Quantitative Research

The traditional, positivist "**scientific method**" refers to a general set of orderly, disciplined procedures used to acquire information. Quantitative researchers use deductive reasoning to generate hunches that are tested in the real world. They typically move in an orderly and systematic fashion from the definition of a problem and the selection of concepts on which to focus, through the design of the study and collection of information, to the solution of the problem. By **systematic,** we mean that the investigator progresses logically through a series of steps, according to a prespecified plan of action.

Quantitative researchers use mechanisms designed to control the study. **Control** involves imposing conditions on the research situation so that biases are minimized and precision and validity are maximized. The problems that are of interest to nurse researchers—for example, obesity, compliance with a regimen, or pain—are highly complicated phenomena, often representing the effects of various forces. In trying to isolate relationships between phenomena, quantitative researchers attempt to control factors that are not under direct investigation. For example, if a scientist is interested in exploring the relationship between diet and heart disease, steps are usually taken to control other potential contributors to coronary disorders, such as stress and cigarette smoking, as well as additional factors that might be relevant, such as a person's age and gender. Control mechanisms are discussed at length in this book.

Quantitative researchers gather **empirical evidence**—evidence that is rooted in objective reality and gathered directly or indirectly through the senses. Empirical evidence, then, consists of observations gathered through sight, hearing, taste, touch, or smell. Observations of the presence or absence of skin inflammation, the heart rate of a patient, or the weight of a newborn infant are all examples of empirical observations. The requirement to use empirical evidence as the basis for knowledge means that findings are grounded in reality rather than in researchers' personal beliefs.

Evidence for a study in the positivist paradigm is gathered according to a specified plan, using formal instruments to collect needed information. Usually (but not always) the information gathered in such a study is **quantitative**—that is, numeric information that results from some type of formal measurement and that is analyzed with statistical procedures.

An important goal of a traditional scientific study is to understand phenomena, not in isolated circumstances, but in a broad, general sense. For example, quantitative researchers are typically not as interested in understanding why Ann Jones has cervical cancer as in understanding what general factors lead to this carcinoma in Ann and others. The desire to go beyond the specifics of the situation is an important feature of the traditional scientific approach. In fact, the degree to which research findings can be generalized to individuals other than those who participated in the study (referred to as the **generalizability** of the research) is a widely used criterion for assessing the quality of quantitative studies.

The traditional scientific approach used by quantitative researchers has enjoyed considerable stature as a method of inquiry, and it has been used productively by nurse researchers studying a wide range of nursing problems. This is not to say, however, that this approach can solve all nursing problems. One important limitation—common to both quantitative and qualitative research—is that research methods cannot be used to answer moral or ethical questions. Many of our most persistent and intriguing questions about the human experience fall into this area—questions such as whether euthanasia should be practiced or abortion should be legal. Given the many moral issues that are linked to health care, it is inevitable that the nursing process will never rely exclusively on scientific information.

The traditional research approach also must contend with problems of measurement. To study a phenomenon, quantitative researchers attempt to measure it. For example, if the phenomenon of interest is patient morale, researchers might want to assess if morale is high or low, or higher under certain conditions than under others. Although there are reasonably accurate measures of physiologic phenomena, such as blood pressure and body temperature, comparably accurate measures of such psychological phenomena as patient morale, pain, or self-image have not been developed.

Another issue is that nursing research tends to focus on human beings, who are inherently complex and diverse. Traditional quantitative methods typically focus on a relatively small portion of the human experience (e.g., weight gain, depression, chemical dependency) in a single study. Complexities tend to be controlled and, if possible, eliminated, rather than studied directly, and this narrowness of focus can sometimes obscure insights.

Finally and relatedly, quantitative research conducted in the positivist paradigm has sometimes been accused of a narrowness and inflexibility of vision, a problem that has been called a **sedimented view** of the world that does not fully capture the reality of human experience.

Naturalistic Methods and Qualitative Research

Naturalistic methods of inquiry attempt to deal with the issue of human complexity by exploring it directly. Researchers in the naturalistic tradition emphasize the inherent complexity of humans, their ability to shape and create their own experiences, and the idea that truth is a composite of realities. Consequently, naturalistic investigations place a heavy emphasis on *understanding* the human experience as it is lived, usually through the careful collection and analysis of **qualitative** materials that are narrative and subjective.

Researchers who reject the traditional "scientific method" believe that a major limitation of the classical model is that it is **reductionist**—that is, it reduces human experience to only the few concepts under investigation, and those concepts are defined in advance by the researcher rather than emerging from the experiences of those under study. Naturalistic researchers tend to emphasize the dynamic, holistic, and individual aspects of human experience and attempt to capture those aspects in their entirety, within the context of those who are experiencing them.

Flexible, evolving procedures are used to capitalize on findings that emerge in the course of the study. Naturalistic inquiry always takes place in the **field** (i.e., in naturalistic settings), often over an extended period of time, while quantitative research takes place both in natural as well as in contrived laboratory settings. In naturalistic research, the collection of information and its analysis typically progress concurrently; as researchers sift through information, insights are gained, new questions emerge, and further evidence is sought to amplify or confirm the insights. Through an inductive process, researchers integrate information to develop a theory or description that helps explicate processes under observation.

Naturalistic studies result in rich, in-depth information that has the potential to elucidate varied dimensions of a complicated phenomenon. Because of this feature—and the relative ease with which qualitative findings can be communicated to lay audiences—it has been argued that qualitative methods will play a more prominent role in health care policy and development in the future (Carey, 1997).

The findings from in-depth qualitative research are rarely superficial, but there are several limitations of the approach. Human beings are used directly as the instrument through which information is gathered, and humans are extremely intelligent and sensitive—but fallible—tools. The subjectivity that enriches the analytic insights of skillful researchers can yield trivial "findings" among less competent inquirers.

The subjective nature of naturalistic inquiry sometimes causes concerns about the idiosyncratic nature of the conclusions. Would two naturalistic researchers studying the same phenomenon in the same setting arrive at the same results? The situation is further complicated by the fact that most naturalistic studies involve a relatively small group of people under study. Questions about the generalizability of findings from naturalistic inquiries sometimes arise.

Multiple Paradigms and Nursing Research

Paradigms should be viewed as lenses that help to sharpen our focus on a phenomenon of interest, not as blinders that limit intellectual curiosity. The emergence of alternative paradigms for the study of nursing problems is, in our view, a healthy and desirable trend in the pursuit of new evidence for practice. Although researchers' world view may be paradigmatic, knowledge itself is not. Nursing knowledge would be thin, indeed, if there were not a rich array of methods available within the two paradigms—methods that are often complementary in their strengths and limitations. We believe that intellectual pluralism should be encouraged and fostered.

Thus far, we have emphasized differences between the two paradigms and their associated methods so that their distinctions would be easy to understand. Subsequent chapters of this book will further elaborate on differences in terminology, methods, and research products. It is equally important, however, to note that these two paradigms have many features in common, only some of which are mentioned here:

- *Ultimate goals.* The ultimate aim of disciplined inquiry, regardless of the underlying paradigm, is to gain understanding about phenomena. Both quantitative and qualitative researchers seek to capture the truth with regard to an aspect of the world in which they are interested, and both groups can make significant contributions to nursing knowledge. Moreover, qualitative studies often serve as a crucial starting point for more controlled quantitative studies.
- *External evidence.* Although the word *empiricism* has come to be allied with the traditional scientific approach, it is nevertheless the case that researchers in both traditions gather and analyze external evidence that is collected through their senses. Neither qualitative nor quantitative researchers are armchair analysts, relying on their own beliefs and views of the world for their conclusions. Information is gathered from others in a deliberate fashion.
- *Reliance on human cooperation.* Because evidence for nursing research comes primarily from human participants, the need for human cooperation is inevitable. To understand people's characteristics and experiences, researchers must persuade them to participate in the investigation *and* to act and speak candidly. For certain

topics, the need for candor and cooperation is a challenging requirement—for researchers in either tradition.

- *Ethical constraints.* Research with human beings is guided by ethical principles that sometimes interfere with research goals. For example, if researchers want to test a potentially beneficial intervention, is it ethical to withhold the treatment from some people to see what happens? As discussed later in the book (see Chapter 7), ethical dilemmas often confront researchers, regardless of their paradigmatic orientation.

- *Fallibility of disciplined research.* Virtually all studies—in either paradigm—have some limitations. Every research question can be addressed in many different ways, and inevitably there are tradeoffs. Financial constraints are universal, but limitations exist even when resources are abundant. This does not mean that small, simple studies have no value. *It means that no single study can ever definitively answer a research question.* Each completed study adds to a body of accumulated knowledge. If several researchers pose the same question and if each obtains the same or similar results, increased confidence can be placed in the answer to the question. The fallibility of any single study makes it important to understand the tradeoffs and decisions that investigators make when evaluating the adequacy of those decisions.

Thus, despite philosophic and methodologic differences, researchers using the traditional quantitative approach or naturalistic methods often share overall goals and face many similar constraints and challenges. The selection of an appropriate method depends on researchers' personal taste and philosophy, and also on the research question. If a researcher asks, "What are the effects of surgery on circadian rhythms (biologic cycles)?" the researcher really needs to express the effects through the careful quantitative measurement of various bodily properties subject to rhythmic variation. On the other hand, if a researcher asks, "What is the process by which parents learn to cope with the death of a child?" the researcher

would be hard pressed to quantify such a process. Personal world views of researchers help to shape their questions.

In reading about the alternative paradigms for nursing research, you likely were more attracted to one of the two paradigms—the one that corresponds most closely to your view of the world and of reality. It is important, however, to learn about and respect both approaches to disciplined inquiry, and to recognize their respective strengths and limitations. In this textbook, we describe methods associated with both qualitative and quantitative research.

THE PURPOSES OF NURSING RESEARCH

The general purpose of nursing research is to answer questions or solve problems of relevance to the nursing profession. Sometimes a distinction is made between basic and applied research. As traditionally defined, **basic research** is undertaken to extend the base of knowledge in a discipline, or to formulate or refine a theory. For example, a researcher may perform an in-depth study to better understand normal grieving processes, without having *explicit* nursing applications in mind. **Applied research** focuses on finding solutions to existing problems. For example, a study to determine the effectiveness of a nursing intervention to ease grieving would be applied research. Basic research is appropriate for discovering general principles of human behavior and biophysiologic processes; applied research is designed to indicate how these principles can be used to solve problems in nursing practice. In nursing, the findings from applied research may pose questions for basic research, and the results of basic research often suggest clinical applications.

The specific purposes of nursing research include identification, description, exploration, explanation, prediction, and control. Within each purpose, various types of question are addressed by nurse researchers; certain questions are more amenable to qualitative than to quantitative inquiry, and vice versa.

Identification and Description

Qualitative researchers sometimes study phenomena about which little is known. In some cases, so little is known that the phenomenon has yet to be clearly identified or named or has been inadequately defined or conceptualized. The in-depth, probing nature of qualitative research is well suited to the task of answering such questions as, "What is this phenomenon?" and "What is its name?" (Table 1-3). In quantitative research, by contrast, the researcher begins with a phenomenon that has been previously studied or defined—sometimes in a qualitative study. Thus, in quantitative research, identification typically precedes the inquiry.

Qualitative example of identification:
Weiss and Hutchinson (2000) investigated people with diabetes and hypertension to discover the basic social problem that affects their adherence

TABLE 1.3 Research Purposes and Research Questions

PURPOSE	TYPES OF QUESTIONS: QUANTITATIVE RESEARCH	TYPES OF QUESTIONS: QUALITATIVE RESEARCH
Identification		What is this phenomenon? What is its name?
Description	How prevalent is the phenomenon? How often does the phenomenon occur? What are the characteristics of the phenomenon?	What are the dimensions of the phenomenon? What variations exist? What is important about the phenomenon?
Exploration	What factors are related to the phenomenon? What are the antecedents of the phenomenon?	What is the full nature of the phenomenon? What is really going on here? What is the process by which the phenomenon evolves or is experienced?
Explanation	What are the measurable associations between phenomena? What factors cause the phenomenon? Does the theory explain the phenomenon?	How does the phenomenon work? Why does the phenomenon exist? What is the meaning of the phenomenon? How did the phenomenon occur?
Prediction	What will happen if we alter a phenomenon or introduce an intervention? If phenomenon X occurs, will phenomenon Y follow?	
Control	How can we make the phenomenon happen or alter its nature or prevalence? Can the occurrence of the phenomenon be prevented or controlled?	

to health care directives. Through in-depth interviews with 21 clients, the researchers identified that *warnings of vulnerability* was the basic problem undermining adherence.

Description of phenomena is another important purpose of research. In a descriptive study, researchers observe, count, delineate, and classify. Nurse researchers have described a wide variety of phenomena. Examples include patients' stress and coping, pain management, adaptation processes, health beliefs, rehabilitation success, and time patterns of temperature readings.

Description can be a major purpose for both qualitative and quantitative researchers. Quantitative description focuses on the prevalence, incidence, size, and measurable attributes of phenomena. Qualitative researchers, on the other hand, use in-depth methods to describe the dimensions, variations, and importance of phenomena. Table 1-3 compares descriptive questions posed by quantitative and qualitative researchers.

Quantitative example of description: Bohachick, Taylor, Sereika, Reeder, and Anton (2002) conducted a study to describe quantitative changes in psychological well-being and psychological resources 6 months after a heart transplantation.

Qualitative example of description: Bournes and Mitchell (2002) undertook an in-depth study to describe the experience of *waiting* in a critical care waiting room.

Exploration

Like descriptive research, exploratory research begins with a phenomenon of interest; but rather than simply observing and describing it, exploratory research investigates the full nature of the phenomenon, the manner in which it is manifested, and the other factors to which it is related. For example, a descriptive quantitative study of patients' preoperative stress might seek to document the degree of stress patients experience before surgery and the percentage of patients who actually experience it. An exploratory study might ask the following: What factors diminish or increase a patient's stress? Is a patient's stress related to behaviors of the nursing staff? Is stress related to the patient's cultural backgrounds?

Qualitative methods are especially useful for exploring the full nature of a little-understood phenomenon. Exploratory qualitative research is designed to shed light on the various ways in which a phenomenon is manifested and on underlying processes.

Quantitative example of exploration: Reynolds and Neidig (2002) studied the incidence and severity of nausea accompanying combinative antiretroviral therapies among HIV-infected patients, and explored patterns of nausea in relation to patient characteristics.

Qualitative example of exploration: Through in-depth interviews, Sadala and Mendes (2000) explored the experiences of 18 nurses who cared for patients who had been pronounced brain dead but kept alive to serve as organ donors.

Explanation

The goals of explanatory research are to understand the underpinnings of specific natural phenomena, and to explain systematic relationships among phenomena. Explanatory research is often linked to **theories**, which represent a method of deriving, organizing, and integrating ideas about the manner in which phenomena are interrelated. Whereas descriptive research provides new information, and exploratory research provides promising insights, explanatory research attempts to offer understanding of the underlying causes or full nature of a phenomenon.

In quantitative research, theories or prior findings are used deductively as the basis for generating explanations that are then tested empirically. That is, based on a previously developed theory or body of evidence, researchers make specific predictions that, if upheld by the findings, add credibility to the explanation. In qualitative studies, researchers may search for explanations about how or why a phenomenon exists or what a phenomenon means as a basis for *developing* a theory that is grounded in rich, in-depth, experiential evidence.

Quantitative example of explanation:
Resnick, Orwig, Maganizer, and Wynne (2002) tested a model to explain exercise behavior among older adults on the basis of social support, age, and self-efficacy expectations.

Qualitative example of explanation:
Hupcey (2000) undertook a study that involved the development of a model explaining the psychosocial needs of patients in the intensive care unit. Feeling safe was the overwhelming need of patients in the intensive care unit.

Prediction and Control

Many phenomena defy explanation. Yet it is frequently possible to make predictions and to control phenomena based on research findings, even in the absence of complete understanding. For example, research has shown that the incidence of Down syndrome in infants increases with the age of the mother. We can predict that a woman aged 40 years is at higher risk of bearing a child with Down syndrome than is a woman aged 25 years. We can partially control the outcome by educating women about the risks and offering amniocentesis to women older than 35 years of age. Note, however, that the ability to predict and control in this example does not depend on an explanation of *why* older women are at a higher risk of having an abnormal child. In many examples of nursing and health-related studies—typically, quantitative ones—prediction and control are key objectives. Studies designed to test the efficacy of a nursing intervention are ultimately concerned with controlling patient outcomes or the costs of care.

Quantitative example of prediction:
Lindeke, Stanley, Else, and Mills (2002) used neonatal data to predict academic performance and the need for special services among school-aged children who had been in a level 3 neonatal intensive care unit.

RESEARCH EXAMPLES

Each chapter of this book presents brief descriptions of actual studies conducted by nurse researchers. The descriptions focus on aspects of the study emphasized in the chapter. A review of the full journal article likely would prove useful.

Research Example of a Quantitative Study

McDonald, Freeland, Thomas, and Moore (2001) conducted a study to determine the effectiveness of a preoperative pain management intervention for relieving pain among elders undergoing surgery. Their report appeared in the journal *Research in Nursing & Health*.

McDonald (who had conducted earlier research on the topic of pain and pain management) and her colleagues developed a preoperative intervention that taught pain management and pain communication skills. The content was specifically geared to older adults undergoing surgery. Forty elders, all older than age 65 years, were recruited to participate in the study. Half of these elders were assigned, at random, to participate in the special intervention; the remaining half got usual preoperative care. Postoperative pain was measured for both groups on the evening of the surgery, on postoperative day 1, and on postoperative day 2. The results supported the researchers' predictions that (a) pain in both groups would decline over time; and (b) those receiving the special intervention would experience greater decreases in pain over time.

The researchers noted that further research is needed to determine whether the intervention's effect resulted from instruction in pain management or in pain communication skills (and, indeed, McDonald reported being in the process of conducting such a study). They also noted that the study was based on elders undergoing certain types of surgery at a single site, acknowledging that the findings need confirmation in other settings and contexts. Nevertheless, this study offers evidence that pain responses of elderly surgical patients can be lowered through a nursing intervention. The strength of this evidence lies in several factors— several of which you will appreciate more as you become familiar with research methods. Most important, this study was quite rigorous. The intervention itself was based on a formal theory of communication accommodation, which addresses how people adjust communication to their own needs. The researchers took care to ensure that the two groups being compared were equivalent in terms of background and medical characteristics, so that group differences in pain responses reflected the intervention and not some spurious factor. The research team members who measured pain responses were not aware of whether the elders were in the intervention group, so as not to bias the measurements. Finally, the findings are more persuasive because the team of researchers who conducted the study have developed a solid program of research on pain, and their research has contributed incrementally to understanding pain responses and appropriate nursing interventions.

Research Example of a Qualitative Study

Cheek and Ballantyne (2001) undertook a study to describe the search and selection process for an aged care facility after discharge of a family member from acute hospital settings in Australia, and to explore the effects the process had on the individuals and their families. Twelve residents and 20 of their sponsors (the primary contact person responsible for the resident) participated in the study. Face-to-face in-depth interviews were conducted with residents in the aged care facilities and with family members in their homes. They were all asked to talk about their personal experiences of the search and selection process and its effect on their well-being.

These interviews were audiotaped and then transcribed. Analysis of the interview transcripts revealed five themes. One theme, for example, was labeled "dealing with the system—cutting through the maze." Dealing with the system was perceived as being in the middle of a war zone. This sense of battle was related to confusion, lack of control, and the feeling of being at the system's mercy. Contributing to this perception of being at war with the system was the stress of having to deal with multiple aged care facilities on an individual basis. A second major theme was labeled "Urgency—moving them on and in." Sponsors felt a sense of urgency in finding a suitable facility to have their family member transferred to from the acute setting. Sponsors felt pressured to make on-the-spot decisions to accept or reject a place in a facility once it had become available.

This thorough and careful study provides a first-hand perspective on the experiences of people going through the process of selecting an appropriate long-term care facility for aging family members. One of the central implications for practice of this study concerns the need to revise the search and selection process to make it more efficient in terms of time and effort of the sponsors and residents. In addition, the study suggests that increased communication—from the acute setting to the aged care facilities being considered could play an important role in decreasing the stress of this guilt-ridden experience. The clinical implications of the study are strengthened by the fact that the researchers took steps to ensure its rigor. For example, the transcripts of these interviews were read by at least two members of the research team who individually identified themes from each interview. The researchers then compared and discussed the themes from all the interviews until consensus was reached. Moreover, the researchers took steps to weigh their evidence for their thematic conclusions against potentially competing explanations of the data.

SUMMARY POINTS

- **Nursing research** is systematic inquiry to develop knowledge about issues of importance to nurses.
- Nurses in various settings are adopting an **evidence-based practice** that incorporates research findings into their decisions and their interactions with clients.
- Knowledge of nursing research enhances the professional practice of all nurses—including both **consumers of research** (who read and evaluate studies) and **producers of research** (who design and undertake research studies).
- Nursing research began with Florence Nightingale but developed slowly until its rapid acceleration in the 1950s. Since the 1970s, nursing research has focused on problems relating to clinical practice.
- The **National Institute of Nursing Research** (NINR), established at the U.S. National Institutes of Health in 1993, affirms the stature of nursing research in the United States.
- Future emphases of nursing research are likely to include **outcomes research**, research utilization projects, **replications** of research, multisite studies, and expanded dissemination efforts.

- Disciplined research stands in contrast to other sources of evidence for nursing practice, such as tradition, voices of authority, personal experience, trial and error, intuition, and logical reasoning; rigorous research is at the pinnacle of the **evidence hierarchy** as a basis for making clinical decisions.
- Disciplined inquiry in nursing is conducted within two broad **paradigms**—world views with underlying **assumptions** about the complexities of reality: the positivist paradigm and the naturalistic paradigm.
- In the **positivist paradigm**, it is assumed that there is an objective reality and that natural phenomena are regular and orderly. The related assumption of **determinism** refers to the belief that phenomena are the result of prior causes and are not haphazard.
- In the **naturalistic paradigm**, it is assumed that reality is not a fixed entity but is rather a construction of human minds—and thus "truth" is a composite of multiple constructions of reality.
- The positivist paradigm is associated with **quantitative research**—the collection and analysis of numeric information. Quantitative research is typically conducted within the traditional "**scientific method**," which is a systematic and controlled process. Quantitative researchers base their findings on **empirical evidence** (evidence collected by way of the human senses) and strive for **generalizability** of their findings beyond a single setting or situation.
- Researchers within the naturalistic paradigm emphasize understanding the human experience as it is lived through the collection and analysis of subjective, narrative materials using flexible procedures that evolve in the **field;** this paradigm is associated with **qualitative research.**
- **Basic research** is designed to extend the base of information for the sake of knowledge. **Applied research** focuses on discovering solutions to immediate problems.
- Research purposes for nursing research include identification, description, exploration, explanation, prediction, and control.

STUDY ACTIVITIES

Chapter 1 of the *Study Guide to Accompany Nursing Research: Principles and Methods, 7th edition,* offers various exercises and study suggestions for reinforcing the concepts presented in this chapter. In addition, the following study questions can be addressed:

1. What are some of the current changes occurring in the health care delivery system, and how could these changes influence nursing research?
2. Is your world view closer to the positivist or the naturalistic paradigm? Explore the aspects of the two paradigms that are especially consistent with your world view.
3. How does the assumption of scientific determinism conflict with or coincide with superstitious thinking? Take, as an example, the superstition associated with four-leaf clovers or a rabbit's foot.
4. How does the ability to predict phenomena offer the possibility of their control?

SUGGESTED READINGS

Methodologic and Theoretical References

American Nurses' Association Cabinet on Nursing Research. (1985). *Directions for nursing research: Toward the twenty-first century.* Kansas City, MO: American Nurses' Association.

Baldwin, K. M., & Nail, L. M. (2000). Opportunities and challenges in clinical nursing research. *Journal of Nursing Scholarship, 32,* 163–166.

Brown, E. L. (1948). *Nursing for the future.* New York: Russell Sage.

Carey, M. A. (1997). Qualitative research in policy development. In J. M. Morse (Ed.) *Completing a qualitative project: Details and dialogue* (pp. 345–354). Thousand Oaks, CA: Sage.

D'Antonio, P. (1997). Toward a history of research in nursing. *Nursing Research, 46,* 105–110.

Donaldson, S. K. (2000). Breakthroughs in scientific research: The discipline of nursing, 1960–1999. *Annual Review of Nursing Research, 18,* 247–311.

French, P. (1999). The development of evidence-based nursing. *Journal of Advanced Nursing, 29,* 72–78.

Goode, C. J. (2000). What constitutes "evidence" in evidence-based practice? *Applied Nursing Research, 13*, 222–225.

Guba, E. G. (Ed.). (1990). *The paradigm dialog.* Newbury Park, CA: Sage.

Lincoln, Y. S., & Guba, E. G. (1985). *Naturalistic inquiry.* Beverly Hills, CA: Sage.

Lindeman, C. A. (1975). Delphi survey of priorities in clinical nursing research. *Nursing Research, 24*, 434–441.

Millenson, M. L. (1997). *Demanding medical evidence.* Chicago: University of Chicago Press.

Nightingale, F. (1859). *Notes on nursing: What it is, and what it is not.* Philadelphia: J. B. Lippincott.

Stetler, C. B., & Marram, G. (1976). Evaluating research findings for applicability in practice. *Nursing Outlook, 24*, 559–563.

Walker, V. H. (1967). *Nursing and ritualistic practice.* New York: Macmillan.

Studies Cited in Chapter 1

Barnard, K. E. (1973). The effects of stimulation on the sleep behavior of the premature infant. In M. Batey (Ed.), *Communicating nursing research* (Vol. 6, pp. 12–33). Boulder, CO: WICHE.

Barnard, K. E. (1976). The state of the art: Nursing and early intervention with handicapped infants. In T. Tjossem (Ed.), *Proceedings of the 1974 President's Committee on Mental Retardation.* Baltimore, MD: University Park Press.

Barnard, K. E., & Collar, B. S. (1973). Early diagnosis, interpretation, and intervention. *Annals of the New York Academy of Sciences, 205*, 373–382.

Barnard, K. E., Wenner, W., Weber, B., Gray, C., & Peterson, A. (1977). Premature infant refocus. In P. Miller (Ed.), *Research to practice in mental retardation: Vol. 3, Biomedical aspects.* Baltimore, MD: University Park Press.

Bohachick, P., Taylor, M., Sereika, S., Reeder, S., & Anton, B. (2002). Social support, personal control, and psychosocial recovery following heart transplantation. *Clinical Nursing Research, 11*, 34–51.

Bournes, D. A., & Mitchell, G. J. (2002). Waiting: The experience of persons in a critical care waiting room. *Research in Nursing & Health, 25*, 58–67.

Brooten, D., Brown, L. P., Munro, B. H., York, R., Cohen, S., Roncoli, M., & Hollingsworth, A. (1988). Early discharge and specialist transitional care. *Image: Journal of Nursing Scholarship, 20*, 64–68.

Brooten, D., Gennaro, S., Knapp, H., Brown, L. P., & York, R. (1989). Clinical specialist pre- and post-discharge teaching of parents of very low birthweight infants. *Journal of Obstetric, Gynecologic, and Neonatal Nursing, 18*, 316–322.

Brooten, D., Kumar, S., Brown, L. P., Butts, P., Finkler, S., Bakewell-Sachs, S., Gibbons, S., & Delivoria Papadopoulos, M. (1986). A randomized clinical trail of early hospital discharge and home follow-up of very low birthweight infants. *New England Journal of Medicine, 315*, 934–939.

Brooten, D., Roncoli, M., Finkler, S., Arnold, L., Cohen, A., & Mennuti, M. (1994). A randomized clinical trial of early hospital discharge and home follow-up of women having cesarean birth. *Obstetrics and Gynecology, 84*, 832–838.

Cheek, J. & Ballantyne, A. (2001). Moving them on and in: The process of searching for and selecting an aged care facility. *Qualitative Health Research, 11*, 221–237.

Doering, L. V., Esmailian, F., Imperial-Perez, F., & Monsein, S. (2001). Determinants of intensive care length of stay after coronary artery bypass graft surgery. *Heart & Lung, 30*, 9–17.

Hupcey, J. E. (2000). Feeling safe: The psychosocial needs of ICU patients. *Journal of Nursing Scholarship, 32*, 361–367.

Lindeke, L. L., Stanley, J. R., Else, B. S., & Mills, M. M. (2002). Neonatal predictors of school-based services used by NICU graduates at school age. *Journal of Maternal—Child Nursing, 27*, 41–46.

Lund, C. H., Kuller, J., Lane, A. T., Lott, J., Raines, D., & Thomas, K. (2001). Neonatal skin care: Evaluation of the AWHONN/NANN research-based practice project on knowledge and skin care practices. *Journal of Obstetric, Gynecologic, and Neonatal Nursing, 30*, 30–40.

Lund, C. H., Osborne, J., Kuller, J., Lane, A. T., Lott, J., & Raines, D. (2001). Neonatal skin care: Clinical outcomes of the AWHONN/NANN evidence-based clinical practice guideline. *Journal of Obstetric, Gynecologic, and Neonatal Nursing, 30*, 41–51.

McDonald, D. D., Freeland, M., Thomas, G., & Moore, J. (2001). Testing a preoperative pain management intervention for elders. *Research in Nursing & Health, 24*, 402–409.

Paterson, J., & Stewart, J. (2002). Adults with acquired brain injury: Perceptions of their social world. *Rehabilitation Nursing, 27*, 13–18.

Quint, J. C. (1962). Delineation of qualitative aspects of nursing care. *Nursing Research, 11*, 204–206.

Quint, J. C. (1963). The impact of mastectomy. *American Journal of Nursing, 63*, 88–91.

Quint, J. C. (1967). *The nurse and the dying patient.* New York: Macmillan.

Resnick, B., Orwig, D., Maganizer, J., & Wynne, C. (2002). The effect of social support on exercise behavior in older adults. *Clinical Nursing Research, 11*, 52–70.

Reynolds, N. R., & Neidig, J. L. (2002). Characteristics of nausea reported by HIV-infected patients initiating combination antiretroviral regimens. *Clinical Nursing Research, 11*, 71–88.

Sadala, M. L. A., & Mendes, H. W. B. (2000). Caring for organ donors: The intensive care unit nurses' view. *Qualitative Health Research, 10*, 788–805.

Samselle, C. M., Wyman, J. F., Thomas, K. K., Newman, D. K., Gray, M., Dougherty, M., & Burns, P. A. (2000a). Continence for women: Evaluation of AWHONN's third research utilization project. *Journal of Obstetric, Gynecologic, and Neonatal Nursing, 29*, 9–17.

Samselle, C. M., Wyman, J. F., Thomas, K. K., Newman, D. K., Gray, M., Dougherty, M., & Burns, P. A. (2000b). Continence for women: A test of AWHONN's evidence-based practice protocol in clinical practice. *Journal of Obstetric, Gynecologic, and Neonatal Nursing, 29*, 18–26.

Swanson, B., Cronin-Stubbs, D., Zeller, J. M., Kessler, H. A., & Bielauskas, L. A. (1993). Characterizing the neuropsychological functioning of persons with human immunodeficiency virus infection. *Archives of Psychiatric Nursing, 7*, 82–90.

Swanson, B., Zeller, J. M., & Spear, G. (1998). Cortisol upregulates HIV p24 antigen in cultured human monocyte-derived macrophages. *Journal of the Association of Nurses in AIDS care, 9*, 78–83.

Weiss, J., & Hutchinson, S. A. (2000). Warnings about vulnerability in clients with diabetes and hypertension. *Qualitative Health Research, 10*, 521–537.

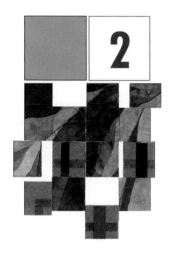

2

Key Concepts and Terms in Qualitative and Quantitative Research

Research, like nursing or any other discipline, has its own language and terminology—its own *jargon*. Some terms are used by both qualitative and quantitative researchers (although in some cases, the connotations differ), whereas others are used predominantly by one or the other group. New terms are introduced throughout this textbook, but we devote this chapter to some fundamental terms and concepts so that more complex ideas can be more readily grasped.

THE FACES AND PLACES OF RESEARCH

When researchers address a problem or answer a question through disciplined research—regardless of the underlying paradigm—they are doing a **study** (or an **investigation** or **research project**). Studies involve various people working together in different roles.

Roles on a Research Project

Studies with humans involve two sets of people: those who do the research and those who provide the information. In a quantitative study, the people who are being studied are referred to as **subjects** or **study participants**, as shown in Table 2-1. (Subjects who provide information to researchers

by answering questions directly—e.g., by filling out a questionnaire—may be called **respondents**.)

The term *subjects* implies that people are *acted upon* by researchers (i.e., are subject to research protocols), and usually is avoided by qualitative researchers. In a qualitative study, the individuals cooperating in the study play an active rather than a passive role in the research, and are usually referred to as study participants, **informants,** or **key informants**. Collectively, both in qualitative and quantitative studies, study participants comprise the **sample**.

The person who undertakes the research is the **researcher** or **investigator** (or sometimes, especially in quantitative studies, the **scientist**). Studies are often undertaken by several people rather than by a single researcher. **Collaborative research** involving a team of nurses with both clinical and methodologic expertise (or involving different members of a health care team) is increasingly common in addressing problems of clinical relevance.

When a study is undertaken by a research team, the person directing the investigation is referred to as the **project director** or **principal investigator (PI)**. Two or three researchers collaborating equally are **co-investigators**. When specialized expertise is needed on a short-term basis (e.g., for statistical analysis), projects may involve one or more **consultants**. In a large-scale project,

TABLE 2.1 Key Terms Used in Quantitative and Qualitative Research

CONCEPT	QUANTITATIVE TERM	QUALITATIVE TERM
Person Contributing Information	Subject Study participant Respondent	— Study participant Informant, key informant
Person Undertaking the Study	Researcher Investigator Scientist	Researcher Investigator —
That Which Is Being Investigated	— Concepts Constructs Variables	Phenomena Concepts — —
System of Organizing Concepts	Theory, theoretical framework Conceptual framework, conceptual model	Theory Conceptual framework, sensitizing framework
Information Gathered	Data (numerical values)	Data (narrative descriptions)
Connections Between Concepts	Relationships (cause-and-effect, functional)	Patterns of association
Quality of the Evidence	Reliability Validity Generalizability Objectivity	Dependability Credibility Transferability Confirmability

dozens of individuals may be involved in planning the study, producing research-related materials, collecting and analyzing the information, and managing the flow of work. The examples of staffing configurations that follow span the continuum from an extremely large project to a more modest one.

Examples of staffing:

Example of Staffing on a Quantitative Study The first author of this book has been involved in a complex, multicomponent 6-year study of poor women living in four major cities (Cleveland, Los Angeles, Miami, and Philadelphia). As part of the study, she and two colleagues prepared a book-length report documenting the health problems and health care concerns of about 4000 welfare mothers who were interviewed in 1998 and again in 2001 (Polit, London, & Martinez, 2001). The total project staff for this research involves well over 100 people, including two co-investigators; lead investigators of the 6 project components (Polit was one of these); a dozen other senior-level researchers; over 50 interviewers; 5 interview supervisors; and dozens of research assistants, computer programmers, secretaries, editors, and other support staff. Several health consultants, including a prominent nurse researcher, were reviewers of the report. The project was funded by a consortium of government agencies and private foundations.

Example of Staffing on a Qualitative Study
Beck (2002) conducted a qualitative study focusing on the experiences of mothers of twins. The team included Beck as the PI (who gathered and analyzed all the information herself); a childbirth educator (who helped to recruit mothers into the study); an administrative assistant (who handled a variety of administrative tasks, like paying stipends to the mothers); a transcriber (who listened to tape-recorded conversations with the mothers and typed them up verbatim); and a secretary (who handled correspondence). This study had some financial support through Beck's university.

In addition to participants and researchers, other parties sometimes are involved in studies. When financial assistance is obtained to pay for research costs, the organization providing the money is the **funder** or **sponsor**. **Reviewers** are sometimes called on to critique various aspects of a study and offer feedback. If these people are at a similar level of experience as the researchers, they may be called **peer reviewers**. Student projects are more likely to be reviewed by faculty advisors. Sometimes students or young researchers get advice and support from **mentors**, who not only give direct feedback but model standards of excellence in research.

Research Settings

Research can be conducted in a wide variety of locales—in health care facilities, in people's homes, in classrooms, and so on. Researchers make decisions about where to conduct a study based on the nature of the research question and the type of information needed to address it.

Generally speaking, the **site** is the overall location for the research—it could be an entire community (e.g., a Haitian neighborhood in Miami) or an institution within a community (e.g., a hospital in Boston). Researchers sometimes engage in **multisite studies** because the use of multiple sites usually offers a larger or more diverse sample of study participants. For example, in a study of a new nursing intervention, researchers may wish to implement the intervention in both public and private hospitals or in urban and rural locations.

Settings are the more specific places where data collection occurs. In some cases, the setting and the site are the same, as when the selected site is a large hospital, and information is collected exclusively within that setting. When the site is a larger community, however, the researcher must decide where data should be collected—in nursing homes, homeless shelters, and so on. Because the nature of the setting can influence the way people behave or feel and how they respond to questions, the selection of an appropriate setting is important.

Some studies take place in **naturalistic settings** (in the *field*), such as in people's homes or offices. In-depth qualitative studies are especially likely to be done in natural settings because qualitative researchers are interested in studying the context of participants' experiences. When researchers go into the field to collect their information, they are engaged in **fieldwork**. In qualitative studies, fieldwork may take months or even years to complete. Qualitative fieldwork often involves studying participants in multiple settings within the selected site (e.g., in their homes, at meetings, and so on).

At the other extreme, studies sometimes are conducted in highly controlled **laboratory settings** that may or may not have elaborate scientific equipment installed. Both human and nonhuman research can occur in laboratory settings.

For nurse researchers, studies are often conducted in quasi-natural settings, such as hospitals or other similar facilities. These are settings that are not necessarily natural to the participants (unless the participants are nurses or other health care personnel), but neither are they highly contrived and controlled research laboratories.

 Example of a study in a naturalistic setting:
Carlisle (2000) studied the search for meaning in the caregiving experience among informal carers of people living with HIV and AIDS. The researcher gathered in-depth information from carers in their homes and in HIV/AIDS volunteer organizations.

Example of a study in a laboratory setting:

Pierce and Clancy (2001) studied the effects of hypoxia on diaphragm activity in anesthetized rats.

THE BUILDING BLOCKS OF A STUDY

Phenomena, Concepts, and Constructs

Research focuses on abstract rather than tangible phenomena. For example, the terms *pain*, *coping*, *grief*, and *resilience* are all abstractions of particular aspects of human behavior and characteristics. These abstractions are referred to as **concepts** or, in qualitative studies, **phenomena**.

Researchers (especially quantitative researchers) also use the term **construct**. Like a concept, a construct refers to an abstraction or mental representation inferred from situations or behaviors. Kerlinger and Lee (2000) distinguish concepts from constructs by noting that constructs are abstractions that are deliberately and systematically invented (or constructed) by researchers for a specific purpose. For example, *self-care* in Orem's model of health maintenance is a construct. The terms *construct* and *concept* are sometimes used interchangeably, although by convention, a construct often refers to a more complex abstraction than a concept.

Theories and Conceptual Models

A **theory** is a systematic, abstract explanation of some aspect of reality. In a theory, concepts are knitted together into a coherent system to describe or explain some aspect of the world. Theories play a role in both qualitative and quantitative research.

In a quantitative study, researchers often start with a theory, **framework**, or **conceptual model** (the distinctions are discussed in Chapter 6). On the basis of theory, researchers make predictions about how phenomena will behave in the real world *if the theory is true*. In other words, researchers use deductive reasoning to develop from the general theory specific predictions that can be tested empirically. The results of the research are used to reject, modify, or lend credence to the theory.

In qualitative research, theories may be used in various ways (Sandelowski, 1993). Sometimes conceptual or **sensitizing frameworks**—derived from various disciplines or qualitative research traditions that will be described in Chapter 3—provide an impetus for a study or offer an orienting world view with clear conceptual underpinnings. In such studies, the framework may help in interpreting information gathered by researchers. In other qualitative studies, theory is the *product* of the research: The investigators use information from the participants inductively as the basis for developing a theory firmly rooted in the participants' experiences. The participants' input is the starting point from which the researcher begins to conceptualize, seeking to explain patterns, commonalities, and relationships emerging from the researcher—participant interactions. The goal in such studies is to arrive at a theory that explains phenomena *as they occur*, not as they are preconceived. Inductively generated theories from qualitative studies are sometimes subjected to more controlled confirmation through quantitative research.

Variables

In quantitative studies, concepts are usually referred to as **variables**. A variable, as the name implies, is something that varies. Weight, anxiety levels, income, and body temperature are all variables (i.e., each of these properties varies from one person to another). To quantitative researchers, nearly all aspects of human beings and their environment are variables. For example, if everyone weighed 150 pounds, weight would not be a variable. If it rained continuously and the temperature was always 70°F, weather would not be a variable, it would be a **constant**. But it is precisely because people and conditions *do* vary that research is conducted. Most quantitative researchers seek to understand how or why things vary, and to learn how differences in one variable are related to differences in another. For example, lung cancer research is concerned with the variable of lung cancer. It is a variable because not everybody has this disease. Researchers have studied what variables might be linked to lung cancer and have discovered that cigarette smoking is related. Smoking is also a variable because not everyone smokes. A variable, then, is any quality of a person, group, or situation that varies or takes on different values.

Variables are the central building blocks of quantitative studies. There are different types of variables, as discussed next.

Continuous, Discrete, and Categorical Variables

Sometimes variables take on a wide range of values. A person's age, for instance, can take on values from zero to more than 100, and the values are not restricted to whole numbers. Such **continuous variables** have values that can be represented on a continuum. In theory, a continuous variable can assume an infinite number of values between two points. For example, consider the continuous variable *weight*: between 1 and 2 pounds, the number of values is limitless: 1.005, 1.7, 1.33333, and so on.

By contrast, a **discrete variable** is one that has a finite number of values between any two points, representing discrete quantities. For example, if people were asked how many children they had, they might answer 0, 1, 2, 3, or more. The value for number of children is discrete, because a number such as 1.5 is not a meaningful value. Between the values 1 and 3, the only possible value is 2.

Other variables take on a small range of values that do not inherently represent a *quantity*. The variable gender, for example, has only two values (male and female). Variables that take on only a handful of discrete nonquantitative values are **categorical variables**. Another example is blood type (A, B, AB, and O). When categorical variables take on only two values, they are sometimes referred to as **dichotomous variables.** Some examples of dichotomous variables are pregnant/not pregnant, HIV positive/HIV negative, and alive/dead.

Active Versus Attribute Variables

Variables are often characteristics of research subjects, such as their age, health beliefs, or weight. Variables such as these are **attribute variables**. In

many research situations, however, the investigator *creates* a variable. For example, if a researcher is interested in testing the effectiveness of patient-controlled analgesia as opposed to intramuscular analgesia in relieving pain after surgery, some patients would be given patient controlled analgesia and others would receive intramuscular analgesia. In the context of this study, method of pain management is a variable because different patients are given different analgesic methods. Kerlinger and Lee (2000) refer to variables that the researcher creates as **active variables**. Note that an active variable in one study could be an attribute variable in another. For example, a researcher might create an "active" salt-intake variable by exposing two groups of people to different amounts of salt in their diets. Another researcher could examine the salt-intake "attributes" of a sample by asking about their consumption of salt.

Dependent Versus Independent Variables

Many studies are aimed at unraveling and understanding causes of phenomena. Does a nursing intervention *cause* more rapid recovery? Does smoking *cause* lung cancer? The presumed cause is the **independent variable**, and the presumed effect is the **dependent variable**. (Note that some researchers use the term **criterion variable** rather than dependent variable. In studies that analyze the consequences of an intervention, it is usually necessary to establish criteria against which the intervention's success can be assessed—hence, the origin of the term *criterion variable*. Others use the term **outcome variable**—the variable capturing the outcome of interest—in lieu of dependent variable. The term *dependent variable,* however, is more general and is the term used throughout this book.)

Variability in the dependent variable is presumed to *depend on* variability in the independent variable. For example, researchers investigate the extent to which lung cancer (the dependent variable) depends on smoking (the independent variable). Or, investigators may be concerned with the extent to which patients' perception of pain (the dependent variable) depends on different nursing actions (the independent variable).

Frequently, the terms *independent variable* and *dependent variable* are used to indicate *direction of influence* rather than causal link. For example, suppose a researcher studied the behaviors of people caring for cognitively impaired elders and found that the patient's age and the caregivers' use of social touch were related: the older the patient, the less social touch the caregiver used. The researcher would likely not conclude that patient age *caused* reductions in social touch. Yet the direction of influence clearly runs from age to touch: it makes *no* sense to suggest that caregivers' social touch influenced elders' age! Although in this example the researcher does not infer a cause-and-effect connection, it is appropriate to conceptualize social touch as the dependent variable and age as the independent variable, because it is the caregivers' use of social touch that the researcher is interested in understanding, explaining, or predicting.

Many dependent variables studied by nurse researchers have multiple causes or antecedents. If we were interested in studying factors that influence people's weight, for example, we might consider their height, physical activity, and diet as independent variables. Multiple *dependent* variables also may be of interest to researchers. For example, an investigator may be concerned with comparing the effectiveness of two methods of nursing care for children with cystic fibrosis. Several dependent variables could be used as criteria of treatment effectiveness, such as length of hospital stay, number of recurrent respiratory infections, presence of cough, and so forth. In short, it is common to design studies with multiple independent and dependent variables.

Variables are not *inherently* dependent or independent. A dependent variable in one study could be an independent variable in another study. For example, a study might examine the effect of nurses' contraceptive counseling (the independent variable) on unwanted births (the dependent variable). Another study might investigate the effect of unwanted births (the independent variable) on the incidence of child abuse (the dependent variable). In short, whether a variable is independent or dependent is a function of the role that it plays in a particular study.

 Example of independent and dependent variables:
Varda and Behnke (2000) asked, What is the effect of the timing of an initial bath on temperature in newborns? Their independent variable was timing of the infant's initial bath (1 hour versus 2 hours after birth). Their dependent variable was axillary temperature.

Heterogeneity

A term frequently used in connection with variables is *heterogeneity*. When an attribute is extremely varied in the group under investigation, the group is said to be **heterogeneous** with respect to that variable. If, on the other hand, the amount of variability is limited, the group is described as relatively **homogeneous**. For example, for the variable height, a group of 2-year-old children is likely to be more homogeneous than a group of 18-year-old adolescents. The degree of **variability** or **heterogeneity** of a group of subjects has implications for study design.

Definitions of Concepts and Variables

Concepts in a study need to be defined and explicated, and dictionary definitions are almost never adequate. Two types of definitions are of particular relevance in a study—conceptual and operational.

The concepts in which researchers are interested are, as noted, abstractions of observable phenomena. Researchers' world view and their outlook on nursing shape how those concepts are defined. A **conceptual definition** presents the abstract or theoretical meaning of the concepts being studied. Conceptual meanings are based on theoretical formulations, on a firm understanding of relevant literature, or on researchers' clinical experience (or on a combination of these). Even seemingly straightforward terms need to be conceptually defined by researchers. The classic example of this is the concept of *caring*. Morse and her colleagues (1990) scrutinized the works of numerous nurse researchers and theorists to determine how *caring* was defined, and identified five different categories of conceptual definitions: as a human trait; a moral imperative; an affect; an interpersonal relationship; and a therapeutic intervention. Researchers undertaking studies concerned with caring need to make clear which conceptual definition of caring they have adopted—both to themselves and to their audience of readers. In qualitative studies, conceptual definitions of key phenomena may be the major end product of the endeavor, reflecting an intent to have the meaning of concepts defined by those being studied.

In quantitative studies, however, researchers need to clarify and define the research concepts at the outset. This is necessary because quantitative researchers must indicate how the variables will be observed and measured in the actual research situation. An **operational definition** of a concept specifies the operations that researchers must perform to collect the required information. Operational definitions should correspond to conceptual definitions.

Variables differ in the ease with which they can be operationalized. The variable weight, for example, is easy to define and measure. We might operationally define weight as follows: the amount that an object weighs in pounds, to the nearest full pound. Note that this definition designates that weight will be determined with one measuring system (pounds) rather than another (grams). The operational definition might also specify that subjects' weight will be measured to the nearest pound using a spring scale with subjects fully undressed after 10 hours of fasting. This operational definition clearly indicates what is meant by the variable *weight*.

Unfortunately, few variables of interest in nursing research are operationalized as easily as weight. There are multiple methods of measuring most variables, and researchers must choose the method that best captures the variables as they conceptualize them. Take, for example, *anxiety*, which can be defined in terms of both physiologic and psychological functioning. For researchers choosing to emphasize physiologic aspects of anxiety, the operational definition might involve a physiologic measure such as the Palmar Sweat Index. If,

on the other hand, researchers conceptualize anxiety as primarily a psychological state, the operational definition might involve a paper-and-pencil measure such as the State Anxiety Scale. Readers of research reports may not agree with how investigators conceptualized and operationalized variables, but precision in defining terms has the advantage of communicating exactly what terms mean within the context of the study.

 Example of conceptual and operational definitions:

Beck and Gable (2001) conceptually defined various aspects of *postpartum depression* and then described how the definitions were linked operationally to a measure Beck developed, the Postpartum Depression Screening Scale (PDSS). For example, one aspect of postpartum depression is *cognitive impairment*, conceptually defined as "a mother's loss of control over her thought processes leaves her frightened that she may be losing her mind." Operationally, the PDSS captured this dimension by having women indicate their level of agreement with such statements as, "I could not stop the thoughts that kept racing in my mind."

Data

Research **data** (singular, datum) are the pieces of information obtained in the course of the investigation.

In quantitative studies, researchers identify the variables of interest, develop operational definitions of those variables, and then collect relevant data from subjects. The actual *values* of the study variables constitute the data for the project. Quantitative researchers collect primarily **quantitative data**—that is, information in numeric form. As an example, suppose we were conducting a quantitative study in which a key variable was depression; we would need to measure how depressed study participants were. We might ask, "Thinking about the past week, how depressed would you say you have been on a scale from 0 to 10, where 0 means 'not at all' and 10 means 'the most possible'?" Box 2-1 presents some quantitative data for three fictitious

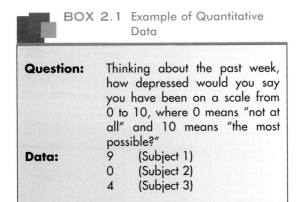

BOX 2.1 Example of Quantitative Data

Question:	Thinking about the past week, how depressed would you say you have been on a scale from 0 to 10, where 0 means "not at all" and 10 means "the most possible?"
Data:	9 (Subject 1)
	0 (Subject 2)
	4 (Subject 3)

respondents. The subjects have provided a number corresponding to their degree of depression—9 for subject 1 (a high level of depression), 0 for subject 2 (no depression), and 4 for subject 3 (little depression). The numeric values for all subjects in the study, collectively, would comprise the data on depression.

In qualitative studies, the researcher collects primarily **qualitative data**, that is, narrative descriptions. Narrative information can be obtained by having conversations with the participants, by making detailed notes about how participants behave in naturalistic settings, or by obtaining narrative records from participants, such as diaries.

Suppose we were studying depression qualitatively. Box 2-2 presents qualitative data for three participants responding conversationally to the question, "Tell me about how you've been feeling lately—have you felt sad or depressed at all, or have you generally been in good spirits?" Here, the data consist of rich narrative descriptions of each participant's emotional state.

Typically, an operation known as **coding** is required to make research data amenable to analysis. In quantitative studies, coding is the process of translating verbal data into numeric form. For example, answers to a question about a subject's gender might be coded "1" for female and "2" for male (or vice versa). In qualitative coding, researchers develop coding categories that represent important themes in the data.

Relationships

Researchers are rarely interested in a single isolated concept or phenomenon, except in descriptive studies. As an example of a descriptive study, a researcher might do research to determine the percentage of patients receiving intravenous (IV) therapy who experience IV infiltration. In this example, the variable is IV infiltration versus no infiltration. Usually, however, researchers study phenomena in relation to other phenomena—that is, they explore

BOX 2.2 Example of Qualitative Data

Question:	Tell me about how you've been feeling lately—have you felt sad or depressed at all, or have you generally been in good spirits?
Data:	Well, actually, I've been pretty depressed lately, to tell you the truth. I wake up each morning and I can't seem to think of anything to look forward to. I mope around the house all day, kind of in despair. I just can't seem to shake the blues, and I've begun to think I need to go see a shrink. (Participant 1)
	I can't remember ever feeling better in my life. I just got promoted to a new job that makes me feel like I can really get ahead in my company. And I've just gotten engaged to a really great guy who is very special. (Participant 2)
	I've had a few ups and downs the past week, but basically things are on a pretty even keel. I don't have too many complaints. (Participant 3)

or test relationships. A **relationship** is a bond or a connection between phenomena. For example, researchers repeatedly have found a *relationship* between cigarette smoking and lung cancer. Both qualitative and quantitative studies examine relationships, but in different ways.

In quantitative studies, researchers are primarily interested in the relationship between the independent variables and dependent variables. The research question focuses on whether variation in the dependent variable is systematically related to variation in the independent variable. Relationships are usually expressed in quantitative terms, such as *more than*, *less than*, and so on. For example, let us consider as our dependent variable a person's body weight. What variables are related to (associated with) a person's weight? Some possibilities are height, caloric intake, and exercise. For each of these independent variables, we can make a prediction about the nature of the relationship to the dependent variable:

Height: Taller people will weigh more than shorter people.
Caloric intake: People with higher caloric intake will be heavier than those with lower caloric intake.
Exercise: The lower the amount of exercise, the greater will be the person's weight.

Each statement expresses a predicted relationship between weight (the dependent variable) and a measurable independent variable. Terms such as *more than* and *heavier than* imply that as we observe a change in one variable, we are likely to observe a corresponding change in weight. If Nate is taller than Tom, we would predict (in the absence of any other information) that Nate is also heavier than Tom. Most quantitative studies are undertaken to determine whether relationships exist among variables.

Quantitative studies typically address one or more of the following questions about relationships:

- Does a relationship between variables *exist*? (e.g., is cigarette smoking related to lung cancer?)
- What is the *direction* of the relationship between variables? (e.g., are people who smoke

more likely or *less* likely to get lung cancer than those who do not?)
- How *strong* is the relationship between the variables? (e.g., how powerful is the relationship between smoking and lung cancer? How probable is it that smokers will be lung cancer victims?)
- What is the *nature* of the relationship between variables? (e.g., does smoking *cause* lung cancer? Does some other factor *cause* both smoking and lung cancer?)

As this last question suggests, quantitative variables can be related to one another in different ways. One type of relationship is referred to as a **cause-and-effect** (or **causal**) **relationship**. Within the positivist paradigm, natural phenomena are assumed not to be random or haphazard; if phenomena have antecedent factors or causes, they are presumably discoverable. For instance, in our example about a person's weight, we might speculate that there is a causal relationship between caloric intake and weight: consuming more calories causes weight gain.

Example of a study of causal relationships: Keller and Treviño (2001) studied whether a regimen of walking (and different frequencies of walking) caused reductions in cardiovascular risk factors, such as obesity and high blood lipids, in Mexican-American women.

Not all relationships between variables can be interpreted as cause-and-effect relationships. There is a relationship, for example, between a person's pulmonary artery and tympanic temperatures: people with high readings on one tend to have high readings on the other. We cannot say, however, that pulmonary artery temperature *caused* tympanic temperature, nor that tympanic temperature *caused* pulmonary artery temperature, despite the relationship that exists between the two variables. This type of relationship is sometimes referred to as a **functional relationship** (or an **associative relationship**) rather than as a causal relationship.

Example of a study of functional relationships: Pressler and Hepworth (2002) examined the relationship between preterm neonate's behavioral competence on the one hand, and the infant's gender and race on the other.

Qualitative researchers are not concerned with quantifying relationships, nor in testing and confirming causal relationships. Rather, qualitative researchers seek patterns of association as a way of illuminating the underlying meaning and dimensionality of phenomena of interest. Patterns of interconnected themes and processes are identified as a means of understanding the whole. In some qualitative studies, theories are generated by identifying relationships between emerging categories. These new connections help to "weave the fractured story back together after the data have been analyzed" (Glaser, 1978, p. 72).

Example of a qualitative study of patterns: Lam and Mackenzie (2002) explored Chinese parents' experiences in parenting a child with Down syndrome. One major theme that emerged in the in-depth interviews was parental acceptance of the child. Although the researchers had not specifically sought to examine differences between mothers and fathers, they noted that mothers and fathers did not accept their child at the same pace.

KEY CHALLENGES OF CONDUCTING RESEARCH

Researchers face numerous challenges in conducting research, including the following:

- Conceptual challenges (How should key concepts be defined? What are the theoretical underpinnings of the study?)
- Financial challenges (How will the study be paid for? Will available resources be adequate?)
- Administrative challenges (Is there sufficient time to complete the study? Can the flow of tasks be adequately managed?)
- Practical challenges (Will there be enough study participants? Will institutions cooperate in the study?)
- Ethical challenges (Can the study achieve its goals without infringing on human or animal rights?)

- Clinical challenges (Will the research goals conflict with clinical goals? What difficulties will be encountered in doing research with vulnerable or frail patients?)
- Methodologic challenges (Will the methods used to address the research question yield accurate and valid results?)

Most of this book provides guidance relating to the last question, and this section highlights key methodologic challenges. However, other challenges are also discussed in this book.*

Reliability, Validity, and Trustworthiness

Researchers want their findings to reflect the *truth*. Research cannot contribute evidence to guide clinical practice if the findings are inaccurate, biased, fail adequately to represent the experiences of the target group, or are based on a misinterpretation of the data. Consumers of research need to assess the quality of evidence offered in a study by evaluating the conceptual and methodologic decisions the researchers made, and producers of research need to strive to make good decisions to produce evidence of the highest possible quality.

Quantitative researchers use several criteria to assess the quality of a study, and two of the most important criteria are reliability and validity. **Reliability** refers to the accuracy and consistency of information obtained in a study. The term is most often associated with the methods used to measure research variables. For example, if a thermometer measured Bob's temperature as 98.1°F one minute and as 102.5°F the next minute, the reliability of the thermometer would be highly suspect. The concept of reliability is also important in interpreting the results of statistical analyses. Statistical reliability refers to the probability that the same results would be obtained with a completely new sample of subjects—that is, that the results are an

---

*The following chapters present relevant materials: conceptual issues—Chapter 6; financial issues—Chapter 25; administrative, practical, and clinical issues—Chapter 4; and ethical issues—Chapter 7.

accurate reflection of a wider group than just the particular people who participated in the study.

Validity is a more complex concept that broadly concerns the *soundness* of the study's evidence—that is, whether the findings are cogent, convincing, and well grounded. Like reliability, validity is an important criterion for assessing the methods of measuring variables. In this context, the validity question is whether there is evidence to support the assertion that the methods are really measuring the abstract concepts that they purport to measure. Is a paper-and-pencil measure of depression *really* measuring depression? Or is it measuring something else, such as loneliness, low self-esteem, or stress? The importance of having solid conceptual definitions of research variables—as well as high-quality methods to operationalize them—should be apparent.

Another aspect of validity concerns the quality of the researcher's evidence regarding the effect of the independent variable on the dependent variable. Did a nursing intervention *really* bring about improvements in patients' outcomes—or were other factors responsible for patients' progress? Researchers make numerous methodologic decisions that can influence this type of study validity.

Qualitative researchers use somewhat different criteria (and different terminology) in evaluating a study's quality. In general, qualitative researchers discuss methods of enhancing the **trustworthiness** of the study's data (Lincoln & Guba, 1985). Trustworthiness encompasses several different dimensions—credibility, transferability (discussed later in the chapter), confirmability, and dependability. **Dependability** refers to evidence that is consistent and stable. **Confirmability** is similar to objectivity; it is the degree to which study results are derived from characteristics of participants and the study context, not from researcher biases.

Credibility, an especially important aspect of trustworthiness, is achieved to the extent that the research methods engender confidence in the truth of the data and in the researchers' interpretations of the data. Credibility in a qualitative study can be enhanced through various approaches (see Chapter 18), but one in particular merits early discussion because it has implications for the design of all

studies, including quantitative ones. **Triangulation** is the use of multiple sources or referents to draw conclusions about what constitutes the truth. In a quantitative study, this might mean having alternative operational definitions of a dependent variable to determine if predicted effects are consistent across the two. In a qualitative study, triangulation might involve trying to understand the full complexity of a poorly understood phenomenon by using multiple means of data collection to converge on the truth (e.g., having in-depth discussions with study participants, as well as watching their behavior in natural settings). Nurse researchers are also beginning to triangulate across paradigms—that is, to integrate both qualitative and quantitative data in a single study to offset the shortcomings of each approach.

Example of triangulation:
Tarzian (2000) used triangulation of data methods in her qualitative study on caring for dying patients with air hunger. Tarzian interviewed 10 nurses who had cared for air-hungry patients and, to complement the nurses' accounts, two family members who witnessed spouses suffering from air hunger. Trustworthiness of the study findings was enhanced because family members confirmed important themes. For example, nurses disclosed that air hunger evoked a physical effect, such as feeling out of breath just watching patients struggling to breathe. Family members supported this theme. One husband recalled, "My chest hurt just watching her, breathing like that all day long" (p. 139).

Nurse researchers need to design their studies in such a way that threats to the reliability, validity, and trustworthiness of their studies are minimized. This book offers advice on how to do this.

Bias

Bias is a major concern in designing a study because it can threaten the study's validity and trustworthiness. In general, a **bias** is an influence that produces a distortion in the study results. Biases can affect the quality of evidence in both qualitative and quantitative studies.

Bias can result from a number of factors, including the following:

- *Study participants' candor.* Sometimes people distort their behavior or their self-disclosures (consciously or subconsciously) in an effort to present themselves in the best possible light.
- *Subjectivity of the researcher.* Investigators may distort information in the direction of their preconceptions, or in line with their own experiences.
- *Sample characteristics.* The sample itself may be biased; for example, if a researcher studies abortion attitudes but includes only members of right-to-life (or pro-choice) groups in the sample, the results would be distorted.
- *Faulty methods of data collection.* An inadequate method of capturing key concepts can lead to biases; for example, a flawed paper-and-pencil measure of patient satisfaction with nursing care may exaggerate or underestimate patients' complaints.
- *Faulty study design.* A researcher may not have structured the study in such a way that an unbiased answer to the research question can be achieved.

To some extent, bias can never be avoided totally because the potential for its occurrence is so pervasive. Some bias is haphazard and affects only small segments of the data. As an example of such **random bias,** a handful of study participants might fail to provide totally accurate information as a result of extreme fatigue at the time the data were collected. **Systematic bias**, on the other hand, results when the bias is consistent or uniform. For example, if a spring scale consistently measured people's weights as being 2 pounds heavier than their true weight, there would be systematic bias in the data on weight. Rigorous research methods aim to eliminate or minimize systematic bias—or, at least, to detect its presence so it can be taken into account in interpreting the data.

Researchers adopt a variety of strategies to address bias. Triangulation is one such approach, the idea being that multiple sources of information or points of view can help counterbalance biases and offer avenues to identify them. Quantitative researchers use various methods to combat the effects of bias, and many of these entail research control.

Research Control

One of the central features of quantitative studies is that they typically involve efforts to control tightly various aspects of the research. **Research control** involves holding constant other influences on the dependent variable so that the true relationship between the independent and dependent variables can be understood. In other words, research control attempts to eliminate contaminating factors that might cloud the relationship between the variables that are of central interest.

The issue of contaminating factors—or **extraneous variables**, as they are called—can best be illustrated with an example. Suppose we were interested in studying whether teenage women are at higher risk of having low-birth-weight infants than are older mothers *because of their age*. In other words, we want to test whether there is something about women's maturational development that causes differences in birth weight. Existing studies have shown that, in fact, teenagers have a higher rate of low-birth-weight babies than women in their 20s. The question here is whether maternal age itself (the independent variable) causes differences in birth weight (the dependent variable), or whether there are other mechanisms that account for the relationship between age and birth weight. We need to design a study so as to control other influences on the dependent variable—influences that are also related to the independent variable.

Two variables of interest are the mother's nutritional habits and her prenatal care. Teenagers tend to be less careful than older women about their eating patterns during pregnancy, and are also less likely to obtain adequate prenatal care. Both nutrition and the amount of care could, in turn, affect the baby's birth weight. Thus, if these two factors are not controlled, then any observed relationship between mother's age and her baby's weight at birth could be caused by the mother's age itself, her diet, or her prenatal care. It would be impossible to know what the underlying cause really is.

These three possible explanations might be portrayed schematically as follows:

1. Mother's age→infant birth weight
2. Mother's age→prenatal care→infant birth weight
3. Mother's age→nutrition→infant birth weight

The arrows here symbolize a causal mechanism or an influence. In examples 2 and 3, the effect of maternal age on infant birth weight is mediated by prenatal care and nutrition, respectively; these variables would be considered **mediating variables** in these last two models. Some research is specifically designed to test paths of mediation, but in the present example these variables are extraneous to the research question. Our task is to design a study so that the first explanation can be tested. Both nutrition and prenatal care must be controlled if our goal is to learn if explanation 1 is valid.

How can we impose such control? There are a number of ways, as discussed in Chapter 9, but the general principle underlying each alternative is the same: *the extraneous variables of the study must be held constant.* The extraneous variables must somehow be handled so that, *in the context of the study,* they are not related to the independent or dependent variable. As an example, let us say we want to compare the birth weights of infants born to two groups of women: those aged 15 to 19 years and those aged 25 to 29 years. We must then design a study in such a way that the nutritional and prenatal health care practices of the two groups are comparable, even though, in general, the two groups are not comparable in these respects. Table 2-2 illustrates how we might deliberately select subjects for the study in such a way that both older and younger mothers had similar eating habits and amounts of prenatal attention; the two groups have been **matched** in terms of the two extraneous variables; one third of both groups have the same nutrition ratings and amount of prenatal care. By building in this comparability, nutrition and prenatal care have been held constant in the two groups. If groups differ in birth weight (as they, in fact, do in Table 2-2), then we might infer that age (and not diet or prenatal care) influenced the infants' birth weights. If the two groups did not differ, however, we might tentatively conclude that it is not mother's age *per se* that causes young women to have a higher percentage of low-birth-weight babies, but rather some other variable, such as nutrition or prenatal care. It is important to note that although we have designated prenatal care and nutrition as extraneous variables in this particular study, they are not at all extraneous to a full understanding of the factors that influence birth weight; in other studies, nutritional practices and frequency of prenatal care might be key independent variables.

By exercising control in this example, we have taken a step toward explaining the relationship between variables. The world is complex, and many

---

TABLE 2.2 Fictitious Example: Control of Two Extraneous Variables

AGE OF MOTHER (YEARS)	NUTRITIONAL PRACTICES	NO. OF PRENATAL VISITS	INFANT BIRTH WEIGHT
15–19	33% rated "good" 33% rated "fair" 33% rated "poor"	33% 1–3 visits 33% 4–6 visits 33% > 6 visits	20% ≤ 2500 g; 80% > 2500 g
25–29	33% rated "good" 33% rated "fair" 33% rated "poor"	33% 1–3 visits 33% 4–6 visits 33% > 6 visits	9% ≤ 2500 g; 91% > 2500 g

variables are interrelated in complicated ways. When studying a particular problem within the positivist paradigm, it is difficult to examine this complexity directly; researchers must usually analyze a couple of relationships at a time and put pieces together like a jigsaw puzzle. That is why even modest studies can make contributions to knowledge. The extent of the contribution in a quantitative study, however, is often directly related to how well researchers control contaminating influences.

In the present example, we identified three variables that could affect birth weight, but dozens of others might be relevant, such as maternal stress, mothers' use of drugs or alcohol during pregnancy, and so on. Researchers need to isolate the independent and dependent variables in which they are interested and then pinpoint from dozens of possible candidates those extraneous variables that need to be controlled.

Example of control through matching:
Mackey, Williams, and Tiller (2000) compared the stress and birth outcomes of women who experienced preterm labor during pregnancy with those who did not. To keep the groups similar, the groups were matched in terms of age, race, parity, gestational age, and method of hospital payment.

It is often impossible to control all variables that affect the dependent variable, and not even necessary to do so. Extraneous variables need to be controlled only if they simultaneously are related to both the dependent and independent variables. This notion is illustrated in Figure 2-1, which has the following elements:

- Each circle represents all the variability associated with a particular variable.
- The large circle in the center stands for the dependent variable, infant birth weight.
- Smaller circles stand for factors contributing to infant birth weight.
- Overlapping circles indicate the degree to which the variables are related to each other.

In this hypothetical example, four variables are related to infant birth weight: mother's age, amount of prenatal care, nutritional practices, and smoking during pregnancy. The first three of these variables are also interrelated; this is shown by the fact that these three circles overlap not only with infant birth weight but also with each other. That is, younger mothers tend to have different patterns of prenatal care and nutrition than older mothers. The mother's prenatal use of cigarettes, however, is unrelated to these three

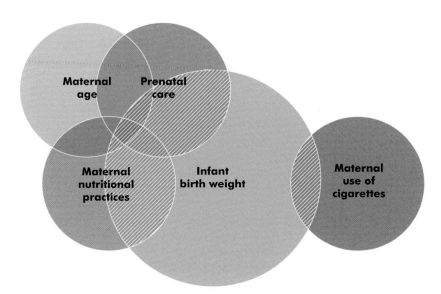

FIGURE 2.1
Hypothetical representation of factors affecting infant birth weight.

variables. In other words, women who smoke during their pregnancies (according to this fictitious representation) are as likely to be young as old, to eat properly as not, and to get adequate prenatal care as not. If this representation were accurate, then maternal smoking would not be need to be controlled to study the effect of maternal age on infant birth weight. If this scheme is incorrect—if teenage mothers smoke more or less than older mothers—then maternal smoking practices should be controlled.

Figure 2-1 does not represent infant birth weight as being totally determined by the four other variables. The darkened area of the birth weight circle designates "unexplained" variability in infant birth weight. That is, other determinants of birth weight are needed for us to understand fully what causes babies to be born weighing different amounts. Genetic characteristics, events occurring during the pregnancy, and medical treatments administered to pregnant women are examples of other factors that contribute to an infant's weight at birth. Dozens, and perhaps hundreds, of circles would need to be sketched onto Figure 2-1 for us to understand factors affecting infant birth weight. In designing a study, quantitative researchers should attempt to control those variables that overlap with both independent and dependent variables to understand fully the relationship between the main variables of interest.

Research control in quantitative studies is viewed as a critical tool for managing bias and for enhancing the validity of researchers' conclusions. There are situations, however, in which too much control can introduce bias. For example, if researchers tightly control the ways in which key study variables can manifest themselves, it is possible that the true nature of those variables will be obscured. When the key concepts are phenomena that are poorly understood or the dimensions of which have not been clarified, then an approach that allows some flexibility is better suited to the study aims—such as in a qualitative study. Research rooted in the naturalistic paradigm does not impose controls. With their emphasis on holism and the individuality of human experience, qualitative researchers typically adhere to the view that to impose controls on a research setting is to remove irrevocably some of the meaning of reality.

Randomness

For quantitative researchers, a powerful tool for eliminating bias concerns the concept of **randomness**—having certain features of the study established by chance rather than by design or personal preference. When people are selected at random to participate in the study, for example, each person has an equal probability of being selected. This in turn means that there are no systematic biases in the make-up of the sample. Men are as likely to be selected as women, for example. Randomness is a compelling method of controlling extraneous variables.

Qualitative researchers almost never consider randomness a desirable tool for fully understanding a phenomenon. Qualitative researchers tend to use information obtained early in the study in a purposive (nonrandom) fashion to guide their inquiry and to pursue information-rich sources that can help them expand or refine their conceptualizations. Researchers' judgments are viewed as indispensable vehicles for uncovering the complexities of the phenomena of interest.

Generalizability and Transferability

Nurses increasingly rely on evidence from disciplined research as a guide in their clinical practice. If study findings are totally unique to the people, places, or circumstances of the original research, can they be used as a basis for changes in practice? The answer, clearly, is no.

As noted in Chapter 1, **generalizability** is the criterion used in a quantitative study to assess the extent to which the findings can be applied to other groups and settings. How do researchers enhance the generalizability of a study? First and foremost, they must design studies strong in reliability and validity. There is little point in wondering whether results are generalizable if they are not accurate or valid. In selecting subjects, researchers must also give thought to the types of people to whom the results might be generalized—and then select them in such a way that a nonbiased sample is obtained. If a study is intended to have implications for male and female patients, then men and women should be included as participants. If an intervention is intended to benefit patients in urban and rural hospitals, then perhaps a multisite study is warranted. Chapter 10 describes other issues to consider in evaluating generalizability.

Qualitative researchers do not specifically seek to make their findings generalizable. Nevertheless, qualitative researchers often seek understandings that might prove useful in other situations. Lincoln and Guba (1985), in their highly influential book on naturalistic inquiry, discuss the concept of **transferability**, the extent to which qualitative findings can be transferred to other settings, as another aspect of a study's trustworthiness. An important mechanism for promoting transferability is the amount of information qualitative researchers provide about the contexts of their studies. **Thick description**, a widely used term among qualitative researchers, refers to a rich and thorough description of the research setting and of observed transactions and processes. Quantitative researchers, like qualitative researchers, need to describe their study participants and their research settings thoroughly so that the utility of the evidence for others can be assessed.

Replication

Virtually every study has flaws or limitations. Even the most rigorous study is likely to contain some bias, or to engender unresolved questions about the validity or trustworthiness of the findings. And few studies are broad enough that findings can be generalized to all groups or settings of interest.

Nursing practice is almost never changed on the basis of a single study, no matter how sound. Evidence-based practice generally builds on accumulated evidence. **Replications** are attempts to validate the findings from one study in an independent inquiry. Replication is, in effect, a form of triangulation—the use of multiple sources and referents (multiple findings) to draw conclusions about the validity or truth of findings. Replication research is critical for the development of nursing science. Yet, remarkably, there is a dearth of replication studies—or, at least, *published* replication studies. This may reflect a strong preference on the part of researchers, editors, and funders for originality and "breaking new ground." "Paving the way," however, is just as critical as breaking new ground, and well-planned and well-executed replication studies are an important paving tool on the road to evidence-based practice. Some strategies for replication are described in Chapter 10.

RESEARCH EXAMPLES

This section presents brief overviews of a quantitative and a qualitative study. These overviews deal primarily with key concepts that were presented in this chapter. You may wish to consult the full research report in thinking about differences in style and content of qualitative and quantitative reports.

Research Example of a Quantitative Study

Health care strategies for urinary incontinence (UI) have emerged and been tested in several studies of community-dwelling women. Dougherty and her co-researchers (2002) noted, however, that health care strategies designed for adults in urban settings do not always transfer well to rural environments. They designed a study to implement and test the efficacy of a behavioral management for continence (BMC) intervention for older women with UI in seven rural counties in north Florida. The intervention involved self-monitoring, bladder training, and pelvic muscle exercise with biofeedback in the women's homes.

Over a 2-year period, 218 women aged 55 years and older who had regular involuntary urine loss were recruited for the study. Half the subjects were selected, at random, to receive the intervention. This procedure permitted a rigorous comparison of the outcomes of the two groups who, because selection into them was random, were presumably alike in all respects—except for receipt of the intervention.

Group membership (i.e., whether a woman was in the BMC group) was the independent variable. Both groups received follow-up visits, during which time outcome data were gathered, every 6 months for up to 2 years. The primary dependent variable was urine loss. This was operationalized as the amount of urine lost in grams per 24 hours, as measured by the change in weight of incontinence pads. Secondary dependent variables relating to urinary outcomes included measures obtained from 3-day bladder diaries that subjects maintained (e.g., micturition frequency and episodes of urine loss). In addition, the researchers assessed the effect of the intervention on subjects' quality of life. This concept was operationalized using a paper-and-pencil instrument known as the Incontinence Impact Questionnaire (IIQ). The IIQ, which involved 26 questions about the extent to which incontinence affected functioning in various areas (e.g., daily living, social interactions, self-perception), previously had been shown to be a reliable and valid indicator of quality of life.

The findings were encouraging. Over the 2 years in which the women were followed, the BMC group sustained UI improvement, whereas those in the other group experienced worsening severity in urine loss. The two groups also differed at follow-up with regard to episodes of urine loss and quality of life.

The study was methodologically strong. Half the women, selected at random, received the special intervention and the other half did not. This is a particularly powerful way to control extraneous variables. Although the number of subjects was fairly small—and therefore replications are clearly needed—it is noteworthy that the sample was drawn from seven different rural counties.

Research Example of a Qualitative Study

Wise (2002) examined the experience of children who received liver transplants from the time before transplantation, through the surgery, and after. The sample consisted of nine children between the ages of 7 and 15 years. Wise conducted all the interviews with the children herself either in their homes or in an outpatient setting. These conversations ranged in length from 20 to 40 minutes. The interviews were audiotaped and transcribed.

Before the interviews, Wise asked the children if they would draw two pictures of themselves, one before the transplantation and one that reflected their present status. The purpose of this artwork was to help the children relax and also to provide an opening for the interviews. An art therapist who interpreted the children's artwork served as a consultant for this qualitative study; the artwork thereby provided an opportunity for triangulation. The qualitative data obtained from the interviews were analyzed and interpreted to discover the underlying themes of the children's experiences.

Wise used thick description in reporting her results. Four themes emerged that described the essence of the phenomenon of pediatric liver transplantation: (1) search for connections with peers before and after transplantation, and also for connections with the donor, (2) ordinary and extraordinary experiences of hospitalization, (3) painful responses and feelings of being out of control, and (4) parents' responses to the illness. The following quote illustrates this fourth theme and is an example of Wise's thick description:

> I will never tell my Mom how I feel about anything. I don't think I would ever tell the truth because I would never want to upset her. I can just see the statement on her face. I know how she feels . . . she has been through so much stuff with me. I basically worry if she is all right instead of me (p. 86).

Wise engaged in a number of activities to establish the rigor of her study. To enhance trustworthiness, for instance, she maintained a journal in which she documented her observations, analysis decisions, and so on. Credibility was established by having an older adolescent validate the themes and also by having an advisor and three colleagues review her findings.

SUMMARY POINTS

• A research **study** (or **investigation** or **research project**) is undertaken by one or more **researchers** (or **investigators** or **scientists**). The people who provide information to the researchers are referred to as **subjects, study participants,** or **respondents** (in quantitative research) or study participants or **informants** in qualitative research; collectively they comprise the **sample**.

- **Collaborative research** involving a team of nurses with both clinical and methodologic expertise is increasingly common in addressing problems of clinical relevance.
- The **site** is the overall location for the research; researchers sometimes engage in **multisite studies**. **Settings** are the more specific places where data collection will occur. Settings for nursing research can range from totally naturalistic environments to formal laboratories.
- Researchers investigate **concepts** and **phenomena** (or **constructs**), which are abstractions or mental representations inferred from behavior or events.
- Concepts are the building blocks of **theories,** which are systematic explanations of some aspect of the real world.
- In quantitative studies, concepts are referred to as *variables*. A **variable** is a characteristic or quality that takes on different values (i.e., a variable varies from one person or object to another).
- Variables that are inherent characteristics of a person that the researcher measures or observes are **attribute variables**. When a researcher actively creates a variable, as when a special intervention is introduced, the variable is an **active variable**.
- Variables that can take on an infinite range of values along a continuum are **continuous variables** (e.g., height and weight). A **discrete variable**, by contrast, is one that has a finite number of values between two points (e.g., number of children). Variables with distinct categories that do not represent a quantity are **categorical variables** (e.g., gender and blood type).
- The **dependent variable** is the behavior, characteristic, or outcome the researcher is interested in understanding, explaining, predicting, or affecting. The **independent variable** is the presumed cause of, antecedent to, or influence on the dependent variable.
- Groups that are highly varied with respect to some attribute are described as **heterogeneous**; groups with limited **variability** are described as **homogeneous**.
- A **conceptual definition** elucidates the abstract or theoretical meaning of the concepts being studied. An **operational definition** is the specification of the procedures and tools required to measure a variable.
- **Data**—the information collected during the course of a study—may take the form of narrative information (**qualitative data**) or numeric values (**quantitative data**).
- Researchers often focus on relationships between two or more concepts. A **relationship** is a bond or connection (or pattern of association) between two phenomena. Quantitative researchers focus on the relationship between the independent variables and dependent variables.
- When the independent variable causes or affects the dependent variable, the relationship is a **cause-and-effect** (or **causal**) **relationship**. In a **functional** or **associative relationship**, variables are related in a noncausal way.
- Researchers face numerous conceptual, practical, ethical, and methodologic challenges. The major methodologic challenge is designing studies that are reliable and valid (quantitative studies) or trustworthy (qualitative studies).
- **Reliability** refers to the accuracy and consistency of information obtained in a study. **Validity** is a more complex concept that broadly concerns the *soundness* of the study's evidence—that is, whether the findings are cogent, convincing, and well grounded.
- **Trustworthiness** in qualitative research encompasses several different dimensions. **Dependability** refers to evidence that is believable, consistent, and stable over time. **Confirmability** refers to evidence of the researcher's objectivity. **Credibility** is achieved to the extent that the research methods engender confidence in the truth of the data and in the researchers' interpretations of the data.
- **Triangulation**, the use of multiple sources or referents to draw conclusions about what constitutes the truth, is one approach to establishing credibility.
- A **bias** is an influence that produces a distortion in the study results. **Systematic bias** results when a bias is consistent or uniform across study participants or situations.

- In quantitative studies, **research control** is used to hold constant outside influences on the dependent variable so that the relationship between the independent and dependent variables can be better understood.
- The external influences the researcher seeks to control are **extraneous variables**—extraneous to the purpose of a specific study. There are a number of ways to control such influences, but the general principle is that the extraneous variables must be held constant.
- For a quantitative researcher, a powerful tool to eliminate bias concerns **randomness**—having certain features of the study established by chance rather than by design or personal preference.
- **Generalizability** is the criterion used in a quantitative study to assess the extent to which the findings can be applied to other groups and settings. A similar concept in qualitative studies is **transferability**, the extent to which qualitative findings can be transferred to other settings. An important mechanism for promoting transferability is **thick description**, the rich and thorough description of the research setting or context so that others can make inferences about contextual similarities
- **Replications**, which are attempts to validate the findings from one study in an independent inquiry, are a crucial form of triangulation. Replication research is essential for the development of nursing science and evidence-based practice.

STUDY ACTIVITIES

Chapter 2 of the *Study Guide to Accompany Nursing Research: Principles and Methods, 7th edition*, offers various exercises and study suggestions for reinforcing concepts presented in this chapter. In addition, the following study questions can be addressed:

1. Suggest ways of conceptually and operationally defining the following concepts: nursing competency, aggressive behavior, pain, home health hazards, postsurgical recovery, and body image.

2. Name five continuous, five discrete, and five categorical variables; identify which, if any, are dichotomous.

3. Identify which of the following variables could be active variables and which are attribute variables (some may be both): height, degree of fatigue, cooperativeness, noise level on hospital units, length of stay in hospital, educational attainment, self-esteem, nurses' job satisfaction.

4. In the following research problems, identify the independent and dependent variables:
   a. How do nurses and physicians differ in the ways they view the extended role concept for nurses?
   b. Does problem-oriented recording lead to more effective patient care than other recording methods?
   c. Do elderly patients have lower pain thresholds than younger patients?
   d. How are the sleeping patterns of infants affected by different forms of stimulation?
   e. Can home visits by nurses to released psychiatric patients reduce readmission rates?

SUGGESTED READINGS
Methodologic References

Glaser, B. (1978). *Theoretical sensitivity*. Mill Valley, CA: The Sociology Press.

Kerlinger, F. N., & Lee, H. B. (2000). *Foundations of behavioral research* (4th ed.). Orlando, FL: Harcourt College Publishers.

Lincoln, Y. S., & Guba, E. G. (1985). *Naturalistic inquiry*. Newbury Park, CA: Sage.

Morse, J. M., Solberg, S. M., Neander, W. L., Bottorff, J. L., & Johnson, J. L. (1990). Concepts of caring and caring as a concept. *Advances in Nursing Science, 13,* 1–14.

Morse, J. M., & Field, P. A. (1995). *Qualitative research methods for health professionals* (2nd ed.). Thousand Oaks, CA: Sage.

Sandelowski, M. (1993). Theory unmasked: The uses and guises of theory in qualitative research. *Research in Nursing & Health, 16,* 213–218.

Studies Cited in Chapter 2

Beck, C. T. (2002). Releasing the pause button: Mothering twins during the first year of life, *Qualitative Health Research, 12*, 593–608.

Beck, C. T., & Gable, R. K. (2001). Ensuring content validity: An illustration of the process. *Journal of Nursing Measurement, 9*, 201–215.

Carlisle, C. (2000). The search for meaning in HIV and AIDS: The carer's experience. *Qualitative Health Research, 10*, 750–765.

Dougherty, M., Dwyer, J., Pendergast, J., Boyington, A., Tomlinson, B., Coward, R., Duncan, R. P., Vogel, B., & Rooks, L. (2002). A randomized trial of behavioral management for continence with older rural women. *Research in Nursing & Health, 25*, 3–13.

Keller, C., & Treviño, R. P. (2001). Effects of two frequencies of walking on cardiovascular risk factor reduction in Mexican American women. *Research in Nursing & Health, 24*, 390–401.

Lam, L., & Mackenzie, A. E. (2002). Coping with a child with Down syndrome. *Qualitative Health Research, 12*, 223–237.

Mackey, M. C., Williams, C. A., & Tiller, C. M. (2000). Stress, pre-term labour and birth outcomes. *Journal of Advanced Nursing, 32*, 666–674.

Pierce, J. D. & Clancy, R. L. (2001). Effects of hypoxia on diaphragm activity in anesthetized rats. *Journal of Perianesthesia Nursing, 16*, 181–186.

Polit, D. F., London, A., & Martinez, J. (2001). *The health of poor urban women.* New York: Manpower Demonstration Research Corporation. (Report available online at: www.mdrc.org.)

Pressler, J. L., & Hepworth, J. T. (2002). A quantitative use of the NIDCAP® tool. *Clinical Nursing Research, 11*, 89–102.

Tarzian, A. J. (2000). Caring for dying patients who have air hunger. *Journal of Nursing Scholarship, 32*, 137–143.

Varda, K. E., & Behnke, R. S. (2000). The effect of timing of initial bath on newborn's temperature. *Journal of Obstetric, Gynecologic, and Neonatal Nursing, 29*, 27–32.

Wise, B. (2002). In their own words: The lived experience of pediatric liver transplantation. *Qualitative Health Research, 12*, 74–90.

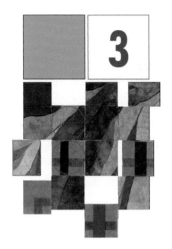

3

Overview of the Research Process in Qualitative and Quantitative Studies

Researchers usually work within a paradigm that is consistent with their world view, and that gives rise to the types of question that excite their curiosity. The maturity of the concept of interest also may lead to one or the other paradigm: when little is known about a topic, a qualitative approach is often more fruitful than a quantitative one.

The progression of activities differs for qualitative and quantitative researchers; we discuss the flow of both in this chapter. First, however, we briefly describe broad categories of quantitative and qualitative research.

MAJOR CLASSES OF QUANTITATIVE AND QUALITATIVE RESEARCH

Experimental and Nonexperimental Studies in Quantitative Research

A basic distinction in quantitative studies is the difference between experimental and nonexperimental research. In **experimental research**, researchers actively introduce an intervention or treatment. In **nonexperimental research**, on the other hand, researchers collect data without making changes or introducing treatments. For example, if a researcher gave bran flakes to one group of subjects and prune juice to another to evaluate which method facilitated elimination more effectively, the

study would be experimental because the researcher intervened in the normal course of things. In this example, the researcher created an "active variable" involving a dietary intervention. If, on the other hand, a researcher compared elimination patterns of two groups of people whose regular eating patterns differed—for example, some normally took foods that stimulated bowel elimination and others did not—there is no intervention. Such a study focuses on existing attributes and is nonexperimental.

Experimental studies are explicitly designed to test causal relationships. Sometimes nonexperimental studies also seek to elucidate or detect causal relationships, but doing so is tricky and usually is less conclusive. Experimental studies offer the possibility of greater control over extraneous variables than nonexperimental studies.

Example of experimental research:
Johnson (2001) tested the effects of a submaximal exercise protocol, in comparison with a near-maximal voluntary contraction protocol, on continence control and muscle contraction strength among women with genuine stress urinary incontinence.

In this example, the researcher intervened by designating that some women would receive the submaximal exercise protocol and others would not. In other words, the researcher *controlled* the independent variable, which in this case was the type of protocol.

Example of nonexperimental research:
Wong and her co-researchers (2002) searched for factors that contributed to hospital readmission in a Hong Kong hospital. A readmitted group was compared with a nonreadmitted group of patients in terms of demographic characteristics and health conditions upon admission.

In this nonexperimental study, the researchers did not intervene in any way; they observed and measured subjects' attributes. They explored whether there were identifiable characteristics and conditions that distinguished the two groups of patients, with the aim of discovering opportunities to reduce readmissions.

Research Traditions in Qualitative Research

Qualitative studies are often rooted in research traditions that originate in the disciplines of anthropology, sociology, and psychology. Three such traditions have had especially strong influences on qualitative nursing research and are briefly describe here. Chapter 11 provides a fuller discussion of alternative research traditions and the methods associated with them.

The **grounded theory** tradition, which has its roots in sociology, seeks to describe and understand the key social psychological and structural processes that occur in a social setting. Grounded theory was developed in the 1960s by two sociologists, Glaser and Strauss (1967). The focus of most grounded theory studies is on a developing social experience—the social and psychological stages and phases that characterize a particular event or episode. A major component of grounded theory is the discovery of a core variable that is central in explaining what is going on in that social scene. Grounded theory researchers strive to generate comprehensive explanations of phenomena that are grounded in reality.

Example of a grounded theory study:
Hauck and Irurita (2002) conducted a grounded theory study to explain the maternal process of managing late stages of breastfeeding and weaning the child from the breast.

Phenomenology, which has its disciplinary roots in both philosophy and psychology and is rooted in a philosophical tradition developed by Husserl and Heidegger, is concerned with the lived experiences of humans. Phenomenology is an approach to thinking about what life experiences of people are like and what they mean. The phenomenological researcher asks the questions: What is the *essence* of this phenomenon as experienced by these people? Or, What is the meaning of the phenomenon to those who experience it?

Example of a phenomenological study:
Sundin, Norberg, and Jansson (2001) conducted a phenomenological study to illuminate the lived experiences of care providers who were highly skilled communicators in their relationships with patients with stroke and aphasia.

Ethnography is the primary research tradition within anthropology, and provides a framework for studying the meanings, patterns, and experiences of a defined cultural group in a holistic fashion. Ethnographers typically engage in extensive fieldwork, often participating to the extent possible in the life of the culture under study. Ethnographic research is in some cases concerned with broadly defined cultures (e.g., Haitian refugee communities), but sometimes focuses on more narrowly defined cultures (e.g., the culture of emergency departments). The aim of ethnographers is to learn from (rather than to study) members of a cultural group, to understand their world view as they perceive and live it.

Example of an ethnographic study:
Powers (2001) undertook an ethnographic analysis of a nursing home residence, focusing on the ethical issues of daily living affecting nursing home residents with dementia.

MAJOR STEPS IN A QUANTITATIVE STUDY

In quantitative studies, researchers move from the beginning point of a study (the posing of a question) to the end point (the obtaining of an answer) in a fairly linear sequence of steps that is broadly similar across studies. In some studies, the steps overlap, whereas in others, certain steps are unnecessary. Still, there is a general flow of activities that is typical of a quantitative study. This section describes that flow, and the next section describes how qualitative studies differ.

Phase 1: The Conceptual Phase

The early steps in a quantitative research project typically involve activities with a strong conceptual or intellectual element. These activities include reading, conceptualizing, theorizing, reconceptualizing, and reviewing ideas with colleagues or advisers. During this phase, researchers call on such skills as creativity, deductive reasoning, insight, and a firm grounding in previous research on the topic of interest.

Step 1: Formulating and Delimiting the Problem

One of the first things a researcher must do is develop a research problem and **research questions**. Good research depends to a great degree on good questions. Without a significant, interesting problem, the most carefully and skillfully designed research project is of little value.

Quantitative researchers usually proceed from the selection of a broad problem area to the development of specific questions that are amenable to empirical inquiry. In developing a research question to be studied, nurse researchers must pay close attention to substantive issues (Is this research question significant, given the existing base of knowledge?); clinical issues (Could findings from this research be useful in clinical practice?); and methodologic issues (How can this question best be studied to yield high-quality evidence?). The identification of research questions must also take into consideration practical and ethical concerns.

TIP: A critical ingredient in developing good research questions is personal interest. We offer this advice to those of you who plan to undertake a research project: Begin with topics that fascinate you or about which you have a passionate interest or curiosity.

Step 2: Reviewing the Related Literature

Quantitative research is typically conducted within the context of previous knowledge. To build on existing theory or research, quantitative researchers strive to understand what is already known about a research problem. A thorough **literature review** provides a foundation on which to base new knowledge and usually is conducted well before any data are collected in quantitative studies. For clinical problems, it would likely also be necessary to learn as much as possible about the "status quo" of current procedures relating to the topic, and to review existing practice guidelines or protocols.

A familiarization with previous studies can also be useful in suggesting research topics or in identifying aspects of a problem about which more research is needed. Thus, a literature review sometimes precedes the delineation of the research problem.

Step 3: Undertaking Clinical Fieldwork

In addition to refreshing or updating clinical knowledge based on written work, researchers embarking on a clinical nursing study benefit from spending time in clinical settings, discussing the topic with clinicians and health care administrators, and observing current practices. Sterling (2001) notes that such clinical fieldwork can provide perspectives on recent clinical trends, current diagnostic procedures, and relevant health care delivery models; it can also help researchers better understand affected clients and the settings in which care is provided. In addition to expanding the researchers' clinical and conceptual knowledge, such fieldwork can be valuable in developing methodologic tools for strengthening the study. For example, in the course of clinical fieldwork researchers might learn what extraneous variables need to be controlled, or might discover the need for Spanish-speaking research assistants.

As with literature reviews, clinical fieldwork may serve as a stimulus for developing research questions and may be the first step in the process for some researchers.

Step 4: Defining the Framework and Developing Conceptual Definitions

Theory is the ultimate aim of science in that it transcends the specifics of a particular time, place, and group of people and aims to identify regularities in the relationships among variables. When quantitative research is performed within the context of a theoretical framework—that is, when previous theory is used as a basis for generating predictions that can be tested through empirical research—the findings may have broader significance and utility.

Even when the research question is not embedded in a theory, researchers must have a clear sense of the concepts under study. Thus, an important task in the initial phase of a project is the development of conceptual definitions.

Step 5: Formulating Hypotheses

A **hypothesis** is a statement of the researcher's expectations about relationships between the variables under investigation. Hypotheses, in other words, are predictions of expected outcomes; they state the relationships researchers expect to find as a result of the study.

The research question identifies the concepts under investigation and asks how the concepts might be related; a hypothesis is the predicted answer. For example, the initial research question might be phrased as follows: Is preeclamptic toxemia in pregnant women associated with stress factors present during pregnancy? This might be translated into the following hypothesis: Pregnant women with a higher incidence of stressful events during pregnancy will be more likely than women with a lower incidence of stress to experience preeclamptic toxemia. Most quantitative studies are designed to test hypotheses through statistical analysis.

Phase 2: The Design and Planning Phase

In the second major phase of a quantitative research project, researchers make decisions about the methods and procedures to be used to address the research question, and plan for the actual collection of data. Sometimes the nature of the question dictates the methods to be used, but more often than not, researchers have considerable flexibility to be creative and make many decisions. These methodologic decisions usually have crucial implications for the validity and reliability of the study findings. If the methods used to collect and analyze research data are seriously flawed, then the evidence from the study may be of little value.

Step 6: Selecting a Research Design

The **research design** is the overall plan for obtaining answers to the questions being studied and for handling some of the difficulties encountered during the research process. A wide variety of research designs is available for quantitative studies, including numerous experimental and nonexperimental designs.

In designing the study, researchers specify which specific design will be adopted and what controls will be used to minimize bias and enhance the interpretability of results. In quantitative studies, research designs tend to be highly structured, with tight controls over extraneous variables. Research designs also indicate other aspects of the research—for example, how often subjects will be measured or observed, what types of comparisons will be made, and where the study will take place. The research design is essentially the architectural backbone of the study.

Step 7: Developing Protocols for the Intervention

In experimental research, researchers actively intervene and create the independent variable, which means that people in the sample will be exposed to different treatments or conditions. For example, if we were interested in testing the effect of biofeedback in treating hypertension, the independent variable would be biofeedback compared with either an alternative treatment (e.g., relaxation therapy), or with no treatment. The **intervention protocol** for the study would need to be developed, specifying exactly what the biofeedback treatment would entail (e.g., who would administer it, how frequently and over how long a period the treatment would last, what specific equipment would be used, and so on) *and* what the alternative condition would be. The goal of well-articulated protocols is to have all subjects in each group treated in the same way. (In nonexperimental research, of course, this step would not be necessary.)

Step 8: Identifying the Population to be Studied

Before selecting subjects, quantitative researchers need to know what characteristics participants should possess. Researchers and others using the findings also need to know to whom study results can be generalized. Thus, during the planning phase of quantitative studies, researchers must identify the population to be studied. The term **population** refers to the aggregate or totality of those conforming to a set of specifications. For example, we might specify nurses (RNs) and residence in the United States as attributes of interest; the study population would then consist of all licensed RNs who reside in the United States. We could in a similar fashion define a population consisting of *all* children younger than 10 years of age with muscular dystrophy in Canada, or *all* the change-of-shift reports for the year 2002 in Massachusetts General Hospital.

Step 9: Designing the Sampling Plan

Research studies almost always rely on a **sample** of subjects, who are a subset of the population. It is clearly more practical and less costly to collect data from a sample than from an entire population. The risk, however, is that the sample might not adequately reflect the population's behaviors, traits, symptoms, or beliefs.

Various methods of obtaining samples are available. These methods vary in cost, effort, and skills required, but their adequacy is assessed by the same criterion: the **representativeness** of the selected sample. That is, the quality of the sample for quantitative studies depends on how typical, or representative, the sample is of the population with respect to the variables of concern in the study. Sophisticated sampling procedures can produce samples that have a high likelihood of being representative. The most sophisticated methods are

probability sampling methods, which use random procedures for selecting subjects. In a probability sample, every member of the population has an equal probability of being included in the sample. With **nonprobability sampling**, by contrast, there is no way of ensuring that each member of the population could be selected; consequently, the risk of a biased (unrepresentative) sample is greater. The design of a **sampling plan** includes the selection of a sampling method, the specification of the sample size (i.e., number of subjects), and the development of procedures for recruiting subjects.

Step 10: Specifying Methods to Measure the Research Variables

Quantitative researchers must develop methods to observe or measure the research variables as accurately as possible. Based on the conceptual definitions, the researcher selects or designs appropriate methods of operationalizing the variables and collecting data. A variety of quantitative data collection approaches exist. **Biophysiologic measurements** often play an important role in clinical nursing research. Through **self-reports**, another popular method of data collection, subjects are asked directly about their feelings, behaviors, attitudes, and personal traits (for example, in an interview with research personnel). Another technique is **observation**, wherein researchers collect data by observing and recording aspects of people's behavior.

Data collection methods vary in the degree of structure imposed on subjects. Quantitative approaches tend to be fairly structured, involving the use of a formal **instrument** that elicits the same information from every subject. Sometimes researchers need to develop their own instruments, but more often they use or adapt measuring instruments that have been developed by others. The task of measuring research variables and developing a **data collection plan** is a complex and challenging process that permits a great deal of creativity and choice. Before finalizing the data collection plan, researchers must carefully evaluate whether the chosen methods capture key concepts accurately.

Step 11: Developing Methods for Safeguarding Human/Animal Rights

Most nursing research involves human subjects, although some studies involve animals. In either case, procedures need to be developed to ensure that the study adheres to ethical principles. For example, forms often need to be developed to document that subjects' participation in the study was voluntary. Each aspect of the study plan needs to be reviewed to determine whether the rights of subjects have been adequately protected. Often that review involves a formal presentation to an external committee.

Step 12: Finalizing and Reviewing the Research Plan

Before actually collecting research data, researchers often perform a number of "tests" to ensure that plans will work smoothly. For example, they may evaluate the readability of any written materials to determine if people with below-average reading skills can comprehend them, or they may need to test whether technical equipment is functioning properly. If questionnaires are used, it is important to know whether respondents understand questions or find certain ones objectionable; this is usually referred to as **pretesting** the questionnaire. During final study preparations, researchers also have to determine the type of training to provide to those responsible for collecting data. If researchers have concerns about their study plans, they may undertake a **pilot study**, which is a small-scale version or trial run of the major study.

Normally, researchers have their research plan critiqued by peers, consultants, or other reviewers to obtain substantive, clinical, or methodologic feedback before implementing the plan. When researchers seek financial support for the study, a **proposal** typically is submitted to a funding source, and reviewers of the proposed plan usually suggest improvements. Students conducting a study as part of a course or degree requirement have their plans reviewed by faculty advisers. Even under other circumstances, however, researchers are well advised to ask individuals external to the project to assess preliminary plans.

Experienced researchers with fresh perspectives can often be invaluable in identifying pitfalls and shortcomings that otherwise might not have been recognized.

Phase 3: The Empirical Phase

The empirical portion of quantitative studies involves collecting research data and preparing those data for **analysis**. In many studies, the empirical phase is one of the most time-consuming parts of the investigation, although the amount of time spent collecting data varies considerably from one study to the next. If data are collected by distributing a written questionnaire to intact groups, this task may be accomplished in a matter of days. More often, however, data collection requires several weeks, or even months, of work.

Step 13: Collecting the Data

The actual collection of data in a quantitative study often proceeds according to a preestablished plan. The researcher's plan typically specifies procedures for the actual collection of data (e.g., where and when the data will be gathered); for describing the study to participants; and for recording information. Technological advances in the past few decades have expanded possibilities for automating data collection.

A considerable amount of both clerical and administrative work is required during data collection. Researchers typically must be sure, for example, that enough materials are available to complete the study; that participants are informed of the time and place that their presence may be required; that research personnel (such as interviewers) are conscientious in keeping their appointments; that schedules do not conflict; and that a suitable system of maintaining confidentiality of information has been implemented.

Step 14: Preparing the Data for Analysis

After data are collected, a few preliminary activities must be performed before data analysis begins. For instance, it is normally necessary to look through questionnaires to determine if they are usable.

Sometimes forms are left almost entirely blank or contain other indications of misinterpretation or noncompliance. Another step is to assign identification numbers to the responses or observations of different subjects, if this was not done previously.

Coding of the data is typically needed at this point. As noted in Chapter 2, coding involves the translation of verbal data into numeric form, according to a specified plan. This might mean assigning numeric codes to categorical variables such as gender (e.g., 1 for females and 2 for males). Coding might also be needed to categorize narrative responses to certain questions. For example, patients' verbatim responses to a question about the quality of nursing care they received during hospitalization might be coded into positive reactions (1), negative reactions (2), neutral reactions (3), or mixed reactions (4). Another preliminary step involves transferring the data from written documents onto computer files for subsequent analysis.

Phase 4: The Analytic Phase

Quantitative data gathered in the empirical phase are not reported in raw form. They are subjected to analysis and interpretation, which occurs in the fourth major phase of a project.

Step 15: Analyzing the Data

The data themselves do not provide answers to research questions. Ordinarily, the amount of data collected in a study is rather extensive; research questions cannot be answered by a simple perusal of numeric information. Data need to be processed and analyzed in an orderly, coherent fashion. Quantitative information is usually analyzed through statistical procedures. **Statistical analyses** cover a broad range of techniques, from simple procedures that we all use regularly (e.g., computing an average) to complex and sophisticated methods. Although some methods are computationally formidable, the underlying logic of statistical tests is relatively easy to grasp, and computers have eliminated the need to get bogged down with detailed mathematic operations.

Step 16: Interpreting the Results

Before the results of a study can be communicated effectively, they must be systematically interpreted. **Interpretation** is the process of making sense of the results and of examining their implications. The process of interpretation begins with an attempt to explain the findings within the context of the theoretical framework, prior empirical knowledge, and clinical experience.

If research hypotheses have been supported, an explanation of the results may be straightforward because the findings fit into a previously conceived argument. If hypotheses are not supported, researchers must explain why this might be so. Is the underlying conceptualization wrong, or was it inappropriate for the research problem? Or do the findings reflect problems with the research methods rather than the framework (e.g., was the measuring tool inappropriate)? To provide sound explanations, researchers not only must be familiar with clinical issues, prior research, and conceptual underpinnings, but must be able to understand methodologic limitations of the study. In other words, the interpretation of the findings must take into account all available evidence about the study's reliability and validity. Researchers need to evaluate critically the decisions they made in designing the study and to recommend alternatives to others interested in the same research problem.

Phase 5: The Dissemination Phase

The analytic phase brings researchers full circle: it provides answers to the questions posed in the first phase of the project. However, researchers' responsibilities are not complete until the study results are disseminated.

Step 17: Communicating the Findings

A study cannot contribute evidence to nursing practice if the results are not communicated. The most compelling hypothesis, the most rigorous study, the most dramatic results are of no value to the nursing community if they are unknown. Another—and often final—task of a research project, therefore, is the preparation of a **research report** that can be shared with others.

Research reports can take various forms: term papers, dissertations, journal articles, presentations at professional conferences, and so on. **Journal articles**—reports appearing in such professional journals as *Nursing Research*—usually are the most useful because they are available to a broad, international audience. There is also a growing number of outlets for research dissemination on the Internet.

Step 18: Utilizing the Findings in Practice

Many interesting studies have been conducted by nurses without having any effect on nursing practice or nursing education. Ideally, the concluding step of a high-quality study is to plan for its utilization in practice settings. Although nurse researchers may not themselves be in a position to implement a plan for utilizing research findings, they can contribute to the process by including in their research reports recommendations regarding how the evidence from the study could be incorporated into the practice of nursing and by vigorously pursuing opportunities to disseminate the findings to practicing nurses.

Organization of a Quantitative Research Project

The steps described in the preceding section represent an idealized conception of what researchers do. The research process rarely follows a neatly prescribed pattern of sequential procedures. Developments in one step, for example, may require alterations in a previously completed activity. Nevertheless, for the quantitative researcher, careful organization is very important.

Almost all research projects are conducted under some time pressure. Students in research courses have end-of-term deadlines; government-sponsored research involves funds granted for a specified time. Those who may not have such formal time constraints (e.g., graduate students working on theses or dissertations) normally have their own goals for project completion. Setting up a timetable in advance may be an important means of

meeting such goals. Having deadlines for tasks—even tentative ones—helps to impose order and delimits tasks that might otherwise continue indefinitely, such as problem selection and literature reviews.

It is not possible to give even approximate figures for the relative percentage of time that should be spent on each task in quantitative studies. Some projects require many months to develop and pretest the measuring instruments, whereas other studies use previously existing ones, for example. The write-up of the study may take many months or only a few days. Clearly, not all steps are equally time-consuming. It would make little sense simply to divide the available time by the number of tasks.

Let us suppose a researcher was studying the following problem: Is a woman's decision to have an annual mammogram related to her perceived susceptibility to breast cancer? Using the organization of steps outlined earlier, here are some of the tasks that might be undertaken:*

1. The researcher, who lost her mother to breast cancer, is concerned that many older women do not get a mammogram regularly. Her specific *research question* is whether mammogram practices are different for women who have different views about their susceptibility to breast cancer.

2. The researcher *reviews the research literature* on mammograms, factors affecting mammography decisions, and interventions designed to promote it.

3. The researcher does *clinical fieldwork* by discussing the problem with nurses and other health care professionals in various clinical settings (health clinics, private obstetrics and gynecology practices) and by informally discussing the problem with women in a support group for breast cancer victims.

4. The researcher *examines frameworks* for conceptualizing the problem. She finds that the

---

*This is, of course, only a partial list of tasks and is designed to illustrate the flow of activities; the flow in this example is more orderly than would ordinarily be true.

Health Belief Model (see Chapter 6) is relevant, and this helps her to develop a conceptual definition of susceptibility to breast cancer.

5. Based on what the researcher has learned, the following *hypothesis is developed*: Women who perceive themselves as not susceptible to breast cancer are less likely than other women to get an annual mammogram.

6. The researcher adopts a nonexperimental *research design* that involves collecting data from subjects at a single point in time. She designs the study to control the extraneous variables of age, marital status, and general health status.

7. There is no *intervention* in this study (the design is nonexperimental) and so this step does not need to be undertaken.

8. The researcher designates that the *population* of interest is women between the ages of 50 and 65 years living in Canada who have not been previously diagnosed as having any form of cancer.

9. The researcher decides to recruit for the *research sample* 200 women living in Toronto; they are identified at random using a telephone procedure known as random-digit dialing.

10. The *research variables will be measured* through self-report; that is, the independent variable (perceived susceptibility), dependent variable (mammogram history), and extraneous variables will be measured by asking the subjects a series of questions. The researcher decides to use existing measures of key variables, rather than developing new ones.

11. A human subjects committee at the researcher's institution is asked to review the research plans to determine whether the study *adheres to ethical standards.*

12. *Plans for the study are finalized*: the methods are reviewed and refined by colleagues with clinical and methodologic expertise; the data collection instruments are pretested; and interviewers who will collect the data are trained.

13. *Data are collected* by conducting telephone interviews with the research sample.

14. *Data are prepared for analysis* by coding them and entering them onto a computer file.

15. *Data are analyzed* using a statistical software package.

16. The results indicate that the hypothesis is supported; however, the researcher's *interpretation* must take into consideration that many women who were asked to participate in the study declined to do so. Moreover, the analysis revealed that mammogram use in the sample was substantially higher than had been reported in earlier studies.

17. The researcher presents an early report on her findings and interpretations at a conference of Sigma Theta Tau International. She subsequently publishes the report in the *Western Journal of Nursing Research.*

18. The researcher seeks out clinicians to discuss how the study findings can be *utilized in practice.*

The researcher in this study wants to conduct this study over a 2-year period. Figure 3-1 presents a hypothetical schedule for the research tasks to be completed. (The selection of the problem is not included because the research topic has already been identified.) Note that many steps overlap or are undertaken concurrently. Some steps are projected to involve little time, whereas others require months of work.

In developing a time schedule of this sort, a number of considerations should be kept in mind, including researchers' level of knowledge and methodologic competence. Resources available to researchers, in terms of research funds and personnel, greatly influence time estimates. In the present example, the researcher almost certainly would have required funding from a sponsor to help pay for the cost of hiring interviewers, unless she were able to depend on colleagues or students.

It is also important to consider the practical aspects of performing the study, which were not all enumerated in the preceding section. Obtaining supplies, securing permissions, getting approval for using

0	2	4	6	8	10	12	14	16	18	20	22	24

Conceptual Phase

Step 2
Step 3
Step 4
Step 5

Planning Phase

Step 6
Step 8*
Step 9
Step 10
Step 11
Step 12

Empirical Phase

Step 13
Step 14

Analytic Phase

Step 15
Step 16

Dissemination Phase

Step 17
Step 18

0	2	4	6	8	10	12	14	16	18	20	22	24

* Note that Step 7 was not necessary because this study did not involve an intervention.

FIGURE 3.1 Project timetable in calendar months.

forms or instruments, hiring staff, and holding meetings are all time-consuming, but necessary, activities.

Individuals differ in the kinds of tasks that appeal to them. Some people enjoy the preliminary phase, which has a strong intellectual component, whereas others are more eager to collect the data, a task that is more interpersonal. Researchers should, however, allocate a reasonable amount of time to do justice to each activity.

ACTIVITIES IN A QUALITATIVE STUDY

As we have just seen, quantitative research involves a fairly linear progression of tasks—researchers plan in advance the steps to be taken to maximize study integrity and then follow those steps as faithfully as possible. In qualitative studies, by contrast, the progression is closer to a circle than to a straight line—qualitative researchers are continually examining and interpreting data and making decisions about how to proceed based on what has already been discovered.

Because qualitative researchers have a flexible approach to the collection and analysis of data, it is impossible to define the flow of activities precisely—the flow varies from one study to another, and researchers themselves do not know ahead of time exactly how the study will proceed. The following sections provide a sense of how qualitative studies are conducted by describing some major activities and indicating how and when they might be performed.

Conceptualizing and Planning a Qualitative Study

Identifying the Research Problem
Like quantitative researchers, qualitative researchers usually begin with a broad topic area to be studied.

However, qualitative researchers usually focus on an aspect of a topic that is poorly understood and about which little is known. Therefore, they do not develop hypotheses or pose highly refined research questions before going into the field. The general topic area may be narrowed and clarified on the basis of self-reflection and discussion with colleagues (or clients), but researchers may proceed with a fairly broad research question that allows the focus to be sharpened and delineated more clearly once the study is underway. (Qualitative researchers may also decide to focus on a topic that has been extensively researched quantitatively, but has had little qualitative attention.)

Doing Literature Reviews

There are conflicting opinions among qualitative researchers about doing a literature review at the outset of a study. At one extreme are those who believe that researchers should not consult the literature before collecting data. Their concern is that prior studies or clinical writings might influence researchers' conceptualization of the phenomena under study. According to this view, the phenomena should be elucidated based on participants' viewpoints rather than on any prior information. Those sharing this viewpoint often do a literature review at the end of the study rather than at the beginning. Others feel that researchers should conduct at least a preliminary up-front literature review to obtain some possible guidance (including guidance in identifying the kinds of biases that have emerged in studying the topic). Still others believe that a full up-front literature review is appropriate. In any case, qualitative researchers typically find a relatively small body of relevant previous work because of the types of question they ask.

Selecting and Gaining Entrée Into Research Sites

During the planning phase, qualitative researchers must also select a site that is consistent with the topic under study. For example, if the topic is the health beliefs of the urban poor, an inner-city neighborhood with a high percentage of low-income residents must be identified. In making such a decision, researchers may need to engage in anticipatory fieldwork (and

perhaps some clinical fieldwork) to identify the most suitable and information-rich environment for the conduct of the study. For a qualitative researcher, an ideal site is one in which (1) entry is possible; (2) a rich mix of people, interactions, and situations relating to the research question is present; and (3) the researcher can adopt—and maintain—an appropriate role vis-à-vis study participants. It is critical to appraise the suitability of the site (and the settings within the site where data will be collecting) before entering the field.

In some cases, researchers may have access to the site selected for the study. In others, however, researchers need to **gain entrée** into the site or settings within it. A site may be well suited to the needs of the research, but if researchers cannot "get in," the study cannot proceed. Gaining entrée typically involves negotiations with **gatekeepers** who have the authority to permit entry into their world. Gaining entrée requires strong interpersonal skills, as well as familiarity with the customs and language of the site. In addition, certain strategies are more likely to succeed than others. For example, gatekeepers might be persuaded to be cooperative if it can be demonstrated that there will be direct benefits to them or their constituents—or if a great humanitarian purpose will be served. Researchers also need to gain the gatekeepers' trust, and that can only occur if researchers are congenial, persuasive, forthright about research requirements (e.g., how much time the fieldwork will require), and—perhaps most important—express genuine interest in and concern for the situations of the people in the site. In qualitative research, gaining entrée is likely to be an ongoing process of establishing relationships and rapport with gatekeepers and others at the site, including prospective informants.

Research Design in Qualitative Studies

As we have seen, quantitative researchers do not collect data until the research design has been finalized. In a qualitative study, by contrast, the research design is often referred to as an **emergent design**—a design that emerges during the course of data collection. Certain design features are guided by the qualitative research tradition within which the researcher is working, but nevertheless few qualitative studies have rigidly structured designs that prohibit changes while in the field. As previously noted, qualitative designs are not concerned with the control of extraneous variables. The full context of the phenomenon is considered an important factor in understanding how it plays out in the lives of people experiencing it.

Although qualitative researchers do not always know in advance exactly how the study will progress in the field, they nevertheless must have some sense of how much time is available for field work and must also arrange for and test needed equipment, such as tape recorders or videotaping equipment. Other planning activities include such tasks as hiring and training interviewers to assist in the collection of data; securing interpreters if the informants speak a different language; and hiring appropriate consultants, transcribers, and support staff.

Addressing Ethical Issues

Qualitative researchers, like quantitative researchers, must also develop plans for addressing ethical issues—and, indeed, there are special concerns in qualitative studies because of the more intimate nature of the relationship that typically develops between researchers and study participants. Chapter 7 describes some of these concerns.

Conducting the Qualitative Study

In qualitative studies, the tasks of sampling, data collection, data analysis, and interpretation typically take place iteratively. Qualitative researchers begin by talking with or observing a few people who have first-hand experience with the phenomenon under study. The discussions and observations are loosely structured, allowing for the expression of a full range of beliefs, feelings, and behaviors. Analysis and interpretation are ongoing, concurrent activities that guide choices about the kinds of people to sample next and the types of questions to ask or observations to make. The actual process of data analysis involves clustering together related types of narrative information into a coherent scheme. The analysis of qualitative data is an intensive, time-consuming activity.

As analysis and interpretation progress, researchers begin to identify **themes** and categories, which are used to build a rich description or theory of the phenomenon. The kinds of data obtained and the people selected as participants tend to become increasingly focused and purposeful as the conceptualization is developed and refined. Concept development and verification shape the sampling process—as a conceptualization or theory develops, the researcher seeks participants who can confirm and enrich the theoretical understandings, as well as participants who can potentially challenge them and lead to further theoretical development.

Quantitative researchers decide in advance how many subjects to include in the study, but qualitative researchers' sampling decisions are guided by the data themselves. Many qualitative researchers use the principle of **data saturation**, which occurs when themes and categories in the data become repetitive and redundant, such that no new information can be gleaned by further data collection.

In quantitative studies, researchers seek to collect high-quality data by using measuring instruments that have been demonstrated to be accurate and valid. Qualitative researchers, by contrast, must take steps to demonstrate the trustworthiness of the data while in the field. The central feature of these efforts is to confirm that the findings accurately reflect the experiences and viewpoints of participants, rather than perceptions of the researchers. One confirmatory activity, for example, involves going back to participants and sharing preliminary interpretations with them so that they can evaluate whether the researcher's thematic analysis is consistent with their experiences. Another strategy is to use triangulation to converge on a thorough depiction of the target phenomena.

An issue that qualitative researchers sometimes need to address is the development of appropriate strategies for leaving the field. Because qualitative researchers may develop strong relationships with study participants and entire communities, they need to be sensitive to the fact that their departure from the field might seem like a form of rejection or abandonment. Graceful departures and methods of achieving closure are important.

Disseminating Qualitative Findings

Qualitative nursing researchers also strive to share their findings with others at conferences and in journal articles. Qualitative findings, because of their depth and richness, also lend themselves more readily to book-length manuscripts than do quantitative findings. Regardless of researchers' position about *when* a literature review should be conducted, they usually include a summary of prior research in their reports as a means of providing context for the study.

Quantitative reports almost never present **raw data**—that is, data in the form they were collected, which are numeric values. Qualitative reports, by contrast, are usually filled with rich verbatim passages directly from participants. The excerpts are used in an evidentiary fashion to support or illustrate researchers' interpretations and theoretical formulations.

Example of raw data in a qualitative report: Scannell-Desch (2000) studied the hardships and personal strategies of 24 female Vietnam war nurses. One of the emotional hardships they experienced had to do with the youth of the patients and the severity of their injuries. The researcher supported this with the following quote from an army nurse:

> I had to amputate the leg of one patient. That was the first time I ever had to do that. His leg was hanging by a tissue band. I was new here, and the doctor yelled at me to "get the damn thing off." Doctors take legs off, nurses don't do that. He yelled at me again and said, "You do it." (pp. 533–534).

Like quantitative researchers, qualitative nurse researchers want their findings used in nursing practice and subsequent research. Qualitative findings often are the basis for formulating hypotheses that are tested by quantitative researchers, and for developing measuring instruments for both research and clinical purposes. Qualitative findings can also provide a foundation for designing effective nursing interventions. Qualitative studies help to shape nurses' perceptions of a problem or situation and their conceptualizations of potential solutions.

RESEARCH EXAMPLES

In this section, we illustrate the progression of activities and discuss the time schedule of two studies (one quantitative and the other qualitative) conducted by the second author of this book.

Project Schedule for a Quantitative Study

Beck and Gable (2001) undertook a study to evaluate the accuracy of the newly developed Postpartum Depression Screening Scale (PDSS) in screening new mothers for this mood disorder.

Phase 1. Conceptual Phase: 1 Month

This phase was the shortest, in large part because much of the conceptual work had been done in Beck and Gable's (2000) first study, in which they actually developed the screening scale. The literature had already been reviewed, so all that was needed was to update the review. The same framework and conceptual definitions that had been used in the first study were used in the new study.

Phase 2. Design and Planning Phase: 6 Months

The second phase was time-consuming. It included not only fine-tuning the research design, but gaining entrée into the hospital where subjects were recruited and obtaining approval of the hospital's human subjects review committee. During this period, Beck met with statistical consultants and an instrument development consultant numerous times to finalize the study design.

Phase 3. Empirical Phase: 11 Months

Data collection took almost a year to complete. The design called for administering the PDSS to 150 mothers who were 6 weeks postpartum, and then scheduling a psychiatric diagnostic interview for them to determine if they were suffering from postpartum depression. Women were recruited into the study during prepared childbirth classes. Recruitment began 4 months before data collection because the researchers had to wait until 6 weeks after delivery to gather data. The nurse psychotherapist, who had her own clinical practice, was able to come to the hospital (a 2-hour drive for her) only 1 day a week to conduct the diagnostic interviews; this contributed to the time required to achieve the desired sample size.

Phase 4. Analytic Phase: 3 Months

Statistical tests were performed to determine a cut-off score on the PDSS above which mothers would be identified as having screened positive for postpartum depression. Data analysis also was undertaken to determine the accuracy of the PDSS in predicting diagnosed postpartum depression. During this phase, Beck met with the statisticians and instrument development consultant to interpret results.

Phase 5. Dissemination Phase: 18 Months

The researchers prepared a research report and submitted the manuscript to the journal *Nursing Research* for possible publication. Within 4 months it was accepted for publication, but it was "in press" (awaiting publication) for 14 months before being published. During this period, the authors presented their findings at regional and international conferences. The researchers also had to prepare a summary report for submission to the agency that funded the research.

Project Schedule for a Qualitative Study

Beck (2002) conducted a grounded theory study on mothering twins during the first year after delivery. Total time from start to finish was approximately 2 years.

Phase 1. Conceptual Phase: 3 Months

Beck became interested in mothers of multiples as a result of her quantitative studies on postpartum depression. The findings of these studies had revealed a much higher prevalence of postpartum depression among mothers of multiples than among those of singletons. Beck had never studied multiple births before, so she needed to review that literature carefully. Gaining entrée into the research site

(a hospital) did not take long, however, because she had previously conducted a study there and was known to the hospital's gatekeepers. The key gatekeeper was a nurse who was in charge of the hospital's support group for parents of multiples—a nurse with whom Beck had developed an excellent rapport in the previous study (the nurse was one of the childbirth educators who had helped recruit mothers for the postpartum depression study).

Phase 2. Design and Planning Phase: 4 Months

After reviewing the literature in the conceptual phase, a grounded theory design was selected. The researcher met with the nurse who headed the support group to plan the best approach for recruiting mothers of twins into the study. Plans were also made for the researcher to attend the monthly meetings of the support group. Once the design was finalized, the research proposal was submitted to and approved by both the hospital's and university's human subjects review committees.

Phase 3. Empirical/Analytic Phases 10 months

Data collection and data analysis phases occurred simultaneously in this grounded theory study. Beck attended the "parents of multiples" support group for 10 months. During that period, she conducted in-depth interviews with 16 mothers of twins in their homes, and analyzed her rich and extensive data. Beck's analysis indicated that "life on hold" was the basic problem mothers of twins experienced during the first year of their twins' lives. As mothers attempted to resume their own lives, they progressed through a four-stage process that Beck called "releasing the pause button."

Phase 4 Dissemination Phase: 6+ Months

A manuscript was written describing this study and submitted for publication in a journal. The manuscript was published in 2002 in the journal *Qualitative Health Research.* In addition to disseminating the results as a journal article, Beck presented the findings at a regional nursing research conference.

SUMMARY POINTS

- A basic distinction in quantitative studies is between experimental and nonexperimental research. In **experimental research**, researchers actively intervene or introduce a treatment, whereas in **nonexperimental research,** researchers make observations of existing situations and characteristics without intervening.
- Qualitative research often is strongly rooted in research traditions that originate in the disciplines of anthropology, sociology, and psychology. Three such traditions have had strong influence on qualitative nursing research: grounded theory, phenomenology, and ethnography.
- **Grounded theory** seeks to describe and understand key social psychological and structural processes that occur in a social setting.
- **Phenomenology** is concerned with the lived experiences of humans and is an approach to thinking about what the life experiences of people are like.
- **Ethnography** provides a framework for studying the meanings, patterns, and experiences of a defined cultural group in a holistic fashion.
- The steps involved in conducting a quantitative study are fairly standard; researchers usually progress in a linear fashion from asking research questions to answering them.
- The main phases and steps in a quantitative study are the conceptual, planning, empirical, analytic, and dissemination phases.
- The **conceptual phase** involves (1) defining the problem to be studied; (2) doing a **literature review;** (3) engaging in **clinical fieldwork** for clinical studies; (4) developing a framework and conceptual definitions; and (5) formulating **hypotheses** to be tested.
- The **planning phase** entails (6) selecting a **research design;** (7) developing **intervention protocols** if the study is experimental; (8) specifying the **population;** (9) developing a **sampling plan;** (10) specifying methods to measure the research variables, through such approaches as **self-report**, **observation**, or the use of **biophysiologic methods**; (11) undertaking

steps to safeguard the rights of subjects; and (12) finalizing the research plan, by conferring with colleagues, **pretesting** instruments, and, in some cases, conducting a **pilot study**.
- The **empirical phase** involves (13) collecting data; and (14) preparing data for analysis.
- The **analytic phase** involves (15) analyzing data through **statistical analysis;** and (16) interpreting the results.
- The **dissemination phase** entails (17) communicating the findings through the preparation of **research reports** that can be presented orally or published in written form, most often as **journal articles**; and (18) efforts to promote the use of the study evidence in nursing practice.
- The conduct of quantitative studies requires careful planning and organization. The preparation of a timetable with expected deadlines for task completion is recommended.
- The flow of activities in a qualitative study is more flexible and less linear.
- Qualitative researchers begin with a broad question regarding the phenomenon of interest, often focusing on a little-studied aspect.
- In the early phase of a qualitative study, researchers select a **site** and seek to **gain entrée** into it and into the specific **settings** in which data collection will occur. Gaining entrée typically involves enlisting the cooperation of **gatekeepers** within the site.
- The research design of qualitative studies is typically an **emergent design**. Once in the field, researchers select informants, collect data, and then analyze and interpret them in an iterative fashion; field experiences help in an ongoing fashion to shape the design of the study.
- Early analysis leads to refinements in sampling and data collection, until **saturation** (redundancy of information) is achieved.
- Qualitative researchers conclude by disseminating findings that can subsequently be used to (1) shape the direction of further studies (including more highly controlled quantitative studies); (2) guide the development of structured measuring tools for clinical and research purposes; and (3) shape nurses' perceptions of a problem or situa-

tion and their conceptualizations of potential solutions.

STUDY ACTIVITIES

Chapter 3 of the *Study Guide to Accompany Nursing Research: Principles and Methods, 7th edition,* offers various exercises and study suggestions for reinforcing concepts presented in this chapter. In addition, the following study questions can be addressed:

1. In quantitative studies, the same measurements are made of all subjects. What do you think researchers are trying to achieve by this degree of structure? Why might such structure not be appropriate in qualitative studies?
2. Which type of research do you think is easier to conduct—qualitative or quantitative research? Defend your response.
3. Suppose you were interested in studying fatigue in patients on chemotherapy. (This could involve either a quantitative or a qualitative approach.) Suggest some possible clinical fieldwork activities that would help you conceptualize the problem and develop a research strategy.

SUGGESTED READINGS

Methodologic References

Creswell, J. W. (1998). *Qualitative inquiry and research design: Choosing among five traditions.* Thousand Oaks, CA: Sage.

Glaser, B. G., & Strauss, A. L. (1967). *The discovery of grounded theory: Strategies for qualitative research.* Chicago: Aldine.

Kerlinger, F. N., & Lee, H. B. (2000). *Foundations of behavioral research.* (4th ed.). Orlando, FL: Harcourt College Publishers.

Sterling, Y. M. (2001). The clinical imperative in clinical nursing research. *Applied Nursing Research, 14,* 44–47.

Studies Cited in Chapter 3

Beck, C. T. (2002). Releasing the pause button: Mothering twins during the first year of life. *Qualitative Health Research, 12,* 593–608.

Beck, C. T., & Gable, R. K. (2000). Postpartum Depression Screening Scale: Development and psychometric testing, *Nursing Research, 49,* 272–282.

Beck, C. T., & Gable, R. K. (2001). Further validation of the Postpartum Depression Screening Scale. *Nursing Research, 50,* 155–164.

Hauck, Y. L., & Irurita, V. F. (2002). Constructing compatibility: Managing breast-feeding and weaning from the mother's perspective. *Qualitative Health Research, 12,* 897–914.

Johnson, V. Y. (2001). Effects of a submaximal exercise protocol to recondition the pelvic floor musculature. *Nursing Research, 50,* 33–41.

Powers, B. A. (2001). Ethnographic analysis of everyday ethics in the care of nursing home residents with dementia. *Nursing Research, 50,* 332–339.

Scannell-Desch, E. A. (2000). Hardships and personal strategies of Vietnam war nurses. *Western Journal of Nursing Research, 22,* 526–550.

Sundin, K., Norberg, A., & Jansson, L. (2001). The meaning of skilled care providers' relationship with stroke and aphasia patients. *Qualitative Health Research, 11,* 308–321.

Wong, F., Ho, M., Chiu, I., Lui, W., Chan, C., & Lee, K. (2002). Factors contributing to hospital readmission in a Hong Kong regional hospital. *Nursing Research, 51,* 40–49.

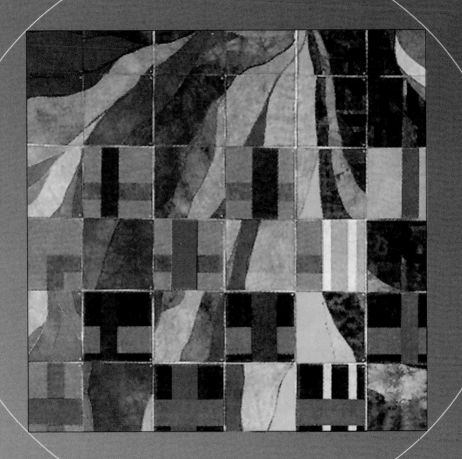

Conceptualizing
a Research Study

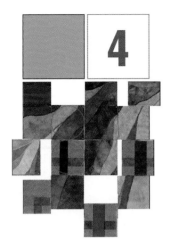

Research Problems, Research Questions, and Hypotheses

OVERVIEW OF RESEARCH PROBLEMS

Studies begin as problems that researchers want to solve or as questions they want to answer. This chapter discusses the formulation and development of research problems. We begin by clarifying some relevant terms.

Basic Terminology

At the most general level, a researcher selects a **topic** or a phenomenon on which to focus. Examples of research topics are adolescent smoking, patient compliance, coping with disability, and pain management. Within each of these broad topics are many potential research problems. In this section, we illustrate various terms using the topic *side effects of chemotherapy*.

A **research problem** is an enigmatic, perplexing, or troubling condition. Both qualitative and quantitative researchers identify a research problem within a broad topic area of interest. The purpose of research is to "solve" the problem—or to contribute to its solution—by accumulating relevant information. A **problem statement** articulates the problem to be addressed and indicates the need for a study. Table 4-1 presents a problem statement related to the topic of side effects of chemotherapy.

Research questions are the specific queries researchers want to answer in addressing the research problem. Research questions guide the types of data to be collected in a study. Researchers who make specific predictions regarding answers to the research question pose **hypotheses** that are tested empirically.

Many reports include a **statement of purpose** (or purpose statement), which is the researcher's summary of the overall goal of a study. A researcher might also identify several **research aims** or **objectives**—the specific accomplishments the researcher hopes to achieve by conducting the study. The objectives include obtaining answers to research questions or testing research hypotheses but may also encompass some broader aims (e.g., developing recommendations for changes to nursing practice based on the study results).

These terms are not always consistently defined in research methods textbooks, and differences between the terms are often subtle. Table 4-1 illustrates the interrelationships among terms as we define them.

Research Problems and Paradigms

Some research problems are better suited for studies using qualitative versus quantitative methods. Quantitative studies usually involve concepts that

TABLE 4.1 Example of Terms Relating to Research Problems

TERM	EXAMPLE
Topic/focus	Side effects of chemotherapy
Research problem	Nausea and vomiting are common side effects among patients on chemotherapy, and interventions to date have been only moderately successful in reducing these effects. New interventions that can reduce or prevent these side effects need to be identified.
Statement of purpose	The purpose of the study is to test an intervention to reduce chemotherapy-induced side effects—specifically, to compare the effectiveness of patient-controlled and nurse-administered antiemetic therapy for controlling nausea and vomiting in patients on chemotherapy.
Research question	What is the relative effectiveness of patient-controlled antiemetic therapy versus nurse-controlled antiemetic therapy with regard to (a) medication consumption and (b) control of nausea and vomiting in patients on chemotherapy?
Hypotheses	(1) Subjects receiving antiemetic therapy by a patient-controlled pump will report less nausea than subjects receiving the therapy by nurse administration; (2) subjects receiving antiemetic therapy by a patient-controlled pump will vomit less than subjects receiving the therapy by nurse administration; (3) subjects receiving antiemetic therapy by a patient-controlled pump will consume less medication than subjects receiving the therapy by nurse administration.
Aims/objectives	This study has as its aim the following objectives: (1) to develop and implement two alternative procedures for administering antiemetic therapy for patients receiving moderate emetogenic chemotherapy (patient controlled versus nurse controlled); (2) to test three hypotheses concerning the relative effectiveness of the alternative procedures on medication consumption and control of side effects; and (3) to use the findings to develop recommendations for possible changes to therapeutic procedures.

are fairly well developed, about which there is an existing body of literature, and for which reliable methods of measurement have been developed. For example, a quantitative study might be undertaken to determine if postpartum depression is higher among women who are employed 6 months after delivery than among those who stay home with their babies. There are relatively accurate measures of postpartum depression that would yield quantitative information about the level of depression in a sample of employed and nonemployed postpartum women.

Qualitative studies are often undertaken because some aspect of a phenomenon is poorly understood, and the researcher wants to develop a rich, comprehensive, and context-bound understanding of it. Qualitative studies are usually initiated to heighten awareness and create a dialogue about a phenomenon. In the example of postpartum depression, qualitative methods would not be well suited to comparing levels of depression among the two groups of women, but they would be ideal for exploring, for example, the *meaning* of postpartum depression among new mothers. Thus, the nature of the research question is closely allied to paradigms and research traditions within paradigms.

SOURCES OF RESEARCH PROBLEMS

Students are sometimes puzzled about the origins of research problems. Where do ideas for research problems come from? How do researchers select topic areas and develop research questions? At the most basic level, research topics originate with researchers' interests. Because research is a time-consuming enterprise, curiosity about and interest in a topic are essential to a project's success. Explicit sources that might fuel researchers' curiosity include experience, the nursing literature, social issues, theories, and ideas from others.

Experience and Clinical Fieldwork

The nurse's everyday clinical experience is a rich source of ideas for research problems. As you are performing your nursing functions, you are bound to find a wealth of research ideas if you are curious about why things are the way they are or about how things could be improved if something were to change. You may be well along the way to developing a research idea if you have ever asked the following kinds of questions: Why are things done this way? What information would help to solve this problem? What is the process by which this situation arose? What would happen if ... ? For beginning researchers in particular, clinical experience (or clinical coursework) is often the most compelling source for topics. Immediate problems that need a solution or that excite the curiosity are relevant and interesting and, thus, may generate more enthusiasm than abstract and distant problems inferred from a theory. Clinical fieldwork before a study may also help to identify clinical problems.

 TIP: Personal experiences in clinical settings are a provocative source of research ideas. Here are some hints on how to proceed:

- Watch for recurring problems and see if you can discern a pattern in situations that lead to the problem.

Example: Why do many patients complain of being tired after being transferred from a coronary care unit to a progressive care unit?

- Think about aspects of your work that are irksome, frustrating, or do not result in the intended outcome—then try to identify factors contributing to the problem that could be changed.

Example: Why is suppertime so frustrating in a nursing home?

- Critically examine some decisions you make in performing your functions. Are these decisions based on tradition, or are they based on systematic evidence that supports their efficacy? Many practices in nursing that have become custom might be challenged.

Example: What would happen if visiting hours in the intensive care unit were changed from 10 minutes every hour to the regularly scheduled hours existing in the rest of the hospital?

Nursing Literature

Ideas for research projects often come from reading the nursing literature. Beginning nurse researchers can profit from regularly reading nursing journals, either clinical specialty journals or research journals such as *Nursing Research* or the *Western Journal of Nursing Research*. Nonresearch articles can be helpful in alerting researchers to clinical trends and issues of importance in clinical settings. Published research reports may suggest problem areas indirectly by stimulating the imagination and directly by specifying further areas in need of investigation.

 Example of a direct suggestion for further research:

Stranahan (2001) studied the relationship between nurse practitioners' attitudes about spiritual care and their spiritual care practices. She made several recommendations for further research in her report, such as the following: "Studies should be conducted to determine reasons why nurse practitioners do not practice spiritual care in the primary care setting" (p. 87).

Inconsistencies in the findings reported in nursing literature sometimes generate ideas for studies. For example, there are inconsistencies regarding which type of tactile stimulation or touch (e.g., gentle touch, stroking, rubbing) has the most beneficial physiologic and behavioral effects on preterm infants. Such discrepancies can lead to the design of a study to resolve the matter.

Researchers may also wonder whether a study similar to one reported in a journal article would yield comparable results if applied in a different setting or with a different population. Replications are needed to establish the validity and generalizability of previous findings.

In summary, a familiarity with existing research, or with problematic and controversial nursing issues that have yet to be understood and investigated systematically, is an important route to developing a research topic. Students who are actively seeking a problem to study will find it useful to read widely in areas of interest. In Chapter 5, we deal more extensively with the conduct of research literature reviews.

TIP: In a pinch, do not hesitate to replicate a study that is reported in the research literature. Replications are a valuable learning experience and can make important contributions if they corroborate (or even if they challenge) earlier findings.

Social Issues

Sometimes, topics are suggested by more global contemporary social or political issues of relevance to the health care community. For example, the feminist movement has raised questions about such topics as sexual harassment, domestic violence, and gender equity in health care and in research. The civil rights movement has led to research on minority health problems, access to health care, and culturally sensitive interventions. Thus, an idea for a study may stem from a familiarity with social concerns or controversial social problems.

Theory

The fourth major source of research problems lies in the theories and conceptual schemes that have been developed in nursing and related disciplines. To be useful in nursing practice, theories must be tested through research for their applicability to hospital units, clinics, classrooms, and other nursing environments.

When researchers decide to base a study on an existing theory, deductions from the theory must be developed. Essentially, researchers must ask the following questions: If this theory is correct, what kind of behavior would I expect to find in certain situations or under certain conditions? What kind of evidence would support this theory? This process, which is described more fully in Chapter 6, would eventually result in a specific problem that could be subjected to systematic investigation.

Ideas From External Sources

External sources can sometimes provide the impetus for a research idea. In some cases, a research topic may be given as a direct suggestion. For example, a faculty member may give students a list of topics from which to choose or may actually assign a specific topic to be studied. Organizations that sponsor funded research, such as government agencies, often identify topics on which research proposals are encouraged. Ideas for research are also being noted on various websites on the internet (see, for example, Duffy, 2001).

Research ideas sometimes represent a response to priorities that are established within the nursing profession, examples of which were discussed in Chapter 1. Priorities for nursing research have been established by many nursing specialty practices. Priority lists can often serve as a useful starting point for exploring research topics.

Often, ideas for studies emerge as a result of a brainstorming session. By discussing possible research topics with peers, advisers or mentors, or researchers with advanced skills, ideas often become clarified and sharpened or enriched and more fully developed. Professional conferences often provide an excellent opportunity for such discussions.

DEVELOPMENT AND REFINEMENT OF RESEARCH PROBLEMS

Unless a research problem is developed on the basis of theory or an explicit suggestion from an external source, the actual procedures for developing a research topic are difficult to describe. The process is rarely a smooth and orderly one; there are likely to be false starts, inspirations, and setbacks in the process of developing a research problem statement. The few suggestions offered here are not intended to imply that there are techniques for making this first step easy but rather to encourage beginning researchers to persevere in the absence of instant success.

Selecting a Topic

The development of a research problem is a creative process that depends on imagination and ingenuity. In the early stages, when research ideas are being generated, it is wise not to be critical of them immediately. It is better to begin by relaxing and jotting down general areas of interest as they come to mind. At this point, it matters little if the terms used to remind you of your ideas are abstract or concrete, broad or specific, technical, or colloquial—the important point is to put some ideas on paper. Examples of some broad topics that may come to mind include nurse—patient communication, pain in patients with cancer, and postoperative loss of orientation.

After this first step, the ideas can be sorted in terms of interest, knowledge about the topics, and the perceived feasibility of turning the topics into a research project. When the most fruitful idea has been selected, the rest of the list should not be discarded; it may be necessary to return to it.

Narrowing the Topic

Once researchers have identified a topic of interest, they need to ask questions that lead to a researchable problem. Examples of question stems that may help to focus an inquiry include the following:

- What is going on with ...?
- What is the process by which ...?
- What is the meaning of ...?
- Why do ...?
- When do ...?
- How do ...?
- What can be done to solve ...?
- What is the extent of ...?
- How intense are ...?
- What influences ...?
- What causes ...?
- What characteristics are associated with ...?
- What differences exist between ...?
- What are the consequences of ...?
- What is the relationship between ...?
- What factors contribute to ...?
- What conditions prevail before ...?
- How effective is ...?

Here again, early criticism of ideas is often counterproductive. Try not to jump to the conclusion that an idea sounds trivial or uninspired without giving it more careful consideration or without exploring it with advisers or colleagues.

Beginning researchers often develop problems that are too broad in scope or too complex and unwieldy for their level of methodologic expertise. The transformation of the general topic into a workable problem is typically accomplished in a number of uneven steps, involving a series of successive approximations. Each step should result in progress toward the goals of narrowing the scope of the problem and sharpening and defining the concepts.

As researchers move from general topics to more specific researchable problems, more than one potential problem area can emerge. Let us consider the following example. Suppose you were working on a medical unit and were puzzled by that fact that some patients always complained about having to wait for pain medication when certain nurses were assigned to them and, yet, these same patients offered no complaints with other nurses. The general problem area is discrepancy in complaints from patients regarding pain medications administered by different nurses. You might ask the following: What accounts for this discrepancy? How can I improve the situation? Such questions are not actual research questions; they are too broad and vague. They may, however, lead you to ask other questions, such as the following: How do the two groups of nurses differ? What characteristics are unique to each group of nurses? What characteristics do the group of complaining patients share? At this point, you may observe that the ethnic background of the patients and nurses appears to be a relevant factor. This may direct you to a review of the literature for studies concerning ethnicity in relation to nursing care, or it may provoke you to discuss the observations with others. The result of these efforts may be several researchable questions, such as the following:

• What is the essence of patient complaints among patients of different ethnic backgrounds?
• What is the patient's experience of waiting for pain medication?
• How do complaints by patients of different ethnic backgrounds get expressed by patients and perceived by nurses?
• Is the ethnic background of nurses related to the frequency with which they dispense pain medication?
• Is the ethnic background of patients related to the frequency and intensity of complaints when waiting for pain medication?
• Does the number of patient complaints increase when patients are of dissimilar ethnic backgrounds as opposed to when they are of the same ethnic background as nurses?
• Do nurses' dispensing behaviors change as a function of the similarity between their own ethnic background and that of patients?

All these questions stem from the same general problem, yet each would be studied differently—for example, some suggest a qualitative approach and others suggest a quantitative one. A quantitative researcher might become curious about nurses' dispensing behaviors, based on some interesting evidence in the literature regarding ethnic differences. Both ethnicity and nurses' dispensing behaviors are variables that can be measured in a straightforward and reliable manner. A qualitative researcher who

noticed differences in patient complaints would likely be more interested in understanding the *essence* of the complaints, the patients' *experience* of frustration, the *process* by which the problem got resolved, or the full *nature* of the nurse—patient interactions regarding the dispensing of medications. These are aspects of the research problem that would be difficult to quantify.

Researchers choose the final problem to be studied based on several factors, including its inherent interest to them and its compatibility with a paradigm of preference. In addition, tentative problems usually vary in their feasibility and worth. It is at this point that a critical evaluation of ideas is appropriate.

Evaluating Research Problems

There are no rules for making a final selection of a research problem. Some criteria, however, should be kept in mind in the decision-making process. The four most important considerations are the significance, researchability, and feasibility of the problem, and its interest to the researcher.

Significance of the Problem

A crucial factor in selecting a problem to be studied is its significance to nursing—especially to nursing practice. Evidence from the study should have the potential of contributing meaningfully to nursing knowledge. Researchers should pose the following kinds of questions: Is the problem an important one? Will patients, nurses, or the broader health care community or society benefit from the evidence that will be produced? Will the results lead to practical applications? Will the results have theoretical relevance? Will the findings challenge (or lend support to) untested assumptions? Will the study help to formulate or alter nursing practices or policies? If the answer to all these questions is "no," then the problem should be abandoned.

Researchability of the Problem

Not all problems are amenable to study through scientific investigation. Problems or questions of a moral or ethical nature, although provocative, are incapable of being researched. Take, for example, the following: Should assisted suicide be legalized? The answer to such a question is based on a person's values. There are no *right* or *wrong* answers, only points of view. The problem is suitable to debate, not to research. To be sure, it is possible to ask related questions that could be researched. For instance, each of the following questions could be investigated in a research project:

- What are nurses' attitudes toward assisted suicide?
- Do oncology nurses hold more favorable opinions of assisted suicide than other nurses?
- What moral dilemmas are perceived by nurses who might be involved in assisted suicide?
- What are the attitudes of terminally ill patients toward assisted suicide?
- Do terminally ill patients living with a high level of pain hold more favorable attitudes toward assisted suicide than those with less pain?
- How do family members experience the loss of a loved one through assisted suicide?

The findings from these hypothetical projects would have no bearing, of course, on whether assisted suicide should be legalized, but the information could be useful in developing a better understanding of the issues.

In quantitative studies, researchable problems are ones involving variables that can be precisely defined and measured. For example, suppose a researcher is trying to determine what effect early discharge has on patient well-being. *Well-being* is too vague a concept for a study. The researcher would have to sharpen and define the concept so that it could be observed and measured. That is, the researcher would have to establish criteria against which patients' progress toward well-being could be assessed.

When a new area of inquiry is being pursued, however, it may be impossible to define the concepts of interest in precise terms. In such cases, it may be appropriate to address the problem using in-depth qualitative research. The problem may then be stated in fairly broad terms to permit full exploration of the concept of interest.

Feasibility of Addressing the Problem

A problem that is both significant and researchable may still be inappropriate if a study designed to address it is not feasible. The issue of feasibility encompasses various considerations. Not all of the following factors are relevant for every problem, but they should be kept in mind in making a final decision.

Time and Timing. Most studies have deadlines or at least goals for completion. Therefore, the problem must be one that can be adequately studied within the time allotted. This means that the scope of the problem should be sufficiently restricted that enough time will be available for the various steps and activities reviewed in Chapter 3. It is wise to be conservative in estimating time for various tasks because research activities often require more time to accomplish than anticipated. Qualitative studies may be especially time-consuming.

A related consideration is the timing of the project. Some of the research steps—especially data collection—may be more readily performed at certain times of the day, week, or year than at other times. For example, if the problem focused on patients with peptic ulcers, the research might be more easily conducted in the fall and spring because of the increase in the number of patients with peptic ulcers during these seasons. When the timing requirements of the tasks do not match the time available for their performance, the feasibility of the project may be jeopardized.

Availability of Study Participants. In any study involving humans, researchers need to consider whether individuals with the desired characteristics will be available and willing to cooperate. Securing people's cooperation may in some cases be easy (e.g., getting nursing students to complete a questionnaire in a classroom), but other situations may pose more difficulties. Some people may not have the time, others may have no interest in a study that has little personal benefit, and others may not feel well enough to participate. Fortunately, people usually *are* willing to cooperate if research demands are minimal. Researchers may need to exert extra effort in recruiting participants—or may have to offer a monetary incentive—if the research is time-consuming or demanding.

An additional problem may be that of identifying and locating people with needed characteristics. For example, if we were interested in studying the coping strategies of people who had lost a family member through suicide, we would have to develop a plan for identifying prospective participants from this distinct and inconspicuous population.

Cooperation of Others. Often, it is insufficient to obtain the cooperation of prospective study participants alone. If the sample includes children, mentally incompetent people, or senile individuals, it would be necessary to secure the permission of parents or guardians, an issue discussed in the chapter on ethics (see Chapter 7). In institutional or organizational settings (e.g., hospitals), access to clients, members, personnel, or records usually requires administrative authorization. Many health care facilities require that any project be presented to a panel of reviewers for approval. As noted in Chapter 3, a critical requirement in many qualitative studies is gaining entrée into an appropriate community, setting, or group, and developing the trust of gatekeepers.

Facilities and Equipment. All studies have resource requirements, although in some cases, needs may be modest. It is prudent to consider what facilities and equipment will be needed and whether they will be available before embarking on a project to avoid disappointment and frustration. The following is a partial list of considerations:

- Will assistants be needed, and are such assistants available?
- If technical equipment and apparatus are needed, can they be secured, and are they functioning properly? Will audiotaping or videotaping equipment be required, and is it of sufficient sensitivity for the research conditions? Will laboratory facilities be required, and are they available?
- Will space be required, and can it be obtained?
- Will telephones, office equipment, or other supplies be required?

- Are duplicating or printing services available, and are they reliable?
- Will transportation needs pose any difficulties?

Money. Monetary requirements for research projects vary widely, ranging from $10 to $20 for small student projects to hundreds of thousands (or even millions) of dollars for large-scale, government-sponsored research. The investigator on a limited budget should think carefully about projected expenses before making the final selection of a problem. Some major categories of research-related expenditures are the following:

- Literature costs—computerized literature search and retrieval service charges, Internet access charges, reproduction costs, index cards, books and journals
- Personnel costs—payments to individuals hired to help with the data collection (e.g., for conducting interviews, coding, data entry, transcribing, word processing)
- Study participant costs—payment to participants as an incentive for their cooperation or to offset their own expenses (e.g., transportation or baby-sitting costs)
- Supplies—paper, envelopes, computer disks, postage, audiotapes, and so forth
- Printing and duplication costs—expenditures for printing forms, questionnaires, participant recruitment notices, and so on
- Equipment—laboratory apparatus, audio- or video-recorders, calculators, and the like
- Computer-related expenses (e.g., purchasing software)
- Laboratory fees for the analysis of biophysiologic data
- Transportation costs

Experience of the Researcher. The problem should be chosen from a field about which investigators have some prior knowledge or experience. Researchers have difficulty adequately developing a study on a topic that is totally new and unfamiliar—although clinical fieldwork before launching the study may make up for certain deficiencies. In addition to substantive knowledge, the issue of technical expertise should not be overlooked. Beginning researchers with limited methodologic skills should avoid research problems that might require the development of sophisticated measuring instruments or that involve complex data analyses.

   Ethical Considerations. A research problem may not be feasible because the investigation of the problem would pose unfair or unethical demands on participants. The ethical responsibilities of researchers should not be taken lightly. People engaged in research activities should be thoroughly knowledgeable about the rights of human or animal subjects. An overview of major ethical considerations concerning human study participants is presented in Chapter 7 and should be reviewed when considering the feasibility of a prospective project.

Interest to the Researcher

Even if the tentative problem is researchable, significant, and feasible, there is one more criterion: the researcher's own interest in the problem. Genuine interest in and curiosity about the chosen research problem are critical prerequisites to a successful study. A great deal of time and energy are expended in a study; there is little sense devoting these personal resources to a project that does not generate enthusiasm.

TIP: Beginning researchers often seek out suggestions on topic areas, and such assistance may be helpful in getting started. Nevertheless, it is rarely wise to be talked into a topic toward which you are not personally inclined. If you do not find a problem attractive or stimulating during the beginning phases of a study—when opportunities for creativity and intellectual enjoyment are at their highest—then you are bound to regret your choice later.

COMMUNICATING THE RESEARCH PROBLEM

It is clear that a study cannot progress without the choice of a problem; it is less clear, but nonetheless true, that the problem and research questions should be carefully stated in writing before proceeding with the design of the study or with field work. Putting one's ideas in writing is often sufficient to illuminate ambiguities and uncertainties. This section discusses the wording of problem statements, statements of purpose, and research questions, and the following major section discusses hypotheses.

Problem Statements

A problem statement is an expression of the dilemma or disturbing situation that needs investigation for the purposes of providing understanding and direction. A problem statement identifies the nature of the problem that is being addressed in the study and, typically, its context and significance. In general, the problem statement should be broad enough to include central concerns, but narrow enough in scope to serve as a guide to study design.

 Example of a problem statement from a quantitative study:

Women account for an increasing percentage of adults with human immunodeficiency virus (HIV).... Most of these HIV-infected women are in their childbearing years. As a result, approximately 7,000 infants are exposed prenatally each year.... All infants exposed to HIV prenatally are at risk for developmental problems.... Little is known about the quality of parental caregiving for infants of mothers with HIV, because few studies have examined parenting in this vulnerable group.... The purpose of this report is to describe the development of infants of mothers with HIV and to determine the extent to which child characteristics, parental caregiver characteristics, family characteristics, and parenting quality influence development (Holditch-Davis, Miles, Burchinal, O'Donnell, McKinney, & Lim, 2001, pp. 5–6).

   In this example, the general topic could be described as infant development among at-risk children. The investigators' more specific focus is on four factors that influence infant development among children exposed to HIV prenatally. The problem statement asserts the nature of the problem (these children are at risk of developmental problems) and indicates its breadth (7000 infants annually). It also provides a justification for conducting a new study: the dearth of existing studies on parenting in this population.

The problem statement for a qualitative study similarly expresses the nature of the problem, its context, and its significance, as in the following example:

 Example of a problem statement from a qualitative study:

Members of cultural minority groups may find themselves surrounded by people whose values, beliefs, and interpretations differ from their own during hospitalization. This is often the case for Canada's aboriginal population, as many live in culturally distinct communities.... To promote healing among clients from minority cultural communities, it is important for nurses to understand the phenomenon of receiving care in an unfamiliar culture. This exploratory study examined how members of the Big Cove Mi'kmaq First Nation Community ... subjectively experienced being cared for in a nonaboriginal institution (Baker & Daigle, 2000, p. 8).

As in the previous example, these qualitative researchers clearly articulated the nature of the problem and the justification for a new study. Qualitative studies that are embedded in a particular research tradition usually incorporate terms and concepts in their problem statements that foreshadow their tradition of inquiry (Creswell, 1998). For example, the problem statement in a grounded theory study might refer to the need to generate a theory relating to social processes. A problem statement for a phenomenological study might note the need to know more about people's experiences (as in the preceding example) or the meanings they attribute to those experiences. And an ethnographer might indicate the desire to describe how cultural forces affect people's behavior.

Problem statements usually appear early in a research report and are often interwoven with a review of the literature, which provides context by documenting knowledge gaps.

Statements of Purpose

Many researchers first articulate their research goals formally as a statement of purpose, worded in the declarative form. The statement captures—usually in one or two clear sentences—the essence of the study. The purpose statement establishes the general direction of the inquiry. The words *purpose* or *goal* usually appear in a purpose statement (e.g., The purpose of this study was..., or, The goal of this study was...), but sometimes the words *intent*, *aim*, or *objective* are used instead. Unfortunately, some research reports leave the statement of purpose implicit, placing an unnecessary burden on readers to make inferences about the goals.

In a quantitative study, a statement of purpose identifies the key study variables and their possible interrelationships, as well as the nature of the population of interest.

 Example of a statement of purpose from a quantitative study:
"The purpose of this study was to determine whether viewing a video of an actual pediatric inhalation induction would reduce the level of parental anxiety" (Zuwala & Barber, 2001, p. 21).

This statement identifies the population of interest (parents whose child required inhalation induction), the independent variable (viewing a video of such an induction, versus not viewing the video), and the dependent variable (parental anxiety).

In qualitative studies, the statement of purpose indicates the nature of the inquiry, the key concept or phenomenon, and the group, community, or setting under study.

 Example of a statement of purpose from a qualitative study:
Gallagher and Pierce (2002) designed their qualitative study for the following two purposes: "to gain the family caregivers' perspective of dealing with UI [urinary incontinence] for the care recipient who lives in a home setting, and to gain care recipients' perspective on the UI care given by family caregivers in the home setting" (p. 25).

This statement indicates that the central phenomenon of interest is perspectives on caregiving and that the groups under study are UI patients in home settings and the family caregivers caring for them. Often, the statement of purpose specifically mentions the underlying research tradition, if this is relevant.

Example of a statement of purpose from a grounded theory study:

The purpose is "to generate a grounded substantive theory of the process of forgiveness in patients with cancer" (Mickley and Cowles, 2001, p. 31).

The statement of purpose communicates more than just the nature of the problem. Through researchers' selection of verbs, a statement of purpose suggests the manner in which they sought to solve the problem, or the state of knowledge on the topic. That is, a study whose purpose is to *explore* or *describe* some phenomenon is likely to be an investigation of a little-researched topic, often involving a qualitative approach such as a phenomenology or ethnography. A statement of purpose for a qualitative study—especially a grounded theory study—may also use verbs such as *understand*, *discover*, *develop*, or *generate*. Creswell (1998) notes that the statements of purpose in qualitative studies often "encode" the tradition of inquiry not only through the researcher's choice of verbs but also through the use of certain terms or "buzz words" associated with those traditions, as follows:

- *Grounded theory*: Processes; social structures; social interactions
- *Phenomenological studies*: Experience; lived experience; meaning; essence
- *Ethnographic studies*: Culture; roles; myths; cultural behavior

Quantitative researchers also suggest the nature of the inquiry through their selection of verbs. A purpose statement indicating that the study purpose is to *test* or *determine* or *evaluate* the effectiveness of an intervention suggests an experimental design, for example. A study whose purpose is to *examine* or *assess* the relationship between two variables is more likely to refer to a nonexperimental quantitative design. In some cases, the verb is ambiguous: a purpose statement indicating that the researcher's intent is to *compare* could be referring to a comparison of alternative treatments (using an experimental approach) or a comparison of two preexisting groups (using a nonexperimental approach). In any event, verbs such as *test*, *evaluate*, and *compare*

suggest an existing knowledge base, quantifiable variables, and designs with tight scientific controls.

Note that the choice of verbs in a statement of purpose should connote objectivity. A statement of purpose indicating that the intent of the study was to *prove*, *demonstrate*, or *show* something suggests a bias.

 TIP: In wording your research questions or statement of purpose, look at published research reports for models. You may find, however, that some reports fail to state unambiguously the study purpose or specific research questions. Thus, in some studies, you may have to infer the research problem from several sources, such as the title of the report. In other reports, the purpose or questions are clearly stated but may be difficult to find. Researchers most often state their purpose or questions at the end of the introductory section of the report.

Research Questions

Research questions are, in some cases, direct rewordings of statements of purpose, phrased interrogatively rather than declaratively, as in the following example:

- The purpose of this study is to assess the relationship between the dependency level of renal transplant recipients and their rate of recovery.
- What is the relationship between the dependency level of renal transplant recipients and their rate of recovery?

The question form has the advantage of simplicity and directness. Questions invite an answer and help to focus attention on the kinds of data that would have to be collected to provide that answer. Some research reports thus omit a statement of purpose and state only research questions. Other researchers use a set of research questions to clarify or lend greater specificity to the purpose statement.

 Example of research questions clarifying a statement of purpose:

Statement of Purpose: The purpose of this study was to explore the relationship between method of pain management during labor and specific labor and birth outcomes.

Research Questions: (1) Are nonepidural and epidural methods of pain relief associated with augmentation during the first stage of labor? (2) Is the length of second stage labor associated with epidural and nonepidural methods of pain relief? (3) Are newborn Apgar scores at 1 minute and 5 minutes associated with method of pain relief? (4) Does epidural anesthesia affect maternal temperature? (Walker & O'Brien, 1999)

In this example, the statement of purpose provides a global message about the researchers' goal to *explore* relationships among several variables. The research questions identified the two methods of pain management (the independent variable) and the specific labor and birth outcomes of interest (the dependent variables).

Research Questions in Quantitative Studies

In quantitative studies, research questions identify the key variables (especially the independent and dependent variables), the relationships among them, and the population under study. The variables are all measurable concepts, and the questions suggest quantification. For example, a descriptive research question might ask about the *frequency* or *prevalence* of variables, or their average values (What percentage of women breastfeed their infants? or What is the average interstitial fluid volume at 60 minutes after intravenous infiltration following treatment with cold applications?).

Most quantitative studies, however, ask questions about relationships between variables. In Chapter 2, we noted that researchers ask various questions about relationships. These can be illustrated with an example of women's emotional responses to miscarriage:

1. *Existence of relationship*: Is there a relationship between miscarriage and depression—that is, are there differences in depression levels of pregnant women who miscarry compared with those who do not?
2. *Direction of relationship*: Do women who miscarry exhibit higher (or lower) levels of depression than pregnant women who do not?

3. *Strength of relationship*: How strong is the risk of depression among women who miscarry?
4. *Nature of relationship*: Does having a miscarriage contribute to depression? Does depression contribute to a miscarriage? Or does some other factor influence both?
5. *Moderated relationship*: Are levels of depression among women who miscarry moderated by whether the woman has previously given birth? (i.e., Is the relationship between depression and miscarriage different for primiparas and multiparas?)
6. *Mediated relationship*: Does a miscarriage directly affect depression or does depression occur because the miscarriage had a negative effect on marital relations?

The last two research questions involve mediator and moderator variables, which are variables of interest to the researcher (i.e., that are not extraneous) and that affect the relationship between the independent and dependent variables. A **moderator variable** is a variable that affects the strength or direction of an association between the independent and dependent variable. The independent variable is said to *interact* with the moderator: the independent variable's relationship with the dependent variable is stronger or weaker for different values of the moderator variable (Bennett, 2000). In the preceding example, it might be that the risk of depression after a miscarriage is low among women who had previously given birth (i.e., when the moderating variable parity is greater than 0), but high among women who do not have children (i.e., when parity equals 0). When all women are considered together without taking parity into account, the relationship between experiencing a miscarriage (the independent variable) and levels of depression (the dependent variable) might appear moderate. Therefore, identifying parity as a key moderator is important in understanding *when* to expect a relationship between miscarriage and depression, and this understanding has clinical relevance.

Research questions that involve mediator variables concern the identification of causal pathways. A **mediator variable** is a variable that intervenes between the independent and dependent variable and helps to explain why the relationship exists. In our hypothetical example, we are asking whether depression levels among women who have experienced a miscarriage are influenced by the negative effect of the miscarriage on marital relations. In research questions involving mediators, researchers are typically more interested in the mediators than in the independent variable, because the mediators are key explanatory mechanisms.

In summary, except for questions of a purely descriptive nature, research questions in quantitative research focus on unraveling relationships among variables.

 Example of a research question from a quantitative study:
Watt-Watson, Garfinkel, Gallop, Stevens, and Streiner (2000) conducted a study about acute care nurses' empathy and its effects on patients. Their primary research question was about the existence and direction of a relationship:
Do nurses with greater empathy have patients experiencing less pain and receiving adequate analgesia than those with less empathy?

Research Questions in Qualitative Studies

Researchers in the various qualitative traditions vary in their conceptualization of what types of questions are important. Grounded theory researchers are likely to ask *process* questions, phenomenologists tend to ask *meaning* questions, and ethnographers generally ask *descriptive* questions about cultures. The terms associated with the various traditions, discussed previously in connection with purpose statements, are likely to be incorporated into the research questions.

 Example of a research question from a phenomenological study:
What is the lived experience of caring for a family member with Alzheimer's disease at home? (Butcher, Holkup, & Buckwalter, 2001)

It is important to note, however, that not all qualitative studies are rooted in a specific research

tradition. Many researchers use naturalistic methods to describe or explore phenomena without focusing on cultures, meaning, or social processes.

 Example of a research question from a qualitative study:
Wilson and Williams (2000) undertook a qualitative study that explored the potential effects of visualism (a prejudice in favor of the seen) on the perceived legitimacy of telephone work in community nursing. Among the specific research questions that guided their in-depth interviews with community nurses were the following:
Is telephone consultation considered real work? Is it considered real communication? Can telephone consultation bring the community and its nursing services into close relationship?

In qualitative studies, research questions sometimes evolve over the course of the study. The researcher begins with a *focus* that defines the general boundaries of the inquiry. However, the boundaries are not cast in stone; the boundaries "can be altered and, in the typical naturalistic inquiry, will be" (Lincoln & Guba, 1985, p. 228). The naturalist begins with a research question that provides a general starting point but does not prohibit discovery; qualitative researchers are often sufficiently flexible that the question can be modified as new information makes it relevant to do so.

RESEARCH HYPOTHESES

A hypothesis is a prediction about the relationship between two or more variables. A hypothesis thus translates a quantitative research question into a precise prediction of expected outcomes. In qualitative studies, researchers do not begin with a hypothesis, in part because there is usually too little known about the topic to justify a hypothesis, and in part because qualitative researchers want the inquiry to be guided by participants' viewpoints rather than by their own. Thus, this discussion focuses on hypotheses used to guide quantitative inquiries (some of which are generated within qualitative studies).

Function of Hypotheses in Quantitative Research

Research questions, as we have seen, are usually queries about relationships between variables. Hypotheses are proposed solutions or answers to these queries. For instance, the research question might ask: Does history of sexual abuse in childhood affect the development of irritable bowel syndrome in women? The researcher might predict the following: Women who were sexually abused in childhood have a higher incidence of irritable bowel syndrome than women who were not.

Hypotheses sometimes follow directly from a theoretical framework. Scientists reason from theories to hypotheses and test those hypotheses in the real world. The validity of a theory is never examined directly. Rather, it is through hypothesis testing that the worth of a theory can be evaluated. Let us take as an example the theory of reinforcement. This theory maintains that behavior that is positively reinforced (rewarded) tends to be learned or repeated. The theory itself is too abstract to be put to an empirical test, but if the theory is valid, it should be possible to make predictions about certain kinds of behavior. For example, the following hypotheses have been deduced from reinforcement theory:

- Elderly patients who are praised (reinforced) by nursing personnel for self-feeding require less assistance in feeding than patients who are not praised.
- Pediatric patients who are given a reward (e.g., a balloon or permission to watch television) when they cooperate during nursing procedures tend to be more obliging during those procedures than nonrewarded peers.

Both of these propositions can be put to a test in the real world. The theory gains support if the hypotheses are confirmed.

Not all hypotheses are derived from theory. Even in the absence of a theory, well-conceived hypotheses offer direction and suggest explanations. Perhaps an example will clarify this point. Suppose we hypothesized that nurses who have received a baccalaureate education are more likely to experience stress in their first nursing job than are nurses with a diploma-school education. We could justify our speculation based on theory (e.g., role conflict theory, cognitive dissonance theory), earlier studies, personal observations, or on the basis of some combination of these.

> The development of predictions in and of itself forces researchers to think logically, to exercise critical judgment, and to tie together earlier research findings.

Now let us suppose the preceding hypothesis is not confirmed by the evidence collected; that is, we find that baccalaureate and diploma nurses demonstrate comparable stress in their first job.

> The failure of data to support a prediction forces researchers to analyze theory or previous research critically, to carefully review the limitations of the study's methods, and to explore alternative explanations for the findings.

The use of hypotheses in quantitative studies tends to induce critical thinking and to facilitate understanding and interpretation of the data.

To illustrate further the utility of hypotheses, suppose we conducted the study guided only by the research question, Is there a relationship between nurses' basic preparation and the degree of stress experienced on the first job? The investigator without a hypothesis is, apparently, prepared to accept any results. The problem is that it is almost always possible to explain something superficially after the fact, no matter what the findings are. Hypotheses guard against superficiality and minimize the possibility that spurious results will be misconstrued.

Characteristics of Testable Hypotheses

Testable research hypotheses state expected relationships between the independent variable (the presumed cause or antecedent) and the dependent variable (the presumed effect or outcome) within a population.

Example of a research hypothesis:
Cardiac patients receiving an intervention involving "vicarious experience" through support

from former patients have (1) less anxiety; (2) higher self-efficacy expectation; and (3) higher self-reported activity than other patients (Parent & Fortin, 2000).

In this example, the independent variable is receipt versus nonreceipt of the intervention, and the dependent variables are anxiety, self-efficacy expectation, and activity. The hypothesis predicts better outcomes among patients who receive the intervention.

Unfortunately, researchers occasionally present hypotheses that fail to make a relational statement. For example, the following prediction is *not* an acceptable research hypothesis:

Pregnant women who receive prenatal instruction regarding postpartum experiences are not likely to experience postpartum depression.

This statement expresses no anticipated relationship; in fact, there is only one variable (postpartum depression), and a relationship by definition requires at least two variables.

When a prediction does not express an anticipated relationship, it cannot be tested. In our example, how would we know whether the hypothesis was supported—what absolute standard could be used to decide whether to accept or reject the hypothesis? To illustrate the problem more concretely, suppose we asked a group of mothers who had been given instruction on postpartum experiences the following question 1 month after delivery: On the whole, how depressed have you been since you gave birth? Would you say (1) extremely depressed, (2) moderately depressed, (3) somewhat depressed, or (4) not at all depressed?

Based on responses to this question, how could we compare the actual outcome with the predicted outcome? Would *all* the women have to say they were "not at all depressed?" Would the prediction be supported if 51% of the women said they were "not at all depressed" *or* "somewhat depressed?" There is no adequate way of testing the accuracy of the prediction.

A test is simple, however, if we modify the prediction to the following: Pregnant women who receive prenatal instruction are less likely to experi-ence postpartum depression than those with no prenatal instruction. Here, the dependent variable is the women's depression, and the independent variable is their receipt versus nonreceipt of prenatal instruction. The relational aspect of the prediction is embodied in the phrase *less than*. If a hypothesis lacks a phrase such as *more than, less than, greater than, different from, related to, associated with,* or something similar, it is not amenable to testing in a quantitative study. To test this revised hypothesis, we could ask two groups of women with different prenatal instruction experiences to respond to the question on depression and then compare the groups' responses. The absolute degree of depression of either group would not be at issue.

Hypotheses, ideally, should be based on sound, justifiable rationales. The most defensible hypotheses follow from previous research findings or are deduced from a theory. When a relatively new area is being investigated, the researcher may have to turn to logical reasoning or personal experience to justify the predictions. There are, however, few problems for which research evidence is totally lacking.

The Derivation of Hypotheses

Many students ask the question, How do I go about developing hypotheses? Two basic processes—induction and deduction—constitute the intellectual machinery involved in deriving hypotheses.

An **inductive hypothesis** is a generalization based on observed relationships. Researchers observe certain patterns, trends, or associations among phenomena and then use the observations as a basis for predictions. Related literature should be examined to learn what is already known on a topic, but an important source for inductive hypotheses is personal experiences, combined with intuition and critical analysis. For example, a nurse might notice that presurgical patients who ask a lot of questions relating to pain or who express many pain-related apprehensions have a more difficult time in learning appropriate postoperative procedures. The nurse could then formulate a hypothesis, such as the following, that could be tested through more rigorous procedures: Patients who are stressed by fears of pain will have more difficulty in deep breathing and coughing after their surgery than patients who are not stressed. Qualitative studies are an important source of inspiration for inductive hypotheses.

Example of deriving an inductive hypothesis: In Beck's (1998) qualitative study of postpartum-onset panic disorder, one of her findings was a theme relating to self-esteem: "As a result of recurring panic attacks, negative changes in women's lifestyles ensued—lowering their self-esteem and leaving them to bear the burden of disappointing not only themselves but also their families" (p. 134). A hypothesis that can be derived from this qualitative finding might be as follows: Women who experience postpartum onset panic disorder have lower self-esteem than women who do not experience this disorder.

The other mechanism for deriving hypotheses is through deduction. Theories of how phenomena behave and interrelate cannot be tested directly. Through deductive reasoning, a researcher can develop hypotheses based on general theoretical principles. Inductive hypotheses begin with specific observations and move toward generalizations; **deductive hypotheses** have as a starting point theories that are applied to particular situations. The following syllogism illustrates the reasoning process involved:

- All human beings have red and white blood cells.
- John Doe is a human being.
- Therefore, John Doe has red and white blood cells.

In this simple example, the hypothesis is that John Doe does, in fact, have red and white blood cells, a deduction that could be verified.

Theories thus can serve as a valuable point of departure for hypothesis development. Researchers must ask: If this theory is valid, what are the implications for a phenomenon of interest? In other words, researchers deduce that if the general theory is true, then certain outcomes or consequences can be expected. Specific predictions derived from general principles must then be subjected to testing through the collection of empirical data. If these data are congruent with hypothesized outcomes, then the theory is strengthened.

The advancement of nursing knowledge depends on both inductive and deductive hypotheses. Ideally, a cyclical process is set in motion wherein observations are made (e.g., in a qualitative study); inductive hypotheses are formulated; systematic and controlled observations are made to test the hypotheses; theoretical systems are developed on the basis of the results; deductive hypotheses are formulated from the theory; new data are gathered; theories are modified, and so forth. Researchers need to be organizers of concepts (think inductively), logicians (think deductively), and, above all, critics and skeptics of resulting formulations, constantly demanding evidence.

Wording of Hypotheses

A good hypothesis is worded in simple, clear, and concise language. Although it is cumbersome to include conceptual or operational definitions of terms directly in the hypothesis statement, it should be specific enough so that readers understand what the variables are and whom researchers will be studying.

Simple Versus Complex Hypotheses

For the purpose of this book, we define a **simple hypothesis** as a hypothesis that expresses an expected relationship between *one* independent and *one* dependent variable. A **complex hypothesis** is a prediction of a relationship between two (or more) independent variables and/or two (or more) dependent variables. Complex hypotheses sometimes are referred to as **multivariate hypotheses** because they involve multiple variables.

We give some concrete examples of both types of hypotheses, but let us first explain the differences in abstract terms. Simple hypotheses state a relationship between a single independent variable, which we will call X, and a single dependent variable, which we will label Y. Y is the predicted effect, outcome, or consequence of X, which is the presumed cause, antecedent, or precondition. The nature of this relationship is presented in Figure 4-1A. The

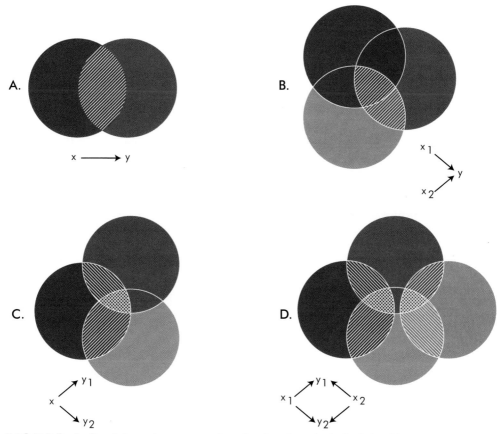

FIGURE 4.1 Schematic representation of various hypothetical relationships.

hatched area of the circles, which represent variables X and Y, signifies the strength of the relationship between them. If there were a one-to-one correspondence between variables X and Y, the two circles would completely overlap, and the entire area would be hatched. If the variables were totally unrelated, the circles would not overlap at all.

Example of a simple hypothesis:
Patients receiving a warmed solution for body cavity irrigation during surgical procedures [X] will maintain a higher core body temperature [Y] than patients receiving a room temperature solution (Kelly, Doughty, Hasselbeck, & Vacchiano, 2000).

Most phenomena are the result not of one variable but of a complex array of variables. A person's

weight, for example, is affected simultaneously by such factors as the person's height, diet, bone structure, activity level, and metabolism. If Y in Figure 4-1A was weight, and X was a person's caloric intake, we would not be able to explain or understand individual variation in weight completely. For example, knowing that Dave Harper's daily caloric intake averaged 2500 calories would not allow us a perfect prediction of his weight. Knowledge of other factors, such as his height, would improve the accuracy with which his weight could be predicted.

Figure 4-1B presents a schematic representation of the effect of two independent variables on one dependent variable. The complex hypothesis would state the nature of the relationship between Y on the one hand and X_1 and X_2 on the other. To pursue the preceding example, the hypothesis might be: Taller people (X_1) and people with higher caloric intake (X_2) weigh more (Y) than shorter people and those with lower caloric intake. As the figure shows, a larger proportion of the area of Y is hatched when there are two independent variables than when there is only one. This means that caloric intake *and* height do a better job in helping us explaining variations in weight (Y) than caloric intake alone. Complex hypotheses have the advantage of allowing researchers to capture some of the complexity of the real world. It is not always possible to design a study with complex hypotheses. Practical considerations (e.g., researchers' technical skills and resources) may make it difficult to test complex hypotheses. An important goal of research, however, is to explain the dependent variable as thoroughly as possible, and two or more independent variables are typically more successful than one alone.

 Example of a complex hypothesis—multiple independent variables:
Among breast cancer survivors, emotional well-being [Y] is influenced by the women's self-esteem [X_1], their resourcefulness [X_2] and their degree of social support [X_3] (Dirksen, 2000).

Just as a phenomenon can result from more than one independent variable, so a single independent variable can have an effect on, or be antecedent to, more than one phenomenon. Figure 4-1C illustrates this type of relationship. A number of studies have found, for example, that cigarette smoking (the independent variable, X), can lead to both lung cancer (Y_1) and coronary disorders (Y_2). This type of complex hypothesis is common in studies that try to assess the impact of a nursing intervention on a variety of criterion measures of patient well-being.

 Example of a complex hypothesis—multiple dependent variables:
The implementation of an evidence-based protocol for urinary incontinence [X] will result in decreased frequency of urinary incontinence episodes (Y_1), decreased urine loss per episode [Y_2], and decreased avoidance of activities [Y_3] among women in ambulatory care settings (Sampselle et al., 2000).

Finally, a more complex type of hypothesis, which links two or more independent variables to two or more dependent variables, is shown in Figure 4-1D. An example might be a hypothesis that smoking *and* the consumption of alcohol during pregnancy might lead to lower birth weights *and* lower Apgar scores in infants.

Hypotheses are also complex if mediator or moderator variables are included in the prediction. For example, it might be hypothesized that the effect of caloric intake (X) on weight (Y) is moderated by gender (Z)—that is, the relationship between height and weight is different for men and women.

 Example of a complex hypothesis with mediator:
The quality of life of a family [Y] during the survivor phase after cancer diagnosis is affected by family resources [X_1] and illness survival stressors such as fear of recurrence [X_2], *through* the mediating variable, the family meaning of the illness [Z] (Mellon & Northouse, 2001).

In general, hypotheses should be worded in the present tense. Researchers make predictions about relationships that exist in the population, and not just about a relationship that will be revealed in a particular sample. Hypotheses can be stated in various ways as long as the researcher specifies or implies the relationship to be tested. Here are examples:

1. Older patients are more at risk of experiencing a fall than younger patients.
2. There is a relationship between the age of a patient and the risk of falling.
3. The older the patient, the greater the risk that she or he will fall.
4. Older patients differ from younger ones with respect to their risk of falling.
5. Younger patients tend to be less at risk of a fall than older patients.
6. The risk of falling increases with the age of the patient.

Other variations are also possible. The important point to remember is that the hypothesis must specify the independent variable (here, patients' age) and the dependent variables (here, risk of falling) and the anticipated relationship between them.

Directional Versus Nondirectional Hypotheses

Sometimes hypotheses are described as being either directional or nondirectional. A **directional hypothesis** is one that specifies not only the existence but the expected direction of the relationship between variables. In the six versions of the hypothesis in the preceding list, versions 1, 3, 5, and 6 are directional because there is an explicit prediction that older patients are at greater risk of falling than younger ones.

A **nondirectional hypothesis**, by contrast, does not stipulate the direction of the relationship. Versions 2 and 4 in the example illustrate the wording of nondirectional hypotheses. These hypotheses state the prediction that a patient's age and the risk of falling are related; they do not stipulate, however, whether the researcher thinks that *older* patients or *younger* ones are at greater risk.

Hypotheses derived from theory are almost always directional because theories explain phenomena, thus providing a rationale for expecting variables to be related in certain ways. Existing studies also offer a basis for directional hypotheses. When there is no theory or related research, when the findings of related studies are contradictory, or when researchers' own experience leads to ambivalence, nondirectional hypotheses may be appropriate. Some people argue, in fact, that nondirectional hypotheses are preferable because they connote a degree of impartiality. Directional hypotheses, it is said, imply that researchers are intellectually committed to certain outcomes, and such a commitment might lead to bias. This argument fails to recognize that researchers typically *do* have hunches about outcomes, whether they state those expectations explicitly or not. We prefer directional hypotheses—when there is a reasonable basis for them—because they clarify the study's framework and demonstrate that researchers have thought critically about the phenomena under study. Directional hypotheses may also permit a more sensitive statistical test through the use of a *one-tailed test*—a rather fine point that is discussed in Chapter 20.

Research Versus Null Hypotheses

Hypotheses are sometimes classified as being either research hypotheses or null hypotheses. **Research hypotheses** (also referred to as *substantive*, *declarative*, or *scientific* hypotheses) are statements of expected relationships between variables. All the hypotheses presented thus far are research hypotheses that indicate researchers' actual expectations.

The logic of statistical inference operates on principles that are somewhat confusing to many beginning students. This logic requires that hypotheses be expressed such that *no* relationship is expected. **Null hypotheses** (or **statistical hypotheses**) state that there is no relationship between the independent and dependent variables. The null form of the hypothesis used in our preceding examples would be a statement such as: "Patients' age is unrelated to their risk of falling" or "Older patients are just as likely as younger patients to fall." The null hypothesis might be compared with the assumption of innocence of an accused criminal in our system of justice: the variables are assumed to be "innocent" of any relationship until they can be shown "guilty" through appropriate statistical procedures. The null hypothesis represents the formal statement of this assumption of innocence.

TIP: If you formulate hypotheses, avoid stating them in null form. When statistical tests are performed, the underlying null hypothesis is assumed without being explicitly stated. Stating hypotheses in the null form gives an amateurish impression.

Hypothesis Testing

Hypotheses are formally tested through statistical procedures; researchers seek to determine through statistics whether their hypotheses have a high probability of being correct. However, hypotheses are never *proved* through hypothesis testing; rather, they are *accepted* or *supported*. Findings are always tentative. Certainly, if the same results are replicated in numerous investigations, then greater confidence can be placed in the conclusions. Hypotheses come to be increasingly supported with mounting evidence.

Let us look more closely at why this is so. Suppose we hypothesized that height and weight are related. We predict that, on average, tall people weigh more than short people. We then obtain height and weight measurements from a sample and analyze the data. Now suppose we happened by chance to choose a sample that consisted of short, heavy people, and tall, thin people. Our results might indicate that there is no relationship between a person's height and weight. Would we then be justified in stating that this study *proved* or *demonstrated* that height and weight in humans are unrelated?

As another example, suppose we hypothesized that tall nurses are more effective than short ones. This hypothesis is used here only to illustrate a point because, in reality, we would expect no relationship between height and a nurse's job performance. Now suppose that, by chance again, we drew a sample of nurses in which tall nurses received better job evaluations than short ones. Could we conclude definitively that height is related to a nurse's performance? These two examples illustrate the difficulty of using observations from a sample to generalize to a population. Other issues, such as the accuracy of the measures, the effects of uncontrolled extraneous variables, and the validity of underlying assumptions prevent researchers from concluding with finality that hypotheses are proved.

TIP: If a researcher uses any statistical tests (as is true in most quantitative studies), it means that there are underlying hypotheses—regardless of whether the researcher explicitly states them—because statistical tests are designed to test hypotheses. In planning a quantitative study of your own, do not be afraid to make a prediction, that is, to state a hypothesis.

RESEARCH EXAMPLES

This section describes how the research problem and research questions were communicated in two nursing studies, one quantitative and one qualitative.

Research Example of a Quantitative Study

Van Servellen, Aguirre, Sarna, and Brecht (2002) studied emotional distress in HIV-infected men and women. The researchers noted that, despite the fact that AIDS rates have been dropping for men but increasing for women, few studies have described the health experiences of HIV-infected women or compared them with those of men. This situation was viewed as especially troubling because of certain evidence indicating that, once HIV infected, women may be at greater risk than men for illness-related morbidity and adverse outcomes.

As stated by the researchers, the purpose of their study was "to describe and compare patterns of emotional distress in men and women with symptomatic HIV seeking care in community based treatment centers" (p. 50). The researchers went on to note that understanding gender differences and similarities in relation to sociodemographic characteristics, health status, and stress-resistant resources could "provide important information in designing gender-specific programs to improve quality of life and reduce emotional distress in clients affected by HIV" (p. 50).

The conceptual framework for the study was attribution theory, which offers explanations of links between life stressors and emotional distress. This framework guided the development of the four study hypotheses, which were as follows:

Hypothesis 1: Sociodemographic vulnerability (less than high school education, etc.) will be associated with emotional distress in both men and women.

Hypothesis 2: Poor physical and functional health status will be associated with emotional distress in both men and women.

Hypothesis 3: Optimism and social support will be associated with positive mental health outcomes ... in both men and women.

Hypothesis 4: Women will have higher levels of emotional distress than men (pp. 53–54).

Data for the study were collected from 82 men and 44 women with HIV disease in Los Angeles. The results indicated that women had greater disruptions in physical and psychosocial well-being than men, consistent with the fourth hypothesis. Physical health and optimism were the primary predictors of emotional distress in both men and women, supporting hypotheses 2 and 3. However, the first hypothesis was not supported in this low-income sample: there were no significant relationships between any sociodemographic vulnerability indicators and the subjects' level of anxiety or depression.

Research Example of a Qualitative Study

Beery, Sommers, and Hall (2002) studied the experiences of women with permanent cardiac pacemakers. The researchers stated that biotechnical devices such as pacemakers are increasingly being implanted into people to manage an array of disorders, yet relatively little research has examined the emotional impact of such an experience. They further noted that women may have distinctive responses to implanted devices because of cultural messages about the masculinity of technology, but little was known about women's unique responses to permanent cardiac pacemakers.

The purpose of Beery and colleagues' study was to explore women's responses to pacemaker implementation, using in-depth interviews to solicit the women's life stories. The researchers identified two specific research questions for their study: "What is the experience of women living with permanent cardiac pacemakers?" and "How do women incorporate permanent cardiac pacemakers into their lives and bodies?" (p. 8).

A sample of 11 women who were patients at the cardiology service of a large hospital participated in the study. During interviews, the women were asked a series of questions regarding life events that led up to, and occurred during and after, their pacemaker's implantation. Each woman participated in two interviews. An example of the questions asked in the initial interview is: "What has living with a pacemaker been like for you?" (p. 12). In the follow-up interviews, more specific questions were asked, such as, "How often do you think about the pacemaker?" and "When might you be reminded of it?" (p. 12).

The researchers' analysis revealed eight themes that emerged from the interview data: relinquishing care, owning the pacemaker, experiencing fears and resistance, imaging their body, normalizing, positioning as caregivers, finding resilience, and sensing omnipotence.

SUMMARY POINTS

- A **research problem** is a perplexing or enigmatic situation that a researcher wants to address through disciplined inquiry.
- Researchers usually identify a broad **topic,** narrow the scope of the problem, and then identify questions consistent with a paradigm of choice.
- The most common sources of ideas for nursing research problems are experience, relevant literature, social issues, theory, and external sources.
- Various criteria should be considered in assessing the value of a research problem. The problem should be clinically significant; researchable (questions of a moral or ethical nature are inappropriate); feasible; and of personal interest.
- Feasibility involves the issues of time, cooperation of study participants and other people, availability of facilities and equipment, researcher experience, and ethical considerations.
- Researchers communicate their aims in research reports as problem statements, statements of purpose, research questions, or hypotheses. The **problem statement** articulates the nature, context, and significance of a problem to be studied.
- A **statement of purpose** summarizes the overall study goal; in both qualitative and quantitative studies, the purpose statement identifies the key concepts (variables) and the study group or population.
- Purpose statements often communicate, through the use of verbs and other key terms, the underlying research tradition of qualitative studies, or whether study is experimental or nonexperimental in quantitative ones.
- A **research question** is the specific query researchers want to answer in addressing the research problem. In quantitative studies, research questions usually are about the existence, nature, strength, and direction of relationships.
- Some research questions are about **moderating variables** that affect the strength or direction of

a relationship between the independent and dependent variables; others are about **mediating variables** that intervene between the independent and dependent variable and help to explain why the relationship exists.

- In quantitative studies, a **hypothesis** is a statement of predicted relationships between two or more variables. A testable hypothesis states the anticipated association between one or more independent and one or more dependent variables.

- **Simple hypotheses** express a predicted relationship between one independent variable and one dependent variable, whereas **complex hypotheses** state an anticipated relationship between two or more independent variables and two or more dependent variables (or state predictions about mediating or moderating variables).

- **Directional hypotheses** predict the direction of a relationship; **nondirectional hypotheses** predict the existence of relationships, not their direction.

- **Research hypotheses** predict the existence of relationships; **statistical** or **null hypotheses** express the absence of a relationship.

- Hypotheses are never proved or disproved in an ultimate sense—they are accepted or rejected, supported or not supported by the data.

STUDY ACTIVITIES

Chapter 4 of the *Study Guide to Accompany Nursing Research: Principles and Methods, 7th edition*, offers various exercises and study suggestions for reinforcing the concepts presented in this chapter. In addition, the following study questions can be addressed:

1. Think of a frustrating experience you have had as a nursing student or as a practicing nurse. Identify the problem area. Ask yourself a series of questions until you have one that you think is researchable. Evaluate the problem in terms of the evaluation criteria discussed in this chapter.

2. Examine the following five problem statements. Are they researchable problems as stated? Why or why not? If a problem statement is not researchable, modify it in such a way that the problem could be studied scientifically.

a. What are the factors affecting the attrition rate of nursing students?

b. What is the relationship between atmospheric humidity and heart rate in humans?

c. Should nurses be responsible for inserting nasogastric tubes?

d. How effective are walk-in clinics?

e. What is the best approach for conducting patient interviews?

3. Examine a recent issue of a nursing research journal. Find an article that does not present a formal, well-articulated statement of purpose. Write a statement of purpose (or research questions) for that study.

4. Below are four hypotheses. For each hypothesis: (1) identify the independent and dependent variables; (2) indicate whether the hypothesis is simple or complex, and directional or nondirectional; and (3) state the hypotheses in null form.

a. Patients who are not told their diagnoses report more subjective feelings of stress than do patients who are told their diagnosis.

b. Patients receiving intravenous therapy report greater nighttime sleep pattern disturbances than patients not receiving intravenous therapy.

c. Patients with roommates call for a nurse less often than patients without roommates.

d. Women who have participated in Lamaze classes request pain medication during labor less often than women who have not taken these classes.

SUGGESTED READINGS

Methodologic References

Bennett, J. A. (2000). Mediator and moderator variables in nursing research: Conceptual and statistical differences. *Research in Nursing & Health, 23*, 415–420.

Creswell, J. W. (1998). *Qualitative inquiry and research design: Choosing among five traditions.* Thousand Oaks, CA: Sage.

Duffy, M. (2001). Getting qualitative research ideas and help on-line. In P. L. Munhall (Ed.), *Nursing Research: A qualitative perspective* (3rd ed., pp. 639–645). Sudbury, MA: Jones & Bartlett.

Kerlinger, F. N., & Lee, H. B. (2000). *Foundations of behavioral research* (4th ed.). Orlando, FL: Harcourt College Publishers.

Lincoln, Y. S., & Guba, E. G. (1985). *Naturalistic inquiry.* Newbury Park, CA: Sage.

Martin, P. A. (1994). The utility of the research problem statement. *Applied Nursing Research, 7*, 47–49.

Studies Cited in Chapter 4

Baker, C., & Daigle, M. C. (2000). Cross-cultural hospital care as experienced by Mi'kmaq clients. *Western Journal of Nursing Research, 22*, 8–28.

Beck, C. T. (1998). Postpartum onset panic disorder. *Image: Journal of Nursing Scholarship, 30*, 131–135.

Beery, T. A., Sommers, M. S., & Hall, J. (2002). Focused life stories of women with cardiac pacemakers. *Western Journal of Nursing Research, 24*, 7–27.

Butcher, H. K., Holkup, P. A., & Buckwalter, K. C. (2001). The experience of caring for a family member with Alzheimer's disease. *Western Journal of Nursing Research, 23*, 33–55.

Dirksen, S. R. (2000). Predicting well-being among breast cancer survivors. *Journal of Advanced Nursing, 32*, 937–943.

Gallagher, M., & Pierce, L. L. (2002). Caregivers' and care recipients' perceptions of dealing with urinary incontinence. *Rehabilitation Nursing, 27*, 25–31.

Holditch-Davis, D., Miles, M. S., Burchinal, M., O'Donnell, K., McKinney, R., & Lim, W. (2001). Parental caregiving and developmental outcomes of infants of mothers with HIV. *Nursing Research, 50*, 5–14.

Kelly, J. A., Doughty, J. K., Hasselbeck, A. N., & Vacchiano, C. (2000). The effect of arthroscopic irrigation fluid warming on body temperature. *Journal of Perianesthesia Nursing, 15*, 245–252.

Mellon, S., & Northouse, L. L. (2001). Family survivorship and quality of life following a cancer diagnosis. *Research in Nursing & Health, 24*, 446–459.

Mickley, J. R., & Cowles, K. (2001). Ameliorating the tension: The use of forgiveness for healing. *Oncology Nursing Forum, 28*, 31–37.

Parent, N., & Fortin, F. (2000). A randomized, controlled trial of vicarious experience through peer support for male first-time cardiac surgery patients. *Heart & Lung, 29*, 389–400.

Sampselle, C. M., Wyman, J., Thomas, K., Newman, D. K., Gray, M., Dougherty, M., & Burns, P. A. (2000). Continence for women: A test of AWHONN's evidence-based protocol in clinical practice. *Journal of Obstetric, Gynecologic, and Neonatal Nursing, 29*, 18–26.

Stranahan, S. (2001). Spiritual perception, attitudes about spiritual care, and spiritual care practices among nurse practitioners. *Western Journal of Nursing Research, 23*, 90–104.

van Servellen, G., Aguirre, M., Sarna, L., & Brecht, M. (2002). Differential predictors of emotional distress in HIV-infected men and women. *Western Journal of Nursing Research, 24*, 49–72.

Walker, N. C., & O'Brien, B. (1999). The relationship between method of pain management during labor and birth outcomes. *Clinical Nursing Research, 8*, 119–134.

Watt-Watson, J., Garfinkel, P., Gallop, R., Stevens, B., & Streiner, D. (2000). The impact of nurses' empathic responses on patients' pain management in acute care. *Nursing Research, 49*, 191–200.

Wilson, K., & Williams, W. A. (2000). Visualism in community nursing: Implications for telephone work with service users. *Qualitative Health Research, 10*, 507–520.

Zuwala R., & Barber K.R. (2001). Reducing anxiety in parents before and during pediatric anesthesia induction. *AANA Journal, 69*, 21–25.

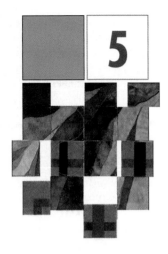

5

Reviewing the Literature

Researchers almost never conduct a study in an intellectual vacuum; their studies are usually undertaken within the context of an existing knowledge base. Researchers undertake a **literature review** to familiarize themselves with that knowledge base—although, as noted in Chapter 3, some qualitative researchers deliberately bypass an in-depth literature search before entering the field to avoid having their inquiries constrained or biased by prior work on the topic.

This chapter discusses the functions that a literature review can play in a research project and the kinds of material covered in a literature review. Suggestions are provided on finding references, reading research reports, recording information, and organizing and drafting a written review. Because research reports are not always easy to digest, a section of this chapter offers suggestions on reading them.

PURPOSES OF A LITERATURE REVIEW

Literature reviews can serve a number of important functions in the research process—as well as important functions for nurses seeking to develop an evidence-based practice. For researchers, acquaintance with relevant research literature and the state of current knowledge can help with the following:

- Identification of a research problem and development or refinement of research questions or hypotheses
- Orientation to what is known and not known about an area of inquiry, to ascertain what research can best make a contribution to the existing base of evidence
- Determination of any gaps or inconsistencies in a body of research
- Determination of a need to replicate a prior study in a different setting or with a different study population
- Identification or development of new or refined clinical interventions to test through empirical research
- Identification of relevant theoretical or conceptual frameworks for a research problem
- Identification of suitable designs and data collection methods for a study
- For those developing research proposals for funding, identification of experts in the field who could be used as consultants
- Assistance in interpreting study findings and in developing implications and recommendations

A literature review helps to lay the foundation for a study, and can also inspire new research ideas. A literature review also plays a role at the end of the study, when researchers are trying to make sense of their findings. Most research reports include summaries of relevant literature in the introduction. A literature review early in the report provides readers with a background for understanding current knowledge on a topic and illuminates the significance of the new study. Written research reviews are also included in research proposals that describe what a researcher is planning to study and how the study will be conducted.

Of course, research reviews are not undertaken exclusively by researchers. Both consumers and producers of nursing research need to acquire skills for reviewing research critically. Nursing students, nursing faculty, clinical nurses, nurse administrators, and nurses involved in policy-making organizations also need to review and synthesize evidence-based information.

SCOPE OF A LITERATURE SEARCH

You undoubtedly have some skills in locating and organizing information. However, a review of research literature differs in many respects from other kinds of term papers that students prepare. In this section, the type of information that should be sought in conducting a research review is examined, and other issues relating to the breadth and depth of the review are considered—including differences among the main qualitative research traditions.

Types of Information to Seek

Written materials vary considerably in their quality, their intended audience, and the kind of information they contain. Researchers performing a review of the literature ordinarily come in contact with a wide range of material and have to decide what to read or what to include in a written review. We offer some suggestions that may help in making such decisions.

The appropriateness of a reference concerns both its content (i.e., its relevance to the topic of the review) and the nature of the information it contains. The most important type of information for a research review are findings from empirical investi-gations. Cumulatively, research reports sum up what is known on a topic, but the information from such reports is of greatest value when the findings are integrated in a critical synthesis.

For a literature review, you should rely mostly on **primary source** research reports, which are descriptions of studies written by the researchers who conducted them. **Secondary source** research documents are descriptions of studies prepared by someone other than the original researcher. Literature review summaries, then, are secondary sources. Such reviews, if they exist and are recent, are an especially good place to begin a literature search because they provide a quick summary of the literature, and the bibliography is helpful. For many clinical topics, the reviews prepared by the Cochrane Collaboration are a particularly good resource.

However, secondary descriptions of studies should not be considered substitutes for primary sources for a new literature review. Secondary sources typically fail to provide much detail about studies, and they are seldom completely objective. Our own values and biases are a filter through which information passes (although we should make efforts to control such biases), but we should not accept as a second filter the biases of the person who prepared a secondary source summary of research studies.

 Examples of primary and secondary sources:

- Secondary source, a review of the literature on patient experiences in the ICU: Stein-Parbury, J. & McKinley, S. (2000). Patients' experiences of being in an intensive care unit: A select literature review. *American Journal of Critical Care, 9*, 20–27.

- Primary source, an original qualitative study on patient experiences in the ICU: Hupcey, J. E. (2000). Feeling safe: The psychosocial needs of ICU patients. *Journal of Nursing Scholarship, 32*, 361–367.

In addition to locating empirical references, you may find in your search various nonresearch references, including opinion articles, case reports, anecdotes, and clinical descriptions. Some qualitative researchers also review relevant literary or artistic work, to gain insights about human experiences. Such materials may serve to broaden understanding of a research problem, illustrate a point, demonstrate a need for research, or describe aspects of clinical practice. Such writings may thus may play a very important role in formulating research ideas—or may even suggest ways to broaden or focus the literature search—but they usually have limited utility in written research reviews because they are subjective and do not address the central question of written reviews: What is the current state of *knowledge* on this research problem?

Depth and Breadth of Literature Coverage

Some students worry about how broad their literature search should be. Of course, there is no convenient formula for the number of references that should be tracked down, or how many pages the written review should be. The extensiveness of the review depends on a number of factors. For written reviews, a major determinant is the nature of the document being prepared. The major types of research reviews include the following:

- *A review included in a research report.* As we discuss later in this chapter, research reports published in journals usually include brief literature reviews in their introductions. These reviews are succinct and have two major goals: to provide readers with a quick overview of the state of knowledge on the research problem being addressed; and to document the need for the new study and demonstrate how it will contribute to existing evidence. These reviews are usually only two to four double-spaced pages, and therefore only a limited number of references can be cited. This does not mean, of course, that researchers have not conducted a more thorough review, but rather that they are summarizing only what readers need to know to understand the study context. (If the report is published in a book or other format, the literature review section may be longer.)

- *A review included in a research proposal.* Research proposals designed to persuade funders (or advisors) about the merits of a proposed study usually include a literature review section. As with a review in a research report, a review in a proposal provides a knowledge context and confirms the need for and significance of new research. In a proposal, however, a review also demonstrates the writer's command of the literature. The length of such reviews may be established in proposal guidelines, but they are often 5 to 10 pages long.

- *A review in a thesis or dissertation.* Doctoral dissertations often include a thorough review covering materials directly and indirectly related to the problem area. Often, an entire chapter is devoted to a summary of the literature, and such chapters are frequently 15 to 25 pages in length.

- *Free-standing literature reviews.* Increasingly, nurses are preparing literature reviews that critically appraise and summarize a body of research on a topic, and such reviews play a powerful role in the development of an evidence-based practice. Students are sometimes asked to prepare a written research review for a course, and nurses sometimes do literature reviews as part of utilization projects. Researchers who are experts in a field also may do integrative reviews that are published as journal articles or that contribute to major evidence-based practice projects. Such integrative reviews are discussed in more detail in Chapter 27. Free-standing literature reviews designed to appraise a body of research critically are usually at least 15 to 25 pages long.

The breadth of a literature review also depends on the topic. For some topics, it may be necessary to review research findings in the non-nursing literature, such as sociology, psychology, biology, or medicine. Breadth of the review may also be affected by how extensive the research on the topic has been. If there have been 15 published studies on a specific problem, it would be difficult to draw conclusions about the current state of knowledge on that topic without reading all 15 reports. However, it is not necessarily true that the literature task is easier for little-researched topics. Literature reviews on new areas of inquiry *may* need to include studies of peripherally related topics to develop a meaningful context. Relevance and quality are the key criteria for including references in a written review of the literature.

With respect to depth in describing studies in a written review, the most important criteria are relevance and type of review. Research that is highly related to the problem usually merits more detailed coverage. Studies that are only indirectly related can often be summarized in a sentence or two, or omitted entirely if there are page restrictions.

Literature Reviews in Qualitative Research Traditions

As indicated in Chapter 3, qualitative researchers have different views about reviewing the literature as part of a new study. Some of the differences reflect viewpoints associated with various qualitative research traditions.

In grounded theory studies, researchers typically collect data in the field before reviewing the literature. As the data are analyzed, the grounded theory begins to take shape. Once the theory appears to be sufficiently developed, researchers then turn to the literature, seeking to relate prior findings to the theory. Glaser (1978) warns that "It's hard enough to generate one's own ideas without the 'rich' detailment provided by literature in the same field" (p. 31). Thus, grounded theory researchers defer the literature review, but then determine how previous research fits with or extends the emerging theory.

Phenomenologists often undertake a search for relevant materials at the outset of a study. In reviewing the literature for a phenomenological study, researchers look for experiential descriptions of the phenomenon being studied (Munhall, 2001). The purpose is to expand the researcher's understanding of the phenomenon from multiple perspectives. Van Manen (1990) suggests that, in addition to past research studies, artistic sources of experiential descriptions should be located such as poetry, novels, plays, films, and art. These artistic sources can offer powerful examples and images of the experience under study.

Even though "ethnography starts with a conscious attitude of almost complete ignorance" (Spradley, 1979, p. 4), a review of the literature that led to the choice of the cultural problem to be studied is often done before data collection. Munhall (2001) points out that this literature review may be more conceptual than data-based. A second, more thorough literature review is often done during data analysis and interpretation so that findings can be compared with previous literature.

LOCATING RELEVANT LITERATURE FOR A RESEARCH REVIEW

The ability to identify and locate documents on a research topic is an important skill that requires adaptability—rapid technological changes, such as the expanding use of the Internet, are making manual methods of finding information from print resources obsolete, and more sophisticated methods of searching the literature are being introduced continuously. We urge you to consult with librarians at your institution or to search the Internet for updated information.

One caveat should be mentioned. You may be tempted to do a search through an Internet search engine, such as Yahoo, Google, or Alta Vista. Such a search might provide you with interesting information about interest groups, support groups, advocacy organizations, and the like. However, such Internet searches are not likely to give you comprehensive bibliographic information on the *research* literature on your topic—and you might become frustrated with searching through the vast number of websites now available.

 TIP: Locating all relevant information on a research question is a bit like being a detective. The various electronic and print literature retrieval tools are a tremendous aid, but there inevitably needs to be some digging for, and a lot of sifting and sorting of, the clues to knowledge on a topic. Be prepared for sleuthing! And don't hesitate to ask your reference librarians for help in your detective work.

Electronic Literature Searches

In most college and university libraries, students can perform their own searches of **electronic databases**—huge bibliographic files that can be accessed by computer. Most of the electronic databases of interest to nurses can be accessed either through an **online search** (i.e., by directly communicating with a host computer over telephone lines or the Internet) or by **CD-ROM** (compact disks that store the bibliographic information). Several competing commercial vendors offer information retrieval services for bibliographic databases. Currently, the most widely used service providers for accessing bibliographic files are the following:

- Aries Knowledge Finder (www.ariessys.com)
- Ebsco Information Services (www.ebsco.com)
- Ovid Technologies (www.ovid.com)
- PaperChase (www.paperchase.com)
- SilverPlatter Information (www.silverplatter.com)

All of these services provide user-friendly retrieval of bibliographic information—they offer menu-driven systems with on-screen support so that retrieval can usually proceed with minimal instruction. However, the services vary with regard to a number of factors, such as number of databases covered, cost, online help, ease of use, special features, methods of access, and mapping capabilities. **Mapping** is a feature that allows you to search for topics in your own words, rather than needing to enter a term that is exactly the same as a subject heading in the database. The vendor's software translates ("maps") the topic you enter into the most plausible subject heading.

TIP: Even when there are mapping capabilities, it may prove useful in your search to learn the subject headings of the database or the **key words** that researchers themselves identify to classify their studies. Subject headings for databases can be located in the database's thesaurus. A good place to find key words is in a journal article once you have found a relevant reference.

Several other electronic resources should be mentioned. First, books and other holdings of libraries can almost always be scanned electronically using **online catalog systems.** Moreover, through the Internet, the catalog holdings of libraries across the country can be searched. Finally, it may be useful to search through Sigma Theta Tau International's Registry of Nursing Research on the Internet. This registry is an electronic research database with over 12,000 studies that can be searched by key words, variables, and researchers' names. The registry provides access to studies that have not yet been published, which cuts down the publication lag time; however, caution is needed because these studies have not been subjected to peer review (i.e., critical review by other experts in the field). Electronic publishing in general is expanding at a rapid pace; librarians and faculty should be consulted for the most useful websites.

TIP: It is rarely possible to identify all relevant studies exclusively through automated literature retrieval mechanisms. An excellent method of identifying additional references is to examine citations in recently published studies or published literature reviews.

Key Electronic Databases for Nurse Researchers

The two electronic databases that are most likely to be useful to nurse researchers are CINAHL (**C**umulative **I**ndex to **N**ursing and **A**llied **H**ealth **L**iterature) and MEDLINE® (**Med**ical Literature On-**Line**). Other potentially useful bibliographic databases for nurse researchers include:

- AIDSLINE (**AIDS** Information On-**Line**)
- CancerLit (**Cancer Lit**erature)
- CHID (**C**ombined **H**ealth **I**nformation **D**atabase)
- EMBASE (the Excerpta Medica database)
- ETOH (Alcohol and Alcohol Problems Science Database)
- HealthSTAR (**Health S**ervices, **T**echnology, **A**dministration, and **R**esearch)
- PsycINFO (**Psy**chology **Info**rmation)
- Rndex (Nursing and managed care database)

The CINAHL Database

The **CINAHL database** is the most important electronic database for nurses. This database covers references to virtually all English-language nursing and allied health journals, as well as to books, book chapters, nursing dissertations, and selected conference proceedings in nursing and allied health fields. References from more than 1200 journals are included in CINAHL.

The CINAHL database covers materials dating from 1982 to the present and contains more than 420,000 records. In addition to providing bibliographic information for locating references (i.e., the author, title, journal, year of publication, volume, and page numbers), this database provides abstracts (brief summaries) of articles for more than 300 journals. Supplementary information, such as names of data collection instruments, is available for many records in the database. Documents of interest can typically be ordered electronically.

CINAHL can be accessed online or by CD-ROM, either directly through CINAHL or through one of the commercial vendors cited earlier. Information about CINAHL's own online service can be obtained through the CINAHL website (www.cinahl.com).

We will use the CINAHL database to illustrate some of the features of an electronic search. Our example relied on the Ovid Search Software for CD-ROM, but similar features are available through other vendors' software.

Most searches are likely to begin with a **subject search** (i.e., a search for references on a specific topic). For such a search, you would type in a word or phrase that captures the essence of the topic (or the subject heading, if you know it), and the computer would then proceed with the search. An important alternative to a subject search is a **textword search** that looks for the words you enter in text fields of each record, including the title and the abstract. If you know the name of a researcher who has worked on the topic, an **author search** might be productive.

TIP: If you want to identify all major research reports on a topic, you need to be flexible and to think broadly about the key words that could be related to your topic. For example, if you are interested in anorexia nervosa, you might look under *anorexia*, *eating disorders*, and *weight loss*, and perhaps under *appetite, eating behavi..., food habits, bulimia,* and *body weight changes.*

In a subject search, after you enter the topic the computer might give you a message through *scope notes* about the definition of the CINAHL subject heading so you could determine whether the mapping procedure produced the right match. For example, if you typed in the subject "baby blues," the software would lead you to the subject heading "postpartum depression," and the scope note would give the following definition: "Any depressive disorder associated with the postpartum period. Severity may range from a mild case of 'baby blues' to a psychotic state." If this is the topic you had in mind, you would then learn the number of "hits" there are in the database for postpartum depression—that is, how many matches there are for that topic.

TIP: If your topic includes independent and dependent variables, you may need to do separate searches for each. For example, if you were interested in learning about the effect of health beliefs on compliance behaviors among patients with AIDS, you might want to read about health beliefs (in general) and about compliance behaviors (in general). Moreover, you might also want to access research on patients with AIDS and their circumstances.

In most cases, the number of hits in a subject search initially is rather large, and you will want to refine the search to ensure that you retrieve the most appropriate references. You can delimit retrieved documents in a number of ways. For example, you can restrict the search to those references for which your topic is the *main focus* of the document. For most subject headings, you also can select from a number of *subheadings* specific to the topic you are searching. You might also want to limit the references to a certain *type* of document (e.g., only research reports); specific *journal subsets* (e.g., only ones published in nursing journals); certain features of the document (e.g., only ones with abstracts); restricted *publication dates* (e.g., only those after 1999); certain *languages* (e.g., only those written in English); or certain *study participant characteristics* (e.g., only adolescents).

n searching a database through a vendor, it is usually possible to find only those references that more topics. For example, if we ...rested in the effect of stress on substance ...ouse, we could do independent searches for the two topics and then combine the searches to identify studies involving both variables.

To illustrate how searches can be delimited with a concrete example, suppose we were interested in recent research on brain injury, which is the term we enter in a subject search. Here is an example of how many hits there were on successive restrictions to the search, using the CINAHL database through June 2001:

Search Topic/Restriction	Hits
Brain injuries	1459
Restrict to main focus	1263
Limit to research reports	481
Limit to nursing journals	28
Limit to 1999 through 2001 publications	12

This narrowing of the search—from 1459 initial references on brain injuries to 12 references for recent nursing research reports on brain injuries—took under 1 minute to perform. Next, we would display the information for these 12 references on the monitor, and we could then print full bibliographic information for the ones that appeared especially promising. An example of one of the CINAHL record entries retrieved through this search on brain injuries is presented in Box 5-1. Each entry shows an accession number that is the unique identifier for each record in the database (the number that can be used to order the full text. Then, the authors and title of the reference are displayed, followed by source information. The source indicates the following:

- Name of the journal (*Critical Care Nursing Quarterly*)
- Volume (23)
- Issue (4)
- Page numbers (42–51)
- Year and month of publication (2001 Feb.)
- Number of cited references (23)

The printout also shows all the CINAHL subject headings that were coded for this particular entry; any of these headings could have been used in the subject search process to retrieve this particular reference. Note that the subject headings include both substantive/topical headings (e.g., brain injuries, quality of life) and methodologic headings (e.g., interviews). Next, when formal, named instruments are used in the study, these are printed under Instrumentation. Finally, the abstract for the study is presented.

Based on the abstract, we would then decide whether this reference was pertinent to our inquiry. Once relevant references are identified, the full research reports can be obtained and reviewed. All the documents referenced in the database can be ordered by mail or facsimile (fax), so it is not necessary for your library to subscribe to the referenced journal. Many of the retrieval service providers (such as Ovid) offer **full text** online services, so that, for certain journals, documents can be browsed directly, linked to other documents, and downloaded.

The MEDLINE®Database

The MEDLINE® database was developed by the U.S. National Library of Medicine (NLM), and is widely recognized as the premier source for bibliographic coverage of the biomedical literature. MEDLINE® incorporates information from Index Medicus, *International Nursing Index*, and other sources. MEDLINE® covers more than 4300 journals and contains more than 11 million records. In 1999, abstracts of reviews from the Cochrane Collaboration became available through MEDLINE® (they are also available directly on the internet at www.hcn.net.au/cochrane).

Because the MEDLINE® database is so large, it is often useful to access a subset of the database rather than the unabridged version that has references dating from 1966 to the present. For example, some subsets of the database cover only references within the previous 5 years. Other subsets include core medical journals, specialty journals, and nursing journals.

The MEDLINE® database can be accessed online or by CD-ROM through a commercial vendor (e.g., Ovid, Aries Knowledge Finder) for a fee. This

BOX 5.1   Example of a Printout From a CINAHL Search

ACCESSION NUMBER

2001035983.

SPECIAL FIELDS CONTAINED

Fields available in this record: abstract.

AUTHORS

DePalma JA.

INSTITUTION

Senior Research Associate, Oncology Nursing Society, Pittsburgh, Pennsylvania.

TITLE

Measuring quality of life of patients of traumatic brain injury.

SOURCE

Critical Care Nursing Quarterly, 23(4):42–51, 2001 Feb. (23 ref)

ABBREVIATED SOURCE

CRIT CARE NURS Q, 23(4):42–51, 2001 Feb. (23 ref)

CINAHL SUBJECT HEADINGS

Brain Injuries/pr [Prognosis]
Brain Injuries/rh [Rehabilitation]
*Brain Injuries/pf [Psychosocial Factors]
Clinical Nursing Research
Data Collection
Family/pf [Psychosocial Factors]
Inpatients
Interviews

*Quality of Life/ev [Evaluation]
Questionnaires
Recovery
Research Instruments
Research Subjects
Survivors/pf [Psychosocial Factors]
Trauma Severity Indices
Treatment Outcomes

INSTRUMENTATION

Sickness Impact Profile (SIP).

ABSTRACT

Quality of life (QOL) is recognized as an important indicator of health care and the patient's ability to cope with illness, treatment, and recuperation. Issues that need to be addressed in any proposed QOL research include a clear definition of QOL, a sound rationale for the choice of a measurement instrument, and the value of qualitative data. Measuring QOL in a patient population that has experienced traumatic brain injury (TBI) raises special concerns associated with the physical, behavioral, and cognitive limitations inherent with the specific TBI population. These pertinent issues are discussed with a focus that should be helpful for persons planning QOL projects and those reading and critiquing related literature. A study conducted by the author with patients with severe trauma injury will be used as an example of the impact of these issues on an actual project. Copyright © 2001 by Aspen Publishers, Inc. (23 ref) database can also be accessed for free through the Internet at various websites, including the following:

- PubMed (http://www.ncbi.nlm.nih.gov/PubMed)
- Infotrieve (http://www4.infotrieve.com/newmed-line/search.asp)

The advantage of accessing the database through commercial vendors is that they offer superior search capabilities and special features.

Print Resources

Print-based resources that must be searched manually are rapidly being overshadowed by electronic databases, but their availability should not be ignored. It is sometimes necessary to refer to printed resources to perform a search to include early literature on a topic. For example, the CINAHL database does not include references to research reports published before 1982.

Print indexes are books that are used to locate articles in journals and periodicals, books, dissertations, publications of professional organizations, and government documents. Indexes that are particularly useful to nurses are the *International Nursing Index*, *Cumulative Index to Nursing and Allied Health Literature* (the "red books"), *Nursing Studies Index*, *Index Medicus*, and *Hospital Literature Index*. Indexes are published periodically throughout the year (e.g., quarterly), with an annual cumulative index. When using a print index, you usually first need to identify the appropriate subject heading. Subject headings can be located in the index's thesaurus. Once the proper subject heading is determined, you can proceed to the subject section of the index, which lists the actual references.

Abstract journals summarize articles that have appeared in other journals. Abstracting services are in general more useful than indexes because they provide a summary of a study rather than just a title. Two important abstract sources for the nursing literature are *Nursing Abstracts* and *Psychological Abstracts*.

TIP: If you are doing a completely manual search, it is a wise practice to begin the search with the most recent issue of the index or abstract journal and then to proceed backward.

(Most electronic databases are organized chronologically, with the most recent references appearing at the beginning of a listing.)

READING RESEARCH REPORTS

Once you have identified potential references, you can proceed to locate the documents. For research literature reviews, relevant information will be found mainly in research reports in professional journals, such as *Nursing Research*. Before discussing how to prepare a written review, we briefly present some suggestions on how to read research reports in journals.

What Are Research Journal Articles?

Research **journal articles** are reports that summarize a study or one aspect of a complex study. Because journal space is limited, the typical research article is relatively brief—usually only 15 to 25 manuscript pages, double-spaced. This means that the researcher must condense a lot of information into a short space.

Research reports are accepted by journals on a competitive basis and are critically reviewed before acceptance for publication. Readers of research journal articles thus have some assurance that the studies have already been scrutinized for their scientific merit. Nevertheless, the publication of an article does not mean that the findings can be uncritically accepted as true, because most studies have some limitations that have implications for the validity of the findings. This is why consumers as well as producers of research can profit from understanding research methods.

Research reports in journals tend to be organized in certain format and written in a particular style. The next two sections discuss the content and style of research journal articles.*

Content of Research Reports

Research reports typically consist of four major sections (introduction, method section, results section, discussion section), plus an abstract and references.

---

*A more detailed discussion of the structure of journal articles is presented in Chapter 24.

The Abstract

The **abstract** is a brief description of the study placed at the beginning of the journal article. The abstract answers, in about 100 to 200 words, the following questions: What were the research questions? What methods did the researcher use to address those questions? What did the researcher find? and What are the implications for nursing practice? Readers can review an abstract to assess whether the entire report is of interest.

Some journals have moved from having traditional abstracts—which are single paragraphs summarizing the main features of the study—to slightly longer, more structured, and more informative abstracts with specific headings. For example, abstracts in *Nursing Research* after 1997 present information about the study organized under the following headings: Background, Objectives, Method, Results, Conclusions, and Key Words.

Box 5-2 presents abstracts from two actual studies. The first is a "new style" abstract for a quantitative study entitled "Family reports of barriers to optimal care of the dying" (Tolle, Tilden, Rosenfeld, & Hickman, 2000). The second is a more traditional abstract for a qualitative study entitled "Families of origin of homeless and never-homeless women" (Anderson & Imle, 2001). These two studies are used as illustrations throughout this section.

BOX 5.2 Examples of Abstracts From Published Research

QUANTITATIVE STUDY

Background: In response to intense national pressure to improve care of the dying, efforts have been made to determine problems or barriers to optimal care. However, prior research is limited by such factors as setting, focus, and sampling.

Objectives: The purpose of this study was to identify barriers to optimal care of a population-based representative sample of decedents across a full range of settings in which death occurred.

Method: Families were contacted 2 to 5 months after decedents' deaths by using data on their death certificates. Over a 14-month period, telephone interviews were conducted with 475 family informants who had been involved in caring for the patient in the last month of life. Interviews were standardized by use of a 58-item structured questionnaire.

Results: Data show a high frequency of advance planning (68%) and a high level of respect by clinicians for patient—family preferences about end-of-life location and treatment decisions. Family satisfaction with care was generally high, even though pain was a problem in one-third of the sample of decedents.

Conclusion: Barriers to optimal care of the dying remain, despite a generally positive overall profile; barriers include level of pain and management of pain, as well as some dissatisfaction with physician availability (Tolle, Tilden, Rosenfeld, & Hickman, 2000).

QUALITATIVE STUDY

Naturalistic inquiry was used to compare the characteristics of families of origin of homeless women with never-homeless women. The women's experiences in their families of origin were explored during in-depth interviews using Lofland and Lofland's conceptions of meanings, practices, episodes, roles, and relationships to guide the analysis. The two groups were similar with respect to family abuse history, transience, and loss. The never-homeless women had support from an extended family member who provided unconditional love, protection, a sense of connection, and age-appropriate expectations, as contrasted with homeless women who described themselves as being without, disconnected, and having to be little adults in their families of origin. The experiences of family love and connection seemed to protect never-homeless women from the effects of traumatic life events in childhood. These findings provide support for the influence of a woman's family of origin as a precursor to homelessness (Anderson & Imle, 2001).

The Introduction

The introduction acquaints readers with the research problem and its context. The introduction, which may or may not be specifically labeled "Introduction," follows immediately after the abstract. This section usually describes the following:

- *The central phenomena, concepts, or variables under study.* The problem area under investigation is identified.
- *The statement of purpose, and research questions or hypotheses to be tested.* The reader is told what the researcher set out to accomplish in the study.
- *A review of the related literature.* Current knowledge relating to the study problem is briefly described so readers can understand how the study fits in with previous findings and can assess the contribution of the new study.
- *The theoretical framework.* In theoretically driven studies, the framework is usually presented in the introduction.
- *The significance of and need for the study.* The introduction to most research reports includes an explanation of why the study is important to nursing.

Thus, the introduction sets the stage for a description of what the researcher did and what was learned.

 Examples from an introductory paragraph:

The homeless in the United States continue to increase in numbers and in diversity.... An estimated 760,000 people experience homelessness at some time during a one-year period.... Women and families make up the fastest-growing segment of the homeless population, and women head an estimated 90% of homeless families. The purpose of this study was to compare the characteristics of families of origin of homeless women with the families of origin of never-homeless women whose childhood experiences placed them at risk for homelessness (Anderson & Imle, 2001, p. 394).

In this paragraph, the researchers described the background of the problem, the population of primary interest (homeless women), and the study purpose.

The Method Section

The method section describes the method the researcher used to answer the research questions. The method section tells readers about major methodologic decisions, and may offer rationales for those decisions. For example, a report for a qualitative study often explains why a qualitative approach was considered to be especially appropriate and fruitful.

In a quantitative study, the method section usually describes the following, which may be presented as labeled subsections:

- *The research design.* A description of the research design focuses on the overall plan for the collection of data, often including the steps the researcher took to minimize biases and enhance the interpretability of the results by instituting various controls.
- *The subjects.* Quantitative research reports usually describe the population under study, specifying the criteria by which the researcher decided whether a person would be eligible for the study. The method section also describes the actual sample, indicating how people were selected and the number of subjects in the sample.
- *Measures and data collection.* In the method section, researchers describe the methods and procedures used to collect the data, including how the critical research variables were operationalized; they may also present information concerning the quality of the measuring tools.
- *Study procedures.* The method section contains a description of the procedures used to conduct the study, including a description of any intervention. The researcher's efforts to protect the rights of human subjects may also be documented in the method section.

Table 5-1 presents excerpts from the method section of the quantitative study by Tolle and her colleagues (2000).

Qualitative researchers discuss many of the same issues, but with different emphases. For example, a qualitative study often provides more information about the research setting and the context of the study, and less information on sampling. Also, because formal instruments are not used to collect qualitative data, there is little discussion about data collection methods, but there may be more information on data collection procedures. Increasingly, reports of qualitative studies are including descriptions of the

TABLE 5.1 Excerpts From Method Section, Quantitative Report

METHODOLOGIC ELEMENT	EXCERPT FROM TOLLE ET AL.'S STUDY, 2000*
Research design	Telephone surveys were conducted with 475 family respondents 2 to 5 months after decedents' deaths (p. 311).
Sample	...Death certificates for all Oregon deaths occurring in the 14 months between November 1996 and December 1997 were systematically randomly sampled, excluding decedents under the age of 18 years and deaths attributable to suicide, homicide, accident, or those undergoing medical examiner review. Out of a sampling frame of N = 24,074, the systematic random sample yielded 1,458 death certificates (p. 311).
Data collection	Family respondents were interviewed by use of a 58-item questionnaire developed by the investigators.... Telephone interviews were conducted by graduate student research assistants, intensively trained to standardize survey administration (pp. 311–312).
Procedure	In the initial telephone call, the study was explained. If the potential respondent gave their informed consent to participate, an appointment for the interview was made for the following week.... Those who agreed to participate were mailed a letter of introduction, an information sheet explaining the study, and a postcard to return if the person subsequently decided to decline participation (p. 311).

* From, Tolle, S. W., Tilden, V. P., Rosenfeld, A. G., & Hickman, S. E. (2000). Family reports of barriers to optimal care of the dying. *Nursing Research, 49,* 310–317.

researchers' efforts to ensure the trustworthiness of the data. Some qualitative reports also have a subsection on data analysis. There are fairly standard ways of analyzing quantitative data, but such standardization does not exist for qualitative data, so qualitative researchers may describe their analytic approach. Table 5-2 presents excerpts from the method section of the study by Anderson and Imle (2001).

The Results Section

The results section presents the **research findings** (i.e., the results obtained in the analyses of the data). The text summarizes the findings, often accompanied by tables or figures that highlight the most noteworthy results.

Virtually all results sections contain basic descriptive information, including a description of the study participants (e.g., their average age). In quantitative studies, the researcher provides basic descriptive information for the key variables, using simple statistics. For example, in a study of the effect of prenatal drug exposure on the birth outcomes of infants, the results section might begin by describing the average birth weights and Apgar scores of the infants, or the percentage who were of low birth weight (under 2500 g).

In quantitative studies, the results section also reports the following information relating to the statistical analyses performed:

- *The names of statistical tests used.* A **statistical test** is a procedure for testing hypotheses and

TABLE 5.2 Excerpts From Method Section, Qualitative Report

METHODOLOGIC ELEMENT	EXCERPT FROM ANDERSON & IMLE'S STUDY, 2001*
Design	Naturalistic inquiry was used to explore the families of origin of homeless and never-homeless women from their perspectives (p. 397).
Sample	The criteria for inclusion in the study were that the women had never been homeless, had experienced traumatic childhoods, were at least 18 years of age and spoke English.... The inclusion criteria for the study of homeless women were that the women had experienced homelessness, had taken steps toward moving away from life on the streets, were age 18 or over, and spoke English. The homeless ($n = 12$) and never-homeless ($n = 16$) women were similar in age, number of persons in the family of origin...education, ethnicity, and abuse histories (p. 398).
Data collection	One to three in-depth interviews, lasting 45 minutes to 2 hours, were conducted with both homeless and never-homeless women. Intensive interviewing is especially well suited to a retrospective study that relies on the participant to recall their memories because the setting described no longer exists.... All interviews were conducted by the author (p. 397).
Data analysis	Social units of analysis...were used to organize and assist in the coding and analysis of the interview data. The 5 social units that emerged during the interviews with the homeless sample were analyzed in the sample of never-homeless women and themes were identified (p. 400).

* From Anderson, D. G. & Imle. (2001). Families of origin of homeless and never-homeless women. *Western Journal of Nursing Research, 23,* 394–413.

evaluating the believability of the findings. For example, if the percentage of low-birth-weight infants in the sample of drug-exposed infants is computed, how probable is it that the percentage is accurate? If the researcher finds that the average birth weight of drug-exposed infants in the sample is lower than that of nonexposed infants, how probable is it that the same would be true for other infants not in the sample? That is, is the relationship between prenatal drug exposure and infant birth weight *real* and likely to be replicated with a new sample of infants—or does the result reflect a peculiarity of the sample? Statistical tests answer such questions. Statistical tests are based on common principles; you do not have to

know the names of all statistical tests (there are dozens) to comprehend the findings.

• *The value of the calculated statistic.* Computers are used to compute a numeric value for the particular statistical test used. The value allows the researchers to draw conclusions about the meaning of the results. The *actual* numeric value of the statistic, however, is not inherently meaningful and need not concern you.

• *The significance.* The most important information is whether the results of the statistical tests were significant (not to be confused with important or clinically relevant). If a researcher reports that the results are **statistically significant,** it means the findings are probably valid and replicable with a new sample of subjects. Research reports also indicate the **level of significance,** which is an index of how probable it is that the findings are reliable. For example, if a report indicates that a finding was significant at the .05 level, this means that only 5 times out of 100 (5 ÷ 100 = .05) would the obtained result be spurious or haphazard. In other words, 95 times out of 100, similar results would be obtained with a new sample. Readers can therefore have a high degree of confidence—but not total assurance—that the findings are reliable.

 Example from the results section of a quantitative study:

Overall, 71% of family respondents reported knowing the decedent's preference for place of death, and 68% of those families believed that the decedent had died in their preferred location. Decedents who got their wish differed significantly by location of death, χ^2 (2, $n = 337$) = 131.2, $p < .001$. Of decedents whose wishes were known, 100% of those who died at home wanted to die at home, and 40% of decedents who died in nursing homes and 45% of those who died in hospitals got their wish for location of death" (Tolle et al., 2000, p. 313).

In this excerpt, the authors indicated that decedents who died at home were much more likely to have died in their preferred location than decedents who died in nursing homes or hospitals, and that the probability (p) that this finding is spurious is less than 1 in 1000 (1 ÷ 1000 = .001). Thus, the finding is *highly* reliable. Note that to comprehend this finding, you do not need to understand what the χ^2 statistic is, nor to concern yourself with the actual value of the statistic, 131.2.

In qualitative reports, the researcher often organizes findings according to the major **themes,** processes, or categories that were identified in the data. The results section of qualitative reports sometimes has several subsections, the headings of which correspond to the researcher's labels for the themes. Excerpts from the raw data are presented to support and provide a rich description of the thematic analysis. The results section of qualitative studies may also present the researcher's emerging theory about the phenomenon under study, although this may appear in the concluding section of the report.

 Example from the results section of a qualitative study:

The homeless people interviewed did not have a sense of connectedness.... In contrast, the never-homeless women had connections to family, friends, and to larger social systems that lasted into adulthood and the foreseeable future.... Many of the never-homeless also described tangible links to their past. Robin, for example, described her dining room set that had belonged to her adopted grandparents: "I was always told that this table came with them on a covered wagon.... They paid $35 for this set; that includes the chairs and buffet.... There are places on here that have [her brother's] teeth marks. I used to play house under here" (Anderson & Imle, 2001, p. 409).

In this excerpt, the researchers illustrate their finding that never-homeless women maintained rich connections with their past with a direct quote from a study participant.

The Discussion Section

In the discussion section, the researcher draws conclusions about the meaning and implications of the findings. This section tries to unravel what the results mean, why things turned out the way they did, and how the results can be used in practice. The discussion in both qualitative and quantitative reports may incorporate the following elements:

- *An interpretation of the results.* The interpretation involves the translation of findings into practical, conceptual, or theoretical meaning.
- *Implications.* Researchers often offer suggestions for how their findings could be used to improve nursing, and they may also make recommendations on how best to advance knowledge in the area through additional research.
- *Study limitations.* The researcher is in the best position possible to discuss study limitations, such as sample deficiencies, design problems, weaknesses in data collection, and so forth. A discussion section that presents these limitations demonstrates to readers that the author was aware of these limitations and probably took them into account in interpreting the findings.

Example from a discussion section of a quantitative report:

Overall, one third of the sample of family respondents indicated moderate to severe decedent pain in the final week of life. Although this rate is somewhat better than rates reported elsewhere, it still raises concern that control of pain for dying patients is simply not good enough.... Interestingly, families had more complaints about the management of pain for decedents who died at home, even though they did not report higher levels of pain. Perhaps this is because in the home setting, family members are more aware of pain management problems and bear more responsibility for direct care of such needs (Tolle et al., 2000, p. 315).

References

Research journal articles conclude with a list of the books, reports, and journal articles that were referenced in the text of the report. For those interested in pursuing additional reading on a substantive topic, the reference list of a current research study is an excellent place to begin.

The Style of Research Journal Articles

Research reports tell a story. However, the style in which many research journal articles are written—especially reports of quantitative studies—makes it difficult for beginning research consumers to become interested in the story. To unaccustomed audiences, research reports may seem stuffy, pedantic, and bewildering. Four factors contribute to this impression:

1. *Compactness.* Journal space is limited, so authors try to compress many ideas and concepts into a short space. Interesting, personalized aspects of the investigation often cannot be reported. And, in qualitative studies, only a handful of supporting quotes can be included.
2. *Jargon.* The authors of both qualitative and quantitative reports use research terms that are assumed to be part of readers' vocabulary, but that may seem esoteric.
3. *Objectivity.* Quantitative researchers normally avoid any impression of subjectivity and thus research stories are told in a way that makes them sound impersonal. For example, most quantitative research reports are written in the passive voice (i.e., personal pronouns are avoided). Use of the passive voice tends to make a report less inviting and lively than the use of the active voice, and it tends to give the impression that the researcher did not play an active role in conducting the study. (Qualitative reports, by contrast, are more subjective and personal, and written in a more conversational style.)
4. *Statistical information.* In quantitative reports, numbers and statistical symbols may intimidate readers who do not have strong mathematic interest or training. Most nursing studies are quantitative, and thus most research reports summarize the results of statistical analyses. Indeed, nurse researchers have become increasingly sophisticated during the past decade and have begun to use more powerful and complex statistical tools.

A major goal of this textbook is to assist nurses in dealing with these issues.

Tips on Reading Research Reports

As you progress through this textbook, you will acquire skills for evaluating various aspects of research reports critically. Some preliminary hints on digesting research reports and dealing with the issues previously described follow.

- Grow accustomed to the style of research reports by reading them frequently, even though you may not yet understand all the technical points. Try to keep the underlying rationale for the style of research reports in mind as you are reading.
- Read from a report that has been photocopied. Then you will be able to use a highlighter, underline portions of the article, write questions or notes in the margins, and so on.
- Read journal articles slowly. It may be useful to skim the article first to get the major points and then read the article more carefully a second time.
- On the second or later reading of a journal article, train yourself to become an *active* reader.

Reading actively means that you are constantly monitoring yourself to determine whether you understand what you are reading. If you have comprehension problems, go back and reread difficult passages or make notes about your confusion so that you can ask someone for clarification. In most cases, that "someone" will be your research instructor or another faculty member, but also consider contacting the researchers themselves. The postal and e-mail addresses of the researchers are usually included in the journal article, and researchers are generally more than willing to discuss their research with others.

• Keep this textbook with you as a reference while you are reading articles initially. This will enable you to look up unfamiliar terms in the glossary at the end of the book, or in the index.

• Try not to get bogged down in (or scared away by) statistical information. Try to grasp the gist of the story without letting formulas and numbers frustrate you.

• Until you become accustomed to the style and jargon of research journal articles, you may want to "translate" them mentally or in writing. You can do this by expanding compact paragraphs into looser constructions, by translating jargon into more familiar terms, by recasting the report into an active voice, and by summarizing the findings with words rather than numbers. As an example, Box 5-3 presents a summary of a fictitious study, written in the style typically found in research reports. Terms that can be looked up in the glossary of this book are underlined, and the notes in the margins indicate the type of information the author is communicating. Box 5-4 presents a "translation" of this summary, recasting the information into language that is more digestible. Note that it is not just the jargon specific to research methods that makes the original version complicated (e.g., "sequelae" is more obscure than "consequences"). Thus, a dictionary might also be needed when reading research reports.

• Although it is certainly important to read research reports with understanding, it is also important to read them critically, especially when you are preparing a written literature review. A critical reading involves an evaluation of the researcher's major conceptual and methodologic decisions. Unfortunately, it is difficult for students to criticize these decisions before they have gained some conceptual and methodologic skills themselves. These skills will be strengthened as you progress through this book, but sometimes common sense and thoughtful analysis may suggest flaws in a study, even to beginning students. Some of the key questions to ask include the following: Does the way the researcher conceptualized the problem make sense—for example, do the hypotheses seem sensible? Did the researcher conduct a quantitative study when a qualitative one would have been more appropriate? In a quantitative study, were the research variables measured in a reasonable way, or would an alternative method have been better? Additional guidelines for critiquing various aspects of a research report are presented in Chapter 26.

PREPARING A WRITTEN LITERATURE REVIEW

A number of steps are involved in preparing a written review, as summarized in Figure 5-1. As the figure shows, after identifying potential sources, you need to locate the references and screen them for their relevancy.

Screening References

References that have been identified through the literature search need to be screened. One screen is totally practical—is the reference readily accessible? For example, although abstracts of dissertations may be easy to retrieve, full dissertations are not; some references may be written in a language you do not read. A second screen is the relevance of the reference, which you can usually (but not always) surmise by reading the abstract. When abstracts are not available, you will need to take a

BOX 5.3 Summary of a Fictitious Study for Translation

	The potentially negative sequelae of having an abortion on the psychological adjustment of adolescents have not been adequately studied.	**Need for the study**
Purpose of the study	The present study sought to determine whether alternative pregnancy resolution decisions have different long-term effects on the psychological functioning of young women.	
Research design	Three groups of low-income pregnant teenagers attending an inner-city clinic were the <u>subjects</u> in this study: those who delivered and kept the baby; those who delivered and relinquished the baby for adoption; and those who had an abortion. There were 25 subjects in each group.	**Study population**
Research instruments	The study <u>instruments</u> included a self-administered <u>questionnaire</u> and a battery of psychological tests measuring depression, anxiety, and psychosomatic symptoms. The instruments were administered upon entry into the study (when the subjects first came to the clinic) and then 1 year after termination of the pregnancy.	**Research sample**
Data analysis procedure	The <u>data</u> were analyzed using <u>analysis of variance (ANOVA)</u>. The ANOVA tests indicated that the three groups did not differ significantly in terms of depression, anxiety, or psychosomatic symptoms at the initial testing. At the <u>post-test</u>, however, the abortion group had significantly higher scores on the depression scale, and these girls were significantly more likely than the two delivery groups to report severe tension headaches. There were no <u>significant</u> differences on any of the <u>dependent variables</u> for the two delivery groups.	**Results**
Implications	The results of this study suggest that young women who elect to have an abortion may experience a number of long-term negative consequences. It would appear that appropriate efforts should be made to follow up abortion patients to determine their need for suitable treatment.	**Interpretation**

BOX 5.4 Translated Version of Fictitious Research Study

As researchers, we wondered whether young women who had an abortion had any emotional problems in the long run. It seemed to us that not enough research had been done to know whether any psychological harm resulted from an abortion.

We decided to study this question ourselves by comparing the experiences of three types of teenagers who became pregnant—first, girls who delivered and kept their babies; second, those who delivered the babies but gave them up for adoption; and third, those who elected to have an abortion. All teenagers in the sample were poor, and all were patients at an inner-city clinic. Altogether, we studied 75 girls—25 in each of the three groups. We evaluated the teenagers' emotional states by asking them to fill out a questionnaire and to take several psychological tests. These tests allowed us to assess things such as the girls' degree of depression and anxiety and whether they had any complaints of a psychosomatic nature. We asked them to fill out the forms twice: once when they came into the clinic, and then again a year after the abortion or the delivery.

We learned that the three groups of teenagers looked pretty much alike in terms of their emotional states when they first filled out the forms. But when we compared how the three groups looked a year later, we found that the teenagers who had abortions were more depressed and were more likely to say they had severe tension headaches than teenagers in the other two groups. The teenagers who kept their babies and those who gave their babies up for adoption looked pretty similar one year after their babies were born, at least in terms of depression, anxiety, and psychosomatic complaints.

Thus, it seems that we might be right in having some concerns about the emotional effects of having an abortion. Nurses should be aware of these long-term emotional effects, and it even may be advisable to institute some type of follow-up procedure to find out if these young women need additional help.

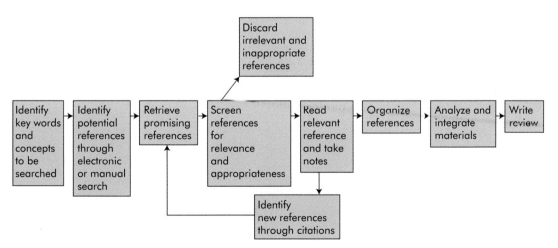

FIGURE 5.1 Flow of tasks in a literature review.

guess about relevance based on the title. For critical integrated reviews (see Chapter 27), a third criterion is the study's methodologic quality—that is, the quality of evidence the study yields.

Abstracting and Recording Notes

Once a document has been determined to be relevant, you should read the entire report carefully and critically, identifying material that is sufficiently important to warrant note taking and observing flaws in the study or gaps in the report. As noted earlier, it is useful to work with photocopied articles so that you can highlight or underline critical information. Even with a copied article, we recommend taking notes or writing a summary of the report's strengths and limitations. A formal protocol is sometimes helpful for recording information in a systematic fashion. An example of such a protocol is presented in Figure 5-2. Although many of the terms on this protocol are probably not familiar to you at this point, you will learn their meaning as you progress through this book.

Organizing the Review

Organization of information is a critical task in preparing a written review. When the literature on a topic is extensive, we recommend preparing a summary table. The table could include columns with headings such as Author, Type of Study (Qualitative versus Quantitative), Sample, Design, Data Collection Approach, and Key Findings. Such a table provides a quick overview that allows you to make sense of a mass of information.

Example of a summary table:
Abercrombie (2001) reviewed research related to strategies that have been found to improve follow-up after an abnormal Papanicolaou (Pap) smear test. Her review included a table that summarized nine studies. The headings in her columns were: Author and date; sample size; objectives; design/intervention; and results.

Most writers find it helpful to work from an outline when preparing a written review. If the review is lengthy and complex, it is useful to write out the outline; a mental outline may be sufficient for shorter reviews. The important point is to work out a structure before starting to write so that the presentation has a meaningful and understandable flow. Lack of organization is a common weakness in students' first attempts at writing a research literature review. Although the specifics of the organization differ from topic to topic, the overall goal is to structure the review in such a way that the presentation is logical, demonstrates meaningful integration, and leads to a conclusion about what is known and not known about the topic.

TIP: An important principle in organizing a review is to figure out a way to cluster and compare studies. For example, you could contrast studies that have similar findings with studies that have conflicting or inconclusive findings, making sure to analyze why the discrepancies may have occurred. Or you might want to cluster studies that have operationalized key variables in similar ways. Other reviews might have as an organizing theme the nature of the setting or the sample if research findings vary according to key characteristics (e.g., comparing research with female subjects and research with male subjects, if the results differ.) Doing a research review is a little bit like doing a qualitative study—you must search for important themes.

Once the main topics and their order of presentation have been determined, a review of the notes is in order. This not only will help you recall materials read earlier but also will lay the groundwork for decisions about where (if at all) a particular reference fits in terms of your outline. If certain references do not seem to fit anywhere, the outline may need to be revised or the reference discarded.

Writing a Literature Review

At this point, you will have completed the most difficult tasks of the literature review process, but that process is not complete until you have drafted and edited a written product. Although it is beyond the scope of this textbook to offer detailed guidance on writing research reviews, we offer a few comments on their content and style. Additional assistance is

Citation: Authors: _____
                       Title: _____
                       Journal: _____
                       Year: _____ Volume _____ Issue _____ Pages: _____

Type of Study: ☐ Quantitative   ☐ Qualitative   ☐ Both

Location/setting: _____

Key Concepts/   Concepts: _____
Variables: Intervention/Independent Variable: _____
                       Dependent Variable: _____
                       Controlled Variables: _____

Design Type: ☐ Experimental   ☐ Quasi-experimental   ☐ Pre-experimental ☐ Nonexperimental
                       Specific Design: _____
                       Descrip. of Intervention: _____
                       _____

                       ☐ Longitudinal/prospective ☐ Cross-sectional   No. of data collection points: _____
                       Comparison group(s): _____

Qual. Tradition: ☐ Grounded theory   ☐ Phenomenology   ☐ Ethnography   ☐ Other: _____

Sample: Size: _____ Sampling method: _____
                       Sample characteristics: _____

Data Sources: Type: ☐ Self-report   ☐ Observational   ☐ Biophysiologic   ☐ Other: _____
                       Description of measures: _____
                       Data Quality: _____

Statistical Tests: Bivariate: ☐ T test   ☐ ANOVA ☐ Chi-square   ☐ Pearson's r ☐ Other: _____
                       Multivariate: ☐ Multiple regression ☐ MANOVA   ☐ Factor analysis   ☐ Other: _____

Findings: _____
                       _____
                       _____

Recommendations: _____
                       _____

Strengths: _____
                       _____

Weaknesses: _____
                       _____

FIGURE 5.2   Example of a literature review protocol.

provided in books such as those by Fink (1998) and Galvan (1999).

Content of the Written Literature Review

A written research review should provide readers with an objective, well-organized summary of the current state of knowledge on a topic. A literature review should be neither a series of quotes nor a series of abstracts. The central tasks are to summarize and critically evaluate the evidence so as to reveal the current state of knowledge on a topic—not simply to describe what researchers have done. The review should point out both consistencies and contradictions in the literature, and offer possible explanations for inconsistencies (e.g., different conceptualizations or data collection methods).

Although important studies should be described in some detail, it is not necessary to provide extensive coverage for every reference (especially if there are page constraints). Reports of lesser significance that result in comparable findings can be summarized together.

Example of grouped studies: McCullagh, Lusk, and Ronis (2002, p. 33) summarized several studies as follows: "Although noise-induced hearing loss is preventable through appropriate use of hearing protection devices, studies among farmers consistently show a low level of use (Broste et al., 1989; Engstrand, 1995; Hallet, 1987; Karlovich et al.,1988; Langsford et al., 1995)."

The literature should be summarized in your own words. The review should demonstrate that consideration has been given to the cumulative significance of the body of research. Stringing together quotes from various documents fails to show that previous research has been assimilated and understood.

The review should be objective, to the extent possible. Studies that conflict with personal values or hunches should not be omitted. The review also should not deliberately ignore a study because its findings contradict other studies. Inconsistent results should be analyzed and the supporting evidence evaluated objectively.

The literature review should conclude with a summary of the state of the art of knowledge on the topic. The summary should recap study findings and indicate how credible they are; it should also make note of gaps or areas of research inactivity. The summary thus requires critical judgment about the extensiveness and dependability of the evidence on a topic. If the literature review is conducted as part of a new study, this critical summary should demonstrate the need for the research and should clarify the context within which any hypotheses were developed.

TIP: The literature review section of a research report (or research proposal) usually includes information not only about what is known about the problem and relevant interventions (if any), but about how prevalent the problem is. In research reports and proposals, the authors are trying to "build a case" for their new study.

As you progress through this book, you will become increasingly proficient in critically evaluating the research literature. We hope you will understand the mechanics of writing a research review once you have completed this chapter, but we do not expect that you will be in a position to write a state-of-the-art review until you have acquired more skills in research methods.

Style of a Research Review

Students preparing their first written research review often have trouble adjusting to the standard style of such reviews. For example, some students accept research results without criticism or reservation, reflecting a common misunderstanding about the conclusiveness of empirical research. You should keep in mind that no hypothesis or theory can be proved or disproved by empirical testing, and no research question can be definitely answered in a single study. Every study has some limitations, the severity of which is affected by the researcher's methodologic decisions. The fact that theories and hypotheses cannot be ultimately proved or disproved does not, of course, mean that we must disregard evidence or challenge every idea

TABLE 5.3 Examples of Stylistic Difficulties for Research Reviews*

INAPPROPRIATE STYLE OR WORDING	RECOMMENDED CHANGE
1. It is known that unmet expectations engender anxiety.	Several experts (Greenberg, 2001; Cameron, 2000) have asserted that unmet expectations engender anxiety.
2. The woman who does not participate in childbirth preparation classes tends to manifest a high degree of stress during labor.	Previous studies have indicated that women who participate in preparation for childbirth classes manifest less stress during labor than those who do not (Klotz, 2002; Mirling, 2000; McTygue, 2001).
3. Studies have proved that doctors and nurses do not fully understand the psychobiologic dynamics of recovery from a myocardial infarction.	The studies by Sacks (2000) and Carter (2001) suggest that doctors and nurses do not fully understand the psychobiologic dynamics of recovery from a myocardial infarction.
4. Attitudes cannot be changed quickly.	Attitudes have been found to be relatively enduring attributes that cannot be changed quickly (Dodge-Hanson, 2000; Woodward, 2001).
5. Responsibility is an intrinsic stressor.	According to Doctor A. Cassard, an authority on stress, responsibility is an intrinsic stressor (Cassard, 2000, 2001).

* All references are fictitious.

we encounter—especially if results have been replicated. The problem is partly a semantic one: hypotheses are not proved, they are *supported* by research findings; theories are not *verified,* but they may be tentatively *accepted* if there a substantial body of evidence demonstrates their legitimacy.

TIP: When describing study findings, you should generally use phrases indicating tentativeness of the results, such as the following:

- Several studies have *found*
- Findings thus far *suggest*
- Results from a landmark study *indicated*
- The data *supported* the hypothesis . . .
- There *appears* to be strong evidence that

A related stylistic problem is an inclination of novice reviewers to interject opinions (their own or someone else's) into the review. The review should include opinions sparingly and should be explicit about their source. Reviewers' own opinions do not belong in a review, with the exception of assessments of study quality.

The left-hand column of Table 5-3 presents several examples of stylistic flaws. The right-hand column offers recommendations for rewording the sentences to conform to a more acceptable form for a research literature review. Many alternative wordings are possible.

RESEARCH EXAMPLES OF RESEARCH LITERATURE REVIEWS

The best way to learn about the style, content, and organization of a research literature review is to read several reviews that appear in the nursing literature. We present two excerpts from reviews here and urge you to read other reviews on a topic of interest to you.

Research Example From a Quantitative Research Report

Teel, Duncan, and Lai (2001) conducted a study about the experiences of 83 caregivers of patients who had had a stroke. A segment of their literature review that was included in their introduction follows (Teel et al., 2001, pp. 53–54).

Over half a million Americans suffer strokes each year. Approximately 75% survive, yet most have residual neurologic impairment that requires supportive care (Gresham et al., 1995)*. Long-term assistance for many stroke patients is provided in home settings, by family caregivers who must acquire a number of new skills to successfully manage the outcomes of stroke... (Biegel et al., 1991; Evans et al., 1992; Jacob, 1991; Matson, 1994). Family home care management after stroke is essential, yet it is often stressful and demanding. The physical care requirements, vigilance, and altered roles that are often part of the stroke sequelae contribute to caregiving stress (Davis & Grant, 1994).

Caregiving demands can have negative emotional and physical consequences for the family caregivers, which can, in turn, have negative implications for continuation of the caregiving role. Because of the potential effects, many caregiver outcomes have been studied. Mental health outcomes, including depression, perceived burden and strain, anxiety, and alternations in mood, have been examined relative to caregiving (Matson, 1994; Periard & Ames, 1993). Stroke caregivers were found to have higher depression scores than noncaregivers, and the elevated levels persisted at 1 year post-stroke (Schultz et al., 1988). For caregiving wives, increased social support was correlated with less depression (Robinson & Kaye, 1994). Physical health outcomes for caregivers have included assessments of general health and chronic illness (George & Gwyther, 1986), number of physician visits or days hospitalized (Cattanach & Tebes, 1991), assessment of immune function (Kiecolt-Glaser et al., 1991), and fatigue (Jensen & Given, 1991; Nygaard, 1988; Rabins et al., 1982; Teel & Press, 1999). Stroke caregivers have reported impaired physical health (Deimling & Bass, 1986), yet Rees and colleagues (1994) found no immunologic alterations in stroke caregivers who had been caring for at least 6 months compared with caregivers in a cross-sectional analysis of immune function.

* Consult the full research report for references cited in this excerpted literature review.

Evans and colleagues (1992) have suggested that the influence of the family also may affect stroke outcome. For example, the family can have a buffering effect on patient coping, with family emotional, informational, and practical support enhancing post-stroke coping ability. Patients categorized as having suboptimal home environments at 1 year after stroke had caregivers who were more likely to be depressed, less likely to be a spouse caregiver, had below average knowledge about stroke care, and reported more family dysfunction than caregivers in the optimal group (Evans et al., 1991). Because each of these variables has been associated with stroke outcome, post-stroke evaluation and treatment should include attention to minimizing caregiver depression and family dysfunction, while promoting knowledge about stroke care (Evans et al., 1991, 1992).

Overall, the research literature is extremely limited in reports of outcomes for caregivers of stroke patients. In particular, studies about caregiving in the first several months after a stroke, a time in which there can be significant change in patient condition and caregiving routine, is virtually absent from the literature.

Research Example From a Qualitative Research Report

Boydell, Goering, and Morrell-Bellai (2000) conducted a study of the experiences of 29 homeless individuals. A portion of the literature review for their research report follows (Boydell et al., 2000, pp. 26–27).

Studies show that homelessness involves much more than not having a place to live. Individuals often lose their sense of identity, self-worth, and self-efficacy (Buckner, Bassuk, & Zima, 1993). Hallebone (1997) studied 38 homeless men ethnographically and found that psychosocial identities tend to be fragmented....

Taylor's (1993) study involving qualitative interviews with 10 homeless women indicates that participants shared experiences of depersonalization and stigmatization and the subsequent effects on their personhood. It was found that being or appearing unclean and having an identity without certification (paper proof) greatly affected the women's sense of self-esteem and personhood.

Snow and Anderson (1993) report that those recently dislocated expressed a strong aversion to other homeless individuals. In contrast, those who had been homeless for extended periods of time were more likely than those recently dislocated to embrace self-concepts such as tramp and bum. These unconventional self-concepts may be acquired and reinforced, at least in part, through social comparisons and identification with other homeless people (Grigsby et al., 1990).... Montgomery (1994) found that homeless women felt that their hard times contributed to the creation of a new and more positive self.... The literature also suggests that there is a spiritual dimension to the experience of homelessness that is often ignored. Matousek (1991) describes how the profound loss of self, which is associated with homelessness, presents a spiritual challenge to define one's very existence.

SUMMARY POINTS

- A research **literature review** is a written summary of the state of existing knowledge on a research problem. The task of reviewing research literature involves the identification, selection, critical analysis, and written description of existing information on a topic.

- Researchers review the research literature to develop research ideas, to determine knowledge on a topic of interest, to provide a context for a study, and to justify the need for a study; consumers review and synthesize evidence-based information to gain knowledge and improve nursing practice.

- The most important type of information for a research review are findings from empirical studies. Various nonresearch references—including opinion articles, case reports, anecdotes, and clinical descriptions—may serve to broaden understanding of a research problem or demonstrate a need for research, but in general they have limited utility in written research reviews.

- A **primary source** with respect to the research literature is the original description of a study prepared by the researcher who conducted it; a **secondary source** is a description of the study by a person unconnected with it. Primary sources should be consulted whenever possible in performing a literature review.

- An important bibliographic development for locating references for a research review is the widespread availability of various **electronic databases,** many of which can be accessed through an **online search** or by way of **CD-ROM.** For nurses, the **CINAHL** and **MEDLINE** ® databases are especially useful.

- In searching a bibliographic database, users usually perform a **subject search** for a topic of interest, but other types of searches (e.g., **textword search, author search**) are available.

- Although electronic information retrieval is widespread, print resources such as **print indexes** and **abstract journals** are also available.

- References that have been identified must be screened for relevance and then read critically. For research reviews, most references are likely to be found in professional journals.

- Research **journal articles** provide brief descriptions of research studies and are designed to communicate the contribution the study has made to knowledge.

- Journal articles often consist of an **abstract** (a brief synopsis of the study) and four major sections: an introduction (explanation of the study problem and its context); method section (the strategies used to address the research problem); results section (the actual study findings); and discussion (the interpretation of the findings).

- Research reports are often difficult to read because they are dense, concise, and contain a lot of jargon. Qualitative research reports are written in a more inviting and conversational style than quantitative ones, which are more impersonal and include information on statistical tests.

- **Statistical tests** are procedures for testing research hypotheses and evaluating the believability of the findings. Findings that are **statistically significant** are ones that have a high probability of being reliable.

- In preparing a written review, it is important to organize materials in a logical, coherent fashion. The preparation of an outline is recommended, and the development of summary charts often helps in integrating diverse studies.

- The written review should not be a succession of quotes or abstracts. The reviewers' role is to point out what has been studied, how adequate and dependable the studies are, what gaps exist in the body of research, and (in the context of a new study), what contribution the study would make.

STUDY ACTIVITIES

Chapter 5 of the *Study Guide to Accompany Nursing Research: Principles and Methods, 7th edition*, offers various exercises and study suggestions for reinforcing the concepts presented in this chapter. In addition, the following study suggestions can be addressed:

1. Read the study by Oermann and her colleagues (2001) entitled, "Teaching by the nurse: How important is it to patients?" *Applied Nursing Research, 14,* 11–17. Write a summary of the problem, methods, findings, and conclusions of the study. Your summary should be capable of serving as notes for a review of the literature.

2. Suppose that you were planning to study counseling practices and programs for rape trauma victims. Make a list of several key words relating to this topic that could be used for identifying previous work.

3. Below are five sentences from literature reviews that require stylistic improvements. Rewrite these sentences to conform to considerations mentioned in the text. (Feel free to give fictitious references.)

   a. Children are less distressed during immunization when their parents are present.

   b. Young adolescents are unprepared to cope with complex issues of sexual morality.

   c. More structured programs to use part-time nurses are needed.

   d. Intensive care nurses need so much emotional support themselves that they can provide insufficient support to patients.

   e. Most nurses have not been adequately educated to understand and cope with the reality of the dying patient.

4. Suppose you were studying factors relating to the discharge of chronic psychiatric patients. Obtain five bibliographic references for this topic. Compare your references and sources with those of other students.

SUGGESTED READINGS

Methodologic References

Allen, M. (1999). Nursing knowledge: Access via bibliographic databases. In L. Q. These (Ed.), *Computers in nursing: Bridges to the future* (pp. 149–170). Philadelphia: Lippincott Williams & Wilkins.

American Psychological Association. (1994). *Publication manual* (4th ed.). Washington, DC: Author.

Cooper, H. M. (1984). *The integrative research review.* Beverly Hills, CA: Sage.

Fink, A. (1998). *Conducting research literature reviews: From paper to the Internet.* Thousand Oaks, CA: Sage.

Fox, R. N., & Ventura, M. R. (1984). Efficiency of automated literature search mechanisms. *Nursing Research, 33,* 174–177.

Galvan, J. L. (1999). *Writing literature reviews.* Los Angeles: Pyrczak.

Ganong, L. H. (1987). Integrative reviews of nursing research. *Research in Nursing & Health, 10,* 1–11.

Glaser, B. G. (1978). *Theoretical sensitivity.* Mill Valley, MA: The Sociology Press.

Light, R. J., & Pillemer, D. B. (1984). *Summing up: The science of reviewing research.* Cambridge, MA: Harvard University Press.

Martin, P. A. (1997) Writing a useful literature review for a quantitative research project. *Applied Nursing Research, 10,* 159–162.

Munhall, P. L. (2001). *Nursing research: A qualitative perspective.* Sudbury, MA: Jones & Bartlett.

Saba, V. K., Oatway, D. M., & Rieder, K. A. (1989). How to use nursing information sources. *Nursing Outlook, 37,* 189–195.

Smith, L. W. (1988). Microcomputer-based bibliographic searching. *Nursing Research, 37,* 125–127.

Spradley, J. (1979). *The ethnographic interview.* New York: Holt, Rinehart, & Winston.

Van Manen, M. (1990). *Researching lived experience.* New York: State University of New York Press.

Studies Cited in Chapter 5

Abercrombie, P. D. (2001). Improving adherence to abnormal Pap smear follow-up. *Journal of Obstetric, Gynecologic, and Neonatal Nursing, 30,* 80–88.

Anderson, D. G., & Imle, M. A. (2001). Families of origin of homeless and never-homeless women. *Western Journal of Nursing Research, 23,* 394–413.

Boydell, K. M., Goering, P., & Morrell-Bellai, T. L. (2000). Narratives of identity: Re-presentation of self in people who are homeless. *Qualitative Health Research, 10*, 26–38.

Hupcey, J. E. (2000). Feeling safe: The psychosocial needs of ICU patients. *Journal of Nursing Scholarship, 32*, 361–367.

McCullagh, M., Lusk, S. L., & Ronis, D. L. (2002). Factors influencing use of hearing protection among farmers. *Nursing Research, 51*, 33–39.

Stein-Parbury, J., & McKinley, S. (2000). Patients' experiences of being in an intensive care unit: A select literature review. *American Journal of Critical Care, 9*, 20–27.

Teel, C. S., Duncan, P., & Lai, S. M. (2001). Caregiving experiences after stroke. *Nursing Research, 50*, 53–60.

Tolle, S. W., Tilden, V. P., Rosenfeld, A. G., & Hickman, S. E. (2000). Family reports of barriers to optimal care of the dying. *Nursing Research, 49*, 310–317.

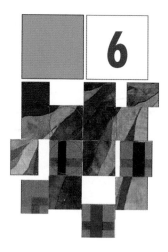

6

Developing a Conceptual Context

Good research usually integrates research findings into an orderly, coherent system. Such integration typically involves linking new research and existing knowledge through a thorough review of prior research on a topic (see Chapter 5) and by identifying or developing an appropriate conceptual framework. Both activities provide an important context for a research project. This chapter discusses theoretical and conceptual contexts for nursing research problems.

THEORIES, MODELS, AND FRAMEWORKS

Many terms have been used in connection with conceptual contexts for research, including theories, models, frameworks, schemes, and maps. There is some overlap in how these terms are used, partly because they are used differently by different writers, and partly because they are interrelated. We offer guidance in distinguishing these terms, but note that our definitions are not universal.

Theories

The term *theory* is used in many ways. For example, nursing instructors and students frequently use the term to refer to the content covered in classrooms, as opposed to the actual practice of performing nursing activities. In both lay and scientific usage, the term theory connotes an *abstraction*.

In research circles, the term theory is used differently by different authors. Classically, scientists have used **theory** to refer to an abstract generalization that offers a systematic explanation about how phenomena are interrelated. The traditional definition requires a theory to embody at least two concepts that are related in a manner that the theory purports to explain.

Others, however, use the term *theory* less restrictively to refer to a broad characterization of a phenomenon. According to this less restrictive definition, a theory can account for (i.e., thoroughly describe) a single phenomenon. Some authors specifically refer to this type of theory as **descriptive theory**. For example, Fawcett (1999) defines descriptive theories as empirically driven theories that "describe or classify specific dimensions or characteristics of individuals, groups, situations, or events by summarizing commonalities found in discrete observations" (p. 15). Descriptive theory plays an especially important role in qualitative studies. Qualitative researchers often strive to develop a conceptualization of the phenomena under study that is grounded in the actual observations made by researchers.

Components of a Traditional Theory
As traditionally defined, scientific theories involve a series of propositions regarding interrelationships

among concepts. The writings on scientific theory include a variety of terms such as *proposition*, *postulate*, *premise*, *axiom*, *law*, *principle*, and so forth, some of which are used interchangeably, and others of which introduce subtleties that are too complex for our discussion. Here, we present a simplified analysis of the components of a theory.

Concepts are the basic building blocks of a theory. Examples of nursing concepts are adaptation, health, anxiety, and nurse–client interaction. Classical theories comprise a set of propositions that indicate a relationship among the concepts. Relationships are denoted by such terms as "is associated with," "varies directly with," or "is contingent on." The propositions form a logically interrelated deductive system. This means that the theory provides a mechanism for logically arriving at new statements from the original propositions.

Let us consider the following example, which illustrates these points. The **Theory of Planned Behavior** (TPB; Ajzen, 1988), which is an extension of an earlier theory called the Theory of Reasoned Action (Ajzen & Fishbein, 1980), provides a framework for understanding people's behavior and its psychological determinants. A greatly simplified construction of the TPB consists of the following propositions:

1. Behavior that is volitional is determined by people's intention to perform that behavior.
2. Intention to perform or not perform a behavior is determined by three factors:

   Attitudes toward the behavior (i.e., the overall evaluation of performing the behavior)
   Subjective norms (i.e., perceived social pressure to perform or not perform the behavior)
   Perceived behavioral control (i.e., anticipated ease or difficulty of engaging in the behavior)

3. The relative importance of the three factors in influencing intention varies across behaviors and situations.

The concepts that form the basis of the TPB include behaviors, intentions, attitudes, subjective norms, and perceived self-control. The theory, which specifies the nature of the relationship among these concepts, provides a framework for generating many hypotheses relating to health behaviors. We might hypothesize on the basis of the TPB, for example, that compliance with a medical regimen could be enhanced by influencing people's attitudes toward compliance, or by increasing their sense of control. The TPB has been used as the underlying theory in studying a wide range of health decision-making behaviors, including contraceptive choice, AIDS prevention behavior, condom use, vaccination behavior, and preventive health screening.

Example of the TPB:
Aminzadeh and Edwards (2000) conducted a study, guided by the TPB, in which they examined factors associated with the use of a cane among community-dwelling older adults. Their results provided further evidence of the utility of the TPB in understanding health behaviors and have implications for the design of theory-based fall prevention interventions.

Types of Traditional Theories

Theories differ in their level of generality. So-called **grand theories** or **macrotheories** purport to describe and explain large segments of the human experience. Some learning theorists, such as Clark Hull, or sociologists, such as Talcott Parsons, developed general theoretical systems to account for broad classes of behavior.

Within nursing, theories are more restricted in scope, focusing on a narrow range of experience. Such **middle-range theories** attempt to explain such phenomena as decision-making, stress, self-care, health promotion, and infant attachment.

Conceptual Models

Conceptual models, **conceptual frameworks**, or **conceptual schemes** (we use the terms interchangeably) represent a less formal attempt at organizing phenomena than theories. Conceptual models, like theories, deal with abstractions (concepts) that are assembled by virtue of their relevance to a common theme. What is absent from conceptual models is the deductive system of propositions that assert and explain a relationship among concepts. Conceptual models provide a perspective regarding interrelated phenomena, but are more loosely structured than theories. A conceptual model broadly presents an understanding of the phenomenon of interest and reflects the assumptions and philosophic views of the model's designer. Conceptual models can serve as springboards for generating research hypotheses.

Much of the conceptual work that has been done in connection with nursing practice falls into the category we call conceptual models. These models represent world views about the nursing process and the nature of nurse—client relationships. A subsequent section of this chapter describes some conceptual models in nursing and illustrates how they have been used in nursing research.

Schematic and Statistical Models

The term *model* is often used in connection with symbolic representations of a conceptualization. There are many references in the research literature to schematic models and mathematic (or statistical) models. These models, like conceptual models, are constructed representations of some aspect of reality; they use concepts as building blocks, with a minimal use of words. A visual or symbolic representation of a theory or conceptual framework often helps to express abstract ideas in a concise and readily understandable form.

Schematic models, which are common in both qualitative and quantitative research, represent phenomena graphically. Concepts and the linkages between them are represented through the use of boxes, arrows, or other symbols. An example of a schematic model (also referred to as a **conceptual map**) is presented in Figure 6-1. This model, known as **Pender's Health Promotion Model**, is "a multivariate paradigm for explaining and predicting the health-promotion component of lifestyle" (Pender, Walker, Sechrist, & Frank-Stromborg, 1990, p. 326). Schematic models of this type can be useful in clarifying associations among concepts.

Statistical models are playing a growing role in quantitative studies. These models use symbols to express quantitatively the nature of relationships among variables. Few relationships in the behavioral sciences can be summarized as elegantly as in the mathematic model $F = ma$ (force = mass $\times$ acceleration). Because human behavior is complex and subject to many influences, researchers typically are able to model it only in a probabilistic manner. This means that we are not able to develop equations, such as the example of force from mechanics, in which a human behavior can be simply described as the product of two other phenomena. What we can do, however, is describe the *probability* that a certain behavior or characteristic will exist, given the occurrence of other phenomena. This is the function of statistical models. An example of a statistical model is shown in the following:

$$Y = \beta_1 X_1 + \beta_2 X_2 + \beta_3 X_3 + \beta_4 X_4 + e$$

where

Y = nursing effectiveness, as measured by a supervisor's evaluation

X_1 = nursing knowledge, as measured by a standardized test of knowledge

X_2 = past achievement, as measured by grades in nursing school

X_3 = decision-making skills, as measured by the Participation in Decision Activities Questionnaire

X_4 = empathy, as measured by the Mehrabian Emotional Empathy Scale

e = a residual, unexplained factor

β_1, β_2, β_3, and β_4 = weights indicating the importance of X_1, X_2, X_3, and X_4, respectively, in determining nursing effectiveness

Each term in this model is quantifiable; that is, every symbol can be replaced by a numeric value, such as an individual's score on a standardized test of knowledge (X_1).

What does this equation mean and how does it work? This model offers a mechanism for understanding and predicting nursing effectiveness. The model proposes that nurses' on-the-job effectiveness

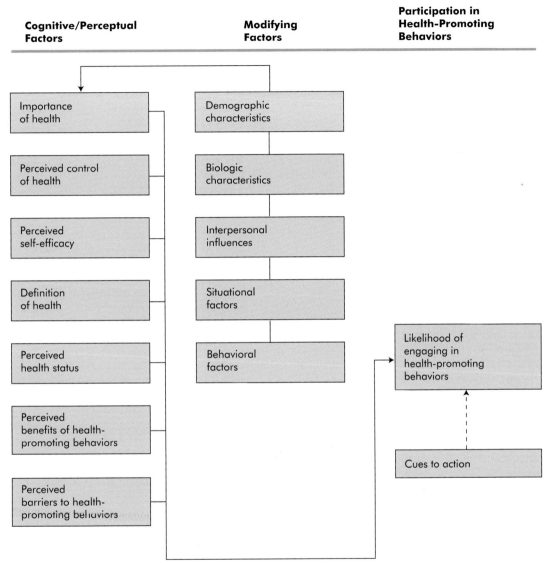

Cognitive/Perceptual Factors

Modifying Factors

Participation in Health-Promoting Behaviors

- Importance of health
- Perceived control of health
- Perceived self-efficacy
- Definition of health
- Perceived health status
- Perceived benefits of health-promoting behaviors
- Perceived barriers to health-promoting behaviors

- Demographic characteristics
- Biologic characteristics
- Interpersonal influences
- Situational factors
- Behavioral factors

- Likelihood of engaging in health-promoting behaviors

- Cues to action

FIGURE 6.1   The Health Promotion Model (From Pender, N. J., Walker, S. N., Sechrist, K. R., & Frank-Stromborg, M. [1990]. Predicting health-promoting lifestyles in the workplace. *Nursing Research, 39*, 331.)

is affected primarily by four factors: the nursing knowledge, past achievement, decision-making skill, and empathy of the nurse. These influences are not presumed to be equally important. The weights (βs) associated with each factor represent a *recipe* for describing the relative importance of each. If empathy were much more important than past achievement, for example, then the weights might be 2 to 1, respectively (i.e., two parts empathy to one part past achievement). The *e* (or **error term**) at the end of the model represents all those unknown or unmeasurable other attributes that affect nurses' performance. This *e* term would be set to a constant value; it would not vary from one nurse to another because it is an unknown element in the equation. Once values for the weights and *e* have been established (through statistical procedures), the model can be used to predict the nursing effectiveness of any nurse for whom we have gathered information on the four Xs (standardized test scores and so forth). Our prediction of who will make an especially effective nurse is probabilistic and thus will not always be perfectly accurate, in part because of the influence of the unknown factors summarized by e. Perfect forecasting is rarely attainable with probabilistic statistical models. However, such a model makes prediction of nursing effectiveness less haphazard than mere guesswork or intuition.

Frameworks

A **framework** is the overall conceptual underpinnings of a study. Not every study is based on a theory or conceptual model, but every study has a framework. In a study based on a theory, the framework is referred to as the **theoretical framework**; in a study that has its roots in a specified conceptual model, the framework is often called the **conceptual framework** (although the terms conceptual framework and theoretical framework are frequently used interchangeably).

In many cases, the framework for a study is not an explicit theory or conceptual model, but rather is implicit—that is, not formally acknowledged or described. The concepts in which researchers are interested are by definition abstractions of observable phenomena, and our world view (and views on nursing) shape how those concepts are defined and operationalized. What often happens, however, is that researchers fail to clarify the conceptual underpinnings of their research variables, thereby making it more difficult to integrate research findings. As noted in Chapter 2, researchers undertaking a study should make clear the conceptual definition of their key variables, thereby providing information about the study's framework.

Waltz, Strickland, and Lenz (1991) describe a five-step process for developing conceptual definitions. These steps include (1) developing a preliminary definition, (2) reviewing relevant literature, (3) developing or identifying exemplary cases, (4)

mapping the meaning of the concept, and (5) stating the developed conceptual definition.

 ### Example of developing a conceptual definition:

Beck (1996) provides an example of developing a conceptual definition of the concept *panic*:

1. *Preliminary definition*: Panic is a sudden, unpredictable rush of overpowering terror that is associated with a marked physiological uproar along with a loss of reasoning capacity and fears of dying and going crazy.
2. *Literature review*: Inter- and intra-disciplinary review of panic is undertaken.
3. *Developing exemplary cases*: Linda is married and the mother of two children, a 3-year-old daughter and 3-month-old son. She is in her late 20s and is a college graduate.... After her first delivery, Linda experienced postpartum panic disorder. With her first child, the panic began 6 weeks postpartum during her daughter's christening. The panic suddenly came out of nowhere. Her heart started racing, her hands got sweaty, and she could not stop crying. For Linda, it was unbearable trying to stay seated in church. She wanted to run outside very badly. Linda shared that the feelings inside her head were so painful she thought she was going crazy and could not focus on anything. As a result of the panic, Linda altered her lifestyle. She spent a tremendous amount of energy trying to appear normal. She went to great lengths to avoid a panic attack. For example, whenever she went to church, she would make sure she sat in the back and at the end of the aisle so she could quickly exit if she felt panic beginning. While experiencing panic, even if only for 5 or 10 minutes, Linda felt minutes were like hours. When panicking, Linda loses herself. She feels like she is not sitting there (pp. 271–272).
4. *Mapping the concept's meaning*: By integrating literature with empirical observations, a conceptual map was developed that organized the various meanings of panic in the literature.
5. *Stating the revised theoretical definition*: Panic is a sudden, unpredictable rush of overpowering terror that has an all-or-nothing quality and is associated with (1) a marked physiological uproar such as palpitations, faintness and sweating; (2) a distortion of time and loss of reasoning capacity, which engenders fearful cognitions of dying, impending doom, losing control, and/or going crazy; and (3) an intense desire to flee the situation and avoid it in the future (Beck, 1996, pp. 271–272).

Quantitative researchers in general are more guilty of failing to identify their frameworks than qualitative researchers. In most qualitative studies, the frameworks are part of the research tradition within which the study is embedded. For example, ethnographers usually begin their work within a theory of culture. Grounded theory researchers incorporate sociologic principles into their framework and their approach to looking at phenomena. The questions that most qualitative researchers ask and the methods they use to address those questions inherently reflect certain theoretical formulations.

THE NATURE OF THEORIES AND CONCEPTUAL MODELS

Theories and conceptual models have much in common, including their origin, general nature, purposes, and role in research. In this section, we examine some general characteristics of theories and conceptual models. We use the term *theory* in its broadest sense, inclusive of conceptual models.

Origin of Theories and Models

Theories and conceptual models are not *discovered*; they are created and invented. Theory building depends not only on the observable facts in our environment but also on the originator's ingenuity in pulling those facts together and making sense of them. Thus, theory construction is a creative and intellectual enterprise that can be engaged in by anyone who is insightful, has a solid knowledge base, and has the ability to knit together observations and evidence into an intelligible pattern.

Tentative Nature of Theories and Models

Theories and conceptual models cannot be proved. A theory is a scientist's best effort to describe and explain phenomena; today's successful theory may be discredited tomorrow. This may happen if new evidence or observations undermine a previously accepted theory. Or, a new theoretical system might integrate new observations with an existing theory to yield a more parsimonious explanation of a phenomenon.

Theories and models that are not congruent with a culture's values and philosophic orientation also may fall into disfavor over time. It is not unusual for a theory to lose supporters because some aspects of it are no longer in vogue. For example, certain psychoanalytic and structural social theories, which had broad support for decades, have come to be challenged as a result of changes in views about women's roles. This link between theory and values may surprise you if you think of science as being completely objective. Remember, though, that theories are deliberately invented by humans; they are not totally free from human values and ideals, which can change over time.

Thus, theories and models are never considered final and verified. There always remains the possibility that a theory will be modified or discarded. Many theories in the physical sciences have received considerable empirical support, and their well-accepted propositions are often referred to as **laws**, such as Boyle's law of gases. Nevertheless, we have no way of knowing the ultimate accuracy and utility of any theory and should, therefore, treat all theories as tentative. This caveat is nowhere more relevant than in emerging sciences such as nursing.

Purposes of Theories and Conceptual Models

Theoretical and conceptual frameworks play several interrelated roles in the progress of a science. Their overall purpose is to make research findings meaningful and generalizable. Theories allow researchers to knit together observations and facts into an orderly scheme. They are efficient mechanisms for drawing together accumulated facts, sometimes from separate and isolated investigations. The linkage of findings into a coherent structure can make the body of accumulated evidence more accessible and, thus, more useful.

In addition to summarizing, theories and models can guide a researcher's understanding of not only the *what* of natural phenomena but also the *why* of their occurrence. Theories often provide a basis for predicting the occurrence of phenomena. Prediction, in turn, has implications for the control of those phenomena. A utilitarian theory has potential to bring about desirable changes in people's behavior or health.

Theories and conceptual models help to stimulate research and the extension of knowledge by providing both direction and impetus. Many nursing studies have been generated explicitly to examine aspects of a conceptual model of nursing. Thus, theories may serve as a springboard for advances in knowledge and the accumulation of evidence for practice.

Relationship Between Theory and Research

The relationship between theory and research is reciprocal and mutually beneficial. Theories and models are built inductively from observations, and an excellent source for those observations is prior research, including in-depth qualitative studies. Concepts and relationships that are validated empirically through research become the foundation for theory development. The theory, in turn, must be tested by subjecting deductions from it (hypotheses) to further systematic inquiry. Thus, research plays a dual and continuing role in theory building and testing. Theory guides and generates ideas for research; research assesses the worth of the theory and provides a foundation for new theories.

It would be unreasonable to assert, however, that research without a formal substantive theory cannot contribute to nursing practice. In nursing research, many facts still need to be accumulated, and purely descriptive inquiries may well form the basis for subsequent theoretical developments. Research that does not test a theory can potentially be linked to one at a later time. Suggestions for linking a study to a conceptual framework are presented later in this chapter.

CONCEPTUAL MODELS USED IN NURSING RESEARCH

Nurse researchers have used both nursing and non-nursing frameworks to provide a conceptual con-text for their studies. This section briefly discusses several frameworks that have been found useful by nurse researchers.

Conceptual Models of Nursing

In the past few decades, several nurses have formulated a number of conceptual models of nursing practice. These models constitute formal explanations of what the nursing discipline is and what the nursing process entails, according to the model developer's point of view. As Fawcett (1995) has noted, four concepts are central to models of nursing: *person*, *environment*, *health*, and *nursing*. The various conceptual models, however, define these concepts differently, link them in diverse ways, and give different emphases to relationships among them. Moreover, different models emphasize different processes as being central to nursing. For example, Sister Calista Roy's Adaptation Model identifies adaptation of patients as a critical phenomenon (Roy & Andrews, 1991). Martha Rogers (1986), by contrast, emphasizes the centrality of the individual as a unified whole, and her model views nursing as a process in which clients are aided in achieving maximum well-being within their potential.

The conceptual models were not developed primarily as a base for nursing research. Indeed, these models have had more impact on nursing education and clinical practice than on nursing research. Nevertheless, nurse researchers have turned to these conceptual frameworks for inspiration in formulating research questions and hypotheses. Table 6-1 (p. 122) lists 10 prominent conceptual models in nursing that have been used by researchers. The table briefly describes the model's key feature and identifies a study that has claimed the model as its framework. Two nursing models that have generated particular enthusiasm among researchers are described in greater detail.

Roy's Adaptation Model
In **Roy's Adaptation Model**, humans are viewed as biopsychosocial adaptive systems who cope with environmental change through the process of

adaptation. Within the human system, there are four subsystems: physiologic needs, self-concept, role function, and interdependence. These subsystems constitute adaptive modes that provide mechanisms for coping with environmental stimuli and change. The goal of nursing, according to this model, is to promote client adaptation; nursing also regulates stimuli affecting adaptation. Nursing interventions usually take the form of increasing, decreasing, modifying, removing, or maintaining internal and external stimuli that affect adaptation.

Example using Roy's model:
Cook, Green, and Topp (2001) explored the incidence and impact of physician verbal abuse on perioperative nurses, using the Roy Adaptation Model as their conceptual framework. The researchers examined how nurses used adaptive coping behaviors and problem-focused skills to deal with the abuse.

Orem's Self-Care Model
Orem's Self-Care Model focuses on each individual's ability to perform self-care, defined as "the practice of activities that individuals initiate and perform on their own behalf in maintaining life, health, and well-being" (1985, p. 35). Ability to care for oneself is referred to as *self-care* agency, and the ability to care for others is referred to as *dependent-care* agency. In Orem's model, the goal of nursing is to help people meet their own therapeutic self-care demands. Orem identified three types of nursing systems: (1) wholly compensatory, wherein the nurse compensates for the patient's total inability to perform self-care activities; (2) partially compensatory, wherein the nurse compensates for the patient's partial inability to perform these activities; and (3) supportive—educative, wherein the nurse assists the patient in making decisions and acquiring skills and knowledge.

Example using Orem's model:
McCaleb and Cull (2000) studied the influence of sociocultural characteristics and economic circumstances on the self-care practices of middle adolescents, using Orem's model as the framework.

Other Models Developed by Nurses

In addition to conceptual models that are designed to describe and characterize the entire nursing process, nurses have developed other models and theories that focus on more specific phenomena of interest to nurses. Two important examples are Pender's Health Promotion Model and Mishel's Uncertainty in Illness Theory.

The Health Promotion Model
Nola Pender's (1996) Health Promotion Model (HPM) focuses on explaining health-promoting behaviors, using a wellness orientation. According to the model (see Figure 6-1), *health promotion* entails activities directed toward developing resources that maintain or enhance a person's well-being. The HPM encompasses two phases: a decision-making phase and an action phase. In the decision-making phase, the model emphasizes seven cognitive/perceptual factors that compose motivational mechanisms for acquiring and maintaining health-promoting behaviors and five modifying factors that indirectly influence patterns of health behavior. In the action phase, barriers and cues to action trigger activity in health-promoting behavior. Nurse researchers have used the HPM in numerous studies of health promoting behaviors.

Example using the HPM:
McCullagh, Lusk, and Ronis (2002) used the Pender HPM to identify factors affecting farmer's use of hearing protection devices. The findings offered further support of the HPM.

Uncertainty in Illness Theory
Mishel's Uncertainty in Illness Theory (Mishel, 1988) focuses on the concept of uncertainty—the inability of a person to determine the meaning of illness-related events. According to this theory, people develop subjective appraisals to assist them in interpreting the experience of illness and treatment. Uncertainty occurs when people are unable to recognize and categorize stimuli. Uncertainty results in the inability to obtain a clear conception of the situation, but a situation appraised as uncertain will

TABLE 6.1 Conceptual Models of Nursing Used by Nurse Researchers

THEORIST AND REFERENCE	NAME OF MODEL/THEORY	KEY THESIS OF THE MODEL	RESEARCH EXAMPLE
Imogene King, 1981	Open Systems Model	Personal systems, interpersonal systems, and social systems are dynamic and interacting, within which transactions occurs.	Doornbos (2000) based her framework on King's model; she tested the prediction that family stressors, coping, and other factors affected family health with young adults with serious mental illness.
Madeline Leininger, 1991	Theory of Culture Care Diversity and Universality	Caring is a universal phenomenon but varies transculturally.	Raines and Morgan (2000) studied the culturally grounded meanings of the concept of comfort, presence, and involvement in the context of the childbirth experience of black women and white women.
Myra Levine, 1973	Conservation Model	Conservation of integrity contributes to maintenance of a person's wholeness.	Deiriggi and Miles (1995) based their study of the effects of waterbeds on heart rate in preterm infants on Levine's concept of conservation.
Betty Neuman, 1989	Health Care Systems Model	Each person is a complete system; the goal of nursing is to assist in maintaining client system stability.	Brauer (2001) described common patterns of person–environment interaction in adults with rheumatoid arthritis, based on Neuman's model.
Margaret Newman, 1994	Health as Expanding Consciousness	Health is viewed as an expansion of consciousness with health and disease parts of the same whole; health is seen in an evolving pattern of the whole in time, space, and movement.	Endo and colleagues (2000) used Newman's theory to study pattern recognition as a caring partnership between nurses and families of ovarian cancer in Japan.
Dorothea Orem, 1985	Self-Care Model	Self-care activities are what people do on their own behalf to maintain health and well-being; the goal of nursing is to help people meet their own therapeutic self-care demands.	Anderson (2001) explored, with a sample of homeless adults, the relationship between self-care, self-care agency, and well-being.

TABLE 6.1 Conceptual Models of Nursing Used by Nurse Researchers (continued)

THEORIST AND REFERENCE	NAME OF MODEL/THEORY	KEY THESIS OF THE MODEL	RESEARCH EXAMPLE
Rosemarie Rizzo Parse, 1992, 1995	Theory of Human Becoming	Health and meaning are co-created by indivisible humans and their environment; nursing involves having clients share views about meanings.	Mitchell and Lawton (2000) studied how diabetic patients' experienced the consequences of personal choices about living with restrictions, and discussed the emerging concepts within Parse's theory.
Martha Rogers, 1970, 1986	Science of Unitary Human Beings	The individual is a unified whole in constant interaction with the environment; nursing helps individuals achieve maximum well-being within their potential.	Using Rogers' framework, Bays (2001) explored the phenomenon of hope and associated factors in older patients who had experienced a stroke.
Sr. Callista Roy, 1984, 1991	Adaptation Model	Humans are adaptive systems that cope with change through adaptation; nursing helps to promote client adaptation during health and illness.	Roy's Adaptation Model provided the framework for John's (2001) study of whether perceptions of quality of life change over time in adults who receive curative radiation therapy.
Jean Watson, 1999	Theory of Caring	Caring is the moral ideal, and entails mind–body–soul engagement with one another.	Using Watson's 10 carative factors, Baldursdottir and Jonsdottir (2002) studied the importance of nurse caring behaviors as perceived by patients receiving care at an emergency department.

mobilize individuals to use their resources to adapt to the situation. Mishel's conceptualization of uncertainty has been used as a framework for both qualitative and quantitative nursing studies.

Example using Uncertainty in Illness Theory: Santacroce (2001) studied uncertainty in 25 mothers during their infants' diagnosis; the infants were HIV seropositive.

Other Models Used by Nurse Researchers

Many phenomena in which nurse researchers are interested involve concepts that are not unique to nursing, and therefore their studies are sometimes linked to conceptual models that are not models from the nursing profession. In addition to the previously described Theory of Planned

Behavior, three non-nursing models or theories have frequently been used in nursing research investigations: the Health Belief Model, Lazarus and Folkman's Theory of Stress and Coping, and Bandura's Social Cognitive Theory.

The Health Belief Model

The **Health Belief Model** (HBM; Becker, 1978) has become a popular conceptual framework in nursing studies focused on patient compliance and preventive health care practices. The model postulates that health-seeking behavior is influenced by a person's perception of a threat posed by a health problem and the value associated with actions aimed at reducing the threat. The major components of the HBM include perceived susceptibility, perceived severity, perceived benefits and costs, motivation, and enabling or modifying factors. Perceived susceptibility is a person's perception that a health problem is personally relevant or that a diagnosis is accurate. Even when one recognizes personal susceptibility, action will not occur unless the individual perceives the severity to be high enough to have serious organic or social implications. Perceived benefits are the patients' beliefs that a given treatment will cure the illness or help prevent it, and perceived costs are the complexity, duration, and accessibility of the treatment. Motivation is the desire to comply with a treatment. Among the modifying factors that have been identified are personality variables, patient satisfaction, and sociodemographic factors.

 Example using the HBM:
Petro-Nustas (2001) used the HBM as the theoretical framework for a study of young Jordanian women's health beliefs toward mammography as a screening procedure for breast cancer.

Lazarus and Folkman's Theory of Stress and Coping

The **Theory of Stress and Coping** (Folkman & Lazarus, 1988; Lazarus, 1966) is an effort to explain people's methods of dealing with stress, that is, environmental and internal demands that tax or exceed a person's resources and endanger his or her well-being. The model posits that coping strategies are learned, deliberate responses used to adapt to or change stressors. According to this model, a person's perception of mental and physical health is related to the ways he or she evaluates and copes with the stresses of living.

Example using the Theory of Stress and Coping:
Maurier and Northcott (2000) used the Lazarus and Folkman theory as the conceptual framework in a study that examined whether job uncertainty, working conditions, cognitive appraisal, and coping strategies affected the health of nurses during the restructuring of health care in Alberta.

Bandura's Social Cognitive Theory

Social Cognitive Theory (Bandura, 1986, 1997) offers an explanation of human behavior using the concepts of self-efficacy, outcome expectations, and incentives. Self-efficacy expectations are focused on people's belief in their own capacity to carry out particular behaviors (e.g., smoking cessation). Self-efficacy expectations, which are context-specific, determine the behaviors a person chooses to perform, their degree of perseverance, and the quality of the performance. Bandura identified four factors that influence a person's cognitive appraisal of self-efficacy: (1) their own mastery experience; (2) verbal persuasion; (3) vicarious experience; and (4) physiologic and affective cues, such as pain and anxiety. The role of self-efficacy has been studied in relation to numerous health behaviors such as weight control, self-management of chronic illness, phobic reactions, and smoking.

Example using Social Cognitive Theory:
Using social cognitive constructs, Resnick (2001) tested a model of factors that influence the exercise behavior of older adults.

Theoretical Contexts and Nursing Research

As previously noted, theory and research have reciprocal, beneficial ties. Fawcett (1978) described the relationship between theory and research as a double helix, with theory as the impetus of scientific investigations, and with findings from research shaping the development of theory. However, this relationship has not always characterized the progress of nursing science. Many have criticized nurse researchers for producing numerous isolated studies that are not placed in a theoretical context.

This criticism was more justified a decade ago than it is today. Many researchers are developing studies on the basis of conceptual models of nursing. Nursing science is still struggling, however, to integrate accumulated knowledge within theoretical systems. This struggle is reflected, in part, in the number of controversies surrounding the issue of theoretical frameworks in nursing.

One of these controversies concerns whether there should be one single, unified model of nursing or multiple, competing models. Fawcett (1989) has argued against combining different models, noting that "before all nurses follow the same path, the competition of multiple models is needed to determine the superiority of one or more of them" (p. 9). Research can play a critical role in testing the utility and validity of alternative nursing models.

Another controversy involves the desirability and utility of developing theories unique to nursing. Some commentators argue that theories relating to humans developed in other disciplines, such as physiology, psychology, and sociology (so-called **borrowed theories**), can and should be applied to nursing problems. Others advocate the development of unique nursing theories, claiming that only through such development can knowledge to guide nursing practice be produced. Fawcett (1995) argues that borrowed theories are sometimes used without considering their adequacy for nursing inquiry. When a borrowed theory is tested and found to be empirically adequate in health-relevant situations of interest to nurses, it becomes **shared theory**.

Until these controversies are resolved, nursing research is likely to continue on its current path of conducting studies within a multidisciplinary and multitheoretical perspective. We are inclined to see the use of multiple frameworks as a healthy and unavoidable part of the development of nursing science.

TESTING, USING, AND DEVELOPING A THEORY OR FRAMEWORK

The manner in which theory and conceptual frameworks are used by qualitative and quantitative researchers is elaborated on in the following section. In the discussion, the term *theory* is used in its broadest sense to include both conceptual models and formal theories.

Theories and Qualitative Research

Theory is almost always present in studies that are embedded in a qualitative research tradition such as ethnography or phenomenology. As previously noted, these research traditions inherently provide an overarching framework that give qualitative studies a theoretical grounding. However, different traditions involve theory in different ways.

Sandelowski (1993) makes a useful distinction between **substantive theory** (conceptualizations of the target phenomena that are being studied) and theory that reflects a conceptualization of human inquiry. Some qualitative researchers insist on an atheoretical stance vis-à-vis the phenomenon of interest, with the goal of suspending *a priori* conceptualizations (substantive theories) that might bias their collection and analysis of data. For example, phenomenologists are in general committed to theoretical naiveté, and explicitly try to hold preconceived views of the phenomenon in check. Nevertheless, phenomenologists are guided in their inquiries by a framework or philosophy that focuses their analysis on certain aspects of a person's lifeworld. That framework is based on the premise that human experience is an inherent property of the experience itself, not constructed by an outside observer.

Ethnographers typically bring a strong cultural perspective to their studies, and this perspective shapes their initial fieldwork. Fetterman (1989) has observed that most ethnographers adopt one of two cultural theories: **ideational theories**, which suggest that cultural conditions and adaptation stem from mental activity and ideas, or **materialistic theories**, which view material conditions (e.g., resources, money, production) as the source of cultural developments.

The theoretical underpinning of grounded theory studies is **symbolic interactionism**, which stresses that behavior is developed through human interactions, through ongoing processes of negotiation and renegotiation. Similar to phenomenologists, however, grounded theory researchers attempt to hold prior substantive theory (existing knowledge and conceptualizations about the phenomenon) in abeyance until their substantive theory begins to emerge. Once the theory starts to take shape, grounded theorists do not ignore the literature; rather, previous literature is used for comparison with the emerging and developing categories of the theory. The goal of grounded theory researchers is to develop a conceptualization of a phenomenon that is *grounded* in actual observations—that is, to explicate an empirically based conceptualization for integrating and making sense of a process or phenomenon. Theory development in a grounded theory study is an inductive process. Grounded theory researchers seek to identify patterns, commonalities, and relationships through the scrutiny of specific instances and events. During the ongoing analysis of data, the researchers move from specific pieces of data to abstract generalizations that synthesize and give structure to the observed phenomenon. The goal is to use the data, grounded in reality, to provide a description or an explanation of events as they occur in reality—not as they have been conceptualized in preexisting theories. Grounded theory methods are designed to facilitate the generation of theory that is *conceptually dense*, that is, with many conceptual patterns and relationships.

 Example of a grounded theory study:
Schreiber, Stern, and Wilson (2000) developed a grounded theory of how black West Indian-Canadian women manage depression and its stigma. These women from a nondominant cultural background used the process they called "being strong" to manage depression. "Being strong" included three subprocesses of "dwelling on it," "diverting myself," and "regaining composure." As illustrated in their graphic model (Figure 6-2), these subprocesses overlap.

In grounded theory studies, theory is produced "from the inside," but theory can also enter a qualitative study "from the outside." That is, some qualitative researchers use existing theory as an interpretive framework. For example, a number of qualitative nurse researchers acknowledge that the philosophic roots of their studies lie in conceptual models of nursing such as those developed by Neuman, Parse, and Rogers. Other qualitative researchers use substantive theories about the target phenomenon as a comparative context for interpreting data *after* the researcher has undertaken a preliminary analysis. Sandelowski (1993) notes that, in this manner, previous substantive theories or conceptualizations are essentially data themselves, and can be taken into consideration, along with study data, as part of an inductively driven new conceptualization.

Example of using existing theory as an interpretive framework:
In Yeh's (2001) qualitative study of the adaptation process of 34 Taiwanese children with cancer, she used Roy's Adaptation Model as a guide for in-depth interviews and also for her data analysis.

An integrative review of qualitative research studies in a specific topic is another strategy that can lead to theory development. In such integrative reviews, qualitative studies are combined to identify their essential elements. These findings from different sources are then used for theory building. Paterson (2001), for example, used the results of 292 qualitative studies that described the experiences of adults with chronic illness to develop the shifting perspectives model of chronic illness. This model depicts living with chronic illness as an ongoing, constantly shifting process in which individuals' perspectives change in the amount to which illness is in the foreground or background in their lives.

Theories in Quantitative Research

Quantitative researchers, like qualitative researchers, link research to theory or models in several ways. The classic approach is to test hypotheses deduced from a previously proposed theory.

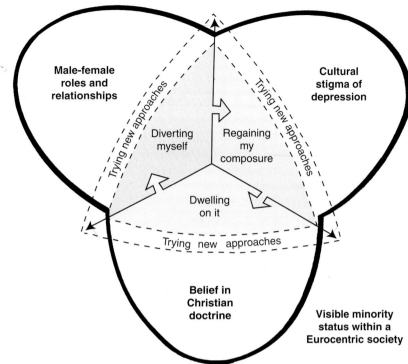

FIGURE 6.2 Being strong: how black West-Indian Canadian women manage depression and its stigma. (Adapted with permission from Schreiber, R., Stern, P. N., & Wilson, C. [2000]. Being strong: How black West-Indian Canadian women manage depression and its stigma. *Journal of Nursing Scholarship, 32*, p. 41.)

Testing a Theory

Theories often stimulate new studies. For example, a nurse might read about Orem's Self-Care Model. As reading progresses, conjectures such as the following might arise: "If Orem's Self-Care Model is valid, then I would expect that nursing effectiveness can be enhanced in environments more conducive to self-care (e.g., a birthing room versus a delivery room)." Such a conjecture, derived from a theory or conceptual framework, can serve as a starting point for testing the theory's adequacy.

In testing a theory, researchers deduce implications (as in the preceding example) and develop research hypotheses, which are predictions about the manner in which variables would be related if the theory were correct. The hypotheses are then subjected to empirical testing through systematic data collection and analysis.

TIP: If you are testing a specific theory or conceptual model, be sure to read about it from a primary source. It is important to understand fully the conceptual perspective of the theorist, and the detailed explication of key constructs.

The focus of the testing process involves a comparison between observed outcomes with those predicted in the hypotheses. Through this process, a theory is continually subjected to potential disconfirmation. If studies repeatedly fail to disconfirm a theory, it gains support and acceptance (e.g., the Theory of Planned Behavior). The testing process continues until pieces of evidence cannot be interpreted within the context of the theory but *can* be explained by a new theory that also accounts for previous findings. Theory-testing studies are most useful when researchers devise logically sound deductions from the theory, design a study that reduces the plausibility of alternative explanations for observed relationships, and use methods that assess the theory's validity under maximally heterogeneous situations so that potentially competing theories can be ruled out.

Researchers sometimes base a new study on a theory in an effort to explain earlier descriptive findings. For example, suppose several researchers had found that nursing home patients demonstrate greater levels of anxiety and noncompliance with nursing staff around bedtime than at other times. These findings shed no light on underlying causes of the problem, and consequently suggest no way to improve it. Several explanations, rooted in models such as Lazarus and Folkman's Stress and Coping Model or Neuman's Health Care Systems Model, may be relevant in explaining nursing home patients' behavior. By directly testing the theory in a new study (i.e., deducing hypotheses derived from the theory), a researcher might learn *why* bedtime is a vulnerable period for the elderly in nursing homes.

 TIP: It may be useful to read research reports of other studies that were based on a theory in which you are interested—even if the research problem is not similar to your own. By reading other studies, you will be better able to judge how much empirical support the theory has received and perhaps how the theory should be adapted.

Tests of a theory sometimes take the form of testing a theory-based intervention. If a theory is correct, it has implications for strategies to influence people's attitudes or behavior, including health-related ones. The impetus for an intervention may be a theory developed within the context of qualitative studies, as in the example of Swanson's theory of caring described later in this chapter. The actual tests of the effectiveness of the intervention—which are also indirect tests of the theory—are usually done in structured quantitative research.

Example of theory testing in an intervention study:
Chang (1999) used Lazarus and Folkman's Theory of Stress and Coping to develop and test an intervention for homebound caregivers of persons with dementia (PWD). According to the theory, the relationship between stress and a person's coping ability is mediated by primary appraisal—the *perception* of an experience as stressful or nonstressful. Chang reasoned that an intervention that affects primary appraisal could positively affect caregiver anxiety and depression. She developed a cognitive-behavioral intervention designed to provide caregivers with knowledge and skills to improve the PWD's eating and dressing abilities, and also to increase caregiver knowledge of coping strategies. In a careful study that compared caregivers who received the intervention with those who did not, Chang found that depression decreased more in the intervention group.

Researchers sometimes combine elements from more than one theory as a basis for generating hypotheses. In doing this, researchers need to be thoroughly knowledgeable about both theories to see if there is an adequate conceptual and empirical basis for conjoining them. If underlying assumptions or conceptual definitions of key concepts are not compatible, the theories should not be combined (although perhaps elements of the two can be used to create a new conceptual framework with its own assumptions and definitions). Two theories that have given rise to combinatory efforts are the HBM and the Theory of Reasoned Action.

Example of testing two combined models: Poss (2001) combined the HBM and the Theory of Reasoned Action to examine the factors associated with the participation by Mexican migrant farm workers in a tuberculosis screening program. Figure 6-3 illustrates how Poss integrated these two models/theories in her study.

Testing Two Competing Theories

Researchers who directly test two competing theories to explain a phenomenon are in a particularly good position to advance knowledge. Almost all phenomena can be explained in alternative ways, as suggested by the alternative conceptual models of nursing. There are also competing theories for such phenomena as stress, child development, and grieving, all of which are important to nursing. Each competing theory suggests alternative approaches to facilitating a positive outcome or minimizing a negative one. In designing effective

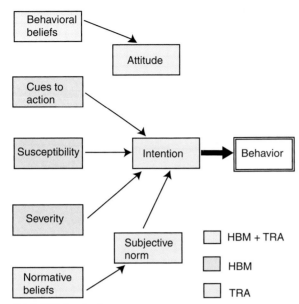

FIGURE 6.3 Combined Health Belief Model and Theory of Reasoned Action. (Adapted with permission from Poss, J. E. [2001]. Developing a new model for cross-cultural research: Synthesizing the Health Belief Model and the Theory of Reasoned Action. *Advances in Nursing Science, 23*, p. 12.)

nursing interventions, it is important to know which explanation has more validity.

Typically, researchers test a single theory (or one combined model) in a study. Then, to evaluate the worth of competing theories, they must compare the results of different studies. Such comparisons are problematic because each study design is unique. For example, one study of stress might use a sample of college students taking an examination, another might use military personnel in a combat situation, and yet another might use terminally ill patients with cancer. Each study might, in addition to having divergent samples, measure stress differently. If the results of these studies support alternative theories of stress to different degrees, it would be difficult to know the extent to which the results reflected differences in study design rather than differences in the validity of the theories.

 TIP: It is often suggested that theories first be evaluated before being used as a basis for

a study—an enterprise that may be difficult for beginning researchers. For advanced students, Chinn and Kramer (1999) and Fawcett (1999) present criteria for assessing conceptual frameworks. Box 6-1 presents a few basic questions that can be asked in a preliminary assessment of a theory or model.

The researcher who directly tests two (or more) competing theories, using a single sample of subjects and comparable measures of the key research variables, is in a position to make powerful and meaningful comparisons. Such a study requires considerable advance planning and the inclusion of a wider array of measures than would otherwise be the case, but such efforts are important. In recent years, several nurse researchers have used this approach to generate and refine our knowledge base and to provide promising new leads for further research.

Example of a test of competing theories: Yarcheski, Mahon, and Yarcheski (1999) tested three alternative theories of anger in early adolescents: one relating anger to stress; another attributing anger to differential emotions; and a third relating anger to personality traits. The findings suggested that all three theories are sound and relevant explanations, but the trait theory provided the most powerful explanation.

Using a Model or Theory as an Organizing Structure

Many researchers who cite a theory or model as their framework are not directly testing the theory. Silva (1986), in her analysis of 62 studies that used 5 nursing models, found that only 9 were direct and explicit tests of the models cited by the researchers. She found that the most common use of nursing models in empirical studies was to provide an organizing structure. In such an approach, a researcher begins with a broad conceptualization of nursing (or stress, health beliefs, and so on) that is consistent with that of the model developers. These researchers *assume* that the models they espouse are valid, and then use the model's constructs or proposed schemas to provide a broad organizational

BOX 6.1 Some Questions for a Preliminary Assessment of a Model or Theory

ISSUE	QUESTIONS
Theoretical clarity	• Are key concepts defined and are the definitions sufficiently clear? • Do all concepts "fit" within the theory? Are concepts used in the theory in a manner compatible with conceptual definitions? • Are basic assumptions consistent with one another? • Are schematic models helpful, and are they compatible with the text? Are schematic models needed but not presented? • Can the theory be followed—is it adequately explained? Are there ambiguities?
Theoretical complexity	• Is the theory sufficiently rich and detailed to explain phenomena of interest? • Is the theory overly complex? • Can the theory be used to explain or predict, or only to describe phenomena?
Theoretical grounding	• Are the concepts identifiable in reality? • Is there an empirical basis for the theory? • Is the empirical basis solid? • Can the theoretical concepts be adequately operationalized?
Appropriateness of the theory	• Does the theory suggest possibilities for influencing nursing practice? • Are the tenets of the theory compatible with nursing's philosophy? • Are key concepts within the domain of nursing?
Importance of the theory	• Will research based on this theory answer critical questions? • How will testing the theory contribute to nursing's evidence base?
General issues	• Are there theories or models that do a better job of explaining phenomenon of interest? • Is the theory compatible with your world view?

or interpretive context. Some use (or develop) data collection instruments that are allied with the model. Silva noted that using models in this fashion can serve a valuable organizing purpose, but such studies offer little evidence about the validity of the theory itself.

 Example of using a model as organizing structure:

Resnick and Jenkins (2000) used Bandura's social cognitive theory as an organizing structure to revise an unpublished instrument to measure self-efficacy barriers to exercise. Focusing on Bandura's construct of self-efficacy, Resnick and Jenkins developed the Self-Efficacy for Exercise Scale. They assessed their new measure with 187 older adults living in a continuing care retirement community.

To our knowledge, Silva's study has not been replicated with a more recent sample of studies. However, we suspect that, even today, most quantitative studies that offer models and theories as their conceptual frameworks are using them primarily as organizational or interpretive tools. Silva (1986) offered seven evaluation criteria for determining whether a study was actually testing a theory, rather than simply identifying an organizational context. Box 6-2, broadly adapted from Silva's criteria, presents a set of evaluative questions to determine if a study was actually testing a theory.

 Example of a study meeting seven theory-testing criteria:

Woods and Isenberg (2001) tested one aspect of a middle-range theory based on the Roy Adaptation

BOX 6.2 Criteria to Determine if a Theory/Model is Being Tested

1. Is the purpose of the study to determine the validity of a theory's assumptions or propositions?
2. Does the report explicitly note that the theory is the framework for the research?
3. Is the theory discussed in sufficient detail that the relationship between the theory on the one hand and the study hypotheses or research questions on the other is clear?
4. Are study hypotheses directly deduced from the theory?
5. Are study hypotheses empirically tested in an appropriate manner, so as to shed light on the validity of the theory?
6. Is the validity of the theory's assumptions or propositions supported (or challenged) based on evidence from the empirical tests?
7. Does the report discuss how evidence from empirical tests supports or refutes the theory, or how the theory explains relevant aspects of the findings?

Adapted from Silva M. C. (1986). Research testing nursing theory: State of the art. *Advances in Nursing Science, 9*, 1–11.

Model. Their purpose was to test the efficacy of adaptation as a mediator of intimate abuse and traumatic stress in battered women. They tested the following two relational statements: "(1) physical abuse, emotional abuse, and risk of homicide are focal stimuli that elicit the response of post traumatic stress disorder (PTSD) in battered women and (2) adaptation in the physiologic, self-concept, role, and interdependence modes acts as a mediator between the focal stimuli of intimate physical abuse, emotional abuse, and risk of homicide and the response of PTSD in women" (p. 215). As a result of empirical testing, Woods and Isenberg reported that adaptation in three of the four modes partially mediated the relationship between intimate abuse, the focal stimuli, and the response of PTSD.

Fitting a Problem to a Theory

The preceding sections addressed the situation in which a researcher *begins* with a specific theory or model and uses it either as the basis for developing hypotheses or for an organizational or interpretive purpose. Circumstances sometimes arise in which the problem is formulated before any consideration is given to a conceptual framework. Even in such situations, researchers sometimes try to devise a theoretical context. Although in some situations such an approach may be appropriate, we nevertheless caution that an after-the-fact linkage of theory to a problem may add little to the study's worth and, of course, no evidence of the theory's validity. (An exception is when the researcher is struggling to make sense of findings, and calls on an existing theory to help explain or interpret them.)

If it is necessary to find a relevant theory after selecting a problem, the search for such a theory must begin by first conceptualizing the problem on an abstract level. For example, take the research question: "Do daily telephone conversations between a psychiatric nurse and a patient for 2 weeks after discharge from the hospital result in lower rates of readmission by short-term psychiatric patients?" This is a relatively concrete research problem, but it might profitably be viewed within the context of Orem's Self-Care Model, a theory of reinforcement, a theory of social influence, or a theory of crisis resolution. Part of the difficulty in finding a theory is that a single phenomenon of interest can be conceptualized in a number of ways and, depending on the manner chosen, may refer the researcher to conceptual schemes from a wide range of disciplines.

TIP: If you begin with a research problem and are trying to identify a suitable framework, it is probably wise to confer with others—especially with people who may be familiar with a broad range of theoretical perspectives. By having an open discussion, you are more likely to become aware of your own conceptual perspectives and are thus in a better position to identify an appropriate framework.

Textbooks, handbooks, and encyclopedias in the chosen discipline usually are a good starting point for the identification of a framework. These sources usually summarize the status of a theoretical position and document the efforts to confirm and disconfirm it. Journal articles contain more current information but are usually restricted to descriptions of specific studies rather than to broad expositions or evaluations of theories. Perhaps our brief overview of frameworks that have been useful to nurses can serve as a starting point for identifying a suitable model or theory.

Fitting a problem to a theory after-the-fact should be done with circumspection. It is true that having a theoretical context can enhance the meaningfulness of a study, but artificially "cramming" a problem into a theory is not the route to scientific utility, nor to enhancing nursing's evidence base. There are many published studies that purport to have a conceptual framework when, in fact, the tenuous *post hoc* linkage is all too evident. In Silva's (1986) previously mentioned analysis of 62 studies that claimed a nursing model as their underpinnings, approximately one third essentially paid only lip service to a model. If a conceptual framework is really linked to a research problem, then the design of the study, the selection of data collection methods, the data analysis, and (especially) the interpretation of the findings *flow* from that conceptualization. We advocate a balanced and reasoned perspective on this issue: *Researchers should not shirk their intellectual duties by ignoring attempts to link their problem to broader theoretical concerns, but there is no point in fabricating such a link when it does not exist.*

TIP: If you begin with a research question and then subsequently identify a theory or

model, be willing to adapt or augment your original research problem as you gain greater understanding of the theory. The linking of theory and research question may involve an iterative approach.

Developing a Framework in a Quantitative Study

Novice researchers may think of themselves as unqualified to develop a conceptual scheme of their own. But theory development depends much less on research experience than on powers of observation, grasp of a problem, and knowledge of prior research. There is nothing to prevent an imaginative and sensitive person from formulating an original conceptual framework for a study. The conceptual scheme may not be a full-fledged formal theory, but it should place the issues of the study into some broader perspective.

The basic intellectual process underlying theory development is induction—that is, the process of reasoning from particular observations and facts to generalizations. The inductive process involves integrating what one has experienced or learned into some conclusion. The observations used in the inductive process need not be personal observations; they may be (and often are) the findings and conclusions from other studies. When relationships among variables are arrived at this way, one has the makings of a theory that can be put to a more rigorous test. The first step in theory development, then, is to formulate a generalized scheme of relevant concepts, that is, to perform a conceptual analysis.

Let us consider the following simple example. Suppose that we were interested in understanding the factors influencing enrollment in a prenatal education program. We might begin by considering two basic sets of forces: those that promote enrollment and those that hinder it. After reviewing the literature, discussing the problem with colleagues, and developing ideas from our own experiences, we might arrive at a conceptual scheme such as the one presented in Figure 6-4. This framework is crude, but it does allow us to study a number of research questions *and* to place those problems in perspective. For example, the conceptual scheme suggests that as the availability of social supports declines, obstacles to participation in a prenatal

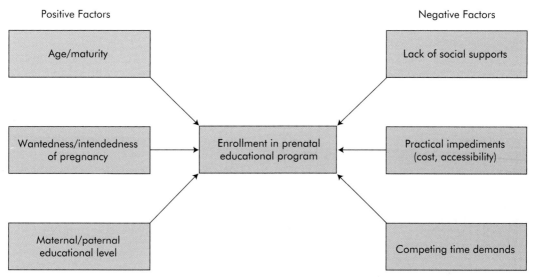

FIGURE 6.4 Conceptual model—factors that influence enrollment in a prenatal education program.

education program increase. We might then make the following hypothesis: "Single pregnant women are less likely to participate in a prenatal education program than married pregnant women," on the assumption that husbands are an important source of social support to women in their pregnancy. (Of course, this example is contrived; in reality, several existing theories such as the HBM or TPB could be used to study enrollment in prenatal care education.) Many nursing studies involve conceptual frameworks developed by the researchers.

Example of model development: Stuifbergen, Seraphine, and Roberts (2000) conducted a study based on their own conceptual model of quality of life in persons with chronic disabling conditions. The model represented "a synthesis of findings from extant literature and a series of preliminary qualitative and quantitative investigations" (p. 123).

RESEARCH EXAMPLES

Throughout this chapter, we have described studies that involved various widely used conceptual and theoretical models. This section presents two examples of the linkages between theory and research from the nursing research literature—one from a quantitative study and the other from a qualitative study.

Research Example From a Quantitative Study: Testing Orem's Self-Care Model

Renker (1999) used Orem's Self-Care Model of nursing to study the relationships between self-care, social support, physical abuse, and pregnancy outcomes of older adolescent mothers and their infants. The study's research variables included measures of the major constructs in Orem's model, including basic conditioning factors, self-care agency, and self-care. Orem's basic conditioning factors (factors that affect people's ability to engage in self-care) include (1) social-environmental factors and (2) resource availability and adequacy factors. In Renker's study, physical abuse represented the key social environmental factor, and social support represented the resource availability and adequacy factor. Denyes' Self-Care Agency Instrument was used to measure pregnancy self-care agency, and Denyes' Self-Care Practice Instrument measured pregnancy self-care.

Based on Orem's model, Renker hypothesized that the absence of physical abuse and the presence of social support increased self-care agency. Increased levels of self-care agency were expected to enhance self-care practices, which in turn were expected to result in increased infant birth weight and decreased pregnancy complications. Renker tested her hypotheses in a sample of 139 pregnant teenagers.

The results lent support to Orem's model. Abused pregnant teenagers gave birth to infants with significantly lower birth weights than the teenagers who were not abused. Social support, self-care agency, and self-care practice were all significantly related to infant birth weight.

A particular strength of this study is that Orem's Self-Care Deficit Model was interwoven throughout its design. Renker developed hypotheses based on the model and included all major constructs of Orem's model as research variables. Moreover, several data collection instruments were specifically developed to assess components of Orem's theory.

Research Example From a Qualitative Study: Development of a Theory of Caring

As noted earlier in this chapter, many qualitative studies have theory development as an explicit goal. Here we describe the efforts of a qualitative researcher who developed an empirically derived theory of caring, and has used the theory in the development of a caring-based counseling intervention (Swanson, 1999). Although the qualitative studies were done over a decade ago, they are an excellent illustration of theory development.

Using data from three separate qualitative investigations, Swanson (1991) inductively derived and then refined a theory of the caring process. Swanson studied caring in three separate perinatal contexts: as experienced by women who miscarried, as provided by parents and professionals in the newborn intensive care unit, and as recalled by at-risk mothers who had received a long-term public health nursing intervention. Data were gathered through in-depth interviews with study participants and also through observations of care provision. Data from the first study led to the identification and preliminary definition of five caring processes. The outcome of the second study was confirmation of the five processes and refinement of their definitions. In the third study, Swanson confirmed the five processes, redefined one of them, developed subdimensions of each process, and derived a definition of the overall concept of caring: *"Caring is a nurtur-*

ing way of relating to a valued other toward whom one feels a personal sense of commitment and responsibility" (p. 165).

According to Swanson's theory, the five caring processes are as follows:

- *Knowing*—striving to understand an event as it has meaning in the life of the other
- *Being With*—being emotionally present to the other
- *Doing For*—doing for the other as he or she would do for the self if it were at all possible
- *Enabling*—facilitating the other's passage through life transitions and unfamiliar events
- *Maintaining Belief*—sustaining faith in the other's capacity to get through an event or transition and face a future with meaning

In presenting her theory, Swanson described the five processes, supporting each with rich excerpts from her in-depth interviews. Here is an example of the excerpt illustrating the process of knowing:

> When things weren't right, I could say that things were fine and it was only a matter of time. I mean the nurse would ask certain questions and there would be no way that I could be consistent without telling the truth. And then we would talk, and pretty soon instead of saying it was fine, I would start out with what was really wrong. (p. 163)

Swanson's theory of caring, in addition to being used in the development and testing of a caring-based nurse counseling program for women who miscarry (Swanson, 1999), has been used by other researchers, including a qualitative study of the interactions of AIDS family caregivers and professional health care providers (Powell-Cope, 1994) and a study of the involvement of relatives in the care of the dying (Andershed & Ternestedt, 1999).

SUMMARY POINTS

- A **theory** is a broad abstract characterization of phenomena. As classically defined, a theory is an abstract generalization that systematically explains relationships among phenomena. **Descriptive theory** thoroughly describes a phenomenon.
- In a research context, the overall objective of theory is to make findings meaningful, to summarize existing knowledge into coherent systems,

to stimulate new research, and to explain phenomena and relationships among them.

- The basic components of a theory are concepts; classically defined theories consist of a set of propositions about the interrelationships among concepts, arranged in a logically interrelated system that permits new statements to be derived from them.
- **Grand theories** (or **macrotheories**) attempt to describe large segments of the human experience. **Middle-range theories** are more specific to certain phenomena.
- Concepts are also the basic elements of **conceptual models**, but concepts are not linked in a logically ordered, deductive system. Conceptual models, like theories, provide context for nursing studies.
- **Schematic models** (sometimes referred to as **conceptual maps**) are representations of phenomena using symbols or diagrams. **Statistical models** use mathematic symbols to express quantitatively the nature and strength of relationships among variables.
- A **framework** is the conceptual underpinning of a study. In many studies, the framework is implicit, but ideally researchers clarify the **conceptual definitions** of key concepts. In qualitative studies, the framework usually springs from distinct research traditions.
- Several conceptual models of nursing have been developed and have been used in nursing research. The concepts central to models of nursing are person, environment, health, and nursing.
- Two major conceptual models of nursing used by nurse researchers are Orem's Self-Care Model and Roy's Adaptation Model.
- Non-nursing models used by nurse researchers (e.g., Lazarus and Folkman's Theory of Stress and Coping) are referred to as **borrowed theories**; when the appropriateness of borrowed theories for nursing inquiry is confirmed, the theories become **shared theories**.
- In some qualitative research traditions (e.g., phenomenology), the researcher strives to suspend previously held substantive conceptualizations of the phenomena under study, but nevertheless there is a rich theoretical underpinning associated with the tradition itself.
- Some qualitative researchers specifically seek to develop **grounded theories,** data-driven explanations to account for phenomena under study through inductive processes.
- In the classical use of theory, researchers test hypotheses deduced from an existing theory. A particularly fruitful approach is the testing of two competing theories in one study.
- In both qualitative and quantitative studies, researchers sometimes use a theory or model as an organizing framework, or as an interpretive tool.
- Researchers sometimes develop a problem, design a study, and *then* look for a conceptual framework; such an after-the-fact selection of a framework is less compelling than the systematic testing of a particular theory.

STUDY ACTIVITIES

Chapter 6 of the *Study Guide to Accompany Nursing Research: Principles and Methods*, 7th edition, offers various exercises and study suggestions for reinforcing concepts presented in this chapter. In addition, the following study questions can be addressed:

1. Read the following article: Liken, M. A. (2001). Caregivers in crisis. *Clinical Nursing Research*, *10*, 52–68. What theoretical basis does the author use in this study? Would you classify the theoretical basis as a theory or as a conceptual framework? Did Liken use the framework to test hypotheses formally, or was the framework used as an organizational structure?

2. Select one of the nursing conceptual frameworks or models described in this chapter. Formulate a research question and two hypotheses that could be used empirically to test the utility of the conceptual framework or model in nursing practice.

3. Four researchable problems follow. Abstract a generalized issue or issues for each of these

problems. Search for an existing theory that might be applicable and appropriate.

   a. What is the relationship between angina pain and alcohol intake?

   b. What effect does rapid weight gain during the second trimester have on the outcome of pregnancy?

   c. Do multiple hospital readmissions affect the achievement level of children?

   d. To what extent do coping mechanisms of individuals differ in health and illness?

4. Read the following article: Kelly-Powell, M. L. (1997). Personalizing choices: Patients' experiences with making treatment decisions. *Research in Nursing & Health, 20*, 219–227. What evidence does the researcher offer to substantiate that her grounded theory is a good fit with her data?

SUGGESTED READINGS

Theoretical References

Andrews, H. A., & Roy, C. (1986). *Essentials of the Roy Adaptation Model*. Norwalk, CT: Appleton-Century-Crofts.

Ajzen, I. (1988). *Attitudes, personality, and behavior*. Milton Keynes, United Kingdom: Open University Press.

Ajzen, I., & Fishbein, M. (1980). *Understanding attitudes and predicting social behavior*. Englewood Cliffs, NJ: Prentice-Hall.

Bandura, A. (1986). *Social foundations of thought and action: A social cognitive theory*. Englewood Cliffs, NJ: Prentice-Hall.

Bandura, A. (1997). *Self-efficacy: The exercise of control*. New York: W. H. Freeman.

Becker, M. (1978). The Health Belief Model and sick role behavior. *Nursing Digest, 6*, 35–40.

Chinn, P. L., & Kramer, M. K. (1999). *Theory and nursing: Integrated knowledge development* (5th ed.). St. Louis: C. V. Mosby.

Craig, S. L. (1980). Theory development and its relevance for nursing. *Journal of Advanced Nursing, 5*, 349–355.

Fawcett, J. (1978). The relationship between theory and research: A double helix. *Advances in Nursing Science, 1*, 49–62.

Fawcett, J. (1989). *Analysis and evaluation of conceptual models of nursing* (2nd ed.). Philadelphia: F. A. Davis.

Fawcett, J. (1995). *Analysis and evaluation of conceptual models of nursing* (3rd ed.). Philadelphia: F. A. Davis.

Fawcett, J. (1999). *The relationship between theory and research* (3rd ed.). Philadelphia: F. A. Davis.

Fetterman, D. M. (1989). *Ethnography: Step by step*. Newbury Park, CA: Sage.

Flaskerud, J. H. (1984). Nursing models as conceptual frameworks for research. *Western Journal of Nursing Research, 6*, 153–155.

Flaskerud, J. H., & Halloran, E. J. (1980). Areas of agreement in nursing theory development. *Advances in Nursing Science, 3*, 1–7.

Folkman, S., & Lazarus, R. S. (1988). Coping as a mediator of emotion. *Journal of Personality and Social Psychology, 54*, 466–475.

Hardy, M. E. (1974). Theories: Components, development, evaluation. *Nursing Research, 23*, 100–107.

King, I. M. (1981). *A theory for nursing: Systems, concepts, and process*. New York: John Wiley and Sons.

Lazarus, R. (1966). *Psychological stress and the coping response*. New York: McGraw-Hill.

Leininger, M. (1991). *Culture care diversity and universality: A theory of nursing*. New York: National League for Nursing.

Levine, M. E. (1973). *Introduction to clinical nursing* (2nd ed.). Philadelphia: F. A. Davis.

Marriner-Tomey, A. (Ed.). (1998). *Nursing theorists and their work* (4th ed.). St. Louis: C. V. Mosby.

Mehrabian, A., & Epstein, N. (1972). A measure of emotional empathy. *Journal of Personality, 40*, 525–543.

Meleis, A. I. (1997). *Theoretical nursing: Development and progress* (3rd ed.). Philadelphia: Lippincott-Raven.[Q2]

Mishel, M. H. (1988), Uncertainty in illness. *Image: Journal of Nursing Scholarship, 20*, 225–232.

Neuman, B. (1989). *The Neuman Systems Model* (2nd ed.). Norwalk, CT: Appleton & Lange.

Newman, M. (1994). *Health as expanding consciousness*. New York: NLN.

Nicoll, L. H. (1996). *Perspectives on nursing theory*. Philadelphia: J. B. Lippincott.

Orem, D. E. (1985). *Concepts of practice* (3rd ed.). New York: McGraw-Hill.

Parse, R. R. (1992). Human becoming: Parse's theory. *Nursing Science Quarterly, 5*, 35–42.

Parse, R. R. (1995). *Illuminations: The Human Becoming Theory in practice and research*. New York: NLN Pub. #15-2670.

Pender, N. (1996). *Health promotion in nursing practice* (3rd ed.). Englewood Cliffs, NJ: Prentice-Hall.

Rogers, M. E. (1970). *An introduction to the theoretical basis of nursing.* Philadelphia: F. A. Davis.

Rogers, M. E. (1986). Science of unitary human beings. In V. Malinski (Ed.), *Explorations on Martha Rogers' science of unitary human beings.* Norwalk, CT: Appleton-Century-Crofts.

Roy, C. (1984). *Introduction to nursing: An adaptation model* (2nd ed.). Englewood Cliffs, NJ: Prentice-Hall.

Roy, C. Sr., & Andrews, H. (1991). *The Roy Adaptation Model: The definitive statement.* Norwalk, CT: Appleton & Lange.

Sandelowski, M. (1993). Theory unmasked: The uses and guises of theory in qualitative research. *Research in Nursing & Health, 16,* 213–218.

Silva, M. C. (1986). Research testing nursing theory: State of the art. *Advances in Nursing Science, 9,* 1–11.

Silva, M. C., & Sorrell, J. M. (1992). Testing of nursing theory: Critique and philosophical expansion. *Advances in Nursing Science, 14,* 12–23.

Stevens, B. J. (1994). *Nursing theory: Analysis, application, evaluation* (4th ed.). Philadelphia: J. B. Lippincott.

Waltz, C., Strickland, O., & Lenz, E. (1991). *Measurement in nursing research.* Philadelphia: F. A. Davis.

Watson, J. (1999). *Postmodern nursing and beyond.* New York: Churchill Livingston.

Studies Cited in Chapter 6

Aminzadeh, F., & Edwards, N. (2000). Factors associated with cane use among community-dwelling older adults. *Public Health Nursing, 17,* 474–483.

Andershed, B., & Ternestedt, B. (1999). Involvement of relatives in care of the dying in different care cultures. *Nursing Science Quarterly, 12,* 45–51.

Anderson, J. A. (2001). Understanding homeless adults by testing the theory of self-care. *Nursing Science Quarterly, 14,* 59–67.

Baldursdottir, G., & Jonsdottir, H. (2002). The importance of nurse caring behaviors as perceived by patients receiving care at an emergency department. *Heart & Lung, 31,* 67–75.

Bays, C. L. (2001). Older adults' descriptions of hope after stroke. *Rehabilitation Nursing, 26,* 18–20.

Beck, C. T. (1996). A concept analysis of panic, *Archives of Psychiatric Nursing, 10,* 265–275.

Brauer, D. J. (2001). Common patterns of person-environment interaction in persons with rheumatoid arthritis. *Western Journal of Nursing Research, 23,* 414–430.

Chang, B. L. (1999). Cognitive-behavioral intervention for homebound caregivers of persons with dementia. *Nursing Research, 48,* 173–182.

Cook, J. K., Green, M., & Topp, R. V. (2001). Exploring the impact of physician abuse on perioperative nurses. *AORN Journal, 74,* 317–327.

Deiriggi, P. M., & Miles, K. E. (1995). The effects of waterbeds on heart rate in preterm infants. *Scholarly Inquiry for Nursing Practice, 9,* 245–262.

Doornbos, M. M. (2000). King's systems framework and family health: The derivation and testing of a theory. *Journal of Theory Construction and Testing, 4,* 20–26.

Endo, E., Nitta., N., Inayoshi, M., Saito, R., Takemura, K., Minegishi, H., Kubo, S., & Kondo, M. (2000). Pattern recognition as a caring partnership in families with cancer. *Journal of Advanced Nursing, 32,* 603–610.

John, L. D. (2001). Quality of life in patients receiving radiation therapy for non-small cell lung cancer. *Oncology Nursing Forum, 28,* 807–813.

Maurier, W. L., & Northcott, H. C. (2000). Job uncertainty and health status for nurses during restructuring of health care in Alberta. *Western Journal of Nursing Research, 22,* 623–641.

McCaleb, A., & Cull, V. V. (2000). Sociocultural influences and self-care practices of middle adolescents. *Journal of Pediatric Nursing, 15,* 30–35.

McCullagh, M., Lusk, S. L., & Ronis, D. L. (2002). Factors influencing use of hearing protection among farmers. *Nursing Research, 51,* 33–39.

Mitchell, G. J., & Lawton, C. (2000). Living with the consequences of personal choices for persons with diabetes. *Canadian Journal of Diabetes Care, 24,* 23–30.

Paterson, B. L. (2001). The shifting perspectives model of chronic illness. *Journal of Nursing Scholarship, 33,* 21–26.

Pender, N. J., Walker, S. N., Sechrist, K. R., & Frank-Stromborg, M. (1990). Predicting health-promoting lifestyles in the workplace. *Nursing Research, 39,* 326–332.

Petro-Nustas, W. (2001). Young Jordanian women's health beliefs about mammography. *Journal of Community Health Nursing, 18,* 177–194.

Poss, J. E. (2001). Developing a new model for cross-cultural research: Synthesizing the Health Belief

Model and the Theory of Reasoned Action. *Advances in Nursing Science, 23,* 1–15.

Powell-Cope, G. M. (1994). Family caregivers of people with AIDS: Negotiating partnerships with professional health care providers. *Nursing Research, 43,* 324–330.

Raines, D. A., & Morgan, Z. (2000). Culturally sensitive care during childbirth. *Applied Nursing Research, 13,* 167–172.

Renker, P. R. (1999). Physical abuse, social support, self-care, and pregnancy outcomes of older adolescents. *Journal of Obstetric, Gynecologic, and Neonatal Nursing, 28,* 377–388.

Resnick, B. (2001). Testing a model of exercise behavior in older adults. *Research in Nursing & Health, 24,* 83–92.

Resnick, B., & Jenkins, L. S. (2000). Testing the reliability and validity of the Self-Efficacy for Exercise Scale. *Nursing Research, 49,* 154–159.

Santacroce, S. J. (2001). Measuring parental uncertainty during the diagnosis phase of serious illness in a child. *Journal of Pediatric Nursing, 16,* 3–12.

Schreiber, R., Stern, P. N., & Wilson, C. (2000). Being strong: How black West-Indian Canadian women manage depression and its stigma. *Journal of Nursing Scholarship, 32,* 39–45.

Stuifbergen, A. K., Seraphine, A., & Roberts, G. (2000). An explanatory model of health promotion and quality of life in chronic disabling conditions. *Nursing Research, 49,* 122–129.

Swanson, K. M. (1991). Empirical development of a middle range theory of caring. *Nursing Research, 40,* 161–166.

Swanson, K. M. (1999). Effects of caring, measurement, and time on miscarriage impact and women's well-being. *Nursing Research, 48,* 288–298.

Woods, S. J., & Isenberg, M. A. (2001). Adaptation as a mediator of intimate abuse and traumatic stress in battered women. *Nursing Science Quarterly, 14,* 215–221.

Yarcheski, A., Mahon, N. E., & Yarcheski, T. J. (1999). An empirical test of alternate theories of anger in early adolescents. *Nursing Research, 48,* 317–323.

Yeh, C. H. (2001). Adaptation in children with cancer: Research with Roy's model. *Nursing Science Quarterly, 14,* 141–148.

PART

3

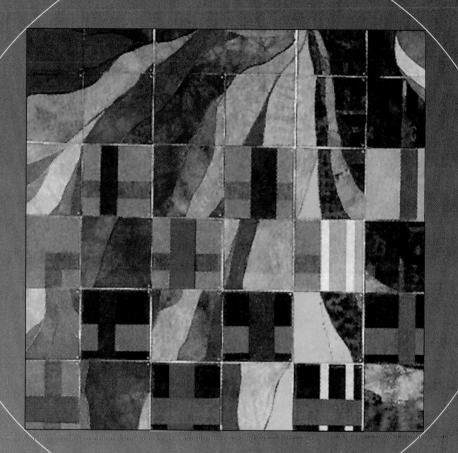

Designs for Nursing Research

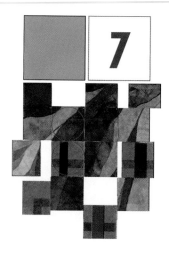

7

Designing Ethical Research

This part of the textbook presents materials relating to the planning and design stage of empirical research. Ethical concerns permeate every aspect of the design of a study and the execution of the design. Therefore, before discussing techniques of research design, we present in this chapter major ethical principles that must be considered in developing research plans.

The proliferation of research has led to growing concerns about the protection of the rights of study participants. Ethical concerns are especially prominent in the field of nursing because the line of demarcation between what constitutes the expected practice of nursing and the collection of research information has become less distinct as research by nurses increases. Furthermore, ethics can create particular challenges to nurse researchers because ethical requirements sometimes conflict with the need to produce evidence of the highest possible quality for practice.

THE NEED FOR ETHICAL GUIDELINES

When humans are used as study participants—as they usually are in nursing research—care must be exercised in ensuring that the rights of those humans are protected. The requirement for ethical conduct may strike you as so self-evident as to

require no further comment, but the fact is that ethical considerations have not always been given adequate attention. In this section, we consider some of the reasons that ethical guidelines became imperative.

Historical Background

As modern, civilized people, we might like to think that systematic violations of moral principles within a research context occurred centuries ago rather than in recent times, but this is not the case. The Nazi medical experiments of the 1930s and 1940s are the most famous example of recent disregard for ethical conduct. The Nazi program of research involved the use of prisoners of war and racial "enemies" in numerous experiments designed to test the limits of human endurance and human reaction to diseases and untested drugs. The studies were unethical not only because they exposed these people to permanent physical harm and even death but because subjects could not refuse participation.

Some recent examples of ethical transgressions have also occurred in the United States. For instance, between 1932 and 1972, a study known as the Tuskegee Syphilis Study, sponsored by the U.S. Public Health Service, investigated the effects of syphilis among 400 men from a poor

African-American community. Medical treatment was deliberately withheld to study the course of the untreated disease. Another well-known case of unethical research involved the injection of live cancer cells into elderly patients at the Jewish Chronic Disease Hospital in Brooklyn, without the consent of those patients. Even more recently, it was revealed in 1993 that U.S. federal agencies had sponsored radiation experiments since the 1940s on hundreds of people, many of them prisoners or elderly hospital patients. Many other examples of studies with ethical transgressions—often much more subtle than these examples—have emerged to give ethical concerns the high visibility they have today.

Ethical Dilemmas in Conducting Research

Research that violates ethical principles is rarely done specifically to be cruel or immoral, but more typically occurs out of a conviction that knowledge is important and potentially life-saving or beneficial to others in the long run. There are research problems in which participants' rights and study demands are put in direct conflict, posing **ethical dilemmas** for researchers. Here are examples of research problems in which the desire for rigor conflicts with ethical considerations:

1. *Research question:* How empathic are nurses in their treatment of patients in the intensive care unit (ICU)?
   Ethical dilemma: Ethics require that participants be cognizant of their role in a study. Yet if the researcher informs nurses participating in this study that their degree of empathy in treating ICU patients will be scrutinized, will their behavior be "normal?" If the nurses' usual behavior is altered because of the known presence of research observers, the findings will not be valid.
2. *Research question:* What are the coping mechanisms of parents whose children have a terminal illness?
   Ethical dilemma: To answer this question, the researcher may need to probe into the psycho-

logical state of the parents at a vulnerable time in their lives; such probing could be painful and even traumatic. Yet knowledge of the parents' coping mechanisms might help to design more effective ways of dealing with parents' grief and anger.

3. *Research question:* Does a new medication prolong life in patients with cancer?
   Ethical dilemma: The best way to test the effectiveness of an intervention is to administer the intervention to some participants but withhold it from others to see if differences between the groups emerge. However, if the intervention is untested (e.g., a new drug), the group receiving the intervention may be exposed to potentially hazardous side effects. On the other hand, the group *not* receiving the drug may be denied a beneficial treatment.
4. *Research question:* What is the process by which adult children adapt to the day-to-day stresses of caring for a terminally ill parent?
   Ethical dilemma: In a qualitative study, which would be appropriate for this research question, the researcher sometimes becomes so closely involved with participants that they become willing to share "secrets" and privileged information. Interviews can become confessions—sometimes of unseemly or even illegal or immoral behavior. In this example, suppose a participant admitted to physically abusing an adult parent—how does the researcher respond to that information without undermining a pledge of confidentiality? And, if the researcher divulges the information to appropriate authorities, how can a pledge of confidentiality be given in good faith to other participants?

As these examples suggest, researchers involved with human participants are sometimes in a bind. They are obligated to advance knowledge and develop the highest-quality evidence for practice, using the best methods available; however, they must also adhere to the dictates of ethical rules that have been developed to protect human rights. Another type of dilemma arises from the fact that nurse researchers may be confronted with conflict-of-interest situations, in which their expected behavior as nurses comes into conflict with the expected behavior of researchers (e.g., deviating from a standard research protocol to give needed assistance to a patient). It is precisely because of such conflicts and dilemmas that **codes of ethics** have been developed to guide the efforts of researchers.

Codes of Ethics

During the past four decades, largely in response to the human rights violations described earlier, various codes of ethics have been developed. One of the first internationally recognized efforts to establish ethical standards is referred to as the **Nuremberg Code**, developed after the Nazi atrocities were made public in the Nuremberg trials. Several other international standards have subsequently been developed, the most notable of which is the **Declaration of Helsinki**, which was adopted in 1964 by the World Medical Association and then later revised, most recently in 2000.

Most disciplines have established their own code of ethics. The American Nurses' Association (ANA) put forth a document in 1995 entitled *Ethical Guidelines in the Conduct, Dissemination, and Implementation of Nursing Research* (Silva, 1995). Box 7-1 presents the nine ethical principles outlined in that document. The American Sociological Association published a revised *Code of Ethics* in 1997. Guidelines for psychologists were published by the American Psychological Association (1992) in *Ethical Principles of Psychologists and Code of Conduct*. Although there is considerable overlap in the basic principles articulated in these documents, each deals with problems of particular concern to their respective disciplines.

In the United States, an important code of ethics was adopted by the National Commission for the Protection of Human Subjects of Biomedical and Behavioral Research (1978). The commission, established by the National Research Act (Public Law 93–348), issued a report in 1978 that served as the basis for regulations affecting research sponsored by the federal government. The report, sometimes referred to as the *Belmont Report*, also served as a model for many of the guidelines adopted by specific disciplines. The *Belmont Report* articulated three primary ethical principles on which standards of ethical conduct in research are based: beneficence, respect for human dignity, and justice.

TIP: The following websites offer information about various codes of ethics and ethical requirements for government-sponsored research:

U.S. federal policy for the protection of human subjects, from the Office of Human Research Protections (OHRP): http://ohrp.osophs.dhhs.gov

Canadian policies, from the Tri-Council Policy Statement of the Natural Sciences and Engineering Research Council of Canada (NSERC): http://www.nserc.ca/programs/ethics/english

American Psychological Association: http://www.apa.org/ethics/code.html

American Sociological Association: http://www.asanet.org/members/ecoderev.html

THE PRINCIPLE OF BENEFICENCE

One of the most fundamental ethical principles in research is that of **beneficence**, which encompasses the maxim: Above all, do no harm. Ethical Principle 2 of the ANA guidelines addresses beneficence. Most researchers consider that this principle contains multiple dimensions.

Freedom From Harm

Study participants can be harmed in a variety of ways, including harm that is physical (e.g., injury, fatigue), psychological (e.g., stress, fear), social (e.g., loss of friends), and economic (e.g., loss of wages). Researchers should strive to minimize all types of harm and discomfort and to achieve insofar as possible a balance between the potential benefits and risks of being a participant.

Clearly, exposing study participants to experiences that result in serious or permanent harm is unacceptable. Research should be conducted only

BOX 7.1 Ethical Principles in Nursing Research

THE INVESTIGATOR . . .

1. Respects autonomous research participants' capacity to consent to participate in research and to determine the degree and duration of that participation without negative consequences.
2. Prevents harm, minimizes harm, and/or promotes good to all research participants, including vulnerable groups and others affected by the research.
3. Respects the personhood of research participants, their families, and significant others, valuing their diversity.
4. Ensures that the benefits and burdens of research are equitably distributed in the selection of research participants.
5. Protects the privacy of research participants to the maximum degree possible.
6. Ensures the ethical integrity of the research process by use of appropriate checks and balances throughout the conduct, dissemination, and implementation of the research.
7. Reports suspected, alleged, or known incidents of scientific misconduct in research to appropriate institutional officials for investigation.
8. Maintains competency in the subject matter and methodologies of his or her research, as well as in other professional and societal issues that affect nursing research and the public good.
9. Involved in animal research maximizes the benefits of the research with the least possible harm or suffering to the animals.

From Silva, M. C. (1995). *Ethical guidelines in the conduct, dissemination, and implementation of nursing research* (pp. v–vi). Washington, DC: American Nurses' Association.

---

by qualified people, especially if potentially dangerous technical equipment or specialized procedures are used. Ethical researchers must be prepared to terminate the research if there is reason to suspect that continuation would result in injury, death, disability, or undue distress to study participants. When a new medical procedure or drug is being tested, it is almost always advisable to experiment with animals or tissue cultures before proceeding to tests with humans. (Ethical guidelines relating to the treatment of animal subjects should be consulted for research on animals; see, for example, the American Psychological Association's *Guidelines for ethical conduct in the care and use of animals* at http://www.apa.org/science/anguide.html.)

Example of risk reduction:
Varda and Behnke (2000) studied the effect of the timing of an initial bath (1 hour versus 2 hours after birth) on newborn temperature. To min-

imize risks, the researchers excluded all infants with conditions (e.g., infection, fetal distress, hypoglycemia) that could predispose them to temperature instability.

Although protecting human beings from physical harm may be straightforward, the psychological consequences of participating in a study are usually subtle and thus require close attention and sensitivity. For example, participants may be asked questions about their personal views, weaknesses, or fears. Such queries might lead people to reveal sensitive personal information. The point is not that researchers should refrain from asking questions but rather that they need to be aware of the nature of the intrusion on people's psyches. Researchers can avoid or minimize psychological harm by carefully phrasing questions, by having **debriefing** sessions that permit participants to ask questions or air complaints after data are collected, and, in some situations, by making referrals to appropriate health, social, or psychological services.

Example of referrals:
In the study by Polit, London, and Martinez (2001) of the health of nearly 4000 poor women in 4 major cities, the 90-minute interviews covered such sensitive topics as substance abuse, depression, parenting stress, and domestic violence. Each interviewer had an information sheet with contact information for local service providers who could assist with any issue about which a participant mentioned a need for help.

The need for sensitivity may be greater in qualitative studies, which often involve in-depth exploration into highly personal areas. In-depth probing may actually expose deep-seated fears and anxieties that study participants had previously repressed. Qualitative researchers, regardless of the underlying research tradition, must thus be especially vigilant in anticipating such problems.

Example of an issue of risk in a qualitative study:
Caelli (2001) conducted a phenomenological study to illuminate nurses' understandings of health, and how such understandings translated into nursing practice. One participant, having explored her experience of health with the researcher over several interview sessions, resigned from her city hospital job as a result of gaining a new recognition of the role health played in her life.

Freedom From Exploitation

Involvement in a research study should not place participants at a disadvantage or expose them to situations for which they have not been prepared. Participants need to be assured that their participation, or information they might provide, will not be used against them in any way. For example, a person describing his or her economic circumstances to a researcher should not be exposed to the risk of losing Medicaid benefits; a person reporting drug use should not fear exposure to criminal authorities.

Study participants enter into a special relationship with researchers, and it is crucial that this relationship not be exploited. Exploitation may be overt and malicious (e.g., sexual exploitation, use of subjects' identifying information to create a mailing list, and use of donated blood for the development of a commercial product), but it might also be more subtle. For example, suppose subjects agreed to participate in a study requiring 30 minutes of their time and that the researcher decided 1 year later to go back to them, to follow their progress or circumstances. Unless the researcher had previously explained to participants that there might be a follow-up study, the researcher might be accused of not adhering to the agreement previously reached and of exploiting the researcher—participant relationship.

Because nurse researchers may have a nurse—patient (in addition to a researcher—participant) relationship, special care may need to be exercised to avoid exploiting that bond. Patients' consent to participate in a study may result from their understanding of the researcher's role as *nurse*, not as *researcher.*

In qualitative research, the risk of exploitation may become especially acute because the psychological distance between investigators and participants typically declines as the study progresses. The emergence of a pseudotherapeutic relationship is not uncommon, which imposes additional responsibilities on researchers—and additional risks that exploitation could inadvertently occur. On the other hand, qualitative researchers typically are in a better position than quantitative researchers to *do good*, rather than just to avoid doing harm, because of the close relationships they often develop with participants. Munhall (2001) has argued that qualitative nurse researchers have the responsibility of ensuring that the "therapeutic imperative of nursing (advocacy) takes precedent over the research imperative (advancing knowledge) if conflict develops" (p. 538).

Benefits From Research

People agree to participate in research investigations for a number of reasons. They may perceive that there are some direct personal benefits. More often, however, any benefits from the research accrue to society in general or to other individuals. Thus, many individuals may participate in a study out of a desire to be helpful. Researchers should strive insofar as possible to maximize benefits and to communicate potential benefits to participants.

The Risk/Benefit Ratio

In designing a study, researchers must carefully assess the risks and benefits that would be incurred. The assessment of risks and benefits that individual participants might experience should be shared with them so that they can evaluate whether it is in their best interest to participate. Box 7-2 summarizes the major risks and benefits of research participation. In evaluating the anticipated **risk/benefit ratio** of a study design, researchers might want to consider how comfortable they would feel if their own family members were participating in the study.

The risk/benefit ratio should also be considered in terms of whether the risks to participants are commensurate with the benefit to society and the nursing profession in terms of the quality of evidence produced. The general guideline is that the degree of risk to be taken by those participating in the research should never exceed the potential humanitarian benefits of the knowledge to be gained. Thus, the selection of a significant topic that has the potential to improve patient care is the first step in ensuring that research is ethical.

All research involves some risks, but in many cases, the risk is minimal. **Minimal risk** is defined as risks anticipated to be no greater than those ordinarily encountered in daily life or during routine physical or psychological tests or procedures. When the risks are not minimal, researchers must proceed with caution, taking every step possible to reduce risks and maximize benefits. If the perceived

BOX 7.2 Potential Benefits and Risks of Research to Participants

MAJOR POTENTIAL BENEFITS TO PARTICIPANTS

- Access to an intervention that might otherwise be unavailable to them
- Comfort in being able to discuss their situation or problem with a friendly, objective person
- Increased knowledge about themselves or their conditions, either through opportunity for introspection and self-reflection or through direct interaction with researchers
- Escape from normal routine, excitement of being part of a study
- Satisfaction that information they provide may help others with similar problems or conditions
- Direct monetary or material gains through stipends or other incentives

MAJOR POTENTIAL RISKS TO PARTICIPANTS

- Physical harm, including unanticipated side effects
- Physical discomfort, fatigue, or boredom
- Psychological or emotional distress resulting from self-disclosure, introspection, fear of the unknown, discomfort with strangers, fear of eventual repercussions, anger or embarrassment at the type of questions being asked
- Social risks, such as the risk of stigma, adverse effects on personal relationships, loss of status
- Loss of privacy
- Loss of time
- Monetary costs (e.g., for transportation, child care, time lost from work)

risks and costs to participants outweigh the anticipated benefits of the study, the research should be either abandoned or redesigned.

In quantitative studies, most of the details of the study are usually spelled out in advance, and therefore a reasonably accurate risk/benefit ratio assessment can be developed. Qualitative studies, however, usually evolve as data are gathered, and it may therefore be more difficult to assess all risks at the outset of a study. Qualitative researchers thus must remain sensitive to potential risks throughout the research process.

THE PRINCIPLE OF RESPECT FOR HUMAN DIGNITY

Respect for human dignity is the second ethical principle articulated in the *Belmont Report*. This principle, which includes the right to self-determination and the right to full disclosure, is covered in the ANA guidelines under principles 1 and 3.

The Right to Self-Determination

Humans should be treated as autonomous agents, capable of controlling their own activities. The principle of **self-determination** means that prospective participants have the right to decide voluntarily whether to participate in a study, without risking any penalty or prejudicial treatment. It also means that people have the right to ask questions, to refuse to give information, to ask for clarification, or to terminate their participation.

A person's right to self-determination includes freedom from coercion of any type. **Coercion** involves explicit or implicit threats of penalty from failing to participate in a study or excessive rewards from agreeing to participate. The obligation to protect people from coercion requires careful thought when the researcher is in a position of authority, control, or influence over potential participants, as might often be the case in a nurse—patient relationship. The issue of coercion may require scrutiny even when there is not a preestablished relationship. For example, a generous monetary incentive (or stipend) offered to encourage the participation of an economically disadvantaged group (e.g., the homeless) might be considered mildly coercive because such incentives may place undue pressure on prospective participants; its acceptability might have to be evaluated in terms of the overall risk/benefit ratio.

TIP: Stipends used to increase the rate of participation in a study appear to be especially effective when the group under study is difficult to recruit or when the study is time-consuming or tedious. Stipends range from $1 to hundreds of dollars, but most are in the $10 to $25 range. Federal agencies that sponsor research sometimes do not allow the payment of an outright stipend but will allow reimbursement of certain expenses (e.g., for participants' travel, child care, or lunch money).

The Right to Full Disclosure

The principle of respect for human dignity encompasses people's right to make informed, voluntary decisions about study participation, which requires full disclosure. **Full disclosure** means that the researcher has fully described the nature of the study, the person's right to refuse participation, the researcher's responsibilities, and likely risks and benefits. The right to self-determination and the right to full disclosure are the two major elements on which informed consent is based. Procedures for obtaining informed consent from participants are discussed later in this chapter.

Although full disclosure is normally provided to participants before they begin a study, there is often a need for further disclosure at a later point, either in debriefing sessions or in written communications. For example, issues that arise during the course of data collection may need to be clarified, or participants may want aspects of the study explained once again. Some researchers offer to send participants summaries of the research findings after the information has been analyzed. In qualitative studies, the consent process may require an ongoing negotiation between researchers and participants.

Issues Relating to the Principle of Respect

Although most researchers would, in the abstract, endorse participants' right to self-determination and full disclosure, these standards are sometimes difficult to adhere to in practice. One issue concerns the inability of some individuals to make well-informed judgments about the risks and benefits of study participation. Children, for example, may be unable to give truly informed consent. The issue of groups that are vulnerable within a research context is discussed later in this chapter.

Another issue is that full disclosure can sometimes create two types of bias: first, a bias resulting if subjects provide inaccurate information, and second, a bias resulting if a representative sample is not recruited. Suppose we were studying the relationship between high school students' substance abuse and their absenteeism from school; we hypothesize that students with a high rate of absenteeism are more likely to be substance abusers than students with a good attendance record. If we approached potential participants and fully explained the purpose of the study, some students might refuse to participate, and nonparticipation would be selective; those least likely to volunteer for such a study might well be students who are substance abusers—the very group of primary interest. Moreover, by knowing the research question, those who do participate might not give candid responses. In such a situation, full disclosure could undermine the study.

One technique that researchers sometimes use in such situations is **covert data collection** or **concealment**—the collection of information without participants' knowledge and thus without their consent. This might happen, for example, if a researcher wanted to observe people's behavior in a real-world setting and was concerned that doing so openly would result in changes in the very behavior of interest. The researcher might choose to obtain the information through concealed methods, such as by observing through a one-way mirror, videotaping with hidden equipment, or observing while pretending to be engaged in other activities. As another example, hospital patients might unwittingly become participants in a study through researchers' use of existing hospital records. In general, covert data collection may be acceptable as long as risks are negligible and participants' right to privacy has not been violated, and if the researcher has arranged to debrief participants about the nature of the study subsequent to data collection. Covert data collection is least likely to be ethically acceptable if the research is focused on sensitive aspects of people's behavior, such as drug use, sexual conduct, or illegal acts.

A more controversial technique is the use of deception. **Deception** can involve deliberately withholding information about the study, or providing participants with false information. For example, in studying high school students' use of drugs we might describe the research as a study of students' health practices, which is a mild form of misinformation.

The practice of deception is problematic ethically because it interferes with participants' right to make a truly informed decision about personal costs and benefits of participation. Some people argue that deception is never justified. Others, however, believe that if the study involves minimal risk to subjects and if there are anticipated benefits to the profession and society, then deception may be justified to enhance the validity of the findings. The ANA guidelines offer this advice about deception and concealment:

> The investigator understands that concealment or deception in research is controversial, depending on the type of research. Some investigators believe that concealment or deception in research can never be morally justified. The investigator further understands that before concealment or deception is used, certain criteria must be met: (1) The study must be of such small risk to the research participant and of such great significance to the advancement of the public good that concealment or deception can be morally justified. . . . (2) The acceptability of concealment or deception is related to the degree of risks to research participants. . . . (3) Concealment or deception are used only as last resorts, when no other approach can ensure the validity of the study's findings. . . . (4) The investigator has a moral responsibility to inform research

participants of any concealment or deception as soon as possible and to explain the rationale for its use. (Silva, 1995, p. 10, Section 4.2).

Another issue relating to the principle of respect that has emerged in this new era of electronic communications concerns the collection of data from people over the Internet. For example, some researchers are analyzing the content of messages posted to chat rooms or on listserves. The issue is whether such messages can be used as data without the authors' permission and their informed consent. Some researchers believe that anything posted electronically is in the public domain and therefore can be used without consent for purposes of research. Others, however, feel that the same ethical standards must apply in cyberspace research and that electronic researchers must carefully protect the rights of individuals who are participants in "virtual" communities. Schrum (1995) has developed some ethical guidelines for use by such researchers. As one example, she advocates that researchers, before collecting electronic data, negotiate their entry into an electronic community (e.g., a chat room) with the list owner. Sixsmith and Murray (2001) also warn researchers that obtaining consent from list moderators does not necessarily mean that every member of the listserve or chat room has provided consent. Researchers should periodically remind members of the on-line group of their presence at the site.

THE PRINCIPLE OF JUSTICE

The third broad principle articulated in the *Belmont Report* concerns justice. Justice, which includes participants' right to fair treatment and their right to privacy, is covered in the ANA guidelines under principles 4 and 5.

The Right to Fair Treatment

Study participants have the right to fair and equitable treatment before, during, and after their participation in the study. Fair treatment includes the following features:

- The fair and nondiscriminatory selection of participants such that any risks and benefits will be equitably shared; participants should be selected based on research requirements and not on the vulnerability or compromised position of certain people
- Respect for cultural and other forms of human diversity
- The nonprejudicial treatment of those who decline to participate or who withdraw from the study after agreeing to participate
- The honoring of all agreements between researchers and participants, including adherence to the procedures described to them and payment of any promised stipends
- Participants' access to research personnel at any point in the study to clarify information
- Participants' access to appropriate professional assistance if there is any physical or psychological damage
- Debriefing, if necessary, to divulge information withheld before the study or to clarify issues that arose during the study
- Courteous and tactful treatment at all times

The Right to Privacy

Virtually all research with humans involves intruding into personal lives. Researchers should ensure that their research is not more intrusive than it needs to be and that participants' privacy is maintained throughout the study.

Participants have the right to expect that any data they provide will be kept in strictest confidence. This can occur either through anonymity or through other confidentiality procedures. **Anonymity** occurs when even the researcher cannot link participants to their data. For example, if questionnaires were distributed to a group of nursing home residents and were returned without any identifying information on them, responses would be anonymous. As another example, if a researcher reviewed hospital records from which all identifying information (e.g., name, address, social security number, and so forth) had been expunged, anonymity would again protect participants' right to privacy. Whenever it is possible to achieve anonymity, researchers should strive to do so.

Example of anonymity:
Thomas, Stamler, Lafrenier, and Dumala (2001) used the Internet to gather data from an international sample of women about their perceptions of breast health education and screening. A website with a questionnaire was established. No identifying information was sought from respondents, and so their anonymity was guaranteed.

When anonymity is impossible, appropriate **confidentiality procedures** need to be implemented. A promise of confidentiality is a pledge that any information participants provide will not be publicly reported in a manner that identifies them and will not be made accessible to others. This means that research information should not be shared with strangers nor with people known to the participants (e.g., family members, physicians, other nurses), unless the researcher has been given explicit permission to share it.

Researchers can take a number of steps to ensure that breaches of confidentiality do not occur, including the following:

- Obtain identifying information (e.g., name, address) from participants only when essential.
- Assign an identification (ID) number to each participant and attach the ID number rather than other identifiers to the actual data.
- Maintain identifying information in a locked file.
- Restrict access to identifying information to a small number of people on a need-to-know basis.
- Enter no identifying information onto computer files.
- Destroy identifying information as quickly as practical.
- Make research personnel sign confidentiality pledges if they have access to data or identifying information.
- Report research information in the aggregate; if information for a specific participant is reported, take steps to disguise the person's identity, such as through the use of a fictitious name.

TIP: Researchers who plan to collect data from study participants on multiple occasions (or who use multiple data forms that need to be connected) might believe that anonymity is not possible. However, a technique that has been successfully used is to have participants themselves generate an ID number. They might be instructed, for example, to use their birth year and the first three letters of their mother's maiden names as their ID code (e.g., 1946CRU). This code would be put on every form participants complete, but researchers would not know participants' identities.

Qualitative researchers may need to take extra steps to safeguard the privacy of their participants. Anonymity is almost never possible in qualitative studies because researchers typically become closely involved with participants. Moreover, because of the in-depth nature of qualitative studies, there may be a greater invasion of privacy than is true in quantitative research. Researchers who spend time in the home of a participant may, for example, have difficulty segregating the public behaviors that the participant is willing to share from the private behaviors that unfold unwittingly during the course of data collection. A final issue is adequately disguising participants in research reports. Because the number of respondents is small, qualitative researchers may need to take considerable precautions to safeguard identities. This may mean more than simply using a fictitious name—it may also mean not sharing detailed information about informants' characteristics, such as their occupation and diagnosis.

TIP: Qualitative researchers may have to slightly distort identifying information in their reports, or provide fairly general descriptions. For example, a 49-year-old antique dealer with ovarian cancer might be described as "a middle-aged cancer patient who works in retail sales" to avoid identification that could occur with the more detailed description.

INFORMED CONSENT

Prospective participants who are fully informed about the nature of the research and its potential risks and benefits are in a position to make rational decisions about participating in the study. **Informed consent** means that participants have adequate information regarding the research, are capable of comprehending the information, and have the power of free choice, enabling them to consent to or decline participation voluntarily. This section discusses procedures for obtaining informed consent.

The Content of Informed Consent

Fully informed consent involves communicating the following pieces of information to participants:

1. *Participant status.* Prospective participants need to understand clearly the distinction between *research* and *treatment.* They should be told which health care activities are routine and which are implemented specifically for the study. They also should be informed that data they provide will be used for research purposes.

2. *Study goals.* The overall goals of the research should be stated, in lay rather than technical terms. The use to which the data will be put should be described.

3. *Type of data.* Prospective participants should be told the type of data that will be collected.

4. *Procedures.* Prospective participants should be given a description of the data collection procedures, and of the procedures to be used in any innovative treatment.

5. *Nature of the commitment.* Information should be provided regarding participants' estimated time commitment at each point of contact, and the number of contacts within specified timeframes.

6. *Sponsorship.* Information on who is sponsoring or funding the study should be noted; if the research is part of an academic requirement, this information should be shared.

7. *Participant selection.* Researchers should explain how prospective participants were selected for recruitment, and how many people will be participating.

8. *Potential risks.* Prospective participants should be informed of any foreseeable risks (physical, psychological, social, or economic) or discomforts that might be incurred as a result of participation, and any efforts that will be taken to minimize risks. The possibility of unforeseeable risks should also be discussed, if appropriate. If injury or damage is possible, treatments that will be made available to participants should be described. When risks are more than minimal, prospective participants should be encouraged to seek the advice of others before consenting.

9. *Potential benefits.* Specific benefits to participants, if any, should be described, as well as information on possible benefits to others.

10. *Alternatives.* If appropriate, researchers should provide information about alternative procedures or treatments that might be advantageous to participants.

11. *Compensation.* If stipends or reimbursements are to be paid (or if treatments are offered without fee), these arrangements should be discussed.

12. *Confidentiality pledge.* Prospective participants should be assured that their privacy will at all times be protected. If anonymity can be guaranteed, this should be noted.

13. *Voluntary consent.* Researchers should indicate that participation is strictly voluntary and that failure to volunteer will not result in any penalty or loss of benefits.

14. *Right to withdraw and withhold information.* Prospective participants should be told that even after consenting they have the right to withdraw from the study and to refuse to provide any specific piece of information. Researchers may, in some cases, need to provide participants with a description of circumstances under which researchers would terminate the overall study.

15. *Contact information.* The researcher should provide information on whom participants could contact in the event of further questions, comments, or complaints.

In some qualitative studies, especially those requiring repeated contact with the same participants, it is difficult to obtain a meaningful informed consent at the outset. Qualitative researchers do not always know in advance how the study will evolve.

Because the research design emerges during the data collection and analysis process, researchers may not know the exact nature of the data to be collected, what the risks and benefits to participants will be, or how much of a time commitment they will be expected to make. Thus, in a qualitative study, consent is often viewed as an ongoing, transactional process, referred to as **process consent**. In process consent, the researcher continually renegotiates the consent, allowing participants to play a collaborative role in the decision-making process regarding ongoing participation.

Example of informed consent:
Wilde (2002) studied the experience of living with a long-term urinary catheter in a community-dwelling sample of adults. Fourteen men and women were recruited for this phenomenological study. Full informed consent was obtained before each interview, and reaffirmed as interviews continued.

Comprehension of Informed Consent

Consent information is normally presented to prospective participants while they are being recruited, either orally or in writing. A written notice should not, however, take the place of spoken explanations. Oral presentations provide opportunities for greater elaboration and for participant questioning.

Because informed consent is based on a person's evaluation of the potential risks and benefits of participation, it is important that the critical information not only be communicated but understood. Researchers must assume the role of teacher in communicating consent information. They should be careful to use simple language and to avoid jargon and technical terms whenever possible; they should also avoid biased language that might unduly influence the person's decision to participate. Written statements should be consistent with the participants' reading levels and educational attainment. For participants from a general population (e.g., patients in a hospital), the statement should be written at about seventh or eighth grade reading level.

For studies involving more than minimal risk, researchers need to make special efforts to ensure that prospective participants understand what participation will involve. In some cases, this might involve testing participants for their comprehension of the informed consent material before deeming them eligible for participation.

Documentation of Informed Consent

Researchers usually document the informed consent process by having participants sign a **consent form**. In the United States, federal regulations covering studies funded by government agencies require written consent of human subjects, except under certain circumstances. In particular, when the study does not involve an intervention and data are collected anonymously (or when existing data from records or specimens are used and identifying information is not linked to the data), regulations requiring written informed consent do not apply.

The consent form should contain all the information essential to informed consent, as described earlier. Prospective participants (or their legally authorized representative) should have ample time to review the written document before signing it. The document should also be signed by the researcher, and a copy should be retained by both parties. An example of a written consent form used in a study of one of the authors is presented in Figure 7-1. The numbers in the margins correspond to the types of information for informed consent outlined earlier. (Note that the form does not indicate how subjects were selected, because this is implied in the study purpose, and prospective participants knew they were recruited from a support group for mothers of multiples.)

 TIP: In developing a consent form, the following guidelines might prove helpful:

1. Organize the form coherently so that prospective participants can follow the logic of what is being communicated. If the form is complex, use headings as an organizational aid.
2. Use a large enough font so that the form can be easily read, and use spacing that avoids making the document appear too dense. Make the form as attractive and inviting as possible.

1 2 3,5 4 12 11 8	I understand that I am being asked to participate in a research study at Saint Francis Hospital and Medical Center. This research study will evaluate: What it is like being a mother of multiples during the first year of the infants' lives. If I agree to participate in the study, I will be interviewed for approximately 30 to 60 minutes about my experience as a mother of multiple infants. The interview will be tape-recorded and take place in a private office at St. Francis Hospital. No identifying information will be included when the interview is transcribed. I understand I will receive $25.00 for participating in the study. There are no known risks associated with this study.
7	I realize that I may not participate in the study if I am younger than 18 years of age or I cannot speak English.
10	I realize that the knowledge gained from this study may help either me or other mothers of multiple infants in the future.
13 14	I realize that my participation in this study is entirely voluntary, and I may withdraw from the study at any time I wish. If I decide to discontinue my participation in this study, I will continue to be treated in the usual and customary fashion.
12	I understand that all study data will be kept confidential. However, this information may be used in nursing publications or presentations.
8	I understand that if I sustain injuries from my participation in this research project, I will not be automatically compensated by Saint Francis Hospital and Medical Center.
15	If I need to, I can contact Dr. Cheryl Beck, University of Connecticut, School of Nursing, any time during the study.
1,2	The study has been explained to me. I have read and understand this consent form, all of my questions have been answered, and I agree to participate. I understand that I will be given a copy of this signed consent form.

_____   _____
Signature of Subject   Date

_____   _____
Signature of Witness   Date

_____   _____
Signature of Investigator   Date

FIGURE 7.1 Example of an informed consent form.

3. In general, simplify. Use clear and consistent terminology, and avoid technical terms if possible. If technical terms are needed, include definitions.
4. If possible, use a **readability formula** to estimate the form's reading level, and make revisions to ensure an appropriate reading level for the group under study. There are several such formulas, the most widely used being the FOG Index (Gunning, 1968), the SMOG index (McLaughlin, 1969), and the Flesch Reading Ease score and Flesch-Kincaid grade level score (Flesch, 1948). Specialized software (e.g., RightWriter) is available, and some word-processing software (e.g., Microsoft Word) also provides readability information.
5. Test the form with people similar to those who will be recruited, and ask for feedback.

If the informed consent information is lengthy, researchers whose studies are funded by U.S. government agencies have the option of presenting the full information orally and then summarizing essential information in a **short form**. If a short form is used, however, the oral presentation must be witnessed by a third party, and the signature of the witness must appear on the short consent form. The signature of a third-party witness is also advisable in studies involving more than minimal risk, even when a long and comprehensive consent form is used.

For studies that are not government sponsored, researchers should err on the side of being conservative. They should implement consent procedures that fully adhere to the principle that prospective participants can make good decisions about participation only if they are fully informed about the study's risks and benefits.

TIP: When the primary means of data collection is through a self-administered questionnaire, some researchers opt not to obtain written informed consent because they assume **implied consent** (i.e., that the return of the completed questionnaire reflects voluntary consent to participate). This assumption, however, may not always be warranted (e.g., if patients feel that their treatment might be affected by failure to cooperate with the researcher).

VULNERABLE SUBJECTS

Adherence to ethical standards is often straightforward. However, the rights of special vulnerable groups may need to be protected through additional procedures and heightened sensitivity. **Vulnerable subjects** (the term used in U.S. federal guidelines) may be incapable of giving fully informed consent (e.g., mentally retarded people) or may be at high risk of unintended side effects because of their circumstances (e.g., pregnant women). Researchers interested in studying high-risk groups should become acquainted with guidelines governing informed consent, risk/benefit assessments, and acceptable research procedures for such groups. In general, research with vulnerable subjects should be undertaken only when the risk/benefit ratio is low or when there is no alternative (e.g., studies of childhood development require child participants).

Among the groups that nurse researchers should consider as being vulnerable are the following:

• *Children.* Legally and ethically, children do not have the competence to give informed consent. Usually, the informed consent of children's parents or legal guardians should be obtained. However, it is appropriate—especially if the child is at least 7 years of age—to obtain the child's assent as well. **Assent** refers to the child's affirmative agreement to participate.

If the child is developmentally mature enough to understand the basic information involved in informed consent (e.g., a 13-year-old), it is advisable to obtain written consent from the child as well, as evidence of respect for the child's right to self-determination. Lindeke, Hauck, and Tanner (2000) and Broome (1999) provide excellent guidance regarding children's assent and consent to participate in research. The U.S. government has issued special regulations for the additional protection of children as study participants (see Code of Federal Regulations, 1991, Subpart D).

• *Mentally or emotionally disabled people.* Individuals whose disability makes it impossible for them to weigh the risks and benefits of participation and make an informed decision (e.g., people affected by mental retardation, senility, mental illness, or unconsciousness) also cannot legally or ethically provide informed consent. In such cases, researchers should obtain the written consent of a legal guardian. Researchers should, however, be aware of the fact that a legal guardian may not necessarily have the person's best interests in mind. In such cases, informed consent should also be obtained from someone whose primary interest is the person's welfare. As in the case of children, informed consent or assent from prospective participants themselves should be sought to the extent possible, in addition to guardians' consent.

- *Severely ill or physically disabled people.* For patients who are very ill or undergoing certain treatments, it might be necessary to assess their ability to make reasoned decisions about study participation. For example, Higgins and Daly (1999) described a process they used to assess the decisional capacity of mechanically ventilated patients. Another issue is that for certain disabilities, special procedures for obtaining consent may be required. For example, with deaf participants, the entire consent process may need to be in writing. For people who have a physical impairment preventing them from writing or for participants who cannot read and write, alternative procedures for documenting informed consent (such as audiotaping or videotaping consent proceedings) should be used.

- *The terminally ill.* Terminally ill people who participate in the study can seldom expect to benefit personally from the research, and thus the risk/benefit ratio needs to be carefully assessed. Researchers must also take steps to ensure that if the terminally ill participate in the study, the health care and comfort of these individuals are not compromised. Special procedures may be required for obtaining informed consent if they are physically or mentally incapacitated.

- *Institutionalized people.* Nurses often conduct studies with hospitalized or institutionalized people. Particular care may be required in recruiting such people because they often depend on health care personnel and may feel pressured into participating or may feel that their treatment would be jeopardized by their failure to cooperate. Inmates of prisons and other correctional facilities, who have lost their autonomy in many spheres of activity, may similarly feel constrained in their ability to give free consent. The U.S. government has issued specific regulations for the protection of prisoners as study participants (see Code of Federal Regulations, 1991, Subpart C). Researchers studying institutionalized groups need to emphasize the voluntary nature of participation.

- *Pregnant women.* The U.S. government has issued stringent additional requirements governing research with pregnant women and fetuses (Code of Federal Regulations, 1991, Subpart B). These requirements reflect a desire to safeguard both the pregnant woman, who may be at heightened physical and psychological risk, and the fetus, who cannot give informed consent. The regulations stipulate that a pregnant woman cannot be involved in a study unless the purpose of the research is to meet the health needs of the pregnant woman and risks to her and the fetus are minimized or there is only a minimal risk to the fetus.

Example of research with a vulnerable group: Anderson, Nyamathi, McAvoy, Conde, and Casey (2001) conducted a study to explore perceptions of risk for human immunodeficiency virus infection/acquired immunodeficiency syndrome among adolescents in juvenile detention. The researchers obtained approval to conduct the study from the presiding judge, the detention facility, and a human subjects committee at their own institution. They structured their protocols to assure teens that their participation would be voluntary and would influence neither the duration of their detention nor their adjudication process. The data were collected in spaces that provided privacy for sound and afforded visual surveillance by probation staff.

It should go without saying that researchers need to proceed with extreme caution in conducting research with people who might fall into two or more vulnerable categories, as was the case in this example.

EXTERNAL REVIEWS AND THE PROTECTION OF HUMAN RIGHTS

Researchers may not be objective in assessing risk/benefit ratios or in developing procedures to protect participants' rights. Biases may arise as a result of the researchers' commitment to an area of knowledge and their desire to conduct a study with as much rigor as possible. Because of the risk of a biased evaluation, the ethical dimensions of a study should normally be subjected to external review.

Most hospitals, universities, and other institutions where research is conducted have established formal committees and protocols for reviewing proposed research plans before they are implemented. These committees are sometimes called *human subjects committees*, *ethical advisory boards*, or *research ethics committees*. If the institution receives funds from the U.S. government to help pay for the costs of research, the committee likely will be called an **Institutional Review Board (IRB).**

TIP: If the research is being conducted within an institution or with its help (e.g., assistance in recruiting subjects), you should find out early what the institution's requirements are regarding ethical issues, in terms of its forms, procedures, and review schedules.

Federally sponsored studies (including fellowships) are subject to strict guidelines for evaluating the treatment of human participants. Before undertaking such a study, researchers must submit research plans to the IRB, and must also go through a formal IRB training process. The duty of the IRB is to ensure that the proposed plans meet the federal requirements for ethical research. An IRB can approve the proposed plans, require modifications, or disapprove the plans. The main requirements governing IRB decisions may be summarized as follows (Code of Federal Regulations, 1991, §46.111):

- Risks to participants are minimized.
- Risks to participants are reasonable in relation to anticipated benefits, if any, and the impor-

tance of the knowledge that may reasonably be expected to result.
- Selection of participants is equitable.
- Informed consent will be sought, as required.
- Informed consent will be appropriately documented.
- Adequate provision is made for monitoring the research to ensure participants' safety.
- Appropriate provisions are made to protect participants' privacy and confidentiality of the data.
- When vulnerable subjects are involved, appropriate additional safeguards are included to protect their rights and welfare.

Example of IRB approval:
Jones, Bond, Gardner, and Hernandez (2002) studied the family planning patterns of immigrant Hispanic women in relation to their acculturation to American culture. The researchers sought and obtained approval for the study from the IRB of both a university and a medical center.

Many research projects require a full IRB review. For a full review, the IRB convenes meetings at which most IRB members are present. An IRB must have five or more members, at least one of whom is not a researcher (e.g., a member of the clergy or a lawyer may be appropriate). One IRB member must be a person who is not affiliated with the institution and is not a family member of a person who is affiliated. To protect against potential biases, the IRB cannot comprise entirely men, women, or members from a single profession.

For certain kinds of research involving no more than minimal risk, the IRB can use expedited review procedures, which do not require a meeting. In an **expedited review**, a single IRB member (usually the IRB chairperson or a member designated by the chairperson) carries out the review. Examples of research activities that qualify for an expedited IRB review, if they are deemed to be minimal-risk, include (1) the collection of blood samples in amounts not exceeding 550 ml in an 8-week period, from healthy, nonpregnant adults weighing at least 110 pounds; and (2) research on individual or group characteristics or behavior or "research employing survey, interview, focus group, program evaluation, human factors evaluation, or quality assurance methodologies" (*Federal Register* notice cited in Code of Federal Regulations, 1991, §46.110).

The federal regulations also allow certain types of research to be totally exempt from IRB review. These are studies in which there are no apparent risks to human participants. The website of the Office of Human Research Protections, in its policy guidance section, includes decision charts designed to clarify whether a study is exempt from the federal regulations.

TIP: Not all research is subject to federal guidelines, and so not all studies are reviewed by formal committees. Nevertheless, researchers must ensure that their research plans are ethically sound and are encouraged to seek outside advice on the ethical dimensions of a study before it gets underway. Advisers might include faculty members, the clergy, representatives from the group being asked to participate, or advocates for that group.

BUILDING ETHICS INTO THE DESIGN OF THE STUDY

Researchers need to give careful thought to ethical requirements during the planning of a research project and to ask themselves continually whether planned safeguards for protecting humans are sufficient. They must persist in being vigilant throughout the implementation of the research plans as well, because unforeseen ethical dilemmas may arise during the conduct of the study. Of course, a first step in doing ethical research is to scrutinize the research questions to determine whether they are clinically significant and whether it is feasible to undertake the study in a manner that conforms to ethical guidelines.

The remaining chapters of the book offer advice on how to design studies that yield high-quality evidence for practice. Methodologic decisions about rigor, however, must factor in ethical considerations. Here are some examples of the kinds of questions that might be posed in thinking about various aspects of study design:

Research design:
- Will participants get allocated to different treatment groups fairly?
- Will research controls add to the risks participants will incur?
- Will the setting for the study be selected to protect against participant discomfort?

Intervention:
- Is the intervention designed to maximize good and minimize harm?
- Under what conditions might a treatment be withdrawn or altered?

Sample:
- Is the population defined so as to unwittingly and unnecessarily exclude important segments of people (e.g., women, minorities)?
- Is the population defined in such a way that especially high-risk people (e.g., unstable patients) could be excused from the study?
- Will potential participants be recruited into the study equitably?

Data collection:
- Will data be collected in such a way as to minimize respondent burden?
- Will procedures for ensuring confidentiality of data be adequate?
- Will data collection staff be appropriately trained to be sensitive and courteous?

Reporting:
- Will participants' identities be adequately protected?

TIP: As a means of enhancing both individual and institutional privacy, research reports frequently avoid giving explicit information about the locale of the study. For example, the report might say that data were collected in a

200-bed, private, for-profit nursing home, without mentioning its name or location.

Once the study procedures have been developed, researchers should undertake a self-evaluation of those procedures to determine if they meet ethical requirements. Box 26-15 in Chapter 26 provides some guidelines for such a self-evaluation.

RESEARCH EXAMPLES

Because researchers usually attempt to report research results as succinctly as possible, they rarely describe in much detail the efforts they have made to safeguard participants' rights. (The absence of any mention of such safeguards does not, of course, imply that no precautions were taken.) Researchers are especially likely to discuss their adherence to ethical guidelines for studies that involve more than minimal risk or when the people being studied are a vulnerable group. Two research examples that highlight ethical issues are presented in the following sections.

Research Example from a Quantitative Study

Willson, McFarlane, Lemmy, and Malecha (2001) conducted a study to evaluate whether abused women's use of the police reduced further violence. The study sought to describe the extent of violence and homicide danger experienced by women before and after filing assault charges against an intimate through the police department.

After obtaining approval for conducting the study from the agency (a special family violence unit in a large metropolitan police department) and the researchers' IRB, the researchers sought to interview a consecutive sample of women who met study criteria (18 years of age or older, English speaking) and who attempted to file assault charges during a 1-month period in 1998. Investigators approached prospective participants and explained the study purpose, research protocols, administration time, and follow-up schedules. Women were paid a $20 stipend for each completed interview. Both verbal and written consent was obtained from a sample of 90 women.

The researchers took care to protect the women's rights during data collection. Data were obtained confidentially in private interview rooms. The women were assigned an ID number to maintain confidentiality. The subjects' safety was ensured for follow-up interviews by establishing a convenient, private, and safe time for the 3- and 6-month follow-up interviews. A total of 83 women completed all three rounds of interviews.

The researchers found that women seeking police help had significantly reduced threats of abuse, actual experiences of abuse, and perceived danger of being killed than before.

Research Example From a Qualitative Study

Wackerbarth (1999) undertook an in-depth study designed to describe the dynamics of caretaker decision making. Wackerbarth's study focused on understanding the decision process among family caregivers of persons with dementia. A local chapter of the Alzheimer's Association mailed out 100 preinterview questionnaires with an introductory letter from the director of the chapter. Caregivers interested in participating in the study mailed back a completed consent form and the preinterview questionnaire. From the pool of 80 caregivers who returned the questionnaire, 28 were selected to be interviewed. The sample was carefully selected to represent a broad viewpoint for developing a decision-making model.

Wackerbarth's article carefully explained the attention that was paid to participants' rights in this study: (1) the study objectives and methods were described orally and in writing to ensure that they were understood; (2) an informed consent form, which highlighted the voluntary nature of participation and indicated the safeguards that would be taken to protect their confidentiality, was signed before data collection began; (3) all preinterview questionnaires, tape recordings, and interview transcripts were kept in a locked file cabinet; (4) no identifying information was appended to study materials; and (5) participants were asked to review written materials and to give permission before publication of quotes and study findings.

On the basis of the interviews, Wackerbarth developed a model charting the caregiving experience over time, and documented decisions made to maintain tolerable situations. The model captured the intrapersonal struggle driving the decision-making efforts of care-givers who care for family members with dementia.

SUMMARY POINTS

- Because research has not always been conducted ethically, and because of the genuine **ethical dilemmas** researchers often face in designing studies that are both ethical and methodologically rigorous, **codes of ethics** have been developed to guide researchers.
- The three major ethical principles incorporated into most guidelines are beneficence, respect for human dignity, and justice.
- **Beneficence** involves the protection of participants from physical and psychological harm, protection of participants from exploitation, and the performance of some good.
- In deciding to conduct a study, researchers must carefully weigh the **risk/benefit ratio** of participation to individuals and also the risks to participants against potential benefits to society.
- **Respect for human dignity** involves the participants' **right to self-determination**, which means participants have the freedom to control their own activities, including study participation.
- Respect for human dignity also encompasses the **right to full disclosure,** which means that researchers have fully described to prospective participants their rights and the full nature of the study. When full disclosure poses the risk of biased results, researchers sometimes use **covert data collection** or **concealment** (the collection of information without the participants' knowledge or consent) or **deception** (either withholding information from participants or providing false information). If deception or concealment is deemed necessary, extra precautions should be used to minimize risks and protect other rights.
- **Justice** includes the **right to fair treatment** (both in the selection of participants and during the course of the study) and the **right to privacy**. Privacy can be maintained through **anonymity** (wherein not even researchers know participants' identities) or through formal **confidentiality pro-**cedures that safeguard the information participants provide.
- **Informed consent** procedures, which provide prospective participants with information needed to make a reasoned decision about participation, normally involve signing a **consent form** to document voluntary and informed participation. In qualitative studies, consent may need to be continually renegotiated with participants as the study evolves, through **process consent**.
- **Vulnerable subjects** require additional protection. These people may be vulnerable because they are not able to make a truly informed decision about study participation (e.g., children); because their circumstances make them believe free choice is constrained (e.g., prisoners); or because their circumstances heighten the risk of physical or psychological harm (e.g., pregnant women, the terminally ill).
- External review of the ethical aspects of a study by a human subjects committee or **Institutional Review Board (IRB)** is highly desirable and may be required by either the agency funding the research or the organization from which participants are recruited.
- In studies in which risks to participants are minimal, an **expedited review** (review by a single member of the IRB) may be substituted for a full board review; in cases in which there are no anticipated risks, the research may be exempted from review.
- Researchers are always advised, even in the absence of an IRB review, to consult with at least one external adviser whose perspective allows an objective evaluation of the ethics of a proposed study.
- Researchers need to give careful thought to ethical requirements throughout the study's planning and implementation and to ask themselves continually whether safeguards for protecting humans are sufficient.

STUDY ACTIVITIES

Chapter 7 of the *Study Guide to Accompany Nursing Research*: *Principles and Methods*, 7th edition, offers various exercises and study suggestions for reinforcing concepts presented in this chapter. In addition, the following study questions can be addressed:

1. Point out the ethical dilemmas that might emerge in the following studies:
   a. A study of the relationship between sleeping patterns and acting-out behaviors in hospitalized psychiatric patients
   b. A study of the effects of a new drug treatment for diabetic patients
   c. An investigation of an individual's psychological state after an abortion
   d. An investigation of the contraceptive decisions of high school students at a school-based clinic
2. For each of the studies described in question 1, indicate whether you think the study would require a full IRB review or an expedited review, or whether it would be totally exempt from review.
3. For the study described in the research example section (Willson et al., 2001), prepare an informed consent form that includes required information, as described in the section on informed consent.

SUGGESTED READINGS

References on Research Ethics

American Nurses' Association. (1975). *Human rights guidelines for nurses in clinical and other research.* Kansas City, MO: Author.

American Nurses' Association. (1985). *Code for nurses with interpretive statements.* Kansas City, MO: Author.

American Psychological Association. (1992). *Ethical principles of psychologists and code of conduct.* Washington, DC: Author.

American Sociological Association. (1997). *Code of ethics.* Washington, DC: Author.

Broome, M. E. (1999). Consent (assent) for research with pediatric patients. *Seminars in Oncology Nursing, 15,* 96–103.

Code of Federal Regulations. (1991). *Protection of human subjects: 45CFR46* (revised as of June 18, 1991). Washington, DC: Department of Health and Human Services.

Cowles, K. V. (1988). Issues in qualitative research on sensitive topics. *Western Journal of Nursing Research, 10,* 163–179.

Damrosch, S. P. (1986). Ensuring anonymity by use of subject-generated identification codes. *Research in Nursing & Health, 9,* 61–63.

Davis, A. J. (1989a). Clinical nurses' ethical decision-making in situations of informed consent. *Advances in Nursing Science, 11,* 63–69.

Davis, A. J. (1989b). Informed consent process in research protocols: Dilemmas for clinical nurses. *Western Journal of Nursing Research, 11,* 448–457.

Flesch, R. (1948). New readability yardstick. *Journal of Applied Psychology, 32,* 221–223.

Gunning, R. (1968). *The technique of clear writing* (Rev. ed.). New York: McGraw-Hill.

Higgins, P. A., & Daly, B. J. (1999). Research methodology issues related to interviewing the mechanically ventilated patient. *Western Journal of Nursing Research, 21,* 773–784.

McLaughlin, G. H. (1969). SMOG grading: A new readability formula. *Journal of Reading, 12,* 639–646.

Meade, C. D. (1999). Improving understanding of the informed consent process and document. *Seminars in Oncology Nursing, 15,* 124–137.

Munhall, P. L. (2001). Ethical considerations in qualitative research. In P. L. Munhall (Ed.), *Nursing research: A qualitative perspective* (pp. 537–549). Sudbury, MA: Jones & Bartlett.

National Commission for the Protection of Human Subjects of Biomedical and Behavioral Research. (1978). *Belmont report: Ethical principles and guidelines for research involving human subjects.* Washington, DC: U.S. Government Printing Office.

Ramos, M. C. (1989). Some ethical implications of qualitative research. *Research in Nursing & Health, 12,* 57–64.

Rempusheski, V. F. (1991a). Elements, perceptions, and issues of informed consent. *Applied Nursing Research, 4,* 201–204.

Rempusheski, V. F. (1991b). Research data management: Piles into files—locked and secured. *Applied Nursing Research, 4,* 147–149.

Sales, B. D., & Folkman, S. (Eds.). (2000). *Ethics in research with human participants.* Washington, DC: American Psychological Corporation.

Schrum, L. (1995). Framing the debate: Ethical research in the information age. *Qualitative Inquiry, 1,* 311–326.

Silva, M. C. (1995). *Ethical guidelines in the conduct, dissemination, and implementation of nursing research.* Washington, DC: American Nurses' Association.

Silva, M. C., & Sorrell, J. M. (1984). Factors influencing comprehension of information for informed consent. *International Journal of Nursing Studies, 21*, 233–240.

Sixsmith, J., & Murray, C. D. (2001). Ethical issues in the documentary data analysis of Internet posts and archives. *Qualitative Health Research, 11*, 423–432.

Lindeke, L., Hauck, M. R., & Tanner, M. (2000). Practical issues in obtaining child assent for research. *Journal of Pediatric Nursing, 15*, 99–104.

Thurber, F. W., Deatrick, J. A., & Grey, M. (1992). Children's participation in research: Their right to consent. *Journal of Pediatric Nursing, 7*, 165–170.

Watson, A. B. (1982). Informed consent of special subjects. *Nursing Research, 31*, 43–47.

Studies Cited in Chapter 7

Anderson, N. L. R., Nyamathi, A., McAvoy, J. A., Conde, F., & Casey, C. (2001) Perceptions about risk for HIV/AIDS among adolescents in juvenile detention. *Western Journal of Nursing Research, 23*, 336–359.

Caelli, K. (2001). Engaging with phenomenology: Is it more of a challenge than it needs to be? *Qualitative Health Research, 11*, 273–281.

Jones, M. E., Bond, M. L., Gardner, S., & Hernandez, M. (2002). Acculturation level and family planning patterns of Hispanic immigrant women. *MCN: The American Journal of Maternal/Child Nursing, 27*, 26–32.

Polit, D. F., London, A. S., & Martinez, J. M. (2001). *The health of poor urban women.* New York: MDRC.

Thomas, B., Stamler, L. L., Lafrenier, K., & Dumala, R. (2001). The Internet: An effective tool for nursing research with women. *Computers in Nursing, 18*, 13–18.

Varda, K. E., & Behnke, R. S. (2000). The effect of timing of initial bath on newborn's temperature. *Journal of Obstetric, Gynecologic, and Neonatal Nursing, 29*, 27–32.

Wackerbarth, S. (1999). Modeling a dynamic decision process: Supporting the decisions of caregivers of family members with dementia. *Qualitative Health Research, 9*, 294–314.

Wilde, M. H. (2002). Urine flowing: A phenomenological study of living with a urinary catheter. *Research in Nursing & Health, 25*, 14–24.

Willson, P., McFarlane, J., Lemmey, D., & Malecha, A. (2001). Referring abused women: Does police assistance decrease abuse? *Clinical Nursing Research, 10*, 69–81.

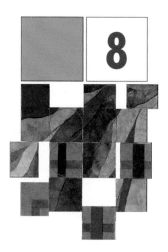

8

Designing Quantitative Studies

The research design of a study spells out the basic strategies that researchers adopt to develop evidence that is accurate and interpretable. The research design incorporates some of the most important methodologic decisions that researchers make, particularly in quantitative studies. Thus, it is important to understand design options when embarking on a research project. This chapter and the two that follow focus on design issues for quantitative research, and Chapter 11 discusses designs for qualitative research.

TIP: If you are doing a study, you will need to make many important decisions about the study's design. These decisions will affect the overall believability of your findings. In some cases, the decisions will affect whether you receive funding (if you are seeking financial support for your study) or whether you are able to publish your research report (if you plan to submit it to a journal). Therefore, a great deal of care and thought should go into these decisions.

ASPECTS OF QUANTITATIVE RESEARCH DESIGN

The overall plan for addressing a research problem encompasses multiple issues, all of which have implications for the quality of evidence the study yields.

Intervention

A fundamental design decision concerns the researcher's role vis-à-vis study participants. In some studies, nurse researchers want to test the effects of a specific intervention (e.g., an innovative program to promote breast self-examination). In such **experimental studies**, researchers play an active role by introducing the intervention. In other studies, referred to as **nonexperimental studies**, the researcher observes phenomena as they naturally occur without intervening. There are numerous specific experimental and nonexperimental designs from which to choose.

Comparisons

In most studies, researchers develop comparisons to provide a context for interpreting results. The most common of types of comparison are as follows:

1. *Comparison between two or more groups.* For example, suppose we wanted to study the emotional consequences of having an abortion. To do this, we might compare the emotional status of women who had an abortion with that of women with an unintended pregnancy who delivered the baby.
2. *Comparison of one group's status at two or more points in time.* For example, we might

want to assess patients' levels of stress before and after introducing a new procedure to reduce preoperative stress. Or we might want to compare coping processes among caregivers of patients with AIDS early and later in the caregiving experience.

3. *Comparison of one group's status under different circumstances.* For example, we might compare people's heart rates during two different types of exercise.

4. *Comparison based on relative rankings.* If, for example, we hypothesized a relationship between level of pain of cancer patients and their degree of hopefulness, we would be asking whether patients with high levels of pain feel less hopeful than patients with low levels of pain. This research question involves a comparison of those with different rankings—high versus low—on both variables.

5. *Comparison with other studies.* Researchers may directly compare their results with results from other studies, sometimes using statistical procedures. This type of comparison typically supplements rather than replaces other types of comparisons. In quantitative studies, this approach is useful primarily when the dependent variable is measured with a widely accepted approach (e.g., blood pressure measures or scores on a standard measure of depression).

 Example of using comparative data from other studies:

Beckie, Beckstead, and Webb (2001) studied quality of life and health of women who had suffered a cardiac event. Women in their sample were administered standard scales for which there were national comparison data, enabling the researchers to evaluate their sample's outcomes relative to national norms in the United States.

Comparisons are often the central focus of a study, but even when they are not, they provide a context for understanding the findings. In the example of studying the emotional status of women who had an abortion, it would be difficult to know whether their emotional status was of concern without comparing it with that of others.

In some studies, a natural comparison group suggests itself. For example, if we were testing the effectiveness of a new nursing procedure for a group of nursing home residents, an obvious comparison group would be nursing home residents who were exposed to the standard procedure rather than to the innovation. In other cases, however, the choice of a comparison group is less clearcut, and the researcher's decision about a comparison group can affect the interpretability of the findings. In the example about the emotional consequences of an abortion, we opted to use women who had delivered a baby as the comparison group. This reflects a comparison focusing on pregnancy *outcome* (i.e., pregnancy termination versus live birth). An alternative comparison group might be women who had a miscarriage. In this case, the comparison focuses not on the outcome (in both groups, the outcome is pregnancy loss) but rather on the *determinant* of the outcome. Thus, in designing a study, researchers must choose comparisons that will best illuminate the central issue under investigation.

Controls for Extraneous Variables

As noted in Chapter 2, the complexity of relationships among human characteristics often makes it difficult to answer research questions unambiguously unless efforts are made to isolate the key research variables and to control other factors extraneous to the research question. Thus, an important feature of the research design of quantitative studies is the steps that will be taken to control extraneous variables. Familiarity with the research literature often helps to identify especially important variables to control. Methods for enhancing research control are discussed in Chapter 9.

Timing of Data Collection

In most studies, data are collected from participants at a single point in time. For example, patients might be asked on a single occasion to describe their health-promoting behaviors. Some designs, however, call for multiple contacts with participants, usually to determine how things have changed over time. Thus, in designing a study, the researcher must decide on the number of data collection points needed to address the research question properly. The research design also designates *when*, relative to other events, data will be collected. For example, the design might call for interviews with pregnant women in the sixteenth and thirtieth weeks of gestation, or for blood samples to be drawn after 10 hours of fasting.

Research Sites and Settings

Research designs also specify the site and setting for the study. As discussed in Chapter 2, sites are the overall locations for the research, and settings are the more specific places where data collection will occur. Sites and settings should be selected so as to maximize the validity and reliability of the data. In designing a study, it may be important to consider whether participants are influenced by being in settings that may be anxiety-provoking or foreign to their usual experiences.

Communication With the Subjects

In designing the study, the researcher must decide how much information to provide to study participants. As discussed in the previous chapter, full disclosure to subjects before obtaining their consent is ethically correct, but can sometimes undermine the value of the research. The researcher should also consider the costs and benefits of alternative means of communicating information to study participants. Among the issues that should be addressed are the following:

- How much information about the study aims will be provided to (and withheld from) prospective subjects while they are being recruited and during the informed consent process?
- How will information be provided—orally or in writing?
- What is the reading and comprehension level of the *least* skilled participants?
- Who will provide the information, and what will that person be expected to say in response to additional questions participants might ask?

- Will there be debriefing sessions after data are collected to explain more fully the study purpose or to answer questions?

The nature of the communication with participants can affect their cooperation and the data they provide, and so these issues should be given careful consideration in designing the study.

TIP: In making design decisions, you will often need to balance various considerations, such as time, cost, ethical issues, and study integrity. Try to get a firm understanding of your "upper limits" before making final design decisions. That is, what is the *most* money that can be spent on the project? What is the *maximal amount* of time available for conducting the study? What is the limit of acceptability with regard to ethical issues, given the risk/benefit ratio of the study? These limits often eliminate some design options. With these constraints in mind, the central focus should be on designing a study that maximizes the validity of the data.

OVERVIEW OF RESEARCH DESIGN TYPES

Quantitative research designs vary along a number of dimensions (some of which relate to factors discussed in the preceding section), as shown in Table 8-1. Some dimensions are independent of the others. For example, an experimental design can be cross-sectional or longitudinal.

Quantitative designs in general share one thing in common: they tend to be fairly structured. Typically, quantitative researchers specify the nature of any intervention, comparisons to be made, methods to be used to control extraneous variables, timing of data collection, the study site and setting, and information to be given to participants—all before a single piece of data is gathered. Once data collection is underway, modifications to the research design are rarely instituted. As discussed in Chapter 11, research design in a qualitative study is more fluid: qualitative researchers often make deliberate modifications that are sensitive to what is being learned as data are gathered.

TABLE 8.1 Dimensions of Research Designs

DIMENSION	DESIGN	MAJOR FEATURES
Degree of structure	Structured	Design is specified before data are collected
	Flexible	Design evolves during data collection
Type of group comparisons	Between-subjects	Subjects in groups being compared are different people
	Within-subjects	Subjects in groups being compared are the same people at different times or in different conditions
Time frame	Cross-sectional	Data are collected at one point in time
	Longitudinal	Data are collected at two or more points in time over an extended period
Control over independent variable	Experimental	Manipulation of independent variable, control group, randomization
	Quasi-experimental	Manipulation of independent variable, but no randomization or no control group
	Preexperimental	Manipulation of independent variable, no randomization or control group, limited control over extraneous variables
	Nonexperimental	No manipulation of independent variable
Measurement of independent and dependent variables	Retrospective	Study begins with dependent variable and looks backward for cause or antecedent
	Prospective	Study begins with independent variable and looks forward for the effect

This section describes several of the dimensions along which quantitative research designs vary. Other dimensions are discussed later in this chapter.

Between-Subjects and Within-Subjects Designs

As previously noted, most quantitative studies involve making comparisons, which are often between separate groups of people. For example, the hypothesis that the drug tamoxifen reduces the rate of breast cancer in high-risk women could be tested by comparing women who received tamoxifen and those who did not. In this example, those getting the drug are not the same people as those not getting it. In another example, if we were interested in comparing the pain tolerance of men and women, the groups being compared would obviously involve different people. This class of design is referred to as **between-subjects designs**.

 Example of a study with a between-subjects design:
Nantais-Smith and her colleagues (2001) examined differences in plasma and nipple aspirate carotenoid 12 months postpartum between women who had and women who had not breastfed their infants.

It is sometimes desirable to make comparisons for the *same* study participants. For example, we might be interested in studying patients' heart rates before and after a nursing intervention, or we might want to compare lower back pain for patients lying in two different positions. These examples both call for a **within-subjects design**, involving comparisons of the same people under two conditions or at two points in time. The nature of the comparison has implications for the type of statistical test used.

 Example of a study with a within-subjects design:

Hill, Kurkowski, and Garcia (2000) examined the effect of oral support (cheek and jaw support) on nutritive sucking patterns of preterm infants during feeding. Twenty preterm infants were observed under two conditions: with the support and without it.

The Time Dimension

Although most studies collect data at a single point in time, there are four situations in which it is appropriate to design a study with multiple points of data collection:

1. *Studying time-related processes.* Certain research problems specifically focus on phenomena that evolve over time (e.g., healing, learning, recidivism, and physical growth).
2. *Determining time sequences.* It is sometimes important to determine the sequencing of phenomena. For example, if it is hypothesized that infertility results in depression, then it would be important to determine that the depression did not precede the fertility problem.
3. *Developing comparisons over time.* Some studies are undertaken to determine if changes have occurred over time. For example, a study might be concerned with documenting trends in the smoking behavior of teenagers over a 10-year period. As another example, an experimental study might examine whether an intervention led to both short-term and long-term effects.
4. *Enhancing research control.* Some research designs for quantitative studies involve the collection of data at multiple points to enhance the interpretability of the results. For example,

when two groups are being compared with regard to the effects of alternative interventions, the collection of data before any intervention occurs allows the researcher to detect—and control—any initial differences between groups.

Studies are often categorized in terms of how they deal with time. The major distinction is between cross-sectional and longitudinal designs.

Cross-Sectional Designs

Cross-sectional designs involve the collection of data at one point in time: the phenomena under study are captured during one period of data collection. Cross-sectional studies are appropriate for describing the status of phenomena or for describing relationships among phenomena at a fixed point in time. For example, we might be interested in determining whether psychological symptoms in menopausal women are correlated contemporaneously with physiologic symptoms.

Cross-sectional designs are sometimes used for time-related purposes, but the results may be ambiguous. For example, we might test the hypothesis, using cross-sectional data, that a determinant of excessive alcohol consumption is low impulse control, as measured by a psychological test. When both alcohol consumption and impulse control are measured concurrently, however, it is difficult to know which variable influenced the other, if either. Cross-sectional data can most appropriately be used to infer time sequence under two circumstances: (1) when there is evidence or logical reasoning indicating that one variable preceded the other (e.g., in a study of the effects of low birth weight on morbidity in school-aged children, there would be no confusion over whether birth weight came first); and (2) when a strong theoretical framework guides the analysis.

Cross-sectional studies can also be designed to permit inferences about processes evolving over time, such as when measurements capture a process at different points in its evolution with different people. As an example, suppose we wanted to study changes in professionalism as nursing students progress through a 4-year baccalaureate program. One way to investigate this would be to gather data from students every year until they graduate; this would be a longitudinal design. On the other hand, we could use a cross-sectional design by gathering data at a single point from members of the four classes, and then comparing the responses of the four classes. If seniors had higher scores on a measure of professionalism than freshmen, it might be inferred that nursing students become increasingly socialized professionally by their educational experiences. To make this kind of inference, we must assume that the seniors would have responded as the freshmen responded had they been questioned 3 years earlier, or, conversely, that freshmen students would demonstrate increased professionalism if they were questioned 3 years later. Such a design, which involves a comparison of multiple age cohorts, is sometimes referred to as a **cohort comparison design**.

The main advantage of cross-sectional designs in such situations is that they are practical: they are easy to do and are relatively economical. There are, however, problems in inferring changes over time using a cross-sectional design. In our example, seniors and freshmen may have different attitudes toward the nursing profession, independent of any experiences during their 4 years of education. The overwhelming number of social and technologic changes in our society frequently makes it questionable to assume that differences in the behaviors, attitudes, or characteristics of different age groups are the result of time passing rather than a reflection of cohort or generational differences. In cross-sectional studies designed to study change, there are frequently several alternative explanations for the research findings—and that is precisely what good research design tries to avoid.

Example of a cross-sectional study:
Mindell and Jacobson (2000) assessed sleep patterns and the prevalence of sleep disorders during pregnancy. With a cross-sectional design, they compared women who were at four points in pregnancy: 8 to 12 weeks, 18 to 22 weeks; 25 to 28 weeks; and 35 to 38 weeks. They concluded that sleep disturbances were especially common in late pregnancy.

Longitudinal Designs

A study in which data are collected at more than one point in time *over an extended period* uses a **longitudinal design**. (A study involving the collection of postoperative patient data on vital signs over a 2-day period would not be described as longitudinal.) There are several types of longitudinal designs.

Trend studies are investigations in which samples from a population are studied over time with respect to some phenomenon. Different samples are selected at repeated intervals, but the samples are always drawn from the same population. Trend studies permit researchers to examine patterns and rates of change over time and to predict future developments. Trend studies typically are based on *surveys*, which are described in further detail in Chapter 10.

Example of a trend study:
Greenfield, Midanik, and Rogers (2000) studied trends in alcohol consumption in the United States over a 10-year period, using data from the 1984, 1990, and 1995 National Alcohol Surveys. They found that rates of heavy drinking had fallen between 1984 and 1990, but had remained unchanged between 1990 and 1995.

Cohort studies are a particular kind of trend study in which specific subpopulations are examined over time. The samples are usually drawn from specific age-related subgroups. For example, the cohort of women born from 1946 to 1950 may be studied at regular intervals with respect to health care utilization. In a design known as a **cross-sequential design**,* two or more age cohorts are studied longitudinally so that both changes over time *and* generational (cohort) differences can be detected.

In **panel studies**, the *same* people are used to supply data at two or more points in time. The term **panel** refers to the sample of subjects providing data. Because the same people are studied over time,

---

*This design is sometimes referred to as a **cohort-sequential design**, or as a *longitudinal cohort comparison design*.

researchers can identify individuals who did and did not change and then examine characteristics that differentiate the two groups. As an example, a panel study could be designed to explore over time the antecedent characteristics of smokers who were later able to quit. Panel studies also allow researchers to examine how conditions and characteristics at time 1 influence characteristics and conditions at time 2. For example, health outcomes at time 2 could be studied among individuals with different health-related behaviors at time 1. Panel studies are intuitively appealing as an approach to studying change but are expensive to manage and can run into difficulties. The most serious challenge is the loss of participants over time—a problem known as **attrition**. Attrition is problematic because those who drop out of the study often differ in important ways from those who continue to participate, resulting in potential biases and lack of generalizability.

Example of a panel study:
Wilson, White, Cobb, Curry, Greene, and Popovich (2000) explored relationships between paternal—and maternal—fetal attachment and infant temperament. They first gathered data from pregnant women and their partners during the third trimester of pregnancy. These parental data were then linked to the infants' temperament 1 year later when they were 8 to 9 months of age.

Follow-up studies are similar to panel studies, but are usually undertaken to determine the subsequent development of individuals who have a specified condition or who have received a specified intervention—unlike panel studies, which have samples drawn from more general populations. For example, patients who have received a particular nursing intervention or clinical treatment may be followed to ascertain the long-term effects of the treatment. As another example, samples of premature infants may be followed to assess their later perceptual and motor development.

Example of a follow-up study:
McFarlane, Soeken, and Wiist (2000) tested three alternative interventions designed to decrease intimate partner violence to pregnant women. A sample of over 300 pregnant, physically abused women were followed up through interviews at 2, 6, 12, and 18 months after delivery.

In sum, longitudinal designs are appropriate for studying the dynamics of a phenomenon over time. Researchers must make decisions about the number of data collection points and the intervals between them based on the nature of study and available resources. When change or development is rapid, numerous time points at short intervals may be needed to document it. Researchers interested in outcomes that may occur years after the original data collection must use longer-term follow-up. However, the longer the interval, the greater the risk of attrition—and, usually, the costlier the study.

 TIP: Try not to make design decisions single-handedly. Seek the advice of professors, colleagues, or research consultants. Once you have made design decisions, it may be useful to write out a rationale for your choices, and share it with those you have consulted to see if they can find any flaws in your reasoning or if they can make suggestions for further improvements.

EXPERIMENTS

A basic distinction in quantitative research design is that between experimental and nonexperimental research. In an **experiment**, researchers are active agents, not passive observers. Early physical scientists learned that although pure observation of phenomena is valuable, complexities occurring in nature often made it difficult to understand important relationships. This problem was handled by isolating phenomena in a laboratory and controlling the conditions under which they occurred. The procedures developed by physical scientists were profitably adopted by biologists during the 19th century, resulting in many achievements in physiology and medicine. The 20th century has witnessed the use of experimental methods by researchers interested in human behavior.

Characteristics of True Experiments

The controlled experiment is considered by many to be an ideal—the gold standard for yielding reliable evidence about causes and effects. Except for purely descriptive research, the aim of many research studies is to understand relationships among phenomena. For example, does a certain drug result in the cure of a disease? Does a nursing intervention produce a decrease in patient anxiety? The strength of true experiments lies in the fact that experimenters can achieve greater confidence in the genuineness of causal relationships because they are observed under controlled conditions. As we pointed out in Chapter 4, hypotheses are never proved or disproved by scientific methods, but true experiments offer the most convincing evidence about the effect one variable has on another.

A true experimental design is characterized by the following properties:

- *Manipulation*—the experimenter *does* something to at least some subjects
- *Control*—the experimenter introduces controls over the experimental situation, including the use of a control group
- *Randomization*—the experimenter assigns subjects to a control or experimental group on a random basis

Each of these features is discussed more fully in the following sections.

Manipulation

Manipulation involves *doing* something to study participants. The introduction of that "something" (i.e., the experimental **treatment** or **intervention**) constitutes the independent variable. The experimenter manipulates the independent variable by administering a treatment to some subjects and withholding it from others (or by administering some other treatment). The experimenter thus consciously *varies* the independent variable and observes the effect on the dependent variable.

For example, suppose we hypothesized that gentle massage is effective as a pain relief measure for elderly nursing home residents. The independent variable (the presumed cause) in this example is receipt of gentle massage, which could be manipulated by giving some patients the massage intervention and withholding it from others. We would then compare patients' pain level (the dependent variable) in the two groups to see if differences in receipt of the intervention resulted in differences in average pain levels.

Control

Control is achieved in an experimental study by manipulating, by randomizing, by carefully preparing the experimental protocols, and by using a control group. This section focuses on the function of the control group in experiments.

Obtaining evidence about relationships requires making at least one comparison. If we were to supplement the diet of premature infants with a particular nutrient for 2 weeks, their weight at the end of 2 weeks would tell us nothing about treatment effectiveness. At a bare minimum, we would need to compare their posttreatment weight with their pretreatment weight to determine if, at least, their weight had increased. But let us assume that we find an average weight gain of 1 pound. Does this gain support the conclusion that the nutritional supplement (the independent variable) caused weight gain (the dependent variable)? No, it does not. Babies normally gain weight as they mature. Without a control group—a group that does *not* receive the nutritional supplements—it is impossible to separate the effects of maturation from those of the treatment. The term **control group** refers to a group of subjects whose performance on a dependent variable is used to evaluate the performance of the **experimental group** or **treatment group** (the group that receives the intervention) on the same dependent variable.

Randomization

Randomization (also called **random assignment**) involves placing subjects in groups at random. *Random* essentially means that every subject has an equal chance of being assigned to any group. If subjects are placed in groups randomly, there is no **systematic bias** in the groups with respect to attributes that could affect the dependent variable.

Let us consider the purpose of random assignment. Suppose we wanted to study the effectiveness of a contraceptive counseling program for multiparous women who have just given birth. Two groups of subjects are included—one will be counseled and the other will not. The women in the sample are likely to differ from one another in many ways, such as age, marital status, financial situation, attitudes toward child-rearing, and the like. Any of these characteristics could affect a woman's diligence in practicing contraception, independent of whether she receives counseling. We need to have the "counsel" and "no counsel" groups equal with respect to these extraneous characteristics to assess the impact of the experimental counseling program on subsequent pregnancies. The random assignment of subjects to one group or the other is designed to perform this equalization function. One method might be to flip a coin for each woman (more elaborate procedures are discussed later). If the coin comes up "heads," the woman would be assigned to one group; if the coin comes up "tails," she would be assigned to the other group.

Although randomization is the preferred scientific method for equalizing groups, there is no *guarantee* that the groups will, in fact, be equal. As an extreme example, suppose the study sample involves 10 women who have given birth to 4 or more children. Five of the 10 women are aged 35 years or older, and the remaining 5 are younger than age 35. We would expect random assignment to result in two or three women from the two age ranges in each group. But suppose that, by chance, the older five women all ended up in the experimental group. Because these women are nearing the end of their childbearing years, the likelihood of their conceiving is diminished. Thus, follow-up of their subsequent childbearing (the dependent variable) might suggest that the counseling program was effective in reducing subsequent pregnancies; however, a higher birth rate for the control group may reflect only age and fecundity differences, not lack of exposure to counseling.

Despite this possibility, randomization remains the most trustworthy and acceptable method of equalizing groups. Unusual or deviant assignments such as this one are rare, and the likelihood of obtaining markedly unequal groups is reduced as the number of subjects increases.

You may wonder why we do not consciously control those subject characteristics that are likely to affect the outcome. The procedure that is sometimes used to accomplish this is known as **matching**. For example, if matching were used in the contraceptive counseling study, we might want to ensure that if there were a married, 38-year-old woman with six children in the experimental group, there would be a married, 38-year-old woman with six children in the control group as well. There are two serious problems with matching, however. First, to match effectively, we must know (and measure) the characteristics that are likely to affect the dependent variable, but this information is not always known. Second, even if we knew the relevant traits, the complications of matching on more than two or three characteristics simultaneously are prohibitive. With random assignment, on the other hand, *all* possible distinguishing characteristics—age, gender, intelligence, blood type, religious affiliation, and so on—are likely to be equally distributed in all groups. Over the long run, the groups tend to be counterbalanced with respect to an infinite number of biologic, psychological, economic, and social traits.

To demonstrate how random assignment is performed, we turn to another example. Suppose we were testing two alternative interventions to lower the preoperative anxiety of children who are about to undergo tonsillectomy. One intervention involves giving structured information about the surgical team's activities (procedural information); the other involves structured information about what the child will feel (sensation information). A third control group receives no special intervention. With a sample of 15 subjects, 5 children will be in each of the 3 groups. With three groups, we cannot use a coin flip to determine group assignments. We could, however, write the children's names on slips of paper, put the slips into a hat, and then draw names. The first five individuals whose names were drawn would be assigned to group I, the second five would be assigned to group II, and the remaining five would be assigned to group III.

Pulling names from a hat involves a lot of work if the sample is big. Researchers typically use a **table of random numbers** in the randomization process. A portion of such a table is reproduced in Table 8-2. In a table of random numbers any digit from 0 to 9 is equally likely to follow any other digit. Going in any direction from any point in the table produces a random sequence.

In our example, we would number the 15 subjects from 1 to 15, as shown in the second column of Table 8-3, and then draw numbers between 01 and 15 from the random number table. A simple procedure for finding a starting point is to close your eyes and let your finger fall at some point on the table. For the sake of following the example, let us assume that our starting point is at number 52, circled on Table 8-2. We can move in any direction in the table from that point, selecting numbers that fall between 01 and 15. Let us move to the right, looking at two-digit combinations (to get numbers

TABLE 8.2 Small Table of Random Digits

46	85	05	23	26		34	67	75	83	00		74	91	06	43	45
69	24	89	34	60		45	30	50	75	21		61	31	83	18	55
14	01	33	17	92		59	74	76	72	77		76	50	33	45	13
56	30	38	73	15		16	**52**	06	96	76		11	65	49	98	93
81	30	44	85	85		68	65	22	73	76		92	85	25	58	66
70	28	42	43	26		79	37	59	52	20		01	15	96	32	67
90	41	59	36	14		33	52	12	66	65		55	82	34	76	41
39	90	40	21	15		59	58	94	90	67		66	82	14	15	75
88	15	20	00	80		20	55	49	14	09		96	27	74	**82**	57
45	13	46	35	45		59	40	47	20	59		43	94	75	16	80
70	01	41	50	21		41	29	06	73	12		71	85	71	59	57
37	23	93	32	95		05	87	00	11	19		92	78	42	63	40
18	63	73	75	09		82	44	49	90	05		04	92	17	37	01
05	32	78	21	62		20	24	78	17	59		45	19	72	53	32
95	09	66	79	46		48	46	08	55	58		15	19	11	87	82
43	25	38	41	45		60	83	32	59	83		01	29	14	13	49
80	85	40	92	79		43	52	90	63	18		38	38	47	47	61
80	08	87	70	74		88	72	25	67	36		66	16	44	94	31
80	89	07	80	02		94	81	33	19	00		54	15	58	34	36
93	12	81	84	64		74	45	79	05	61		72	84	81	18	34
82	47	42	55	93		48	54	53	52	47		18	61	91	36	74
53	34	24	42	76		75	12	21	17	24		74	62	77	37	07
82	64	12	28	20		92	90	41	31	41		32	39	21	97	63
13	57	41	72	00		69	90	26	37	42		78	46	42	25	01
29	59	38	86	27		94	97	21	15	98		62	09	53	67	87
86	88	75	50	87		19	15	20	00	23		12	30	28	07	83
44	98	91	68	22		36	02	40	08	67		76	37	84	16	05
93	39	94	55	47		94	45	87	42	84		05	04	14	98	07
52	16	29	02	86		54	15	83	42	43		46	97	83	54	82
04	73	72	10	31		75	05	19	30	29		47	66	56	43	82

Reprinted from *A Million Random Digits with 100,000 Normal Deviates*. New York: The Free Press, 1955. Used with permission of the Rand Corporation, Santa Monica, CA.

TABLE 8.3 Example of Random Assignment Procedure		
NAME OF SUBJECT	**NUMBER**	**GROUP ASSIGNMENT**
Kristina N.	1	I
Trevor S.	2	III
Adeline B.	3	III
Lauren C.	4	II
Rebecca C.	5	II
Nathan O.	6	I
Lindsey S.	7	III
Thomas N.	8	III
Sean S.	9	II
Amy D.	10	III
Alana M.	11	I
Emily B.	12	II
Gabriel B	13	II
Taylor M.	14	I
Christopher R.	15	I

TABLE 8.4 Breakdown of the Gender Composition of the Three Groups			
GENDER	**GROUP I**	**GROUP II**	**GROUP III**
Boys	3	2	2
Girls	2	3	3

appeared four times during the randomization procedure. This is perfectly normal because the numbers are random. After the first time a number appears and is used, subsequent appearances can be ignored.

It might be useful to look at the three groups to see if they are about equal with respect to one readily discernible characteristic, that is, the subjects' gender. We started out with eight girls and seven boys in all. As Table 8-4 shows, randomization did a good job of allocating boys and girls about equally across the three research groups. We must accept on faith the probability that other characteristics (e.g., family income, health status, preoperative anxiety) are fairly well distributed in the randomized groups as well.

TIP: Researchers usually do not have the full sample assembled when the study begins, but rather take subjects into the sample on a "rolling enrollment" basis. However, the same system as just described can be used *without knowing any names* if sample size is predetermined. Thus, using the assignments shown in Table 8-3, in a study of 15 subjects and three groups, the first person to enter the study would be assigned to Group I, the second and third person would be assigned to Group III, and so on. This method ensures that the sample sizes for the groups being compared are equal.

greater than 9, i.e., from 10 to 15). The number to the right of 52 is 06. The person whose number is 06, Nathan O., is assigned to group I. Moving along in the table, the next number within the range of 01 to 15 is 11. (To find numbers in the required range, we have to bypass numbers between 16 and 99.) Alana M., whose number is 11, is also assigned to group I. When we get to the end of the row, we move down to the next row, and so forth. The next three numbers are 01, 15, and 14. Thus, Kristina N., Christopher R., and Taylor M. are all put into group I. The next five numbers between 01 and 15 that emerge in the random number table are used to assign five individuals to group II in the same fashion, as shown in the third column of Table 8-3. The remaining five people in the sample are put into group III. Note that numbers that have already been used often reappear in the table before the task is completed. For example, the number 15

Note that in the previous discussion we did not say that the five subjects in group I would be assigned to the procedural information group. This is because it is a good strategy to randomly assign groups to treatments, as well as individuals to groups. Let us give the procedural information, sensation information, and control conditions the numbers 1, 2, and 3, respectively. Finding a new starting point in the random number table, we look for the numbers 1, 2, or 3. This time we can look at one digit at a time because 3 is the biggest number. We will start at number 8 in the ninth row of the table, indicated by a rectangle. Reading *down* this time, we find the number 1. We therefore assign group I to the procedural information condition. Further along in the same column we come to the number 3. Group III, therefore, is assigned to the second condition, sensation information, and the remaining group, group II, is assigned to the control condition.

In most cases, as just discussed, randomization involves the random assignment of individual subjects to different groups. However, an alternative is **cluster randomization**, which involves randomly assigning *clusters* of individuals to different treatment groups (Hauck, Gilliss, Donner, & Gortner, 1991). Cluster randomization may sometimes enhance the feasibility of conducting a true experiment. Groups of patients who enter a hospital unit at the same time, or groups of patients from different medical practices, can be randomly assigned to a treatment condition as a unit—thus ruling out, in some situations, some practical impediments to randomization. This approach also reduces the possibility of **contamination** between two different treatments, that is, the mingling of subjects in the groups, which could reduce the effectiveness of the manipulation. The main disadvantages of cluster randomization are that the statistical analysis of data obtained through this approach is more complex, and sample size requirements are usually greater for a given level of accuracy.

Researchers usually assign subjects to groups in proportion to the number of groups being compared. For example, a sample of 300 subjects in a 2-group design would generally have 150 people in the experimental group and 150 in the control group. If there were 3 groups being compared, there would be 100 per group. However, it is also possible (and sometimes desirable ethically) to have a different allocation. For example, if an especially promising treatment for a serious illness were developed, we could assign 200 to the treatment group and 100 to the control group. Such an allocation does, however, make it more difficult to detect treatment effects at statistically significant levels.

Experimental Designs

There are numerous experimental designs; the most widely used designs are described in this section and summarized in Table 8-5.

Basic Experimental Designs

At the beginning of this chapter, we described a study that tested the effect of gentle massage on the pain levels of elderly nursing home residents. This example illustrates a simple design that is sometimes referred to as an **after-only design** or a **posttest-only design** because data on the dependent variable are collected only once—after random assignment is completed and the experimental treatment has been introduced.

 Example of a posttest-only experimental design:

Milne (2000) used a posttest-only design to study the effect of an educational intervention relating to urinary incontinence on the subsequent help-seeking behavior of older adults. One group received individualized instruction and written information, and the other received written information alone. Two months later, Milne determined how many subjects in each group sought professional help for urinary incontinence.

A second basic design is the most widely used experimental design by nurse researchers. Suppose we hypothesized that convective airflow blankets are more effective than conductive water-flow blankets in cooling critically ill patients with fever. We decide to use a design that involves assigning patients to the two different types of blankets (the independent variable) and measuring the dependent variable (body temperature) twice, before and after the intervention. This scheme permits us to examine whether one blanket type is more effective that the other in *reducing* fever—that is, with this design researchers can examine *change*. This design, because of its two measurement points, is referred to as a

TABLE 8.5 Experimental Designs

NAME OF DESIGN	PREINTERVENTION DATA?	WITHIN- OR BETWEEN-GROUPS	FEATURES
Posttest-only (after-only)	No	Between	One data collection point after the intervention; not appropriate for measuring *change*
Pretest–posttest (before–after)	Yes	Between	Data collection both before and after the intervention; appropriate for measuring change; can determine differences between groups (experimental) and change within groups (quasi- experimental)
Solomon four-group	For some subjects	Between	Data collection before and after the intervention for one experimental and one control group, but after only for a second experimental and control group, to assess pretest effects
Factorial	Optional	Between	Experimental manipulation of more than one independent variable; permits a test of *main effects* for each manipulated variable and *interaction effects* for combinations of manipulated variables
Randomized block	Optional	Between	Random assignment to groups within different levels of a blocking variable that is not under experimental control (e.g., gender)
Crossover/repeated measures	Optional	Within	Subjects are exposed to all treatments but are randomly assigned to different orderings of treatments; subjects serve as their own controls

before—after design or a **pretest—posttest design**. In such designs, the initial measure of the dependent variable is often referred to as the **baseline measure**, and the posttest measure of the dependent variable may be referred to as the **outcome measure**—that is, the measure that captures the outcome of the experimental intervention.

 TIP: When using an experimental design that involves the collection of data both before and after the intervention, it is considered good practice to collect the pretest data *before* randomization to groups. This ensures that subjects (and researchers) will not be biased in any way by knowledge of the group assignments.

 Example of a pretest—posttest experimental design:

Sandgren, McCaul, King, O'Donnell, and Foreman (2000) conducted an experiment to test the effectiveness of a cognitive-behavioral telephone therapy intervention for patients with breast cancer. Women in the study were randomly assigned to the intervention or to a control group. The dependent variables (e.g., psychological distress, coping, and quality of life) were measured at baseline and at follow-up, and changes over time were determined.

Solomon Four-Group Design

When data are collected both before and after an intervention, as in a pretest—posttest design, the posttest measure of the dependent variable may be affected not only by the treatment but also by exposure to the pretest. For example, if the intervention was a workshop to improve nurses' attitudes toward patients with AIDS, a pretest attitudinal measure may in itself constitute a sensitizing treatment that could mask the workshop's effectiveness. Such a situation calls for the **Solomon four-group design**, which involves two experimental groups and two control groups. One experimental group and one control group are administered the pretest and the other groups are not, thereby allowing the effects of the pretest measure and intervention to be segregated. Figure 8-1 illustrates this design.

 Example of a Solomon four-group design:

Swanson (1999) used a Solomon four-group design in her study of the effects of a caring-based counseling intervention on the emotional well-being of women who had had a miscarriage. Swanson adopted this design because of a concern that "the potential existed that participating in a longitudinal control group with early focused attention on loss might, in itself, serve as a form of recognition, support, and validation" (p. 290).

Group	Data Collection Before	Data Collection After
Experimental—with pretest	X	X
Experimental—without pretest		X
Control—with pretest	X	X
Control—without pretest		X

FIGURE 8.1 Solomon four-group experimental design.

Factorial Design

The three designs described thus far are ones in which the experimenter manipulates only one independent variable. It is possible, however, to manipulate two or more variables simultaneously. Suppose we were interested in comparing two therapeutic strategies for premature infants: tactile stimulation versus auditory stimulation. At the same time, we are interested in learning if the daily *amount* of stimulation (15, 30, or 45 minutes) affects infants' progress. The dependent variables for the study are measures of infant development (e.g., weight gain and cardiac responsiveness). Figure 8-2 illustrates the structure of this experiment.

This **factorial design** permits the testing of multiple hypotheses in a single experiment. In this example, the three research questions being addressed are as follows:

1. Does auditory stimulation have a more beneficial effect on the development of premature infants than tactile stimulation, or vice versa?

Type of stimulation

		Auditory A1		Tactile A2	
Daily exposure	15 Min. B1	A1	B1	A2	B1
	30 Min. B2	A1	B2	A2	B2
	45 Min. B3	A1	B3	A2	B3

FIGURE 8.2 Example of a factorial design.

2. Is the duration of stimulation (independent of type) related to infant development?
3. Is auditory stimulation most effective when linked to a certain dose and tactile stimulation most effective when coupled with a different dose?

The third question demonstrates the strength of factorial designs: they permit us to evaluate not only **main effects** (effects resulting from experimentally manipulated variables, as exemplified in questions 1 and 2) but also **interaction effects** (effects resulting from combining treatments). We may feel that it is insufficient to say that auditory stimulation is preferable to tactile stimulation (or vice versa) and that 45 minutes of stimulation per day is more effective than 15 or 30 minutes per day. How these two variables interact (how they behave in combination) is also of interest. Our results may indicate that 15 minutes of tactile stimulation and 45 minutes of auditory stimulation are the most beneficial treatments. We could not have learned this by conducting two separate experiments that manipulated only one independent variable and held the second one constant.

In factorial experiments, subjects are assigned at random to a specific combination of conditions. In the example that Figure 8-2 illustrates, premature infants would be assigned randomly to one of six cells. A **cell** in experimental research refers to a treatment condition; it is represented in a schematic diagram as a box (cell) in the design.

Figure 8-2 can also be used to define some design terminology. The two independent variables in a factorial design are the **factors**. Type of stimulation is factor A and amount of daily exposure is factor B. Each factor must have two or more **levels** (if there were only one level, the factor would not be a variable). Level 1 of factor A is auditory and level 2 of factor A is tactile. When describing the dimensions of the design, researchers refer to the number of levels. The design in Figure 8-2 is 2×3 design: two levels in factor A times three levels in factor B. If a third source of stimulation, such as visual stimulation, were added, and if a daily dosage of 60 minutes were also added, the design would be a 3×4 design. Factorial experiments can be performed with three or more independent variables (factors), but designs with more than three factors are rare.

Example of a factorial design:
Schultz, Ashby-Hughes, Taylor, Gillis, and Wilkins (2000) used a 2×2 factorial design to study treatments to reduce diarrhea among critically ill tube-fed patients receiving antibiotics. One factor was fiber-containing versus fiber-free tube feedings. The second was administration of pectin versus a placebo. The researchers found a trend toward less diarrhea in the fiber/pectin group.

Randomized Block Design

A design that looks similar to a factorial design in structure is the **randomized block design**.* In such a design, there are two factors (independent variables), but one factor is *not* experimentally manipulated. Suppose that we were interested in comparing the effects of tactile versus auditory stimulation for male versus female infants. We could structure this as a 2×2 experiment, with type of stimulation as one factor and gender as the other. The variable gender, which we cannot manipulate, is known as a **blocking variable**. In an experiment to test the effectiveness of alternative stimulation therapies, we obviously could not randomly assign subjects to one of four cells, as in a factorial experiment, because infants' gender is a given. We can, however, randomly assign male and female subjects separately to the two stimulation methods. Suppose there are 40 male infants and 40 female infants available for the study. We would *not* randomly assign half the 80 infants to tactile stimulation and the other half to auditory stimulation. Rather, we would randomize boys and girls separately to the two treatments, thereby guaranteeing 20 subjects in each cell of this 4-cell design.

The inclusion of a blocking variable in a study design enhances the researcher's control over sample composition (i.e., to ensure that sufficient numbers of subjects with specific characteristics are included) and over extraneous variables. That is, if we consider gender a confounding variable because we believe that male and female infants will respond differently to the two therapies, then a randomized block design is

---

*The terminology for this design varies from text to text. Some authors refer to this as a *factorial design*; others call it a *levels-by-treatment design*.

needed. In randomized block designs, as in factorial designs, interaction effects can be examined.

Example of a randomized block design: Harrison, Williams, Berbaum, Stem, and Leeper (2000) used a randomized block design in their study of the effects of gentle human touch on such outcomes as behavioral distress, sleep, and motor activity in preterm infants. The infants were randomly assigned to an experimental or control group within blocks based on gestational age. The blocking variable divided the sample into three gestational age groups: 27 to 28 weeks; 29 to 31 weeks, and 32 to 33 weeks.

The design can be extended to include more than one blocking variable. For example, we could add infant birth weight as a blocking variable in our study of alternative stimulation therapies. It is also possible to include more than one manipulated variable, thereby creating a design that is both a randomized block and a factorial design. In theory, the number of blocking and manipulated variables is unlimited, but practical concerns usually dictate a relatively small number of each. Expansion of the design usually requires that more subjects be used. As a general rule of thumb, a minimum of 20 subjects per cell is recommended to achieve stability within cells. This means that, whereas a minimum of 80 subjects would be needed for a 2×2 design, 160 subjects would be needed for a $2 \times 2 \times 2$ design.

Example of a combined randomized block and factorial design: Metzger, Jarosz, and Noureddine (2000) studied the effects of two experimentally manipulated factors (high-fat versus low-fat diet and forced exercise versus sedentary condition) on obesity in rats. The blocking variable in this study was the genetic obesity of the rats: both genetically obese and lean rats were randomly assigned to the four treatment conditions, yielding a $2 \times 2 \times 2$ design.

Crossover Design

Thus far, we have described experimental studies in which subjects who are randomly assigned to different treatments are different people. For instance, in the previous example, the infants exposed to auditory stimulation were not the same infants as those exposed to tactile stimulation. A **crossover design** (also known as a **repeated measures design**) involves the exposure of the same subjects to more than one experimental treatment. This type of within-subjects design has the advantage of ensuring the highest possible equivalence among subjects exposed to different conditions— the groups being compared are equal with respect to age, weight, health, and so on because they are composed of the same people.

In a crossover experimental design, subjects are randomly assigned to different orderings of treatments. For example, if a crossover design were used to compare the effects of auditory and tactile stimulation on infant development, some infants would be randomly assigned to receive auditory stimulation first, and others would be assigned to receive tactile stimulation first. In such a study, the three conditions for an experiment have been met: there is manipulation, randomization, and a control group, with subjects serving as their own controls.

Although crossover designs are extremely powerful, they are inappropriate for certain research questions because of the problem of **carry-over effects**. When subjects are exposed to two different treatments or conditions, they may be influenced in the second condition by their experience in the first condition. As one example, drug studies rarely use a crossover design because drug B administered *after* drug A is not necessarily the same treatment as drug B administered *before* drug A.

Example of a crossover design: Winkelman (2000) used a randomized crossover design to examine the effect of two alternative backrest positions (flat/horizontal versus 30-degree elevation) on intracranial and cerebral perfusion pressures in brain-injured adults. The elevated position resulted in significant and clinically important improvements.

Experimental and Control Conditions

In designing experimental studies, researchers make many decisions about what the experimental and control conditions entail, and these decisions can affect the researchers' conclusions.

The Experimental Condition

To give an experimental intervention a fair test, researchers need to carefully design an intervention that is appropriate to the problem and of sufficient intensity and duration that effects might reasonably be expected. The full nature of the intervention must be clearly delineated in formal protocols that spell out exactly what the treatment is. Among the questions researchers need to address are the following:

- What *is* the intervention, and how does it differ from usual methods of care?
- If there are two alternative interventions, how exactly do they differ?
- What are the specific procedures to be used with those receiving the intervention?
- What is the dosage or intensity of the intervention?
- Over how long a period will the intervention be administered, how frequently will it be administered, and when will the treatment begin (e.g., 2 hours after surgery)?
- Who will administer the intervention? What are their credentials, and what type of special training will they receive?
- Under what conditions will the intervention be withdrawn or altered?

The goal in most experimental studies is to have a comparable intervention for all subjects in the treatment group. This goal is difficult to achieve without careful advance planning and clear written protocols.

TIP: Qualitative studies can provide valuable information in helping researchers develop interventions to be tested in experimental studies. Gamel, Grypdonck, Hengeveld, and Davis (2001) examined research findings from qualitative studies to develop a nursing intervention for women with gynecologic cancer. Their intervention focused on sexual adaptation and qualitative data helped bring the patient perspective into this treatment.

The Control Condition

The control group condition used as a basis of comparison in a study is referred to as the **counterfactual**. Researchers have choices about what to use as the counterfactual. Their decision is sometimes based on theoretical or substantive grounds, but may also be driven by practical or ethical concerns. In some research, control group subjects receive no treatment at all—they are merely observed with respect to performance on the dependent variable. This kind of situation is not always feasible for nursing research projects; if we wanted to evaluate the effectiveness of a nursing intervention on hospital patients, we would not devise an experiment in which patients in the control group received no nursing care at all. Among the possibilities for the counterfactual are the following:

1. An alternative intervention; for example, in our example of infant stimulation, subjects were exposed to alternative therapies.
2. A **placebo** or pseudointervention presumed to have no therapeutic value; for example, in studies of the effectiveness of drugs, some patients get the experimental drug and others get an innocuous substance, as in the previously described study by Schultz et al. (2000) that compared pectin with a placebo. Placebos are used to control for the nonpharmaceutical effects of drugs, such as the attention being paid to subjects (although there can be **placebo effects**—changes in the dependent variable attributable to the placebo condition—because of subjects' expectations).
3. Standard methods of care—the normal procedures used to treat patients; for example, in Parent and Fortin's (2000) study of an intervention for cardiac surgery patients, described later in this chapter, control group subjects were treated according to the usual hospital procedures for such patients.
4. Different doses or intensities of treatment wherein all subjects get some type of intervention, but the experimental group gets an intervention that is richer, more intense, or longer; for example, in Milne's (2000) study of an educational intervention regarding urinary incontinence for community-dwelling elders, one group got written instruction and the other got written instruction *plus* individual support.

5. Delayed treatment; that is, the control group eventually receives the full experimental treatment, but treatment is deferred.

Example of delayed treatment:
Garcia de Lucio, Gracia Lopez, Marin Lopez, Mas Hesse, and Camana Vaz (2000) tested the effectiveness of an intervention designed to improve the communication skills of nurses when interacting with relatives of seriously ill patients. The experimental group received immediate training; control group training was delayed 6 months. The communication skills of both groups were compared after the initial training, but before control subjects were trained.

Methodologically, the best possible test is between two conditions that are as different as possible, as when the experimental group receives a strong treatment and the control group gets no treatment at all. Ethically, however, the most appealing counterfactual is probably the "delay of treatment" approach (number 5), which may be difficult to do pragmatically. Testing two competing interventions (number 1) also has ethical appeal, but the risk is that the results will be inconclusive because it is difficult to detect differential effects, especially if both interventions are at least moderately effective.

Whatever decision is made about a control group strategy, researchers need to be as careful in spelling out the counterfactual as in delineating the intervention. In research reports, researchers sometimes say that the control group got the "usual methods of care" without explaining what that condition was and how different it was from the intervention being tested. In drawing on an evidence base for practice, nurses need to understand exactly what happened to study participants in different conditions.

TIP: Some researchers elect to combine two or more comparison strategies. For example, they might test two alternative treatments (option 1) against usual methods of care (option 3). Such an approach is attractive but, of course, adds to the cost and complexity of the study.

Strengths and Limitations of Experiments

Controlled experiments are often considered the ideal of science. In this section, we explore the reasons why experimental methods are held in high esteem and examine some of their limitations.

Experimental Strengths
True experiments are the most powerful method available for testing hypotheses of cause-and-effect relationships between variables. Studies using an experimental design are in general thought to yield the highest-quality evidence regarding the effects of specific interventions and nursing actions. Because of their special controlling properties, experiments offer greater corroboration than any other research approach that, *if* the independent variable (e.g., diet, drug dosage, or teaching approach) is manipulated in a specified way, *then* certain consequences in the dependent variable (e.g., weight loss, recovery of health, or learning) may be expected to ensue. This "if... then" type of relationship is important because of its implications for prediction and control. The great strength of experiments, then, lies in the confidence with which causal relationships can be inferred.

Lazarsfeld (1955), whose thinking reflects the ideas of John Stuart Mill, identified three criteria for causality. The first criterion is temporal: a cause must precede an effect in time. If we were testing the hypothesis that saccharin causes bladder cancer, it would be necessary to demonstrate that subjects had not developed cancer before exposure to saccharin. In experiments, researchers manipulate the independent variable and then measure subsequent outcomes, and so the sequence is under their control. The second requirement is that there be an empirical relationship between the presumed cause and the presumed effect. In the saccharin and cancer example, we would have to demonstrate an association between saccharin consumption and the presence of a carcinoma, that is, that a higher percentage of saccharin users than nonusers developed cancer. In an experiment, this empirical relationship between the independent and dependent variables is put to a direct test. The final criterion for establishing a causal relationship is that the relationship cannot be explained as being caused by a third variable. Suppose, for instance, that people who elect to use saccharin tend also to drink more coffee than nonusers of saccharin. There would then be a possibility that any relationship between saccharin use and bladder cancer reflects an underlying causal relationship between a substance in coffee and bladder cancer. It is particularly because of this third criterion that the experimental approach is so strong. Through the controls imposed by manipulation, comparison, and randomization, alternative explanations to a causal interpretation can often be ruled out or discredited.

Experimental Limitations

Despite the benefits of experimental research, this type of design also has limitations. First of all, there are often constraints that make an experimental approach impractical or impossible. These constraints are discussed later in this chapter.

Experiments are sometimes criticized for their artificiality. Part of the difficulty lies in the requirements for randomization and then equal treatment within groups. In ordinary life, the way we interact with people is not random. For example, certain aspects of a patient (e.g., age, physical appearance, or severity of illness) may cause us to modify our behavior and our care. The differences may be subtle, but they undoubtedly are not random. Another aspect of experiments that is sometimes considered artificial is the focus on only a handful of variables while holding all else constant. This requirement has been criticized as being reductionist and as artificially constraining human experience. Experiments that are undertaken without a guiding theoretical framework are sometimes criticized for being able to establish a causal connection between an independent and dependent variable without providing any causal explanation for *why* the intervention resulted in the observed outcomes.

A problem with experiments conducted in clinical settings is that it is often clinical staff, rather than researchers, who administer an intervention, and therefore it can sometimes be difficult to determine if subjects in the experimental group actually received the treatment, and if those in the control group did not. It may be especially difficult to maintain the integrity of the intervention and control conditions if the study period extends over time. Moreover, clinical studies are usually conducted in environments over which researchers have little control—and control is a critical factor in experimental research. McGuire and her colleagues (2000) describe some issues relating to the challenges of testing interventions in clinical settings.

Sometimes a problem emerges if subjects themselves have discretion about participation in the treatment. Suppose, for example, that we randomly assigned patients with HIV infection to a special support group intervention or to a control group. Experimental subjects who elect not to participate in the support groups, or who participate infrequently, actually are in a "condition" that looks more like the control condition than the experimental one. The treatment is diluted through nonparticipation, and it may become difficult to detect any effects of the treatment, no matter how effective it might otherwise have been. Such issues need to be taken into consideration in designing the study.

Another potential problem is the **Hawthorne effect**, which is a placebo effect. The term is derived from a series of experiments conducted at the Hawthorne plant of the Western Electric Corporation in which various environmental conditions, such as light and working hours, were varied to determine their effects on worker productivity. Regardless of what change was introduced, that is, whether the light was made better or worse, productivity increased. Knowledge of being included in the study appears to have affected people's behavior, thereby obscuring the effect of the variable of interest. In a hospital situation, researchers might have to contend with a double Hawthorne effect. For example, if an experiment to investigate the effect of a new postoperative patient routine were conducted, nurses and hospital staff, as well as patients, might be aware of their participation in a study, and both groups might alter their actions accordingly. It is precisely for this reason that **double-blind experiments**, in which neither subjects nor those who administer the treatment know who is in the experimental or control group, are so powerful. Unfortunately, the double-blind approach is not feasible for most nursing studies because nursing interventions are more difficult to disguise than drugs.

 Example of a double-blind experiment: McCormick, Buchman, and Maki (2000) used a double-blind approach (with a before—after design) to test the effectiveness of two alternative hand-care treatments (an oil-containing lotion and a novel barrier skin cream) for health care workers with severe hand irritation. Subjects in both groups experienced marked improvements.

In sum, despite the clearcut superiority of experiments in terms of their ability to test causal hypotheses, they are subject to a number of limitations, some of which may make them difficult to apply to real-world problems. Nevertheless, with the growing demand for evidence-based practice, true experimental designs are increasingly being used to test the effects of nursing practices and procedures.

Research Example of an Experimental Study

Parent and Fortin (2000) used an experimental design to test an intervention for reducing anxiety and increasing postoperative activity in male cardiac surgery patients. The intervention involved "vicarious experience," in which patients about to undergo elective coronary artery bypass graft (CABG) surgery were linked to volunteers who had recovered from similar surgery. The linkage, which involved three supportive visits during the hospitalization and recovery period, was designed to demonstrate the active lives former patients were leading.

A sample of 56 first-time male patients undergoing CABG surgery were randomly assigned to the experimental vicarious experience group or to a control group not receiving the special intervention. Patients in both groups were given routine information on surgery and recovery by health professionals. A coin flip was used to assign subjects to groups. The two groups were found to be comparable before the intervention in terms of a wide range of background characteristics (age, occupa-tional category, smoking status, number of bypass grafts). However, the average baseline anxiety level of those in the experimental group was significantly higher than that of control group members. Thus, randomization equalized the two groups on most, but not all, characteristics. By chance alone, more high-anxiety patients were assigned to the treatment group.

A before—after design was used to assess declines in patient anxiety. Anxiety was measured at 48 hours and 24 hours before surgery, and again at 5 days and 4 weeks after surgery. Data collection after surgery also involved questions about activities and about self-efficacy expectations.

Despite the initially higher anxiety levels of the men who received the vicarious experience treatment, the experimental group had significantly lower anxiety levels after the intervention than the control group. Only men in the experimental group showed a significant decline in anxiety during hospitalization; moreover, they reported higher levels of self-efficacy and self-reported activity after surgery than men in the control group. The researchers concluded that vicarious experience provided through dyadic support is an effective strategy to help cardiac patients cope with surgical anxiety.

TIP: In general, it is wise to randomize whenever possible, to reduce the possibility of biases. In an experiment, this means randomly assigning subjects to groups, groups to treatments, and conditions to subjects (in a repeated measures design). It also means, in general, looking for other opportunities to randomize whenever conditions vary across subjects, such as randomly assigning patients to rooms or nursing staff to patients.

QUASI-EXPERIMENTS

Quasi-experiments, like true experiments, involve the manipulation of an independent variable, that is, an intervention. However, quasi-experimental designs lack randomization to treatment groups, which characterizes true experiments, as shown in Figure 8-3.

Quasi-Experimental Designs

Quasi-experiments are not as powerful as experiments in establishing causal connections between interventions and outcomes. Before showing why

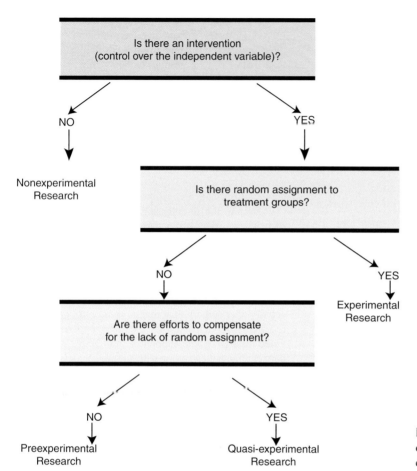

FIGURE 8.3 Characteristics of different quantitative research designs.

this is so, it is useful to introduce some notation based on Campbell and Stanley's (1963) classic monograph. Figure 8-4 presents a symbolic representation of a pretest—posttest experimental design. In this figure, R means random assignment to groups; O represents an observation (i.e., the collection of data on the dependent variable); and X stands for exposure to an intervention. Thus, the top line in this figure represents the experimental group that had subjects randomly assigned to it (R), had both a pretest (O_1) and a posttest (O_2), and has been exposed to an experimental intervention (X). The second row represents the control group, which differs from the experimental group only by absence of the treatment (X). We are now equipped to examine some quasi-experimental designs and to better understand their limitations relative to experimental designs.

Nonequivalent Control Group Designs

The most frequently used quasi-experimental design is the **nonequivalent control group pretest—posttest design**, which involves an experimental treatment and two groups of subjects observed before and after its implementation. Suppose, for example, we wished to study the effect of introducing primary nursing on staff morale in a large metropolitan hospital. Because the new system of nursing

R	O_1	X	O_2
R	O_1		O_2

R = Randomization
O = Observation or measurement
X = Treatment or intervention

FIGURE 8.4 Symbolic representation of a pretest–posttest (before–after) experimental design.

$$O_1 \qquad\qquad X \qquad\qquad O_2$$
$$O_1 \qquad\qquad\qquad\qquad\quad O_2$$

FIGURE 8.5 Nonequivalent control group pretest–posttest design (quasi-experimental).

$$\qquad\qquad X \qquad\qquad\qquad O$$
$$\qquad\qquad\qquad\qquad\qquad\quad O$$

FIGURE 8.6 Nonequivalent control group only posttest design (preexperimental).

care delivery is being implemented throughout the hospital, randomization is not possible. Therefore, we decide to collect comparison data from nurses in another similar hospital that is not instituting primary nursing. Data on staff morale is collected in both hospitals before the change is made (the pretest) and again after the new system is implemented in the first hospital (the posttest).

Figure 8-5 depicts this study symbolically. The top row is our experimental (primary nursing) hospital; the second row is the hospital using traditional nursing. A comparison of this diagram with the one in Figure 8-4 shows that they are identical, *except* that subjects have not been randomly assigned to treatment groups in the second diagram. The design in Figure 8-5 is the weaker of the two because *it can no longer be assumed that the experimental and comparison groups are equivalent at the outset.* Because there was no randomization, this study is quasi-experimental rather than experimental. The design is nevertheless strong, because the pretest data allow us to determine whether the groups had similar morale initially. If the comparison and experimental groups are similar on the pretest, we could be relatively confident that any posttest difference in self-reported morale was the result of the new system of nursing care. If the morale of the two groups is very different initially, however, it will be difficult to interpret any posttest differences, although there are statistical procedures that can help. Note that in quasi-experiments, the term **comparison group** is usually used in lieu of *control group* to refer to the group against which outcomes in the treatment group are evaluated.

Now suppose we had been unable to collect pretest data. This design, diagramed in Figure 8-6, has a flaw that is difficult to remedy. We no longer have information about the initial equivalence of the two nursing staffs. If we find that staff morale in the experimental hospital is lower than that in the con-trol hospital at the posttest, can we conclude that the new method of delivering care *caused* a decline in staff morale? There could be alternative explanations for the posttest differences. In particular, it might be that the morale of the employees in the two hospitals differed even at the outset. Campbell and Stanley (1963) call the *nonequivalent control group posttest-only design* in Figure 8-6 **preexperimental** rather than quasi-experimental because of its fundamental weakness. Thus, although quasi-experiments lack the controlling properties of true experiments, the hallmark of quasi-experiments is the effort to introduce strategies to compensate for the absence of either randomization or control groups.

Example of a nonequivalent control group pretest—posttest design:
Johnson, Budz, Mackay, and Miller (1999) evaluated the effect of a nurse-delivered smoking cessation intervention on smoking status and smoking self-efficacy among patients hospitalized with cardiac disease. Experimental subjects were admitted to one cardiac unit, and comparison subjects were admitted to another. The researchers preferred this approach to randomization within units because information sharing among patients in the same unit could have contaminated treatment conditions. By collecting pretest data, the researchers learned that the two groups were comparable with regard to demographic characteristics and preintervention smoking histories.

Time Series Designs

In the designs just described, a control group was used but randomization was not, but some studies involving an intervention have neither. Let us suppose that a hospital is adopting a requirement that all its nurses accrue a certain number of continuing education units before being eligible for a promotion or raise. The nursing administrators want to assess the consequences of this mandate on turnover rate,

$$O_1 \qquad X \qquad O_2$$

FIGURE 8.7 One group pretest–posttest design (preexperimental).

absentee rate, number of raises and promotions awarded, and so on. For the purposes of this example, assume there is no other hospital that can serve as a good comparison for this study. In such a case, the only kind of comparison that can be made is a before—after contrast. If the requirement were inaugurated in January, one could compare the turnover rate, for example, for the 3-month period before the new rule with the turnover rate for the subsequent 3-month period. The schematic representation of such a study is shown in Figure 8-7.

This **one-group pretest—posttest design** seems straightforward, but it has weaknesses. What if either of the 3-month periods is atypical, apart from the new regulation? What about the effects of any other hospital rules inaugurated during the same period? What about the effects of external factors that influence employment decisions, such as changes in the local economy? This preexperimental design cannot control these factors.*

This one-group pretest—posttest design could be modified so that at least some alternative explanations for change in nurses' turnover rate could be ruled out. One such design is the **time series design**, (sometimes referred to as the **interrupted time series design**) and is diagramed in Figure 8-8. In a time series design, information is collected over an extended period and an intervention is introduced during that period. In the figure, O_1 through O_4 represent four separate instances of data collection on a dependent variable before treatment; X represents the treatment (the introduction of the independent variable); and O_5 through O_8 represent four post-

treatment observations. In our present example, O_1 might be the number of nurses who left the hospital in January through March in the year before the new continuing education rule, O_2 the number of resignations in April through June, and so forth. After the rule is implemented, data on turnover are similarly collected for four consecutive 3-month periods, giving us observations O_5 through O_8.

Even though the time series design does not eliminate all problems of interpreting changes in turnover rate, the extended time period strengthens the ability to attribute change to the intervention. Figure 8-9 demonstrates why this is so. The two diagrams (A and B) in the figure show two possible outcome patterns for eight turnover observations. The vertical dotted line in the center represents the timing of the continuing education rule. Patterns A and B both reflect a feature common to most time series studies—fluctuation from one data point to another. These fluctuations are normal. One would not expect that, if 48 nurses resigned from a hospital in a year, the resignations would be spaced evenly with 4 resignations per month. It is precisely because of these fluctuations that the design shown in Figure 8-7, with only one observation before and after the experimental treatment, is so weak.

Let us compare the kind of interpretations that can be made for the outcomes reflected in Figure 8-9, patterns A and B. In both cases, the number of resignations increased between O_4 and O_5, that is, immediately after the new continuing education requirement. In B, however, the number of resignations fell at O_6 and continued to fall at O_7. The increase at O_5 looks similar to other apparently haphazard fluctuations in the turnover rate at other periods. Therefore, it probably would be erroneous to conclude that the new rule affected resignations. In A, on the other hand, the number of resignations increases at O_5 and remains relatively high for all subsequent observations. Of course, there may be other explanations for a change in turnover rate from one year to the next. The time series design, however, does permit us to rule out the possibility that the data reflect unstable measurements of resignations at only two points in time. If we had used the design in Figure 8-7, it would have been

---

*One-group before—after designs are not always unproductive. For example, if the intervention involved a brief teaching intervention, with baseline knowledge data obtained immediately before the intervention and posttest knowledge data collected immediately after it, it may be reasonable to conclude that the intervention caused gains in knowledge. This is because the intervention is the most plausible—and perhaps the only—explanation for knowledge gains.

$$O_1 \qquad O_2 \qquad O_3 \qquad O_4 \qquad X \qquad O_5 \qquad O_6 \qquad O_7 \qquad O_8$$

FIGURE 8.8 Time series design (quasi-experimental).

analogous to obtaining the measurements at O_4 and O_5 of Figure 8-9 only. The outcomes in both A and B look similar at these two points in time. Yet the broader time perspective leads us to draw different conclusions about two patterns of outcomes.

Example of a time series design:
Nahm and Poston (2000) used a time series design to assess the effect of an integrated point-of-case computer system on the quality of nurses' documentation. Measurements of the quality of documentation were made before the intervention was implemented, and again at 6-, 12-, and 18-months after implementation. The researchers found that quality of nursing documentation increased, and variability in charting decreased.

A particularly powerful quasi-experimental design results when the time series and non-equivalent control group designs are combined, as diagramed in Figure 8-10. In the example just described, **a time series nonequivalent control group design** would involve collecting data over an extended period from both the hospital introducing the continuing education mandate and another hospital not imposing the mandate. This use of information from another hospital with similar characteristics would make any inferences regarding the effects of the mandate more convincing because trends influenced by external factors would presumably be observed in both groups.

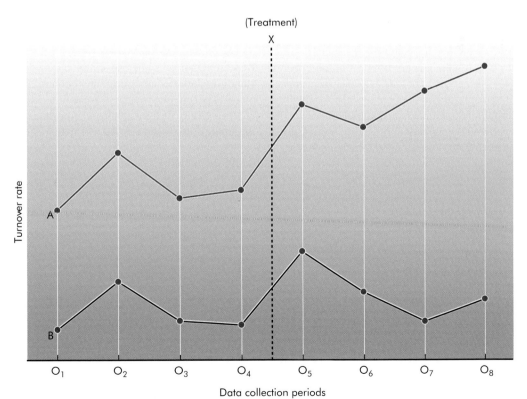

FIGURE 8.9 Two possible time series outcome patterns.

$$O_1 \quad O_2 \quad O_3 \quad O_4 \quad X \quad O_5 \quad O_6 \quad O_7 \quad O_8$$

$$O_1 \quad O_2 \quad O_3 \quad O_4 \quad \quad O_5 \quad O_6 \quad O_7 \quad O_8$$

FIGURE 8.10 Time series nonequivalent control group design (quasi-experimental).

 Example of a time series nonequivalent control group design:
Song, Daly, Rudy, Douglas, and Dyer (1997) examined rates of absenteeism and turnover among nurses working in a nurse-managed special care unit compared with nurses working in a traditional intensive care unit. The two units were compared over a 4-year period.

Numerous variations on the simple time series design are possible and are being used by nurse researchers. For example, additional evidence regarding the effects of a treatment can be achieved by instituting the treatment at several different points in time, strengthening the treatment over time, or instituting the treatment at one point in time and then **withdrawing** the treatment at a later point, sometimes with **reinstitution of treatment**. These three designs are diagramed in Figures 8-11 through 8-13. Clinical nurse researchers are often in a good position to use such time series designs because measures of patient functioning are usually routinely made at multiple points over an extended period.

A particular application of a time series approach sometimes used in clinical studies is called **single-subject experiments** (sometimes referred to as *N-of-1 studies*). Single-subject studies use time series designs to gather information about an intervention based on the responses of a single patient (or a small number of patients) under controlled conditions. In the literature on single-subject methods, the most basic design involves a baseline phase of data gathering (A) and an intervention phase (B), yielding what is referred to as an **AB design** (the design diagrammed in Fig. 8-8). If the treatment is withdrawn, it would be an ABA design; and if a withdrawn treatment is reinstituted (as diagramed in Fig. 8-13) it would be an ABAB design. Portney and Watkins (2000) offer valuable guidance about single-subject studies in clinical settings.

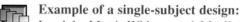 **Example of a single-subject design:**
Landolt, Marti, Widner, and Meuli (2002) used a single-subject experiment (with multiple patients) to test whether cartoon movie viewing is effective in decreasing burned children's pain behavior.

Experimental and Comparison Conditions

Researchers using a quasi-experimental approach, like those adopting an experimental design, should strive to develop strong interventions that provide an opportunity for a fair test, and must develop protocols documenting what the interventions entail. Researchers need to be especially careful in understanding and documenting the counterfactual in quasi-experiments. In the case of nonequivalent control group designs, this means understanding the conditions to which the comparison group is exposed. In our example of using a hospital with traditional nursing systems as a comparison for the new primary nursing system, the nature of that traditional system should be fully understood. In time series designs, the counterfactual is the condition existing before implementing the intervention.

Strengths and Limitations of Quasi-Experiments

A great strength of quasi-experiments is that they are practical. In the real world, it may be difficult, if not impossible, to conduct true experiments.

$$O_1 \quad O_2 \quad X \quad O_3 \quad O_4 \quad X \quad O_5 \quad O_6 \quad X \quad O_7 \quad O_8$$

FIGURE 8.11 Time series with multiple institutions of treatment (quasi-experimental).

$$O_1 \quad O_2 \quad X \quad O_3 \quad O_4 \quad X+1 \quad O_5 \quad O_6 \quad X+2 \quad O_7 \quad O_8$$

FIGURE 8.12 Time series with intensified treatment (quasi-experimental).

Nursing research usually occurs in real-life settings, where it is difficult to deliver an innovative treatment randomly to some people but not to others. Quasi-experimental designs introduce some research control when full experimental rigor is not possible.

Researchers using quasi-experimental designs need, however, to be acquainted with their weaknesses, and take these weaknesses into account in interpreting results. When a quasi-experimental design is used, there may be several **rival hypotheses** competing with the experimental manipulation as explanations for the results. (This is discussed further in Chapter 9.) Take as an example the case in which we administer certain medications to a group of babies whose mothers are heroin addicts to assess whether this treatment results in a weight gain in these typically low-birth-weight babies. If we use no comparison group or if we use a nonequivalent control group and then observe a weight gain, we must ask the questions: Is it *plausible* that some other factor caused or influenced the gain? Is it *plausible* that pretreatment differences between the experimental and comparison groups of babies resulted in differential gain? Is it *plausible* that the babies gained the weight simply as a result of maturation? If the answer is "yes" to any of these questions, then the inferences that can be made about the effect of the experimental treatment are weakened considerably. The plausibility of any one threat cannot, of course, be answered unequivocally. It is usually a situation in which judgment must be exercised. Because the conclusions from quasi-experiments ultimately depend in part on human judgment, rather than on more objective criteria, cause-and-effect inferences may be less convincing.

Research Example of a Quasi-Experimental Study

Bull, Hansen, and Gross (2000) used a strong quasi-experimental design to evaluate the effects of implementing a professional–patient partnership model of discharge planning with elders hospitalized with heart failure. The intervention was designed to facilitate identification of the elderly patients' needs for follow-up care and to identify those requiring more in-depth assessments.

The discharge planning model was implemented in one hospital, and a nonequivalent control group was secured through a different hospital that did not adopt the new model. The two hospitals were matched in terms of size, type, and the discharge planning practices used in the hospitals' cardiac units. Data on a range of measures (including health status, client satisfaction, and health locus of control) were collected from patients and caregivers before the intervention, and then again at 2 weeks and 2 months postdischarge. Moreover, data were gathered in both hospitals both before the intervention and then again after it was implemented, thus combining features of a nonequivalent control group design with that of a mini—time series. Unfortunately, however, data from the comparison group in the second hospital were contaminated by the fact that this hospital introduced an innovation that weakened comparisons. Thus, postintervention data from the experimental group were compared with two rather than three comparison groups, as originally planned: comparison groups from both hospitals before the new model being implemented. The three groups of elders were found to be comparable in terms of demographics and predischarge measures of health. The two comparison groups were combined for the analysis because of the absence of any significant differences.

The findings indicated that elders in the treatment group felt better prepared to manage care, reported more continuity of information about care management,

$$O_1 \quad O_2 \quad X \quad O_3 \quad O_4 \quad (-X) \quad O_5 \quad O_6 \quad X \quad O_7 \quad O_8$$

FIGURE 8.13 Time series with withdrawn and reinstituted treatment (quasi-experimental).

and felt they were in better health than elders in the comparison group. Moreover, elders in the treatment group who were readmitted to the hospital spent fewer days in the hospital than their comparison group counterparts. The strength of the design makes it possible to draw inferences about the effectiveness of the innovative discharge planning model, even in the absence of randomization.

NONEXPERIMENTAL RESEARCH

Many research problems cannot be addressed with an experimental or quasi-experimental design. For example, suppose we were interested in studying the effect of widowhood on health status. Our independent variable is widowhood versus nonwidowhood. Clearly, we cannot manipulate widowhood; people lose their spouses by a process that is neither random nor subject to research control. Thus, we would have to proceed by taking two groups (widows and nonwidows) as they naturally occur and comparing them in terms of health status.

Reasons for Undertaking Nonexperimental Research

Most studies involving human subjects, including nursing studies, are **nonexperimental**. One reason for using a nonexperimental design is that a vast number of human characteristics are inherently not subject to experimental manipulation (e.g., blood type, personality, health beliefs, medical diagnosis); the effects of these characteristics on other phenomena cannot be studied experimentally.

A second issue is that in nursing research, as in other fields, there are many variables that could technically be manipulated but could not be manipulated ethically. If manipulating the independent variable could cause physical or mental harm to subjects, then the variable should not be controlled experimentally. For example, if we were studying the effect of prenatal care on infant mortality, it would be unethical to provide such care to one group of pregnant women while deliberately depriving a second group. We would need to locate a naturally occurring group of pregnant women who

had not received prenatal care. Their birth outcomes could then be compared with those of women who had received appropriate care. The problem, however, is that the two groups of women are likely to differ in terms of many other characteristics, such as age, education, nutrition, and health, any of which individually or in combination could affect infant mortality, independent of the absence or presence of prenatal care. This is precisely why experimental designs are so strong in demonstrating cause-and-effect relationships.

Third, there are many research situations in which it is simply not practical to conduct a true experiment. Constraints might involve insufficient time, lack of administrative approval, excessive inconvenience to patients or staff, or lack of adequate funds.

Fourth, there are some research questions for which an experimental design is not appropriate. This is especially true for descriptive studies, which seek to document the characteristics, prevalence, intensity, or full nature of phenomena. As we discuss in Chapter 11, qualitative studies are nonexperimental. Manipulation is neither attempted nor considered desirable; the emphasis is on the normal experiences of humans.

Finally, nonexperimental research is usually needed before an experimental study can be planned. Experimental interventions are developed on the basis of nonexperimental research documenting the scope of a problem and describing critical relationships between relevant variables.

Ex Post Facto/Correlational Research

There are two broad classes of nonexperimental research, the first of which has been called **ex post facto research**. The literal translation of the Latin term *ex post facto* is "from after the fact." This means that the study has been conducted *after* variations in the independent variable have occurred. Ex post facto research attempts to understand relationships among phenomena as they naturally occur, without any intervention. Ex post facto research is more often referred to as **correlational research**. Basically, a **correlation** is an interrelationship or

GROUP A		X		O	Nonequivalent control group
GROUP B				O	(preexperimental) design

GROUP A			O	
GROUP B			O	Ex post facto design

FIGURE 8.14 Schematic diagram comparing nonequivalent control group and ex post facto designs.

association between two variables, that is, a tendency for variation in one variable to be related to variation in another. For example, in human adults, height and weight are correlated because there is a tendency for taller people to weigh more than shorter people.

Correlational studies often share some structural characteristics with experimental, quasi-experimental, and preexperimental research. If we use the notation scheme described in the previous section to represent symbolically the hypothetical study of the effects of widowhood, we find that it bears a strong resemblance to the nonequivalent control group posttest-only design. Both designs are presented in Figure 8-14. As these diagrams show, the preexperimental design is distinguished from the correlational study only by the presence of an X, the introduction of an intervention.

The purpose of correlational research, like experimental research, is to understand relationships among variables. It is, however, riskier to infer *causal* relationships in correlational research because of the lack of control over the independent variable. In experiments, investigators make a prediction that deliberate variation of X, the independent variable, will result in a change to Y, the dependent variable. For example, they might predict that if a new medication is administered, patient improvement will result. Experimenters have direct control over the X; the experimental treatment can be administered to some and withheld from others, and the two groups can be equalized with respect to everything except the independent variable through randomization.

In correlational research, on the other hand, investigators do not control the independent variable, which has already occurred. The examination of the independent variable—the presumed causative factor—is done after the fact. As a result, attempts to draw any cause-and-effect conclusions

are problematic. For example, we might hypothesize that there is a correlation between smoking and lung cancer, and empirical data would likely corroborate this expectation: smokers are more likely than nonsmokers to develop lung cancer. The inference we would like to make is that cigarette smoking *causes* cancer. This kind of inference, however, is subject to a fallacy called *post hoc, ergo propter hoc* ("after this, therefore caused by this"). The fallacy lies in the assumption that one thing has caused another merely because it occurred before the other.

To illustrate why a cause-and-effect conclusion might not be warranted, let us assume (strictly for the sake of an example) that there is a preponderance of cigarette smokers in urban areas, and people in rural areas are largely nonsmokers. Let us further assume that lung cancer is actually caused by poor environmental conditions in cities. Therefore, we would be incorrect to conclude that cigarette smoking causes lung cancer, despite the strong relationship shown to exist between the two variables. This is because there is *also* a strong relationship between cigarette smoking and the "real" causative agent, living in a polluted environment. Of course, cigarette smoking/lung cancer studies in reality have been replicated in so many different places with so many different groups of people that causal inferences are justified. This hypothetical example illustrates a famous research dictum: *Correlation does not prove causation*. The mere existence of a relationship—even a strong one—between variables is not enough to warrant the conclusion that one variable caused the other.

Although correlational studies are inherently weaker than experimental studies in elucidating cause-and-effect relationships, different designs offer different degrees of supportive evidence.

Retrospective Designs

Studies with a **retrospective design** are ones in which a phenomenon existing in the present is linked to phenomena that occurred in the past, before the study was initiated. That is, the researcher is interested in a present outcome and attempts to determine antecedent factors that caused it. Most of the early epidemiologic studies of the link between cigarette smoking and lung cancer were retrospective. In such a study, the researcher begins with groups of people with and without lung cancer (the dependent variable). The researcher then looks for differences between the two groups in antecedent behaviors or conditions. Retrospective studies are often cross-sectional, with data on both the dependent and independent variables collected once, simultaneously.

Researchers can sometimes strengthen a retrospective design by taking certain steps. For example, one type of retrospective design, referred to as a **case—control design**, involves the comparison of **cases** (subjects with a certain illness or condition, such as lung cancer victims) with controls (e.g., people without lung cancer). In conducting a strong case—control study, researchers find the cases and obtain from them (or *about* them, if records are available) information about the history of the presumed cause. Then the researchers must find controls without the disease or condition *who are as similar as possible to the cases with regard to key extraneous variables* (e.g., age, gender) and also obtain historical information about the presumed cause. If controls are well chosen, the only difference between them and the cases is exposure to the presumed cause. Researchers sometimes use **matching** or other techniques (described in Chapter 9) to control for extraneous variables. To the degree that researchers can demonstrate comparability between cases and controls with regard to extraneous traits, inferences regarding the presumed cause of the disease are enhanced.

Example of a retrospective study:
Heitkemper, Jarrett, Taylor, Walker, Landenburger, and Bond (2001) used a retrospective design in their study of factors contributing to

the onset of irritable bowel syndrome (IBS). They compared samples of women with and without IBS in terms of their history of sexual and physical abuse, and found that abusive experiences were more prevalent among women with IBS.

Prospective Nonexperimental Designs

A nonexperimental study with a **prospective design** (sometimes called a *prospective cohort design*) starts with a presumed cause and then goes forward in time to the presumed effect. For example, we might want to test the hypothesis that the incidence of rubella during pregnancy (the independent variable) is related to infant abnormalities (the dependent variable). To test this hypothesis prospectively, we would begin with a sample of pregnant women, including some who contracted rubella during their pregnancy and others who did not. The subsequent occurrence of congenital anomalies would be assessed for all subjects, and we would examine whether women with rubella were more likely than other women to bear malformed infants. Prospective designs are often longitudinal, but may also be cross-sectional (from the subjects' point of view) if reliable information about the independent variable is available in records or existing data sources.

TIP: Not all longitudinal studies are prospective, because sometimes the independent variable has occurred long before the initial wave of data collection. And not all prospective studies are longitudinal in the classic sense. For example, an experimental study that collects data at 2, 4, and 6 hours after an intervention would be considered prospective but not longitudinal (i.e., data are not collected over an extended period of time.)

Prospective studies are more costly than retrospective studies. For one thing, a substantial follow-up period may be necessary before the dependent variable manifests itself, as is the case in prospective studies of cigarette smoking and lung cancer. Also, prospective designs may require large samples, particularly if the dependent variable of interest is rare, as in the example of malformations associated with maternal rubella. Another issue is that in a good prospective study, researchers take steps to confirm that all subjects are free from the effect (e.g., the disease) at the time the independent variable is measured, and this may in some cases be difficult or expensive to do. For example, in prospective smoking/lung cancer studies, lung cancer may be present initially but not yet diagnosed.

Despite these issues, prospective studies are considerably stronger than retrospective studies. In particular, any ambiguity about whether the presumed cause occurred before the effect is resolved in prospective research if the researcher has confirmed the initial absence of the effect. In addition, samples are more likely to be representative, and investigators may be in a position to impose controls to rule out competing explanations for the results.

Some prospective studies are exploratory. That is, the researcher measures a wide range of possible "causes" at one point in time, and then examines an outcome of interest at a later point (e.g., length of stay in hospital). Such studies are usually stronger than retrospective studies if it can be determined that the outcome was not present initially because time sequences are clear. However, they are not as powerful as prospective studies that involve specific *a priori* hypotheses and the comparison of cohorts known to differ on a presumed cause. Researchers doing exploratory retrospective or prospective studies are sometimes accused of going on "fishing expeditions" that can lead to erroneous conclusions because of spurious or idiosyncratic relationships in a particular sample of subjects.

 Example of a prospective nonexperimental study:

Brook, Sherman, Malen, and Kollef (2000) conducted a prospective cohort study to examine clinical and cost outcomes of early versus late tracheostomy in patients who require prolonged mechanical ventilation. Early tracheostomy was found to be associated with shorter lengths of hospital stay and lower hospital costs.

Natural Experiments

Researchers are sometimes able to study the outcomes of a "**natural experiment**" in which a group exposed to natural or other phenomena that have important health consequences are compared with a nonexposed group. Such natural experiments are nonexperimental because the researcher does not intervene but simply observes the outcome of an external event or circumstance. However, they are called "natural *experiments*" when people are affected essentially at random. For example, the psychological well-being of people living in a community struck with a natural disaster (e.g., a hurricane) could be compared with the well-being of people living in a similar but unaffected community to determine the toll exacted by the disaster (the independent variable). Note that the independent variable does not need to be a "natural" phenomenon. It could, for example, be an act of terrorism. Moreover, the groups being compared do not need to be different people—if pre-event measures had been obtained, before—after comparisons might be profitable. Natural experiments can offer strong evidence about the effect of an independent variable on outcomes of interest if the comparison is carefully selected to achieve equivalence of groups being compared with regard to everything but the event.

Example of a natural experiment:

Keane, Jepson, Pickett, Robinson, and McCorkle (1996) studied the experiences of fire survivors, and attributed high levels of distress to those experiences 14 weeks after the fires, even among victims who did not sustain physical injury. Although there were no prefire measures of distress, it seems reasonable to attribute much of the stress to the "intervention" (the fires).

Path Analytic Studies

Researchers interested in testing theories of causation based on nonexperimental data are increasingly using a technique known as **path analysis** (or similar techniques). Using sophisticated statistical procedures, the researcher tests a hypothesized causal chain among a set of independent variables, mediating variables, and a dependent variable. Path analytic procedures, which are described more fully in Chapter 21, allow researchers to test whether nonexperimental data conform sufficiently to the underlying model to justify causal inferences.

 Example of a path analytic study:
Horsburgh, Beansland, Locking-Cusolito, Howe and Watson (2000) used path analysis to test a model to predict self-care in adults awaiting renal transplantation in Ontario. Their analyses tested hypothesized causal pathways between personality traits, health status, self-care abilities, and self-care behavior.

Descriptive Research

The second broad class of nonexperimental studies is **descriptive research**. The purpose of descriptive studies is to observe, describe, and document aspects of a situation as it naturally occurs and sometimes to serve as a starting point for hypothesis generation or theory development.

Descriptive Correlational Studies

Although researchers often focus on understanding the causes of behaviors, conditions, and situations, sometimes they can do little more than describe relationships without comprehending causal pathways. Many research problems are cast in noncausal terms. We ask, for example, whether men are less likely than women to bond with their newborn infants, not whether a particular configuration of sex chromosomes *caused* differences in parental attachment. Unlike other types of correlational research—such as the cigarette smoking and lung cancer investigations—the aim of **descriptive correlational research** is to describe the relationship among variables rather than to infer cause-and-effect relationships. Descriptive correlational studies are usually cross-sectional.

 Example of a descriptive correlational study:
Morin, Brogan, and Flavin (2002) described the relationship between body image perceptions of postpartum African-American women on the one hand, and their weight (based on the body mass index) on the other. Irrespective of body mass

category, women usually considered themselves larger than they were.

Univariate Descriptive Studies

Some descriptive studies are undertaken to describe the frequency of occurrence of a behavior or condition rather than to study relationships. For example, an investigator may wish to describe the health care and nutritional practices of pregnant teenagers. **Univariate descriptive studies** are not necessarily focused on only one variable. For example, a researcher might be interested in women's experiences during menopause. The study might describe the frequency of various symptoms, the average age at menopause, the percentage of women seeking formal health care, and the percentage of women using medications to alleviate symptoms. There are multiple variables in this study, but the primary purpose is to describe the status of each and not to relate them to one another.

Two types of descriptive study from the field of epidemiology are especially worth noting. **Prevalence studies** are done to determine the prevalence rate of some condition (e.g., a disease or a behavior, such as smoking) at a particular point in time. Prevalence studies rely on cross-sectional designs in which data are obtained from the population at risk of the condition. The researcher takes a "snapshot" of the population at risk to determine the extent to which the condition of interest is present. The formula for a **point prevalence rate** (PR) is:

$$\frac{\text{Number of cases with the condition or disease at a given point in time}}{\text{Number in the population at risk of being a case}} \times K$$

K is the number of people for whom we want to have the rate established (e.g., per 100 or per 1000 population). When data are obtained from a sample (as would usually be the case), the denominator is the size of the sample, and the numerator is the number of cases with the condition, as identified in the study.

If we sampled 500 adults aged 21 years and older living in a community, administered a measure of depression, and found that 80 people met the criteria for clinical depression, then the estimated point prevalence rate of clinical depression per 100 adults in that community would be 16 per 100.

Incidence studies are used to measure the frequency of developing *new* cases. Longitudinal designs are needed to determine incidence because the researcher must first establish who is at risk of becoming a new case—that is, who is free of the condition at the outset. The formula for an **incidence rate** (IR) is:

$$\frac{\text{Number of new cases with the condition}}{\text{or disease over a given time period}} \times K$$
$$\frac{}{\substack{\text{Number at risk of becoming a new case} \\ \text{(free of the condition at the outset)}}}$$

If we continued with our previous example, suppose in October, 2001 we found that 80 in a sample of 500 people were clinically depressed (PR = 16 per 100). To determine the 1-year incidence rate, we would reassess the sample in October, 2002. Suppose that, of the 420 previously deemed *not* to be clinically depressed in 2001, 21 were now found to meet the criteria for depression. In this case, the estimated 1-year incidence rate would be 5 per 100 ((21 ÷ 420) × 100 = 5).

Prevalence and incidence rates can be calculated for subgroups of the population (e.g., for men versus women). When this is done, it is possible to calculate another important descriptive index. **Relative risk** is an estimate of risk of "caseness" in one group compared with another. Relative risk is computed by dividing the rate for one group by the rate for another. Suppose we found that the 1-year incidence rate for depression was 6 per 100 women and 4 per 100 men. Women's relative risk for developing depression over the 1-year period would be 1.5, that is, women would be estimated to be 1.5 times more likely to develop depression than men. Relative risk is an important index in determining the contribution of risk factors to a disease or condition (e.g., by comparing the relative risk for lung cancer for smokers versus nonsmokers).

 Example of an incidence and prevalence study:

Whittington, Patrick, and Roberts (2000) conducted a national study involving 116 acute care facilities in 34 states to determine the incidence and prevalence of pressure ulcers. Prevalence for 17,650 patients in medical-surgical or intensive care units was measured during a 24-hour period at each facility. Incidence was measured over the average length of hospital stay for each facility.

Strengths and Limitations of Correlational Research

The quality of a study is not necessarily related to its approach; there are many excellent nonexperimental studies as well as flawed experiments. Nevertheless, nonexperimental studies have several drawbacks, and we focus here on the weaknesses of correlational studies.

Limitations of Correlational Research

As already noted, the major disadvantage of nonexperimental studies is that, relative to experimental and quasi-experimental research, they are weak in their ability to reveal causal relationships. Correlational studies are susceptible to faulty interpretations. This situation arises because the researcher works with preexisting groups that were not formed at random, but rather by a self-selecting process. Kerlinger and Lee (2000) offer the following description of **self-selection**:

> Self-selection occurs when the members of the groups being studied are in the groups, in part, because they differentially possess traits or characteristics extraneous to the research problem, characteristics that possibly influence or are otherwise related to the variables of the research problem (p. 560).

A researcher doing a correlational study, unlike an experimental study, cannot assume that the groups being compared are similar before the occurrence of the independent variable. Thus, preexisting differences may be a plausible alternative explanation for any group differences on the dependent variable.

To illustrate this problem, let us consider a hypothetical study in which a researcher is examining the relationship between type of nursing program a person attended (the independent variable) and job satisfaction 1 year after graduation. If the investigator finds that diploma school graduates are more satisfied with their work than baccalaureate graduates, the conclusion that the diploma school program leads to increased job satisfaction may or may not be accurate. The students in the two programs undoubtedly differed to begin with in terms of a number of important characteristics, such as personality, career goals, personal values, and so forth. Students selected themselves into one of the two programs and selection traits may have caused different job expectations and satisfactions.

The difficulty of interpreting correlational findings stems from the fact that, in the real world, behaviors, states, attitudes, and characteristics are interrelated (correlated) in complex ways. Another example may help to clarify the problems of interpreting results from correlational studies. Suppose we conducted a cross-sectional study that examined the relationship between level of depression in cancer patients and their social support (i.e., assistance and emotional sustenance through a social network). We hypothesize that social support (the independent variable) affects levels of depression (the dependent variable). Suppose we find that the patients without social support are significantly more depressed than the patients with adequate social support. We could interpret this finding to mean that people's emotional states are influenced by the adequacy of their social supports. This relationship is diagrammed in Figure 8-15A. There are, however, alternative explanations. Perhaps there is a third variable that influences *both* social support and depression, such as the patients' family configuration (e.g., whether they are married or have children). It may be that the availability or quantity of significant others is a powerful influence on how depressed cancer patients feel *and* on the quality of their social support. This set of relationships is diagramed in Figure 8-15B. A third possibility may be reversed causality, as shown in Figure 8-15C. Depressed cancer patients may find it more difficult to elicit needed social support from others than patients who are more cheerful or sociable. In this interpretation, the person's depression causes the amount of received social support, and not the other way around. You may be able to invent other alternatives. The point is that interpretations of most correlational results should be considered tentative, particularly if the research has no theoretical basis.

Strengths of Correlational Research

Earlier, we discussed constraints that limit the possibility of applying experimental designs to some research problems. Correlational research will continue to play a crucial role in nursing, medical, and social science research precisely because many interesting problems in those fields are not amenable to experimentation.

Despite our emphasis on causal relationships, it has already been noted that some kinds of research, such as descriptive research, do not focus on understanding causal networks. Furthermore, if the study is testing a causal hypothesis that has

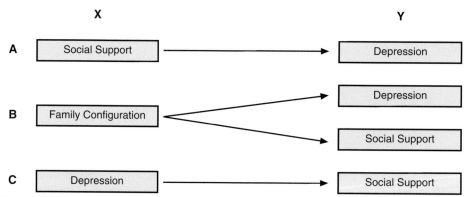

FIGURE 8.15 Alternative explanations for relationship between depression and social support in cancer patients.

been deduced from an established theory, causal inferences may be possible, especially if strong designs (e.g., a prospective design) have been used.

Correlational research is often an efficient means of collecting a large amount of data about a problem. For example, it would be possible to collect extensive information about the health histories and eating habits of a large number of individuals. Researchers could then examine which health problems were associated with which diets, and could thus discover a large number of interrelationships in a relatively short amount of time. By contrast, an experimenter looks at only a few variables at a time. One experiment might manipulate foods high in cholesterol, whereas another might manipulate protein consumption, for example.

Finally, correlational research is often strong in realism and therefore has an intrinsic appeal for solving practical problems. Unlike many experimental studies, correlational research is seldom criticized for its artificiality.

TIP: It is usually advantageous to design a study with as many relevant comparisons as possible. Preexperimental designs are weak in part because the comparative information they yield is limited. In nonexperimental studies, multiple comparison groups can be effective in dealing with self-selection, especially if the comparison groups are selected to address competing biases. For example, in case—control studies of patients with lung cancer, one comparison group could comprise people with a respiratory disease other than lung cancer and a second could comprise those with no respiratory disorder.

Research Example of a Nonexperimental Study

Faulkner, Hathaway, Milstead, and Burghen (2001) noted that there was little evidence about the onset or trajectory of cardiovascular autonomic deterioration in people with type 1 diabetes. To help fill this void, they conducted a cross-sectional nonexperimental study to examine whether age (adolescent versus adult) and diabetes status were associated with differences in measures of heart rate variability. Their descriptive correlational design involved four groups of subjects: adults with type 1 diabetes and renal failure, healthy similar-aged adult control subjects, adolescents with type 1 diabetes, and healthy adolescent control subjects. Most of the adult patients with diabetes had been diagnosed during childhood or adolescence.

The researchers conducted reflex tests to measure subjects' short-term R-R (beat-to-beat) heart rate variability, with deep breathing and with the Valsalva maneuver, in a temperature-controlled and noise-controlled laboratory environment. In addition, 24-hour ambulatory heart rate monitoring with power spectral analysis was obtained. The researchers then examined differences among subjects in the four groups in evoked, frequency, and time domain measures for heart rate variability.

The results indicated that adult patients with type 1 diabetes had significantly poorer heart rate variability measures than subjects in the other three groups. Adult control subjects had significantly lower average values than either of the two adolescent groups. Although most long-term R-R variability measures were lower in adolescents with diabetes than those without the disease, only one measure was significantly lower. Nevertheless, the researchers noted that the trends were important because they provide evidence that autonomic neuropathy begins relatively early in the course of diabetes.

In this example, the researchers were able to describe differences in heart rate variability in relation to two independent variables, age and diabetes status. Neither of these variables could have been experimentally manipulated and so a nonexperimental study was required.

DESIGNS AND RESEARCH EVIDENCE

Evidence for nursing practice depends on descriptive, correlational, and experimental research. There is often a logical progression to knowledge expansion that begins with rich description, including description from qualitative research. Descriptive studies can be invaluable in documenting the prevalence, nature, and intensity of health-related conditions and behaviors, and are critical in the development of effective interventions. Descriptive studies that contribute to the development of descriptive theories can make a particularly valuable contribution.

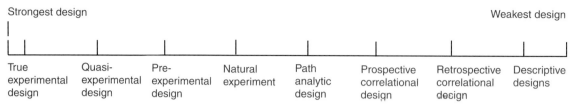

FIGURE 8.16 Continuum of designs for inferring causality.

Correlational studies are often undertaken in the next phase of developing a knowledge base. Exploratory retrospective studies may pave the way for more rigorous case—control studies, and for prospective studies. As the knowledge base builds, conceptual models may be developed and tested using path analytic designs and other nonexperimental theory-testing strategies. These studies can provide hints about how to structure an intervention, who can most profit from it, and when it can best be instituted. Thus, the next important phase is to develop interventions to improve health outcomes.

During the design and early testing of an intervention, it is often appropriate to conduct a **pilot study** (sometimes called a **feasibility study**). Rigorous experimental tests of interventions are expensive, and so it is often useful to begin with a small-scale test to determine the feasibility of a larger study and to ascertain whether a proposed approach shows promise. Feasibility can be assessed in terms of various considerations, including acceptability of the intervention to clients and to staff administering it; costs of the intervention; and ease of integrating it into clinical settings. Pilot studies can provide clues about the likely success of the intervention, and about ways in which the intervention can be strengthened or modified. Pilot studies also provide methodologic guidance (e.g., in determining sample size requirements for a full test, or strategies for recruiting subjects).

TIP: A pilot study is *not* the same as a small-scale study. The term *pilot study* has been misused by some researchers who appear to use it as an excuse for not using a bigger sample (King, 2001). The purpose of a pilot study is not so much to test research hypotheses, but rather to test

protocols, data collection instruments, sample recruitment strategies, and other aspects of a study in preparation for a larger study.

Example of a pilot study:
Zust (2000) described a pilot study that explored the feasibility of a future large-scale experiment to test the effectiveness of a 20-week cognitive therapy intervention on depressed battered women. The pilot test used an experimental before—after design with a sample of 18 rural women. The results supported an expanded test of the intervention.

The progression of evidence-building from descriptive studies to rigorous experimental ones is related to the ability of designs to reveal causal relationships, which may viewed on a continuum. True experimental designs are at one end of that continuum, and descriptive studies are at the other end, as shown in Figure 8-16.

SUMMARY POINTS

- The **research design** is the researcher's overall plan for answering the research question. In quantitative studies, the design indicates whether there is an intervention; the nature of any comparisons; methods used to control **extraneous variables;** timing and location of data collection; and information to be provided to subjects.
- **Between-subjects designs,** in which different groups of people are compared, contrast with **within-subjects designs** that involve comparisons of the same subjects.
- **Cross-sectional designs** involve the collection of data at one point in time, whereas **longitudinal**

designs involve data collection at two or more points over an extended period.

- Longitudinal studies, which are used to study trends, changes, or development over time, include **trend studies** (multiple points of data collection with different samples from the same population), and **panel studies** and **follow-up studies** (which gather data from the *same* subjects more than once).

- Longitudinal studies are typically expensive, time-consuming, and subject to the risk of **attrition** (loss of participants over time), but can produce extremely valuable information.

- **Experiments** involve **manipulation** (the researcher manipulates the independent variable by introducing a **treatment** or **intervention**); control (including the use of a **control group** that is not given the intervention and is compared to the experimental group); and **randomization** or **random assignment** (with subjects allocated to experimental and control groups at random to make the groups comparable at the outset).

- Random assignment is done by methods that give every subject an equal chance of being included in any group, such as by flipping a coin or using a **table of random numbers**. Randomization is the most reliable method for equating groups on all possible characteristics that could affect study outcomes.

- A **posttest-only** (or **after-only**) **design** involves collecting data only once—after the introduction of the treatment.

- In a **pretest—posttest** (or **before—after**) **design**, data are collected both before and after the experimental manipulation, thereby permitting an analysis of change.

- **Factorial designs**, in which two or more variables are manipulated simultaneously, allow researchers to test both **main effects** (effects from the experimentally manipulated variables) and **interaction effects** (effects resulting from combining the treatments).

- In a **randomized block design**, subjects are randomly assigned to groups in different levels of a **blocking variable** that is not manipulated (e.g., gender).

- In a **crossover** (or **repeated measures**) **design**, research subjects are exposed to more than one experimental condition and serve as their own controls.

- Researchers can expose the control group to various conditions, including no treatment; an alternative treatment; a **placebo** or pseudointervention; standard treatment; different doses of the treatment; and delayed treatment.

- True experiments are considered by many to be the ideal of science because they come closer than any other type of research approach to meeting the criteria for inferring causal relationships.

- **Quasi-experimental designs** involve manipulation but lack a comparison group or randomization. In quasi-experiments, control strategies are introduced to compensate for these missing components. By contrast, **preexperimental designs** have no such safeguards.

- The **nonequivalent control group before—after design** involves the use of a **comparison group** that was not created through random assignment and the collection of pretreatment data that permit an assessment of initial group equivalence.

- In a **time series design**, there is no comparison group; information on the dependent variable is collected over a period of time before and after the treatment.

- In evaluating the results of quasi-experiments, it is important to ask whether it is plausible that factors other than the intervention caused or affected the outcomes (i.e., whether there are **rival hypotheses** for explaining the results).

- **Nonexperimental research** includes **descriptive research**—studies that summarize the status of phenomena—and **ex post facto** (or **correlational**) studies that examine relationships among variables but involve no manipulation of the independent variable.

- Nonexperimental research is undertaken because (1) a number of independent variables, such as height and gender, are not amenable to randomization; (2) some variables are technically manipulable but cannot ethically be manipulated; (3) there are sometimes practical constraints to manipulating variables; and (4) researchers sometimes deliberately choose not to manipulate variables, to achieve a more realistic understanding of phenomena as they exist in naturalistic settings.

- There are various designs for correlational studies, including **retrospective designs** (which begin with the outcome and look back in time for antecedent causes); **case—control studies** (retrospective studies that test hypotheses about antecedent causes by comparing **cases** that have a disease or condition with controls that do not); **prospective designs** (longitudinal studies that begin with a presumed cause and look forward in time for its effect); **natural experiments** (comparisons of groups in which one group is affected by a seemingly random event, such as a disaster, and the other is not); and **path analytic studies** (which test causal models developed on the basis of theory).

- Descriptive studies include both **descriptive correlational studies** (which describe how phenomena are interrelated without inferring causality) and **univariate descriptive studies** (which examine the occurrence, frequency, or average value of variables without examining interrelationships).

- Descriptive studies include **prevalence studies** that document the prevalence rate of some condition at a particular point in time, and **incidence studies** that document the frequency of *new* cases, over a given time period. When the incidence rates for two groups are determined, it is possible to compute the **relative risk** of "caseness" for the two.

- The primary weakness of ex post facto or correlational studies is that they can harbor biases due to **self-selection** into groups being compared.

STUDY ACTIVITIES

Chapter 8 of the *Study Guide to Accompany Nursing Research: Principles and Methods, 7th edition*, offers various exercises and study suggestions for reinforcing the concepts presented in this chapter. In addition, the following study questions can be addressed:

1. Suppose you wanted to study how nurses' attitudes toward death change in relation to years of nursing experience. Design a cross-sectional study to research this question, specifying the samples that you would want to include. Now design a longitudinal study to research the same problem. Identify the problems and strengths of each approach.

2. A researcher is interested in studying the effect of sensitivity training for nurses on their behavior in crisis intervention situations. Describe how you would set up an experiment to study this. Now describe two quasi-experimental or preexperimental designs that could be used to study the same problem. Discuss what the weaknesses of each would be.

3. Assume that you have 10 individuals—Z, Y, X, W, V, U, T, S, R, and Q—who are going to participate in an experiment you are conducting. Using a table of random numbers, assign five individuals to group I and five to group II. Then randomly assign the groups to an experimental or control treatment.

4. Using the notation presented in Figures 8-5 to 8-13, diagram a few of the research examples described in the text that are not already shown.

5. A nurse researcher is interested in studying the success of several different approaches to feeding patients with dysphagia. Can the researcher use a correlational design to examine this problem? Why or why not? Could an experimental or quasi-experimental approach be used? How?

6. A nurse researcher is planning to investigate the relationship between the level of economic disadvantage of hospitalized children and the frequency and content of child-initiated communications with the nursing staff. Which is the independent variable, and which is the dependent variable? Would you classify this research as basically experimental or correlational, or could both approaches be used?

SUGGESTED READINGS

Methodologic References

Campbell, D. T., & Stanley, J. C. (1963). *Experimental and quasi-experimental designs for research*. Chicago: Rand McNally.

Christensen, L. M. (1991). *Experimental methodology* (5th ed.). Boston: Allyn and Bacon.

Clinton, J., Beck, R., Radjenovic, D., Taylor, L., Westlake, S., & Wilson, S. E. (1986). Time series designs in clinical nursing research. *Nursing Research, 35,* 188–191.

Conn, V. S., Rantz., M. J., Wipke-Tevis, D. D., & Maas, M. L. (2001). Designing effective nursing interventions. *Research in Nursing & Health, 24,* 433–442.

Cook, T., & Campbell, D. T. (1979). *Quasi-experimental design and analysis issues for field settings.* Chicago: Rand McNally.

Given, B. A., Keilman, L. J., Collins, C., & Given, C. W. (1990). Strategies to minimize attrition in longitudinal studies. *Nursing Research, 39,* 184–186.

Hauck, W. W., Gilliss, C. L., Donner, A., & Gortner, S. (1991). Randomization by cluster. *Nursing Research, 40,* 356–358.

Kerlinger, F. N., & Lee, H. B. (2000). *Foundations of behavioral research* (4th ed.). Orlando, FL: Harcourt College Publishers.

King, K. M. (2001). The problem of under-powering in nursing research. *Western Journal of Nursing Research, 23,* 334–335.

Kirchoff, K. T., & Dille, C. A. (1994). Issues in intervention research: Maintaining integrity. *Applied Nursing Research, 7,* 32–37.

Lazarsfeld, P. (1955). Foreword. In H. Hyman (Ed.), *Survey design and analysis.* New York: The Free Press.

Lipsey, M. W. (1990). *Design sensitivity: Statistical power for experimental research.* Newbury Park, CA: Sage.

McGuire, D.B., DeLoney, V., Yeager, K., Owen, D., Peterson, D., Lin, L., & Webster, J. (2000). Maintaining study validity in a changing clinical environment. *Nursing Research, 49,* 231–235.

Montgomery, D. C. (2000). *Design and analysis of experiments* (5th ed.). New York: John Wiley & Sons.

Motzer, S. A., Moseley, J. R., & Lewis, F. M. (1997). Recruitment and retention of families in clinical trials with longitudinal designs. *Western Journal of Nursing Research, 19,* 314–333.

Page, R. M., Cole, G. E., & Timmreck, T. C. (1995). *Basic epidemiological methods and biostatistics.* Boston: Jones and Bartlett.

Sidani, S., & Stevens, B. Alternative therapies and placebos: Conceptual clarification and methodologic implications. *Canadian Journal of Nursing Research, 31,* 73–86.

Studies Cited in Chapter 8

Beckie, T. M., Beckstead, J. W., & Webb, M. S. (2001). Modeling women's quality of life after cardiac events. *Western Journal of Nursing Research, 23,* 179–194.

Brook, A.D., Sherman, G., Malen, J., & Kollef, M. H. (2000). Early versus late tracheostomy in patients who require prolonged mechanical ventilation. *American Journal of Critical Care, 9,* 352–359.

Bull, M. J., Hansen, H. E., & Gross, C. R. (2000). A professional–patient partnership model of discharge planning with elders hospitalized with heart failure. *Applied Nursing Research, 13,* 19–28.

Faulkner, M. S., Hathaway, D. K., Milstead, E. J., & Burghen, G. A. (2001). Heart rate variability in adolescents and adults with type I diabetes. *Nursing Research, 50,* 95–104.

Gamel, C., Grypdonck, M., Hengeveld, M., & Davis, B. (2001). A method to develop a nursing intervention: The contribution of qualitative studies to the process. *Journal of Advanced Nursing, 33,* 806–819.

Garcia de Lucio, L., Gracia Lopez, F., Marin Lopez, M., Mas Hesse, M., & Camana Vaz, M. (2000). Training programme in techniques of self-control and communication skills to improve nurses' relationships with relatives of seriously ill patients. *Journal of Advanced Nursing, 32,* 425–431.

Greenfield, T. K., Midanik, L. T., and Rogers, J. D. (2000). A 10-year national trend study of alcohol consumption, 1984–1995. *American Journal of Public Health, 90,* 47–52.

Harrison, L. L., Williams, A. K., Berbaum, M. L., Stem, J. T., & Leeper, J. (2000). Physiologic and behavioral effects of gentle human touch on preterm infants. *Research in Nursing & Health, 23,* 435–446.

Heitkemper, M., Jarrett, M., Taylor, P., Walker, E., Landenburger, K., & Bond, E.F. (2001). Effect of sexual and physical abuse on symptom experiences in women with irritable bowel syndrome. *Nursing Research, 50,* 15–23.

Hill, A. S., Kurkowski, T. B., & Garcia, J. (2000). Oral support measures used in feeding the preterm infant. *Nursing Research, 49,* 2–10.

Horsburgh, M. E., Beansland, H., Locking-Cusolito, H., Howe, A., & Watson, D. (2000). Personality traits and self-care in adults awaiting renal transplant. *Western Journal of Nursing Research, 22,* 407–437.

Johnson, J. L., Budz, B., Mackay, M., & Miller, C. (1999). Evaluation of a nurse-delivered smoking cessation intervention for hospitalized patients with cardiac disease. *Heart & Lung, 28,* 55–64.

Keane, A., Jepson, C., Pickett, M., Robinson, L., & McCorkle, R. (1996). Demographic characteristics, fire experiences, and distress of residential fire survivors. *Issues in Mental Health Nursing, 17,* 487–501.

Landolt, M. A., Marti, D., Widner, J., & Meuli, M. (2002). Does cartoon movie distraction decrease burned children's pain behavior. *Journal of Burn Care & Rehabilitation, 23,* 61–65.

McCormick, R. D., Buchman, T. L., & Maki, D. G. (2000). Double-blind, randomized trial of scheduled use of a novel barrier cream and an oil-containing lotion for protecting the hands of health care workers. *American Journal of Infection Control, 28,* 302–310.

McFarlane, J., Soeken, K., & Wiist, W. (2000). An evaluation of interventions to decrease intimate partner violence to pregnant women. *Public Health Nursing, 17,* 443–451.

Metzger, B. L., Jarosz, P. A., & Noureddine, S. (2000). The effect of high-fat diet and exercise on the expression of genetic obesity. *Western Journal of Nursing Research, 22,* 736–748.

Milne, J. (2000). The impact of information on health behaviors of older adults with urinary incontinence. *Clinical Nursing Research, 9,* 161–176.

Mindell, J. A., & Jacobson, B. J. (2000). Sleep disturbances in pregnancy. *Journal of Obstetric, Gynecologic, and Neonatal Nursing, 29,* 590–597.

Morin, K. H., Brogan, S., & Flavin, S. K. (2002). Attitudes and perceptions of body image in postpartum African American women. *MCN: The Journal of Maternal Child/Nursing, 27,* 20–25.

Nahm, R., & Poston, I. (2000). Measurement of the effects of an integrated, point-of-care computer system on quality of nursing documentation and patient satisfaction. *Computers in Nursing, 18,* 220–229.

Nantais-Smith, L. M., Covington, C., Nordstrom-Klee, B., Grubbs, C. J., Eto, I., Lawson, D., Pieper, B., & Northouse, L. (2001). Differences in plasma and nipple aspirate carotenoid by lactation status. *Nursing Research, 50,* 172–177.

Parent, N., & Fortin, F. (2000). A randomized, controlled trial of vicarious experience through peer support for male first-time cardiac surgery patients. *Heart & Lung, 29,* 389–400.

Sandgren, A. K., McCaul, K. D., King, B., O'Donnell, S., & Foreman, G. (2000). Telephone therapy for patients with breast cancer. *Oncology Nursing Forum, 27,* 683–688.

Schultz, A. A., Ashby-Hughes, B., Taylor, R., Gillis, D., & Wilkins, M. (2000). Effects of pectin on diarrhea in critically ill tube-fed patients receiving antibiotics. *American Journal of Critical Care, 9,* 403–411.

Song, R., Daly, B. J., Rudy, E. B., Douglas, S., & Dyer, M. A. (1997). Nurses' job satisfaction, absenteeism, and turnover after implementing a special care unit practice model. *Research in Nursing & Health, 20,* 443–452.

Swanson, K. M. (1999). Effects of caring, measurement, and time on miscarriage impact and women's well-being. *Nursing Research, 48,* 288–298.

Whittington, K., Patrick, M., & Roberts, J. L. (2000). A national study of pressure ulcer prevalence and incidence in acute care hospitals. *Journal of Wound Ostomy and Continence Nursing, 27,* 209–215.

Wilson, M. E., White, M. A., Cobb, B., Curry, R., Greene, D., & Popovich, D. (2000). Family dynamics, parental-fetal attachment, and infant temperament. *Journal of Advanced Nursing, 31,* 204–210.

Winkelman, C., (2000). Effect of backrest position on intracranial and cerebral perfusion pressures in traumatically brain-injured adults. *American Journal of Critical Care, 9,* 373–382.

Zust, B. L. (2000). Effect of cognitive therapy on depression in rural, battered women. *Archives of Psychiatric Nursing, 14,* 51–63.

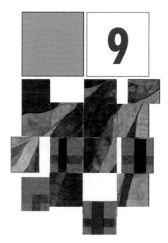

9

Enhancing Rigor in Quantitative Research

This chapter describes methods that can be used to strengthen a wide array of quantitative research designs, including ways to enhance rigor through control over extraneous variables. There are two basic types of extraneous variables: those that are intrinsic to subjects and those that are external, stemming from the research situation. We begin by discussing methods to control situational factors.

CONTROLLING THE RESEARCH SITUATION

In quantitative studies, researchers often take steps to minimize situational contaminants to make the conditions under which data are collected as similar as possible for all subjects. The control that researchers impose by attempting to maintain **constancy of conditions** probably represents one of the earliest forms of scientific control. The environment has been found to exert a powerful influence on people's emotions and behavior, and so, in designing quantitative studies, researchers need to pay attention to environmental context.

Control over the environment is most easily achieved in laboratory experiments in which subjects are brought into environments arranged by the experimenter. Researchers have less control over the environment in studies that occur in natural settings. This does not mean that researchers should

forego efforts to make environments similar. For example, in conducting a nonexperimental study in which data are gathered through an interview, researchers ideally should conduct all interviews in basically the same kind of environment. That is, it is not considered a good practice to interview some respondents in their own homes, some in their places of work, and some in the researcher's office. In each of these settings, participants assume different roles (e.g., wife, husband, parent; employee; client), and responses to questions may be influenced to some degree by those roles.

In real-life settings, even when subjects are randomly assigned to groups, differentiation between groups may be difficult to control. As an example, suppose we were planning to teach nursing students a unit on dyspnea, and we have used a lecture-type approach in the past. If we were interested in trying a computerized autotutorial approach to cover the same material and wanted to evaluate its effectiveness before adopting it for all students, we might randomly assign students to one of the two methods. But now, suppose students in the two groups talk to one another about their experiences. Some lecture-group students might go through parts of the computer program. Some students in the autotutorial group might sit in on some lectures. In short, field experiments are often subject to the problem of **contamination of treatments**. In the same study, it would also be difficult to control other variables, such as the place where learning occurs for the individualized group.

Another external factor to consider is *time*. Depending on the study topic, the dependent variable may be influenced by the time of day or time of year in which the data are collected. In such cases, it would be desirable to strive for constancy of times across subjects. If an investigator were studying fatigue or perceptions of physical well-being, it would matter a great deal whether the data were gathered in the morning, afternoon, or evening, or in the summer as opposed to the winter. Although time constancy is not always critical, it should be considered in designing the study because it is often relatively easy to control.

TIP: If constancy of research conditions cannot be achieved, you should consider controlling external factors by another method. For example, if you suspect that time of day may influence measurement of the dependent variable but cannot collect all the data at the same time of day, perhaps you could assign subjects randomly to morning versus afternoon sessions.

Another issue concerns constancy of communications to subjects. In most studies, researchers inform participants about the study purpose, the use that will be made of the data, under whose auspices the study is being conducted, and so forth. This information should be prepared ahead of time, and the same message should be delivered to all subjects. In general, there should be as little ad-libbing as possible in a quantitative study.

In studies involving an intervention, care should be taken to adhere to intervention protocols. For example, in experiments to test the effectiveness of a new drug to cure a medical problem, researchers would have to ensure that subjects in the experimental group received the same chemical substance and the same dosage, that the substance was administered in the same way, and so forth. When treatments are "fuzzier" than in the case of administering a drug (as is the case for most nursing interventions), researchers should spell out in detail the exact behaviors required of those responsible for administering the treatment.

TIP: Achieving constancy of conditions is not always easy, especially in clinical studies, but various steps can be taken. For example, in addition to having standard protocols, it is important to thoroughly train the people who will be collecting the data and, in the case of an experiment or quasi-experiment, the personnel responsible for implementing the intervention. The extent to which the protocols are followed should be monitored.

In nonexperimental research, researchers do not manipulate the independent variable, so there is no means of ensuring constancy of conditions. Let us take as an example a correlational study that explores whether there is a relationship between people's knowledge of nutrition and their eating habits. Suppose we find no relationship between nutritional knowledge and eating patterns. That is, the results indicate that people who are well informed about nutrition are just as likely as uninformed people to maintain inadequate diets. In this case, however, we had no control over the source of a person's nutritional knowledge (the independent variable). This knowledge was measured after the fact, and the conditions under which the information was obtained cannot be assumed to be constant or even similar. We might conclude from the study that it is not important to teach nutrition to people because knowledge has no impact on their eating behavior. It may be, however, that different methods of providing nutritional information vary in their ability to motivate people to alter their eating habits. Thus, the ability to control or manipulate the independent variable may be critical in understanding relationships between variables, or the absence of relationships.

Example of controlling external factors: Wipke-Tevis, Stotts, Williams, Froelicher, and Hunt (2001) conducted a quasi-experimental study in which great care was taken to ensure constancy of conditions. The study purpose was to compare tissue oxygenation in four body positions among people with venous ulcers. As an example of how the researchers controlled environmental factors, all measurements were made in the early morning; subjects had been instructed to fast so that a fasting blood sample could be drawn; subjects were then provided the same breakfast. After breakfast all subjects rested in bed supine for 30 minutes before testing began.

CONTROLLING INTRINSIC SUBJECT FACTORS

Participant characteristics almost always need to be controlled for quantitative findings to be interpretable. This section describes six ways of controlling extraneous subject characteristics.

Randomization

We have already discussed the most effective method of controlling individual extraneous variables—randomization. The primary function of randomization is to secure comparable groups, that is, to equalize groups with respect to extraneous variables. A distinct advantage of random assignment, compared with other control methods, is that randomization controls *all* possible sources of extraneous variation, *without any conscious decision on the researcher's part about which variables need to be controlled.*

Suppose we were assessing the effect of a physical training program on cardiovascular functioning among nursing home residents. Characteristics such as age, gender, smoking history, diet, and length of stay in the nursing home could all affect a patient's cardiovascular system, independently of the special program. The effects of these other variables are extraneous to the research problem and should be controlled to understand the intervention's effectiveness. Through randomization, we could expect that an experimental group (receiving the training program) and control group (not receiving the program) would be comparable in terms of these as well as any other factors that influence cardiovascular functioning.

Example of randomization:
Kelleher (2002) studied whether the timing of removing indwelling urinary catheters after surgery affected outcomes. Half of the 160 subjects were randomly assigned to have their catheters removed at midnight and the other half had them removed at 6:00 AM, the time traditionally used in England, where the study was conducted. Patients in the midnight removal group passed a greater volume of urine with both their first and second voids, which permitted earlier discharge from the hospital.

Repeated Measures

Randomization in the context of a crossover design is an especially powerful method of ensuring equivalence between groups being compared. However, such a design is not appropriate for all studies because of the problem of carry-over effects. When subjects are exposed to two different conditions, they may be influenced in the second condition by their experience in the first. In our example of the physical training program, a crossover design is unsuitable because the "no-program-followed-by-program" condition would not be the same as the "program-followed-by-no-program" condition: Subjects who were in the program in the first condition might decide to exercise more during the time they are not in the program, for example.

Because treatments are not applied simultaneously in repeated measures designs, the order of the treatment may be important in affecting subjects' performance. The best approach is to use randomized ordering. When there are only two conditions in a repeated measures design, the researcher simply designates that half the subjects, at random, will receive treatment A first and that the other half will receive treatment B first. When there are three or more conditions to which each subject will be exposed, the procedure of **counterbalancing** can be used to rule out ordering effects. For example, if there were three conditions (A, B, C), subjects would be randomly assigned to six different orderings in a counterbalanced scheme:

A, B, C   A, C, B
B, C, A   B, A, C
C, A, B   C, B, A

Note that, in addition to their great potential for control over extraneous subject traits, crossover designs offer another advantage: fewer subjects are needed. Fifty subjects exposed to two treatments in random order yield 100 pieces of data (50 × 2); 50 subjects randomly assigned to two different treatment groups yield only 50 pieces of data (25 × 2).

In sum, a crossover design can be powerful and efficient for eliminating extraneous variables. When carry-over effects from one condition to another are anticipated, however, as might be the case in many nursing interventions, the researcher will need to seek other designs.

Example of counterbalancing:
Stevens, Johnston, Franck, Petryshen, Jack, and Foster (1999) exposed 122 low-birth-weight infants to four different pain-relieving interventions during a heel lance procedure. The interventions included (a) prone positioning; (b) receipt of a pacifier with sterile water; (c) receipt of a pacifier with sucrose; and (d) the standard treatment. The order in which the infants received the four treatments was completely randomized.

Homogeneity

When randomization and repeated measures are not feasible, alternative methods of controlling extraneous characteristics should be used. One such method is to use only subjects who are homogeneous with respect to confounding variables. The extraneous variables, in this case, are not allowed to vary. In our example of the physical training program, suppose our subjects were in two different nursing homes; those in one nursing home will receive the physical training program and those in the other nursing home will not receive it. If gender were considered to be an important confounding variable (and if the two nursing homes had different proportions of men and women), we could control gender by using only men (or only women) as subjects. Similarly, if we were concerned about the confounding effects of subjects' age on cardiovascular functioning, participation could be limited to those within a specified age range.

Using a homogeneous sample is easy and offers considerable control. The limitation of this approach lies in the fact that research findings can be generalized only to the type of subjects who participated in the study. If the physical training program were found to have beneficial effects on the cardiovascular status of a sample of men 65 to 75 years of age, its usefulness for improving the cardiovascular status of women in their 80s would be strictly a matter of conjecture. Indeed, one noteworthy criticism of this approach is that researchers sometimes exclude subjects who are extremely ill or incapacitated, which means that the findings cannot be generalized to the very people who perhaps are most in need of scientific breakthroughs.

Example of control through homogeneity:
Zauszniewski and Chung (2001) studied the effects of depressive symptoms and learned resourcefulness on the health practices of diabetic patients. They restricted their sample to adult women with type 2 diabetes who had no other medical disorder and no history of a mental disorder.

Blocking

A fourth approach to controlling extraneous variables is to include them in the research design as independent variables. To pursue our example of the physical training program, if gender were thought to be a confounding variable, we could build it into the study in a randomized block design. In such a design, elderly men and women would be randomly assigned separately to the treatment group or control group. This approach has the advantage of enhancing the likelihood of detecting differences between our experimental and control groups because we can eliminate the effect of the blocking variable (gender) on the dependent variable. In addition, if the blocking variable is of interest substantively, this approach gives researchers the opportunity to study differences in groups created by the blocking variable (e.g., men versus women).

The design can be extended to include more than one blocking variable, as shown in Figure 9-1. In this design, subjects' age has been included to control for this second extraneous variable. Once again, we would randomly assign subjects from each block to either the experimental or control

Program status

Gender	Age group	Physical training program (Experimental)	No physical training program (Control)
Male			
	66–70		
	71–75		
	76–80		
Female			
	66–70		
	71–75		
	76–80		

FIGURE 9.1 Schematic diagram of a $2 \times 2 \times 3$ randomized block design.

conditions. In other words, half the men 66 to 70 years of age would randomly be assigned to the program, as would half the men 71 to 75 years of age, and so forth. Although in theory the number of blocks that could be added is unlimited, practical concerns usually dictate a relatively small number of blocks (and, hence, a small number of extraneous variables that can be controlled).

Strictly speaking, a blocking design is appropriate only in experiments, but in reality it is used commonly in quasi-experimental and correlational studies as well. If we were studying the effects of a physical training program on cardiovascular functioning after the fact (i.e., subjects self-selected themselves into one of the two groups, and we had no control over who was included in each group), we could set up the analysis in such a way that differential program effects for men and women would be analyzed. The design structure would look similar to the randomized block design, but the conclusions that could be drawn would be different than if we had been able to randomly assign subjects to groups.

Example of control through blocking:
Jones, Jaceldo, Lee, Zhang, and Meleis (2001) studied role integration and perceived health in Asian-American women who were caregivers of aging parents. Relationships among the research variables were examined separately for Chinese and Filipino women.

Matching

A fifth method of dealing with extraneous variables is matching. **Matching** (also known as **pair matching**) involves using knowledge of subject characteristics to form comparison groups. If matching were to be used in our physical training program example, and age and gender were the extraneous variables, we would need to match each subject in the physical training group with one in the comparison group with respect to age and gender.

Despite the intuitive appeal of such a design, there are reasons why matching is problematic. First, to match effectively, researchers must know in advance what the relevant extraneous variables are. Second, after two or three variables, it often becomes impossible to pair match adequately. Suppose we were interested in controlling for subjects' age, gender, race, and length of nursing home stay. Thus, if subject 1 in the physical training program were an 80-year-old African-American woman whose length of stay was 5 years, we would need to seek another woman with these same or similar characteristics as her comparison group counterpart. With more than three variables, matching becomes cumbersome, if not impossible. Yet there are usually far more than three extraneous variables that could affect researchers' dependent variables. For these reasons, matching as a technique for controlling extraneous variables should, in general, be used only when other, more powerful procedures are not feasible, as might be the case for some correlational studies (e.g., case—control designs).

Sometimes, as an alternative to pair matching, in which subjects are matched on a one-to-one basis for each matching variable, researchers use a **balanced design** with regard to key extraneous variables. In such situations, researchers attempt only to ensure that the composition of the groups being compared have proportional representation with regard to extraneous variables. For example, if gender and race were the two extraneous variables of concern in our example of the physical training program, in adopting a balanced design we would strive to ensure that the same percentage of men and women (and the same percentage of white and African-American subjects) were in the physical training and comparison groups. Such an approach is much less cumbersome than pair matching, but it has similar limitations. Nevertheless, both pair matching and balancing are preferable to failing to control subject characteristics at all.

Example of control through matching:
Bliss, McLaughlin, Jung, Lowry, Savik, and Jensen (2000) compared the dietary intake of 39 people with fecal incontinence to that of 39 comparison group members who had normal bowel function. The groups were matched in terms of age and gender.

Statistical Control

A sixth method of controlling extraneous variables is through statistical analysis. Some of you likely are unfamiliar with basic statistical procedures, let alone the sophisticated techniques referred to here. Therefore, a detailed description of powerful **statistical control** mechanisms will not be attempted. If you have a background in statistics, you should consult Chapter 21 or a textbook on advanced statistics for fuller coverage of this topic. Because the notion of statistical control may mystify readers, however, we explain underlying principles with a simple illustration of a procedure called **analysis of covariance**.

Returning to the physical training program example, suppose we had one group participating in the program and a comparison group not participating (e.g., residents of two different nursing homes, only one of which is offering the program). Suppose we used resting heart rate as one of our measures of cardiovascular functioning in this quasi-experimental study. There undoubtedly will be individual differences in heart rate—that is, it will vary from one person to the next. The research question is, Can some of the individual differences be attributed to a person's participation in the physical training program? We know that differences in cardiovascular functioning are also related to other, extraneous characteristics, such as subjects' age. In Figure 9-2, the large circles may be taken to represent total variability (extent of individual differences) for subjects' resting heart rate. A certain amount of variability can be explained by virtue of the subjects' age, which is shown in the figure as the small circle on the left in Figure 9-2A. Another part of the variability can be explained by subjects' participation or nonparticipation in the training program, represented as the small circle on the right in A. The fact that the two small circles (age and program participation) overlap indicates that there is a relationship between those two variables. In other words,

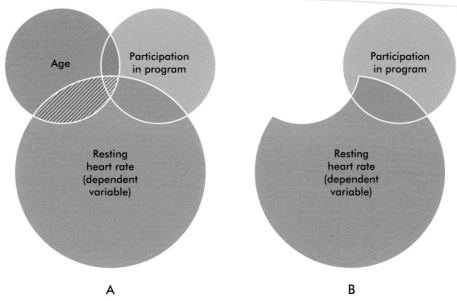

FIGURE 9.2   Schematic diagram illustrating the principle of analysis of covariance.

subjects in the group receiving the physical training program are, on average, either older or younger than members of the comparison group. Therefore, age should be controlled. Otherwise, it will be impossible to determine whether differences in resting heart rate should be attributed to differences in age or program participation.

Analysis of covariance accomplishes this by statistically removing the effect of extraneous variables on the dependent variable. In the illustration, the portion of heart rate variability attributable to age (the hatched area of the large circle in A) is removed through analysis of covariance. Figure 9-2B illustrates that the final analysis examines the effect of program participation on heart rate *after removing the effect of age*. By controlling heart rate variability resulting from age, we get a more accurate estimate of the effect of the training program on heart rate. Note that even after removing variability due to age, there is still individual variation not associated with the program treatment—the bottom half of the large circle in B. This means that the study can probably be further enhanced by controlling additional extraneous variables, such as gender, smoking history, and so forth. Analysis of covariance

and other sophisticated procedures can control multiple extraneous variables.

Pretest measures of the dependent variables, when available, are an excellent choice for control variables; controlling them statistically greatly improves estimates of the effect of the intervention or independent variable. In our example, controlling preprogram measures of cardiovascular functioning through analysis of covariance would be especially powerful because it would remove the effect of individual variation stemming from many other extraneous factors.

Example of statistical control:
Moore and Dolansky (2001) used a pretest—posttest experimental design to test the effectiveness of an audiotaped intervention for patients who had coronary artery bypass graft (CABG) surgery. A taped message describing the typical recovery experiences of CABG patients was given to treatment group patients, both in the hospital and to take home. Control group members were given usual discharge instructions. In the analysis of treatment effectiveness on physical functioning and psychological distress, baseline

TABLE 9.1 Methods of Research Control

METHOD	BENEFITS	LIMITATIONS
Randomization	• Controls all extraneous variables • Does not require advance knowledge of which variables to control	• Ethical and practical constraints on variables that can be manipulated. • Possible artificiality of conditions
Repeated measures	• If done with randomization, strongest possible approach • Reduces sample size requirements	• Cannot be used if there are possible carry-over effects from one condition to the next
Homogeneity	• Easy to achieve in all types of research • Enhances interpretability of relationships	• Limits the generalizability of the results • Requires knowledge of which variables to control
Blocking	• Enhances the ability to detect and interpret relationships • Offers opportunity to examine blocking variable as an independent variable	• Usually restricted to a few blocking variables • Requires knowledge of which variables to control
Matching	• Enhances ability to detect and interpret relationships • May be easy if there is a large "pool" of potential available controls	• Usually restricted to a few matching variables • Requires knowledge of which variables to match • May be difficult to find comparison group matches, especially if there are more than two matching variables
Statistical control	• Enhances ability to detect and interpret relationships • Relatively economical means of controlling numerous extraneous variables	• Requires knowledge of which variables to control, and requires measurement of those variables • Requires statistical sophistication

measures of the outcomes were statistically controlled, as were age, comorbidity, and presurgical cardiac functional status. Moreover, the researchers did separate analyses for men and women. Thus, they used randomization, statistical control, and blocking to control extraneous variables.

TIP: The extraneous variables that need to be controlled vary from one study to another, but we can nevertheless offer some guidance. The best variable is the dependent variable itself, measured before the introduction of the independent variable. Major demographic variables—age, race/ethnicity, gender, education, income, marital status—are good candidates to measure and control because they correlate with many nursing outcomes (as well as with willingness to participate and remain in a study). When the dependent variable is biophysiologic, measures of health status, medication, hospitalization history, and so on are likely to be important. Extraneous variables that are particular to the research problem should be identified through a literature review.

Evaluation of Control Methods

Table 9-1 summarizes the benefits and drawbacks of the six control mechanisms. Overall, random assignment of subjects to groups is the most effective approach to managing extraneous variables because randomization tends to cancel out individual variation on all possible extraneous variables. Crossover designs, although an extremely useful supplement to randomization, cannot be applied to most nursing research problems. The remaining alternatives—homogeneity, blocking, matching, and analysis of covariance—have one disadvantage in common: researchers must know or predict in advance the relevant extraneous variables. To select homogeneous samples, develop a blocking design, match, or perform analysis of covariance, researchers must know which variables need to be measured and controlled. This constraint may limit the degree of control possible, particularly because researchers can seldom deal explicitly with more than two or three

extraneous variables at one time (except in the case of statistical control).

Although we have repeatedly hailed randomization as the ideal mechanism for controlling extraneous subject characteristics, it is clear that randomization is not always possible. For example, if the independent variable cannot be manipulated, then other techniques must be used. In correlational and quasi-experimental studies, the control options available to researchers include homogeneity, blocking, matching, and analysis of covariance. In quantitative research, the use of any of the control procedures discussed here is preferable to the absence of any attempt to control intrinsic extraneous variables.

TIP: This section offered various strategies for controlling a key source of extraneous variation: study participants themselves. These alternative strategies are not mutually exclusive; whenever possible, multiple methods should be used (as was the case in Moore and Dolansky's study). For example, statistical methods of control can be used in conjunction with blocking or matching. Even when randomization has been used, analysis of covariance increases the precision of the design.

CHARACTERISTICS OF GOOD DESIGN

In selecting a research design, researchers should be guided by one overarching consideration: whether the design does the best possible job of providing trustworthy answers to the research questions. Usually, a given research question can be addressed with a number of different designs, and researchers have flexibility in selecting one. Yet many designs are completely unsuitable for dealing with certain research problems. For example, a loosely structured design, such as those used in qualitative studies, would be inappropriate to address the question of whether non-nutritive sucking opportunities among premature infants facilitate early oral feedings. On the other hand, a tightly controlled study may unnecessarily restrict researchers interested in understanding the processes by which nurses make diagnoses. There are many research questions of interest to nurses for which highly structured designs are unsuitable.

TIP: Although techniques of research control are mechanisms for controlling bias, there are situations in which too much control can introduce bias. For example, if researchers tightly control the ways in which key study variables can manifest themselves, it is possible that the true nature of those variables will be obscured. When the key concepts are phenomena that are poorly understood or dimensions of which have not been clarified, then a design that allows some flexibility is better suited to the study aims.

Cook and Campbell (1979), in their classic book on research design, describe four considerations that are important in evaluating research design for studies that focus on relationships among variables. The questions that must be addressed by researchers (and evaluated by research consumers) regarding research design are as follows:

1. What is the strength of the evidence that a relationship exists between two variables?
2. If a relationship exists, what is the strength of the evidence that the independent variable of interest (e.g., an intervention), rather than extraneous factors, caused the outcome?
3. If the relationship is plausibly causal, what are the theoretical constructs underlying the related variables?
4. If the relationship is plausibly causal, what is the strength of evidence that the relationship is generalizable across people, settings, and time?

These questions, respectively, correspond to four aspects of a study's validity: (1) statistical conclusion validity, (2) internal validity, (3) construct validity, and (4) external validity. In this section we discuss certain aspects of statistical conclusion validity, internal validity, and external validity, and factors that can undermine validity. Construct validity, which concerns the measurement of variables, is discussed in Chapter 18.

Statistical Conclusion Validity

As noted in Chapter 8, the first criterion for establishing causality is demonstrating that there is, in fact, an empirical relationship between the independent and dependent variable. Statistical methods are used to determine if such a relationship exists. Design decisions can influence whether statistical tests will actually detect true relationships, and so researchers need to make decisions that protect against reaching false statistical conclusions. Although we cannot at this point in the text discuss all aspects of **statistical conclusion validity**, we can describe a few design issues that can be threats to making valid statistical inferences.

Low Statistical Power

Statistical power refers to the ability of the design to detect true relationships among variables. Adequate statistical power can be achieved in various ways, the most straightforward of which is to use a sufficiently large sample. When small samples are used, statistical power tends to be low, and the analyses may fail to show that the independent and dependent variables are related, even when they are. Power and sample size are discussed in Chapters 13 and 20.

Another aspect of a powerful design concerns the construction or definition of the independent variable, and the counterfactual. Both statistically and substantively, results are clearer when differences between groups and treatments being compared are large. Researchers should usually aim to maximize group differences on the dependent variables by maximizing differences on the independent variable. In other words, the results are likely to be more clearcut if the groups are as different as possible. Conn, Rantz, Wipke-Tevis, and Maas (2001) offer excellent suggestions for strengthening the power and effectiveness of nursing intervention.

Advice about strengthening group differences is more easily followed in experimental than in nonexperimental research. In experiments, investigators can devise treatment conditions that are distinct and as strong as time, money, ethics, and practicality permit. Even in nonexperimental research, however, there are frequently opportunities to operationalize independent variables in such a way that power to detect differences is enhanced.

Inadequate Precision

Quantitative researchers usually try to design a study to achieve the highest possible **precision**, which is achieved through accurate measuring tools, controls over extraneous variables, and powerful statistical methods. Precision can best be understood through a specific example.

Suppose we were studying the effect of admission into a nursing home on depression by comparing elders who were or were not admitted. Depression varies from one elderly person to another for a various reasons. In the present study, we are interested in isolating—as precisely as possible—the portion of variation in depression attributable to nursing home admission. Mechanisms of research control that reduce variability attributable to extraneous factors can be built into the research design, thereby enhancing precision.

In a quantitative study, the following ratio expresses what researchers wish to assess:

$$\frac{\text{Variation in depression}}{\text{Variation in depression due to other factors}}$$
(e.g., age, pain, medical prognosis, social support)

This ratio, although greatly simplified here, captures the essence of many statistical tests. We want to make variability in the numerator (the upper half) as large as possible relative to variability in the denominator (the lower half), to evaluate clearly the relationship between nursing home admission and levels of depression. The smaller the variability in depression due to extraneous variables (e.g., age, prognosis), the easier it will be to detect differences in depression between elders who were or were not admitted to a nursing home. Designs that enable researchers to reduce variability caused by extraneous variables increase the precision of the research. As a purely hypothetical

illustration of why this is so, we will attach some numeric values* to the ratio as follows:

$$\frac{\text{Variability due to nursing home admission}}{\text{Variability due to extraneous variables}} = \frac{10}{4}$$

If we can make the bottom number smaller, say by changing it from 4 to 2, then we will have a purer and more precise estimate of the effect of nursing home admission on depression, relative to other influences. All of the control mechanisms described in the previous section help to reduce variability caused by extraneous variables, and so should be considered in designing studies. We illustrate this by continuing our example. The total variability in levels of depression can be conceptualized as having three components:

Total variability in depression = Variability due to nursing home admission + Variability due to age + Variability due to other extraneous variables.

This equation can be taken to mean that part of the reason why some elderly individuals are depressed and others are not is that some were admitted to a nursing home and others were not; some were older and some were younger; and other factors, such as level of pain, medical prognosis, availability of social supports, also had an effect on depression.

One way to increase the precision in this study would be to control age, thereby removing the variability in depression that results from age differences. We could do this, for example, through homogeneity (i.e., by including in our sample only elderly people within a fairly narrow age range), by using age as a blocking variable, or by statistically controlling age. With any of these methods, the variability in depression due to age would be reduced or eliminated. As a result, the effect of nursing home admission on depression becomes greater, relative to the remaining extraneous variability. Thus, we can say that these designs enabled

---

*At this point, you should not be concerned with how these numbers can be obtained. The procedure is explained in Chapter 20.

us to get a more precise estimate of the effect of nursing home admission on level of depression. Research designs differ considerably in the sensitivity with which effects under study can be detected with statistical tools. Lipsey (1990) has prepared an excellent guide to assist researchers in enhancing the sensitivity of research designs.

Unreliable Implementation of a Treatment

The strength of an intervention (and hence statistical power) can be undermined if the intervention is not as powerful in reality as it is "on paper." An intervention can be weakened by a number of factors, most of which can be influenced to some degree by the researcher.

One issue concerns the extent to which the intervention is similar from one subject to the next. Lack of standardization (constancy of conditions) adds extraneous variation and can diminish the full force of the intervention. Using the notions just described, when standard protocols are not used or not followed, variability due to the intervention (i.e., in the numerator) can be suppressed and variability due to extraneous factors (i.e., in the denominator) can be inflated, possibly leading to the erroneous conclusion that the intervention was ineffective. This suggests the need for careful standardization, adequate training of personnel, and vigilant monitoring to ensure that the intervention is being implemented as planned. Training and monitoring are especially important when double-blind procedures are not used, because the staff administering (or withholding) the treatment may inadvertently send out inappropriate signals or blur the treatment conditions. Of course, in clinical settings there may be pressures on researchers to administer the treatment to some controls, which can threaten the design.

Example of problems with standardization: Winterburn and Fraser (2000) tested the effect of postnatal hospital stay on breastfeeding rates in a teaching hospital in northern England. Women in their third trimester were randomly assigned to a short postnatal stay (6 to 48 hours) or a longer stay (more than 48 hours). The study design was compromised by the fact that some women in the long-stay group were reluctant to stay in the hospital, resulting in relatively small group differences in hospital stay.

Subjects may be exposed to different conditions than were planned if, for example, those in the experimental group elect not to participate fully in the treatment (e.g., they stop going to treatment sessions), or if those in the control group seek and gain access to the treatment. Researchers should design the study to enhance the integrity of the treatment conditions, taking steps in particular to encourage participation among members of the experimental group. As an example, researchers using an experimental design can sometimes affect participation by the timing of random assignment. If subjects are randomly assigned before treatment conditions are explained to them, they may drop out immediately after learning what the conditions will entail; random assignment after the explanation may result in less subject loss among those randomly assigned. Nonparticipation in an intervention is rarely random, so researchers should document which subjects got what amount of treatment so that individual differences in "dose" can be taken into account in the analysis or interpretation of results.

Example of monitoring participation: Cowan, Pike, and Budzynski (2001) conducted a rigorous experimental study of the effectiveness of a psychosocial nursing therapy in reducing mortality for patients who experienced sudden cardiac arrest. Subjects were randomly assigned to the intervention (11 individual therapeutic sessions) or to a control group. Those administering the intervention protocol were trained extensively. Subject adherence to the intervention was carefully monitored (e.g., therapists completed a checklist for each subject), and deemed to be excellent.

When subjects withdraw from a study, both statistical conclusion validity and internal validity (discussed next) can be compromised. In analyzing data from such studies, researchers are in a dilemma about whom to "count" as being "in" a condition. A procedure that is sometimes used is an

on-protocol analysis, which includes members in a treatment group only if they actually received the treatment. Such an analysis is problematic, however, because the sample is no longer representative of the entire group of interest, and self-selection into a nonintervention condition nullifies the comparability of groups. This type of analysis will almost always be biased toward finding positive treatment effects. A more conservative approach is to use a principle known as **intention to treat**, which involves an analysis that assumes that each person received the treatment to which he or she was assigned. This, however, may yield an underestimate of the effects of a treatment if many subjects did not actually get the assigned treatment. If data are analyzed both ways and the outcomes are the same, researchers can have more confidence in the results. Another alternative is to include measures of the "dose" of treatment received into the analysis (Sidani, 1998).

Example of intention to treat:
Dougherty and her colleagues (2002) used an experimental design to test an intervention to manage symptoms of urinary incontinence among older rural women. They used the intention-to-treat approach: women in the experimental group remained in that group even if they failed to comply with the study protocol; and control group members remained in the control group even if they learned a technique that was part of the intervention and practiced it on their own.

Internal Validity

Internal validity refers to the extent to which it is possible to make an inference that the independent variable is truly causing or influencing the dependent variable and that the relationship between the two is not the spurious effect of an extraneous variable. The control mechanisms reviewed earlier in this chapter are all strategies for improving internal validity. If researchers are not careful in managing extraneous variables and in other ways controlling the design of the study, there may be reason to challenge the conclusion that the subjects' perfor-

mance on the dependent measure was caused by the independent variable.

Threats to Internal Validity
True experiments possess a high degree of internal validity because the use of manipulation, randomization, and a control group usually enables the researcher to rule out most alternative explanations for the results. Researchers who use quasi-experimental, preexperimental, or correlational designs must always contend with competing explanations for obtained results. A few of these competing explanations (**threats to internal validity**) are examined here.

History. The threat of **history** refers to the occurrence of external events that take place concurrently with the independent variable that can affect the dependent variables. For example, suppose we were studying the effectiveness of a county-wide nurse outreach program to encourage pregnant women in rural areas to improve their health-related practices before delivery (e.g., better nutritional practices, cessation of smoking, earlier prenatal care). The program might be evaluated by comparing the average birth weight of infants born in the 12 months before the outreach program with the average birth weight of those born in the 12 months after the program was introduced, using a time series design. However, suppose that 1 month after the new program was launched, a highly publicized docudrama regarding the inadequacies of prenatal care for poor women was aired on national television. Infants' birth weight might now be affected by both the intervention and the messages in the docudrama, and it becomes impossible to disentangle the two effects.

In a true experiment, history usually is not a threat to a study's internal validity because we can often assume that external events are as likely to affect the experimental as the control group. When this is the case, group differences on the dependent variables represent effects over and above those created by external factors. There are, however, exceptions. For example, when a crossover design is used, an external event may occur during the first half (or second half) of the experiment, and so treatments would be contaminated by the effect of that event. That is, some people would receive treatment A with the event and others would receive treatment A without it, and the same would be true for treatment B.

Selection. **Selection** encompasses biases resulting from preexisting differences between groups. When individuals are not assigned randomly to groups, there is always a possibility that the groups are nonequivalent. They may differ in ways that are subtle and difficult to detect. If the groups are nonequivalent, differences on outcomes may result from initial differences rather than from the effect of the independent variable. For example, if we found that women with a fertility problem were more likely to be depressed than women who were mothers, it would be impossible to conclude that the two groups differed in depression *because* of differences in reproductive status; women in the two groups might have been different in terms of psychological adjustment from the start. The problem of selection is reduced if researchers can collect data on subject characteristics before the occurrence of the independent variable. In our example of infertility, the best design would be to collect data on women's depression before they attempted to become pregnant. Selection bias is one of the most problematic and frequently encountered threats to the internal validity of studies not using an experimental design. But selection can also enter into experimental designs if some subjects elect not to receive the treatment; these subjects would select themselves into the control condition.

Selection biases also often interact with other biases to compound the threat to the internal validity. For example, if the comparison group is different from the treatment group or main group of interest, then the characteristics of the members of the comparison group could lead them to have different intervening experiences, thereby introducing both history and selection biases into the design.

Maturation. In a research context, **maturation** refers to processes occurring within subjects during the course of the study as a result of the passage of time rather than as a result of a treatment or independent variable. Examples of such processes include physical growth, emotional maturity, fatigue, and the like. For instance, if we wanted to evaluate the effects of a special sensorimotor development program for developmentally delayed children, we would have to consider that progress does occur in these children even without special assistance. A design such as a one-group pretest—posttest design (see Figure 8–7 in Chapter 8), for example, would be highly susceptible to this threat to internal validity.

Maturation is a relevant consideration in many areas of nursing research. Remember that maturation here does not refer to aging or development exclusively but rather to any change that occurs as a function of time. Thus, wound healing, postoperative recovery, and many other bodily changes that can occur with little or no nursing or medical intervention must be considered as an explanation for outcomes that rivals an explanation based on the effects of the independent variable.

Testing. **Testing** refers to the effects of taking a pretest on subjects' performance on a posttest. It has been documented in several studies, particularly in those dealing with opinions and attitudes, that the mere act of collecting data from people changes them. Suppose we administered to a group of nursing students a questionnaire about their attitudes toward assisted suicide. We then acquaint them with various arguments that have been made for and against assisted suicide, outcomes of court cases, and the like. At the end of instruction, we give them the same attitude measure and observe whether their attitudes have changed. The problem is that the first administration of the questionnaire might sensitize students, resulting in attitude changes regardless of whether instruction follows. If a comparison group is not used in the study, it becomes impossible to segregate the effects of the instruction from the effects of taking the pretest. In true experiments, testing may not be a problem because its effects would be expected to be about equal in all groups, but the Solomon four-group design (discussed in Chapter 8) could be used if researchers wanted to isolate intervention effects from pretest effects.

Sensitization, or testing, problems are more likely to occur when pretest data come from self-reports (e.g., through a questionnaire), especially if subjects are exposed to controversial or novel material in the pretest. For some nursing studies (e.g., those that involve biophysiologic data), testing effects are not a major concern.

Instrumentation. Another threat related to measurements is the threat of **instrumentation**. This bias reflects changes in measuring instruments or methods of measurement between two points of data collection. For example, if we used one measure of stress at baseline and a revised measure at follow-up, any differences might reflect changes in the measuring tool rather than the effect of an independent variable. Instrumentation effects can occur even if the same measure is used. For example, if the measuring tool yields more accurate measures on the second administration (e.g., if the people collecting the data are more experienced) or less accurate measures the second time (e.g., if subjects become bored or fatigued), then these differences could bias the results.

Mortality. **Mortality** is the threat that arises from differential attrition in groups being compared. The loss of subjects during the course of a study may differ from one group to another because of *a priori* differences in interest, motivation, health, and so on. For example, suppose we used a nonequivalent control group design to assess the morale of nurses from two different hospitals, one of which was initiating primary nursing. The dependent variable, nursing staff morale, is measured in both hospitals before and after the intervention. Comparison group members, who may have no particular commitment to the study, may decline to complete a posttest questionnaire because of lack of incentive. Those who do fill it out may be unrepresentative of the group as a whole—they may be those who are especially critical of their work environment, for example. It might thus appear that nurses' morale in the comparison hospital had declined over time, but the decline might only be an artifact of biased attrition.

The risk of attrition is especially great when the length of time between points of data collection is long. A 12-month follow-up of subjects, for example, tends to produce higher rates of attrition than a 1-month follow-up. In clinical studies, the problem of attrition may be especially acute because of patient death or disability.

If attrition is random (i.e., those dropping out of a study are similar to those remaining in it with respect to extraneous characteristics), then there would not be bias. However, attrition is rarely totally random. In general, the higher the rate of attrition, the greater the likelihood of bias. Although there is no absolute standard for acceptable attrition rates, biases are usually of concern if the rate exceeds 20%.

TIP: In longitudinal studies, a good method to reduce attrition is to use procedures to help relocate subjects. Attrition often occurs because researchers cannot find participants, rather than because of their refusal to continue in the study. There are many sophisticated (and costly) methods of **tracing** subjects, but a simple and effective strategy is to obtain **contact information** from participants at each point of data collection. Contact information includes, at a minimum, the names, addresses, and telephone numbers of two or three people with whom the subject is close (e.g., parents, siblings, or good friends)—people who would be likely to know how to contact subjects if they moved.

Internal Validity and Research Design

Quasi-experimental, preexperimental, and correlational studies are especially susceptible to threats to internal validity. Table 9-2 lists the specific types of designs that are *most* vulnerable to the threats just described (although it should not be assumed that the threats do not emerge in designs not listed). These threats represent alternative explanations (rival hypotheses) that compete with the independent variable as a cause of the dependent variable. The aim of a strong research design is to rule out these competing explanations.

A good experimental design normally rules out rival hypotheses, but even in true experiments researchers may need to attend to them. For example,

TABLE 9.2 Research Designs and Threats to Internal Validity

THREAT	DESIGNS MOST LIKELY TO BE AFFECTED
History	One-group pretest–posttest Time series Prospective cohort Crossover/repeated measures
Selection	Nonequivalent control group (especially, posttest-only) Case–control "Natural" experiments
Maturation	One-group pretest–posttest
Testing	All pretest–posttest designs
Instrumentation	All pretest–posttest designs
Mortality	Prospective cohort Longitudinal experiments and quasi-experiments

if constancy of conditions is not maintained for experimental and control groups, then history might be a rival explanation for any group differences. Mortality might also be a salient threat in true experiments. Because the experimenter does things differently with the experimental and control groups, subjects in the groups may drop out of the study differentially. This is particularly apt to happen if the experimental treatment is painful, inconvenient, or time-consuming, or if the control condition is boring or bothersome. When this happens, subjects remaining in the study may differ from those who left in important ways, thereby nullifying the initial equivalence of the groups.

In short, in designing a study, researchers should consider how best to guard against and detect all possible threats to internal validity, no matter what design is used.

TIP: In designing a study, try to anticipate negative findings and consider whether design adjustments might affect the results. For example, suppose we hypothesized that environ-mental factors such as light and noise affect the incidence of acute confusion among the hospitalized elderly. With a preliminary design in mind, try to imagine findings that *fail* to support the hypothesis. Then ask yourself what could be done to decrease the possibility of these negative results. Can power be increased by making differences in environmental conditions sharper? Can precision be increased by controlling additional extraneous variables? Can bias be eliminated by better training of research personnel?

Internal Validity and Data Analysis

The best strategy for enhancing internal validity is to use a strong research design that includes the use of control mechanisms discussed earlier in this chapter. Even when this is possible (and, certainly, when this is *not* possible), it is highly advisable to analyze the data to determine the nature and extent of biases that arose. When biases are detected, the information can be used to interpret substantive results; in some cases, biases can be statistically controlled.

Researchers need to be self-critics. They need to consider fully and objectively the types of biases that could have arisen within their chosen design—and then systematically search for evidence of their existence (while hoping, of course, that no evidence can be found). A few examples should illustrate how to proceed.

Selection biases are the most prevalent threat to internal validity and should be examined whenever possible. Typically, this involves comparing subjects on pretest measures, when pretest data have been collected. For example, if we were studying depression in women who delivered a baby by cesarean delivery versus those who delivered vaginally, an ideal way to evaluate selection bias would be to compare depression in these two groups during or before the pregnancy. If there are significant predelivery differences, then postdelivery differences would have to be interpreted with initial differences in mind (or with differences controlled). In posttest-only designs or in cross-sectional correlational studies in which there is no pretest measure of the dependent variable, researchers should nevertheless search for selection biases by comparing groups with respect to important background variables, such as age, gender, ethnicity, social class, health status, and so on. Selection biases should be analyzed even when random assignment has been used to form groups because there is no absolute guarantee that randomization will yield perfectly comparable groups.

Whenever the research design involves multiple points of data collection, researchers should analyze attrition biases. This is typically achieved through a comparison of those who did and did not complete the study with regard to baseline measures of the dependent variable or other characteristics measured at the first point of data collection.

 Example of an examination of attrition and selection bias:
Moser and Dracup (2000) studied the effect of two alternative cardiopulmonary resuscitation (CPR) training interventions against a control condition among 219 spouses of cardiac patients recovering from an acute cardiac event. At the 1-month follow-up, 196 subjects provided outcome data, for a response rate of 89.5%. The researchers noted that there were no significant differences in background characteristics (e.g., race, education) between subjects completing or not completing the study, nor between subjects in the three treatment groups.

In a repeated measures design, history is a potential threat both because an external event could differentially affect subjects in different treatment orderings and because the different orderings are in themselves a kind of differential history. The *substantive* analysis of the data involves comparing the dependent variable under treatment A versus treatment B. The analysis for evidence of bias, by contrast, involves a comparison of subjects in the different orderings (e.g., A then B versus B then A). If there are significant differences between the two orderings, then this is evidence of an ordering bias.

In summary, efforts to enhance the internal validity of a study should not end once the design strategy has been put in place. Researchers should seek additional opportunities to understand (and possibly to correct) the various threats to internal validity that can arise.

TIP: It is important to build in opportunities to analyze bias. This means giving careful consideration to variables that should be measured. For example, information on characteristics that help identify a selection problem should be collected. In a longitudinal study, variables that are likely to be related to attrition should be measured.

External Validity

The term **external validity** refers to the generalizability of the research findings to other settings or samples. Research is almost never conducted to discover relationships among variables for a specific group of people at one point in time. The aim of research typically is to reveal enduring relationships, the understanding of which can be used to improve human health and well-being. If a nursing intervention under investigation is found to be successful, others will want to adopt it. Therefore, an important question is whether the intervention will work in another setting and with different patients. A study is externally valid to the extent that the sample is representative of the broader population, and the study setting and experimental arrangements are representative of other environments.

External Validity and Sampling

One aspect of a study's external validity concerns the adequacy of the sampling design. If the research sample is representative of the population, then generalization is straightforward. Sampling designs are described in Chapter 13.

Strictly speaking, study findings can be safely generalized only to the population from which a sample has been selected at random. If we were studying the effects of a newly developed therapeutic treatment for heroin addicts, we might begin with a population of addicts in a particular drug treatment center in Detroit. From this population, a random sample of drug users could be selected as subjects, who would then be randomly assigned to the treatment or control condition. If the results revealed that the treatment was effective in reducing recidivism in this sample of addicts, could it be concluded that all addicts in North America would benefit from the treatment? Unfortunately, no. The population of heroin addicts undergoing treatment in one particular facility may not be representative of all addicts. For example, drug users from certain ethnic, socioeconomic, or age groups might use the facility in question. Perhaps the new treatment is effective only with individuals from such groups.

Of relevance here is Kempthorne's (1961) distinction between accessible and target populations. The **accessible population** is the population available for a particular study. In our example, heroin addicts enrolled at that Detroit treatment center would be the accessible population. When random procedures have been used to select a sample from an accessible population, there is no difficulty generalizing the results to that group.

The **target population** is the total group of subjects about whom a researcher is interested and to whom results could *reasonably* be generalized. This second type of generalization is more risky and cannot be done with as much confidence as

when generalizing to the accessible population. The appropriateness of such an inference hinges on the similarity of characteristics in the two populations. Thus, researchers must be aware of the characteristics of the accessible population and, in turn, define the target population to be like it. In the drug treatment example, the accessible population might predominantly comprise voluntarily admitted white men in their twenties living in Detroit. Although we might ideally like to generalize our results to all drug addicts, we would be on much safer ground if we defined our target population as young, urban, white men who present themselves for treatment.

Threats to External Validity

In addition to characteristics of the sample that limit the generalizability of research findings, there are various aspects of the research situation that affect the study's representativeness and, hence, its external validity. These characteristics should be taken into consideration in designing a study and in interpreting results. Among the most noteworthy threats to the external validity of studies—particularly those involving an intervention—are the following five effects:

1. *Expectancy effects.* As discussed in Chapter 8, subjects may behave in a particular manner largely because they are aware of their participation in a study (i.e., the Hawthorne effect). If a certain type of behavior is elicited specifically because of the research context, then the results cannot be generalized to more natural settings. Similarly, a placebo effect occurs when subjects administered a pseudointervention show changes or improvements. That same placebo might not, however, have any benefits when not administered in the context of a study. (There are also examples of a so-called **nocebo effect**, which involves adverse side effects experienced by those getting the placebo.)

 Example of a study with possible Hawthorne effect:

Hundley, Milne, Leighton-Beck, Graham, and Fitmaurice (2000) designed an intervention aimed at raising research awareness among midwives and nurses. The treatment group got an educational program, whereas the control group did not. Both groups showed a knowledge gain from pretest to posttest, which the researchers interpreted as a Hawthorne effect (it might also have been the results of a testing effect).

2. *Novelty effects.* When a treatment is new, subjects and research agents alike might alter their behavior in various ways. People may be either enthusiastic or skeptical about new methods of doing things. Results may reflect reactions to the novelty rather than to the intrinsic nature of an intervention; once the treatment is more familiar, results might be different.

3. *Interaction of history and treatment effect.* The results may reflect the impact of the treatment *and* some other events external to the study. When the treatment is implemented again in the absence of the other events, different results may be obtained. For example, if a dietary intervention for people with high cholesterol levels was being evaluated shortly after extensive media coverage of research demonstrating a link between oat bran consumption and reduced cholesterol levels, it would be difficult to know whether any observed effects would be found again if the intervention were implemented several months later with a new group of people.

4. *Experimenter effects.* Subjects' behavior may be affected by characteristics of the researchers. The investigators often have an emotional or intellectual investment in demonstrating that their hypotheses are correct and may unconsciously communicate their expectations to subjects. If this is the case, the results in the original study might be difficult to replicate in a more neutral situation.

5. *Measurement effects.* Researchers collect a considerable amount of data in most studies, such as pretest information, background data, and so forth. The results may not apply to another group of people who are not also exposed to the same data collection (and attention-giving) procedures.

Issues in Achieving Study Validity

Researcher strive to design studies that are strong with respect to all four types of study validity. In some instances, however, the requirements for ensuring one type of validity interfere with the possibility of achieving others.

As one example, consider researchers who use homogeneity to enhance the internal validity of a study. By controlling extraneous variables through selection of a homogeneous sample, researchers strengthen internal validity but limit external validity (i.e., the ability to generalize the study results to an entire population of interest).

As another example, if researchers exert a high degree of control over a study through constancy of conditions in an effort to maximize internal validity, the setting may become highly artificial and pose a threat to the generalizability of the findings to more naturalistic environments. Thus, it is often necessary to reach a compromise by introducing sufficient controls while maintaining some semblance of realism.

When there is a conflict between internal and external validity, it is often preferable to opt for stronger internal validity. Indeed, it can be argued that if findings are not internally valid, they cannot possibly be externally valid. That is, it makes little sense to generalize findings if the findings are themselves ambiguous. Whenever a compromise is necessary, the concept of replication, or the repetition of a study in a new setting with new subjects, is critical. Much greater confidence can be placed in study findings if it can be demonstrated that the results can be replicated in other settings and with new subjects.

RESEARCH EXAMPLE

We conclude this chapter with an example of a study that was especially careful in exercising research control and establishing internal validity.

Knebel, Bentz, and Barnes (2000) conducted a study to determine whether short-term oxygen administration might decrease dyspnea and improve exercise performance among middle-aged adults with a deficiency of the circulating protein alpha$_1$-antitrypsin, a condition that can lead to pulmonary disease. They used an experimental crossover design in which 33 subjects were exposed, in randomized sequence, to an experimental condition (6-minute walks with administration of oxygen) and a control condition (walks with compressed air). A table of random numbers was used to determine order of administration. Both gases were delivered by nasal cannula, and both subjects and research agents were blind to which gas was being used, ruling out any experimenter effect or a placebo effect.

The research protocols were standardized to ensure constancy of conditions. For example, a standardized message of encouragement was given. Subjects were instructed not to talk and to cover as much distance on a 140-foot circular track as possible. All walks occurred at least 2 hours after meals or waking. To control for learning effects, subjects completed three practice walks (without any treatment) before the double-blind tests. The dependent variables in this study included walk distance (to measure activity tolerance), pulse oximetry saturation (to measure oxygen saturation), heart rate and breathing frequency (to measure response to exercise), and a self-assessment of dyspnea intensity.

In addition to testing the research hypotheses, the researchers did some analyses to rule out possible threats to validity. For example, they examined the threat of history by testing for ordering effects (i.e., whether getting oxygen first resulted in different outcomes than getting oxygen last) on walk distance and dyspnea intensity. No ordering effects were found. They also did meticulous tests to rule out learning effects. In brief, they determined that most of the changes in the dependent variables over time occurred during the three practice walks and not during the experimental tests. There was no attrition in this study; both tests were done on the same day and all patients were hospitalized.

With regard to the primary research questions, statistical tests revealed that subjects in the two conditions performed significantly differently with regard to oxygen saturation, but not with regard to other dependent variables. Oxygen saturation was significantly higher with oxygen compared with compressed air.

In addition to using randomization and a crossover design to control for extraneous variables, the researchers also used blocking to increase the precision of their analyses and to test possible interaction effects. Specifically, data for men and women were analyzed separately. The results indicated that for men, dyspnea was not different in the two conditions, but women had a significantly lower dyspnea score with oxygen than with compressed air.

SUMMARY POINTS

- **Research control** is used to remove the effect of situational factors that could affect the study outcomes (e.g., the environment) and intrinsic subject characteristics extraneous to the research question.
- Quantitative researchers strive to achieve **constancy of conditions** under which a study is performed, as a means of controlling situational factors.
- The ideal method of controlling intrinsic subject characteristics is random assignment of subjects to groups, which effectively controls for all possible extraneous variables.
- In some studies, subjects can be exposed to more than one level of a treatment and thus serve as their own controls, although such crossover (repeated measures) designs may be unsuitable because of potential carry-over effects.
- A third control technique is **homogeneity**—the use of a homogeneous sample of subjects to eliminate variability on characteristics that could affect study outcomes.
- Extraneous variables can also be built into the design of a study as independent (blocking) variables, as in the case of a randomized block design.
- Matching involves efforts to make groups comparable by matching subjects (either through **pair-matching** or **balancing** groups) on the basis of one or more extraneous variables.
- Another technique is to control extraneous variables through **statistical control**. One such procedure is known as **analysis of covariance**.
- Homogeneity, blocking, matching, and statistical control share one disadvantage: Researchers must know in advance which variables to control.
- Four types of validity that affect the rigor of a quantitative study include statistical conclusion validity, construct validity, internal validity, and external validity.

- **Statistical conclusion validity** concerns the strength of evidence that a relationship exists between two variables. Threats to statistical conclusion validity include low **statistical power** (the ability to detect true relationships among variables); low **precision** (the exactness of the relationships revealed after controlling extraneous variables); and factors that undermine a strong treatment.
- **Internal validity** concerns the degree to which the results of a study can be attributed to the independent variable. **Threats to internal validity** include **history** (the occurrence of events external to an independent variable that can affect outcomes); **selection** (preexisting group differences; **maturation** (changes resulting from the passage of time); **testing** (effects of a pretest on outcomes); **instrumentation** (changes in the way data are gathered over time); and **mortality** (effects attributable to subject attrition).
- **External validity** refers to the generalizability of study findings to other samples and settings. External validity is increased to the extent that the sample is representative of the population, and the study setting and experimental arrangements are representative of other environments.
- The **accessible population** is the population from which a sample is drawn, and the **target population** represents a larger group of interest. Researchers should define the target population in terms of characteristics that are present in the accessible population.
- **Threats to external validity** include **expectancy effects** (Hawthorne effect, placebo effect, **nocebo effect**); **novelty effects**; **interaction of treatment and history effects**; **experimenter effects**; and **measurement effects**.
- A research design must balance the need for various types of validity, which sometimes compete with each other.

STUDY ACTIVITIES

Chapter 9 of the *Study Guide to Accompany Nursing Research: Principles and Methods, 7th edition*, offers various exercises and study suggestions for reinforc-

ing the concepts presented in this chapter. In addition, the following study questions can be addressed:

1. How do you suppose the use of identical twins in a study could enhance control?
2. Read a research report suggested under the Studies Cited references in Chapter 8. Assess the adequacy of the control mechanisms used by the investigator, and recommend additional controls if appropriate.
3. For each of the following examples, indicate the types of design that could be used to study the problem (experimental, quasi-experimental, and so forth), the design you would recommend using, and how you would go about controlling extraneous variables.
   a. What effect does the presence of the newborn's father in the delivery room have on the mother's subjective report of pain?
   b. What is the effect of different types of bowel evacuation regimes on quadriplegic patients?
   c. Does the reinforcement of intensive care unit nonsmoking behavior in smokers affect postintensive care unit behaviors?
   d. Is the degree of change in body image of surgical patients related to their need for touch?

SUGGESTED READINGS

Methodologic References

Beck, S. L. (1989). The crossover design in clinical nursing research. *Nursing Research, 38,* 291–293.

Braucht, G. H., & Glass, G. V. (1968). The external validity of experiments. *American Educational Research Journal, 5,* 437–473.

Clark, A. J. (1996). Optimizing the intervention in research studies. *Advanced Practice Nursing Quarterly, 2,* 1–4.

Conlon, M., & Anderson, G. C. (1991). Three methods of random assignment: Comparison of balance achieved on potentially confounding variables. *Nursing Research, 39,* 376–378.

Conn, V. S., Rantz, M. J., Wipke-Tevis, D. D., & Maas, M. L. (2001). Designing effective nursing interventions. *Research in Nursing & Health, 24,* 433–442.

Cook, T. D., & Campbell, D. T. (1979). *Quasi-experimental: Design and analysis issues for field settings.* Boston: Houghton, Mifflin.

Fogg, L., & Gross, D. (2000). Threats to validity in randomized clinical trials. *Research in Nursing & Health, 23*, 79–87.

Gilliss, C. L., & Kulkin, I. L. (1991). Technical notes: Monitoring nursing interventions and data collection in a randomized clinical trial. *Western Journal of Nursing Research, 13*, 416–422.

Kempthorne, O. (1961). The design and analysis of experiments with some reference to educational research. In R. O. Collier & S. M. Elan (Eds.), *Research design and analysis* (pp. 97–126). Bloomington, IN: Phi Delta Kappa.

Kerlinger, F. N., & Lee, H. B. (2000). *Foundations of behavioral research* (4th ed.). Orlando, FL: Harcourt College Publishers.

Kwekkeboom, K. L. (1997). The placebo effect in symptom management. *Oncology Nursing Forum, 24*, 1393–1399.

Lipsey, M. W. (1990). *Design sensitivity: Statistical power for experimental research.* Newbury Park, CA: Sage.

McGuire, D. B., DeLoney, V., Yeager, K., Owen, D., Peterson, D., Lin, L., & Webster, J. (2000). Maintaining study validity in a changing clinical environment. *Nursing Research, 49*, 231–235.

Motzer, S. A., Moseley, J. R., & Lewis, F. M. (1997). Recruitment and retention of families in clinical trials with longitudinal designs. *Western Journal of Nursing Research, 19*, 314–333.

Rosenthal, R. (1976). *Experimenter effects in behavioral research.* New York: Halsted Press.

Sidani, S. (1998). Measuring the intervention in effectiveness research. *Western Journal of Nursing Research, 20*, 621–635.

Studies Cited in Chapter 9

Bliss, D. Z., McLaughlin, J., Jung, H., Lowry, A., Savik, K., & Jensen, L. (2000). Comparison of the nutritional composition of diets of persons with fecal incontinence and that of age- and gender-matched controls. *Journal of Wound, Ostomy, and Continence Nursing, 27*, 90–97.

Cowan, M. J., Pike, K. C., & Budzynski, H. K. (2001). Psychosocial nursing therapy following sudden cardiac arrest: Impact on two-year survival. *Nursing Research, 50*, 68–76.

Dougherty, M., Dwyer, J., Pendergast, J., Boyington, A., Tomlinson, B., Coward, R., Duncan, R. P., Vogel, B., & Rooks, L. (2002). A randomized trial of behavioral management for continence with older rural women. *Research in Nursing & Health, 25*, 3–13.

Hundley, V., Milne, J., Leighton-Beck, L., Graham, W., & Fitmaurice, A. (2000). Raising research awareness among midwives and nurses. *Journal of Advanced Nursing, 31*, 78–88.

Jones, P. S., Jaceldo, K. B., Lee, J. R., Zhang, X. E., & Meleis, A. I. (2001). Role integration and perceived health in Asian American women caregivers. *Research in Nursing & Health, 24*, 133–144.

Kelleher, M. M. (2002). Removal of urinary catheters: Midnight vs. 0600 hours. *British Journal of Nursing, 11*, 84–90.

Knebel, A. R., Bentz, E., & Barnes, P. (2000). Dyspnea management in alpha-1 antitrypsin deficiency: Effect of oxygen administration. *Nursing Research, 49*, 333–338.

Moore, S. M., & Dolansky, M. A. (2001). Randomized trial of a home recovery intervention following coronary artery bypass surgery. *Research in Nursing & Health, 24*, 94–104.

Moser, D. K., & Dracup, K. (2000). Impact of cardiopulmonary resuscitation training on perceived control in spouses of recovering cardiac patients. *Research in Nursing & Health, 23*, 270–278.

Stevens, B., Johnston, C., Franck, L., Petryshen, P., Jack, A., & Foster, G. (1999). The efficacy of developmentally sensitive interventions and sucrose for relieving procedural pain in very low birth weight neonates. *Nursing Research, 48*, 35–43.

Winterburn, S., & Fraser, R. (2000). Does the duration of postnatal stay influence breast-feeding rates at one month in women giving birth for the first time? *Journal of Advanced Nursing, 32*, 1152–1157.

Wipke-Tevis, D. D., Stotts, N. A., Williams, D. A., Froelicher, E. S., & Hunt, T. K. (2001). Tissue oxygenation, perfusion, and position in patients with venous leg ulcers. *Nursing Research, 50*, 24–32.

Zauszniewski, J. A., & Chung, C. W. (2001). Resourcefulness and health practices of diabetic women. *Research in Nursing & Health, 24*, 113–121.

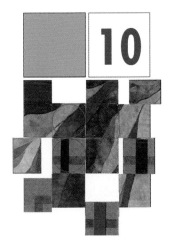

10

Quantitative Research for Various Purposes

All studies can be categorized as either experimental, quasi-experimental/preexperimental, or nonexperimental in design. This chapter describes types of quantitative research that vary according to the study's purpose rather than along the intervention/control dimensions discussed in Chapter 8. The research described here is usually quantitative, but it is important to note that for certain types of research (e.g., evaluation research), qualitative methods may also be used.

STUDIES THAT ARE TYPICALLY EXPERIMENTAL OR QUASI-EXPERIMENTAL

In this section we describe types of research that usually involve an experimental or quasi-experimental design. In other words, the studies—or certain components of them—involve testing an intervention to determine its effects.

Clinical Trials

Clinical trials are studies designed to assess the effectiveness of clinical interventions. Methods associated with clinical trials were developed for medical and epidemiologic research, but nurse researchers are increasingly adopting these methods to test nursing interventions.

Phases of a Full Clinical Trial

Clinical trials undertaken to test a new drug or an innovative therapy often are designed in a series of phases.

- *Phase I* of the trial occurs after the initial development of the drug or therapy, and is designed primarily to determine things like drug dose (or strength of the therapy) and safety. This phase typically uses preexperimental designs (e.g., before—after without a control group). The focus is not on efficacy, but on developing the best possible (and safest) treatment.
- *Phase II* of the trial involves seeking preliminary evidence of the effectiveness of the treatment as it has been designed in phase I, typically using preexperimental or quasi-experimental designs. During this phase, researchers ascertain the feasibility of launching a more rigorous test, seek evidence that the treatment holds promise, and look for signs of possible side effects. This phase is sometimes considered a pilot test of the treatment. There have been clinical trials of drug therapies that have shown such powerful effects during this phase that further phases were considered unnecessary (and even unethical), but this would rarely be the case in nursing studies.

Example of an early phase clinical trial:
In preparation for a phase II trial for a cancer treatment, Schutta and Burnett (2000) gathered data that were useful for assessing the trial's feasibility. The researchers focused on factors influencing patients' decision not to participate in the phase I portion of the study.

- *Phase III* is a full experimental test of the treatment, involving random assignment to an experimental or control group (or to orderings of treatment conditions). The objective of this phase is to arrive at a decision about whether the innovation is more effective than the standard treatment (or an alternative counterfactual). In addition to data about treatment effectiveness, however, researchers may collect data about safety and side effects. Any of the experimental designs discussed in Chapter 8 can be used in this phase of a trial. When the term *clinical trial* is used in the nursing literature, it most often is referring to a phase III trial, which may also be referred to as a **randomized clinical trial** or **RCT.** Phase III clinical trials often involve the use of a large and heterogeneous sample of subjects, frequently selected from multiple, geographically dispersed sites to ensure that findings are not unique to a single setting, and to increase the sample size and hence the power of the statistical tests. Multisite clinical trials are challenging administratively, requiring strong oversight and good systems of communication, staff supervision, and data management.
- *Phase IV* of the trial occurs after the decision to adopt an innovative treatment has been made. In this phase, researchers focus primarily on long-term consequences of the intervention, including both benefits and side effects. This phase might use a nonexperimental, preexperimental, or quasi-experimental design (less often a true experimental design). In nursing, phase IV studies may be part of a utilization project (see Chapter 27).

Example of a multisite randomized clinical trial:
A nurse-managed intervention called the Women's Initiative for Nonsmoking (WINS), developed on the basis of a well-tested smoking-cessation intervention, was tailored specifically to meet the needs of women (Martin, Froelicher, & Miller, 2000). Ten hospitals in the San Francisco area participated in the trial. In each hospital, 50% of the subjects were assigned to the 3-month experimental condition or to a "usual care" group. Follow-up data are being collected at 6, 12, 24, and 30 months after baseline (Froelicher & Christopherson, 2000).

Sequential Clinical Trials

Traditional phase III clinical trials have important drawbacks in certain situations. In particular, it may take many months to recruit and randomize a sufficiently large sample; this is especially problematic if the population being treated is relatively small (e.g., people with a rare disease). Relatedly, in a standard clinical trial it may take months or years to draw conclusions about the intervention's effectiveness (i.e., until all data have been collected and analyzed).

An alternative is the **sequential clinical trial** in which experimental data are continuously analyzed as they become available. Results accumulate over time, so that the experiment can be stopped as soon as the evidence is strong enough to support a conclusion about the intervention's efficacy.

The design for this approach involves a series of "mini-experiments." When the first patient becomes available for the study, he or she is randomly assigned (e.g., by a coin toss) to either the experimental (E) or control (C) condition. The next patient is then automatically assigned to the alternative condition, thereby creating a series of randomized paired comparisons. Most sequential trials use measures indicating preference for either the E or C condition. **Preference** can be defined qualitatively or quantitatively on the basis of clinically meaningful outcomes. Preference measures can include such indicators as survived/did not survive; showed improvement/showed no improvement; resulted in an increase of 20 degrees or more in range of motion/showed smaller or no increase in range of motion. Preference measures are dichotomous (i.e., have two possible outcomes). Using such preference measures, each pair is compared, and there are three possibilities: E is preferred; C is preferred; or the two are tied. Ties are usually thrown out, and all remaining paired comparisons are plotted on graphs for which there are pre-established boundaries with decision rules.

An example of such a graph is presented in Figure 10-1. The horizontal axis in the middle of this graph represents the number of randomized pairs (here, from 1 to 30 pairs, or 60 subjects). The vertical axis is used to indicate which way the "preference" comparison turned out. When the preference for a given pair favors E, the plotted line goes up; when it favors C, the plotted line goes down. The curved butterfly-shaped lines designate decision boundaries. In this example, the first comparison resulted in a preference for the experimental intervention, and so the graph plots a line from the origin to one unit up. The second comparison favored the control condition, and so the plot goes down where the number of pairs equals two. This procedure continues until the plot crosses one of the boundaries, which designate three **stopping rules**. When the upper boundary

(U) is crossed, we would make a terminal decision to conclude that the experimental treatment is more effective. When the lower boundary (L) is crossed, the conclusion is that the control condition is more effective. Finally, when the middle boundary (M) is crossed, the decision is reached that the two treatments are equally effective (or ineffective). In this example, we tested a total of 18 non-tied pairs (for a total sample size of 36) and were then able to conclude that the experimental treatment was significantly superior to the control condition.

Sequential trials have considerable appeal for clinical studies, because decisions typically can be reached much earlier than with traditional designs. However, these trials are not always appropriate (e.g., when three conditions are being compared), or are ambiguous if there are many ties. They may also be complicated if there are multiple outcomes of interest for which preferences have to be plotted separately. For more information about sequential trials, consult Portney and Watkins (2000) or Armitage (1975).

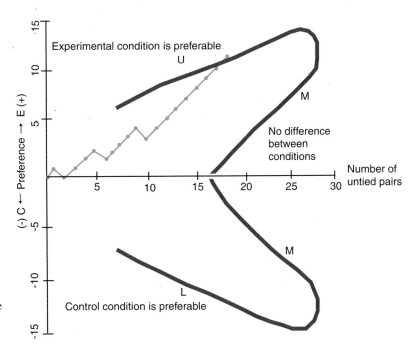

FIGURE 10.1 Example of a sequential clinical trial graph.

Evaluation Research

Evaluation research is an applied form of research that involves finding out how well a specific program, practice, procedure, or policy is working. In evaluations, the research objective is utilitarian—the purpose is to answer the practical questions of people who must make decisions: Should a new program be adopted or an existing one discontinued? Do current practices need to be modified, or should they be abandoned altogether? Do the costs of implementing a new program outweigh the benefits?

Clinical trials are sometimes evaluations. The multisite clinical trial of the WINS program used earlier as an example is also an evaluation of that program. The clinical trial is being used to determine if the WINS program is meeting the objective of reducing smoking. In general, the term *evaluation research* is used when researchers are trying to determine the effectiveness of a rather complex program, rather than when they are evaluating a specific entity (e.g., alternative drugs or sterilizing solutions). Thus, not all clinical trials would be called evaluations, and not all evaluations use methods associated with clinical trials. Moreover, evaluations often try to answer broader questions than simply whether an intervention is more effective clinically than care as usual. Evaluations often involve determining whether the intervention is cost-effective, for example.

Evaluation research plays an important role both locally and nationally. Evaluations are often the cornerstone of an area of research known as **policy research.** Nurses have become increasingly aware of the potential contribution their research can make to the formulation of national and local health policies and thus are undertaking evaluations that have implications for policies that affect the allocation of funds for health services (Wood, 2000).

In doing an evaluation, researchers often confront problems that are organizational, interpersonal, or political. Evaluation research can be threatening. Even when the focus of an evaluation is on a nontangible entity, such as a program, it is *people* who are implementing it. People tend to think that they, or their work, are being evaluated and may feel that their jobs or reputation are at stake. Thus, evaluation researchers need to have more than methodologic skills—they need to be diplomats, adept in interpersonal relations with people,

Evaluation Research Models

Various schools of thought have developed concerning the conduct of evaluation research. The traditional strategy for an evaluation consists of four broad phases: determining program objectives, developing a means to measure the attainment of those objectives, collecting the data, and interpreting the data in terms of the objectives.

It is often not easy to spell out program objectives. There may be many objectives, some of which are vague. The classic evaluation model stresses the importance of developing behavioral objectives. A **behavioral objective** is an intended program outcome stated in terms of the behavior of the people at whom the program is aimed, that is, the behavior of the beneficiaries, rather than the agents, of the program. Thus, if the goal is to have patients ambulate after surgery, the behavioral objective might be stated as, "The patient will walk the length of the corridor within 3 days after surgery." The objective should *not* be stated as, "The nurse will *teach* the patient to walk the length of the corridor within 3 days after surgery." An emphasis on behavioral objectives can be taken to extremes, however. An evaluation may be concerned with psychological dimensions such as morale or an emotion (e.g., anxiety) that do not always manifest themselves in behavioral terms.

An alternative evaluation model is the **goal-free approach.** Proponents of this model argue that programs may have a number of consequences besides accomplishing their official objectives and that the classic model is handicapped by its inability to investigate these other effects. Goal-free evaluation represents an attempt to evaluate the outcomes of a program in the absence of information about intended outcomes. The job of the evaluator—a demanding one—is basically that of describing the repercussions of a program or practice on various components of the overall system. The goal-free model can often be a profitable approach but, in many cases, the model may not be practical because there are seldom unlimited resources (personnel, time, or money) for an evaluation. Decision-makers may need to know whether objectives are being met so that immediate decisions can be made.

Types of Evaluation

Evaluations are undertaken to answer a variety of questions about a program or policy. Some questions involve the use of an experimental (or quasi-experimental) design, but others do not. In evaluations of large-scale interventions (sometimes called **demonstrations** if they are implemented on a trial basis), evaluators may well undertake all the evaluation activities discussed here.

Process or Implementation Analysis. A **process** or **implementation analysis** is undertaken when there is a need for descriptive information about the process by which a program gets implemented and how it actually functions. A process analysis is typically designed to address such questions as the following: Does the program operate the way its designers intended? What are the strongest and weakest aspects of the program? What exactly *is* the treatment, and how does it differ (if at all) from traditional practices? What were the barriers to implementing the program successfully? How do staff and clients feel about the intervention? A process analysis may be undertaken with the aim of improving a new or ongoing program; in such a situation, it might be referred to as a **formative evaluation**. In other situations, the purpose of the process analysis is primarily to describe a program carefully so that it can be replicated by others—or so that people can better understand why the program was or was not effective in meeting its objectives. In either case, a process analysis involves an in-depth examination of the operation of a program, often involving the collection of both qualitative and quantitative data. This type of evaluation is descriptive and therefore nonexperimental.

Example of a process analysis:
Root (2000) described the process of implementing a shared governance model in a California hospital's surgical services department. The goal of the new model was to improve efficiency and morale by transferring decision-making to the staff level.

Outcome Analysis. Evaluations typically focus on whether a program or policy is meeting its objectives. Evaluations that assess the worth of a program are sometimes referred to as **summative evaluations**, in contrast to formative evaluations. The intent of such evaluations is to help people decide whether the program should be discarded, replaced, modified, continued, or replicated. Many evaluation researchers distinguish between an outcome analysis and an impact analysis. An **outcome analysis** tends to be descriptive and does not use a rigorous experimental design. Such an analysis simply documents the extent to which the goals of the program are attained, that is, the extent to which positive outcomes occur. For example, a program may be designed to encourage women in a poor rural community to obtain prenatal care. An outcome analysis would document outcomes without rigorous comparisons. For example, the researchers might document the percentage of pregnant women in the community who had obtained prenatal care, the average month in which prenatal care was begun, and so on, and perhaps compare this information to existing preintervention community data.

Example of an outcome analysis:
Prozialeck and Pesole (2000) evaluated clinical outcomes for clients of a Family Case Management (FCM) program. They compared the birth outcomes (e.g., birth weight, gestational age, and public health nurse contacts) for women who had previously had a low-birth-weight infants and then became pregnant again and used FCM family services.

Impact Analysis. An **impact analysis** attempts to identify the **net impacts** of a program, that is, the impacts that can be attributed exclusively to the program over and above the effects of the counterfactual (e.g., standard treatment). It might be said that whereas outcomes analysis can describe *effectiveness*, impact analysis can demonstrate relative *efficiency*. Impact analyses use an experimental or quasi-experimental design because the aim of such evaluations is to attribute a causal influence to the special program. In the example cited earlier, let us suppose that the program to encourage prenatal care involved having nurses make home visits to women in the rural community to explain the benefits of early care during pregnancy. If the visits could be made to pregnant women on a random basis, the labor and delivery outcomes of the group of women receiving the home visits and of those not receiving them could be compared to determine the net impacts of the intervention, that is, the percentage *increase* in receipt of prenatal care among the experimental group relative to the control group. Many nursing evaluations are impact analyses, although they are not necessarily labeled as such.

Impact analyses often involve **subgroup analyses** to determine the types of people for whom a program is most (and least) effective. For example, in our example of the rural outreach program, the researcher might compare program impacts for teenage mothers and older mothers, for multiparas and nulliparas, and so on. This would be done by comparing experimental and control group members for each subgroup.

> **Example of an impact analysis:**
> Ritz and co-researchers (2000) used a pretest–posttest experimental design to evaluate the effects of advanced practice nursing (APN) care on the quality of life and well-being of women diagnosed with breast cancer. The control group received standard medical care and the intervention group received standard care plus APN interventions. Impacts were assessed both for the overall sample and for subgroups (e.g., married and unmarried women).

Cost Analysis. New programs or policies are often expensive to implement, but existing programs also may be expensive to operate. In our current situation of spiraling health care costs, program evaluations increasingly include a **cost analysis** to determine whether the benefits of the program outweigh the monetary costs. Administrators and public policy officials make decisions about resource allocations for health services not only on the basis of whether something "works," but also on the basis of whether it is economically viable. Cost—benefit analyses are typically done in connection with impact analyses and phase III clinical trials, that is, when researchers establish solid evidence regarding program effectiveness.

As described by Chang and Henry (1999), there are several different types of cost analyses, the two most common of which are the following:

- **Cost–benefit analysis**, in which monetary estimates are established for both costs and benefits. One difficulty with such an analysis is that it is sometimes difficult to quantify benefits of health services in monetary terms. There is also controversy about methods of assigning dollar amounts to the value of human life. Cost–benefit analyses are, however, the most widely used approach to cost analysis.
- **Cost-effectiveness analysis**, which is used to compare health outcomes and resource costs of alternative interventions. Costs are measured in monetary terms, but outcome effectiveness is not. The point of such analyses is to estimate what it costs to produce impacts on outcomes that cannot easily be valued in dollars. This approach avoids the pitfalls of assigning dollar values to such outcomes as quality of life. However, without information on monetary benefits, such research faces more challenges in persuading decision-makers to make changes.

Researchers doing such cost analyses need to document what it costs to operate both the new intervention and its alternative. For complex programs, cost analyses may need to show costs for individual program components. It may also be useful to identify costs for different subgroups whose resource requirements are expected to vary.

In doing cost–benefit analyses, researchers need to think carefully about an array of possible short-term benefits (e.g., clients' days of work missed in 6 months after the intervention) and long-term benefits (e.g., years of productive work life). Often the cost–benefit analyst examines economic gains and losses from several different accounting perspectives—for example, for the target group; the hospital or facility implementing the program; third-party payers; employers; taxpayers; and society as a whole (i.e., the target group and taxpayers combined). Distinguishing these different perspectives is crucial if a particular program effect is a loss for one group (e.g., taxpayers) but a gain for another (e.g., the target group).

Nurse researchers increasingly will be called on to become involved in such economic analyses. Duren-Winfield and her colleagues (2000) provide an excellent description of the methods used in a cost-effectiveness analysis of an exercise intervention for patients with chronic obstructive pulmonary disease.

Example of a cost analysis:
Wilson (2000) did a cost–benefit analysis of a city-wide, school-based hepatitis B vaccination program. The percentage of fully immunized sixth-grade students rose from 8% to over 80%. School-based administration of the vaccine was estimated as costing $1.46 less per dose than traditional methods. Wilson also estimated that over $20 million of health care costs could potentially be avoided through such a program.

Intervention Research

Both clinical trials and evaluations usually involve *interventions*. However, the term **intervention research*** is increasingly being used to describe a research approach distinguished not so much by a particular research methodology as by a distinctive *process* of planning, developing, implementing, testing, and disseminating interventions. The approach is being espoused by researchers and planners in different disciplines, including nursing (Rothman & Thomas, 1994; Sidani & Braden, 1998).

---

*The term *intervention research* is not used uniformly. It is often use to refer to any study involving an intervention, or to any study using an experimental design.

Proponents of the process are critical of the rather simplistic and atheoretical approach that is often used to design and evaluate nursing interventions. The recommended process for intervention research involves careful, collaborative planning at all steps, and the development of an intervention theory to guide the inquiry. More specifically, the process includes the following:

1. *Project planning* begins by putting together a project team with diverse clinical, research, and dissemination skills. The team may also include members of the target population or the affected community, resulting in what is sometimes called **participatory research**. The team's initial job is to clearly define the problem to be solved, gather relevant information about the problem and prior solutions and interventions, and then develop an **intervention theory** that clearly articulates what must be done to achieve desired outcomes. The theory indicates, based on the best available knowledge, the nature of the clinical intervention, factors that would mediate the effects of clinical procedures on expected outcomes, and extraneous variables that would need to be controlled or considered as part of a test.

2. *Intervention design* flows from the intervention theory. The design of the intervention is done incrementally, building on early tests and refinements. The intervention design specifies not only what the clinical inputs would be but also such aspects as duration and intensity of the intervention.

3. *Implementation of a data collection system* begins before the intervention is introduced. Such advance data collection might detect aspects of the community or population of relevance to the intervention and possibly lead to further refinements of the intervention and its test.

4. *Testing the intervention* occurs in stages that are not dissimilar to the four phases of a clinical trial. An intervention prototype is developed, pilot tested, and then formally evaluated,

most often using experimental designs. If the intervention's effectiveness is established, advanced testing focuses on identifying the subgroups for whom and settings in which effectiveness is strongest (and weakest). The final phase involves field tests in clinical settings.

5. *Dissemination* is a built-in feature of this model of research, which involves such activities as establishing standards for using the intervention, identifying possible markets, creating demand for the intervention, and making provisions to offer technical assistance.

This model of intervention research is, at this point, more of an ideal than an actual practice. A few research teams have begun to implement portions of the model, and efforts are likely to expand. However, undertaking such a long-term, ambitious research agenda is clearly expensive. The ultimate effectiveness (both in terms of cost and in terms of health outcomes) of the full process—as opposed to more traditional approaches to designing and evaluating interventions—has yet to be established.

Example of intervention research:
Riesch and her colleagues (Riesch, Tosi, & Thurston, 1999; Riesch, Tosi, Thurston, Forsythe, Kuenning, & Kestly, 1993) undertook an intervention project that involved years of careful advance planning and collaboration with members of the community in which the intervention was implemented. The intervention involved communication skills training for adolescents and their parents.

STUDIES THAT CAN BE EITHER EXPERIMENTAL OR NONEXPERIMENTAL

The studies described in the previous section sometimes have a nonexperimental *component*, but, because they involve an intervention, almost always involve an experimental or quasi-experimental design as well. In this section we look at three types of research that *can* be experimental, but just as often are not.

Outcomes Research

Outcomes research, designed to document the effectiveness of health care services, is gaining momentum as a research enterprise in nursing and health care fields. Outcomes research overlaps in some instances with evaluation research, but evaluation research more typically focuses on an appraisal of a specific new intervention, whereas outcomes research represents a more global assessment of nursing and health care services. The impetus for outcomes research comes from the quality assessment and quality assurance functions that grew out of the professional standards review organizations in the 1970s. Outcomes research represents a response to the increasing demand from policy makers, insurers, and the public to justify care practices and systems in terms of both improved patient outcomes and costs. The focus of outcomes research in the 1980s was predominantly on patient health status and costs associated with medical care, but there is a growing interest in studying broader patient outcomes in relation to nursing care.

Although many nursing studies are concerned with examining patient outcomes and patient satisfaction, specific efforts to appraise and document the quality of nursing care—as distinct from the care provided by the overall health care system—are not numerous. A major obstacle is attribution—that is, linking patient outcomes to specific nursing actions or interventions, distinct from the actions of other members of the health care team. It is also difficult in some cases to determine a causal connection between outcomes and health care interventions because factors outside the health care system (e.g., patient characteristics) affect outcomes in complex ways. Nevertheless, outcomes research will likely gain momentum in this new century.

Outcomes research has used a variety of traditional designs, sampling strategies, and data collection and analysis approaches, but is also developing a rich array of methods that are not within the traditional research framework. The complex and multidisciplinary nature of outcomes research suggests that this evolving area will offer opportunities for methodologic creativity in the years ahead.

Models of Health Care Quality

In appraising quality in health care and nursing services, various factors need to be considered. Donabedian (1987), whose pioneering efforts created a framework for outcomes research, emphasized three factors: structure, process, and outcomes. The *structure* of care refers to broad organizational and administrative features. Structure can be appraised in terms of such attributes as size, location, range of services, type of facilities, technology, organization structure, and organizational climate. Nursing skill mix and nursing autonomy in decision-making are two structural variables that have been found to be related to patient outcomes. *Processes* involve aspects of clinical management, decision making, and clinical interventions. *Outcomes* refer to the specific clinical end results of patient care. Mitchell, Ferketich, and Jennings (1998) note that "the emphasis on evaluating quality of care has shifted from structures (having the right things) to processes (doing the right things) to outcomes (having the right things happen)" (p. 43).

There have been several suggested modifications to Donabedian's framework for appraising health care quality (e.g., Holzemer, 1994; Mitchell, Ferketich, & Jennings, 1998). Mitchell and her colleagues (1998), for example, have offered a model that is less linear and more dynamic than the original framework, and that takes client characteristics into account. Their model does not link interventions and processes to outcomes, but rather the effects of interventions are seen as mediated by client and system characteristics.

Outcomes studies usually concentrate on various linkages within such models, rather than on testing an overall model. For example, researchers have studied the effect of health care structures on various health care processes and outcomes, although this has not been a major focus among nurses. Efforts have also begun on ways to accurately measure aspects of organizational structures from a nursing perspective (Aiken & Patrician,

2000; Brennan and Anthony, 2000). Most outcomes research in nursing, however, has focused on the process–patient–outcomes nexus.

Example of research on structure: Lichtig, Knauf, and Milholland (1999) used data from California and New York to examine the effect of different nursing staffing patterns on patients' length of stay in hospitals.

Nursing Processes and Interventions

To demonstrate nurses' effects on health outcomes, researchers need to carefully describe and document (quantitatively and qualitatively) nurses' clinical actions and behaviors. Examples of nursing process variables include macrolevel and microlevel nursing actions such as the following:

- Nurses' problem-solving skills
- Clinical decision-making
- Clinical competence
- Nurses' autonomy
- Nursing intensity
- Clinical leadership
- Specific actions or interventions (e.g., communication, touch, clinical actions)

There is increasing interest in describing the work that nurses do in terms of established classification systems and taxonomies, and there is also interest in maintaining complete, accurate, and systematic records of nursing actions in computerized data sets (often referred to as **nursing minimal data sets** or **NMDS**). A number of research-based classification systems of nursing interventions are being developed, refined, and tested, including the following:

- Nursing Diagnoses Taxonomy of the North American Nursing Diagnosis Association or NANDA (North American Nursing Diagnosis Association, 1992);
- Omaha System, a classification originally designed by the Omaha Visiting Nurse Association for community health nursing (Martin & Norris, 1996);
- Nursing Intervention Classification (NIC), developed at the University of Iowa (Iowa Intervention Project, 1993);

- Home Health Care Classification or HHCC (Saba, 1992);
- Ozbolt's Patient Care Data Set (Ozbolt, Fruchtnight, & Hayden, 1994);
- Perioperative Nursing Data Set (Kleinbeck, 1999); and
- Nursing Management Minimum Data Set or NMMDS (Huber, Schumacher, & Delaney, 1997)

We expect that many studies in the future will link processes from these classification systems to health outcomes. Studies with these classification systems have thus far focused on descriptions of patient problems and nursing interventions, and assessments of the utility of these systems.

Example of classification system research: Bowles (2000) used two parts of the Omaha System (the Problem Classification Scheme and Intervention Scheme) to describe the types and frequency of problems in hospitalized elders and the interventions used by nurses. The study described the most frequently experienced problems and linked them to the most common nursing interventions.

A major focus of outcomes research involves studies of the effects of nursing interventions on patient outcomes. When an intervention is new or has not been formally tested, outcomes studies can adopt a quasi-experimental or experimental design within an evaluation research framework.

Patient Risk Assessment

Variations in patient outcomes depend not only on the care patients receive, but also on differences in patient conditions and comorbidities. Adverse outcomes can occur no matter what nursing intervention is used. Thus, in evaluating the effects of nursing interventions on outcomes, there needs to be some way of controlling or taking into account patients' risks for poor outcomes, or the mix of risks in a caseload.

Risk adjustments have been used in a number of studies of the outcomes of medical care, and are only beginning to emerge in nursing outcomes studies. These studies typically involve the use of global measures of patient risks, such as the Case Mix Index

(Anderson, Su, Hsieh, Allred, Owensby, & Joiner-Rogers, 1999), or the APACHE III Acute Physiology Scale (Bakken, Dolter, & Holzemer, 1999).

Outcomes

Measuring outcomes and linking them to nursing actions is critical in developing an evidence-based practice and in launching high-quality improvement efforts. Outcomes of relevance to nursing can be defined in terms of physical or physiologic function (e.g., heart rate, blood pressure, complications), psychological function (e.g., comfort, life quality, satisfaction), or social function (e.g., relations with family members). Outcomes of interest to nurses may be either short term and temporary (e.g., postoperative body temperature) or more long term and permanent (e.g., return to regular employment). Furthermore, outcomes may be defined in terms of the end-results to individual patients receiving care, or to broader units such as a community or our entire society, and this would include cost factors.

Just as there have been efforts to develop classifications of nursing interventions, work has begun on developing outcome classification systems. Of particular note is the Nursing-Sensitive Outcomes Classification (NOC), which has been developed by nurses at the University of Iowa College of Nursing to complement the Nursing Intervention Classification (Maas, Johnson, & Moorhead, 1996).

Example of outcomes research: Greenberg (2000) studied the use of telephone nursing and telephone triage on such outcomes as client satisfaction, reduction in drop-in clinic visits, and unnecessary emergency department and urgent care visits associated with an outpatient pediatric clinic population.

Replication Studies

Replication studies are direct attempts to determine if findings obtained in an original piece of research can be duplicated in another independent study. Replications are appropriate for both experimental/quasi-experimental and nonexperimental research.

A strong evidence-based practice requires replications. Practice cannot be altered on the basis of a single isolated study, but must rely instead on an accumulation of evidence. Evidence can accumulate through a series of "close-enough-to-compare" studies, but deliberate replications offer special advantages in both establishing the credibility of research findings and extending their generalizability. There are, however, relatively few *published* replication studies in the nursing literature, perhaps reflecting a bias for original research on the part of both researchers and editors (and perhaps research funders).*

As discussed by Beck (1994), there have been several attempts to classify replication strategies. One strategy is known as **identical replication** (or *literal* replication), which is an exact duplication of the original methods (e.g., sampling, measurement, analysis). Such exact duplication is rare, except in the case of a subsequent study by the original researcher. More common is **virtual replication** (or *operational* replication), which involves attempts to approximate the methods used in the reference study as closely as possible, but precise duplication is not sought. A third strategy is **systematic extension replication** (or *constructive* replication), in which methods are not duplicated, but there are deliberate attempts to test the implications of the original research. Many nursing studies that build on earlier research could be described as extension replications, but they usually are not so labeled and are not necessarily conceptualized as systematic extensions.

Beck's (1994) analysis of the nursing literature for the years 1983 through 1992 revealed very few examples of replications, and in the examples she found, there was considerable fuzziness about how the studies replicated the original ones. In addition to pointing out the need for more replication studies, she made several important recommendations:

• Reports on replication studies should provide specific detail about what was replicated, and how. They should also make clear how the replication was similar to or different from the original.
• The original research being replicated should be thoroughly critiqued, especially if modifications were made on the basis of any shortcoming.
• Benchmarking—comparing the results of the original and replicated study—is essential. The comparison should be accompanied by conclusions about both the internal and external validity of the study findings.

Many nurse researchers have called for more deliberate replication studies; the push for an evidence-based practice may strengthen their legitimacy as important scientific endeavors.

 Example of a replication study:
Gaffney, Barndt-Maglio, Myers, and Kollar (2002) conducted a three-wave longitudinal study of the relationship between mothers' experiences of discipline as children and their own disciplinary intentions with their own children. Their study replicated a study conducted in 1996 and extended the study by examining maternal *behaviors* as well as intentions.

Methodologic Research

Methodologic research refers to investigations of the ways of obtaining, organizing, and analyzing data. Methodologic studies address the development, validation, and evaluation of research tools or methods. Nurse researchers in recent years have become increasingly interested in methodologic research. This is not surprising in light of growing demands for sound and reliable outcome measures and for sophisticated procedures for obtaining and analyzing data.

Most methodologic studies are descriptive and nonexperimental, often focusing on instrument development and testing. Suppose, for example, we developed and evaluated an instrument to accurately measure patients' satisfaction with nursing care. In such a study, we would not examine levels of patient satisfaction or how satisfaction relates to

---

*Interestingly, a textword search for the word "replication" in the CINAHL database yielded far more studies *calling for* replications in their conclusions than actual replication studies.

characteristics of nurses, hospitals, or patients. Our goals are to develop an effective and trustworthy instrument that can be used by others, and to determine our success in accomplishing this. Instrument development research is becoming increasingly important, and it often involves complex and sophisticated research designs and analyses. Those interested in more information on instrument development can consult a book such as that by Gable and Wolf (1993).

Occasionally researchers use an experimental or quasi-experimental design to test competing methodologic strategies. For example, a researcher might test whether a financial incentive increases the number of volunteers willing to participate in a study. Prospective subjects could be randomly assigned to an incentive or no-incentive condition. The dependent variable in this case is whether people agree to participate.

Methodologic research may appear less exciting than substantive research, but it is virtually impossible to conduct high-quality and useful research on a substantive topic with inadequate research methods. Studies of a methodologic nature are indispensable in any scientific discipline, and perhaps especially so in fields that deal with highly complex, intangible phenomena such as human behavior, as is the case with nursing.

Example of a methodologic study:
Mahon, Yarcheski, and Yarcheski (2002) administered the Personal Lifestyle Questionnaire (PLQ), a widely used measure of positive health practices for adults, to a sample of 222 adolescents to evaluate its reliability and validity with young people. Their study concluded that a subscale of the PLQ yielded an adequate measure of general health practices with adolescents.

STUDIES THAT ARE TYPICALLY NONEXPERIMENTAL

In the types of study described in the following sections, researchers typically do not have an option of controlling independent variables, and so the studies are nonexperimental.

Survey Research

A **survey** is designed to obtain information about the prevalence, distribution, and interrelations of variables within a population. The decennial census of the U.S. population is one example of a survey. Political opinion polls, such as those conducted by Gallup or Harris, are other examples. When surveys use samples of individuals, as they usually do, they may be referred to as **sample surveys** (as opposed to a **census**, which covers the entire population). Surveys obtain information from a sample of people by means of **self-report**—that is, study participants respond to a series of questions posed by investigators. Surveys, which tend to yield quantitative data primarily, may be cross-sectional or longitudinal (e.g., panel studies).

The greatest advantage of survey research is its flexibility and broadness of scope. It can be applied to many populations, it can focus on a wide range of topics, and its information can be used for many purposes. The information obtained in most surveys, however, tends to be relatively superficial: surveys rarely probe deeply into such complexities as contradictions of human behavior and feelings. Survey research is better suited to extensive rather than intensive analysis. Although surveys can be conducted within the context of large-scale experiments, surveys are usually done as nonexperimental studies.

Survey Content

The content of a self-report survey is essentially limited only by the extent to which respondents are able and willing to report on the topic. Any information that can reliably be obtained by direct questioning can be gathered in a survey, although surveys include mostly questions that require brief responses (e.g., yes/no, always/sometimes/never). Often, surveys focus on what people do or how they feel: what they eat, how they care for their health, their compliance in taking medications, how anxious they are, and so forth. In some instances, the emphasis is on what people plan to do—how they plan to vote, for example. Surveys also collect information on people's knowledge, opinions, attitudes, and values.

Survey Administration

Survey data can be collected in a number of ways, but the most respected method is through **personal interviews** (or *face-to-face interviews*), in which interviewers meet in person with respondents to ask them questions. In general, personal interviews are rather costly: They require considerable planning and interviewer training and tend to involve a lot of personnel time. Nevertheless, personal interviews are regarded as the best method of collecting survey data because of the quality of information they yield. A further advantage of personal interviews is that relatively few people refuse to be interviewed in person.

Example of a survey with personal interviews: Polivka, Nickel, Salsberry, Kuthy, Shapiro, and Slack (2000) conducted in-person interviews with a sample of 474 low-income women with preschool-age children to explore factors associated with the children's hospitalizations and emergency department use. The interviews, conducted in clinics or human service agency offices, lasted about 20 to 25 minutes.

Telephone interviews are a less costly, but often less effective, method of gathering survey information. When the interviewer is unknown, respondents may be uncooperative in a telephone situation. Telephoning can, however, be a convenient method of collecting information if the interview is short, specific, and not too personal, or if researchers have had prior personal contact with respondents. As the following example shows, telephone interviews may be difficult for certain groups of respondents, including low-income people (who do not always have a telephone) or the elderly (who may have hearing problems).

Example of a telephone survey: Pesata, Pallija, and Webb (1999) conducted a telephone survey to determine why some children missed their clinic appointments, and to explore barriers to health care. A sample of 200 parents with a history of missed appointments were selected for the survey. Of these 200, nearly half (95) did not have a telephone.

Because of the expense of collecting in-person data, researchers sometimes adopt what is referred to as a **mixed-mode strategy** to collecting survey data. In this approach, an interviewer first attempts to interview a sample member by telephone. If attempts at conducting a telephone interview fail (either because there is no telephone or the person refuses to be interviewed by phone), an interviewer then attempts a personal interview to collect the data (or goes to the subject's home with a cellular telephone and personally asks the person to complete the interview by phone).

Questionnaires differ from interviews in that they are self-administered. (They are sometimes referred to as **SAQs**, that is, self-administered questionnaires.) Respondents read the questions on a written form and give their answers in writing. Because respondents differ in their reading levels and in their ability to communicate in writing, questionnaires are *not* merely a printed form of an interview schedule. Great care must be taken in developing questionnaires to word questions clearly, simply, and unambiguously. Self-administered questionnaires are economical but are not appropriate for surveying certain populations (e.g., the elderly, children). In survey research, questionnaires are often distributed through the mail, but may also be distributed in other ways (e.g., through the Internet).

Example of a mailed survey: Havens (2000) studied factors associated with the execution or nonexecution of advance directives for health care (i.e., living wills or durable powers of attorney). She collected her data from a sample of community-dwelling adults through mailed questionnaires.

Needs Assessments

As the name implies, a **needs assessment** is a study in which researchers collect data to estimate the needs of a group, community, or organization. The aim of such a study is to determine if there is a need for a special intervention or outreach effort, or if a program is meeting the needs of those who are supposed to benefit from it. Nursing educators may wish to assess the needs of their clients (students); hospital nurses may wish to learn the needs of those they serve (patients); public health nurses may wish to gather information on the needs of some target population (e.g., adolescents in the community). Because resources are seldom limitless, information that can help in establishing priorities can be valuable.

There are various methods of doing a needs assessment, and these methods are not mutually exclusive. The **key informant approach** collects information about a group's needs from people who are in a key position to know those needs. These key informants could be community leaders, prominent health care workers, agency directors, or other knowledgeable individuals. Questionnaires or interviews are usually used to collect the data. (In some cases, key informant interviews are used to collect narrative, qualitative information rather than quantitative data.)

Needs assessments most often use a **survey approach**, which involves collecting data from a sample of the group whose needs are being assessed. In a survey, questioning would not be restricted to people who have special expertise. A representative sample from the group or community would be asked about their needs.

Another alternative is to use an **indicators approach**, which relies on facts and statistics available in existing reports or records. For example, a nurse-managed clinic that is interested in analyzing the needs of its clients could examine over a 5-year period the number of appointments that were kept, the employment rate of its clients, the changes in risk appraisal status, methods of payment, and so forth. The indicators approach is cost-effective because the data are available but need organization and interpretation.

Needs assessments almost always involve the development of recommendations. Researchers conducting a needs assessment usually offer judgments about priorities based on their results (taking costs and feasibility into consideration), and may also offer advice about the means by which the most highly prioritized needs can be addressed.

Example of a needs assessment:
Patterson, Moylan, Bannon, and Salih (2000) used a survey approach to investigate the need for and level of interest in five types of cancer-related information (medical, psychological, and so on). A questionnaire was distributed to a cancer population and their families in South Western Sydney. The needs assessment resulted in the development of a cancer education program.

Secondary Analysis

Secondary analysis involves the use of data gathered in a previous study to test new hypotheses or explore new relationships. In a typical study, researchers collect far more data than are actually analyzed. Secondary analysis of existing data is efficient and economical because data collection is typically the most time-consuming and expensive part of a research project. Nurse researchers have used a secondary analysis approach with both large national data sets and smaller, more localized sets.

A number of avenues are available for making use of an existing set of quantitative data:

1. Variables and relationships among variables that were previously unanalyzed can be examined (e.g., an dependent variable in the original study could become the independent variable in the secondary analysis).
2. Data that were collected for nonresearch purposes can be used to answer research questions.
3. The secondary analysis can focus on a particular subgroup rather than on the full original sample (e.g., survey data about health habits from a national sample could be analyzed to study smoking among urban teenagers).
4. The unit of analysis can be changed. A **unit of analysis** is the basic unit that yields data for an analysis; in nursing studies, each individual subject is typically the unit of analysis. However, data are sometimes aggregated to yield information about larger units (e.g., a study of individual nurses from 25 hospitals could be converted to aggregated data about the hospitals).

Researchers interested in performing secondary analyses must undertake several preparatory activities. After determining the research question and identifying data needs, researchers must identify, locate, and gain access to appropriate databases. They should then do a thorough assessment of the identified data sets in terms of their appropriateness for the research question, adequacy of data quality, and technical usability of the data.

An important source of data for secondary analysis are the various clinical nursing databases that are available as management and policy tools. Nail and Lange (1996) note that such databases have great potential for research on the processes and outcomes of nursing care.

A number of groups, such as university institutes and federal agencies, have made efforts to make survey data available to researchers for secondary analysis. The policies regulating public use of data vary from one organization to another, but it is not unusual for a researcher to obtain a data set at roughly the cost of duplicating data files and documentation. Thus, in some cases in which data collection originally cost hundreds of thousands of dollars, reproduced materials may be purchased for less than 1% of the initial costs. Some universities and research institutes in universities maintain libraries of data sets from large national surveys.

Surveys sponsored by the National Center for Health Statistics (NCHS) and other government agencies are an important resource for secondary analysis. For example, NCHS periodically conducts such national surveys as the National Health Interview Survey, the Health Promotion and Disease Prevention Survey, and the National Comorbidity Survey, which gather health-related information from thousands of people all over the United States.

The use of available data makes it possible to bypass time-consuming and costly steps in the research process, but there are some noteworthy disadvantages in working with existing data. In particular, if researchers do not play a role in collecting the data, the chances are fairly high that the data set will be deficient in one or more ways, such as in the sample used, the variables measured, and

so forth. Researchers may continuously face "if only" problems: if only they had asked questions on a certain topic or had measured a particular variable differently. Nevertheless, opportunities for secondary analysis are worth exploring.

Example of a secondary analysis:
Clarke, Frasure-Smith, Lespérance, and Bourassa (2000) used existing data from clinical trials sponsored by the U.S. National Heart, Lung, and Blood Institute (Studies of Left Ventricular Dysfunction Prevention and Treatment). Their analysis, which combined members of the original experimental and control groups, focused on psychosocial and other factors that were predictors of 1-year functional status.

Meta-Analysis

Chapter 5 described the function of a literature review as a preliminary step in a research project. However, careful and systematic integration of research findings constitutes an important scholarly endeavor that can contribute new knowledge—knowledge that can play a key role in developing an evidence-based practice. The procedure known as **meta-analysis** represents an application of statistical procedures to findings from research reports. In essence, meta-analysis treats the findings from one study as a single piece of data: The study is itself the unit of analysis. The findings from multiple studies on the same topic can be combined to yield a data set that can be analyzed in a manner similar to that obtained from individual subjects.

Traditional narrative reviews of the literature are handicapped by several factors. The first is that if the number of studies on a topic is large and if the results are inconsistent, then it is difficult to draw conclusions. Moreover, narrative reviews are often subject to potential biases. Researchers may unwittingly give more weight to findings that are congruent with their own viewpoints. Meta-analytic procedures provide an objective method of integrating a large body of findings and of observing patterns and relationships that might otherwise have gone undetected. Furthermore, meta-analysis provides information about the *magnitude* of differences and relationships. Meta-analysis can thus serve as an important scholarly tool in theory development as well as in research utilization. Because of the importance of meta-analyses, we present more information on how to do them in Chapter 27.

Meta-analytic techniques can be used in contexts other than integrative literature reviews. For example, if a clinical trial was implemented in 15 sites, a meta-analysis could be conducted, using results from each site as one piece of data. This is particularly useful if pooling of the raw data across all sites is not possible (e.g., if the intervention was not implemented the same way in the different sites).

Example of a meta-analysis:
Evans (2002) conducted a meta-analysis of the effectiveness of music as an intervention for hospital patients. All 19 studies included in the meta-analysis were clinical trials. The results indicated that music played through headphones reduces patient anxiety during normal care delivery.

Delphi Surveys

Delphi surveys were developed as a tool for short-term forecasting. The technique involves a panel of experts who are asked to complete a series of questionnaires focusing on their opinions, predictions, or judgment about a topic of interest.

The Delphi technique differs from other surveys in several respects. In a Delphi survey, each expert is asked to complete several rounds of questionnaires. Multiple iterations are used to achieve consensus, without the necessity of face-to-face discussion. A second feature is the use of feedback to panel members. Responses to each round of questionnaires are analyzed, summarized, and returned to the experts with a new questionnaire. The experts can then reformulate their opinions with the group's viewpoint in mind. The process of response—analysis—feedback—response is usually repeated at least three times until a general consensus is obtained.

The Delphi technique is an efficient means of combining the expertise of a large, geographically dispersed group for planning and prediction purposes. The experts are spared the necessity of being brought together for a formal meeting, thus saving time and expense. Another advantage is that a persuasive or prestigious expert cannot have an undue influence on the opinions of others, as could happen in a face-to-face situation. All panel members are on an equal footing. Anonymity probably encourages greater frankness than might be expressed in a formal meeting. The feedback—response loops allow for multichannel communication without any risk of the members being sidetracked from their mission.

However, the Delphi technique is time-consuming for researchers. Experts must be solicited, questionnaires prepared and mailed, responses analyzed, results summarized, new questionnaires prepared, and so forth. The cooperation of the panel members may wane in later rounds of the questionnaire mailings. The problem of bias through attrition is a constant concern. Another concern is how to define consensus (i.e., how many participants have to agree before researchers conclude that consensus has been achieved). Recommendations range from a liberal 51% to a more cautious 70%. On the whole, the Delphi technique represents a significant methodologic tool for problem-solving, planning, and forecasting.

Example of a Delphi survey:
Scheffer and Rubenfeld (2000) conducted a five-round Delphi survey, involving an international panel of experts from nine countries, to define critical thinking in nursing. A consensus definition of critical thinking in nursing was achieved; the panel also identified 7 skills and 10 habits of the mind that contribute to critical thinking.

RESEARCH EXAMPLES OF VARIOUS TYPES OF QUANTITATIVE STUDIES

Studies of each type of research presented in this chapter have already been noted. Two studies are described in greater detail in the following sections.

Research Example of a Clinical Trial

Simpson, Parsons, Greenwood, and Wade (2001) noted that many pregnant women consume raspberry leaf herb because of the widespread belief that it shortens labor and makes labor easier. Although the use of the herb is promoted by some midwives and doctors, there is little scientific evidence about its effectiveness or safety. The researchers undertook a randomized clinical trial to address questions about whether regular intake of raspberry leaf tablets has adverse effects on the mother or baby, and whether it is effective in shortening labor.

The researchers were careful in estimating how many subjects would be needed to achieve adequate statistical power in their analyses. Based on their calculations, a total of 240 low-risk nulliparous women were recruited from a hospital in Sydney, Australia. Women who agreed to participate were randomly assigned to either the treatment group or a control group, which received a placebo. Because this was the first study of its kind, a conservative dose of the raspberry herb (2.4 grams per day) was tested. Raspberry herb was added to the mixture in the placebo tablets (calcium phosphate and other constituents). Women in both groups were given tablets, which they were instructed to ingest twice daily (with breakfast and the evening meal) beginning in their thirty-second week of gestation. Tablets were distributed in a double-blind manner, with neither subjects nor those giving the pills aware of which women were in the experimental group.

Some 48 subjects withdrew from the study for various reasons, leaving 192 subjects (96 per group). The two treatment groups were compared with regard to demographic characteristics and found to be comparable in terms of age, weight, and ethnicity. The investigators also examined compliance with tablet consumption and found that the average rate of compliance was 89% (i.e., 89% of the prescribed tablets were consumed).

The researchers began their analyses by examining the safety of ingesting the raspberry leaf tablets. The two groups were compared in terms of such factors as maternal blood loss, maternal diastolic blood pressure prebirth and postbirth, length of gestation, infant birth weight, and infant Apgar score at 5 minutes. The researchers also explored whether there might be side effects of the herb, and so asked subjects to report various symptoms (e.g., vomiting, nausea, dizziness) at each antenatal visit. The researchers found no adverse effects of the herb for mother or baby.

The main outcome variable was length of time in labor. Contrary to popular belief, the raspberry leaf tablets did not shorten the first stage of labor, but the experimental group did have a significantly shorter second stage of labor than the control group (a difference of about 10 minutes). There was also a lower rate of forceps delivery among those in the treatment group (19% versus 30%), perhaps the result of the shorter second stage.

The researchers concluded that although the tablets did not result in anticipated effects on the length of first-stage labor, their effects on second-stage labor duration and on the need for artificial rupture of membranes were clinically significant. They recommend further clinical trials, with an emphasis on finding the optimal dose that will maintain safety while producing beneficial effects.

Research Example of a Methodologic Study Within a Survey

Neumark, Stommel, Given, and Given (2001) were involved in the conduct of a longitudinal survey of older families with cancer and their caregivers, the Family Care Study. Survey respondents were interviewed by telephone four times over the first year after a cancer diagnosis, and also completed four rounds of self-administered questionnaires. Subjects for the study were recruited over a 3-year period in multiple hospitals and cancer treatment centers in two states.

The researchers undertook a methodologic study within the context of this survey research, to identify factors that could account for loss of subjects in the earliest phases of sample accrual. They compared three groups: eligible patients who declined to participate (nonconsenters), patients who originally consented to participate but then later declined (early dropouts), and subjects who actually took part in the study (participants). The researchers examined two broad types of factors that might help to explain nonparticipation in the study: subject characteristics and research design characteristics. The aim was to obtain information that would benefit others in designing studies and recruiting subjects.

The researchers had recruited subjects in facilities that were fortunately able to provide basic demographic and illness-related characteristics of all subjects eligible for the study (e.g., age, race, gender, cancer diagnosis). In addition, the researchers carefully maintained records about aspects of the research design for each eligible person who was recruited. For example, they had information about the type of recruiter used, whether recruiters were reimbursed for obtaining consent, whether a family caregiver was involved, and in what phase of data collection the recruitment occurred.

The researchers found that both subject and research design factors contributed to nonparticipation. Older patients, for example, were significantly less likely to consent (but not more likely to be an early dropout once they had consented). In terms of design features, the most powerful factor was whether a family caregiver was approached to participate. Patients were more likely to give consent and less likely to drop out early when caregivers were also approached. Also, paid recruiters were notably more successful in getting subjects' consent than unpaid recruiters—but these subjects were more likely to drop out early, neutralizing the effect of recruiter payment. The researchers concluded that predicting nonparticipation "may help target recruitment and retention efforts, particularly in reducing the extent to which study-related factors contribute to attrition" (p. 368).

SUMMARY POINTS

- Quantitative studies vary according to purpose as well as design. Studies that almost always involve an experimental or quasi-experimental design include clinical trials, evaluations, and intervention research.
- **Clinical trials**, which are studies designed to assess the effectiveness of clinical interventions, are often designed in a series of phases.
- *Phase I* of a clinical trial is designed to finalize the features of the intervention. *Phase II* involves seeking preliminary evidence of the effectiveness of the treatment as designed in phase I. *Phase III* is a full experimental test of the treatment, often referred to as a **randomized clinical trial**. In *phase IV*, the researcher focuses primarily on long-term consequences of the intervention, including both benefits and side effects.
- In a **sequential clinical trial**, experimental data from paired "mini-experiments" are continu-

ously analyzed; the experiment is stopped as soon as the evidence supports a conclusion about the efficacy of the intervention.

- Most sequential trials use measures indicating **preference** for either the experimental or control condition for each pair of observations. Preferences are plotted on special graphs until the plot crosses one of the boundaries, which designate **stopping rules** for the experiment.
- **Evaluation research** assesses the effectiveness of a program, policy, or procedure to assist decision-makers in choosing a course of action.
- The classic evaluation model assesses the congruence between the goals of the program and actual outcomes; the **goal-free model** attempts to understand all the effects of a program, regardless of whether they were intended.
- Evaluations can answer a variety of questions. **Process** or **implementation analyses** describe the process by which a program gets implemented and how it functions in practice. **Outcome analyses** *describe* the status of some condition after the introduction of an intervention. **Impact analyses** test whether an intervention caused any **net impacts** relative to the counterfactual. **Cost analyses** seek to determine whether the monetary costs of a program are outweighed by benefits and include both **cost–benefit analyses** and **cost-effectiveness analyses**.
- **Intervention research** is a term sometimes used to refer to a distinctive *process* of planning, developing, implementing, testing, and disseminating interventions. A key feature of this process is the development of an **intervention theory** from which the design and evaluation of an intervention flow.
- **Outcomes research** is undertaken to document the quality and effectiveness of health care and nursing services. A model of health care quality encompasses several broad concepts, including: *structure* (factors such as accessibility, range of services, facilities, and organizational climate); *process* (nursing interventions and actions); client risk factors (e.g., severity of illness and case mix of the caseload); and *outcomes* (the

specific end-results of patient care in terms of patient functioning).

- Replication studies include **identical replications** (exact duplication of methods of an earlier study in a new study); **virtual replication** (close approximation but not exact duplication of methods); and **systematic extension replication** (deliberate attempts to test the implications of the original research).

- In **methodologic research**, the investigator is concerned with the development, validation, and assessment of methodologic tools or strategies.

- **Survey research** examines people's characteristics, behaviors, attitudes, and intentions by asking them to answer a series of questions.

- The preferred survey method is through **personal interviews**, in which interviewers meet respondents face-to-face and question them. **Telephone interviews** are more economical, but are not recommended if the interview is long or detailed or if the questions are sensitive or personal. **Questionnaires** are self-administered (i.e., questions are read by respondents, who then give written responses).

- **Needs assessments** are studies to document the needs of a group or community. The three main techniques used to conduct needs assessments include the **key informant**, survey, or **indicator approach**.

- **Secondary analysis** refers to studies in which researchers analyze previously collected data. The secondary analyst may examine unanalyzed variables, test unexplored relationships, focus on a particular subsample, or change the **unit of analysis**.

- **Meta-analysis** is a method of integrating the findings of prior research using statistical procedures, counting each study as one unit of analysis.

- The **Delphi technique** is a method of problem solving in which several rounds of questionnaires are mailed to a panel of experts. Feedback from previous questionnaires is provided with each new questionnaire so that the experts can converge on a consensus opinion in subsequent rounds.

STUDY ACTIVITIES

Chapter 10 of the *Study Guide to Accompany Nursing Research: Principles and Methods, 7th edition*, offers various exercises and study suggestions for reinforcing concepts presented in this chapter. In addition, the following study questions can be addressed:

1. Suppose you were interested in doing a survey of nurses' attitudes toward caring for cancer patients. Would you use a personal interview, telephone interview, or questionnaire to collect your data? Defend your decision.

2. A psychiatric nurse therapist working with emotionally disturbed children is interested in evaluating a program of play therapy. Explain how you might proceed if you were to use (a) the classic evaluation model and (b) a goal-free approach. Which approach do you think would be more useful, and why?

3. Explain how you would use the key informant, survey, and indicator approaches to assess the need to teach Spanish to nurses in a given community.

4. In the research example by Neumark and colleagues (2001), what were the dependent and independent variables? How might other researchers benefit from this research?

SUGGESTED READINGS

Methodologic References

Armitage, P. (1975). *Sequential medical trials* (2nd ed.). New York: John Wiley.

Beck, C. T. (1994). Replication strategies for nursing research. *Image: The Journal of Nursing Scholarship, 26*, 191–194.

Brown, J. S., & Semradek, J. (1992). Secondary data on health-related subjects: Major sources, uses, and limitations. *Public Health Nursing, 3*, 162–171.

Brown, S. A. (1991). Measurement of quality of primary studies for meta-analysis. *Nursing Research, 40*, 352–355.

Chang, W., & Henry, B. M. (2000). Methodologic principles of cost analyses in the nursing, medical, and health services literature, 1990–1996. *Nursing Research, 48*, 94–104.

Crisp, J., Pelletier, D., Duffield, C., Adams, A., & Nagy, S. (1997). The Delphi method? *Nursing Research, 46*, 116–118.

Dillman, D. (1978). *Mail and telephone surveys: The Total Design Method.* New York: John Wiley and Sons.

Donabedian, A. (1987). Some basic issues in evaluating the quality of health care. In L. T. Rinke (Ed.), *Outcome measures in home care* (Vol. I, pp. 3–28). New York: National League for Nursing.

Duren-Winfield, V., Berry, M. J., Jones, S. A., Clark, D. H., & Sevick, M. A. (2000). Cost-effectiveness analysis methods for the REACT study. *Western Journal of Nursing Research, 22*, 460–474.

Fetter, M. S., Feetham, S. L., D'Apolito, K., Chaze, B. A., Fink, A., Frink, B., Hougart, M., & Rushton, C. (1989). Randomized clinical trials: Issues for researchers. *Nursing Research, 38,* 117–120.

Fowler, F. J. (1993). *Survey research methods* (2nd ed.). Beverly Hills, CA: Sage.

Gable, R., & Wolf, M. (1993). *Instrument development in the affective domain* (2nd ed.). Hingham, MA: Kluwer Academic Publishers.

Glass, G. V., McGaw, B., & Smith, M. L. (1981). *Meta-analysis of social research.* Beverly Hills, CA: Sage.

Hasson, F., Keeney, S., & McKenna, H. (2000). Research guidelines for the Delphi survey technique. *Journal of Advanced Nursing, 32*, 1008–1015.

Holzemer, W. L. (1994). The impact of nursing care in Latin America and the Caribbean: A focus on outcomes. *Journal of Advanced Nursing, 20*, 5–12.

Huber, D., Schumacher, L., & Delaney, C. (1997). Nursing Management Minimum Data Set. *Journal of Nursing Administration, 27*, 42–48.

Iowa Intervention Project. (1993). The NIC taxonomy. *Image: The Journal of Nursing Scholarship, 25*, 187–192.

Jacobson, A. F., Hamilton, P., & Galloway, J. (1993). Obtaining and evaluating data sets for secondary analysis in nursing research. *Western Journal of Nursing Research, 15*, 483–494.

Kirchoff, K. T., & Dille, C. A. (1994). Issues in intervention research: Maintaining integrity. *Applied Nursing Research, 7*, 32–37.

Kleinbeck, S. V. M. (1999). Development of the perioperative nursing data set. *AORN Journal, 70*, 15–28.

Maas, M. L., Johnson, M., & Moorhead, S. (1996). Classifying nursing-sensitive patient outcomes. *Image: The Journal of Nursing Scholarship, 28*, 295–301.

Martin, K. S., & Norris, J. (1996). The Omaha System: A model for describing practice. *Holistic Nursing Practice, 11*, 75–83.

McCain, N. L., Smith, M. C., & Abraham, I. L. (1986). Meta-analysis of nursing interventions. *Western Journal of Nursing Research, 8,* 155–167.

McKillip, J. (1986). *Needs analysis: Tools for the human services and education.* Beverly Hills, CA: Sage.

Mitchell, P. H., Ferketich, S., & Jennings, B. M. (1998). Quality health outcomes model. *Image: The Journal of Nursing Scholarship, 30*, 43–46.

Nail, L. M., & Lange, L. L. (1996). Using computerized clinical nursing data bases for nursing research. *Journal of Professional Nursing, 12*, 197–206.

Neuliep, J. W. (Ed.). (1990). *Handbook of replication research in the behavioral and social sciences* [Special issue]. *Journal of Social Behavior and Personality, 15* (4).

North American Nursing Diagnosis Association. (1992). *NANDA nursing diagnoses: Definitions and classification, 1992.* Philadelphia: Author.

Ozbolt, J., Fruchtnight, J. N., & Hayden, J. (1994). Toward clinical standards for clinical nursing information. *Journal of the American Medical Informatics Association, 1*, 175–185.

Pocock, S. J. (1996). *Clinical trials: A practical approach.* New York: John Wiley.

Portnoy, L. G., & Watkins, M. P. (2000). *Foundations of clinical research: Applications to practice* (2nd ed.). Upper Saddle River, NJ: Prentice-Hall Heath.

Reynolds, N. R., Timmerman, G., Anderson, J., & Stevenson, J. S. (1992). Meta-analysis for descriptive research. *Research in Nursing & Health, 15*, 467–475.

Rossi, P. H., & Freeman, H. E. (1993). *Evaluation: A systematic approach* (5th ed.). Beverly Hills, CA: Sage.

Rothman, J. & Thomas, E. J. (Eds.). (1994). *Intervention research: Design and development for human service.* New York: Haworth Press.

Saba, V. (1992). The classification of home health care nursing: Diagnoses and interventions. *Caring, 11*, 50–57.

Sidani, S. (1996). Methodological issues in outcomes research. *Canadian Journal of Nursing Research, 28*, 87–94.

Sidani, S., & Braden, C. J. (1998). *Evaluating nursing interventions: A theory driven approach.* Thousand Oaks, CA: Sage.

Stewart, D. W., & Kamins, M. A. (1993). *Secondary research: Information sources and methods.* (2nd ed.). Thousand Oaks, CA: Sage.

Warheit, G. J., Bell, R. A., & Schwab, J. J. (1975). *Planning for change: Needs assessment approaches.* Washington, DC: National Institute of Mental Health.

Witkin, B. R., & Altschuld, J. W. (1995). *Planning and conducting needs assessments.* Thousand Oaks, CA: Sage.

Wood, M. J. (2000). Influencing health policy through research. *Clinical Nursing Research, 9,* 2113–216.

Studies Cited in Chapter 10

Aiken, L. H., & Patrician, P. A. (2000). Measuring organizational traits of hospitals: The Revised Nursing Work Index. *Nursing Research, 49,* 146–153.

Anderson, R. A., Su, H., Hsieh, P., Allred, C. A., Owensby, S., & Joiner-Rogers, G. (1999). Case mix adjustment in nursing systems research. *Research in Nursing & Health, 22,* 271–283.

Bakken, S., Dolter, K. J., & Holzemer, W. L. (1999). A comparison of three strategies for risk-adjustment of outcomes for AIDS patients hospitalized for *Pneumocystis carinii* pneumonia. *Journal of Advanced Nursing, 30,* 1424–1431.

Bowles, K. H. (2000). Patient problems and nurse interventions during acute care and discharge planning. *Journal of Cardiovascular Nursing, 14,* 29–41.

Brennan, P. F., & Anthony, M. K. (2000). Measuring Nursing Practice Models using multi-attribute utility theory. *Research in Nursing & Health, 23,* 372–382.

Clarke, S. P., Frasure-Smith, N., Lespérance, F., & Bourassa, M. G. (2000). Psychosocial factors as predictors of functional status at 1 year in patients with left ventricular dysfunction. *Research in Nursing & Health, 23,* 290–300.

Evans, D. (2002). The effectiveness of music as an intervention for hospital patients: A systematic review. *Journal of Advanced Nursing, 37,* 8–18.

Froelicher, E. S., & Christopherson, D. J. (2000). Women's Initiative for Nonsmoking (WINS) I: Design and methods. *Heart & Lung, 29,* 429–437.

Gaffney, K. F., Barndt-Maglio, B., Myers, S., & Kollar, S. J. (2002). Early clinical assessment for harsh child discipline strategies. *MCN: American Journal of Maternal-Child Nursing, 27,* 34–40.

Greenberg, M. E. (2000). Telephone nursing: Evidence of client and organizational benefits. *Nursing Economics, 18,* 117–123.

Havens, G. A. D. (2000). Differences in the execution/nonexecution of advance directives by community-dwelling adults. *Research in Nursing & Health, 23,* 319–333.

Lichtig, L. K., Knauf, R. A., & Milholland, D. K. (1999). Some impacts of nursing on acute care hospital outcomes. *Journal of Nursing Administration, 29,* 25–53.

Mahon, N. E., Yarcheski, A., & Yarchesky, T. J. (2002). Psychometric evaluation of the Personal Lifestyle Questionnaire for adolescents. *Research in Nursing & Health, 25,* 68–75.

Martin, K., Froelicher, E. S., & Miller, N. H. (2000). Women's Initiative for Nonsmoking (WINS) I: The intervention. *Heart & Lung, 29,* 438–445.

Neumark, D. E., Stommel, M., Given, C. W., & Given, B. A. (2001). Research design and subject characteristics predicting nonparticipation in a panel survey of older families with cancer. *Nursing Research, 50,* 363–368.

Patterson, P., Moylan, E., Bannon, S., & Salih, F. (2000). Needs analysis of a cancer education program in South Western Sydney. *Cancer Nursing, 23,* 186–192.

Pesata, V., Pallija, G., & Webb, A. A. (1999). A descriptive study of missed appointments: Families' perceptions of barriers to care. *Journal of Pediatric Health Care, 13,* 178–182.

Polivka, B. J., Nickel, J. T., Salsberry, P. J., Kuthy, R., Shapiro, N., & Slack, C. (2000). Hospital and emergency department use by young low-income children. *Nursing Research, 49,* 253–261.

Prozialeck, L. L., & Pesole, L. (2000). Performing a program evaluation in a family case management program: Determining outcomes for low birthweight deliveries. *Public Health Nursing, 17,* 195–201.

Riesch, S. K., Tosi, C. B., & Thurston, C. A. (1999). Accessing young adolescents and their families for research. *Image: The Journal of Nursing Scholarship, 31,* 323–326.

Riesch, S. K., Tosi, C. B., Thurston, C. A., Forsythe, D. M., Kuenning, T. S., & Kestly, J. (1993). Effects of communication training on parents and young adolescents. *Nursing Research, 42,* 10–16.

Ritz, L. J., Nissen, M. J., Swenson, K. K., Farrell, J. B., Sperduto, P. W., Sladek, P. W., Lally, R. M., & Schroeder, L. M. (2000). Effects of advanced nursing care on quality of life and cost outcomes of women diagnosed with breast cancer. *Oncology Nursing Forum, 27,* 923–932.

Root, S. D. (2000). Implementing a shared governance model in the perioperative setting. *AORN Journal, 72,* 95–102.

Scheffer, B. K., & Rubenfeld, M. G. (2000). A consensus statement on critical thinking in nursing. *Journal of Nursing Education, 39,* 352–359.

Schutta, K. M., & Burnett, C. B. (2000). Factors that influence a patient's decision to participate in a phase I cancer clinical trial. *Oncology Nursing Forum, 27,* 1435–1438.

Simpson, M., Parsons, M., Greenwood, J., & Wade, K. (2001). Raspberry leaf in pregnancy: Its safety and efficacy in labor. *Journal of Midwifery & Women's Health, 46,* 51–59.

Wilson, T. (2000). Economic evaluation of a metropolitan-wide, school-based hepatitis B vaccination program. *Public Health Nursing, 17,* 222–227.

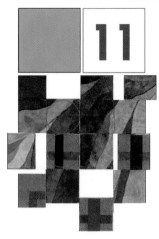

11

Qualitative Research Design and Approaches

THE DESIGN OF QUALITATIVE STUDIES

As we have seen, quantitative researchers carefully specify a research design before collecting even one piece of data, and rarely depart from that design once the study is underway. In qualitative research, by contrast, the study design typically evolves over the course of the project. Decisions about how best to obtain data, from whom to obtain data, how to schedule data collection, and how long each data collection session should last are made in the field as the study unfolds. Qualitative studies use an **emergent design**—a design that emerges as researchers make ongoing decisions reflecting what has already been learned. As noted by Lincoln and Guba (1985), an emergent design in qualitative studies is not the result of sloppiness or laziness on the part of researchers, but rather a reflection of their desire to have the inquiry based on the realities and viewpoints of those under study—realities and viewpoints that are not known or understood at the outset.

Characteristics of Qualitative Research Design

Qualitative inquiry has been guided by different disciplines, and each has developed methods for ad-

dressing questions of particular interest. However, some general characteristics of qualitative research design tend to apply across disciplines. In general, qualitative design:

- Often involves a merging together of various data collection strategies;
- Is flexible and elastic, capable of adjusting to what is being learned during the course of data collection;
- Tends to be holistic, striving for an understanding of the whole;
- Requires researchers to become intensely involved, often remaining in the field for lengthy periods of time;
- Requires the researcher to become the research instrument; and
- Requires ongoing analysis of the data to formulate subsequent strategies and to determine when field work is done.

With regard to the first characteristic, qualitative researchers tend to put together a complex array of data, derived from a variety of sources and using a variety of methods. This tendency has sometimes been described as **bricolage**, and the qualitative researcher has been referred to as a **bricoleur**, a person who "is adept at performing a large number of diverse tasks, ranging from interviewing to observing, to interpreting personal and historical documents, to intensive reflection and introspection" (Denzin & Lincoln, 1994, p. 2).

Qualitative Design and Planning

Although design decisions are not specified in advance, qualitative researchers typically do considerable advance planning that supports their flexibility in developing an emergent design. In the total absence of planning, design choices might actually be constrained. For example, researchers initially might anticipate a 6-month period for data collection, but may need to be prepared (financially and emotionally) to spend even longer periods of time in the field to pursue data collection opportunities that could not have been foreseen. In other words, qualitative researchers plan for broad contingencies that may be expected to pose decision opportunities once the study has begun. Examples of the areas in which advanced planning is especially useful include the following:

- Selecting a broad framework or tradition (described in the next section) to guide certain design decisions
- Identifying potential study collaborators and reviewers of the research plans
- Developing a broad data collection strategy (e.g., will interviews be conducted?), and identifying opportunities for enhancing credibility (e.g., through triangulation)
- Selecting the site where the study will take place and identifying the types of settings
- Identifying any "gatekeepers" who can provide (or deny) access to important sources of data, and can make arrangements for gaining entrée
- Collecting relevant written or photographic materials about the site (e.g., maps, organizational charts, resource directories.)
- Determining the maximum amount of time available for the study, given costs and other constraints
- Identifying the types of equipment that could aid in the collection and analysis of data in the field (e.g., audio and video recording equipment, laptop computers)
- Determining the number and type of assistants needed (if any) to complete the project

- Training any assistants—and self-training
- Identifying appropriate informed consent procedures, including contingencies for dealing with ethical issues as they present themselves during data collection
- Developing plans for assessing the trustworthiness of the data and the overall inquiry

Thus, a qualitative researcher needs to plan for a variety of potential circumstances, but decisions about how he or she will deal with them must be resolved when the social context of time, place, and human interactions are better understood. By both allowing for and anticipating an evolution of strategies, qualitative researchers seek to make their research design responsive to the situation and to the phenomenon under study.

One further task that qualitative researchers typically undertake before collecting data is an analysis of their own biases and ideology. Qualitative researchers tend to accept that research is subjective and may be ideologically driven. Decisions about research design and research approaches are not value-free. Qualitative researchers, then, are more inclined to take on as an early research challenge the identification of their own biases and presuppositions. Such an identification is particularly important in qualitative inquiry because of the intensely personal nature of the data collection and data analysis experience.

 Example illustrating self-disclosure of possible bias:

Rashid (2001) studied women's views about the use of the Norplant contraceptive implant in rural Bangladesh. She wrote: "My writing on this subject is influenced by my position as a native (born in Bangladesh) and as an outsider (I grew up overseas from 1979 to 1993). The kind of fieldwork I carried out was influenced by my cultural background, Muslim identity, status as an unmarried Bengali woman, and mixed cultural upbringing..." (p. 89).

Phases in Qualitative Design

Although the exact form of a qualitative study cannot be known and specified in advance, Lincoln and Guba (1985) have noted that a naturalistic inquiry typically progresses through three broad phases while in the field:

1. *Orientation and overview.* Quantitative researchers usually believe that they know what they do not know—that is, they know exactly what type of knowledge they expect to obtain by doing a study, and then strive to obtain it. Qualitative researchers, by contrast, enter the study not knowing what is not known—that is, not knowing what it is about the phenomenon that will drive the inquiry forward. Therefore, the first phase of many qualitative studies is to get a handle on what *is* salient about the phenomenon of interest.

2. *Focused exploration.* The second phase of the study is a more focused scrutiny and in-depth exploration of those aspects of the phenomenon that are judged to be salient. The questions asked and the types of people invited to participate in the study are shaped by the understandings developed in the first phase.

3. *Confirmation and closure.* In the final phase, qualitative researchers undertake efforts to establish that their findings are trustworthy, often by going back and discussing their understanding with study participants.

The three phases are not discrete events. Rather, they overlap to a greater or lesser degree in different projects. For example, even the first few interviews or observations are typically used as a basis for selecting subsequent informants, even though the researcher is still striving to understand the full scope of the phenomenon and to identify its major dimensions. The various phases may take many months or even years to complete.

Qualitative Design Features

Some of the design features of quantitative studies (see Chapter 8) also apply to qualitative ones. However, qualitative design features are often post hoc characterizations of what happened in the field rather than features specifically planned in advance. To further contrast qualitative and quantitative research design, we refer the reader to the design elements identified in Table 8-1.

Control Over the Independent Variable

Qualitative research is almost always nonexperimental (although, as discussed in the next chapter, a qualitative study sometimes is embedded in an experimental project). Researchers conducting a study within the naturalistic paradigm do not normally conceptualize their studies as having independent and dependent variables, and they rarely control or manipulate any aspect of the people or environment under study. The goal of most qualitative studies is to develop a rich understanding of a phenomenon as it exists in the real world and as it is constructed by individuals in the context of that world.

Type of Group Comparisons

Qualitative researchers typically do not plan in advance to make group comparisons because the intent of most qualitative studies is to thoroughly describe and explain a phenomenon. Nevertheless, patterns emerging in the data sometimes suggest that certain comparisons are relevant and illuminating. Sometimes, of course, comparisons *are* planned in qualitative studies (e.g., comparisons of two different cultures).

Example of qualitative comparisons: Draucker and Stern (2000) conducted a grounded theory study to describe women's responses to sexual violence by male intimates. They labeled the central process for these women as *forging ahead,* but discovered that there were variants to this process for three subgroups of women who experienced different types of sexual violence.

Number of Data Collection Points

Qualitative research, like quantitative research, can be either cross-sectional, with one data collection point, or longitudinal, with multiple data collection points over an extended time period, to observe the evolution of some phenomenon. Sometimes qualitative researchers plan in advance for a longitudinal design, but, in other cases, the decision to study a phenomenon longitudinally may be made in the field after preliminary data have been collected and analyzed.

Examples of the time dimension in qualitative studies:

- *Cross-sectional:* Dewar and Lee (2000) examined how people with a catastrophic illness or injury managed their circumstances. In a single interview, the researchers asked participants (who had endured their condition for between 3 and 25 years) to describe their coping processes over time.
- *Longitudinal:* Reising (2002) conducted a longitudinal study of the early socialization processes of critical care nurses. New critical care nurses were interviewed multiple times and kept a journal over a 5-month period.

Occurrence of the Independent and Dependent Variables

Qualitative researchers typically would not apply the terms *retrospective* or *prospective* to their studies. Nevertheless, in trying to elucidate the full nature of a phenomenon, they may look back retrospectively (with the assistance of study participants) for antecedent events leading to the occurrence of a phenomenon. Qualitative researchers may also study the effects of a phenomenon prospectively.

 Examples of exploring influences on phenomena in qualitative designs:

- *Retrospective exploration:* Hawley (2000) studied hospitalized patients' accounts of their physical and emotional well-being in relation to their descriptions of comforting strategies their nurses had used.
- *Prospective exploration:* Williams, Schutte, Evers, and Holkup (2000) conducted a prospective study to explore the short- and longer-term effects of getting normal test results from predictive gene testing for neurodegenerative disorders such as Huntington disease.

Research Setting

Qualitative researchers collect their data in real-world, naturalistic settings. And, whereas a quantitative researcher usually strives to collect data in one type of setting to maintain constancy of conditions (e.g., conducting all interviews in study participants' homes), qualitative researchers may deliberately strive to study their phenomena in a variety of natural contexts.

 Example of variation in settings:
Long, Kneafsey, Ryan, and Berry (2002) conducted a 2-year qualitative study to examine the nurse's role within multiprofessional rehabilitation teams in the United Kingdom. Forty-nine clients were recruited. Their pathways through rehabilitation services were observed for 6 months in a variety of settings, including homes, outpatient clinics, hospital wards, and nursing homes.

QUALITATIVE RESEARCH TRADITIONS

Despite the fact that there are some features common to many qualitative research designs, there is nevertheless a wide variety of overall approaches. Unfortunately, there is no readily agreed-upon classification system or taxonomy for the various approaches. Some authors have categorized qualitative studies in terms of analysis styles, others have classified them according to their broad focus. One useful system is to describe various types of qualitative research according to disciplinary traditions. These traditions vary in their conceptualization of what types of questions are important to ask in understanding the world in which we live. The section that follows provides an overview of several qualitative research traditions (some of which we have previously introduced), and subsequent sections describe in greater detail four traditions that have been especially useful for nurse researchers.

Overview of Qualitative Research Traditions

The research traditions that have provided a theoretical underpinning for qualitative studies come primarily from the disciplines of anthropology, psychology, and sociology. As shown in Table 11-1, each discipline has tended to focus on one or two broad domains of inquiry.

TABLE 11.1 Overview of Qualitative Research Traditions

DISCIPLINE	DOMAIN	RESEARCH TRADITION	AREA OF INQUIRY
Anthropology	Culture	Ethnography Ethnoscience (cognitive anthropology)	Holistic view of a culture Mapping of the cognitive world of a culture; a culture's shared meanings, semantic rules
Psychology/ philosophy	Lived experience	Phenomenology Hermeneutics	Experiences of individuals within their lifeworld Interpretations and meanings of individuals' experiences
Psychology	Behavior and events	Ethology Ecologic psychology	Behavior observed over time in natural context Behavior as influenced by the environment
Sociology	Social settings	Grounded theory Ethnomethodology Symbolic interaction (semiotics)	Social structural processes within a social setting Manner by which shared agreement is achieved in social settings Manner by which people make sense of social interactions
Sociolinguistics	Human communication	Discourse analysis	Forms and rules of conversation
History	Past behavior, events, and conditions	Historical analysis	Description and interpretation of historical events

The discipline of anthropology is concerned with human cultures. **Ethnography** (discussed more fully later in this chapter) is the primary research tradition in anthropology. Ethnographers study cultural patterns and experiences in a holistic fashion. **Ethnoscience** (sometimes referred to as **cognitive anthropology**) focuses on the cognitive world of a culture, with particular emphasis on the semantic rules and shared meanings that shape behavior.

Phenomenology has its disciplinary roots in both philosophy and psychology. As noted in Chapter 3, phenomenology focuses on the meaning of lived experiences of humans. A closely related research tradition is **hermeneutics**, which uses lived experiences as a tool for better understanding the social, cultural, political, or historical context in which those experiences occur. Hermeneutic inquiry almost always focuses on meaning and interpretation—how socially and historically conditioned individuals interpret their world within their given context.

The discipline of psychology has several other qualitative research traditions that focus on *behavior*.

Human **ethology**, which is sometimes described as the biology of human behavior, studies behavior as it evolves in its natural context. Human ethologists use primarily observational methods in an attempt to discover universal behavioral structures. **Ecological psychology** focuses more specifically on the influence of the environment on human behavior, and attempts to identify principles that explain the interdependence of humans and their environmental context.

Example of an ethologic study:
Morse, Penrod, Kassab, and Dellasega (2000) studied comforting behaviors of trauma team practitioners and their effect on successful completion of the uncomfortable procedure of nasogastric tube insertion. Thirty-two attempts at nasogastric insertion from 193 videotaped trauma cases were analyzed in detail.

Sociologists study the social world in which we live and have developed several research traditions of importance to qualitative researchers. The **grounded theory** tradition (described briefly earlier and elaborated upon later in this chapter) seeks to describe and understand key social psychological and structural processes in social settings.

Ethnomethodology seeks to discover how people make sense of their everyday activities and interpret their social worlds so as to behave in socially acceptable ways. Within this tradition, researchers attempt to understand a social group's norms and assumptions that are so deeply ingrained that the members no longer think about the underlying reasons for their behaviors.

Example of an ethnomethodologic study:
Wakefield (2000) conducted an ethnomethodologic study to examine the practicalities of organizing surgical nurses' work in the United Kingdom health service. Wakefield made detailed observations of nurses working on a 32-bed general surgical unit.

Unlike most other qualitative researchers, ethnomethodologists occasionally engage in **ethnomethodologic experiments**. During such experiments, researchers disrupt ordinary activity by doing something that violates the group's norms

and assumptions. They then observe what group members do and how they try to make sense of what is happening. An example is observing what happens when a nurse violates expectations of appropriate behavior at nurses' change of shift report on a medical intensive care unit. For example, a nurse might be enlisted to start her day shift by deliberately taking out a novel and reading it while the charge nurse from nights is reporting on the status of critically ill patients. The researcher would then observe how the rest of the unit staff deals with this departure from expected behavior.

Symbolic interaction is a sociologic and social-psychological tradition with roots in American pragmatism. Like other qualitative frameworks, symbolic interaction has been defined and specified in various ways and is therefore difficult to describe briefly. Basically, symbolic interaction focuses on the manner in which people make sense of social interactions and the interpretations they attach to social symbols, such as language. There are three basic premises underlying this tradition: first, that people act and react on the basis of the meanings that objects and other people in their environment have for them; second, that these meanings are based on social interaction and communication; and third, that these meanings are established through an interpretive process undertaken by each individual. Symbolic interactionists sometimes use **semiotics**, which refers to the study of signs and their meanings. A sign is any entity or object that carries information (e.g., a diagram, map, or picture).

Example of an symbolic interaction study:
Rehm (2000) studied Mexican-American parents' perceptions of family relationships influenced by their children's chronic physical conditions. The researcher believed that symbolic interaction, which focuses on the interaction between family members and the meaning shared through this social interaction, was a useful framework for studying families' coping.

The domain of inquiry for sociolinguists is human communication. The tradition often referred to as **discourse analysis** (sometimes called *conversation analysis*) seeks to understand the rules, mechanisms, and structure of conversations. Discourse analysts are interested in understanding the action that a given kind of talk "performs." The data for discourse analysis typically are transcripts from naturally occurring conversations, such as those between nurses and their patients. In discourse analysis, the texts are situated in their social, cultural, political, and historical context. Parker (1992) and Potter and Wetherall (1994) offer suggestions on how to approach a discourse analysis.

Example of a discourse analysis:
Hallett, Austin, Caress, and Luker (2000) used discourse analysis to study community nurses' perceptions of patient compliance in wound care. Sixty-two nurses in the United Kingdom were interviewed. The texts of their interview transcripts were analyzed to identify hidden meanings in the nurses' narratives.

Finally, **historical research**—the systematic collection and critical evaluation of data relating to past occurrences—is also a tradition that relies primarily on qualitative data. Nurses have used historical research methods to examine a wide range of phenomena in both the recent and more distant past.

Researchers in each of these traditions have developed methodologic guidelines for the design and conduct of relevant studies. Thus, once a researcher has identified what aspect of the human experience is of greatest interest, there is typically a wealth of advice available about methods likely to be productive and design issues that need to be handled in the field.

TIP: Sometimes a research report identifies more than one tradition as having provided the framework for a qualitative inquiry (e.g., a phenomenological study using the grounded theory method). However, such "method slurring" (Baker, Wuest, & Stern, 1992) has been criticized because each research tradition has different intellectual assumptions and methodologic prescriptions.

Ethnography

Ethnography is a type of qualitative inquiry that involves the description and interpretation of cultural behavior. Ethnographies are a blend of a process and a product, field work, and a written text. Field work is the process by which the ethnographer inevitably comes to understand a culture, and the ethnographic text is how that culture is communicated and portrayed. Because culture is, in itself, not visible or tangible, it must be constructed through ethnographic writing. Culture is inferred from the words, actions, and products of members of a group.

Ethnographic research is in some cases concerned with broadly defined cultures (e.g., a Samoan village culture), in what is sometimes referred to as a **macroethnography.** However, ethnographies sometimes focus on more narrowly defined cultures in a **microethnography**. Microethnographies are exhaustive, fine-grained studies of either small units in a group or culture (e.g., the culture of homeless shelters), or of specific activities in an organizational unit (e.g., how nurses communicate with children in an emergency department). An underlying assumption of the ethnographer is that every human group eventually evolves a culture that guides the members' view of the world and the way they structure their experiences.

Ethnographers seek to learn from (rather than to study) members of a cultural group—to understand their world view. Ethnographic researchers sometimes refer to "emic" and "etic" perspectives (terms that originate in linguistics, i.e., phon*emic* versus phon*etic*). An **emic perspective** refers to the way the members of the culture envision their world—it is the insiders' view. The emic is the local language, concepts, or means of expression that are used by the members of the group under study to name and characterize their experiences. The **etic perspective**, by contrast, is the outsiders' interpretation of the experiences of that culture; it is the language used by those doing the research to refer to the same phenomena. Ethnographers strive to acquire an emic perspective of a culture under study. Moreover, they strive to reveal what has been referred to as **tacit knowledge**, information about the culture that is so deeply embedded in cultural experiences that members do not talk about it or may not even be consciously aware of it. Although it is important to grasp the insider's perspective, it is also important for the ethnographer to illuminate the connection between the emic and the second-order, integrative and interpretational concepts that advance the aims of knowledge.

Ethnographers almost invariably undertake extensive field work to learn about the cultural group in which they are interested. Ethnographic research typically is a labor-intensive endeavor that requires long periods of time in the field—years of field work may be required. In most cases, researchers strive to participate actively in cultural events and activities. The study of a culture requires a certain level of intimacy with members of the cultural group, and such intimacy can be developed only over time and by working directly with those members as active participants. The concept of **researcher as instrument** is frequently used by anthropologists to describe the significant role ethnographers play in analyzing and interpreting a culture.

Three broad types of information are usually sought by ethnographers: cultural behavior (what members of the culture do), cultural artifacts (what members of the culture make and use), and cultural speech (what people say). This implies that ethnographers rely on a wide variety of data sources, including observations, in-depth interviews, records, charts, and other types of physical evidence (e.g., photographs, diaries, letters).

The product of ethnographic research usually is a rich and holistic description of the culture under study. Ethnographers also make interpretations of the culture, describing normative behavioral and social patterns. Among health care researchers, ethnography provides access to the health beliefs and health practices of a culture or subculture. Ethnographic inquiry can thus help to facilitate understanding of behaviors affecting health and illness.

A rich array of ethnographic methods have been developed and cannot be fully explicated in this general textbook, but more information may be found in Hammersley and Atkinson (1983),

Spradley and McCurdy (1972), Fetterman (1989), and Goetz and LeCompte (1984). Two variants of ethnographic research (ethnonursing research and ethnoscience) are described here, and a third (critical ethnography) is described later in this chapter.

Example of an ethnographic study:
Lipson (2001) conducted an ethnographic study about the experiences of people with multiple chemical sensitivity. She gathered her data (which included in-depth interviews and observations) in two U.S. and two Canadian settings. Her report includes a particularly valuable discussion of issues relating to the conduct of **autoethnography** (or **insider research**), in which ethnographers study their own culture or group.

Ethnonursing Research

Many nurse researchers have undertaken ethnographic studies. Indeed, Leininger has coined the phrase **ethnonursing research**, which she defines as "the study and analysis of the local or indigenous people's viewpoints, beliefs, and practices about nursing care behavior and processes of designated cultures" (1985, p. 38). In conducting an ethnonursing study, the investigator uses a broad theoretical framework to guide the research, such as Leininger's theory of culture care.

Leininger (1991) developed a number of enablers to help guide researchers in conducting ethnonursing research. *Enablers* are ways to help discover complex phenomena like human care. Some of her enablers include her Stranger—Friend Model, Observation—Participation—Reflection Model, and Acculturation Enabler Guide.

Example of an ethnonursing study:
Wittig (2001) conducted an ethnonursing study focusing on organ donation beliefs of African-American women living in rural Mississippi. Wittig made numerous visits to the site and conducted in-depth interviews with 10 African-American women.

Ethnoscience

In cognitive anthropology, culture is defined in purely mentalistic terms. This type of ethnography concentrates on understanding cultural knowledge through an emphasis on relationships between words. Cognitive anthropologists assume that a group's cultural knowledge is reflected in its language. One of the purposes of cognitive anthropology is to produce a map of the cognitive world of a culture that addresses its semantic rules. Ethnoscience often relies on quantitative as well as qualitative data. Findings of ethnoscience are often displayed in taxonomic trees.

Example of an ethnoscience study:
Banister (1999) investigated midlife women's perceptions of their changing bodies in Western culture using an ethnoscience approach. Eleven women 40 to 53 years of age were interviewed and their transcripts were analyzed using Spradley and McCurdy's (1972) method.

Phenomenology

Phenomenology, rooted in a philosophical tradition developed by Husserl and Heidegger, is an approach to discovering the meaning of people's life experiences. Phenomenological researchers ask: What is the *essence* of this phenomenon as experienced by these people and what does it *mean*? Phenomenologists assume there is an essence—an essential invariant structure—that can be understood, in much the same way that ethnographers assume that cultures exist. Phenomenologists investigate subjective phenomena in the belief that critical truths about reality are grounded in people's lived experiences.

There are two "schools" of phenomenology: descriptive phenomenology and interpretive phenomenology (hermeneutics). Descriptive phenomenology was developed first by Husserl (1962), who was primarily interested in the question: What do we know as persons? His philosophy emphasized descriptions of the meaning of human experience. Heidegger, a student of Husserl, moved away from his professor's philosophy into interpretive phenomenology. To Heidegger (1962), the critical question is: What is Being? He stressed interpreting and understanding—not just describing—

human experience. The focus of phenomenological inquiry, then, is the meaning of people's experience in regard to a phenomenon (descriptive phenomenology), and how those experiences are interpreted (hermeneutics).

Phenomenologists believe that lived experience gives meaning to each person's perception of a particular phenomenon. The goal of phenomenological inquiry is to fully describe lived experience and the perceptions to which it gives rise. Four aspects of lived experience that are of interest to phenomenologists are **lived space** or **spatiality; lived body** or **corporeality; lived time** or **temporality; and lived human relation** or **relationality.**

Phenomenologists believe that human existence is meaningful and interesting because of people's consciousness of that existence. The phrase **being-in-the-world** (or **embodiment**) is a concept that acknowledges people's physical ties to their world—they think, see, hear, feel, and are conscious through their bodies' interaction with the world.

In a phenomenological study, the main data source is in-depth conversations, with researchers and informants as full coparticipants. The researcher helps the informant to describe lived experiences without leading the discussion. Through in-depth conversations, the researcher strives to gain entrance into the informants' world, to have full access to their experiences as lived. Sometimes two separate interviews or conversations may be needed. For some phenomenological researchers, the inquiry includes not only gathering information from informants, but also efforts to experience the phenomenon in the same way, typically through participation, observation, and introspective reflection.

Although there are a number of methodologic interpretations of phenomenology, a descriptive phenomenological study often involves the following four steps: bracketing, intuiting, analyzing, and describing. **Bracketing** refers to the process of identifying and holding in abeyance preconceived beliefs and opinions about the phenomenon under study. Although bracketing can never be achieved totally, researchers bracket out the world and any presuppositions, to the extent possible, so as to confront the data in pure form. Bracketing is an iterative process that involves preparing, evaluating, and providing systematic, ongoing feedback about the effectiveness of the bracketing. Porter (1993) believes that bracketing can result in more productive use of researchers' time if they attempt to understand the effects of their experiences rather than expending energy trying to eliminate them. Ahern (1999) provides 10 tips to help qualitative researchers with bracketing through notes in a **reflexive journal**:

1. Make note of interests that, as a researcher, you may take for granted (i.e., gaining access).
2. Clarify your personal values and identify areas in which you know you are biased.
3. Identify areas of possible role conflict.
4. Recognize gatekeepers' interest and make note of the degree to which they are favorably or unfavorably disposed toward your research.
5. Identify any feelings you have that may indicate a lack of neutrality.
6. Describe new or surprising findings in collecting and analyzing data.
7. Reflect on and profit from methodologic problems that occur during your research.
8. After data analysis is complete, reflect on how you write up your findings.
9. Reflect on whether the literature review is truly supporting your findings, or whether it is expressing the similar cultural background that you have.
10. Consider whether you can address any bias in your data collection or analysis by interviewing a participant a second time or reanalyzing the transcript in question.

Intuiting, the second step in descriptive phenomenology, occurs when researchers remain open to the meanings attributed to the phenomenon by those who have experienced it. Phenomenological researchers then proceed to the analysis phase (i.e., extracting significant statements, categorizing, and making sense of the essential meanings of the phenomenon). (Chapter 23 provides further information regarding the analysis of data collected in phenomenological studies.) Finally, the descriptive

phase occurs when the researcher comes to understand and define the phenomenon. Note that an important distinction between descriptive and interpretive phenomenology is that in an interpretive phenomenological study, bracketing does not occur. For Heidegger, it was not possible to bracket one's being-in-the-world. Hermeneutics presupposes prior understanding on the researcher's part.

The phenomenological approach is especially useful when a phenomenon of interest has been poorly conceptualized. The topics appropriate to phenomenology are ones that are fundamental to the life experiences of humans; for health researchers, these include such topics as the meaning of stress, the experience of bereavement, and quality of life with a chronic illness.

A wealth of resources are available on phenomenological methods. Interested readers may wish to consult Spiegelberg (1975), Giorgi (1985), Colaizzi (1978), or Van Manen (1990).

Example of a phenomenological study: Rungreangkulkij and Chesla (2001) conducted a phenomenological study of Thai mothers' experiences caring for a child with schizophrenia. In-depth interviews were conducted with 12 Thai mothers who had adult schizophrenic children. Findings centered on the mothers' attempts to smooth their hearts with lots of water. In Thai culture, the metaphor of water and fire is used to help people calm down when experiencing negative emotions such as anger or frustration.

Grounded Theory

Grounded theory has become an important research method for the study of nursing phenomena, and has contributed to the development of many middle-range theories of phenomena relevant to nurses. Grounded theory began more as a systematic method of qualitative research than as a philosophy. Grounded theory was developed in the 1960s by two sociologists, Glaser and Strauss (1967), whose own theoretical links were in symbolic interactionism. One of their earliest studies (Glaser & Strauss, 1965) was a grounded theory study on dying in hospitals, in which the "prime controllable" variable was characterized as *awareness context* (i.e., who knows what about the patient's dying).

Grounded theory is an approach to the study of social processes and social structures. The focus of most grounded theory studies is the development and evolution of a social experience—the social and psychological stages and phases that characterize a particular event or episode. As noted in Chapter 6, the primary purpose of the grounded theory approach is to generate comprehensive explanations of phenomena that are grounded in reality.

In-depth interviews and observation are the most common data source in grounded theory studies, but existing documents and other data sources may also be used. Grounded theory research can involve the analysis of quantitative as well as qualitative data (Glaser & Strauss, 1967), but this rarely happens in practice.

Grounded theory methods constitute an entire approach to the conduct of field research. For example, a study that truly follows Glaser and Strauss's precepts does not begin with a highly focused research problem; the problem emerges from the data. One of the fundamental features of the grounded theory approach is that data collection, data analysis, and sampling of study participants occur simultaneously. Grounded theory methods are inherently nonlinear in nature, and therefore difficult to characterize. The process is recursive: researchers must systematically collect data, categorize them, describe the central phenomenon, and recycle earlier steps.

A procedure referred to as **constant comparison** is used to develop and refine theoretically relevant categories. Categories elicited from the data are constantly compared with data obtained earlier in the data collection process so that commonalities and variations can be determined. As data collection proceeds, the inquiry becomes increasingly focused on emerging theoretical concerns. Data analysis in a grounded theory framework is described in greater depth in Chapter 23.

 TIP: Beginning qualitative researchers should be aware that if they have constraints

in the amount of time they can devote to conducting a study, a grounded theory study is a much lengthier process than a phenomenological study.

Example of a grounded theory study:
Knobf (2002) sought to develop a substantive theory to explain women's responses to chemotherapy-induced premature menopause within the context of breast cancer. *Vulnerability* was identified as the women's basic social problem, and *carrying on* is the basic social process explaining how women respond to vulnerability.

Formal Grounded Theory

Glaser and Strauss (1967) distinguished two types of grounded theory: substantive and formal. **Substantive theory** is grounded in data on a specific substantive area, such as postpartum depression. It can serve as a springboard for **formal grounded theory**, which involves developing a higher, more abstract level of theory from a compilation of substantive grounded theory studies regarding a particular phenomenon. Glaser and Strauss' (1971) theory of status passage is an example of a formal grounded theory.

Kearney (1998) used an interesting analogy to differentiate substantive theories (custom-tailored clothing) and formal theory (ready-to-wear clothing). Formal grounded theories were likened to clothing sold in department stores that can fit a wider variety of users. Formal grounded theory is not personally tailored like substantive theory, but rather provides a conceptualization that applies to a broader population experiencing a common phenomenon. Formal grounded theories are not situation specific. The best data for constructing formal grounded theories are substantive grounded theories.

Example of a formal grounded theory:
Kearney (2001a) developed a formal grounded theory of women's response to violent relationships, based on 13 studies of women's experiences with domestic violence. The formal grounded theory described women's basic process of *enduring love.*

Alternate Views of Grounded Theory

In 1990, Strauss and Corbin published what was to become a controversial book, *Basics of Qualitative Research: Grounded Theory Procedures and Techniques.* Strauss and Corbin stated that the purpose of the book was to provide beginning grounded theory students with a more concrete description of the procedures involved in building theory at the substantive level.

Glaser, however, disagreed with some of the procedures advocated by Strauss (his original coauthor) and Corbin (a nurse researcher). Glaser published a rebuttal in 1992, *Emergence Versus Forcing: Basics of Grounded Theory Analysis.* Glaser believed that Strauss and Corbin developed a method that is not grounded theory but rather what he calls "full conceptual description." According to Glaser, the purpose of grounded theory is to generate concepts and theories about their relationships that explain, account for, and interpret variation in behavior in the substantive area under study. *Conceptual description*, in contrast, is aimed at describing the full range of behavior of what is occurring in the substantive area, "irrespective of relevance and accounting for variation in behavior" (Glaser, 1992, p. 19).

Nurse researchers have conducted grounded theory studies using both the original Glaser and Strauss and the Strauss and Corbin approaches.

 Example of grounded theory alternatives: Kendall (1999) provided an excellent comparison of the two approaches to grounded theory from her own research on families with a child with attention deficit—hyperactivity disorder. She described study results two ways—first, results obtained using Strauss and Corbin's approach, and second, the findings that emerged using Glaser and Strauss' original grounded theory approach. Kendall felt that Strauss and Corbin's coding procedure was a distraction that hindered her ability to reach the higher level of abstract thinking needed in grounded theory analysis.

Historical Research

Historical research is the systematic collection, critical evaluation, and interpretation of historical evidence (i.e., data relating to past occurrences). In general, historical research is undertaken to answer questions about causes, effects, or trends relating to past events that may shed light on present behaviors or practices. An understanding of contemporary nursing theories, practices, or issues can often be enhanced by an investigation of a specified segment of the past. Historical data are usually qualitative, but quantitative data are sometimes used (e.g., historical census data).

Historical research can take many forms. For example, many nurse researchers have undertaken *biographical histories* that study the experiences or contributions of individuals, such as nursing leaders. Currently, some historians are focusing on the history and experience of the ordinary person, often studying such issues as gender, race, and class. Other historical researchers undertake *social histories* that focus on a particular period in attempts to understand prevailing values and beliefs that may have helped to shape subsequent developments. Still others undertake what might be called *intellectual histories*, where historical ideas or ways of thinking are scrutinized.

Historical research should not be confused with a review of the literature about historical events. Like other types of research, historical inquiry has as its goal the discovery of *new* knowledge, not the summary of existing knowledge. One important difference between historical research and a literature review is that historical researchers are often guided by specific hypotheses or questions, or by a theoretical orientation or ideology (e.g., feminism). Hypotheses in historical research represent attempts to explain and interpret the conditions, events, or phenomena under investigation. Such hypotheses are not tested statistically; rather, they are broadly stated conjectures about relationships among historical events, trends, and phenomena.

Example of a hypothesis in historical research:
Lusk (2000) analyzed images of nurses in advertisements from 1930 to 1950. She hypothesized that nurses' relative status in advertisements would be higher in 1940 (when women were encouraged to enter nursing as a patriotic duty) than in 1930 or 1950. Her hypothesis was supported.

After research questions or hypotheses are developed, researchers must determine what types of data are available. Historical researchers typically need to devote considerable effort to identifying and evaluating data sources on events and situations that occurred in the past.

Collecting Historical Data

Data for historical research are usually in the form of written records: diaries, letters, notes, newspapers, minutes of meetings, medical or legal documents, and so forth. However, nonwritten materials may also be of interest. For example, physical remains and objects are potential sources of information. Visual materials, such as photographs and films, are forms of data, as are audio materials, such as records and tapes. In some cases, it is possible to conduct interviews with people who participated in historical events (e.g., nurses who served in Vietnam).

Many historical materials may be difficult to obtain and, in many cases, have been discarded. Historically significant materials are not always conveniently indexed by subject, author, or title. The identification of appropriate historical materials usually requires a considerable amount of time, effort, and detective work. Fortunately, there are several archives of historical nursing documents, such as the collections at several universities (e.g., Archives of Nursing Leadership, University of Connecticut; The Nursing Archives, Mugar Memorial Library, Boston University; Teachers College Milbank Memorial Library, Columbia University; Sterling Memorial Library, Yale University; South West Center for Nursing History, University of Texas, Austin; Center for the Study of the History of Nursing, University of Pennsylvania), as well as collections at National Library of Medicine, the American Journal of Nursing Company, the National League for Nursing, and the New York Public Library. Useful sources for identifying archives in the United States include the *National Inventory of Documentary Sources in the United States* and the *Directory of Archives and Manuscript Repositories in the United States*. Finally, the American Association for the History of Nursing, which publishes the *Nursing History Review*, is a potential source for locating public and private manuscript collections.

TIP: Archives are different from libraries. Archives contain unpublished materials that are accessed through **finding aids** rather than card catalogs. A finding aid is a resource that tells researchers what is in the archive. Archival materials do not circulate; researchers are almost always required to use the material on site (although sometimes microfiches are available). Typically, because of the fragile nature of the material, it cannot be photocopied, so researchers must take detailed notes (laptop computers are invaluable). Sometimes gloves are required when touching original materials. Access to archives may be limited to researchers who present a description of a proposed project to archivists.

Historical materials usually are classified as either primary or secondary sources. A **primary source** is first-hand information, such as original documents, relics, or artifacts. Examples are the diaries and writings of Sophronia Bucklin (1869), minutes of American Nurses Association meetings, hospital records, and so forth. Written primary sources are authored by people directly *involved* in a described event. Primary sources represent the most direct link with historical events or situations: Only the narrator (in the case of written materials) intrudes between original events and the historical researcher.

Secondary sources are second- or third-hand accounts of historical events or experiences. For example, textbooks, other reference books, and newspaper articles are secondary sources. Secondary sources, in other words, are discussions of events written by individuals who did not participate in them, but are often summarizing or interpreting primary source materials. Secondary sources may be historical (e.g., newspaper accounts contemporaneous with the events under study), or more modern interpretations of past events. Primary sources should be used whenever possible in historical research. The further removed from the historical event the information is, the less reliable, objective, and comprehensive the data are likely to be. However, secondary sources can be useful in identifying primary sources. It is particularly important in reading secondary source material to pay careful attention to footnotes, which often provide important clues about primary sources.

Evaluating Historical Data

Historical evidence is subjected to two types of evaluation, which historians refer to as external and internal criticism. **External criticism** is concerned with the data's authenticity. For example, a nursing historian might have a diary presumed to be written by Dorothea Dix. External criticism would involve asking such questions as: Is this the handwriting of Ms. Dix? Is the diary's paper of the right age? Are the writing style and ideas expressed consistent with her other writings? There are various scientific techniques available to determine the age of materials, such as x-ray and radioactive procedures. Other flaws, however, may be less easy to detect. For example, there is the possibility that material of interest may have been written by a ghost writer, that is, by someone other than the person of interest. There are also potential problems of mechanical errors associated with transcriptions, translations, or typed versions of historical materials.

Internal criticism of historical data refers to an evaluation of the worth of the evidence. The focus of internal criticism is not on the physical aspects of the materials but on their content. The key issue is the accuracy or truth of the data. For example, researchers must question whether a writer's representations of historical events are unbiased. It may also be appropriate to ask if the author of a document was in a position to make a valid report of an event or occurrence, or whether the writer was competent as a recorder of fact. Evidence bearing on the accuracy of historical data often includes comparisons with other people's accounts of the same event to determine the degree of agreement, knowledge of the time at which the document was produced (reports of events or situations tend to be more accurate if

they are written immediately after the event), and knowledge of the writers' point of view or biases and their competence to record events authoritatively and accurately.

TIP: Tuchman (1994) offers this useful advice: "Ask questions of all data, primary and secondary sources. Do not assume anything about the data is 'natural,' inevitable, or even true. To be sure, a datum has a physical presence: One may touch the page ... one has located. But that physical truth may be radically different from the interpretive truth..." (p. 321).

Analyzing and Interpreting Historical Data

In historical research, data analysis and data collection are usually ongoing, concurrent activities. The analysis of historical data is broadly similar to other approaches to qualitative analysis (see Chapter 23), in that researchers search for themes. In historical research, however, the thematic analysis is often guided by underlying hypotheses or theoretical frameworks. Within the selected framework, researchers concentrate on particular issues present in the data.

Historical research is usually interpretive. Historical researchers try to describe what happened, and also how and why it happened. Relationships between events and ideas, between people and organizations, are explored and interpreted within both their historical context and within the context of new viewpoints about what is historically significant.

There are many resources available for those interested in historical nursing research, including Lewenson (2003), Fitzpatrick (2001), and Lusk (1997).

Example of a historical study:
Dunphy (2001a, b) examined the stories of nurses and patients about the iron lung (the so-called "steel cocoon") between 1929 and 1955. She used a variety of sources such as photographs, drawings, procedural pamphlets from the March of Dimes and American Red Cross, first-person accounts, and a website called "Virtual Museum of the Iron Lung."

TIP: Avoid jumping to conclusions about the qualitative research tradition of a study based on the report's title. For example, the study "Hardships and personal strategies of Vietnam War nurses" (Scannell-Desch, 2000) is not a historical study, but rather a phenomenological study. As another example, despite the title's reference to a cultural group, "Hearing and caring for Haitian adolescents" (Colin, 2001) is a phenomenological study, not an ethnography.

OTHER TYPES OF QUALITATIVE RESEARCH

Qualitative studies typically can be characterized and described in terms of the disciplinary research traditions discussed in the previous section. However, several other important types of qualitative research also deserve mention. This section discusses qualitative research that is not associated with any particular discipline.

Case Studies

Case studies are in-depth investigations of a single entity or a small number of entities. The entity may be an individual, family, group, institution, community, or other social unit. In a case study, researchers obtain a wealth of descriptive information and may examine relationships among different phenomena, or may examine trends over time. Case study researchers attempt to analyze and understand issues that are important to the history, development, or circumstances of the entity under study.

One way to think of a case study is to consider what is center stage. In most studies, whether qualitative or quantitative, a certain phenomenon or variable (or set of variables) is the core of the inquiry. In a case study, the *case* itself is central. As befits an intensive analysis, the focus of case studies is typically on determining the dynamics of *why* an individual thinks, behaves, or develops in a particular manner rather than on *what* his or her status, progress, or actions are. It is not unusual for probing research of this type to require detailed study

over a considerable period. Data are often collected that relate not only to the person's present state but also to past experiences and situational factors relevant to the problem being examined. The data for in-depth case studies are usually qualitative, but may also be quantitative.

A distinction is sometimes drawn between an intrinsic and instrumental case study. In an *intrinsic case study,* researchers do not have to select the case. For instance, a process evaluation is often a case study of the implementation of a particular program; the "case" is a given. In an *instrumental case study*, researchers begin with a research question or perplexity, and seek out a case that offers illumination. The aim of such a case study is to use the case to understand something else, some phenomenon of interest. In such a situation, a case is usually selected not because it is typical, but rather because it can maximize what can be learned about the phenomenon.

Although the foremost concern of a case study is to understand the particular case, case studies are sometimes a useful way to explore phenomena that have not been rigorously researched. The information obtained in case studies can be used to develop hypotheses to be tested more rigorously in subsequent research. The intensive probing that characterizes case studies often leads to insights concerning previously unsuspected relationships. Furthermore, in-depth case studies may serve the important role of clarifying concepts or of elucidating ways to capture them.

The greatest strength of case studies is the depth that is possible when a limited number of individuals, institutions, or groups is being investigated. Case studies provide researchers with opportunities of having an intimate knowledge of a person's condition, thoughts, feelings, actions (past and present), intentions, and environment. On the other hand, this same strength is a potential weakness because researchers' familiarity with the person or group may make objectivity more difficult—especially if the data are collected by observational techniques for which the researchers are the main (or only) observers. Perhaps the biggest criticism of case studies concerns generalizability: If researchers discover important relationships, it is difficult to know whether the same relationships would occur with others. However, case studies can often play a critical role in challenging generalizations based on other types of research.

It is important to recognize that case study research is not simply anecdotal descriptions of a particular incident or patient. Case study research is a disciplined process and typically requires an extended period of systematic data collection. Two excellent resources for further reading on case study methods are the books by Yin (1994) and Stake (1995).

Example of a case study:
Porter, Ganong, and Armer (2000) presented a case study of an older rural African-American woman's support network and preferences for care providers. Based on their analysis, the researchers discussed implications for appraising the appropriateness of rural elders' in-home services.

Narrative Analyses

Narrative analysis focuses on *story* in studies in which the purpose is to determine how individuals make sense of events in their lives (Riessman, 1993). What distinguishes narrative analysis from other types of qualitative research designs, such as ethology, is its focus on the broad contours of a narrative. Stories are not fractured and dissected. The broad underlying premise of narrative research in the social sciences (as opposed to literary analysis) is the belief that people most effectively make sense of their world—and communicate these meanings—by constructing, reconstructing, and narrating stories. Individuals construct stories when they wish to understand specific events and situations that require linking an inner world of desire and motive to an external world of observable actions.

Muller (1999) has delineated five primary dimensions of the narrative approach:

1. People organize significant events in terms of stories and, through the telling of these stories, they make meaning of these experiences in their lives.

2. Time and plot are structural properties of narratives. Events in a story follow a sequence.
3. Narratives have a cultural contextual; they do not occur by themselves.
4. Narratives are relational. Stories are told to other people.
5. Narratives have power to shape human behavior. Narratives can be used to produce a moral story of how people are supposed to behave.

There is no standard approach to narrative analysis. Mishler (1995) has proposed a typology of models of narrative analysis. This three-category typology centers on the type of problem that is the central concern of the narrative analysis. Models in the first category focus on the temporal order of events in the discourse. The second set of models is concerned with the structure and coherence of how narratives are organized. Models in the third set of the typology focus on the cultural, social, and psychological contexts and functions of narratives.

Example of a narrative analysis:
Using narrative analysis, Ashida (2000) investigated women's experiences of smoking relapse after giving birth to a child. Twenty-seven women in Canada told their stories of smoking relapse. Analysis of the transcribed interviews involved reading the narratives closely, preparing brief summaries of each narrative, and identifying the central story lines.

Qualitative Outcome Analysis

Qualitative researchers have made considerable contributions to understanding health phenomena and people's experiences of health, illness, injury, and caretaking. However, qualitative researchers have not focused much attention on the development, implementation, and evaluation of interventions derived from qualitative research.

Morse, Penrod, and Hupcey (2000) believe that qualitative researchers have lacked procedural guidelines for moving from theory development to the identification and evaluation of specific clinical interventions. They developed a procedure that they call

qualitative outcome analysis (QOA) to address the theory—practice gap in qualitative research.

Qualitative researchers typically focus on a comprehensive understanding of a phenomenon in a specific context. Nursing strategies that served as interventions during the experience may not be documented or incorporated into the researchers' conceptual scheme because the interventions were not the project's focus. Additional data relevant to interventions can, however, be collected in subsequent QOA projects. QOA builds on an already-completed qualitative study in which a clinical problem has been examined. Table 11-2 presents a comparison of the purpose, focus, and outcome of the original qualitative study and the QOA project.

Morse and her colleagues outlined a series of steps that researchers can follow in planning and undertaking a QOA project. Two preliminary steps are critical, namely, assessing clinical settings for possible implementation of an intervention, and building an appropriate research team. After completing these steps and receiving administrative and institutional review board approval, the following procedures are undertaken:

Step 1: Outline the program of intervention strategies. The original theory is used to conceptualize the dynamics of the clinical problem and to identify appropriate interventions.

Step 2: Identify types of data to be collected. All types of data that could assist in interpreting and evaluating the intervention should be considered, but observation is likely to be especially important.

Step 3: Devise data collecting protocols. Data recording forms for recording strategies and insights of those implementing them are developed.

Step 4: Analyze data. Data are analyzed qualitatively according to both process and outcome.

Step 5: Disseminate findings. QOA project results must be published if they are to be significant for nursing practice.

Example of a QOA project:

In their initial qualitative project, Morse and Doberneck (1995) discovered seven stages in the process of *hoping* in four groups of patients: breast cancer, heart transplantation, spinal cord injury, and breastfeeding after returning back to work. Next, a Hope Assessment Guide was developed to assist nurses in identifying the stage of hope that a patient was in (Morse, Hutchinson, & Penrod, 1998; Penrod & Morse, 1997). The QOA project was designed to evaluate the feasibility of using the Hope Assessment Guide in clinical settings.

Secondary Analysis

In the preceding chapter, we noted that original quantitative studies sometimes involve an analysis of previously collected data, in what is referred to as a *secondary analysis*. Qualitative researchers,

TABLE 11.2 Comparison of an Initial Clinical Qualitative Study and a Qualitative Outcome Analysis (QOA) Project

TYPE OF PROJECT	PURPOSE	FOCUS	OUTCOME
Initial study	To understand a patient's experience	A clinical phenomenon or problem	A theory explaining patient experiences
QOA project	To identify strategies and evaluate their implementation	Intervention strategies	Efficacy of intervention strategies

Adapted from Morse, J. M., Penrod, J., & Hupcey, J. E. (2000). Qualitative outcome analysis: Evaluating nursing interventions for complex clinical phenomena. *Image: The Journal of Nursing Scholarship, 32,* 125–130.

like quantitative researchers, typically collect far more data than are analyzed originally. Secondary analyses of qualitative data provide opportunities to exploit rich data sets.

There are, however, some impediments to secondary analysis with qualitative data. The first is difficulty in identifying a suitable database. The availability of large quantitative data sets (especially from government-sponsored surveys) is widely publicized. There are a few repositories of qualitative data sets (e.g., the Murray Research Center at Radcliffe College, which has especially rich resources in the area of mental health). Identifying a suitable dataset usually means doing a lot of investigation. Probably the most typical method is to approach a researcher or team of researchers whose qualitative data appear to be of interest, based on reports they have written. (Not all qualitative researchers, however, are willing to share their data, because they themselves may intend to do further analyses.)

Another issue is that data from quantitative studies are easy to maintain in computer files, and there are standard protocols for documenting what is in the data set. Qualitative data are more voluminous, and there are few established conventions for maintaining, documenting, and encoding the data in computer files. This situation is beginning to change, however, as researchers have come to recognize the value of facilitating use of rich qualitative data sets for varied purposes by multiple users (Manderson, Kelaher, & Woelz-Stirling, 2001).

Thorne (1994) has identified five types of qualitative secondary analysis:

1. Analytic expansion. Original researchers use their own data to answer new questions as the theory base increases or to ask questions at a higher level of analysis.
2. Retrospective interpretation. The original database is used to examine new questions that were not thoroughly assessed in the original study
3. Armchair induction. This type is used for theory development where inductive approaches to the existing data sets are used.
4. Amplified sampling. Broader theories are developed by comparing different databases.

5. Cross-validation. Existing data sets are used in an effort to confirm new results and identify patterns beyond the ability of the original samples.

Thorne warned of potential hazards in secondary analysis of qualitative studies such as the possibility of exaggerating the effects of the original researcher's biases, and ethical questions regarding the use of the original data sets. Another challenge concerns evaluating the quality of the data set from the primary study. Hinds, Vogel, and Clarke-Steffen (1997) developed an assessment tool for just such a purpose. This assessment tool addresses such criteria as determining the fit of secondary research questions, completeness of the data set, and training of the primary team.

 Example of a secondary analysis of qualitative data:

Butcher, Holkup, and Buckwalter's (2001) study involved secondary analysis of 103 transcribed interviews describing the experience of caring for a family member with Alzheimer's disease. These interviews had been obtained from a larger, 4-year longitudinal study that tested a community-based psychoeducational nursing intervention. Butcher and colleagues conducted a secondary analysis of these interviews, conducted before the nursing intervention took place, using a phenomenological method.

Metasynthesis

As discussed in Chapter 10, the need to integrate knowledge across studies is growing—partly in response to the evidence-based movement—and this is true for both qualitative and quantitative research. Efforts are underway to develop techniques for qualitative metasynthesis (the qualitative analogue of meta-analysis).

An interpretive metasynthesis is more than just a narrative integration and summary of qualitative findings (i.e., a traditional literature review). **Metasynthesis** has been defined as "the theories, grand narratives, generalizations, or interpretive translations produced from the integration or comparison of findings from qualitative studies" (Sandelowski, Docherty, and Emden, 1997, p. 366).

Metasynthesis is described in greater detail in Chapter 27.

It might be noted that the terminology for qualitative synthesis approaches can be confusing. Researchers use different terms to label qualitative synthesis, such as qualitative meta-analysis, metaethnography, metainterpretation, or aggregating qualitative findings. Kearney's (2001b) "meta family" helps to clear up some of the confusion by placing current approaches to qualitative synthesis on a continuum from most theorizing to most interpretive. Starting with the theorizing end of the continuum and going to the interpretive end, Kearney orders these approaches as follows: grounded theory, metainterpretation, aggregated analysis, metastudy, metasynthesis, and metaethnography.

Example of a metasynthesis:
Beck (2001) conducted a metasynthesis of 14 qualitative studies on the meaning of caring in nursing education. The metasynthesis revealed five themes that permeated caring in nursing education, whether it was faculty caring for each other or their students, or nursing students caring for each other or their clients. These themes centered on reciprocal connecting, which consisted of presencing, sharing, supporting, competence, and the uplifting effects of caring.

Descriptive Qualitative Studies

Most qualitative researchers acknowledge a link to one of the research traditions or types of studies discussed in this chapter. Some qualitative studies, however, claim no particular disciplinary or methodologic roots. The researchers may simply indicate that they have conducted a qualitative study or a naturalistic inquiry, or they may say that they have done a **content analysis** of their qualitative data (i.e., an analysis of themes and patterns that emerge). Thus, some qualitative studies do not have a formal name or do not fit into the typology we have presented in this chapter. We refer to these as **descriptive qualitative studies**.

Sandelowski (2000) notes that in doing such descriptive qualitative studies, researchers tend not to penetrate their data in any interpretive depth.

These studies present comprehensive summaries of a phenomenon or of events in everyday language. Qualitative descriptive designs tend to be eclectic and are based on the general premises of naturalistic inquiry. Sandelowski stresses that researchers should not be ashamed to "just" use qualitative description as their research design. It is the method of choice if what they want is straight description of an event or phenomenon.

Example of a descriptive qualitative study:
Stubblefield and Murray (2001) interviewed 15 parents whose children had undergone lung transplantation to study the effect of the procedure on the parents' interpersonal relationships. The authors wrote that they "conducted a content analysis to formulate a narrative description of the parents' relationships with others" (p. 58).

RESEARCH WITH IDEOLOGICAL PERSPECTIVES

Some researchers, who have relied predominantly on qualitative data, conduct inquiries within an ideological framework, typically to draw attention to certain social problems or the needs of certain groups. These approaches represent important investigative avenues and are briefly described in this section.

Critical Theory

Critical theory originated with a group of Marxist-oriented German scholars in the 1920s, collectively referred to as the Frankfurt School. Variants of critical theory abound in the social sciences. Essentially, a critical researcher is concerned with a critique of society and with envisioning new possibilities.

Critical social science is typically action-oriented. Its broad aim is to integrate theory and practice such that people become aware of contradictions and disparities in their beliefs and social practices, and become inspired to change them. Critical researchers reject the idea of an objective and disinterested inquirer and are oriented toward a transformation process. An important feature of critical theory is that it calls for inquiries that foster enlightened self-knowledge and sociopolitical action. Moreover, critical theory involves a self-reflexive aspect. To prevent a critical theory of society from becoming yet another self-serving ideology, critical theorists must account for their own transformative effects.

The design of research in critical theory often begins with a thorough analysis of certain aspects of the problem. For example, critical researchers might analyze and critique taken-for-granted assumptions that underlie the problem, the language used to depict the situation, and the biases of prior researchers investigating the problem. Critical researchers often triangulate multiple methodologies, and emphasize multiple perspectives (e.g., alternative racial or social class perspectives) on problems. Critical researchers typically interact with study participants in ways that emphasize participants' expertise.

Critical theory has been applied in a number of disciplines, and has played an especially important role in ethnography. **Critical ethnography** focuses on raising consciousness and aiding emancipatory goals in the hope of effecting social change. Critical ethnographers address the historical, social, political and economic dimensions of cultures and their value-laden agendas. An assumption in critical ethnographic research is that actions and thoughts are mediated by power relationships (Hammersley, 1992). Critical ethnographers attempt to increase the political dimensions of cultural research and undermine oppressive systems (Giroux, 1992).

Some of the features that distinguish more traditional qualitative research and critical research are summarized in Table 11-3. Morrow and Brown (1994) and Carspecken and Apple (1992) provide useful accounts of critical theory methodology.

Example of a critical ethnography:
Herdman (2000) described a critical ethnography that focused on institutional discrimination in a hospital regarding health care to people with HIV/AIDS. The study sought to identify structures in the hospital that contributed to discrimination, so that these structures could be transformed. The

TABLE 11.3 Comparison of Traditional Qualitative Research and Critical Research

ISSUE	TRADITIONAL QUALITATIVE RESEARCH	CRITICAL RESEARCH
Research aims	Understanding; reconstruction of multiple constructions	Critique; transformation; consciousness-raising; advocacy
View of knowledge	Transactional/subjective; knowledge is created in interaction between investigator and participants	Transactional/subjective; value-mediated and value-dependent; importance of historical insights
Methods	Dialectic: truth is arrived at logically through conversations	Dialectic and didactic: dialogue designed to transform naivety and misinformation
Evaluative criteria for inquiry quality	Authenticity; trustworthiness	Historical situatedness of the inquiry; erosion of ignorance; stimulus for change
Researcher's role	Facilitator of multivoice reconstruction	Transformative agent; advocate; activist

publication of the research report gave rise to heated debates, including objections by the hospital's institutional ethics committee and a defensive reaction by some health care professionals.

Feminist Research

Feminist research approaches are similar to critical theory research, but the focus is sharply on gender domination and discrimination within patriarchal societies. Similar to critical researchers, feminist researchers seek to establish collaborative and nonexploitative relationships with their informants, to place themselves within the study to avoid objectification, and to conduct research that is transformative.

Gender is the organizing principle in feminist research, and investigators seek to understand how gender and a gendered social order have shaped women's lives and their consciousness. The aim is to ameliorate the "invisibility and distortion of female experience in ways relevant to ending women's unequal social position" (Lather, 1991, p. 71).

Although feminist researchers generally agree that it is important to focus on women's diverse situations and the institutions and relationships that frame those situations, there are many variants of feminist inquiry. Three broad models (within each of which there is diversity) have been identified: (1) *feminist empiricism*, whose adherents usually work within fairly standard norms of qualitative inquiry but who seek to portray more accurate pictures of the social realities of women's lives; (2) *feminist standpoint research*, which holds that inquiry ought to begin in and be tested against the lived everyday sociopolitical experiences of women, and that women's views are particular and privileged; and (3) *feminist postmodernism*, which stresses that "truth" is a destructive illusion, and views the world as endless stories, texts, and narratives. In nursing and health care, feminist empiricism and feminist standpoint research have been most prevalent.

The scope of feminist research ranges from studies of the particular and subjective views of individual women, to studies of social movements, structures, and broad policies that affect (and often

exclude) women. Olesen (1994), a sociologist who studied nurses' career patterns and definitions of success, has noted that some of the best feminist research on women's subjective experiences has been done in the area of women's health.

Feminist research methods typically include in-depth, interactive, and collaborative individual interviews or group interviews that offer the possibility of reciprocally educational encounters. Feminists usually seek to negotiate the meanings of the results with those participating in the study, and to be self-reflexive about what they themselves are experiencing and learning.

Feminist research, like other research that has an ideological perspective, has raised the bar for the conduct of ethical research. With the emphasis on trust, empathy, and nonexploitative relationships, proponents of these newer modes of inquiry view any type of deception or manipulation as abhorrent. As Punch (1994) has noted in speaking about ethics and feminist research, "you do not rip off your sisters" (p. 89).

Those interested in feminist methodologies may wish to consult such writers as Lather (1991) or Reinharz (1992).

Example of feminist research:
Gustafson (2000) collaborated with 10 other nurses in a study of nurses' job displacement in Canadian hospitals during the 1990s. She adopted a method that was "intended to be political in standpoint, gendered in focus, reflexive in process, and transformative in outcome" (p. 717). Gustafson described in some detail the benefits and limitations of using a feminist, collaborative research method, and how her "best laid plans" regarding the research were not always easy to sustain.

Participatory Action Research

A type of research known as participatory action research is closely allied to both critical research and feminist research. **Participatory action research** (PAR), one of several types of *action research* that originated in the 1940s with social psychologist Kurt Lewin, is based on a recognition that the production of knowledge can be political and can be used to exert power. Researchers in this approach typically work with groups or communities that are vulnerable to the control or oppression of a dominant group or culture.

Participatory action research is, as the name implies, participatory. There is collaboration between researchers and study participants in the definition of the problem, the selection of an approach and research methods, the analysis of the data, and the use to which findings are put. The aim of PAR is to produce not only knowledge, but action and consciousness-raising as well. Researchers specifically seek to empower people through the process of constructing and using knowledge. The PAR tradition has as its starting point a concern for the powerlessness of the group under study. Thus, a key objective is to produce an impetus that is directly used to make improvements through education and sociopolitical action.

In PAR, the research methods take second place to emergent processes of collaboration and dialogue that can motivate, increase self-esteem, and generate community solidarity. Thus, the "data-gathering" strategies used are not only the traditional methods of interview and observation (including both qualitative and quantitative approaches), but may include storytelling, sociodrama, drawing and painting, plays and skits, and other activities designed to encourage people to find creative ways to explore their lives, tell their stories, and recognize their own strengths.

Useful resources for learning more about PAR include Whyte (1990), Elden and Chisholm (1993), Morrison and Lilford (2001), and Holter and Schwartz-Barcott (1993). The multidisciplinary journal *Collaborative Inquiry* is specifically devoted to PAR and related modes of research.

Example of PAR:

Anderson, Nyamathi, McAvoy, Conde, and Casey (2001) used PAR to examine the perceptions of adolescents in juvenile detention regarding risks for HIV and other health problems. The researchers chose PAR because it involved the adolescents in a shared partnership in the research endeavor. PAR facilitated the empowerment of the detained adolescents by providing them with knowledge and skills generated from the research findings.

RESEARCH EXAMPLES

Nurse researchers have conducted studies in all of the qualitative research traditions described in this chapter, and several examples have been described. In the following sections we present more detailed descriptions of three qualitative nursing studies.

Research Example of a Critical/Feminist Ethnography

Brown and Fiske (2001) conducted a critical ethnography, drawing on feminist approaches, to explore First Nations (Aboriginal) women's experiences with mainstream health care services. The study addressed two central questions: How do First Nations women describe their encounters with local mainstream health care services, and how are these encounters shaped by social, political, and economic factors?

The research was conducted in partnership with a First Nations reserve community with a population of 600 in a rural area of northwest Canada. The community believed that it would benefit from a thorough description of the women's encounters as it developed plans for improving health and health care for its members. Women from the community (including one of the researchers) were renowned locally as First Nations leaders in health, and yet First Nations people were rarely invited to join nearby mainstream health boards or decision-making bodies.

Using input from community leaders and elders, the researchers selected 10 women to participate in two rounds of interviews. Each woman was interviewed separately for 1 to 2 hours. The second interviews were used to clarify and verify information from the first interviews. Participants were asked to describe both positive encounters (model cases) and negative encounters (contrary cases) with the health care establishment. An interpretive thematic analysis was conducted with transcripts from these interviews. The initial analysis was subjected to critical questioning, reflection, and discussions with participants.

The narratives revealed that the "women's encounters were shaped by racism, discrimination, and structural inequalities that continue to marginalize and disadvantage First Nations women" (p. 126). Participants described situations in which their health concerns or reported symptoms were not taken seriously or were trivialized. Encounters that revealed health care workers' discriminatory attitudes and behaviors were found to be pervasive.

Research Example of a Phenomenological Study

McInnis and White (2001) conducted a phenomenological study to explore the meaning of loneliness for 20 older adults living in the community. Before data collection, the researchers made every effort to bracket their presuppositions. For example, one of the researchers bracketed her extensive experience as a geropsychiatric nurse.

In-depth interviews were conducted with each older adult. The two main questions asked were, "Tell me about your loneliness" and "Describe the circumstances around this experience" (p. 132). The interviews were recorded, transcribed, and then analyzed using Giorgi's phenomenological method. This method entailed (1) reading and rereading the transcripts to dwell with the data, (2) identifying meaning units from each transcript, (3) expressing the psychological insight contained in each meaning unit, and (4) synthesizing all the formulated meanings into the essence of the experience.

The essence of the experience of loneliness for these elders consisted of five themes. One such theme was that loneliness is a state of anxiety or fear, influenced by dependency or the fear of it, and the decreased level of functioning. An excerpt illustrating this theme is as follows:

> You are so alone and you don't have anybody, you're almost afraid, don't want the night to come ... you see, during the day you might go out to the store or things like that ... but at night you sit and a woman is not going to be running around at night. (p. 134)

McInnis and White took great care to enhance and document the rigor of their study. For instance, a field journal was kept throughout the study to help with bracketing. The researchers also provided a piece of the documentation they maintained to give readers a concrete example of their research procedures.

Research Example of a Grounded Theory Study

Sayre (2000) conducted a grounded theory study of adults' perceptions of being psychiatric patients. She conducted biweekly interviews, from admission to discharge, with 35 patients diagnosed with schizophrenia who had been hospitalized in psychiatric units of an urban public facility. The central question of the inquiry was: How do individuals explain their admission to a psychiatric facility? Subquestions included: What contextual and intervening experiences influenced their explanation? What strategies resulted? and What were the consequences of those strategies?

Sayre strategically combined data from multiple sources to develop a thorough and comprehensive understanding of the patients' perceptions and strategies. Data were collected through in-depth interviews with the patients, observations, review of medical records, and informal conversations with staff. Two hundred hours of interview data were obtained.

The constant comparative method of data analysis revealed that *managing self-worth* was the process inpatients used to cope with the stigma of being a psychiatric patient. Factors that affected individual responses to psychiatric hospitalization included substance abuse, lack of social capital (especially lack of stable housing), and medication noncompliance. Six attribution styles, rated on a continuum from acceptance to rejection of the psychiatric treatment model, emerged from the analysis: problem, disease, crisis, punishment, ordination, and violation. These attribution styles helped the patients to maintain their sense of self-worth during the stigmatizing process of psychiatric hospitalization.

SUMMARY POINTS

- Qualitative research involves an **emergent design**—a design that emerges in the field as the study unfolds.
- As **bricoleurs**, qualitative researchers tend to be creative and intuitive, putting together an array of data drawn from many sources to arrive at a holistic understanding of a phenomenon.
- Although qualitative design is elastic and flexible, qualitative researchers nevertheless can plan for broad contingencies that can be expected to pose decision opportunities for study design in the field.

- A naturalistic inquiry typically progresses through three broad phases: an orientation and overview phase to determine salient aspects of the phenomenon under study; a focused exploration phase that closely examines important aspects of the phenomenon; and a confirmation and closure phase to confirm findings.
- Qualitative research traditions have their roots in anthropology (e.g., **ethnography** and **ethnoscience**); philosophy (**phenomenology** and **hermeneutics**); psychology (**etiology** and **ecological psychology**); sociology (**grounded theory, ethnomethodology,** and **symbolic interaction**); sociolinguistics (**discourse analysis**); and history (**historical research**).
- Ethnography focuses on the culture of a group of people and relies on extensive field work. Ethnographers strive to acquire an **emic** (insider's) perspective of a culture rather than an **etic** (outsider's) perspective. Nurses sometimes refer to their ethnographic studies as **ethnonursing research**.
- The concept of **researcher as instrument** is frequently used by ethnographers to describe the significant role researchers play in analyzing and interpreting a culture.
- Phenomenology seeks to discover the *essence* and *meaning* of a phenomenon as it is experienced by people. In descriptive phenomenology, researchers strive to **bracket** out preconceived views and to **intuit** the essence of the phenomenon by remaining open to meanings attributed to it by those who have experienced it. Bracketing is not a feature of interpretive (hermeneutical) phenomenology.
- **Grounded theory**, an approach to studying social psychological processes and social structures, aims to discover theoretical precepts grounded in the data. This approach uses **constant comparison**: categories elicited from the data are constantly compared with data obtained earlier so that shared themes and variations can be determined.
- There are two types of grounded theory: **substantive theory**, which is grounded in data on a specific substantive area, and **formal grounded theory** (often using data from substantive theory studies), which is at a higher level of abstraction.
- A major controversy among grounded theory researchers concerns whether to follow the original Glaser and Strauss procedures or to use the adapted procedures of Strauss and Corbin; Glaser has argued that the latter approach does not result in *grounded theories* but rather in *conceptual descriptions*.
- **Historical research** is the systematic attempt to establish facts and relationships about past events. Historical data are normally subjected to **external criticism**, which is concerned with the authenticity of the source, and **internal criticism**, which assesses the worth of the evidence.
- **Case studies** are intensive investigations of a single entity or a small number of entities, such as individuals, groups, organizations, families, or communities; such studies usually involve collecting data over an extended period.
- **Narrative analysis** focuses on *story* in studies in which the purpose is to determine how individuals make sense of events in their lives.
- **Qualitative outcome analysis (QOA)** is a systematic means of confirming the applicability of clinical strategies suggested by a qualitative study and to evaluate clinical outcomes.
- Secondary analyses of qualitative data offer special opportunities, but researchers interested in such studies face several challenges.
- Qualitative **metasyntheses** are interpretive translations produced from the integration of findings from qualitative studies.
- A number of descriptive qualitative studies have no formal name or do not fit into any disciplinary tradition. Such studies may simply be referred to as qualitative studies, naturalistic inquiries, or as qualitative **content analyses**.
- Research is sometimes conducted within an ideological perspective, and such research tends to rely primarily on qualitative research.
- **Critical theory** is concerned with a critique of existing social structures; critical researchers strive to conduct inquiries that involve collaboration

with participants and foster enlightened self-knowledge and transformation. **Critical ethnography** uses the principles of critical theory in the study of cultures.

- **Feminist research**, like critical research, is designed to be transformative, but the focus is sharply on how gender domination and discrimination shape women's lives and their consciousness.

- **Participatory action research** (PAR) produces knowledge through close collaboration with groups or communities that are vulnerable to control or oppression by a dominant culture; in PAR research, methods take second place to emergent processes that can motivate people and generate community solidarity.

STUDY ACTIVITIES

Chapter 11 of the *Study Guide to Accompany Nursing Research: Principles and Methods, 7th edition*, offers various exercises and study suggestions for reinforcing concepts presented in this chapter. In addition, the following study questions can be addressed:

1. Develop a research question for a nursing research macroethnography. Then develop a research question that would be appropriate for a microethnography.
2. Suppose a researcher goes to a hospital waiting room and deliberately sits next to other people, even though there are many empty seats, and observes the behavior of those people. What type of study would this be?
3. Which of the following topics is best suited to a phenomenological inquiry? To an ethnography? To a grounded theory study? Provide a rationale for each response.
   a. The passage through menarche among Haitian refugees.
   b. The process of coping among AIDS patients.
   c. The experience of having a child with leukemia
   d. Rituals relating to dying among nursing home residents

   e. The experience of waiting for service in a hospital emergency department
   f. The decision-making process among nurses regarding do-not-resuscitate orders
4. Why is it that most qualitative researchers do not know in advance how many weeks or months will be required in the field to complete an investigation?
5. Choose a clinical problem that you see occurring in a specific patient population. Develop a research question related to this clinical problem that can be answered by conducting a phenomenological study. Develop another research question, but this time one that can be answered by conducting critical research or participatory action research.

SUGGESTED READINGS

Methodologic References

Ahern, K. J. (1999). Ten tips for reflexive bracketing. *Qualitative Health Research, 9*, 407–411.

Baker, C., Wuest, J., & Stern, P. N. (1992). Method slurring: The grounded theory/phenomenology example. *Journal of Advanced Nursing, 17*, 1355–1360.

Carspecken, P. F., & Apple, M. (1992). Critical qualitative research: Theory, methodology, and practice. In M. L. LeCompte, W. L. Millroy, & J. Preissle (Eds.), *The handbook of qualitative research in education*. San Diego, CA: Academic Press.

Chenitz, W. C., & Swanson, J. (Eds.). (1985). *Qualitative research in nursing: From practice to grounded theory*. Menlo-Park, CA: Addison-Wesley.

Cohen, M. Z., Kahn, D. L., & Steeves, R. H. (2000). *Hermeneutic phenomenological research: A practical guide for nurses*. Thousand Oaks, CA: Sage.

Colaizzi, P. F. (1978). Psychological research as the phenomenologist views it. In R. Valle & M. King (Eds.), *Existential phenomenological alternative for psychology*. New York: Oxford University Press.

Crabtree, B. C., & Miller, W. L. (Eds.). (1999). *Doing qualitative research* (2nd ed.). Thousand Oaks, CA: Sage.

Creswell, J. W. (1998). *Qualitative inquiry and research design: Choosing among five traditions*. Thousand Oaks, CA: Sage.

Denzin, N. K. (1989). *The research act* (3rd ed.). Englewood Cliffs, NJ: Prentice-Hall.

Denzin, N. K., & Lincoln, Y. S. (Eds.). (1994). *Handbook of qualitative research*. Thousand Oaks, CA: Sage.

Elden, M., & Chisholm, R. (Eds.). (1993). Varieties of action research [Special issue]. *Human Relations, 46*(2).

Fetterman, D. M. (1989). *Ethnography: Step by step*. Newbury Park, CA: Sage.

Fitzpatrick, M. L. (2001). Historical research: The method. In P. L. Munhall & C. J. Oiler (Eds.), *Nursing research: A qualitative perspective* (pp. 403–415). Norwalk, CT: Appleton-Century-Crofts.

Giorgi, A. (1985). *Phenomenology and psychological research*. Pittsburgh: Duquesne University Press.

Giroux, H. (1992). *Border crossings: Cultural workers and the politics of education*. New York: Routledge.

Glaser, B., & Strauss, A. (1971). *Status passage: A formal theory*. Chicago: Aldine.

Glaser, B. G. (1978). *Theoretical sensitivity*. Mill Valley, CA: Sociology Press.

Glaser, B. G. (1992). *Emergence versus forcing: Basics of grounded theory analysis*. Mill Valley, CA.: Sociology Press.

Glaser, B. G., & Strauss, A. L. (1967). *The discovery of grounded theory: Strategies for qualitative research*. Chicago: Aldine.

Goetz, J. P., & LeCompte, M. D. (1984). *Ethnography and qualitative design in educational research*. Orlando, FL: Academic Press.

Hammersley, M. (1992). *What's wrong with ethnography? Methodological explorations*. London: Routledge.

Hammersley, M., & Atkinson, P. (1983). *Ethnography: Principles in practice*. London: Tavistock.

Heidegger, M. (1962). *Being and time*. New York: Harper & Row.

Hinds, P. S., Vogel, R. J., & Clarke-Steffen, L. (1997). The possibilities and pitfalls of doing a secondary analysis of a qualitative data set. *Qualitative Health Research, 7*, 408–424.

Holter, I. M., & Schwartz-Barcott, D. (1993). Action research: What is it? How has it been used and how can it be used in nursing? *Journal of Advanced Nursing, 18*, 298–304.

Husserl, E. (1962). *Ideas: General introduction to pure phenomenology*. New York: Macmillan.

Kearney, M. H. (1998). Ready-to-wear: Discovering grounded formal theory. *Research in Nursing & Health, 21*, 179–186.

Kearney, M. H. (2001b). New directions in grounded formal theory. In R. S. Schreiber & P. N. Stern (Eds.), *Using grounded theory in nursing* (pp. 227–246). New York: Springer.

Lather, P. (1991). *Getting smart: Feminist research and pedagogy with/in the postmodern*. New York: Routledge.

Leininger, M. M. (Ed.). (1985). *Qualitative research methods in nursing*. New York: Grune and Stratton.

Leininger, M. M. (1991). *Culture care diversity and universality: A theory of nursing*. New York: NLN Press.

Lewenson, S. B. (2003). Historical research approach. In Speziale, H. J., & D. R. Carpenter (Eds.), *Qualitative research in nursing: Advancing the humanistic perspective* (pp. 207–233). Philadelphia: Lippincott Williams & Wilkins.

Lincoln, Y. S., & Guba, E. G. (1985). *Naturalistic inquiry*. Newbury Park, CA: Sage.

Lusk, B. (1997). Historical methodology for nursing research. *Image: The Journal of Nursing Scholarship, 29*, 355–359.

Manderson, L., Kelaher, M., & Woelz-Stirling, N. (2001). Developing qualitative databases for multiple users. *Qualitative Health Research, 11*, 149–160.

Mishler, E. G. (1995). Model of narrative analysis: A typology. *Journal of Narrative and Life History, 5*, 87–123.

Morrison, B., & Lilford, R. (2001). How can action research apply to health services? *Qualitative Health Research, 11*, 436–449.

Morrow, R. A., & Brown, D. D. (1994) *Critical theory and methodology*. Thousand Oaks, CA: Sage.

Morse, J. M. (1991). *Qualitative nursing research: A contemporary dialogue*. Newbury Park, CA: Sage.

Morse, J. M., & Field, P. A. (1995). *Qualitative research methods for health professionals* (2nd ed.). Thousand Oaks, CA: Sage.

Morse, J. M., Penrod, J., & Hupcey, J. E. (2000). Qualitative outcome analysis: Evaluating nursing interventions for complex clinical phenomena. *Journal of Nursing Scholarship, 32*, 125–130.

Muller, J. H. (1999). Narrative approaches to qualitative research in primary care. In B. F. Crabtree & W. L. Miller (Eds.), *Doing qualitative research* (pp. 221–238). Thousand Oaks, CA: Sage.

Olesen, V. (1994). Feminism and models of qualitative research. In N. K. Denzin & Y. S. Lincoln (Eds.), *Handbook of qualitative research* (pp. 158–174). Thousand Oaks, CA: Sage.

Parker, I. (1992). *Discourse dynamics: Critical analysis for social and individual psychology*. London: Routledge.

Porter, S. (1993). Nursing research conventions: Objectivity or obfuscation? *Journal of Advanced Nursing, 18*, 137–143.

Potter, J., & Wetherell, M. (1994). Analyzing discourse. In A. Bryman, & R. G. Burgess (Eds.), *Analyzing qualitative data* (pp. 83–97). London: Routledge.

Punch, M. (1994). Politics and ethics in qualitative research. In N. K. Denzin & Y. S. Lincoln (Eds.), *Handbook of qualitative research*. Thousand Oaks, CA: Sage.

Reinharz, S. (1992). *Feminist methods in social research.* New York: Oxford University Press.

Riessman, C. K. (1993). *Narrative analysis.* Newbury Park, CA: Sage.

Sandelowski, M. (2000). Whatever happened to qualitative description? *Research in Nursing & Health, 23,* 334–340.

Sandelowski, M., Docherty, S., & Emden, C. (1997). Qualitative metasynthesis: Issues and techniques. *Research in Nursing & Health, 20,* 365–371.

Spiegelberg, H. (1975). *Doing phenomenology.* The Hague: Nijhoff.

Spradley, J. P., & McCurdy, D. W. (1972). *The cultural experience: Ethnography in complex society.* Prospect Heights, IL: Waveland Press.

Stake, R. (1995). *The art of case study research.* Thousand Oaks, CA: Sage.

Strauss, A., & Corbin, J. (1990). *Basics of qualitative research: Grounded theory procedures and techniques.* Newbury Park, CA: Sage.

Speziale, H. J., & Carpenter, D. R. (2001). *Qualitative research in nursing: Advancing the humanistic imperative.* Philadelphia: Lippincott Williams & Wilkins.

Szabo, V., & Strang, V. (1997). Secondary analysis of qualitative data. *Advances in Nursing Science, 20,* 66–74.

Thorne, S. (1994). Secondary analysis in qualitative research: Issues and implications. In J. M. Morse (Ed.), *Critical issues in qualitative research methods.* Thousand Oaks, CA: Sage.

Tuchman, G. (1994). Historical social science: Methodologies, methods, and meanings. In N. K. Denzin & Y. S. Lincoln (Eds.), *Handbook of qualitative research* (pp. 306–323). Thousand Oaks, CA: Sage.

Van Manen, M. (1990). *Researching lived experience: Human science for an action sensitive pedagogy.* London, Ontario: Althouse.

Whyte, W. F. (Ed.). (1991). *Participatory action research.* Newbury Park, CA: Sage.

Yin, R. (1994). *Case study research: Design and methods* (2nd ed.). Thousand Oaks, CA: Sage.

Studies Cited in Chapter 11

Ashida, C. (2000). Narratives of smoking relapse: The stories of postpartum women. *Research in Nursing & Health, 23,* 126–134.

Anderson, N. L., Nyamathi, A., McAvoy, J. A., Conde, F., & Casey, C. (2001). Perceptions about risk for HIV/AIDS among adolescents in juvenile detention. *Western Journal of Nursing Research, 23,* 336–359.

Banister, E. M. (1999). Women's midlife experience of their changing bodies. *Qualitative Health Research, 9,* 520–537.

Beck, C. T. (2001). Caring within nursing education. *Journal of Nursing Education, 40,* 101–109.

Browne, A. J., & Fiske, J. (2001). First Nations women's encounters with mainstream health services. *Western Journal of Nursing Research, 23,* 126–147.

Butcher, H. K., Holkup, P. A., & Buckwalter, K. C. (2001). The experience of caring for a family member with Alzheimer's disease. *Western Journal of Nursing Research, 23,* 33–55.

Colin, J. M. (2001). Voices of hope: Hearing and caring for Haitian adolescents. *Journal of Holistic Nursing, 19,* 187–211.

Dewar, A. L., & Lee, E. A. (2000). Bearing illness and injury. *Western Journal of Nursing Research, 22,* 912–926.

Draucker, C. B., & Stern, P. N. (2000). Women's responses to sexual violence by male intimates. *Western Journal of Nursing Research, 22,* 385–406.

Dunphy, L. M. (2001a). "The steel cocoon": Tales of the nurses and patients of the iron lung, 1929–1955. *Nursing History Review, 9,* 3–33.

Dunphy, L. M. (2001b). "Constant and relentless": The nursing care of patients in iron lungs, 1928–1955. In P. Munhall (Ed.), *Nursing research: A qualitative perspective* (pp. 417–438). Sudbury, MA: Jones & Bartlett.

Glaser, B., & Strauss, A. (1965). *Awareness of dying.* Chicago: Aldine.

Gustafson, D. L. (2000). Best laid plans: Examining contradictions between intent and outcome in a feminist, collaborative research project. *Qualitative Health Research, 10,* 717–733.

Hallett, C. E., Austin, L., Caress, A., & Luker, K. A. (2000). Community nurses' perceptions of patient 'compliance' in wound care: A discourse analysis, *Journal of Advanced Nursing, 32,* 115–123.

Hawley, M. P. (2000). Nurse comforting strategies. *Clinical Nursing Research, 9,* 441–459.

Herdman, E. (2000). Reflections on "Making somebody angry." *Qualitative Health Research, 10,* 691–702.

Kearney, M. H. (2001a). Enduring love: A grounded formal theory of women's experience of domestic violence. *Research in Nursing & Health, 24,* 270–282.

Kendall, J. (1999). Axial coding and the grounded theory controversy. *Western Journal of Nursing Research, 21,* 743–757.

Knobf, M. T. (2002). Carrying on: The experience of premature menopause in women with early stage breast cancer. *Nursing Research, 51,* 9–17.

Lipson, J. G. (2001). We are the canaries: Multiple chemical sensitivity sufferers. *Qualitative Health Research, 11,* 103–116.

Long, A. F., Kneafsey, R., Ryan, J., and Berry, J. (2002). The role of the nurse within the multi-professional rehabilitation team. *Journal of Advanced Nursing, 37,* 70–78.

Lusk, B. (2000). Pretty and powerless: Nurses in advertisements, 1930–1950. *Research in Nursing & Health, 23,* 229–236.

McInnis, G. J., & White, J. H. (2001). A phenomenological exploration of loneliness in the older adult. *Archives of Psychiatric Nursing, 15,* 128–139.

Morse, J. M., & Doberneck, B. (1995). Delineating the concept of hope. *Image: The Journal of Nursing Scholarship, 27,* 283–291.

Morse, J. M., Hutchinson, S., & Penrod, J. (1998). From theory of practice: The development of assessment guides from qualitatively derived theory. *Qualitative Health Research, 8,* 329–340.

Morse, J. M., Penrod, J., Kassab, C., & Dellasega, C. (2000). Evaluating the efficiency and effectiveness of approaches to nasogastric tube insertion during trauma care. *American Journal of Critical Care, 9,* 325–333.

Penrod, J. & Morse, J. (1997). Strategies for assessing and fostering hope: The Hope Assessment Guide. *Oncology Nursing Forum, 24,* 1055–1063.

Porter, E. J., Ganong, L. H., & Armer, J. M. (2000). The church family and kin: An older rural black woman's support network and preferences for care providers. *Qualitative Health Research, 10,* 452–470.

Rashid, S. F. (2001). Indigenous notions of the workings of the inner body: Conflicts and dilemmas with Norplant use in rural Bangladesh. *Qualitative Health Research, 11,* 85–102.

Rehm, R. S. (2000). Parental encouragement, protection, and advocacy for Mexican-American children with chronic conditions. *Journal of Pediatric Nursing, 15,* 89–98.

Reising, D. L. (2002). Early socialization of new critical care nurses. *American Journal of Critical Care, 11,* 19–26.

Rungreangkulkij, S., & Chesla, C. (2001). Smooth a heart with water: Thai mothers care for a child with schizophrenia. *Archives of Psychiatric Nursing, 15,* 120–127.

Sayre, J. (2000). The patient's diagnosis: Explanatory models of mental illness, *Qualitative Health Research, 10,* 71–83

Scannell-Desch, E. A. (2000). Hardships and personal strategies of Vietnam war nurses. *Western Journal of Nursing Research, 22,* 526–550.

Stubblefield, C., & Murray, R. L. (2001). Pediatric lung transplantation: Families' need for understanding. *Qualitative Health Research, 11,* 58–68.

Wakefield, A. (2000). Ethnomethodology: The problems of unique adequacy. *NT Research, 5,* 46–53.

Williams, J. K., Schutte, D. L., Evers, C., & Holkup, P. A. (2000). Redefinition: Coping with normal results from predictive gene testing for neurodegenerative disorders. *Research in Nursing & Health, 23,* 260–269.

Wittig, D. R. (2001). Organ donation beliefs of African American women residing in a small Southern community. *Journal of Transcultural Nursing, 12,* 203–210.

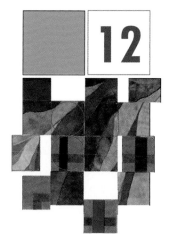

12

Integration of Qualitative and Quantitative Designs

Until recently, nursing research was dominated by quantitative studies. Consistent with the overall expansion of nursing research inquiry and with increased appreciation of methodologic pluralism, qualitative studies have gained considerable ground since the 1980s. A growing trend is the blending of qualitative and quantitative data within single studies or coordinated clusters of studies. This chapter discusses some strategies for using such integrated designs.

RATIONALE FOR MULTIMETHOD RESEARCH

The dichotomy between quantitative and qualitative data represents the key epistemologic and methodologic distinction within the social, behavioral, and health sciences. Some people argue that qualitative and quantitative research are based on totally incompatible paradigms. Thus, there are people who likely disagree with the fundamental premise of this chapter, namely, that some areas of inquiry can be enriched through the judicious blending of qualitative and quantitative data—that is, by undertaking what is usually referred to as **multimethod** (or **mixed-method**) **research**. It would be foolish to argue that all research problems could be enhanced by such integration or that all (or most) researchers should strive to collect and

blend both types of data. However, we believe there are many noteworthy advantages of combining various types of data in an investigation.

Complementarity

One argument for blending qualitative and quantitative data in a study is that they are complementary; they represent words and numbers, the two fundamental languages of human communication. Researchers address problems with methods and measures that are fallible. By integrating different methods and modes of analysis, the weaknesses of a single approach may be diminished or overcome.

Quantitative data from large or representative samples have many strengths. Quantitative studies are often strong in generalizability, precision, and control over extraneous variables. However, sometimes the validity of such research is called into question. By introducing tight controls, quantitative studies may fail to capture situational context. Moreover, by reducing complex human experiences, behavior, and characteristics to numbers, such studies sometimes seem superficial. The use of tightly structured methods can sometimes lead to biases in capturing constructs under study. All these weaknesses are aspects of the study's ability to yield valid, meaningful answers to research questions.

Qualitative research, by contrast, has strengths and weaknesses that are diametrically opposite. The strength of qualitative research lies in its flexibility and its potential to yield insights into the true nature of complex phenomena through in-depth scrutiny. However, qualitative research is almost always based on small, unrepresentative samples. It is often undertaken by a single researcher or small research team, using data collection and analytic procedures that rely on subjective judgments. Thus, qualitative research is sometimes criticized for problems with reliability and generalizability.

This discussion suggests that *neither of the two styles of research can fully deliver on its promise to establish the truth about phenomena of interest to nurse researchers.* However, the strengths and weaknesses of quantitative and qualitative data are complementary. Combined shrewdly in a single study, qualitative and quantitative data can "supply each other's lack." By using multiple methods, researchers can allow each method to do what it does best, with the possibility of avoiding the limitations of a single approach.

Enhanced Theoretical Insights

Most theories do not have paradigmatic boundaries. As discussed in Chapter 6, the major nursing theories embrace four broad concepts: (1) person, (2) environment, (3) health, and (4) nursing. There is nothing inherent in these concepts that demands (or excludes) a qualitative or quantitative orientation.

The world in which we live is complex and multidimensional, as are most theories developed to make sense of it. Qualitative and quantitative research constitute alternative ways of viewing and interpreting the world. These alternatives are not necessarily correct or incorrect; rather, they reflect and reveal different aspects of reality. To be maximally useful, nursing research should strive to understand these multiple aspects. We believe that the blending of quantitative and qualitative data in a single analysis can lead to insights on these multiple aspects that might be unattainable without such integration. Denzin (1989), who has been a staunch advocate of combining methods, coined the term

triangulation to refer to the use of multiple sources to converge on the truth. He expressed the value of triangulation eloquently:

> Each method implies a different line of action toward reality—and hence each will reveal different aspects of it, much as a kaleidoscope, depending on the angle at which it is held, will reveal different colors and configurations of objects to the viewer. Methods are like the kaleidoscope: depending on how they are approached, held, and acted toward, different observations will be revealed. This is not to imply that reality has the shifting qualities of the colored prism, but that it too is an object that moves and that will not permit one interpretation to be stamped upon it (p. 235).

Incrementality

It is sometimes argued that different approaches are especially appropriate for different phases in the evolution of knowledge. In particular, it has been said that qualitative methods are well suited to exploratory or hypothesis-generating research early in the development of a problem area, and quantitative methods are needed as the problem area matures for the purposes of verification. However, the evolution of a theory or problem area is rarely linear and unidirectional. The need for exploration and in-depth insights is rarely confined to the beginning of an area of research inquiry, and subjective insights may need to be evaluated early and continually.

Thus, progress in developing a body of evidence for nursing practice tends to be incremental and to rely on multiple feedback loops. It can be productive to build a loop into the design of a single study, potentially speeding the progress toward understanding. This point is illustrated by inquiry in the area of work-related stress and coping. Bargagliotti and Trygstad (1987) conducted two separate studies of job stress among nurses, one using quantitative procedures and the other using qualitative procedures. The quantitative study identified discrete events as sources of stress, and the qualitative study revealed stress-related processes over time. The discrepant findings, because they were derived from different samples of nurses working in different settings, could not be easily integrated and reconciled. The investigators noted, "Comparison of findings from the two studies suggests that the questions raised by the findings in each study might have been more fully addressed by using a combined quantitative/qualitative methodology" (p. 172).

Enhanced Validity

Another advantage of designing multimethod research lies in the potential for enhancing the validity of study findings. When researchers' hypotheses or models are supported by multiple and complementary types of data, they can be more confident about the validity of the results. Scientists are basically skeptics, constantly seeking evidence to validate their theories and models. Evidence derived from different approaches can be especially persuasive. As Brewer and Hunter (1989) noted, "Although each type of method is relatively stronger than the others in certain respects, none of the methods is so perfect even in its area of greatest strength that it cannot benefit from corroboration by other methods' findings" (p. 51).

In Chapter 9, we discussed various types of validity problems in quantitative studies—such problems as rival explanations of the results (internal validity), and difficulties of generalizing beyond the study (external validity). In Chapter 18, we discuss validity problems of measures that fail to capture the constructs under investigation. The use of a single approach can leave the study vulnerable to at least one (and often more than one) validity problem. The integration of qualitative and quantitative data can provide better opportunities for testing alternative interpretations of the data, for examining the extent to which the context helped to shape the results, and for arriving at convergence in tapping a construct. For example, Ersek, Ferrell, Dow, and Melancon (1997), in their study of quality of life in women with ovarian cancer, used qualitative data to validate their quantitative quality-of-life measures.

Creating New Frontiers

Researchers sometimes find that qualitative and quantitative data are inconsistent with each other. This lack of congruity—when it happens in the context of a single investigation—can lead to insights that can push a line of inquiry further than would otherwise have been possible.

When separate investigations yield inconsistent results, the differences are difficult to reconcile and interpret because they may reflect differences in the people being studied and in the circumstances under which they were studied, rather than theoretically meaningful distinctions that merit further investigation. In a single study, discrepancies can be tackled head on. By probing into the reasons for any observed incongruities, researchers can help to rethink the constructs under investigation and possibly to redirect the research process. The incongruent findings, in other words, can be used as a springboard for exploring reasons for discrepancies and for a thoughtful analysis of the study's methodologic and theoretical underpinnings.

APPLICATIONS OF MULTIMETHOD RESEARCH

Researchers make decisions about the types of data to collect and analyze based on the specific objectives. In this section, we illustrate how multimethod research can be used to address a variety of research goals.

Instrument Development

Qualitative data are sometimes collected for the development and validation of formal, quantitative instruments for research or clinical purposes. When researchers become aware of the need for a new measuring tool, they sometimes derive the questions for a formal instrument from clinical experience, theory, or prior research. When a construct is new, however, these mechanisms may be inadequate to capture its full complexity and dimensionality. No matter how rich the researcher's experience or knowledge base, this base is personal and biased by the researcher's values and world view. Thus, many nurse researchers have begun to use data obtained from qualitative inquiries as the basis for generating questions for quantitative instruments that are subsequently subjected to rigorous quantitative assessment.

Example of instrumentation:
Beck and Gable (2000) developed the Postpartum Depression Screening Scale (PDSS), a quantitative instrument that screens new mothers for this mood disorder. Scale items were based on in-depth interviews with mothers suffering from postpartum depression in a grounded theory study and two phenomenological studies. Here is an example of how items on the PDSS were developed from mothers' quotes. The quote "I was extremely obsessive with my thoughts. They would never stop. I could not control them" was developed into the item: I could not control the thoughts that kept coming into my mind (Beck and Gable, 2001).

Qualitative inquiries can also be used to refine research instruments or to assess the validity of existing ones. Such inquiries can play an important role in identifying problems in the use of quantitative instruments for certain populations or within certain contexts.

 Example of qualitative inquiry on a quantitative instrument:
Barroso and Sandelowski (2001) recorded qualitatively the problems experienced in administering the widely-used Beck Depression Inventory (BDI) to a sample of human immunodeficiency virus—infected patients. The researchers concluded that their experiences with the BDI "show the importance of incorporating qualitative techniques of interviewing and observation in all phases of the process of instrument utilization" (p. 501).

Explicating and Validating Constructs

Multimethod research is often used to develop a comprehensive understanding of a construct, or to validate the construct's dimensions. Such research may be undertaken when a little-researched phenomenon has been identified as worthy of further scrutiny (usually in an in-depth qualitative study), or when there is a body of existing research in which some serious gaps have been identified or doubts have been raised about the prevailing conceptualization.

Example of validating constructs:
Reece and Harkless (1996) conducted a multimethod study to examine the maternal experiences of women older than 35 years. The researchers administered an existing quantitative measure of maternal experience, the revised "What Being the Parent of a Baby is Like" (WPL-R) scale, which involves three subscales: Self-Evaluation in Parenting, Centrality, and Life Change. The researchers also asked respondents broad, probing questions about their motherhood experience and qualitatively analyzed the themes that emerged. The investigators found that several new dimensions arose in the qualitative portion of the research, including loss of control, fatigue and the need to heal, and the sense of mortality and the passage of time.

Hypothesis Generation

In-depth qualitative studies are often fertile with insights about constructs or relationships among them. These insights then can be tested and confirmed in quantitative studies, and the generalizability of the insights can be assessed. This most often happens in the context of discrete investigations. One problem, however, is that it usually takes years to do a study and publish the results, which means that considerable time may elapse between the qualitative insights and the formal quantitative testing of hypotheses based on those insights. A research team interested in a phenomenon might wish to collaborate in a research program that has hypothesis generation and testing as an explicit goal.

Example of hypothesis generation:
Wendler (2001) described how the use of a **meta-matrix** can be used to facilitate pattern recognition across data from different sources, including qualitative and quantitative sources, and to generate hypotheses and new research questions. In Wendler's example of a mixed-method study of Tellington touch (t-touch), use of a meta-matrix led to a discovery of the relationship between the administration of t-touch and the practitioner's physical state (e.g., caffeine intake).

Illustration, Clarification, and Amplification

Qualitative data are sometimes combined with quantitative data to illustrate the meaning of constructs or relationships. Such illustrations often help to clarify important results or to corroborate the understandings gleaned from the statistical analysis. In this sense, these illustrations often help to illuminate the analyses and give guidance to the interpretation of results.

Qualitative materials can be used to illustrate specific statistical findings or can also be used to provide more global and dynamic views of the phenomena under study, often in the form of illustrative case studies.

 Example of illustrating with qualitative data:

Polit, London, and Martinez (2000, 2001) used data from the ethnographic part of a multimethod study of poor urban families to illustrate how food insecurity—which was reported by 51% of the women in the survey sample—was experienced and managed. The following excerpt illustrated the food-related problems some women had: "It was hard, especially when you got kids at home saying, 'I'm hungry.'... I started working at the church as a babysitter. I was getting paid $20 a week and a bag of food every Thursday... . Then I was doing very odd jobs that most people would not dare to do. I was making deliveries on pizza in bad neighborhoods where most people wouldn't go. I mean, I literally took my life in my own hands." (2001, p. 58).

In this example, the qualitative materials added a rich perspective that the quantitative results alone could not provide. On the other hand, the survey results made it clear that such experiences with hunger and food insecurity were not just the problems of a small minority of poor families, but rather affected half of them.

In addition to offering possibilities of illustration, qualitative data can also be used to clarify an issue or amplify dimensions of the problem. As an example from the same multimethod study, Polit and her colleagues learned from the ethnographic

data that when *families* (the unit used in the survey) were confronted with hunger and food insecurity, the mothers often went to great lengths to shield children, adding to their own distress. Here is one of the many excerpts that provided this insight: "I'll go maybe three days at a time without eating just so my kids can have their three meals a day" (Polit et al., 2000, p. 18).

Understanding Relationships and Causal Processes

Quantitative methods often demonstrate that variables are systematically related to one another, but they often fail to provide insights about *why* variables are related. This situation is especially likely to occur with correlational research.

The discussion section of research reports typically is devoted to an interpretation of the findings. In quantitative studies, interpretations are often speculative, representing researchers' best guess (a guess that may, of course, be built on solid theory or prior research) about what the findings mean. In essence, the interpretations represent a new set of hypotheses that could be tested in another study. When a study integrates both qualitative and quantitative data, however, researchers may be in a much stronger position to derive meaning immediately from the statistical findings through the analysis of qualitative material.

 Example of illuminating with qualitative data:

Tilden, Tolle, Nelson, and Field (2001) collected both qualitative and quantitative data about family members' decision to withdraw life-sustaining treatments from hospitalized patients. The quantitative data indicated that family members had lower scores on a measure of stress if the patient had left advance directives. The qualitative data provided rich information about how people with low stress scores were more convinced that they made the right decision, because they knew what the patient wanted.

In some quantitative studies, it may be useful to collect qualitative data to help identify study weaknesses that can be used in interpreting results. For example, if a researcher is concerned with biases that could result from attrition in a longitudinal survey, it might be profitable to undertake a small number of in-depth interviews with nonrespondents to evaluate the direction and magnitude of such biases.

Quantitative analyses can also help to clarify and give shape to findings obtained in qualitative analyses. For example, a thematic analysis of interviews with infertile couples could reveal various aspects of the emotional consequences of infertility and shed light on the meaning of those consequences to individuals; the administration of a standardized scale (such as the Center for Epidemiological Studies—Depression, or CES-D, Scale) to the same subjects could indicate more precisely the distribution of depressive symptoms and their magnitude among the infertile couples.

Example of confirming with quantitative data:

Roe (2000) conducted case studies of two health authorities in England that differed in management strategies for dealing with incontinence. The primary means of data collection involved in-depth interviews with incontinent patients in the two authorities about their experience with incontinence and its management. Quantitative data were collected after the qualitative interviews using the Incontinent Impact Questionnaire, which provided better comparative data.

TIP: In many situations, researchers come to the final stage of a study—the interpretation of the findings—realizing that interpretation is hampered by the absence of information on some issue, suggesting that many studies would benefit from additional planning. It is often wise to consider in advance a wide variety of scenarios with regard to the findings (especially in studies that are primarily quantitative, which tend to be somewhat less flexible once the study is underway). For example, if you knew in advance that your hypotheses would *not* be supported, what else might you want to ask respondents? If you knew that the hypotheses would be supported only for certain types of people, or in certain types of conditions, what kinds of data would you like to

have to help explain this pattern? Integrated methods can be an excellent strategy to help with interpretive ambiguities.

Theory Building, Testing, and Refinement

The most ambitious application of multimethod research is in the area of theory development. As we have pointed out, a theory is neither proved nor confirmed but rather is supported to a greater or lesser extent. A theory gains acceptance as it escapes disconfirmation. The use of multiple methods provides greater opportunity for potential disconfirmation of the theory. If the theory can survive these assaults, it can provide a substantially stronger context for the organization of our clinical and intellectual work. Brewer and Hunter (1989), in their discussion of the role of multimethod research in theory development, made the following observation:

> Theory building and theory testing clearly require variety. In building theories, the more varied the empirical generalizations to be explained, the easier it will be to discriminate between the many possible theories that might explain any one of the generalizations. And in testing theories, the more varied the predictions, the more sharply the ensuing research will discriminate among competing theories (p. 36).

Example of theory building:

Salazar and Carter (1993) conducted a study that promotes the development of theory in the area of decision making. They sought to identify factors that influence women's decision to practice breast self-examination (BSE). The first phase of the study involved in-depth interviews with 19 women, selected on the basis of how frequently the women practiced BSE. The transcribed interviews were qualitatively analyzed and led to the development of a hierarchical scheme of factors influencing the BSE decision. In the next phase of the research, the researchers used the hierarchy as the basis for developing a survey questionnaire, which was administered to 52 women. BSE performers and nonperformers were compared, and a powerful statistical analysis was used to identify factors in the decision hierarchy that best distinguished the two groups.

MULTIMETHOD RESEARCH DESIGNS

Green and Caracelli (1997) have identified several types of research designs that involve a multi-method approach. The designs cluster into two broad categories that they label *component designs* and *integrated designs*.

Multimethod Component Designs

In studies with a **component design**, the qualitative and quantitative aspects are implemented as discrete components of the overall inquiry, and remain distinct during data collection and analysis. Combining the qualitative and quantitative components occurs during the interpretation and reporting phases of the project. (Miller and Crabtree [1994] refer to such designs as *concurrent designs*.)

Green and Caracelli (1997) describe three types of component designs. In a **triangulated design,** both qualitative and quantitative methods are used to capture the same phenomenon, with a focus on convergence and increased validity. This design fits the application described in the previous section as "explicating and validating constructs." Second, in **complementarity designs,** the results from one method type are enhanced or clarified by results from the other type. Polit and her colleagues (2000) used a complementarity design in their previously described study of food insecurity. The third component design is the **expansion design,** in which different methods are used for distinct inquiry components—as might be the case in an evaluation that involved both a process and an impact analysis. The results from such studies are often presented in a side-by-side fashion, rather than woven together into a single story.

Example of a component design:
Elliot, Quinless, and Parietti (2000) conducted a multimethod participatory needs assessment of a Hispanic neighborhood in Newark, New Jersey. Surveys were used to collect quantitative information about perceived needs from a sample of nearly 800 community residents. Qualitative data were obtained through 10 in-depth group interviews. The results, which were substantially similar in both components, were used to promote community activism and to introduce a number of programs in response to identified needs.

Multimethod Integrated Designs

In studies that Green and Caracelli (1997) refer to as having an **integrated design**, there is greater integration of the method types at all phases of the project, from the development of research questions, through data collection and analysis, to the interpretation of the results. The blending of data occurs in ways that integrate the elements from the different paradigms and offers the possibility of yielding more insightful understandings of the phenomenon under study.

Four types of integrated designs have been identified. **Iterative designs** involve a dynamic in which the findings from one method are used as a basis for moving forward with further research using the alternative method (as is typically the case with instrument development and refinement). In some studies, there is a single iteration, moving from qualitative to quantitative (or vice versa); in other studies, there might be multiple iterations, with a progressive reconfiguration of data collection, data analysis, and interpretation in a spiraling pattern of findings and insights. (Miller and Crabtree [1994] call such a design a *sequential design*.)

In **embedded designs** (or **nested designs**), one methodologic approach is embedded in the other, "interlocking contrasting inquiry characteristics in a framework of creative tension" (Green & Caracelli, 1997, p. 24). **Holistic designs** feature the essential interdependence of alternative methods for gaining a full understanding of complex phenomena. In holistic designs, the methods are integrated simultaneously rather than hierarchically. Finally, in **transformative designs,** the emphasis is on blending the value commitments of different research traditions to arrive at a better representation of the multiple interests in the larger social context. In general, integrated designs are better suited to theory building and testing than are component designs.

Example of an integrated design:
Chesler and Parry (2001) used an iterative multimethod design to explore the experiences of fathers of children with cancer. They collected survey data from several hundred parents of children with cancer, and used the survey to select 52 fathers with whom they conducted in-depth qualitative interviews.

Timing and Design

Sandelowski (2000) has offered an alternative typology of multimethod designs. Her scheme focuses on which approach (qualitative or quantitative) has priority, and how the approaches are ordered in a study. She developed a useful matrix that indicates the kinds of objectives that can be addressed with alternative design configurations. For example, in her Template Design #1, the qualitative approach is the dominant one and quantitative data are viewed as an adjunct. The quantitative data, which are collected concurrently with or after the qualitative data, are used to provide measured description, validation, and formal generalizations. Template Design #4, by contrast, involves qualitative data occurring before (and as an adjunct to) the quantitative portion of the study. Such a design is used when the aim is to generate questions for a quantitative instrument, or to generate hypotheses to be tested formally.

Sandelowski's scheme makes clear that most multimethod studies involve decisions about how to order data collection. In some cases (especially in component studies), data collection for the two approaches occurs more or less simultaneously. In others, however, there are important advantages to timing the approaches so that the second phase builds on knowledge gained in the first.

TIP: Many multimethod studies are conducted in two or more phases, such as conducting in-depth interviews with a subsample of patients from whom biophysiologic data were obtained after analysis of those data has been done. If there is a possibility that you *might* go back to study participants to obtain more data, be sure to structure your consent form in such a way that they are aware of any potential future demands on their time. Also, be sure to obtain contact information to facilitate finding them at a later date.

STRATEGIES FOR MULTIMETHOD RESEARCH

The ways in which researchers might choose to combine qualitative and quantitative methods in a single study are almost limitless—or rather, are limited only by the researchers' ingenuity, and by their views about the value of multimethod research.

Researchers who do primarily quantitative research tend to be more likely to see the value of incorporating qualitative approaches into their designs than vice versa. Phenomenological researchers, in particular, seldom build a quantitative component into their studies. Indeed, a number of qualitative researchers argue that true integration is not even possible. Massé (2000), for example, believes that "the quest for *meaning* and the quest for *measurement* are incommensurable" (p. 411, emphasis added).

Nevertheless, examples of multimethod research abound. Although it is not possible to develop a catalog of multimethod strategies, Table 12-1 illustrates (with hypothetical questions) ways in which qualitative research can be used to enhance knowledge in several types of quantitative studies, and vice versa. Some specific scenarios are discussed further in this section.

Clinical Trials

Although phase III clinical trials almost always use an experimental design with structured, quantitative outcome measures, qualitative inquiries embedded in the trials can prove valuable in all phases. For example, in phase I, when the intervention is being fine-tuned, in-depth discussions with clinical staff and with patients can provide critical insights into how to develop the best possible intervention. Sandelowski (1996) has argued that qualitative methods used as a component of quantitative research can increase the meaningfulness of experimental studies by placing them more firmly in the real world (Sandelowski, 1996).

Even in a formal phase III evaluation of a clinical trial, many questions can be addressed qualitatively. Why did some patients drop out of the study? How did staff and patients feel about the intervention? Why didn't certain patients improve as a result of the intervention? What contextual factors constrained (or enabled) the intervention's success?

TABLE 12.1 Examples of Integration Possibilities

TYPE	EXAMPLE OF QUESTION FOR QUANTITATIVE COMPONENT	EXAMPLE OF QUESTION FOR QUALITATIVE COMPONENT
Clinical trial	Are boomerang pillows more effective than straight pillows in improving the respiratory capacity of hospitalized patients?	Why did some patients complain about the boomerang pillows? How did the pillows feel?
Evaluation	How effective and cost-effective is a nurse-managed special care unit compared with traditional intensive care units?	How accepting were other health care workers of the special unit, and what problems of implementation ensued?
Outcomes research	What effect do alternative levels of nursing intensity have on the functional ability of elderly residents in long-term care facilities?	How do elderly long-term care residents interact with nurses in environments with different nursing intensity?
Needs assessments	What percentage of Haitian immigrants have unmet health care needs, and what are the highest-priority needs?	What are the barriers that prevent Haitian immigrants from getting needed health services?
Survey	How prevalent is asthma among inner-city children, and how is it treated?	How is asthma experienced by inner-city children and their parents?
Methodologic research	How accurate is a new measure of loneliness for hospitalized psychiatric patients?	Does the new measure adequately capture the dimensions and manifestations of loneliness of psychiatric patients?
Ethnography	What percentage of women in rural Appalachia seek and obtain prenatal care, and what are their birth outcomes?	How do women in rural Appalachia view their pregnancies and how do they prepare for childbirth?
Historical research	What were the trends in treating breast cancer through radical mastectomy from 1900 to 1980?	What roles did nurses play in addressing the needs of women undergoing radical mastectomies, and how did the roles evolve?
Case study	How have the demographic characteristics of the caseload of St. Jude's Homeless Shelter changed over a 10-year period?	How are social, health, and psychological services integrated in St. Jude's Homeless Shelter?
Feminist research	What percentage of nurses in an urban hospital have experienced sex discrimination and sexual harassment?	What are the ways in which sex discrimination is manifested and experienced in the hospital, and what changes are needed to correct the situation?

Example of a multimethod clinical trial:
Whittemore, Rankin, Callhan, Leder, and Carroll (2000) were involved in a clinical trial of alternative social support interventions, administered by nurse versus peer advisors, for patients who had had a myocardial infarction. Subjects, who were randomly assigned to three groups (nurse advisors, peer advisors, or control group), were compared in terms of health outcomes. The qualitative part of the study, which was designed to understand better the *experiences* of the peer advisors, was based on written logs and individual and group interviews.

Evaluation Research

Evaluation research often involves both quantitative components (e.g., impact analyses and cost analyses) and qualitative components (e.g., process analyses). In some cases, the components are "stand-alone" features of the study and are not linked in a systematic fashion. However, the most powerful and useful evaluations *do* use data from one component to inform findings in other components.

Qualitative data collection methods are especially useful when the researcher is evaluating complex interventions. When a new treatment is straightforward (e.g., a new drug), it is usually easy to interpret the results: post-treatment group differences usually can be attributed to the intervention. However, many nursing interventions are not so straightforward. They may involve new ways of interacting with patients or new approaches to organizing the delivery of care. Sometimes, the intervention is multidimensional, involving several distinct features. At the end of the evaluation, even when hypothesized results are obtained, people may ask, What *was* it that really caused the group differences? (If there were no group differences, then the important question would be, *Why* was the intervention unsuccessful?) In-depth qualitative interviews with subjects could help to address these questions. In other words, qualitative data may help researchers to address the **black box** question—understanding what it is about the complex intervention that drove observed effects. This knowledge can be helpful for theoretical purposes, and can also help to strengthen an intervention or to streamline it and make it more efficient and cost-effective.

Another reason for gathering qualitative data in evaluations of complex interventions is that there is often a need to understand exactly what the intervention was like in practice and how people reacted to it. Unstructured observations and interviews with people with different perspectives (e.g., nurses, physicians, hospital administrators, patients, or patients' family members) are especially well suited for such process evaluations.

Use of qualitative methods in evaluations can also have salvaging power. Weinholtz, Kacer, and Rocklin (1995) illustrated how the use of supplemental qualitative data about an intervention itself can help prevent quantitative researchers from obtaining ambiguous or erroneous findings. Qualitative data can provide insights in studies that yield nonsignificant findings by identifying subtleties in the intervention procedure that can be used to interpret the research findings. Between- and within-subject variation on research outcomes can be further explained by qualitative data.

Example of a multimethod evaluation:
Hecker (2000) collected both qualitative and quantitative data in an evaluation of a community-wide health fair held in a suburb of Mexico City. A collaborative research team gathered qualitative information about the planning and implementation of the health fair, and quantitative data about the outcomes of the fair. The researchers used both types of data to develop recommendations for program replication and modification.

Surveys

The most common data collection method currently used by nurse researchers is structured self-reports, which are discussed at some length in Chapter 15. Once researchers have gained the cooperation of a sample in a survey, they are in a good position to gather in-depth data from a subset of initial respondents. The qualitative portion might involve such approaches as in-depth individual or group interviews or unstructured observations in a naturalistic environment such as a hospital or nursing home.

From a practical point of view, it is efficient to collect both types of data simultaneously. For example, researchers could administer a structured questionnaire and then conduct an in-depth interview on the same day to a subsample of survey respondents. In some studies, this procedure is likely to work well, but a two-stage (iterative) approach has two distinct advantages. First, if the second-stage data collection can be postponed until after the quantitative data have been collected and analyzed, researchers will have greater opportunity to probe deeply into reasons for any obtained results. This is especially likely to be beneficial if the quantitative analyses did not confirm the researchers' hypotheses or if there were any inconsistent results. Second-stage respondents, in other words, can be used as informants to help researchers interpret outcomes. A second reason for using an iterative approach is that researchers can use information from the first stage to select a useful subsample for the second. For example, they might want to use data from the first round to select informants with certain characteristics, such as those who are most knowledgeable about the phenomena under investigation, those who represent "typical" cases, or those who are at opposite extremes with regard to the key constructs.

 Example of a qualitative study after a survey:

Wilson and Williams (2000) were involved in a three-phase study on telephone consultation among community nurses in England. The first phase involved a national survey of community nurses by mailed questionnaire. In the second phase, which involved in-depth interviews with a subset of 14 survey respondents, nurses were probed about their experiences with telephone consultations. The third phase involved a survey of clients from the interviewees' caseload who had used telephone services.

Ethnographies

Ethnographic research has a long history of using multiple methods of data collection. The methods used in ethnographic field studies usually yield a rich array of data amenable to qualitative analysis, such as notes from qualitative observations, in-depth interviews, and narrative documents such as diaries and letters. Ethnographers can, in some cases, profit from the collection of more structured information from a larger or more representative sample than is possible in collecting the qualitative data. The secondary data might be in the form of structured self-reports from a survey, or quantifiable records. For example, if the field work focused on family violence in an inner-city neighborhood, police and hospital records could be used to gather data amenable to statistical analysis.

As field work progresses, ethnographers typically gain considerable insight into the cultures under study. With this knowledge, researchers can generate hypotheses that can be subjected to more systematic scrutiny through structured data collection methods. Alternatively, the quantitative portion of the study could be used to gather descriptive information about the characteristics of the community or organization so that qualitative findings could be understood in a broader context. In either case, having already gained entrée into the community and the trust and cooperation of its members, ethnographers may be in an ideal position to pursue a survey or record-extraction activity.

Example of a multimethod ethnography:

Clark (2002) conducted a focused ethnography of Mexican-origin mothers' experiences of obtaining and using health services for their children in an urban Latino community in the United States. In addition to gathering in-depth ethnographic data through multiple interviews and participant observation, Clark gathered and analyzed quantitative information from the children's medical records (e.g., number of emergency department visits, number of well-child visits).

OBSTACLES TO MULTIMETHOD RESEARCH

Throughout this chapter, we have stressed the advantages of designing studies that blend qualitative and quantitative data in a single investigation. We believe that the potential for advancing nursing science through such integration is great and is as yet relatively untapped. We also believe that integration efforts such as those proposed are inevitable because, at the level of the problem, almost all research topics are inherently multimethod.

Nevertheless, we recognize that there are obstacles that may constrain the gathering of qualitative and quantitative data in a single investigation. Among the most salient are the following:

- *Epistemologic biases.* Qualitative and quantitative researchers often operate with a different set of assumptions about the world and ways of learning about it. For those with a hard-line, purist view, these assumptions may be seen as inevitably irreconcilable. According to a survey of nurses with doctorates, however, extreme positions of this type are atypical among nurse researchers (Damrosch & Strasser, 1988).
- *Costs.* A major obstacle facing researchers who would like to gather qualitative and quantitative data is that multimethod research is usually expensive. Agencies that sponsor research activities may need to be "educated" about the contribution that multimethod designs can make. In addition to the many substantive advantages that integration offers, it can also be argued that blending qualitative and quantitative data in a single study is actually less costly and more efficient than two discrete research projects on the same topic.
- *Researcher training.* Most researchers obtain graduate-level training that stresses either qualitative or quantitative research methods. Thus, investigator skills may pose an obstacle to multimethod research. All phases of a study, however, do not have to be done by a single researcher. Collaboration among researchers might be an important by-product of the decision to use a multimethod approach. Such collaboration provides opportunities for triangulation in terms of both methods and investigator perspectives.

TIP: If you are considering the possibility of doing a multimethod research study, try to find someone whose research skills complement yours to collaborate with you. It is almost always useful to have two (or more) minds working on a common problem, and this is especially true when methods are diverse. Top-notch qualitative researchers are rarely top-notch quantitative researchers, and vice versa. It is usually wise to do what you do best and to brainstorm with a person whose talents are different.

- *Analytic challenges.* Despite the many advantages of doing multimethod research, it is nevertheless true that a successful integrated data analysis is a challenging task. The researcher may be confronted with issues about how best to combine numeric and narrative data or about how to resolve and interpret inconsistent or contradictory findings. However, the outcome of such challenges may well be more refined conceptualizations of the phenomenon under study.
- *Publication biases.* Some journals have a distinct preference for studies that are qualitative, and others lean toward quantitative studies. Because of this, researchers might be concerned that they would need to write up the qualitative and quantitative results separately, foregoing many of the advantages of multimethod research. However, publication biases are much less evident today than they were a decade ago. All the major nursing journals devoted to research publish qualitative and quantitative studies, and they are increasingly publishing reports of multimethod studies.

In conclusion, although there are various obstacles to multimethod research, we believe that the simultaneous use of qualitative and quantitative data to address problems of interest to the nursing profession represents a powerful methodologic strategy. We are confident that nurse researchers will develop mechanisms for dealing with the obstacles.

RESEARCH EXAMPLES

We have provided examples of multimethod studies throughout this chapter in an effort to demonstrate the advantages of such an approach as well as to illustrate different applications to which such integration has been put. Two additional examples are described here in greater detail.

Research Example of a Survey and Ethnography

Polit, London, and Martinez (2001) are part of a multi-disciplinary team of researchers working on a research project known as Urban Change. The project is designed to study the lives of poor, urban, mother-headed families who were faced with new policies affecting their public assistance. Polit and her colleagues analyzed data from the survey and ethnographic components of the study to examine the health and health care of these families.

The study gathered data from poor women in four large cities (where about 14% of the U.S. welfare caseload lives): Cleveland, Los Angeles, Miami, and Philadelphia. A sample of nearly 4000 survey respondents were selected randomly from among the May 1995 public assistance recipients residing in high-poverty neighborhoods in each city. The women were first interviewed in 1998–1999, and second-round interviews were conducted in 2001. Longitudinal ethnographic interview and observational data were collected from about 160 families living in selected neighborhoods in each site (about 40 per site). None of the ethnographic respondents was in the survey sample.

Polit and her colleagues examined a rich array of health issues in the lives of these women, including health-related material hardships (e.g., unsafe housing, homelessness), physical health, mental health, domestic violence, substance abuse, health care, and health insurance. Many of these women endured multiple health problems. One survey question asked them to rate their health as being "excellent, very good, good, fair, or poor." Some 26% of the women responded that their health was either fair or poor, compared with only 8% of same-aged women nationally.

However, the ethnographic data suggested that health problems were even more pervasive than the survey results indicated. Several ethnographic respondents who said they were in "good" health revealed during the in-depth interview that they were, in fact, in very poor health. The following excerpt is from an ethnographic interview with a woman who said her health was "pretty good." Later in the interview, the interviewer probed about an injury the woman had had:

> *Respondent*: I was standing on the third shelf. Lost my footing, smashed my ankle into the shelf. A ganglioid cyst tumor developed in the soft tissue. It started growing

through the tendons and the nerves before they [Medicaid] okayed the surgery. And now I have nerve damage.
> *Interviewer*: You said you had also injured your back before. Is that better?
> *Respondent*: No, it's not better, but I just keep going. I don't let it get me down. Even the asthma, I don't let it stop me.
> *Interviewer*: Do you have asthma, too?
> *Respondent*: Yeah. I mean, I try not to think about it. ... I just got over a really bad case of bronchitis. And I just had breast surgery done in May. They removed a cyst. Thank God it wasn't cancerous (p. 91).

Another woman who said her health was good later admitted that she had been to the doctors for some tests because they suspected she had cervical cancer—but she did not return to learn the test results. Another woman who had said she was "very healthy" later admitted that she had leg cancer. Thus, the ethnographic data suggest that a direct question about health status may mask problems that are revealed only through in-depth discussions that are not necessarily focused on health issues. These findings led to a number of revisions to the second-round survey; also, later rounds of the ethnography incorporated some health measures from the survey.

Research Example of Theory Building Integration

Connelly, Bott, Hoffart, and Taunton (1997) conducted a multimethod research project that focused on the retention of staff nurses. Their study was primarily quantitative, and involved the development of a sophisticated statistical model designed to predict nurse retention. The researchers measured four types of factors that they believed could predict retention: characteristics of the managers (e.g., leadership style); characteristics of the organization (e.g., promotional opportunity); work characteristics (e.g., group cohesion); and characteristics of the nurses themselves (e.g., education, marital status). The variables in the model had all been verified in the research literature. Nevertheless, cumulative predictive power of these variables was relatively low.

In the final year of the project, the researchers did a qualitative study to examine whether a different research approach might produce an additional construct that belonged in the retention model. A total of 21 staff nurses who had low scores on an "Intent to

Stay" scale that had been administered to them in the first year of the project—but who had nevertheless remained working in the same hospital—were interviewed in depth about their reasons for staying, their possible reasons for leaving, and the positive and negative aspects of their employment.

The researchers found that there was some correspondence between the information obtained through the in-depth interviews and the variables included in their model, thereby validating aspects of the model. However, new themes also emerged during the qualitative interviews—for example, such variables as location close to home, fringe benefits, ability to provide high-quality care, and ability to transfer among units within the hospital. The advantages of having used a multimethod design were described as follows:

> Triangulation helped us attain three benefits. First, the careful comparison of quantitative and qualitative data added support for the variables in the retention model. Second, the comparison also showed new dimensions about nurse retention, thereby contributing to a more complete understanding of nurse retention... . Third, the researchers were able to make suggestions for revision of the quantitative instrument (p. 301).

SUMMARY POINTS

- **Multimethod** (or **mixed-method**) **research,** the blending of qualitative and quantitative data in a single project, can be advantageous in developing an evidence base for nursing practice.
- Advantages include: (1) the two methods have complementary strengths and weaknesses; (2) an integrated approach can lead to theoretical and substantive insights into the multidimensional nature of reality; (3) multimethod research can provide feedback loops that augment the incremental gains in knowledge from a single-method study; (4) confirmation of hypotheses through multiple types of data can strengthen study validity; and (5) if findings are inconsistent, a careful scrutiny of the discrepancies could push the line of inquiry further.
- In nursing, one of the most frequent uses of multimethod research has been in the area of instrument development and refinement.

- Qualitative data are also used to illustrate, clarify, or amplify the meaning of quantified descriptions or relationships.
- Multimethod studies can help to explicate constructs or to interpret and give shape to relationships and causal processes; they can also be used to generate and test hypotheses.
- The most ambitious application of an integrated approach is in the area of theory development.
- In multimethod studies with a **component design**, the qualitative and quantitative aspects of the study are implemented as discrete components, and are distinct during data collection and data analysis. Examples of component designs include **triangulated designs**, **complementarity designs**, and **expansion designs**.
- The second broad category is **integrated designs**, in which there is greater integration of methods throughout the research process. The four major types of integrated designs are **iterative designs**, **embedded (nested) designs**, **holistic designs**, and **transformative designs**.
- In some studies, the simultaneous collection and analysis of qualitative and quantitative data may address the objectives of integration, but in many studies, a multistage approach is likely to yield more insights.
- Researchers can implement a multimethod study in a variety of ways, including the use of qualitative data as an adjunct in clinical trials, experimental evaluations, and surveys.
- The collection of quantitative data in the context of a primarily qualitative study is somewhat less common, but is most likely to happen in an ethnography (or in qualitative studies not done within another specific tradition).
- Despite the advantages of multimethod research, there are several potential obstacles. These include epistemologic biases, high costs, inadequate researcher training, and publication biases

STUDY ACTIVITIES

Chapter 12 of the *Study Guide to Accompany Nursing Research: Principles and Methods, 7th edition,* offers various exercises and study suggestions for reinforcing concepts presented in this chapter. In addition, the following study questions can be addressed:

1. Suppose you were interested in studying the psychological consequences of a miscarriage. Suggest ways in which qualitative and quantitative data could be gathered for such a study.
2. Read an article in a recent issue of a nursing research journal in which the researcher collected only quantitative data. Suggest some possibilities for how qualitative data might have enhanced the validity or interpretability of the findings.
3. Read one of the studies included in the Studies Cited references section at the end of this chapter. To what extent were the qualitative and quantitative analyses integrated? Describe how the absence of either the quantitative or qualitative portions of the study might have affected the study quality and the study conclusions.

SUGGESTED READINGS

Methodologic References

Brewer, J., & Hunter, A. (1989). *Multimethod research: A synthesis of styles.* Newbury Park, CA: Sage.

Bryman, A. (1988). *Quantity and quality in social research.* London: Unwin Hyman.

Carey, J. W. (1993). Linking qualitative and quantitative methods: Integrating cultural factors into public health. *Qualitative Health Research, 3,* 298–318.

Chesla, C. A. (1992). When qualitative and quantitative findings do not converge. *Western Journal of Nursing Research, 14,* 681–685.

Damrosch, S. P., & Strasser, J. A. (1988). A survey of doctorally prepared academic nurses on qualitative and quantitative research issues. *Nursing Research, 37,* 176–180.

Denzin, N. K. (1989). *The research act* (3rd ed.). Englewood Cliffs, NJ: Prentice-Hall.

Duffy, M. (1987). Methodological triangulation: A vehicle for merging quantitative and qualitative research methods. *Image: The Journal of Nursing Scholarship, 19,* 130–133.

Ford-Gilboe, M., Campbell, J., & Berman, H. (1995). Stories and numbers: Coexistence without compromise. *Advances in Nursing Science, 18,* 14–26.

Green, J. C., & Caracelli, V. J. (Eds.). (1997). *Advances in mixed method evaluation: The challenges and ben-efits of integrating diverse paradigms.* San Francisco: Jossey-Bass.

Haase, J. E., & Myers, S. T. (1988) Reconciling paradigm assumptions of qualitative and quantitative research. *Western Journal of Nursing Research, 10,* 128–137.

Jicks, T. D. (1979). Mixing qualitative and quantitative methods: Triangulation in action. *Administrative Science Quarterly, 24,* 602–611.

Massé, R. (2000). Qualitative and quantitative analyses of psychological distress: Methodological complementarity and ontological incommensurability, *Qualitative Health Research, 10,* 411–423.

Miller, W. L., & Crabtree, B. F. (1994). Clinical research. In N. K. Denzin & Y. S. Lincoln (Eds.), *Handbook of qualitative research* (pp. 340–352). Thousand Oaks, CA: Sage.

Mitchell, E. S. (1986). Multiple triangulation: A methodology for nursing science. *Advances in Nursing Science, 8,* 18–26.

Morse, J. M. (1991). Approaches to qualitative-quantitative methodological triangulation. *Nursing Research, 40,* 120–122.

Murphy, S. A. (1989). Multiple triangulation: Applications in a program of nursing research. *Nursing Research, 38,* 294–298.

Myers, S. T., & Haase, J. E. (1989). Guidelines for integration of quantitative and qualitative approaches. *Nursing Research, 38,* 299–301.

Ragin, C. C. (1987). *The comparative method: Moving beyond qualitative and quantitative strategies.* Berkeley, CA: University of California Press.

Rossman, G. B., & Wilson, B. L. (1985). Numbers and words: Combining quantitative and qualitative methods is a single large-scale evaluation study. *Evaluation Review, 9,* 627–643.

Sandelowski, M. (1996). Using qualitative methods in intervention studies. *Research in Nursing & Health, 19,* 359–364.

Sandelowski, M. (2000). Combining qualitative and quantitative sampling, data collection, and analysis techniques in mixed-method studies. *Research in Nursing & Health, 23,* 246–255.

Tashakkori, A., & Teddlie, C. (1998). *Mixed methodology: Combining qualitative and quantitative approaches.* Thousand Oaks, CA: Sage.

Tilden, V. P., Nelson, C. A., & May, B. A. (1990). Use of qualitative methods to enhance content validity. *Nursing Research, 39,* 172–175.

Tripp-Reimer, T. (1985). Combining qualitative and quantitative methodologies. In M. Leininger (Ed.),

Qualitative research methods in nursing (pp. 179–194). New York: Grune & Stratton.

Weinhholtz, D., Kacer, B., & Rocklin, T. (1995). Salvaging quantitative research with qualitative data. *Qualitative Health Research, 5,* 388–397.

Studies Cited in Chapter 12

Bargagliotti, L. A., & Trygstad, L. N. (1987). Differences in stress and coping findings: A reflection of social realities or methodologies. *Nursing Research, 36,* 170–173.

Barroso, J., & Sandelowski, M. (2001). In the field with the Beck Depression Inventory. *Qualitative Health Research, 11,* 491–504.

Beck, C. T., & Gable, R. K (2000). Postpartum Depression Screening Scale: Development and psychometric testing. *Nursing Research, 49,* 272–282.

Beck, C. T., & Gable, R. K. (2001). Ensuring content validity: An illustration of the process. *Journal of Nursing Measurement, 9,* 201–215.

Chesler, M. A., & Parry, C. (2001). Gender roles and/or styles in crisis: An integrative analysis of the experiences of children with cancer. *Qualitative Health Research, 11,* 363–384.

Clark, L. (2002). Mexican-origin mothers' experiences using children's health care services. *Western Journal of Nursing Research, 24,* 159–179.

Connelly, L. M., Bott, M., Hoffart, N., & Taunton, R. L. (1997). Methodological triangulation in a study of nurse retention. *Nursing Research, 46,* 299–302.

Elliot, N. L., Quinless, F. W., & Parietti, E. S. (2000). Assessment of a Newark neighborhood. *Journal of Community Health Nursing, 17,* 211–224.

Ersek, M., Ferrell, B. R., Dow, K. H., & Melancon, C. H. (1997). Quality of life in women with ovarian cancer. *Western Journal of Nursing Research, 19,* 334–350.

Hecker, E. J. (2000). Feria de Salud: Implementation and evaluation of a community-wide health fair. *Public Health Nursing, 17,* 247–256.

Polit, D. F., London, A. S., & Martinez, J. M. (2000). *Food security and hunger in poor, mother-headed families in four U. S. cities.* New York: MDRC (available at www.mdrc.org).

Polit, D. F., London, A. S., & Martinez, J. M. (2001). *The health of poor urban women.* New York: MDRC (available at www.mdrc.org).

Reece, S. M., & Harkless, G. (1996). Divergent themes in maternal experience in women older than 35 years of age. *Applied Nursing Research, 9,* 148–153.

Roe, B. (2000). Effective and ineffective management of incontinence issues around illness trajectory and health care. *Qualitative Health Research, 10,* 677–690.

Salazar, M. K., & Carter, W. B. (1993). Evaluation of breast self-examination beliefs using a decision model. *Western Journal of Nursing Research, 15,* 403–418.

Tilden, V. P., Tolle, S. W., Nelson, C. A., & Fields, J. (2001). Family decision-making to withdraw life-sustaining treatments from hospitalized patients. *Nursing Research, 50,* 105–115.

Wendler, M. C. (2001). Triangulation using a meta-matrix. *Journal of Advanced Nursing, 35,* 521–525.

Whittemore, R., Rankin, S. H., Callhan, C. D., Leder, M. C., & Carroll, D. L. (2000). The peer advisor experience providing social support. *Qualitative Health Research, 10,* 260–276.

Wilson, K., & Williams, A. (2000). Visualism in community nursing: Implications for telephone work with service users. *Qualitative Health Research, 10,* 507–520.

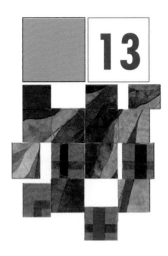

13

Sampling Designs

Sampling is a complex and technical topic. Yet at the same time, sampling is familiar to us all. In the course of our daily activities, we get information, make decisions, and develop predictions through sampling. A nursing student may select an elective course by sampling two or three classes on the first day of the semester. Patients may generalize about nurses' friendliness in a particular hospital based on the care they received from a sample of nurses. We all come to conclusions about phenomena based on exposure to a limited portion of those phenomena.

Researchers, too, usually obtain data from samples. For example, in testing the efficacy of a new asthma medication, researchers reach conclusions without administering the drug to all asthmatic patients. Researchers, however, cannot afford to draw conclusions about the effectiveness of interventions or the validity of relationships based on a sample of only three or four subjects. The consequences of making erroneous decisions are more momentous in disciplined inquiries than in private decision making.

Quantitative and qualitative researchers have different approaches to sampling. Quantitative researchers seek to select samples that will allow them to generalize their results to broader groups. They therefore develop a **sampling plan** that specifies in advance how study participants are to be selected and how many to include. Qualitative researchers are not concerned with issues of generalizability but rather with a holistic understanding of the phenomenon of interest. They make sampling decisions during the course of data collection based on informational and theoretical needs, and typically do not develop a formal sampling plan in advance. This chapter discusses sampling issues for both quantitative and qualitative research.

BASIC SAMPLING CONCEPTS IN QUANTITATIVE STUDIES

Sampling is a critical part of the design of quantitative research. Let us first consider some terms associated with sampling—terms that are used primarily (but not exclusively) with quantitative studies.

Populations

A **population** is the entire aggregation of cases in which a researcher is interested. For instance, if a nurse researcher were studying American nurses with doctoral degrees, the population could be defined as all U.S. citizens who are registered nurses (RNs) and who have acquired a Ph.D., D.N.Sc., Ed.D., or other doctoral-level degree. Other possible populations might be all male patients who underwent cardiac surgery in St. Peter's Hospital during 2002, all women currently in treatment for breast cancer in Boston, or all children in Canada with cystic fibrosis. As this list illustrates, a population may be broadly defined, involving thousands of individuals, or may be narrowly specified to include only several hundred people.

Populations are not restricted to human subjects. A population might consist of all the hospital records on file in a particular hospital, all the blood samples taken from clients of a health maintenance organization, or all the high schools in the United States with a school-based clinic that dispenses contraceptives. Whatever the basic unit, the population always comprises the entire aggregate of elements in which the researcher is interested.

As noted in Chapter 9, it is sometimes useful to make a distinction between target and accessible populations. The **accessible population** is the aggregate of cases that conform to the designated criteria *and* that are accessible as a pool of subjects for a study. The **target population** is the aggregate of cases about which the researcher would like to make generalizations. A target population might consist of all diabetic people in the United States, but the accessible population might consist of all diabetic people who are members of a particular health plan. Researchers usually sample from an accessible population and hope to generalize to a target population.

TIP: A serious issue for the development of an evidence-based practice is information about the populations on whom research has been conducted. Many quantitative researchers fail to identify their target population, or discuss the issue of the generalizability of the results. The population of interest needs to be carefully considered in planning and reporting a study.

Eligibility Criteria

Researchers should be specific about the criteria that define who is included in the population. Consider the population of American nursing students. Does this population include students in all types of nursing programs? How about RNs returning to school for a bachelor's degree? Or students who took a leave of absence for a semester? Do foreign students enrolled in American nursing programs qualify? Insofar as possible, the researcher must consider the exact criteria by which it could be decided whether an individual would or would not be classified as a member of the population. The criteria that specify population characteristics are referred to as **eligibility criteria** or **inclusion criteria**. Sometimes, a population is defined in terms of characteristics that people must *not* possess (i.e., stipulating the **exclusion criteria**). For example, the population may be defined to exclude people who cannot speak English.

Inclusion or exclusion criteria for a study often reflect considerations other than substantive or theoretical interests. The eligibility criteria may reflect one or more of the following issues:

- *Costs.* Some criteria result from cost constraints. For example, when non–English-speaking people are excluded, this does not necessarily mean researchers are not interested in non–English speakers, but may mean that they cannot afford to hire translators and multilingual data collectors.
- *Practical concerns.* Sometimes, there are other practical constraints, such as difficulty in including people from rural areas, people who are hearing impaired, and so on.
- *People's ability to participate in a study.* The health condition of some people may preclude their participation. For example, people with mental impairments, who are in a coma, or who are in an unstable medical condition may need to be excluded.
- *Design considerations.* As noted in Chapter 9, it is sometimes advantageous to define a fairly homogeneous population as a means of controlling extraneous variables.

The criteria used to define a population for a research project have implications for both the interpretation of the results and the generalizability of the findings.

Example of inclusion and exclusion criteria: Keele-Smith and Price-Daniel (2001) used an experimental design to examine the effect of crossing legs on blood pressure measurements. Study participants were seniors, and could be either normotensive or hypertensive. People were excluded if they were taking antihypertensive medications and had not taken their medication that day; had a diagnosis of peripheral vascular disease; had lower leg amputations; had had surgery within the 2 prior weeks; or could not cross their legs.

Samples and Sampling

Sampling is the process of selecting a portion of the population to represent the entire population. A **sample**, then, is a subset of population elements. An **element** is the most basic unit about which information is collected. In nursing research, the elements are usually humans.

Samples and sampling plans vary in quality. *The overriding consideration in assessing a sample in a quantitative study is its representativeness.* A **representative sample** is one whose key characteristics closely approximate those of the population. If the population in a study of blood donors is 50% male and 50% female, then a representative sample would have a similar gender distribution. If the sample is not representative of the population, the external validity (generalizability) of the study is at risk.

Unfortunately, there is no way to make sure that a sample is representative without obtaining the information from the population. Certain sampling procedures are less likely to result in biased samples than others, but a representative sample can never be guaranteed. This may sound discouraging, but it must be remembered that researchers operate under conditions in which error is possible. Quantitative researchers strive to minimize those errors and, if possible, to estimate their magnitude.

Sampling designs are classified as either probability sampling or nonprobability sampling. **Probability sampling** involves random selection in choosing the elements. The hallmark of a probability sample is that researchers can specify the probability that each element of the population will be included in the sample. Probability sampling is the more respected of the two approaches because greater confidence can be placed in the representativeness of probability samples. In **nonprobability samples**, elements are selected by nonrandom methods. There is no way to estimate the probability that each element has of being included in a nonprobability sample, and every element usually does *not* have a chance for inclusion.

Strata

Sometimes, it is useful to think of populations as consisting of two or more subpopulations, or **strata**. A stratum is a mutually exclusive segment of a population, established by one or more characteristics. For instance, suppose our population was all RNs currently employed in the United States. This population could be divided into two strata based on gender. Alternatively, we could specify three strata consisting of nurses younger than 30 years of age, nurses aged 30 to 45 years, and nurses 46 years or older. Strata are often used in the sample selection process to enhance the sample's representativeness.

Sampling Bias

Researchers work with samples rather than with populations because it is more cost-effective to do so. Researchers typically have neither the time nor the resources to study all members of a population. Furthermore, it is unnecessary to gather data from an entire population; it is usually possible to obtain reasonably accurate information from a sample.

Still, data from samples *can* lead to erroneous conclusions. Finding 100 people willing to participate in a study seldom poses difficulty. It is considerably more problematic to select 100 subjects who are not a biased subset of the population. **Sampling bias** refers to the systematic over-representation or under-representation of some segment of the population in terms of a characteristic relevant to the research question.

As an example of consciously biased selection, suppose we were investigating patients' responsiveness to nurses' touch and decide to use as our sample the first 50 patients meeting eligibility criteria in a specific hospital unit. We decide to omit Mr. Z from the sample because he has shown hostility to nurses. Mrs. X, who has just lost a spouse, is also excluded from the study because she is under stress. We have made conscious decisions to exclude certain individuals, and the decisions do not reflect bona fide eligibility criteria. This can lead to bias because responsiveness to nurses' touch (the dependent variable) may be affected by patients' feelings about nurses or their emotional state.

Sampling bias usually occurs unconsciously, however. If we were studying nursing students and systematically interviewed every 10th student who entered the nursing library, the sample of students would be biased in favor of library-goers, even if we are conscientious about including every 10th entrant regardless of the person's appearance, gender, or other traits.

Sampling bias is partly a function of population homogeneity. If population elements were all identical with respect to key attributes, then any sample would be as good as any other. Indeed, if the population were completely homogeneous, that is, exhibited no variability at all, then a *single* element would be a sufficient sample to draw conclusions about the population. For many physiologic attributes, it may be safe to assume a reasonably high degree of homogeneity. For example, the blood in a person's veins is relatively homogeneous and so a single blood sample chosen haphazardly is adequate. For most human attributes, however, homogeneity is the exception rather than the rule. Age, health condition, stress, attitudes, habits—all these attributes reflect the heterogeneity of humans. When variation occurs in the population, then similar variation ideally should be reflected in a sample.

TIP: One straightforward way to increase the generalizability of a study is to select study participants from two or more sites, such as from different hospitals, nursing homes, communities, and so on. Ideally, the two different sites would be sufficiently divergent that broader representation of the population would be obtained.

NONPROBABILITY SAMPLING

Nonprobability sampling is less likely than probability sampling to produce accurate and representative samples. Despite this fact, most research samples in nursing and other disciplines are nonprobability samples. Three primary methods of nonprobability sampling are convenience, quota, and purposive.

Convenience Sampling

Convenience sampling entails using the most conveniently available people as study participants. A faculty member who distributes questionnaires to nursing students in a class is using a convenience sample, or an **accidental sample**, as it is sometimes called. The nurse who conducts an observational study of women delivering twins at the local hospital is also relying on a convenience sample. The problem with convenience sampling is that available subjects might be atypical of the population of interest with regard to critical variables.

Convenience samples do not necessarily comprise individuals known to the researchers. Stopping people at a street corner to conduct an interview is sampling by convenience. Sometimes, researchers seeking people with certain characteristics place an advertisement in a newspaper, put up signs in clinics or supermarkets, or post messages in chat rooms on the Internet. These approaches are subject to bias because people select themselves as pedestrians on certain streets or as volunteers in response to posted notices.

Snowball sampling (also called **network sampling** or **chain sampling**) is a variant of convenience sampling. With this approach, early sample members are asked to identify and refer other people who meet the eligibility criteria. This method of sampling is often used when the research population is people with specific traits who might otherwise be difficult to identify (e.g., people who are afraid of hospitals). Snowballing begins with a few eligible study participants and then continues on the basis of referrals from those participants until the desired sample size has been obtained.

Convenience sampling is the weakest form of sampling. It is also the most commonly used sampling method in many disciplines. In heterogeneous populations, there is no other sampling approach in which the risk of sampling bias is greater.

Example of a convenience sample:
Board and Ryan-Wenger (2002) prospectively examined the long-term effects of the pediatric intensive care unit experience on parents and on family adaptation. The researchers used convenience sampling to recruit three groups of parents: those with a hospitalized child in the pediatric intensive care unit, those with a child in a general care unit, and those with nonhospitalized ill children.

Quota Sampling

A **quota sample** is one in which the researcher identifies population strata and determines how many participants are needed from each stratum. By using information about population characteristics, researchers can ensure that diverse segments are represented in the sample, preferably in the proportion in which they occur in the population.

Suppose we were interested in studying nursing students' attitude toward working with AIDS patients. The accessible population is a school of nursing with an undergraduate enrollment of 1000 students; a sample of 200 students is desired. The easiest procedure would be to use a convenience sample by distributing questionnaires in classrooms or catching students as they enter or leave the library. Suppose, however, we suspect that male and female students have different attitudes toward working with AIDS victims. A convenience sample might result in too many men or women. Table 13-1 presents fictitious data showing the gender distribution for the population and for a convenience sample in the first two columns. In this example, the convenience sample over-represents women and under-represents men. We can, however, guide the selection of study participants so that the sample includes the correct number of cases from both strata. The far-right panel of Table 13-1 shows the number of men and women required for a quota sample for this example.

If we pursue this same example a bit further, you may better appreciate the dangers of a biased sample. Suppose that one of the key questions in this study was, "Would you be willing to work on a unit that cared exclusively for AIDS patients?" The percentage of students in the population who would respond "yes" to this inquiry is shown in the first column of Table 13-2. Of course, we would not know these values; they are displayed to illustrate a point. Within the population, men are more likely than women to be willing to work on a unit with AIDS patients, yet men were seriously under-represented in the convenience sample. As a result, there is a discrepancy between the population and sample values on the outcome variable: about 27% more students in the population are favorable toward working with AIDS victims (14.0%) than we would conclude based on results from the convenience sample (11.0%). The quota sample, on the other hand, does a better job of reflecting the viewpoint of the population (14.5%). In actual research situations, the distortions from a convenience sample may be smaller than in this example, but could be larger as well.

Quota sampling does not require sophisticated skills or a lot of effort—and it is surprising that so

TABLE 13.1 Numbers and Percentages of Students in Strata of a Population, Convenience Sample, and Quota Sample

STRATA	POPULATION	CONVENIENCE SAMPLE	QUOTA SAMPLE
Male	200 (20%)	10 (5%)	40 (20%)
Female	800 (80%)	190 (95%)	160 (80%)
Total	1000 (100%)	200 (100%)	200 (100%)

TABLE 13.2 Students Willing to Work on an AIDS Unit, in the Population, Convenience Sample, and Quota Sample

	NUMBER IN POPULATION	NUMBER IN CONVENIENCE SAMPLE	NUMBER IN QUOTA SAMPLE
Male	55	3	12
Female	85	19	17
Total Number of Willing Students	140	22	29
Total Number of All Students	1000	200	200
Percentage Willing	14.0%	11.0%	14.5%

few researchers use this strategy. Many researchers who use a convenience sample could probably design a quota sampling plan, and it would be advantageous to do so. Stratification should be based on one or more variables that would reflect important differences in the dependent variable under study. Such variables as age, gender, ethnicity, educational attainment, and medical diagnosis are often good stratifying variables.

Except for identifying the strata and the desired representation for each, quota sampling is procedurally similar to convenience sampling. The subjects in any particular cell constitute, in essence, a convenience sample from that stratum of the population. Referring back to the example in Table 13-1, the initial sample of 200 students constituted a convenience sample from the population of 1000. In the quota sample, the 40 men constitute a convenience sample of the 200 men in the population. Because of this fact, quota sampling shares many of the same weaknesses as convenience sampling. For instance, if a researcher is required by a quota sampling plan to interview 10 men between the ages of 65 and 80 years, a trip to a nursing home might be the most convenient method of obtaining those subjects. Yet this approach would fail to represent the many senior citizens who live independently in the community. Despite its prob-

lems, quota sampling represents an important improvement over convenience sampling and should be considered by quantitative researchers whose resources prevent the use of probability sampling.

Example of a quota sample:
Williams, Soetjiningsih, and Williams (2000) studied Balinese mothers' expectations for children's development. The researchers used quota sampling to ensure an equal number of urban and rural Balinese mothers, and an equal number of male and female children.

Purposive Sampling

Purposive sampling or **judgmental sampling** is based on the belief that researchers' knowledge about the population can be used to hand-pick sample members. Researchers might decide purposely to select subjects who are judged to be typical of the population or particularly knowledgeable about the issues under study. Sampling in this subjective manner, however, provides no external, objective method for assessing the typicalness of the selected subjects. Nevertheless, this method can be used to advantage in certain situations. Newly developed instruments can be effectively pretested and evaluated with a purposive sample of diverse types of people. Purposive sampling is often used when researchers want a sample of experts, as in the case of a needs assessment using the key informant approach or in Delphi surveys. Also, as discussed later in this chapter, purposive sampling is frequently used by qualitative researchers.

Example of purposive sampling:
Friedemann, Montgomery, Rice, and Farrell (1999) studied family members' involvement in the nursing home. The first stage of their sampling plan involved purposively sampling 24 nursing homes with a diversity of policies related to family involvement, based on a survey of 208 nursing homes in southern Michigan. In the second stage, all family members of residents admitted to these nursing homes during a 20-month window were invited to participate.

Evaluation of Nonprobability Sampling

Although a nonprobability sample is often acceptable for pilot, exploratory, or in-depth qualitative research, for most quantitative studies, the use of nonprobability samples is problematic. Nonprobability samples are rarely representative of the population. When every element in the population does not have a chance of being included in the sample, it is likely that some segment of it will be systematically underrepresented.

Why, then, are nonprobability samples used in most nursing studies? Clearly, the advantage of these sampling designs lies in their convenience and economy. Probability sampling, discussed next, requires skill and resources. There is often no option but to use a nonprobability approach or to abandon the project altogether. Even hard-nosed research methodologists would hesitate to advocate the abandonment of an idea in the absence of a random sample. Quantitative researchers using nonprobability samples out of necessity must be cautious about the inferences and conclusions drawn from the data. With care in the selection of the sample, a conservative interpretation of the results, and replication of the study with new samples, researchers may find that nonprobability samples work reasonably well.

TIP: If you use a convenience sample, you can still take steps to enhance the sample's representativeness. First, identify important extraneous variables—factors that affect variation in the dependent variable. For example, in a study of the effect of stress on health, family income would be an important extraneous variable because poor people tend to be less healthy (*and* more stressed) than more affluent ones. Then, decide how to account for this source of variation in the sampling design. One solution is to eliminate variation from extraneous variables, as discussed in Chapter 9. In the stress and health example, we might restrict the population to middle-class people. Alternatively, we could select the convenience sample from two communities known to differ socioeconomically so that our sample would reflect the experiences of both lower- and middle-class subjects. This approaches using a quota sampling method. In other words, if the population is known to be heterogeneous, you should take steps either to make it more homogeneous (thereby redefining the population) or to capture the full variation in the sample.

PROBABILITY SAMPLING

Probability sampling involves the random selection of elements from a population. Random selection should not be (although it often is) confused with random assignment, which was described in connection with experimental designs in Chapter 8. Random assignment refers to the process of allocating subjects to different treatment conditions at random. Random *assignment* has no bearing on how subjects in an experiment were selected in the first place. **Random sampling** involves a selection process in which each element in the population has an equal, independent chance of being selected. The four most commonly used probability sampling methods are simple random, stratified random, cluster, and systematic sampling.

Simple Random Sampling

Simple random sampling is the most basic probability sampling design. Because the more complex probability sampling designs incorporate features of simple random sampling, the procedures involved are described here in some detail.

In simple random sampling, researchers establish a **sampling frame,** the technical name for the list of the elements from which the sample will be chosen. If nursing students at the University of Connecticut were the accessible population, then a roster of those students would be the sampling frame. If the sampling unit were 500-bed (or larger) hospitals in Canada, then a list of all such hospitals would be the sampling frame. In practice, a population may be defined in terms of an existing sampling frame rather than starting with a population and developing a list of elements. For example, if we wanted to use a telephone directory as a sampling frame, we would have to define the population as community residents who are customers of the telephone company *and* who had a number listed at the time the directory was published. Because not all members of a community own a telephone and others do not have listed numbers, it would not be appropriate to consider a telephone directory as the sampling frame for the entire population.

Once a sampling frame has been developed, elements are numbered consecutively. A table of random numbers would then be used to draw a sample of the desired size. An example of a sampling frame for a population of 50 people is presented in Table 13-3. Let us assume we want to select randomly a sample of 20 people. As in the case of random assignment, we would find a starting place in a table of random numbers by blindly placing our finger at some point on the page. To include all numbers between 1 and 50, two-digit combinations would be read. Suppose, for the sake of the example, that we began random selection with the first number in the random number table of Table 8-2 (p 171), which is 46. The person corresponding to that number, D. Abraham, is the first subject selected to participate in the study. Number 05, C. Eldred, is the second selection, and number 23, R. Yarinsky, is the third. This process would continue until the 20 subjects were chosen. The selected elements are circled in Table 13-3.

TABLE 13.3	Sampling Frame for Simple Random Sampling Example	
(1) N. Alexander	(26) G. Berlin
2. T. Brock	27. C. Coulton
3. H. Collado	28. R. De los Santos
4. F. Doolittle	29. D. Edelstein
(5) C. Eldred	(30) B. Fink
(6) R. Fellerath	(31) J. Gueron
7. B. Goldman	32. J. Hunter
8. G. Hamilton	(33) R. Joyce
9. R. Ivry	(34) Y. Kim
10. S. James	35. A. London
11. V. Knox	36. J. Martinez
12. S. Lynn	37. C. Nicholson
(13) C. Michalopoulos	(38) R. Ortega
(14) L. Nelson	39. K. Paget
15. J. O'Brien	40. G. Queto
16. M. Price	41. J. Riccio
(17) J. Quint	42. E. Scott
(18) D. Romm	(43) L. Traeger
19. R. Seupersad	44. E. Vallejo
20. P. Tang	(45) J. Wallace
(21) N. Verma	(46) D. Abraham
22. R. Widom	47. D. Butler
(23) R. Yarinsky	48. O. Cardenas
(24) M. Zaslow	49. F. Derocher
25. M. Agudelo	(50) K. Edin

It should be clear that a sample selected randomly in this fashion is not subject to researchers' biases. Although there is no guarantee that a randomly drawn sample will be representative, random selection does ensure that differences in the attributes of the sample and the population are purely a function of chance. The probability of selecting a markedly deviant sample is low, and this probability decreases as the size of the sample increases.

Simple random sampling tends to be laborious. Developing the sampling frame, numbering all the elements, and selecting sample elements are time-consuming chores, particularly if the population is large. Imagine enumerating all the telephone subscribers listed in the New York City telephone directory! If the elements can be arranged in computer-readable form, then the computer can be programmed to select the sample automatically. In actual practice, simple random sampling is not used frequently because it is a relatively inefficient procedure. Furthermore, it is not always possible to get a listing of every element in the population, so other methods may be required.

Example of a simple random sample: Yoon and Horne (2001) studied the use of herbal products for medicinal purposes in a sample of older women. A random sample of 86 women aged 65 or older who lived independently in a Florida County was selected, using a sampling frame compiled from information from the state motor vehicle agency.

Stratified Random Sampling

In **stratified random sampling,** the population is first divided into two or more strata. As with quota sampling, the aim of stratified sampling is to enhance representativeness. Stratified sampling designs subdivide the population into homogeneous subsets from which an appropriate number of elements are selected at random.

Stratification is often based on such demographic attributes as age, gender, and income level. One difficulty is that the stratifying attributes must be known in advance and may not be readily discernible. If you were working with a telephone directory, it would be risky to guess a person's gender, and age, ethnicity, or other personal information could not be used as stratifying variables. Patient listings, student rosters, or organizational directories might contain information for a meaningful stratification. Quota sampling does not have the same problem because researchers can ask prospective subjects questions that determine their eligibility for a particular stratum. In stratified sampling, however, a person's status in a stratum must be known before random selection.

The most common procedure for drawing a stratified sample is to group together elements belonging to a stratum and to select randomly the desired number of elements. Researchers can either select an equal number of elements from each stratum or select unequal numbers, for reasons discussed later. To illustrate the procedure used in the simplest case, suppose that the list in Table 13-3 consisted of 25 men (numbers 1 through 25) and 25 women (numbers 26 through 50). Using gender as the stratifying variable, we could guarantee a sample of 10 men and 10 women by randomly sampling 10 numbers from the first half of the list and 10 from the second half. As it turns out, our simple random sampling did result in 10 elements being chosen from each half of the list, but this was purely by chance. It would not have been unusual to draw, say, 8 names from one half and 12 from the other. Stratified sampling can guarantee the appropriate representation of different segments of the population.

Stratifying variables usually divide the population into unequal subpopulations. For example, if the person's race were used to stratify the population of U. S. citizens, the subpopulation of white people would be larger than that of African-American and other nonwhite people. The researcher might decide to select subjects in proportion to the size of the stratum in the population, using **proportionate stratified sampling**. If the population was students in a nursing school that had 10% African-American students, 10% Hispanic students, and 80% white students, then a proportionate stratified sample of 100 students, with racial/ethnic background as the stratifying variable, would consist of 10, 10, and 80 students from the respective strata.

When researchers are interested in understanding differences among strata, proportionate sampling may result in insufficient numbers for making comparisons. In the previous example, would the researcher be justified in drawing conclusions about the characteristics of Hispanic nursing students based on only 10 cases? It would be unwise to do so. For this reason, researchers often adopt a **disproportionate sampling design** when comparisons are sought between strata of greatly unequal size. In the example, the sampling proportions might be altered to select 20 African-American students, 20 Hispanic students, and 60 white students. This design would ensure a more adequate representation of the two racial/ethnic minorities. When disproportionate sampling is used, however, it is necessary to make an adjustment to the data to arrive at the best estimate of *overall* population values. This adjustment process, known as **weighting**, is a simple mathematic computation described in textbooks on sampling.

Stratified random sampling enables researchers to sharpen the precision and representativeness of the final sample. When it is desirable to obtain reliable information about subpopulations whose memberships are relatively small, stratification provides a means of including a sufficient number of cases in the sample by oversampling for that stratum. Stratified sampling, however, may be impossible if information on the critical variables is unavailable. Furthermore, a stratified sample requires even more labor and effort than simple random sampling because the sample must be drawn from multiple enumerated listings.

Example of stratified random sampling: Bath, Singleton, Strikas, Stevenson, McDonald, and Williams (2000) conducted a survey to determine the extent to which hospitals with labor and delivery services had policies about screening pregnant women for hepatitis B. A stratified random sample of 968 hospitals (stratified by number of beds and affiliation with a medical school) was selected.

Cluster Sampling

For many populations, it is impossible to obtain a listing of all elements. For example, the population of full-time nursing students in the United States would be difficult to list and enumerate for the purpose of drawing a simple or stratified random sample. It might also be prohibitively expensive to sample students in this way because the resulting sample would include only one or two students per institution. If personal interviews were involved, the interviewers would have to travel to students scattered throughout the country. Large-scale surveys almost never use simple or stratified random sampling; they usually rely on cluster sampling.

In **cluster sampling**, there is a successive random sampling of units. The first unit is large groupings, or clusters. In drawing a sample of nursing students, we might first draw a random sample of nursing schools and then draw a sample of students from the selected schools. The usual procedure for selecting samples from a general population is to sample successively such administrative units as states, cities, census tracts, and then households. Because of the successive stages in cluster sampling, this approach is often called **multistage sampling**. The resulting design is usually described in terms of the number of stages (e.g., three-stage cluster sampling).

The clusters can be selected either by simple or stratified methods. For instance, in selecting clusters of nursing schools, it may be advisable to stratify on program type. The final selection from within a cluster may also be performed by simple or stratified random sampling.

For a specified number of cases, cluster sampling tends to be less accurate than simple or stratified random sampling. Despite this disadvantage, cluster sampling is more economical and practical than other types of probability sampling, particularly when the population is large and widely dispersed.

Example of cluster/multistage sampling: Trinkoff, Zhou, Storr, and Soeken (2000) studied nurses' substance abuse, using data from a two-stage cluster sample. In the first stage, 10 states in the United States were selected using a complex stratification procedure. In the second stage, RNs were selected from each state (a total sample of 3600) by simple random sampling.

Systematic Sampling

The final sampling design can be either probability or nonprobability sampling, depending on the exact procedure used. **Systematic sampling** involves the selection of every *k*th case from a list or group, such as every 10th person on a patient list or every 100th person in a directory of American Nurses Association members. Systematic sampling is sometimes used to sample every *k*th person entering a bookstore, or passing down the street, or leaving a hospital, and so forth. In such situations, unless the population is narrowly defined as all those people entering, passing by, or leaving, the sampling is nonprobability in nature.

Systematic sampling can be applied so that an essentially random sample is drawn. If we had a list, or sampling frame, the following procedure could be adopted. The desired sample size is established at some number (*n*). The size of the population must be known or estimated (*N*). By dividing *N* by *n,* the sampling interval width (*k*) is established. The **sampling interval** is the standard distance between elements chosen for the sample. For instance, if we were seeking a sample of 200 from a population of 40,000, then our sampling interval would be as follows:

$$k = \frac{40,000}{200} = 200$$

In other words, every 200th element on the list would be sampled. The first element should be selected randomly, using a table of random numbers. Let us say that we randomly selected number 73 from a table. The people corresponding to numbers 73, 273, 473, 673, and so forth would be sampled. Alternatively, we could randomly select a number from 1 to the number of elements listed on a page, and then randomly select every *k*th unit on all pages (e.g., number 38 on every page).

Systematic sampling conducted in this manner yields essentially the same results as simple random sampling, but involves far less work. Problems would arise if the list were arranged in such a way that a certain type of element is listed at intervals coinciding with the sampling interval. For instance, if every 10th nurse listed in a nursing personnel roster were a head nurse and the sampling interval was 10, then head nurses would either always or never be included in the sample. Problems of this type are rare, fortunately. In most cases, systematic sampling is preferable to simple random sampling because the same results are obtained in a more efficient manner. Systematic sampling can also be applied to lists that have been stratified.

Example of a systematic sample:
Tolle, Tilden, Rosenfeld, and Hickman (2000) explored barriers to optimal care of the dying by surveying family members of decedents. Their sampling frame was 24,074 death certificates in Oregon, from which they sampled, through systematic sampling, 1458 certificates. They then traced as many family members of the decedents as possible and conducted telephone interviews.

Evaluation of Probability Sampling

Probability sampling is the only viable method of obtaining representative samples. If all the elements in the population have an equal probability of being selected, then the resulting sample is likely to do a good job of representing the population. A further advantage is that probability sampling allows researchers to estimate the magnitude of sampling error. **Sampling error** refers to differences between population values (such as the average age of the population) and sample values (such as the average age of the sample). It is a rare sample that is perfectly representative of a population; probability sampling permits estimates of the degree of error. Advanced textbooks on sampling elaborate on procedures for making such estimates.

The great drawbacks of probability sampling are its inconvenience and complexity. It is usually beyond the scope of most researchers to sample using a probability design, unless the population is narrowly defined—and if it *is* narrowly defined, probability sampling may seem like "overkill." Probability sampling is the preferred and most respected method of obtaining sample elements, but it may in some cases be impractical.

TIP: Whenever possible, it is useful to compare sample characteristics with population characteristics. Published information about the characteristics of many groups of interest to nurses may be available to help provide a context for evaluating sampling bias. For example, if you were studying low-income children in Detroit, you could obtain information on the Internet about salient characteristics (e.g., race/ethnicity, age distribution) of low-income American children from the U. S. Bureau of the Census. Population characteristics could then be compared with sample characteristics, and differences taken into account in interpreting the findings.

SAMPLE SIZE IN QUANTITATIVE STUDIES

Quantitative researchers need to pay careful attention to the number of subjects needed to test research hypotheses adequately. A sophisticated procedure known as **power analysis** can be used to estimate sample size needs, but some statistical knowledge is needed before this procedure can be explained. In this section we offer guidelines to beginning researchers; advanced

students can read about power analysis in Chapter 20 or consult a sampling or statistical textbook.

There are no simple formulas that can tell you how large a sample is needed in a given quantitative study, but we can offer a simple piece of advice: You should use the largest sample possible. The larger the sample, the more representative of the population it is likely to be. Every time researchers calculate a percentage or an average based on sample data, they are estimating a population value. Smaller samples tend to produce less accurate estimates than larger ones. In other words, the larger the sample, the smaller the sampling error.

Let us illustrate this with an example of monthly aspirin consumption in a nursing home facility (Table 13-4). The population consists of 15 residents whose aspirin consumption averages 16 aspirins per month, as shown in the top row of the table. Eight simple random samples—two each with sample sizes of 2,

TABLE 13.4 Comparison of Population and Sample Values and Averages: Nursing Home Aspirin Consumption Example

NUMBER OF PEOPLE IN GROUP	GROUP	INDIVIDUAL DATA VALUES (NUMBER OF ASPIRINS CONSUMED, PRIOR MONTH)	AVERAGE
15	Population	2, 4, 6, 8, 10, 12, 14, 16, 18, 20, 22, 24, 26, 28, 30	16.0
2	Sample 1A	6, 14	10.0
2	Sample 1B	20, 28	24.0
3	Sample 2A	16, 18, 8	14.0
3	Sample 2B	20, 14, 26	20.0
5	Sample 3A	26, 14, 18, 2, 28	17.6
5	Sample 3B	30, 2, 26, 10, 4	14.4
10	Sample 4A	22, 16, 24, 20, 2, 8, 14, 28, 20, 4	15.8
10	Sample 4B	12, 18, 8, 10, 16, 6, 28, 14, 30, 22	16.4

3, 5, and 10—have been drawn. Each sample average represents an estimate of the population average (16). Under ordinary circumstances, of course, the population value would be unknown, and we would draw only one sample. With a sample size of two, our estimate might have been wrong by as many as eight aspirins (sample 1B, average of 24), which is a 50% error. As the sample size increases, the averages get closer to the true population value, *and* the differences in the estimates between samples A and B get smaller as well. As the sample size increases, the probability of getting a markedly deviant sample diminishes. Large samples provide an opportunity to counterbalance atypical values. Unless a power analysis can be done, the safest procedure is to obtain data from as large a sample as is practically feasible.

Large samples are no assurance of accuracy, however. When nonprobability sampling methods are used, even a large sample can harbor extensive bias. The famous example illustrating this point is the 1936 presidential poll conducted by the magazine *Literary Digest,* which predicted that Alfred M. Landon would defeat Franklin D. Roosevelt by a landslide. About 2.5 million individuals participated in this poll—a substantial sample. Biases resulted from the fact that the sample was drawn from telephone directories and automobile registrations during a depression year when only the well-to-do (who preferred Landon) had a car or telephone. Thus, a large sample cannot correct for a faulty sampling design.

Because practical constraints such as time, subject availability, and resources often limit sample size, many nursing studies are based on relatively small samples. In a survey of nursing studies published over four decades (the 1950s to the 1980s), Brown, Tanner and Padrick (1984) found that the average sample size was under 100 subjects in all four decades, and similar results were reported in a more recent analysis (Moody, Wilson, Smyth, Schwartz, Tittle, & VanCott, 1988). In many cases, a small sample can lead to misleading or inconclusive results. Below we discuss some considerations that affect sample size requirements in quantitative studies.

Homogeneity of the Population

If there is reason to believe that the population is relatively homogeneous, a small sample may be adequate. Let us demonstrate that this is so. The top half of Table 13-5 presents hypothetical population values for three different populations, with only 10 people in each population. These values could

TABLE 13.5 Three Populations of Different Homogeneity

GROUP	INDIVIDUAL DATA VALUES	LOWEST VALUE	HIGHEST VALUE	AVERAGE
Population A	100 110 105 95 90 110 105 95 90 100	90	110	100.0
Population B	110 120 105 85 80 120 115 85 80 100	80	120	100.0
Population C	100 130 125 75 70 130 125 75 70 100	70	130	100.0
Sample A	110 90 95	90	110	98.3
Sample B	120 80 85	80	120	95.0
Sample C	125 70 75	70	125	90.0

reflect, for example, scores on a measure of anxiety. In all three populations, the average anxiety score is 100. In population A, however, the individuals have similar anxiety scores, ranging from a low of 90 to a high of 110. In population B, the scores are more variable, and in population C, the scores are more variable still, ranging from 70 to 130.

The second half of Table 13-5 presents three sample values from the three populations. In the most homogeneous population (A), the average anxiety score for the sample is 98.3, which is close to the population average of 100. As the population becomes less homogeneous, the average sample values less accurately reflect population values. In other words, there is greater sampling error when the population is heterogeneous on the key variable. By increasing the sample size, the risk of sampling error would be reduced. For example, if sample C consisted of five values rather than three (say, all the even-numbered population values), then the sample average would be closer to the population average (i.e., 102 rather than 90).

For clinical studies that deal with biophysiologic processes in which variation is limited, a small sample may adequately represent the population. For most nursing studies, however, it is safer to assume a fair degree of heterogeneity, unless there is evidence from prior research to the contrary.

Effect Size

Power analysis builds on the concept of an **effect size**, which expresses the strength of relationships among research variables. If there is reason to expect that the independent and dependent variables will be strongly related, then a relatively small sample should be adequate to demonstrate the relationship statistically. For example, if we were testing a powerful new drug to treat AIDS, it might be possible to demonstrate its effectiveness with a small sample. Typically, however, interventions have modest effects, and variables are usually only moderately correlated with one another. When there is no *a priori* reason for believing that relationships will be strong (i.e., when the effect size is expected to be modest), then small samples are risky.

Attrition

In longitudinal studies, the number of subjects usually declines over time. This is most likely to occur if the time lag between data collection points is great; if the population is mobile or hard to locate; or if the population is a vulnerable one at risk of death or disability. If resources are devoted to tracing subjects, or if the researcher has an ongoing relationship with them (as might be true in clinical studies), then the rate of attrition might be low. It is a rare longitudinal study, however, that maintains the full research sample. Therefore, in estimating sample size needs, researchers should factor in anticipated loss of subjects over time.

Attrition problems are not restricted to longitudinal studies. People who initially agree to cooperate in a study may be subsequently unable or unwilling to participate for various reasons, such as death, deteriorating health, early discharge, discontinued need for an intervention, or simply a change of heart. Researchers should expect a certain amount of subject loss and recruit accordingly.

Subgroup Analyses

Researchers are sometimes interested in testing hypotheses not only for an entire population but for subgroups. For example, we might be interested in determining whether a structured exercise program is effective in improving infants' motor skills. After testing the general hypothesis with a sample of infants, we might wish to test whether the intervention is more effective for certain infants (e.g., low-birth-weight versus normal-birth-weight infants). When a sample is divided to test for **subgroup effects**, the sample must be large enough to support these divisions of the sample.

Sensitivity of the Measures

Instruments vary in their ability to measure key concepts precisely. Biophysiologic measures are usually very sensitive—they measure phenomena accurately, and can make fine discriminations in values. Psychosocial measures often contain a fair amount of error and lack precision. When measuring tools are imprecise and susceptible to errors, larger samples are needed to test hypotheses adequately.

IMPLEMENTING A SAMPLING PLAN IN QUANTITATIVE STUDIES

Once decisions are made about the sampling design and sample size, the plan must be implemented. This section provides some practical information about implementation of a sampling plan.

Steps in Sampling in Quantitative Studies

The steps to be undertaken in drawing a sample vary somewhat from one sampling design to the next, but a general outline of procedures can be described.

1. *Identify the population.* It is good to begin with a clear idea about the target population to which you would ideally like to be able to generalize your results. Unless you have extensive resources, you are unlikely to have access to the entire target population, and so you will also need to identify the portion of the target population that is accessible to you. Researchers often *begin* by identifying an accessible population, and then decide how best to define the target population.

2. *Specify the eligibility criteria.* The criteria for eligibility in the sample should then be spelled out. The criteria should be as specific as possible with respect to characteristics that might exclude potential subjects (e.g., extremes of poor health, inability to read English). The criteria might lead you to redefine your target population.

3. *Specify the sampling plan.* Once the accessible population has been identified, you must decide (a) the method of drawing the sample and (b) how large it will be. Sample size specifications should consider the aspects of the study discussed in the previous section. If you can perform a power analysis to determine the desired number of subjects, it is highly recommended that you do so. Similarly, if probabil-

ity sampling is an option for selecting a sample, that option should be exercised. If you are not in a position to do either, we recommend using as large a sample as possible and taking steps to build representativeness into the design (e.g., by using quota sampling).

4. *Recruit the sample.* Once the sampling design has been specified, the next step is to recruit prospective study participants according to the plan (after any needed institutional permissions have been obtained) and ask for their cooperation. Issues relating to subject recruitment are discussed next.

Sample Recruitment

Recruiting subjects to participate in a study involves two major tasks: identifying eligible candidates and persuading them to participate. Researchers may in some cases need to spend time early in the project deciding the best sources for recruiting potential participants. Researchers must ask such questions as, Where do people with the characteristics I want live or obtain care in large numbers? Will I have direct access to subjects, or will I need administrative approval? Will there be sufficiently large numbers in one location, or will multiple sites be necessary? During the recruitment phase, it may be necessary to develop a **screening instrument**, which is a brief interview or form that allows researchers to determine whether a prospective subject meets all eligibility criteria for the study.

The next task involves actually gaining the cooperation of people who have been deemed eligible for the study. It is critical to have an effective recruitment strategy. Most people, given the right circumstances, will agree to cooperate, but some are hesitant. Researchers should ask themselves, What will make this research experience enjoyable, worthwhile, convenient, pleasant, and nonthreatening for subjects? Factors over which researchers have control that can influence the rate of cooperation include the following:

• *Recruitment method.* Face-to-face recruitment is usually more effective than solicitation by a telephone call or a letter.

- *Courtesy*. Successful recruitment depends on using recruiters who are pleasant, courteous, respectful, and nonthreatening. Cooperation sometimes is enhanced if characteristics of recruiters are similar to those of prospective subjects—particularly with regard to gender, race, and ethnicity.
- *Persistence*. Although high-pressure tactics are never acceptable, persistence may sometimes be needed. When prospective subjects are first approached, their initial reaction may be to decline participation, because they might be taken off guard. If a person hesitates or gives an equivocal answer at the first attempt, recruiters should ask if they could come back at a later time.
- *Incentives*. Gifts and monetary incentives have been found to increase participation rates.
- *Research benefits*. The benefits of participating to the individual and to society should be carefully explained, without exaggeration or misleading information.
- *Sharing results*. Sometimes it is useful to provide people with tangible evidence of their contribution to the study by offering to send them a brief summary of the study results.
- *Convenience*. Every effort should be made to collect data at a time and location that is convenient for subjects. In some cases, this may mean making arrangements for transportation or for the care of young children.
- *Endorsements*. It may be valuable to have the study endorsed or acknowledged by a person, group, or organization that has prospective subjects' confidence, and to communicate this to them. Endorsements might come from the institution serving as the research setting, from a funding agency, or from a respected community group or person, such as a church leader. Press releases in advance of recruitment are sometimes advantageous.
- *Assurances*. Prospective subjects should be told who will see the data, what use will be made of the data, and how confidentiality will be maintained.

TIP: Subject recruitment often proceeds at a slower pace than researchers anticipate. Once you have determined your sample size needs,

it is a good idea to develop contingency plans for recruiting more subjects, should the initial plan prove overly optimistic. For example, a contingency plan might involve relaxing the eligibility criteria, identifying another institution through which participants could be recruited, offering incentives to make participation more attractive, or the lengthening the recruitment period. When contingency plans are developed at the outset, it reduces the likelihood that you will have to settle for a less-than-desirable sample size.

Generalizing From Samples

Ideally, the sample is representative of the accessible population, and the accessible population is representative of the target population. By using an appropriate sampling plan, researchers can be reasonably confident that the first part of this ideal has been realized. The second part of the ideal entails greater risk. Are the unemployed nurses in Atlanta representative of all unemployed nurses in the United States? Researchers must exercise judgment in assessing the degree of similarity.

The best advice is to be realistic and conservative, and to ask challenging questions: Is it reasonable to assume that the accessible population is representative of the target population? In what ways might they differ? How would such differences affect the conclusions? If differences are great, it would be prudent to specify a more restricted target population to which the findings could be meaningfully generalized.

TIP: As you recruit your sample, it is wise to document thoroughly. The more information you have about who the sample is and who it is not, the better able you will be to identify potential biases. Biases can occur even in probability sampling because the *selection* of elements that are representative of the population does not guarantee the *participation* of all those elements, and refusal to participate in a study is rarely random. Thus, you should calculate a **response rate** (the number of people participating in the study relative to the number of people sampled) and document the

nonresponse bias, that is, differences between the characteristics of participants and those of people who refused to participate in the study. Also, those who remain in a study should be compared with those who drop out to document any attrition biases. It may also be useful to document the reasons people give for not cooperating (or not continuing to cooperate) in a study.

SAMPLING IN QUALITATIVE RESEARCH

Qualitative studies almost always use small, non-random samples. This does not mean that qualitative researchers are unconcerned with the quality of their samples, but rather that they use different criteria for selecting study participants. This section examines considerations that apply to sampling in qualitative studies.

The Logic of Qualitative Sampling

Quantitative research is concerned with measuring attributes and relationships in a population, and therefore a representative sample is needed to ensure that the measurements accurately reflect and can be generalized to the population. The aim of most qualitative studies is to discover *meaning* and to uncover multiple realities, and so generalizability is not a guiding criterion.

Qualitative researchers begin with the following types of sampling question in mind: Who would be an information-rich data source for my study? Whom should I talk to, or what should I observe first, so as to maximize my understanding of the phenomenon? A critical first step in qualitative sampling is selecting settings with high potential for information richness.

As the study progresses, new sampling questions emerge, such as the following: Who can I talk to or observe that would confirm my understandings? Challenge or modify my understandings? Enrich my understandings? Thus, as with the overall design in qualitative studies, sampling design is an emergent one that capitalizes on early learning to guide subsequent direction.

Types of Qualitative Sampling

Qualitative researchers usually eschew probability samples. A random sample is not the best method of selecting people who will make good informants, that is, people who are knowledgeable, articulate, reflective, and willing to talk at length with researchers. Various nonprobability sampling designs have been used by qualitative researchers.

Convenience Sampling

Qualitative researchers sometimes use or begin with a convenience sample, which is sometimes referred to in qualitative studies as a **volunteer sample.** Volunteer samples are especially likely to be used when researchers need to have potential participants come forward and identify themselves. For example, if we wanted to study the experiences of people with frequent nightmares, we might have difficulty readily identifying a sufficient number of potential participants. In such a situation, we might recruit sample members by placing a notice on a bulletin board, in a newspaper, or on the Internet, requesting people with frequent nightmares to contact us. In this situation, we would be less interested in obtaining a representative sample of people with nightmares, than in obtaining a broad and diverse group representing various experiences with nightmares.

Sampling by convenience may be easy and efficient, but it is not in general a preferred sampling approach, even in qualitative studies. The key in qualitative studies is to extract the greatest possible information from the few cases in the sample, and a convenience sample may not provide the most information-rich sources. However, a convenience sample may be an economical and easy way to *begin* the sampling process, relying on other methods as data are collected.

Example of a convenience sample: Young, Lynam, Valach, Novak, Brierton, and Christopher (2001) studied parent and adolescent conversations about health. Participants of Indo-Canadian and Euro-Canadian descent were recruited by posting notices in community centers, schools, health units, doctors' offices, and through visits to community agencies. Thirty-five parent—adolescent dyads volunteered.

Snowball Sampling

Qualitative researchers also use snowball sampling, asking early informants to make referrals to other study participants. This method is sometimes referred to as **nominated sampling** because it relies on the nominations of others already in the sample. Researchers may use this method to gain access to people who are difficult to identify. Snowball sampling has distinct advantages over convenience sampling. The first is that it may be more cost-efficient and practical. Researchers may spend less time screening people to determine if they are appropriate for the study, for example. Furthermore, with an introduction from the referring person, researchers may have an easier time establishing a trusting relationship with new participants. Finally, researchers can more readily specify the characteristics that they want new participants to have. For example, in the study of people with nightmares, we could ask early respondents if they knew anyone else who had the same problem *and* who was articulate. We could also ask for referrals to people who would add other dimensions to the sample, such as people who vary in age, race, socioeconomic status, and so on.

A weakness of this approach is that the eventual sample might be restricted to a rather small network of acquaintances. Moreover, the quality of the referrals may be affected by whether the referring sample member trusted the researcher and truly wanted to cooperate.

Example of a snowball sample:
Meadows, Thurston, and Berenson (2001) studied the messages that rural midlife women get about preventive health care. Study participants were recruited through convenience sampling at first, and subsequently through snowball sampling. A sample of 24 midlife women were interviewed.

Purposive Sampling

Qualitative sampling may begin with volunteer informants and may be supplemented with new participants through snowballing, but most qualitative studies eventually evolve to a purposive (or *purposeful*) sampling strategy—that is, hand-picking cases that will most benefit the study.

Example of a purposive sample:
Gebbie, Wakefield, and Kerfoot (2000) purposefully selected 27 American nurses currently active in public health policy to describe their experiences in policy development.

In purposive sampling, several strategies have been identified (Patton, 2002), only some of which are mentioned here. Note that researchers themselves do not necessarily refer to their sampling plans with Patton's labels; his classification shows the kind of diverse strategies qualitative researchers have adopted to meet the theoretical needs of their research:

- **Maximum variation sampling** involves purposefully selecting cases with a wide range of variation on dimensions of interest. By selecting participants with diverse views and perspectives, researchers invite challenges to preconceived or emerging conceptualizations. Maximum variation sampling might involve ensuring that people with diverse backgrounds are represented in the sample (ensuring that there are men and women, poor and affluent people, and so on). It might also involve deliberate attempts to include people with different viewpoints about the phenomenon under study. For example, researchers might use snowballing to ask early participants for referrals to people who hold different points of view.
- **Homogeneous sampling** deliberately reduces variation and permits a more focused inquiry. Researchers may use this approach if they wish to understand a particular group of people especially well. Homogeneous sampling is often used to select people for group interviews.
- **Extreme (deviant) case sampling** provides opportunities for learning from the most unusual and extreme informants (e.g., outstanding successes and notable failures). The assumption underlying this approach is that extreme cases are rich in information because they are special

in some way. In some cases, more can be learned by intensively studying extreme cases, but extreme cases can also distort understanding of a phenomenon.

- **Intensity sampling** is similar to extreme case sampling, but with less emphasis on the extremes. Intensity samples involve information-rich cases that manifest the phenomenon of interest intensely, but not as extreme or potentially distorting manifestations. Thus, the goal in intensity sampling is to select rich cases that offer strong examples of the phenomenon.
- **Typical case sampling** involves the selection of participants who illustrate or highlight what is typical or average. The resulting information can be used to create a qualitative profile illustrating typical manifestations of the phenomenon being studied.
- **Critical case sampling** involves selecting important cases regarding the phenomenon of interest. With this approach, researchers look for the particularly good story that illuminates critical aspects of the phenomenon.
- **Criterion sampling** involves studying cases that meet a predetermined criterion of importance. Criterion sampling is sometimes used in multimethod studies in which data from the quantitative component are used to select cases meeting certain criteria for in-depth study. Sandelowski (2000) offers a number of helpful suggestions for combining sampling strategies in mixed-method research.
- **Theory-based sampling** involves the selection of people or incidents on the basis of their potential representation of important theoretical constructs. Theory-based sampling is a very focused approach that is usually based on an *a priori* theory that is being examined qualitatively.
- **Sampling confirming and disconfirming cases** is often used toward the end of data collection in qualitative studies. As researchers note trends and patterns in the data, emerging conceptualizations need to be checked. **Confirming cases** are additional cases that fit researchers' conceptualizations and offer enhanced credibility. **Disconfirming cases** are examples that do not

fit and serve to challenge researchers' interpretations. These "negative" cases may offer new insights about how the original conceptualization needs to be revised or expanded.

It is important to note that almost all of these sampling strategies require that researchers have some knowledge about the setting in which the study is taking place. For example, to choose extreme cases, typical cases, or critical cases, researchers must have information about the range of variation of the phenomenon and how it manifests itself. Early participants may be helpful in implementing these sampling strategies.

Theoretical Sampling

The method of sampling used in grounded theory is called *theoretical sampling*. Glaser (1978, p. 36) defined this sampling as "the process of data collection for generating theory whereby the analyst jointly collects, codes, and analyzes his data and decides what data to collect next and where to find them, in order to develop his theory as it emerges." The process of theoretical sampling is controlled by the developing grounded theory. Theoretical sampling is not envisioned as a single, unidirectional line. This complex sampling technique requires researchers to be involved with multiple lines and directions as they go back and forth between data and categories as the theory emerges.

Glaser stressed that theoretical sampling is not the same as purposive sampling. Theoretical sampling's purpose is to discover categories and their properties and to offer interrelationships that occur in the substantive theory. "The basic question in theoretical sampling is: what groups or subgroups does one turn to next in data collection?" (Glaser, 1978, p. 36). These groups are not chosen before the research begins but only as they are needed for their theoretical relevance for developing further emerging categories.

Example of a theoretical sampling:
Beck (2002) used theoretical sampling in her grounded theory study of mothering twins during the first year of life, in which 16 mothers of

twins were interviewed in their homes. A specific example of theoretical sampling concerned what the mothers kept referring to as the "blur period"—the first few months of caring for the twins. Initially, Beck interviewed mothers whose twins were around 1 year of age. Her rationale was that these mothers would be able to reflect back over the entire first year of mothering the multiples. When these mothers referred to the "blur period," Beck asked them to describe this period more fully. The mothers said they could not provide many details about this period because it was "such a blur!" Beck then chose to interview mothers whose twins were 3 months of age or younger, to ensure that mothers were still immersed in the "blur period" and would be able to provide rich detail about what this phase of mothering twins was like.

Sample Size in Qualitative Research

There are no criteria or rules for sample size in qualitative research. Sample size is largely a function of the purpose of the inquiry, the quality of the informants, and the type of sampling strategy used. For example, a larger sample is likely to be needed with maximum variation sampling than with typical case sampling.

In qualitative studies, sample size should be determined based on informational needs. Hence, a guiding principle in sampling is **data saturation**—that is, sampling to the point at which no new information is obtained and redundancy is achieved. Morse (2000) has noted that the number of participants needed to reach saturation depends on a number of factors. For example, the broader the scope of the research question, the more participants will likely be needed. Data quality can also affect sample size. If participants are good informants who are able to reflect on their experiences and communicate effectively, saturation can be achieved with a relatively small sample. Also, if longitudinal data are collected, fewer participants may be needed, because each will provide a greater amount of information.

TIP: Sample size ambiguities sometimes create practical dilemmas when you are planning a study, or if you are seeking approval or funding for a project. Patton (2002) recommends specifying *minimum* samples that would reasonably be adequate for understanding the phenomenon. Additional cases can then be added, as necessary, to achieve saturation.

Evaluating Qualitative Samples

In a qualitative study, the sampling plan is evaluated in terms of *adequacy* and *appropriateness* (Morse, 1991). Adequacy refers to the sufficiency and quality of the data the sample yields. An adequate sample provides researchers with data without any "thin" spots. When researchers have truly attained saturation, informational adequacy has been achieved and the resulting description or theory is richly textured and complete. Appropriateness concerns the methods used to select the sample. An appropriate sample is one resulting from the identification and use of participants who can best supply information according to the conceptual requirements of the study. For example, a sampling plan that does not include disconfirming cases may not meet the information needs of the research.

TIP: No matter what type of qualitative sampling you use, you should keep a journal or notebook to jot down ideas and reminders regarding the sampling process (e.g., who you should interview next). Memos to yourself will help you remember valuable ideas about your sample.

Sampling in the Three Main Qualitative Traditions

There are similarities among the various qualitative traditions with regard to sampling: samples are usually small, probability sampling is almost never used, and final sampling decisions usually take place in the field during data collection. However, there are some differences as well.

Sampling in Ethnography

Ethnographers may begin by initially adopting a "big net" approach—that is, mingling with and having conversations with as many members of the culture under study as possible. Although they may converse with many people (usually 25 to 50), they often rely heavily on a smaller number of **key informants**, who are highly knowledgeable about the culture and who develop special, ongoing relationships with the researcher. These key informants are often the researcher's main link to the "inside."

Key informants are chosen purposively, guided by the ethnographer's theoretically informed judgments. Developing a pool of potential key informants often depends on ethnographers' prior theoretical knowledge to construct a relevant framework. For example, an ethnographer might make decisions about different types of key informants to seek out based on roles (e.g., physicians, nurse practitioners) or on some other theoretically meaningful distinction. Once a pool of potential key informants is developed, key considerations for final selection are their level of knowledge about the culture, and how willing they are to collaborate with the ethnographer in revealing and interpreting the culture.

It might be noted that there is some controversy among ethnographers about the use of "stranger" versus "insider" samples. It has been argued that ethnographers should not sample people whom they know or in whom they have a vested interest. According to this argument, it is not possible to do a valid ethnography "in your own backyard" (Glesne & Peshkin, 1992), despite the obvious advantage of having access to a lot of information and being able to gain people's cooperation. The problem is that if ethnographers are part of the culture under study, it may be difficult to get a handle on ingrained norms and values. Moreover, ethnographers who study people known to them have established relationships that can interfere with objective questioning and observation.

Although ethnographies have traditionally entailed studies of cultures in which researchers are strangers, not everyone agrees that this is essential. Field (1991), for example, has described the unique issues involved in nurse researchers studying their own culture and settings.

Sampling in ethnography typically involves more than selecting informants because observation and other means of data collection play a big role in helping researchers understand a culture. Ethnographers have to decide not only *whom* to sample, but *what* to sample as well. For example, ethnographers have to make decisions about observing *events* and *activities*, about examining *records* and *artifacts*, and about exploring *places* that provide clues about the culture. Key informants can play an important role in helping ethnographers decide what to sample.

Example of an ethnographic sample:
Hoga, Alcantara, and deLima (2001) explored the involvement of men in reproductive health in a low-income community in Brazil. These ethnographers used Leininger's ethnonursing research method to collect data. Their sample consisted of 15 adult men, 7 of whom were key informants. "The key informants were selected based on their full knowledge about the domain of inquiry and the observations during the observation-participation-reflection process that they dictate their norms, values, and beliefs during social and mainly in their familiar examples and conversations with children and relatives" (p. 110).

Sampling in Phenomenological Studies

Phenomenologists tend to rely on very small samples of participants—typically 10 or fewer. There is one guiding principle in selecting the sample for a phenomenological study: all participants must have experienced the phenomenon under study and must be able to articulate what it is like to have lived that experience. It might thus be said that phenomenologists use a criterion sampling method, the criterion being experience with the phenomenon under study. Although phenomenological researchers seek participants who have had the targeted experiences, they also want to explore diversity of individual experiences. Thus, as described by Porter (1999), they may specifically look for people with demographic or other differences who have shared a common experience.

Example of a sample in a phenomenological study:

Orne, Fishman, Manka, and Pagnozzi (2000) studied the lived experience of being a medically uninsured working person. They purposively sampled 12 people who were working but lacked health insurance. The participants varied in terms of gender, occupation, and income.

Sampling in Grounded Theory Studies

Grounded theory research is typically done with samples of about 20 to 30 people, using theoretical sampling. The goal in a grounded theory study is to select informants who can best contribute to the evolving theory. Sampling, data collection, data analysis, and theory construction occur concurrently, and so study participants are selected serially and contingently (i.e., contingent on the emerging conceptualization). Sampling might evolve as follows:

1. The researcher begins with a general notion of where and with whom to start. The first few cases may be solicited purposively, by convenience, or through snowballing.
2. In the early part of the study, a strategy such as maximum variation sampling might be used, to gain insights into the range and complexity of the phenomenon under study.
3. The sample is adjusted in an ongoing fashion. Emerging conceptualizations help to focus the sampling process.
4. Sampling continues until saturation is achieved.
5. Final sampling often includes a search for confirming and disconfirming cases to test, refine, and strengthen the theory.

Example of sampling in a grounded theory study:

Patterson and Thorne (2000) studied how people with long-standing type 1 diabetes make decisions in relation to unanticipated blood glucose levels. Initial participants were selected to ensure variation with regard to attributes known to influence self-care decision-making (e.g., cohabitation).

Subsequently, recruitment was directed on the basis of concepts that had relevance to the evolving theory. A total of 22 diabetic patients participated in the study.

RESEARCH EXAMPLES

In the following sections, we describe in some detail the sampling plans of two nursing studies, one quantitative and the other qualitative.

Research Example From a Quantitative Study

Holland and Carruth (2001) conducted a telephone survey to examine the risk factors of farm women who engage in activities that could exposed them to tetanus, and to study the circumstances related to tetanus immunization.

The researchers first used a purposive sampling method to select 10 parishes (counties) in southeast Louisiana. The counties were hand-picked to reflect agricultural and geographic diversity. The researchers had access to a sampling frame of 4804 farm owners in these 10 parishes (a list maintained by Louisiana State University Agricultural Centers and Farm Service Agency).

Next, a stratified random sample of farm owners was drawn, with parish as the stratifying variable. That is, in each parish, a random sample of farm owners was selected. (The research report did not indicate whether proportionate or disproportionate sampling was used.) Sampled farm owners were screened to determine whether an eligible woman lived in the household. Women were deemed eligible if they were 18 years or older and were members of a family participating in a farming operation. If the household included two or more such women, the woman who had the greatest involvement with farming was invited to participate.

A total of 1141 farms were determined to have an eligible sample member. Interviews were completed with 657 women, for a response rate of 57.6% among known eligible farms. The report did not indicate whether an analysis was done to evaluate response bias—although the absence of such information does not mean that such an analysis was not undertaken.

The results indicated that only 54% of the women had had a tetanus booster within the prior 10 years.

Older women were much less likely than younger women to be up to date on their immunizations.

Research Example From a Qualitative Study

Rillstone and Hutchinson (2001) conducted a grounded theory study to examine parents' experiences and feelings when faced with a potentially stressful pregnancy: a pregnancy subsequent to a prior pregnancy which the parents decided to terminate due to a fetal abnormality.

The initial sample was obtained from an urban community in northeastern Florida, where parents were recruited through obstetricians and reproductive endocrinologists. Because only 4 local parents were recruited, Rillstone and Hutchinson sought additional participants through an Internet support network, which yielded 18 additional parents. Sampling continued for an 8-month period. The total sample consisted of 13 women and 9 of their partners from across the nation, plus 2 local health care providers. After 20 interviews, the researchers felt they had achieved data saturation. To assess the validity of their developing grounded theory, two additional women and two health care providers (a nurse and a physician) were interviewed, either by telephone or in person.

The parents who participated in the study had confronted a wide range of diagnoses with the pregnancies where they had to choose whether to terminate the pregnancy. These varied diagnoses included Down syndrome, spina bifida, trisomy 18, bilateral renal agenesis, Prader-Willi syndrome, and autosomal recessive polycystic kidney disease.

The researchers concluded that their sample was not representative of all parents confronting such circumstances. Parents in the sample were in higher-than-average socioeconomic circumstances, were older than 24 years of age, and had high educational levels. Such a bias is consistent with the fact that Internet use is higher among more affluent and better-educated families.

Data analysis revealed that the basic problem these parents had to contend with was the reemergence of mental anguish. Parents coped with this mental anguish by developing emotional armor, limiting disclosure to others about both their past and present pregnancies, delaying attachment to the baby, and becoming increasingly attached to their health care providers.

SUMMARY POINTS

- **Sampling** is the process of selecting a portion of the **population,** which is an entire aggregate of cases.
- An **element** is the basic unit about which information is collected—usually humans in nursing research.
- The criteria that specify population characteristics are the **eligibility criteria** (or **inclusion criteria**).
- Researchers usually sample from an **accessible population**, but should identify the **target population** to which they would like to generalize their results.
- The main consideration in assessing a sample in a quantitative study is its **representativeness**— the extent to which the sample is similar to the population and avoids bias. **Sampling bias** refers to the systematic over-representation or under-representation of some segment of the population.
- The principal types of **nonprobability sampling** (wherein elements are selected by non-random methods) are convenience, quota, and purposive sampling. Nonprobability sampling designs are convenient and economical; a major disadvantage is their potential for bias.
- **Convenience sampling** (or **accidental sampling**) uses the most readily available or most convenient group of people for the sample. **Snowball sampling** is a type of convenience sampling in which referrals for potential participants are made by those already in the sample.
- **Quota sampling** divides the population into homogeneous **strata** (subpopulations) to ensure representation of the subgroups in the sample; within each stratum, subjects are sampled by convenience.
- In **purposive** (or **judgmental**) **sampling,** participants are hand-picked to be included in the sample based on the researcher's knowledge about the population.
- **Probability sampling** designs, which involve the random selection of elements from the population, yield more representative samples than

nonprobability designs and permit estimates of the magnitude of **sampling error**.

- **Simple random sampling** involves the random selection of elements from a **sampling frame** that enumerates all the elements; **stratified random sampling** divides the population into homogeneous subgroups from which elements are selected at random.

- **Cluster sampling** (or **multistage sampling**) involves the successive selection of random samples from larger to smaller units by either simple random or stratified random methods.

- **Systematic sampling** is the selection of every *k*th case from a list. By dividing the population size by the desired sample size, the researcher establishes the **sampling interval,** which is the standard distance between the selected elements.

- In quantitative studies, researchers should ideally use a **power analysis** to estimate **sample size** needs. Large samples are preferable to small ones because larger samples tend to be more representative, but even a large sample does not *guarantee* representativeness.

- Qualitative researchers use the theoretical demands of the study to select articulate and reflective informants with certain types of experience in an emergent way, capitalizing on early learning to guide subsequent sampling decisions.

- Qualitative researchers most often use purposive or, in grounded theory studies, **theoretical sampling** to guide them in selecting data sources that maximize information richness.

- Various purposive sampling strategies have been used by qualitative researchers. One strategy is **maximum variation sampling,** which entails purposely selecting cases with a wide range of variation.

- **Criterion sampling** involves studying cases that meet a predetermined criterion of importance.

- Another important strategy is **sampling confirming and disconfirming cases**, that is, selecting cases that enrich and challenge the researchers' conceptualizations.

- Other types of qualitative sampling include **homogeneous sampling** (deliberately reducing variation); **extreme case sampling** (selecting the most unusual or extreme cases); **intensity sampling** (selecting cases that are intense but not extreme); **typical case sampling** (selecting cases that illustrate what is typical); **critical case sampling** (selecting cases that are especially important or illustrative); and **theory-based sampling** (selecting cases on the basis of their representation of important constructs).

- Samples in qualitative studies are typically small and based on information needs. A guiding principle is **data saturation**, which involves sampling to the point at which no new information is obtained and redundancy is achieved.

- Criteria for evaluating qualitative sampling are informational adequacy and appropriateness.

- Ethnographers make numerous sampling decisions, including not only *whom* to sample but *what* to sample (e.g., activities, events, documents, artifacts); decision making is often aided by their **key informants** who serve as guides and interpreters of the culture.

- Phenomenologists typically work with a small sample of people (10 or fewer) who meet the criterion of having lived the experience under study.

- Grounded theory researchers typically use theoretical sampling and work with samples of about 20 to 30 people.

STUDY ACTIVITIES

Chapter 13 of the *Study Guide to Accompany Nursing Research: Principles and Methods, 7th edition,* offers various exercises and study suggestions for reinforcing concepts presented in this chapter. In addition, the following study questions can be addressed:

1. Draw a simple random sample of 15 people from the sampling frame of Table 13-3, using the table of random numbers that appears in Table 8-2 on page 171. Begin your selection by blindly placing your finger at some point on the table.

2. Suppose you have decided to use a systematic sampling design for a research project. The known population size is 5000, and the sample size desired is 250. What is the sampling interval? If the first element selected is 23, what would be the second, third, and fourth elements selected?

3. Suppose you were interested in studying the attitude of clinical specialists toward autonomy in work situations. Suggest a possible target and accessible population. What strata might be identified if quota sampling were used?

4. What type of sampling design was used to obtain the following samples?
   a. 25 experts in critical care nursing
   b. 60 couples attending a particular prenatal class
   c. 100 nurses from a list of nurses registered in the state of Pennsylvania, using a table of random numbers
   d. 20 adult patients randomly selected from a random selection of 10 hospitals located in one state
   e. Every fifth article published in *Nursing Research* during the 1980s, beginning with the first article.

5. Suppose you wanted to study the experiences of nursing students during their first clinical assignment. Describe what you would need to do to select a sample using maximum variation sampling, critical case sampling, typical case sampling, and homogeneous sampling.

SUGGESTED READINGS

Methodologic References

Babbie, E. (1990). *Survey research methods* (2nd ed.). Belmont, CA: Wadsworth.

Brown, J. S., Tanner, C. A., & Padrick, K. P. (1984). Nursing's search for scientific knowledge. *Nursing Research, 33*, 26–32.

Cochran, W. G. (1977). *Sampling techniques* (3rd ed.). New York: John Wiley & Sons.

Cohen, J. (1977). *Statistical power analysis for the behavioral sciences* (rev. ed.). New York: Academic Press.

Diekmann, J. M., & Smith, J. M. (1989). Strategies for accessment and recruitment of subjects for nursing research. *Western Journal of Nursing Research, 11*, 418–430.

Field, P. A. (1991). Doing fieldwork in your own culture. In J. M. Morse (Ed.), *Qualitative nursing research: A contemporary dialogue*. Newbury Park, CA: Sage.

Glaser, B. G. (1978). *Theoretical sensitivity*. Mill Valley, CA: Sociology Press.

Glesne, C., & Peshkin, A. (1992). *Becoming qualitative researchers: An introduction*. White Plains, NY: Longman.

Kish, L. (1965). *Survey sampling*. New York: John Wiley & Sons.

Levey, P. S., & Lemeshow, S. (1980). *Sampling for health professionals*. New York: Lifetime Learning.

MacDougall, C., & Fudge, E. (2001). Planning and recruiting the sample for focus groups and in-depth interviews. *Qualitative Health Research, 11*, 117–126.

Moody, L. E., Wilson, M. E., Smyth, K., Schwartz, R., Tittle, M., & VanCott, M. L. (1988). Analysis of a decade of nursing practice research: 1977–1986. *Nursing Research, 37*, 374–379.

Morse, J. M. (1991). Strategies for sampling. In J. M. Morse (Ed.), *Qualitative nursing research: A contemporary dialogue*. Newbury Park, CA: Sage.

Morse, J. M. (2000). Determining sample size. *Qualitative Health Research, 10*, 3–5.

Patton, M. Q. (2002). *Qualitative evaluation and research methods* (3rd ed.). Thousand Oaks, CA: Sage.

Polit, D. F., & Sherman, R. (1990). Statistical power analysis in nursing research. *Nursing Research, 39*, 365–369.

Porter, E. J. (1999). Defining the eligible, accessible population for a phenomenological study. *Western Journal of Nursing Research, 21*, 796–804.

Sandelowski, M. (1995). Sample size in qualitative research. *Research in Nursing & Health, 18*, 179–183.

Sandelowski, M. (2000). Combining qualitative and quantitative sampling, data collection, and analysis techniques in mixed-method studies. *Research in Nursing & Health, 23*, 246–255.

Sudman, S. (1976). *Applied sampling*. New York: Academic Press.

Trinkoff, A. M., & Storr, C. L. (1997). Incorporating auxiliary variables into probability sampling designs. *Nursing Research, 46*, 182–185.

Williams, B. (1978). *A sampler on sampling*. New York: John Wiley & Sons.

Studies Cited in Chapter 13

Bath, S., Singleton, J., Strikas, R., Stevenson, J., McDonald, L., & Williams, W. (2000). Performance of U.S. hospitals on recommended screening and immunization practices for pregnant and postpartum women. *American Journal of Infection Control, 28*, 327–332.

Beck, C. T. (2002). Releasing the pause button: Mothering twins during the first year of life. *Qualitative Health Research 12*, 593–608.

Board, R., & Ryan-Wenger, N. (2002). Long-term effects of pediatric intensive care unit hospitalization on families with young children. *Heart & Lung, 31*, 53–66.

Friedemann, M., Montgomery, R. J., Rice, C., & Farrell, L. (1999). Family involvement in the nursing home. *Western Journal of Nursing Research, 21*, 549–567.

Gebbie, K. M., Wakefield, M., & Kerfoot, K. (2000). Nursing and health policy. *Journal of Nursing Scholarship, 32*, 307–315.

Hoga, L. A., Alcantara, A. C., & deLima, V. M. (2001). Adult male involvement in reproductive health: An ethnographic study in a community of Sao Paulo City, Brazil. *Journal of Transcultural Nursing, 12*, 107–114.

Holland, C., & Carruth, A. K. (2001). Exposure risks and tetanus immunization in women of family owned farms. *AAOHN Journal, 49*, 130–136.

Keele-Smith, R., & Price-Daniel, C. (2001). Effects of crossing legs on blood pressure measurement. *Clinical Nursing Research, 10*, 202–213.

Meadows, L. M., Thurston, W. E., & Berenson, C. A. (2001). Health promotion and preventive measures: Interpreting messages at midlife. *Qualitative Health Research, 11*, 450–463.

Orne, R. M., Fishman, S. J., Manka, M., & Pagnozzi, M. E. (2000). Living on the edge: A phenomenological study of medically uninsured working Americans. *Research in Nursing & Health, 23*, 204–212.

Patterson, B., & Thorne, S. (2000). Expert decision-making in relation to unanticipated blood glucose levels. *Research in Nursing & Health, 23*, 147–157.

Rillstone, P., & Hutchinson, S. A. (2001). Managing the reemergence of anguish: Pregnancy after a loss due to anomalies. *Journal of Obstetric, Gynecologic, and Neonatal Nursing, 30*, 291–298.

Tolle, S. W., Tilden, V. P., Rosenfeld, A. G., & Hickman, S. E. (2000). Family reports of barriers to optimal care of the dying. *Nursing Research, 49*, 310–317.

Trinkoff, A. M., Zhou, Q., Storr, C. L., & Soeken, K. L. (2000). Workplace access, negative proscriptions, job strain, and substance use in registered nurses. *Nursing Research, 49*, 83–90.

Williams, P. D., Soetjiningsih, & Williams, A. R. (2000). Balinese mothers' developmental timetables for young children. *Western Journal of Nursing Research, 22*, 717–735.

Yoon, S. L., & Horne, C. H. (2001). Herbal products and conventional medicines used by community-residing older women. *Journal of Advanced Nursing, 33*, 51–59.

Young, R. A., Lynam, M. J., Valach, L., Novak, H., Brierton, I., & Christopher, A. (2001). Joint actions of parents and adolescents in health conversations. *Qualitative Health Research, 11*, 40–57.

PART

4

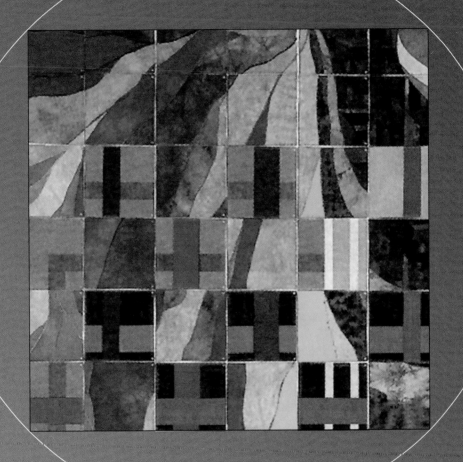

Measurement
and Data
Collection

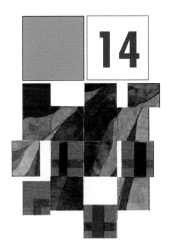

14

Designing and Implementing a Data Collection Plan

The phenomena in which researchers are interested must ultimately be translated into data that can be analyzed. In quantitative studies, the tasks of defining research variables and selecting or developing appropriate methods for collecting data are among the most challenging in the research process. Without high-quality data collection methods, the accuracy and robustness of the conclusions are subject to challenge.

As in the case of research designs and sampling plans, researchers must often choose from an array of alternative data collection methods. This chapter provides an overview of various methods of data collection for qualitative and quantitative studies, and discusses the development of a **data collection plan**.

EXISTING DATA VERSUS ORIGINAL DATA

One of the first decisions that investigators make with regard to research data concerns whether to use existing data or to collect data generated specifically for the study. Most researchers develop original data, but they often can take advantage of existing information.

Existing **records** are an important data source for nurse researchers. A wealth of data gathered for non-research purposes can be fruitfully exploited to answer research questions. Hospital records, patient charts, physicians' order sheets, care plan statements, and the like all constitute rich data sources to which nurse researchers may have access. The use of records data is discussed at greater length in Chapter 17.

Example of a study using records:
Christensen, Janson, and Seago (2001) examined differences in rates of pulmonary complications in head-injured patients with and without concomitant alcohol intoxication. Data for the study were the medical records of 98 consecutive patients admitted to a level I trauma center.

Historical research also typically relies on available data. As noted in Chapter 11, data for historical research are usually in the form of written historical documents: periodicals, diaries, letters, newspapers, minutes of meetings, medical documents, reports, and so forth. Historical researchers must locate the available documents, evaluate the authenticity and accuracy of the data, and then assemble the data set of historical information.

As another example, researchers sometimes perform a secondary analysis (see Chapter 10), which is the use of data gathered in a previous study—often by other researchers—to test new hypotheses or address new research questions. The difference between using records and doing secondary analyses is that researchers doing a secondary analysis typically have a ready-to-analyze data set, whereas researchers using records have to assemble the data set, and considerable coding and data manipulation usually are necessary.

Finally, meta-analyses and metasyntheses make use of existing data—data derived from available research reports. As with records information, researchers doing such integrative studies do not have to collect new data but must ferret out appropriate data, code or transform them, and assemble them into a data set for analysis.

The primary advantages of using existing data are that they are economical and time-saving. On the other hand, it may be difficult to find existing data that are ideally suited to answering a research question.

DIMENSIONS OF DATA COLLECTION APPROACHES

If existing data are not available for the research question, researchers must collect original data. Many methods of collecting new data are used for nursing studies. For example, study participants can be interviewed, observed, or tested with measures of physiologic functioning. Regardless of what specific approach is used, data collection methods vary along four important dimensions: structure, quantifiability, researcher obtrusiveness, and objectivity.

Structure

Research data for quantitative studies are often collected according to a structured plan that indicates what information is to be gathered and how to gather it. For example, most self-administered questionnaires are highly structured: They include a fixed set of questions to be answered in a specified sequence and with predesignated response options (e.g., agree or disagree). Structured methods give participants limited opportunities to qualify their answers or to explain the underlying meaning of their responses.

In some studies it is more appropriate to impose little or no structure and to provide participants with opportunities to reveal information in a naturalistic way. Most qualitative studies rely almost exclusively on unstructured or loosely structured methods of data collection.

There are advantages and disadvantages to both approaches. Structured methods often take considerable effort to develop and refine, but they yield data that are relatively easy to analyze. Structured methods are seldom appropriate for an in-depth examination of a phenomenon, however. Consider the following two methods of asking people about their levels of stress:

Structured: During the past week, would you say you felt stressed:
1. rarely or none of the time,
2. some or a little of the time,
3. occasionally or a moderate amount of the time, or
4. most or all of the time?

Unstructured: How stressed or anxious have you been this past week? Tell me about the kinds of tensions and stresses you have been experiencing.

The structured approach would allow the researcher to compute exactly what percentage of respondents felt stressed most of the time but would provide no information about the intensity, cause, or circumstances of the stress. The unstructured question allows for deeper and more thoughtful responses, but may pose difficulties for people who are not good at expressing themselves verbally. Moreover, the unstructured question yields data that are considerably more difficult to analyze.

When data are collected in a highly structured fashion, the researcher must develop (or borrow) what is referred to as the data collection **instrument**, which is the formal written document used to collect and record information, such as a questionnaire. When unstructured methods are used, there is typically no formal instrument, although there may be a list of the types of information needed.

Quantifiability

Data that will be subjected to statistical analysis must be gathered in such a way that they can be quantified. For statistical analysis, all variables must be quantitatively measured—even though the variables are abstract and intangible phenomena that represent *qualities* of humans, such as hope, loneliness, pain, and body image. Data that are to be analyzed qualitatively are typically collected in narrative form.

Structured data collection approaches usually yield data that are easily quantified. It may be possible (and it is sometimes useful), however, to quantify unstructured information as well. For example, responses to the unstructured question concerning stress could be categorized after the fact according to the four levels of stress indicated in the structured question. Whether it is *wise* to do so depends on the research problem, the researcher's philosophic orientation, and the nature of the responses. This is an issue to which we return later in this chapter.

Researcher Obtrusiveness

Data collection methods differ in the degree to which people are aware of their status as participants. If people are aware of their role in a study, their behavior and responses may not be "normal," and distortions can undermine the value of the research. When data are collected unobtrusively, however, ethical problems may emerge, as discussed in Chapter 7.

Study participants are most likely to distort their behavior and their responses to questions under certain circumstances. In particular, researcher obtrusiveness is likely to be most problematic when: (1) a program is being evaluated and participants have a vested interest in the evaluation outcome; (2) participants are engaged in socially unacceptable or atypical behavior; (3) participants have not complied with medical and nursing instructions; and (4) participants are the type of people who have a strong need to "look good." When researcher obtrusiveness is unavoidable under these circumstances, researchers should make an effort to put participants at ease, to stress the importance of candor and naturalistic behavior, and to train research personnel to convey a neutral and nonjudgmental demeanor.

Objectivity

Objectivity refers to the degree to which two independent researchers can arrive at similar "scores" or make similar observations regarding the concepts of interest, that is, make judgments regarding participants' attributes or behavior that are not biased by personal feelings or beliefs. Some data collection approaches require more subjective judgment than others, and some research problems require a higher degree of objectivity than others.

Researchers whose paradigmatic orientation lies in positivism usually strive for a reasonable amount of objectivity. However, in research based on the naturalistic paradigm, the subjective judgment of investigators is considered an asset because subjectivity is viewed as essential for understanding human experiences.

MAJOR TYPES OF DATA COLLECTION METHODS

In addition to making decisions regarding these four dimensions, researchers must select the form of data collection to use. Three types of approach have been used most frequently by nurse researchers: self-reports, observation, and biophysiologic measures. This section presents an overview of these methods, and subsequent chapters provide more in-depth guidance.

Researchers' decisions about research design usually are independent of decisions about data collection methods. Researchers using an experimental crossover design can rely on self-report data—as can a researcher doing an ethnography, for example. Moreover, the three main data collection methods—self-reports, observation, and biophysiologic measures—can involve either existing data or original data created for research purposes. The research *question* may dictate which specific method of data collection to use—and where along the four continua described in the previous section the methods should lie. Often, however, researchers have great latitude in designing a data collection plan.

Self-Reports

A good deal of information can be gathered by questioning people, a method known as **self-report**. If, for example, we were interested in learning about patients' perceptions of hospital care, their preoperative fears, or their health-promoting habits, we would likely talk to them and ask them questions. The unique ability of humans to communicate verbally on a sophisticated level makes direct questioning a particularly important part of nurse researchers' data collection repertoire. The vast majority of nursing studies involve data collected by self-report.

The self-report method is strong in directness and versatility. If we want to know what people think, feel, or believe, the most efficient means of gathering information is to ask them about it. Perhaps the strongest argument that can be made for the self-report method is that it frequently yields information that would be difficult, if not impossible, to gather by any other means. Behaviors can be observed, but only if participants engage in them publicly. For example, it is usually impossible for researchers to observe such behaviors as child abuse, contraceptive practices, or "road rage." Furthermore, observers can observe only those behaviors occurring at the time of the study. Through self-reports, researchers can gather retrospective data about activities and events occurring in the past or gather projections about behaviors in which people plan to engage in the future. Information about feelings, values, opinions, and motives can sometimes be inferred through observation, but behaviors and feelings do not always correspond exactly. People's actions do not always indicate their state of mind. Here again, self-report methods can be used to capture psychological characteristics through direct communication with participants.

Despite these advantages, verbal report methods have some weaknesses. The most serious issue concerns the validity and accuracy of self-reports: How can we really be sure that respondents feel or act the way they say they do? How can we trust the information that respondents provide, particularly if the true answers would reveal illegal or socially unacceptable behavior? Investigators often have no alternative but to assume that their respondents have been frank. Yet we all have a tendency to want to present ourselves in the best light, and this may conflict with the truth. Researchers who gather self-report data should recognize the limitations of this method, and should be prepared to take these shortcomings into consideration when interpreting the results.

Example of a study using self-reports: Eliott and Olver (2002) analyzed in-depth self-report data in an effort to develop a definitive definition of *hope*. They interviewed 23 oncology clinic outpatients on do-not-resuscitate issues, and 12 spontaneously talked about hope.

Observation

For certain research problems, an alternative to self-reports is **observation** of people's behavior. Information required by nurse researchers as evidence of nursing effectiveness or as clues to improving nursing practices often can be obtained through direct observation. Suppose, for instance, that we were interested in studying mental patients' methods of defending their personal territory, or children's reactions to the removal of a leg cast, or a patient's mode of emergence from anesthesia. These phenomena are all amenable to observation. Observational methods can be used to gather a variety of information, including information on characteristics and conditions of individuals (e.g., the sleep—wake state of patients); verbal communication (e.g., exchange of information during medication administration); nonverbal communication (e.g., facial expressions); activities (e.g., geriatric patients' self-grooming activities); and environmental conditions (e.g., architectural barriers in the homes of disabled people).

Observations can be made in laboratory or in natural settings. In addition, observation can be done directly through the human senses or with the aid of technical apparatus, such as video equipment and tape recorders. Thus, observation is a versatile data collection approach.

Like self-report techniques, observational methods can vary in degree of structure. That is, a researcher could observe nurses' methods of touching patients in an unstructured manner, taking detailed narrative notes regarding their use of touch. Alternatively, the researcher could tabulate the frequency of the nurses' use of specific types of touching, according to a predesignated classification system.

Observational research is particularly well suited to nursing. Nurses are in an advantageous position to observe, relatively unobtrusively, the behaviors and activities of patients, their families, and hospital staff. Moreover, nurses may, by training, be especially sensitive observers. Many nursing problems are better suited to an observational approach than to self-report techniques. Whenever people cannot be expected to describe adequately their own behaviors, observational methods may be needed. This may be the case when people are unaware of their own behavior (e.g., manifesting preoperative symptoms of anxiety), when people are embarrassed to report their activities (e.g., displays of aggression or hostility), when behaviors are emotionally laden (e.g., grieving behavior among widows), or when people are not capable of articulating their actions (e.g., young children or the mentally ill). Observation is intrinsically appealing in its ability to capture directly a record of behaviors and events. Furthermore, with an observational approach, humans—the observers—are used as measuring instruments and provide a uniquely sensitive and intelligent tool.

Several of the shortcomings of the observational approach include possible ethical difficulties, distorted behavior on the part of the person being observed when the observer is conspicuous, and a high rate of refusal to cooperate. Another pervasive problems is the vulnerability of observational data to **observer biases**. A number of factors interfere with objective observations, including the following:

- Emotions, prejudices, attitudes, and values of observers may result in faulty inference.
- Personal interest and commitment may color what is seen in the direction of what observers want to see.
- Anticipation of what is to be observed may affect what *is* observed.
- Hasty decisions before adequate information is collected may result in erroneous classifications or conclusions.

Observational biases probably cannot be eliminated completely, but they can be minimized through careful training.

Example of a study using observation:
Kisida, Holditch-Davis, Miles, and Carlson (2001) examined unsafe caregiving practices to 3-year-old children born prematurely. Observational data were collected in the children's homes in two separate 2-hour sessions.

Biophysiologic Measures

The trend in nursing research has been toward increased clinical, patient-centered investigations. One result of this trend is an expanded use of measures to assess the physiologic status of subjects—typically through quantitative **biophysiologic measures**. Physiologic and physical variables typically require specialized technical instruments and equipment for their measurement and, usually, specialized training for the interpretation of results. Settings in which nurses operate are usually filled with a wide variety of technical instruments for measuring physiologic functions. In comparison with other types of data collection tools, the equipment for obtaining physiologic measurements is costly. Because such equipment is generally available in health care settings, however, the costs to nurse researchers may be small or nonexistent.

A major strength of biophysiologic measures is their objectivity. Nurse A and nurse B, reading from the same spirometer output, are likely to record the same tidal volume measurements. Furthermore, barring the possibility of equipment malfunctioning, two different spirometers are likely to produce identical tidal volume readouts. Another advantage of physiologic measurements is the relative precision and sensitivity they normally offer. By *relative*, we are implicitly comparing physiologic instruments with measures of psychological phenomena, such as self-report measures of anxiety or pain.

Physiologic measures also have some disadvantages. For example, because of the technical nature of the equipment, nonengineers may fail to understand the limitations of the instruments, which may result in greater faith in their accuracy than is warranted. Nevertheless, biophysiologic measures usually yield data of exceptionally high quality.

Example of a study using physiologic measures:

George, Hofa, Boujoukos, and Zullo (2002) studied the effect of three body positions (supine, lateral with allograft lung down, and lateral with native lung down) on oxygenation, ventilation, and blood flow in single-lung transplant recipients.

CONVERTING QUANTITATIVE AND QUALITATIVE DATA

As noted earlier, it is possible to convert qualitative data to numeric codes that can be analyzed quantitatively. It is also possible to treat data collected in a quantitative study qualitatively. In thinking about data collection, researchers might wish to consider whether either of these options would enhance their study, particularly if they are doing multi-method research.

Using Quantitative Data Qualitatively

Most data that are analyzed quantitatively actually begin as qualitative data. If we ask respondents if they have been severely depressed, moderately depressed, somewhat depressed, or not at all depressed in the previous week, they answer in words, not numbers. The words are transformed, through the process of coding, into quantitative categories. Then the numbers are analyzed statistically to determine, for example, what percentage of respondents were severely depressed in the prior week, or whether people diagnosed with cancer are more likely than others to be depressed.

However, it is possible to go back to the data and "read" them qualitatively, a process that Sandelowski (2000) calls **qualitizing** data. For example, an entire survey interview can be read to get a glimpse of the life circumstances, problems, and experiences of individual respondents. In such a situation, researchers can create a mini—case study designed to "give life" to the patterns emerging in the quantitative analysis, to extract more information from the data, and to aid in interpreting them.

As an example, Polit, Widom, and Edin (2001), using data from 90-minute survey interviews with several thousand women, studied the employment patterns and barriers to employment of women who had been welfare recipients. Health problems of the women and their children emerged as important impediments that forced some women to leave their jobs and return to welfare. The researchers identified a survey respondent who typified the experiences of those who could not sustain employment, and prepared this profile:

 Example of qualitizing survey data:

Miranda, a 26-year-old Mexican-American woman from Los Angeles, had had a fairly steady work record until 4 months before we spoke with her, when she had left her job as a bank cashier because her son (age 4) had serious health problems. She also had a 2-year-old daughter and her husband, from whom she was separated, no longer lived nearby to help with child care. The bank job had paid her $210 a week before taxes, without health insurance, sick pay, or paid vacation. At the bank job, she had worked 36 hours a week, working daily from early afternoon until 8 p.m Although at the time of the interview she was getting cash welfare assistance, food stamps, and SSI (disability) benefits on behalf of her son, her relatively high rent and utility costs (over $700 per month) without housing assistance made it difficult for her to make ends meet, and she reported that she sometimes couldn't afford to feed her children balanced meals (Polit, Widom, & Edin, 2001, p. 2).

The survey data in this study were aggregated and used *quantitatively* to describe such things as the women's average weekly pay, the percentage who had employer-provided health insurance and sick pay, and the percentage who left work because of health problems. The data were used *qualitatively* (as in the preceding example) to translate these statistics into what they meant to actual respondents.

When this type of undertaking is done, researchers must be clear about what it is they wish to portray. Often, as in the example just cited, the intent is to illustrate a typical case. In such a situation, researchers look for an individual case whose quantitative values are near the average for the entire sample. However, researchers might also want to illustrate ways in which the averages fail to capture important aspects of a problem, in which case atypical (and often extreme) cases are identified to show the limitations of looking just at averages in the quantitative analysis.

Using Qualitative Data Quantitatively

A somewhat more controversial issue is the use of numbers in qualitative studies. Some qualitative researchers believe that **quantitizing** qualitative data is inappropriate. Sandelowski (2001), however, has argued that some amount of quantitizing is almost inevitable. She noted that every time qualitative researchers use terms such as *a few, some, many,* or *most,* they are implicitly conveying quantitative information about the frequency of occurrence of a theme or pattern. In addition to being inevitable, quantification of qualitative data can in some cases offer distinct benefits. Sandelowski has described how this strategy can be used to achieve several important goals:

1. *Generating meaning from qualitative data.* If qualitative data are displayed in a quantitative fashion (e.g., by displaying frequencies of certain phenomena), patterns sometimes emerge with greater clarity than they might have had the researchers simply relied on their impressions. Tabular displays can also reveal unsuspected patterns that can help in the development of hypotheses to be further tested qualitatively. Sandelowski provides an excellent example in which this procedure enabled her to see her data in a new way, and to better understand the characteristics of her sample. Whenever qualitative data are categorized, researchers are creating data that can be analyzed quantitatively (e.g., to examine the relationship between two phenomena).
2. *Documenting and confirming conclusions.* The use of numbers can assure readers that researchers' assertions are valid. If researchers can document the extent to which the emerging patterns were observed (and not observed), readers will have confidence that the data are fully accounted for. Sandelowski notes that quantitizing in this fashion can address some of the major pitfalls of qualitative analysis, which include (1) giving too much weight to dramatic or vivid accounts; (2) giving too little weight to disconfirming cases; and (3) smoothing out variation, to clean up some of the "messiness" of human experience. Thus, the use of numbers can sometimes help to confirm impressions. A procedure known as *quasi-statistics,* used in some qualitative studies for this purpose, is explained in Chapter 23.
3. *Re-presenting data and lives.* Qualitative researchers are especially likely to use numbers to describe important features of their samples. Thus, qualitative reports may contain tables that show characteristics of the sample as a whole (e.g., the average age, or percentage male and female), or characteristics of each individual participant.

Sandelowski also offers good advice on avoiding the misuse of numbers (e.g., overcounting, or counting that is misleading).

Example of quantitizing qualitative data: Mallory and Stern (2000) studied women who engaged in "survival sex" and thereby exposed themselves to the risk of HIV infection. They presented a table that showed, for each of their 11 informants, whether they were injection drug users, whether they had had sex with injecting drug users, how many partners each had had in the prior year, and whether they had had a sexually transmitted disease. Their table documented the extent to which the women were at risk for contracting HIV.

DEVELOPING A DATA COLLECTION PLAN IN A QUANTITATIVE STUDY

Data collection plans for quantitative studies should ideally yield accurate, valid, and meaningful data that are maximally effective in answering research questions. These are rigorous requirements,

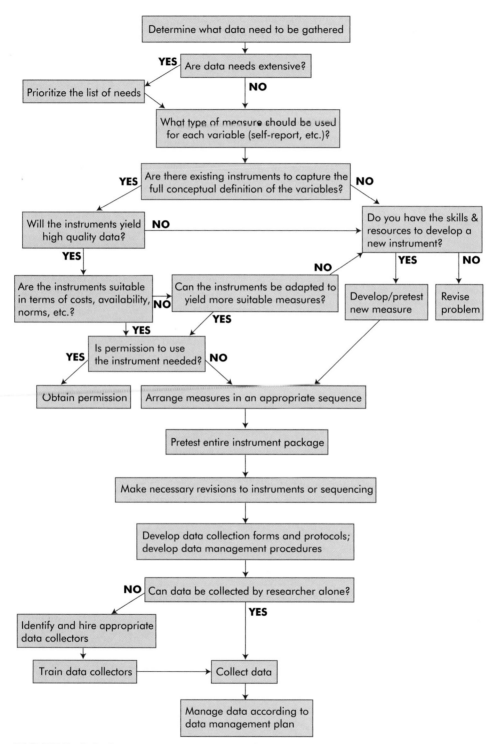

FIGURE 14.1 Developing a data collection plan for quantitative studies.

typically requiring considerable time and effort to achieve. This section discusses steps that are often undertaken in the development of a data collection plan in quantitative studies. Figure 14-1 provides an overview of the procedures used in developing such a plan.

TIP: Although the flow chart in Figure 14-1 suggests a fairly linear process, the development of a data collection plan is often an iterative one. Be prepared to backtrack and make adjustments, recognizing that the ultimate goal is not to get to the bottom of the list of steps but rather to ensure that the process yields conceptually relevant data of the highest possible quality.

Identifying Data Needs

Researchers must usually begin by identifying the types of data needed to complete the study successfully. Typically, researchers gather information about more than just the main study variables. Advance planning may help to avoid "if only" disappointments at the analysis stage.

In a quantitative study, researchers may need to identify data requirements for accomplishing the following:

1. *Testing the hypotheses or addressing the research questions.* Researchers must include one or more measures of all the independent and dependent variables. Multiple measures of some variables may be required if a variable is complex and multifaceted or if there are concerns about the accuracy of a single measure.
2. *Describing sample characteristics.* Information should be gathered about major demographic and health characteristics of the sample. We advise gathering data about participants' age, gender, race or ethnicity, educational background, marital status, and income level. This information is critical in interpreting results and understanding the population to whom the findings can be generalized. If the sample includes participants with a health problem, data on the nature of that problem also should be gathered (e.g., length of illness, severity of

health problem, types of treatment obtained, length of stay in hospital).
3. *Controlling extraneous variables.* As discussed in Chapter 9, various approaches can be used to control extraneous variables, and many of them require the measurement of those variables. For example, when analysis of covariance is used, each variable that is statistically controlled must be measured.
4. *Analyzing potential biases.* Ideally, data that can help the researcher to identify potential biases should be collected. For example, researchers should gather information that would help to identify selection biases in a nonequivalent control group design. Researchers should give some thought to potential biases and then determine how they could be assessed.
5. *Understanding subgroup effects.* It is often desirable to answer the research questions not only for the entire sample but also for certain subgroups of participants. For example, we may wish to know if a special intervention for indigent pregnant women is equally effective for primiparas and multiparas. In such a situation, we would need to collect information about the participants' childbearing history so that we could divide the sample and analyze for separate subgroup effects.
6. *Interpreting results.* Researchers should try to anticipate alternative results, and then determine what types of data would best help in interpreting them. For example, if we hypothesized that the presence of school-based clinics in high schools would lower the incidence of sexually transmitted diseases among students but found that the incidence remained constant after the clinic was established, what type of information would we want to help us interpret this result (information about the students' frequency of intercourse, number of partners, use of condoms, and so on)?
7. *Checking the manipulation.* When researchers manipulate the independent variable, it is sometimes useful to determine if the manipulation actually occurred. Such a **manipulation check** can help in interpreting negative results.

As an example, if a researcher were studying the impact of a new hospital policy on the morale of the nursing staff, it might be important to determine the nurses' level of awareness of the new policy; if the results indicate no change in staff morale, this could reflect lack of awareness of the policy rather than indifference to it.

8. *Obtaining administrative information.* It is almost always necessary to gather administrative information to help in project management. For example, if there are multiple data collectors, identification numbers for each one should be recorded. Other administrative information might include participant identification numbers, dates of attempted contact with participants, dates of actual data collection, where data collection occurred, when the data collection session began and ended, reasons that a potential subject did not participate in the study, and contact information if the study is longitudinal.

The list of possible data needs may seem daunting, but many categories overlap. For example, participant characteristics (for sample description) are often key extraneous variables, or useful in creating subgroups. If time or resource constraints make it impossible to collect the full range of variables, then researchers should prioritize data needs and be aware of how the absence of certain variables could affect the study's integrity. The important point is that researchers should understand their data needs and take steps to ensure the fullest possible coverage.

TIP: In developing instruments, it may be necessary to evaluate tradeoffs between data quality and data quantity. If compromises have to be made, it is usually preferable to forego quantity. For example, it is better to have an excellent measure of the dependent variable without supplementary measures for interpreting outcomes than to have mediocre measures of all desired variables. When data quality for key variables is poor, the results cannot be trusted, so additional information cannot possibly help to clarify the findings.

Selecting Types of Measures

After data needs have been identified, the next step is to select a data collection method for each variable. It is common, and often advantageous, to combine self-reports, observations, or physiologic measures in a single study. Researchers also combine measures that vary in terms of the four basic dimensions. In reviewing data needs, researchers should determine how best to capture each variable in terms of its conceptual or theoretical definition.

Research considerations are not the only factors that drive decisions about methods to use in collecting data. The decisions must also be guided by ethical considerations, cost constraints, the availability of appropriate staff to help with data collection, time pressures, and the anticipated burden to participants and others, such as hospital staff or participants' families.

Data collection is typically the costliest and most time-consuming portion of a study. Because of this, researchers often have to make a number of compromises about the type or amount of data collected.

Selecting and Developing Instruments

Once preliminary decisions have been made regarding the basic data collection methods to be used, researchers should determine if there are instruments available for constructs of interest. For most constructs, existing instruments are available and should be considered. In the next three chapters, we provide sources for locating existing self-report, observational, and other measures.

After potential data collection instruments have been identified, they should be assessed to determine their appropriateness. The primary consideration is whether the instrument is conceptually relevant: Does the instrument capture your conceptual definition of the variable? The next factor to consider is whether the instrument will yield data of sufficiently high quality. Approaches to evaluating data quality are discussed in Chapter 18. In addition to data quality, criteria that may affect researchers' decisions in selecting an instrument are as follows:

1. *Resources.* Resource constraints sometimes prevent the use of the highest-quality measures.

There may be some direct costs associated with the measure (e.g., some psychological tests must be purchased, or physiologic equipment may have to be rented), but the biggest data collection cost involves compensation to data collectors if you cannot do it single-handedly (e.g., hired interviewers or observers). In such a situation, the instrument's length and administration time may determine whether it can be used. Also, if the data collection procedures are burdensome, it may be necessary to pay a subject stipend. Data collection costs should be carefully considered, especially if the use of expensive methods means that you will be forced to cut costs elsewhere (e.g., using a smaller sample).

2. *Availability and familiarity.* In selecting measures, you may need to consider how readily available or accessible various instruments are, especially biophysiologic ones. Similarly, data collection strategies with which you have had experience are in general preferable to new measures because administration is usually smoother and more efficient in such cases.

3. *Norms and comparability.* You may find it desirable to select a measure for which there are relevant norms. **Norms** indicate the "normal" values and distribution of values on the measure for a specified population. Many standardized tests and scales (e.g., the SF-36 Health Survey from the Medical Outcomes Study) have national norms. The availability of norms is useful because norms offer, in essence, a built-in comparison group. For similar reasons, you may find it advantageous to adopt an instrument because it was used in other similar studies and therefore provides a supplementary context for your findings. Indeed, when a study is an intentional replication, it is often essential to use the same instruments as in the original study, even if higher-quality measures are available.

4. *Population appropriateness.* The measure should be chosen with the characteristics of the target population in mind. Characteristics of special importance include participants'

age, their intellectual abilities or reading skills, and their cultural or ethnic backgrounds. If there is concern about participants' reading skills, it may be necessary to calculate the readability of a prospective instrument using procedures described in Chapter 7. If participants include members of minority groups, you should strive to find instruments that are not culturally biased. If non–English-speaking participants are included in the sample, then the selection of a measure may be based, in part, on the availability of a translated version of the measure.

TIP: If you are translating an instrument into another language, you will need to make sure that the content of items is relevant in the new culture. Then you will need to ensure semantic equivalence, that is, that the meaning of each item remains the same after translation. The most acceptable procedure is to do the translation, **back-translate** it into English, and then compare the back-translation with the original (Brislin, 1970). Brislin's widely used methods have recently been adapted by cross-cultural nurse researchers (Jones, Lee, Phillips, Zhang, & Jaceldo, 2001).

Example of a translation:
Beck, Bernal, and Froman (2003) translated the Postpartum Depression Screening Scale (PDSS) into standard Spanish. The process involved eight translators representing the four predominant Hispanic groups in the United States, two each from Puerto Rico, Mexico, Cuba, and other Spanish-speaking Latin American countries. For the back-translation process, the eight translators were paired (e.g., the two Cuban translators were considered a pair). In each pair, one translator translated the first half of the PDSS into standard Spanish and the other person translated the second half, working independently. Each was then given the other pair member's translation to back-translate into English. Blinding translators to the original English version during back-translation prevented them from attempting to infer meaning or make sense of a poor Spanish translation. Next, similarities

8   □   PART 4 Measurement and Data Collection

and differences in the English and Spanish translations among the four Hispanic pairs were summarized. Finally, a meeting with all translators was held
to discuss problematic areas of the back-translation.
A consensus version of the PDSS-Spanish Version
was decided on at this meeting.

   5. *Administration issues.* Some instruments have
      special requirements that need to be consid-
      ered. For example, obtaining information
      about the developmental status of children
      sometimes requires the skills of a professional
      psychologist. Another administration issue is
      that some instruments require or assume strin-
      gent conditions with regard to the time of ad-
      ministration, privacy of the setting, and so on.
      In such a case, requirements for obtaining
      valid measures must match attributes of the
      research setting.
   6. *Reputation.* Instruments designed to measure
      the same construct often differ in the reputa-
      tion they enjoy among specialists working in a
      field, even if they are comparable with regard
      to quality. Therefore, it may be useful to seek
      the advice of knowledgeable people, prefer-
      ably ones with personal, direct experience
      using the instruments.

   Based on such considerations, you may conclude that existing instruments are not suitable for
all research variables. In such a situation, you will
be faced with either adapting an existing instrument
to make it more appropriate, or developing a new
one. Creating a new instrument should be considered a last resort, especially for novice researchers,
because it is difficult to develop accurate and valid
measuring tools. However, there are situations in
which there may not be an acceptable alternative. In
the next few chapters, we provide some guidance
about constructing instruments, but it sometimes
may make more sense to modify the research question so that existing instruments can be used.

   If you are fortunate in identifying a suitable instrument, your next step likely will be to obtain
written permission from the author (or the publisher, if it is a commercially distributed instrument) to use or adapt it. In general, copyrighted

materials always require permission. Instruments
that have been developed under a federal grant are
usually in the public domain, and so do not require
permission because they have been supported with
taxpayers' dollars. When in doubt, however, it is
best to obtain permission. By contacting the author
of an instrument to obtain permission, you can also
request more information about the instrument and
its quality than was available in a published report.

Pretesting the Data Collection Package

Researchers who develop a new instrument almost
always subject it to rigorous **pretesting** (often in a
stand-alone methodologic study) so that it can be
evaluated and refined. However, even when the
data collection plan involves existing instruments,
it is usually wise to conduct a small pretest.

   One purpose of a pretest is to determine how
much time it takes to administer the entire instrument package and whether participants find it
burdensome. Typically, researchers use multiple
instruments when there are many variables to be
measured. It may be difficult to estimate how long
it will take to administer the complete set of instruments, and such estimates may be required for
informed consent purposes or for developing a project budget. If the pretest instruments require more
time than is acceptable, it may be necessary to
eliminate certain variables or instruments, guided
by the prioritization list established earlier.

   Pretests can serve many other purposes, including the following:

   • Identifying parts of the instrument package that
     are difficult for pretest subjects to read or un-
     derstand or that may have been misinterpreted
     by them
   • Identifying any instruments or questions that
     participants find objectionable or offensive
   • Determining whether the sequencing of instru-
     ments is sensible
   • Determining needs for training data collection
     staff
   • Determining if the measures yield data with
     sufficient variability

The last purpose requires explanation. For most research questions, the instruments ideally discriminate among participants with different levels of an attribute. If we are asking, for example, whether women experience greater depression than men when they learn of a cancer diagnosis, we need an instrument capable of distinguishing between people with higher and lower levels of depression. If an instrument yields data with limited variability, then it will be impossible to detect a difference in depression between men and women—even when such a difference actually exists. Thus, researchers should look at pretest variation on key research variables. If, to pursue the example, the entire pretest sample looks very depressed (or not at all depressed), it may be necessary to modify the instruments.

Developing Data Collection Forms and Procedures

After the instrument package has been finalized, researchers face a number of administrative tasks. First, appropriate forms must be developed. In some studies, many forms are required: forms for screening potential participants to determine their eligibility, informed consent forms, records of attempted contacts with participants, forms for recording the actual data, contact information sheets, and administrative logs for recording the receipt of data. It is prudent to design forms that are attractively formatted, legible, and inviting to use, especcially if they are to be used by subjects themselves. Care should also be taken to design forms to ensure confidentiality. For example, identifying information (e.g., names, addresses) is often recorded on a page that can be detached and kept separate from other data.

In most quantitative studies, researchers also develop **data collection protocols** that spell out the procedures to be used in data collection. These protocols describe such things as the following:

- Conditions that must be met for collecting the data (e.g., Can others be present at the time of data collection? Where must data collection occur?)

- Specific procedures for collecting the data, including requirements for sequencing instruments and recording information
- Standard information to provide participants who ask routine questions about the study. These questions may include the following: How will the information from this study be used? How did you get my name, and why are you asking me? How long will this take? Who will have access to this information? What are the possible benefits and risks?
- Procedures to follow in the event that a participant becomes distraught or disoriented, or for any other reason cannot complete the data collection

Finally, procedures and forms may be required for managing collected data, especially if data are being gathered from multiple sites or over an extended period. For example, in an observational study, a data management form might record, for each case, the date the observation was scheduled to take place, the date it actually took place, the date the observation form was received back in some central location, and the date the data were coded and entered onto a computer file.

TIP: Whenever possible, try to avoid reinventing the wheel. It is inefficient and unnecessary to start from scratch—not only in developing instruments but also in creating forms, protocols, training materials, and so on. Ask seasoned researchers if they have materials you could borrow or adapt. Most materials relating to data collection are *not* available in published research articles (although they may be available in dissertations or research reports to funding agencies).

Large-scale surveys are increasingly relying on new technologies to assist in data collection. Most major telephone surveys now use **computer-assisted telephone interviewing (CATI)**, and growing numbers of in-person surveys use **computer-assisted personal interviewing (CAPI)** with laptop computers. Both procedures involve developing computer programs that present interviewers with the questions to be asked on the computer screen;

the interviewers then enter coded responses directly onto a computer file. CATI and CAPI surveys greatly facilitate data collection and usually improve data quality because there is less opportunity for interviewer error. However, it requires considerable resources to substitute a computer program for paper-and-pencil forms.

Example of CATI:
Holland and Carruth (2001) conducted a survey of women living on farms to determine their exposure to risk for tetanus. The telephone interviews were complete using CATI technology.

Audio-CASI (computer-assisted self-interview) technology is the state-of-the-art approach for giving respondents more privacy than is possible in an interview (e.g., to collect information about drug use), and is especially useful for populations with literacy problems. With audio-CASI, respondents sit at a computer and listen to questions over headphones. Respondents enter their responses (usually simple codes like 1 or 2) directly onto the keyboard, without the interviewer having to see the responses.

TIP: Document everything you do as you develop and implement your data collection plan, and save your documentation. You may need the information later when you write your research report, request funding for a follow-up study, or help other researchers.

IMPLEMENTING A DATA COLLECTION PLAN IN A QUANTITATIVE STUDY

Data quality in a quantitative study is affected by decisions that shape the data collection plan. Data quality is also affected by how the plan is implemented.

Selecting Research Personnel

An important decision concerns who will actually collect the research data. In small studies, the researchers in charge often collect the data themselves. In larger studies, however, this may not be feasible. When data are collected by others, it is important to select appropriate people. In general, they should be neutral agents through whom data passes—that is, their characteristics or behavior should not affect the substance of the data. Some considerations that should be kept in mind when selecting research personnel are as follows:

- *Experience.* Research staff ideally have had prior experience collecting data. For example, for a self-report study, it is advantageous to use people with interviewing experience. If it is necessary to use those without experience, look for people who can readily acquire the necessary skills (e.g., an interviewer should have good verbal and social skills).
- *Congruity with sample characteristics.* To the extent possible, data collectors should match study participants with respect to such characteristics as racial or cultural background and gender. In some studies, this is an absolute requirement (e.g., hiring a person who speaks the language of an immigrant sample). The greater the sensitivity of the questions, the greater the desirability of matching characteristics. For example, in a study of the sexual behavior of pregnant African-American teenagers, the interviewers would ideally be African-American women.
- *Unremarkable appearance.* Extremes of appearance should be avoided because participants may react to extremes and alter their behavior or responses accordingly. For example, data collectors should in general not be very old or very young. They should not dress extremely casually (e.g., in shorts and tee shirts), nor very formally (e.g., with elaborate jewelry). While on the job, data collectors should never wear anything that conveys their political, social, or religious views (e.g., political buttons, jewelry with peace symbols).
- *Personality.* Data collectors should be pleasant (but not effusive), sociable (but not overly talkative or overbearing), and nonjudgmental (but not apathetic or unfeeling about participants' lives). The goal is to have nonthreatening staff who can encourage candor and put participants at ease without interjecting their own values and biases.

• *Availability.* Data collectors should ideally be available for the entire data collection period to avoid having to recruit and train new staff. If the study is longitudinal, it is advantageous to hire people who could potentially be available for subsequent rounds of data collection.

In some situations, researchers cannot select research personnel. For example, the data collectors may be staff nurses employed at a hospital or graduate students in a school of nursing. Training of the data collection staff is particularly important in such situations.

 Example of care in selecting research personnel:

Nyamathi, Leake, Keenan, and Gelberg (2000) studied health behaviors and the use of health services among homeless women in Los Angeles. Participants were recruited by African-American or Latina nurses who were trained in working with this population. Data were collected in face-to-face interviews done in English and Spanish by nurses and outreach workers of the same ethnicity as participants.

Training Data Collectors

Depending on the prior experience of data collectors, training will need to cover both general procedures (e.g., how to conduct a research interview) and ones specific to the study (e.g., how to administer a particular set of questions or make certain observations). Training can often be accomplished in a single day, but in complex projects, it may require more time. The lead researcher is usually the best person to conduct the training and to develop training materials.

The data collection protocols, discussed in the previous section, usually are a good foundation for a **training manual**. The manual normally includes background materials (e.g., the study aims), general instructions, specific instructions, and copies of all the data collection and administrative forms. Table 14-1 presents an example of a table of contents for a training manual in a quantitative interview study.

The agenda for the training should cover the content of the training manual, elaborating on any portion that is especially difficult or complex. The training usually includes demonstrations of ficti-

tious data collection sessions, performed either live or on videotape. Finally, the training usually involves having the trainees do trial runs of data collection in front of the trainers to demonstrate their understanding of the instructions.

TABLE 14.1 Example of a Table of Contents: Training Manual for an Interview Study

I. Introduction
   A. Background and Purpose of the Study
   B. The Research Team/Organizational Structure

II. Initial Study Procedures
   A. Tracing and Locating Respondents
   B. Initial Contact With Respondents and Arranging Appointments
   C. Answering Respondents' Questions
   D. Privacy and the Research Setting
   E. Avoiding Refusals and Nonresponse
   F. Informed Consent

III. The Role of the Interviewer
   A. Establishing an Appropriate Interviewing Relationship
   B. Knowing the Interview
   C. Avoiding Bias
   D. Obtaining Full Responses
   E. Recording Information

IV. Instructions for Conducting the Study Interview
   A. Guide to the Use of the Study Instruments
   B. Conventions and Abbreviations Used in the Instruments
   C. Question-by-Question Specifications
   D. Concluding the Interview

V. Administrative Forms and Procedures
   A. Obtaining Interviewing Assignments
   B. Pledge of Confidentiality
   C. Editing Completed Interviews
   D. Submitting Completed Interviews to the Project Director
   E. Errors and Missing Information
   F. Time Forms and Payment

Appendices: Data Collection and Administrative Forms

Example of interviewer training:

In the survey of nearly 4000 welfare mothers that provided data for the report by Polit, London, and Martinez (2001), about 100 interviewers were trained in 4 research sites. Each training session lasted 3 days, and included a half day of training on the use of CAPI. During the training, several trainees were let go because they did not appear sufficiently skilled to master their assignments.

DATA COLLECTION ISSUES IN QUALITATIVE STUDIES

In qualitative studies, data collection usually is more fluid than in quantitative research, and decisions about what to collect evolve in the field. For example, as the researcher begins to gather and digest information, it may become apparent that it would be fruitful to pursue a line of questioning that had not originally been anticipated. However, even while allowing for and profiting from this flexibility, qualitative researchers make a number of up-front decisions about data collection. Moreover, qualitative researchers need to be prepared for problematic situations that can arise in the field. The best prearranged plans for data collection sometimes fall through. Creativity for workable solutions and new strategies is often needed.

Example of need for flexibility in a qualitative study:

Wismont (2000), who undertook a phenomenological study of the pregnancy experience of women in prison, had obtained permission to tape-record interviews with pregnant inmates. When it came time to begin the interviews, the warden informed her that prison rules prohibited her from removing taped interviews from the prison. Wismont needed to come up with an alternate plan for recording the data. She provided all pregnant inmates with a hard-bound notebook to use as a journal for recording their thoughts and feelings.

Types of Data for Qualitative Studies

Qualitative researchers typically go into the field knowing the most likely sources of data, while not ruling out other possible data sources that might come to light as data collection progresses. The primary method of collecting qualitative data is through self-report, that is, by interviewing study participants. Observation is often a part of many qualitative studies as well. Physiologic data are rarely collected in a naturalistic inquiry, except perhaps to describe participants' characteristics or to ascertain eligibility for the sample.

Table 14-2 compares the types of data used by researchers in the three main qualitative traditions, as well as other aspects of the data collection process for each tradition. Ethnographers almost always collect a wide array of data, with observation and interviews being the most important methods. Ethnographers also gather or examine products of the culture under study, such as documents, records, artifacts, photographs, and so on. Phenomenologists and grounded theory researchers rely primarily on in-depth interviews with individual participants, although observation also plays an important role in some grounded theory studies.

The adopted approach also has implications for how the researcher as "self" is used (Lipson, 1991). Researchers conducting phenomenological studies use themselves to collect rich description of human experiences and to develop relationships in which intensive interviews are done with a small number of people. Grounded theorists use themselves not only to collect data but also to process the data and generate categories for the emerging theory. Ethnographers use themselves as observers who collect data not only through informal interviews but also through active participation in field settings.

In qualitative studies, there are usually relatively few forms and protocols developed in advance of going into the field. However, a form might be needed for gathering demographic and administrative information. Also, a preliminary list of questions to be asked or observations to be made during the initial data collection may be useful.

Recording and Storing Qualitative Data

In addition to thinking about the types of data to be gathered, qualitative researchers need to plan ahead for how data will be recorded and stored. Interview

TABLE 14.2 Comparison of Data Collection Issues in Three Qualitative Traditions

ISSUE	ETHNOGRAPHY	PHENOMENOLOGY	GROUNDED THEORY
Types of data	Primarily observation and interviews, plus artifacts, documents, photographs, genealogies, maps, social network diagrams	Primarily in-depth interviews, sometimes diaries, other written materials	Primarily individual interviews, sometimes group interviews, observation, participant journals, documents
Unit of data collection	Cultural systems	Individuals	Individuals
Data collection points	Mainly longitudinal	Mainly cross-sectional	Cross-sectional or longitudinal
Length of time for data collection	Typically long, many months or years	Typically moderate	Typically moderate
Data recording	Field notes, logs, interview notes/recordings	Interview notes/recordings	Interview notes/recordings, memoing, observational notes
Salient field issues	Gaining entrée, reactivity, determining a role, learning how to participate, encouraging candor and other interview logistics, loss of objectivity, premature exit, reflexivity	Bracketing one's views, building rapport, encouraging candor, listening while preparing what to ask next, keeping "on track," handling emotionality	Building rapport, encouraging candor, listening while preparing what to ask next, keeping "on track," handling emotionality

data, common to all qualitative traditions, can be recorded in two ways: by taking detailed notes of what participants say, or by audio recording (or video recording) what they say. To ensure that interview data are the actual verbatim responses of study participants, it is strongly recommended that qualitative interviews be recorded and subsequently transcribed, rather than relying on interviewer notes. Notes tend to be incomplete, and may be biased by the interviewer's memory or personal views. Moreover, note-taking can distract researchers, who must listen intently and direct the flow of questioning based on what has already been said.

Environmental distractions are a common pitfall in recording interviews. A quiet setting with as little noise as possible is ideal, but this is not always possible for clinical nurse researchers. The second author of this book (Beck) has conducted many challenging interviews. As an example, a mother of three children was interviewed in her living room about her experience with postpartum depression. A time had been prearranged to conduct the interview while her two toddlers were napping. When Beck arrived, the mother apologized: her toddlers had napped earlier than usual, so they would be up during the visit. Beck placed the tape recorder as high up on the couch as possible to keep it out of the reach of the toddlers who kept trying to get it during most of the interview. The television was on to occupy the toddlers, and the

6-week old baby was especially fussy that day, crying through most of the interview. The noise level in the background of the tape made accurate transcription difficult.

When observations are made, detailed observational notes must be maintained, unless it is possible to videotape. Observational notes should be made shortly after an observational session and are often entered onto a computer. Whatever method is used to record observations, researchers need to go into the field with the equipment or supplies needed to record their data, and to be sure that the equipment is functioning properly.

Grounded theory researchers write analytic memos to themselves. These memos can vary in length from a sentence to multiple pages. These memos document researchers' ideas about how the theory is developing (e.g., how some themes are interrelated).

TIP: It is wise to use good-quality equipment to ensure proper audio and video recording. For example, for recording interviews, make sure that the microphone is adequately sensitive for the acoustics of the environment, or use lapel microphones for both respondents and interviewers.

If assistants are used to collect the data, qualitative researchers need to be as concerned as quantitative researchers about hiring appropriate staff, and training them to collect high-quality data. Because the data collectors not only collect the data but also are the instruments through which data are collected, it is important that they elicit rich and vivid descriptions. For example, qualitative interviewers need to be good listeners; they need to hear all that is being said, rather than trying to anticipate what is coming next. A good data collector must have both self-awareness and an awareness of the participant (e.g., by paying attention to nonverbal behavior). Qualitative data collectors must be able to create an atmosphere that safely allows for the sharing of experiences and feelings. Respect and authentic caring for participants are critical.

Storage of data while in the field can be problematic because researchers may not have a safe or secure storage space. When this is the case, they often devise a way to keep the data physically with them at all times until it can be secured (e.g., in a fanny pack). Of course, all data such as tapes or forms should be carefully labeled with an identification number, the date the data were collected, and (if relevant) the name or identification number of the data collector.

With regard to final storage of qualitative data, an important issue to consider is how the analysis will be done—manually, or with the assistance of computers. Increasingly, qualitative researchers are using computer programs to facilitate the organization of vast amounts of narrative information, and this has implications for how the data should be stored. Thus, researchers should ideally be familiar with the computer program to be used before deciding on how to store their data.

TIP: It is a wise strategy to have back-up copies of your data. Backing up files is imperative (and easy) for data stored on computers, but if computers are not being used, photocopies of written or transcribed materials should be maintained in a separate location. If you expect a delay between taping and transcribing an interview, you should also consider making back-up copies of the tapes, which can sometimes get erased through static electricity.

Field Issues in Qualitative Studies

Data collection in qualitative studies is complex, and often involves the collection and analysis of multiple data sources. This section discusses some of the issues that can arise in the field while collecting qualitative data. Field issues are especially critical in ethnographies. Ethnographic researchers, in addition to the matters discussed in this section, must deal with such issues as gaining entrée into the field, negotiating for space and privacy for interviewing and recording data, deciding on an appropriate role (i.e., the extent to which they will actually participate in the culture's activities), and taking care not to exit from the field prematurely. Ethnographers also need to be able to cope with culture shock and should have a high tolerance for uncertainty and ambiguity (Agar, 1980).

Gaining Trust

Researchers who do qualitative research must, to an even greater extent than quantitative researchers, gain and maintain a high level of trust with participants. Researchers need to develop strategies in the field to establish credibility among those being studied. This may in some cases be a delicate balancing act, because researchers must try as much as possible to "be like" the people being studied while at the same time keeping a certain distance. "Being like" participants means that researchers should be sensitive to such issues as styles of dress, modes of speech, customs, and schedules. In ethnographic research, it is important not to take sides on any controversial issue and not to appear too strongly affiliated with a particular subgroup of the culture—especially with leaders or prominent members of the culture. It is not usually possible to gain the trust of the group if researchers appear close to those in power.

The Pace of Data Collection

In qualitative studies, data collection is often an intense and exhausting experience, especially if the phenomenon being studied concerns an illness experience or other stressful life event (e.g., caregiving, mourning). Moreover, collecting high-quality qualitative data requires intense concentration and energy. Regardless of the type of data being collected, the process can be an emotional strain for which researchers need to be prepared. One way to deal with this is to collect data at a pace that minimizes the emotional impact. For example, in an interview study it may be prudent to limit interviewing to no more than one a day, and to engage in emotionally releasing activities (e.g., exercising) in between interviews. It may also be helpful to debrief about any feelings of distress with a co-researcher, colleague, or advisor.

Emotional Involvement With Participants

Qualitative researchers need to guard against getting too emotionally involved with participants, a pitfall that has been referred to as **going native**. Researchers who get too close to participants run several risks, including compromising their ability to collect objectively the most meaningful and trust-worthy data, and becoming overwhelmed with participants' suffering. It is important, of course, to be supportive and to listen carefully to people's concerns and difficulties, but it usually is not advisable to intervene and try to solve participants' problems, or to share personal problems with them. If participants need help, it is better to give advice about where they can get it than to give it directly.

Reflexivity

Reflexivity is an important concept in qualitative data collection. **Reflexivity** refers to researchers' awareness of themselves as part of the data they are collecting. Researchers need to be conscious of the part they play in their own study, and reflect on their own behavior and how it can affect the data they obtain.

Example of reflexivity:
Hutchinson, Marsiglio, and Cohan (2002), who were studying young men's developing procreative identity, described their reflexive analysis of the challenges of conducting in-depth interviews with young men. The researchers pondered, for example, how language they used as researchers could affect the kind of data they got from participants. They discovered in their analysis the importance of "turning points" in the young men's experiences, but reflexively demanded: "Under what interview conditions, if any, is it useful to use the words *turning point* if participants had not yet introduced it themselves?" (p. 52).

RESEARCH EXAMPLES

Data collection procedures are often not described in detail in research reports owing to space constraints in journals. Information about the data collection plan for a quantitative and a qualitative study as reported in two research reports follow.

Research Example of Data Collection in a Quantitative Study

Holditch-Davis, Miles, Burchinal, O'Donnell, McKinney, and Lim (2001) studied the developmental outcomes for infants exposed prenatally to HIV, and factors associated with especially poor outcomes.

Their data collection plan was very complex, involving structured self-report measures, developmental tests, and in-home observations. Existing data from medical records were also used. Data were collected longitudinally, first when the infants were about 2 to 5 months of age, and then at 6, 12, 18, and 24 months.

The researchers took care to develop an efficient data collection plan; for example, demographic and medical data were obtained through the child's medical records, rather than by asking the mothers. The research team selected self-report measures with solid reputations and strong records for yielding high-quality data. For example, the caregivers' depressive symptoms were measured with the widely used Center for Epidemiological Studies Depression Scale. Moreover, the researchers tested data quality with these measures within their own research sample, and found evidence of acceptably good quality.

The research report described in some detail the procedures for gathering observational measures. For example, at 12, 18, and 24 months, observers spent 1 hour observing mother—infant interactions, recording negative interactions, positive interactions, play, touch, and so on. Well-trained observers were used to collect data: Before making real observations, the observers had to achieve a high level of agreement in their categorization of behaviors with one of the investigators. A full 3 to 6 months of practice was required to achieve acceptable performance standards.

The dependent variables were measures of the infants' mental and motor development. One test was a respected scale of language development, the Preschool Language Scale. This test was administered by research assistants who had been trained by a doctorally prepared speech pathologist. Another measure was the Bayley Scales of Infant Development, considered the premier measure of its type. Because this scale must be professionally administered, clinical psychologists who had no knowledge of the infants' performance on other tests administered it.

In summary, the researchers' report documented the attention they paid to ensuring the highest possible quality data. These data were used to examine substantive questions, control extraneous variables, test for bias, and describe the research sample. The report described child and caretaker characteristics, relying mainly on records data (e.g., 44% of the mothers were single). Attrition bias was scrutinized by comparing families remaining in and withdrawing from the study, using primarily demographic data. In the analyses that examined the effect of caregiver behaviors on developmental outcomes, a number of variables were statistically controlled (e.g., prematurity, maternal education). The analyses revealed that quality of caregiving had a positive effect on all developmental outcomes, even when background variables were controlled.

Research Example of Data Collection in a Qualitative Study

Davis and Magilvy (2000) conducted an ethnographic study to explore how chronic illness was experienced and managed by older rural adults and their families. Forty-two older adults living in seven rural communities in Colorado participated in the study. The communities were in one of Colorado's most economically depressed areas. The researchers collected data during multiple trips to rural Colorado over a 1-year period, staying for about a week on each trip.

A variety of data collection methods was used. Data sources included in-depth audiotaped interviews, observations, documents, artifacts, and photographs. The in-depth interviews were conducted with 21 primary participants who were noninstitutionalized persons (both Hispanic and white, non-Hispanic) who had one or more chronic illnesses. Less intensive interviews were conducted with 21 secondary participants who were identified by the primary participants as being significant in their lives. These secondary participants included such persons as elders' family members, religious leaders, and health care providers. Most of the participants were interviewed in their homes and these interviews lasted from 30 to 90 minutes.

Interview data were supplemented with observations. Observational data were collected in the elders' homes, and also at church services, community meetings, and other social events. The ethnographers used photography to illustrate community life in this rural Colorado setting. The photographs were used to help participants generate additional understanding of the experience of living with chronic illness. Field notes were written throughout the data collection period.

To increase the trustworthiness of their findings, the researchers maintained a high level of involvement in the community over a 1-year period. They kept detailed records of all their study activities, ideas, and insights. They also relied on triangulation of their multiple data sources to enhance the credibility of their findings.

SUMMARY POINTS

- Some researchers use existing data in their studies—for example, those doing historical research, meta-analyses, secondary analyses, or an analysis of **records**—but most studies involve the collection of original data.
- Data collection methods vary along four dimensions: structure, quantifiability, researcher obtrusiveness, and objectivity.
- Most nursing research studies involve the use of **self-reports**, that is, data obtained by directly questioning people about the phenomena of interest. Self-reports are strong with respect to their directness and versatility; the major drawback is the potential for respondents' deliberate or unconscious misrepresentations.
- **Observational methods** involve obtaining data through the direct observation of phenomena. A wide variety of human activity and traits are amenable to observation, but observation is subject to various **observer biases** and to distorted behavior by study participants.
- **Biophysiologic measures** tend to yield data that are objective and valid, but they are not immune from various technical problems.
- For highly structured data, the researcher often uses formal data collection **instruments**.
- It is sometimes useful for quantitative researchers to **qualitize** their data to provide a richer understanding of phenomena or test their interpretations; and qualitative researchers can sometimes profit from **quantitizing** their data to generate new meaning or to document and confirm their conclusions.
- Quantitative researchers typically develop a detailed **data collection plan** before they actually begin to collect their data.
- An early step in developing such a plan is the identification and prioritization of all data needs. In addition to addressing research questions, data may be needed to describe the sample, control extraneous variables, analyze biases, understand subgroup effects, interpret results, perform **manipulation checks**, and obtain administrative information.

- After data needs have been identified, existing measures of the variables should be sought for use or adaptation. The construction of new instruments requires considerable time and skill and should be undertaken only as a last resort.
- The selection of existing instruments should be based on such considerations as conceptual suitability, expected data quality, cost, population appropriateness, and reputation.
- Even when existing instruments are used, the instrument package should be pretested to determine its length, clarity, and overall adequacy.
- When researchers cannot collect the data without assistance, they should carefully select and train data collection staff.
- Qualitative studies typically adopt data collection plans that are flexible and that evolve as the study progresses.
- Self-reports are the most frequently used type of data collection method in qualitative studies, followed by observation. Ethnographies are especially likely to combine these two data sources with others such as the products of the culture (e.g., photographs, documents, artifacts).
- Qualitative researchers need to plan in advance for how their data will be recorded and stored. If technical equipment is used (e.g., audio recorders, video recorders), care must be taken to select high-quality equipment that functions properly in the field.
- Qualitative researchers are confronted with a number of special fieldwork issues. These include gaining participants' trust, pacing data collection to avoid being overwhelmed by the intensity of data, avoiding emotional involvement with participants (**going native**), and maintaining **reflexivity** (awareness of the part they play in the study and possible effects on their data).

STUDY SUGGESTIONS

Chapter 14 of the *Study Guide to Accompany Nursing Research*: *Principles and Methods, 7th edition*, offers various exercises and study suggestions for reinforcing concepts presented in this chapter. In addition, the following study questions can be addressed:

1. Indicate which method of data collection (self-report, observation, and so forth.) you would use to operationalize the following variables, and why you have made that choice; also indicate where on the four dimensions of structure, quantifiability, researcher obtrusiveness, and objectivity the data collection method would likely lie:
   a. Stress in hospitalized children
   b. Activity level among the noninstitutionalized elderly
   c. Pain in cancer patients
   d. Body image among obese individuals
   e. Decision-making about an unwanted pregnancy
2. Read a recent research report in a nursing journal, paying especially close attention to the data collection plan. What information about procedures that may affect data quality is missing from the report? How, if at all, does this absence affect your acceptance of the researchers' conclusions?
3. Read the following article and indicate which types of data (according to those listed under Identifying Data Needs) were collected:

   Miller, A. M., & Chandler, P. J. (2002). Acculturation, resilience, and depression in midlife women from the former Soviet Union. *Nursing Research, 51*, 26–32.

4. Choose a clinical problem that you would like to investigate. Describe the different types of data collection you would use if you conducted a phenomenological study, a grounded theory study, and an ethnographic study.

SUGGESTED READINGS

Methodologic References

Agar, M. (1980). *The professional stranger: An informal introduction to ethnography*. New York: Academic Press.

Brislin, R. W. (1970). Back-translation for cross-cultural research. *Journal of Cross-Cultural Psychology, 1*, 185–216.

Collins, C., Given, B., Given, C. W., & King, S. (1988). Interviewer training and supervision. *Nursing Research, 37*, 122–124.

Davis, L. L. (1992). Instrument review: Getting the most from a panel of experts. *Applied Nursing Research, 5*, 194–197.

Jacobson, S. F. (1997). Evaluating instruments for use in clinical nursing research. In M. Frank-Stromberg & S. Olsen (Eds.), *Instruments for clinical health care research*. Sudbury, MA: Jones & Bartlett.

Jones, P. S., Lee, J. W., Phillips, L., Zhang, X., & Jaceldo, K. (2001). An adaptation of Brislin's translation model for cross-cultural research. *Nursing Research, 50*, 300–304.

Lipson, J. G. (1991). The use of self in ethnographic research. In J. M. Morse (Ed.). *Qualitative nursing research: A contemporary dialogue* (pp. 73–89). Newbury Park, CA: Sage.

Marlowe, D. P., & Crowne, D. (1960). A new scale of social desirability independent of psychopathology. *Journal of Consulting Psychology, 24*, 349–354.

Martin, P. A. (1993). Data management for surveys. *Applied Nursing Research, 6*, 142–144.

Reineck, C. (1991). Nursing research instruments: Pathway to resources. *Applied Nursing Research, 4*, 34–45.

Rew, L., Bechtel, D., & Sapp, A. (1993). Self-as-instrument in qualitative research. *Nursing Research, 42*, 300–301.

Sandelowski, M. (2000). Combining qualitative and quantitative sampling, data collection, and analysis techniques in mixed-method studies. *Research in Nursing & Health, 23*, 246–255.

Sandelowski, M. (2001). Real qualitative researchers do not count: The use of numbers in qualitative research. *Research in Nursing & Health, 24*, 230–240.

Studies Cited in Chapter 14

Beck, C. T., Bernal, H., & Froman, R. (2003). Methods to document semantic equivalence of a translated scale. *Research in Nursing & Health, 26*, 1–10.

Christensen, M. A., Janson, S., & Seago, J. A. (2001). Alcohol, head injury, and pulmonary complications. *Journal of Neuroscience Nursing, 33*, 184–189.

Davis, R., & Magilvy, J. K. (2000). Quiet pride: The experience of chronic illness by rural older adults. *Image: The Journal of Nursing Scholarship, 32*, 385–390.

Eliott, J., & Olver, I. (2002). The discursive properties of "hope": A qualitative analysis of cancer patients' speech. *Qualitative Nursing Research, 12*, 173–193.

George, E. L., Hofa L. A., Boujoukos, A., & Zullo, T. G. (2002). Effect of positioning on oxygenation in single-lung transplant recipients. *American Journal of Critical Care, 11*, 66–75.

Holditch-Davis, D., Miles, M. S., Burchinal, M., O'Donnell, K., McKinney, R., & Lim, W. (2001). Parental caregiving and developmental outcomes of infants of mothers with HIV. *Nursing Research, 50*, 5–14.

Holland, C., & Carruth, A. K. (2001). Exposure risks and tetanus immunization in women of family owned farms. *AAOHN Journal, 49*, 130–136.

Hutchinson, S., Marsiglio, W., & Cohan, M. (2002). Interviewing young men about sex and procreation: Methodological issues. *Qualitative Health Research, 12*, 42–60.

Kisida, N., Holditch-Davis, D., Miles, M. S., & Carlson, J. (2001). Unsafe caregiving practices experienced by 3-year-old children born prematurely. *Pediatric Nursing, 27*, 13–18.

Mallory, C., & Stern, P. N. (2000). Awakening as a change process among women at risk for HIV who engage in survival sex. *Qualitative Health Research, 10*, 581–594.

Nyamathi, A., Leake, B., Keenan, C., & Gelberg, L. (2000). Type of social support among homeless women. *Nursing Research, 49*, 318–326.

Polit, D. F., London, A. S., & Martinez, J. M. (2001). *The health of poor urban women*. New York: MDRC (available at www.mdrc.org).

Polit, D. F., Widom, R., & Edin, K. (2001). *Is work enough: Experiences of current and former welfare mothers who work*. New York: MDRC (available at www.mdrc.org).

Wismont, J. M. (2000). The lived pregnancy experience of women in prison. *Journal of Midwifery & Women's Health, 45*, 292–300.

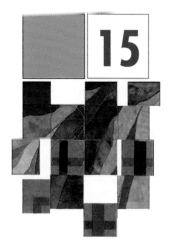

15

Collecting Self-Report Data

elf-report is the most widely used data collection method by both qualitative and quantitative nurse researchers. Self-report data can be gathered either orally in an interview, or in writing in a written questionnaire. Interviews (and, to a lesser extent, questionnaires) vary in their degree of structure, their length and complexity, and their administration. We begin by reviewing various options and procedures for collecting qualitative self-report data.

QUALITATIVE SELF-REPORT TECHNIQUES

Unstructured or loosely structured self-report methods provide narrative data for qualitative analysis. Qualitative researchers usually do not have a specific set of questions that must be asked in a particular order and worded in a given way. Instead, they start with some general questions or topics and allow respondents to tell their stories in a narrative fashion. Unstructured or semistructured interviews, in other words, tend to be conversational.

Unstructured interviews encourage respondents to define the important dimensions of a phenomenon and to elaborate on what is relevant to them, rather than being guided by investigators' *a priori* notions of relevance. Researchers in virtually all qualitative traditions gather unstructured or loosely structured self-report data.

Types of Qualitative Self-Reports

Researchers use various approaches in collecting qualitative self-report data. The main methods are described here.

Unstructured Interviews

When researchers proceed without a preconceived view of the content or flow of information to be gathered, they may conduct completely **unstructured interviews**. Unstructured interviews are conversational and interactive. Unstructured interviews are the mode of choice when researchers do not have a clear idea of what it is they do not know. Researchers using unstructured interviews do not begin with a series of prepared questions because they do not yet know what to ask or even where to begin. In conducting unstructured interviews, it is critical to let participants tell their stories, with little interruption. Phenomenological, grounded theory, and ethnographic studies usually rely heavily on unstructured interviews.

Researchers using a completely unstructured approach often begin by informally asking a broad question (sometimes called a **grand tour question**) relating to the research topic, such as, "What happened when you first learned you had AIDS?" Subsequent questions are more focused and are guided by responses to the broad question. Some respondents may request direction after the initial broad question is posed, perhaps asking, "Where should I begin?" Respondents should be encouraged to begin wherever they wish.

Van Manen (1990) provides suggestions for guiding a phenomenological interview to produce rich descriptions of the experience under study:

- "Describe the experience from the inside, as it were; almost like a state of mind: the feelings, the mood, the emotions, etc.
- Focus on a particular example or incident of the object of experience: describe specific events, an adventure, a happening, a particular experience.
- Try to focus on an example of the experience which stands out for its vividness, or as it was the first time.
- Attend to how the body feels, how things smell(ed), how they sound(ed), etc." (pp. 64–65).

Kahn (2000), discussing unstructured interviews in hermeneutic phenomenological studies, aims for interviews that resemble conversations. If the experience under study is ongoing, Kahn suggests obtaining as much detail as possible about the participant's daily life. For example, a question that can be used is, "Pick a normal day for you and tell me what happened" (p. 62). Repeated interviews over time with the same participant are essential in this prospective approach. If the experience being studied is primarily in the past, then Kahn (2000) uses a retrospective approach. The interviewer begins with a general question such as, "What does this experience mean to you?" (p. 63), and then probes for more detail until the experience is thoroughly described.

 Example of unstructured interviews in a hermeneutic study:

Cohen, Ley, and Tarzian (2001) explored the experience of isolation in 20 patients who had bone marrow transplantation. Unstructured interviews were conducted in the patients' hospital rooms. The opening question for each interview was "What was it like to have a bone marrow transplant?" Common follow-up questions included, "What did that mean to you?" and "How did you feel about that?" (p. 595).

In grounded theory, the interviewing technique changes as the theory is developed. At the outset, interviews are similar to open-ended conversations using unstructured interviews. Glaser and Strauss (1967) suggested researchers initially should just sit back and listen to participants' stories. Later, as the theory emerges, researchers ask more direct questions related to categories in the grounded theory. The more direct questions can be answered rather quickly, and so the length of an interview tends to get shorter as the grounded theory develops.

Ethnographic interviews are also unstructured. Spradley (1979) describes three types of question used to guide interviews: descriptive, structural, and contrast questions (Spradley, 1979). **Descriptive questions** ask participants to describe their experiences in their own language, and are the backbone of ethnographic interviews. **Structural questions** are more focused and help to develop the range of terms in a category or domain. Last are **contrast questions,** which are asked to distinguish differences in the meaning of terms and symbols.

 Example of ethnographic interviewing:

Bannister (1999) conducted an ethnographic study of midlife women's experience of their changing bodies using Spradley's method. An example of a descriptive question was, "I wonder if you could tell me about your experience of your changing body?" (p. 524). An example of a structural question was, "Corinne, you said, 'I see myself getting older.' Are there other phrases you might use to describe this?" (p. 524). Last, an example of one of Bannister's contrast questions was "Mary, how would you describe the difference between your comments, 'How others view me' and 'How I view myself?'" (p. 524).

Semistructured Interviews

Researchers sometimes want to be sure that a specific set of topics is covered in their qualitative interviews. They know what they want to ask, but cannot predict what the answers will be. Their role in the process is somewhat structured, whereas the participants' is not. In such focused or **semistructured interviews**, researchers prepare in advance a written **topic guide**, which is a list of areas or questions to be covered with each respondent. The interviewer's function is to encourage participants to talk freely about all the topics on the list, and to tell stories in their own words. This technique ensures that researchers will obtain all the information required, and gives respondents the freedom to respond in their own words, provide as much detail as they wish, and offer illustrations and explanations.

In preparing the list of questions, care needs to be taken to order questions in a logical sequence, perhaps chronologically, or perhaps from the general to the specific. (However, interviewers need to be attentive because sometimes respondents spontaneously give information about questions that are later on the list.) The list of questions might include suggestions for follow-up questions or **probes** designed to elicit more detailed information. Examples of such probes include, "Please explain what you mean by that," "What happened next?" and "When that happened, how did you feel?" Care should be taken not to include questions that require one- or two-word responses, such as "yes" or "no." The goal is to ask questions that give respondents an opportunity to provide rich, detailed information about the phenomenon under study.

In deciding whether to use a semistructured or unstructured interview, it is important to consider not only the research tradition, but also the state of knowledge on a topic. Gibson (1998) conducted a study of the experiences and expectations of patients discharged from an acute psychiatric hospital using, and compared the richness of data yielded by the two approaches. Gibson found that unstructured interviews resulted in greater depth and detail than semistructured interviews, and that respondents preferred unstructured interviews.

Example of a semistructured interview: Åsbring and Närvänen (2002) studied women's experiences of stigma in relation to chronic fatigue syndrome and fibromyalgia. Their topic guide for semistructured interviews with 25 women included questions about such issues as the women's views of the illness, encounters with health care providers, and the consequences for daily life of encounters with health care providers.

Focus Group Interviews

Focus group interviews are becoming increasingly popular in the study of health problems. In a focus group interview, a group of four or more people is assembled for a discussion. The interviewer (often called a **moderator**) guides the discussion according to a written set of questions or topics to be covered, as in a semistructured interview. Focus group sessions are carefully planned discussions that take advantage of group dynamics for accessing rich information in an efficient manner.

Typically, the people selected for a group (usually through purposive or snowball sampling) are a fairly homogeneous group, to promote a comfortable group dynamic. People usually feel more at ease expressing their views when they share a similar background with other group members. Thus, if the overall sample is diverse, it is usually best to have people with similar characteristics, in terms of race/ethnicity, age, gender, or experience, participating in separate focus groups.

Several writers have suggested that the optimal group size for focus groups is 6 to 12 people, but Côté Arsenault and Morrison-Beedy (1999) advocate smaller groups of about 5 participants when the topic is emotionally charged or sensitive. Groups of four or fewer may not generate sufficient interaction, however, particularly because not everyone is equally comfortable in expressing their views.

TIP: In recruiting group members, it is usually wise to recruit one or two more people than is considered optimal, because of the risk of no-shows. Monetary incentives can help reduce this risk. It is also important to call the recruits the night before the group session to remind them of the appointment and confirm attendance.

The setting for the focus group sessions should be selected carefully and, ideally, should be a neutral one. Churches, hospitals, or other settings that are strongly identified with particular values or expected behaviors may not be suitable, depending on the topic. The location should be one that is comfortable, not intimidating, accessible, and easy to find. It should also be acoustically amenable to audiotape recording.

Moderators play a critical role in the success of focus group interviews. Nurses often already possess the skills and abilities needed to lead focus groups effectively. For example, they are able to elicit detailed and sometimes sensitive information from clients, and often understand the intricacies of group processes. An important job of moderators is to solicit input from all group members, and not let a few vocal people dominate the discussion. It is sometimes useful to have more than one moderator, so that particular cues can be followed up by more than one listener. Researchers other than the moderator should be present, to take detailed notes about each session.

A major advantage of a group format is that it is efficient—researchers obtain the viewpoints of many individuals in a short time. Moreover, focus groups capitalize on the fact that members react to what is being said by others, thereby potentially leading to richer or deeper expressions of opinion. Also, focus group interviews are usually stimulating to respondents. One disadvantage is that some people are uncomfortable about expressing their views in front of a group. Another possible concern is that the dynamics of the session may foster a group culture that could inhibit individual expression as "group think" takes hold. Studies of focus groups have shown, however, that they are similar to individual interviews in terms of number or quality of ideas generated (Kidd & Parshall, 2000).

Focus groups have been used by researchers in many qualitative research traditions, and can play a particularly important role in feminist, critical theory, and participatory action research.

Example of focus group interviews:
Freeman, O'Dell, and Meola (2000) studied the needs of families of children with brain tumors during six stages of the illness. Data were collected in 11 focus group sessions with 4 homogeneous groups: parents and guardians, siblings, affected children younger than 10 years, and affected children age 10 years and older. The moderator asked questions from a topic guide while an assistant moderator took detailed notes. All group meetings were audiotaped and transcribed.

Joint Interviews

Nurse researchers are sometimes interested in phenomena that involve a relationship between two or three people, or that require understanding the perspective of more than one person. For example, the phenomenon might be the grief that mothers *and* fathers experience on losing a child, or the experiences of AIDS patients *and* their caretakers. In such cases, it can be productive to conduct **joint interviews** in which two or more parties are simultaneously questioned, using either an unstructured or semistructured format. Unlike focus group interviews, which typically involve group members who do not know each other, joint or dyadic interviews are done with people who are often intimately related.

Joint interviews usually supplement rather than replace individual interviews, because there are things that cannot readily be discussed in front of the other party (e.g., criticisms of the other person's behavior). However, joint interviews can be especially helpful when researchers want to *observe* the dynamics between two key actors. Morris (2001) provides some useful guidelines and raises important issues in the conduct of joint interviews.

Example of joint interviews:
The purpose of Kalischuk and Davies' (2001) study was to develop a substantive grounded theory to explain how family members heal after a youth suicide. The researchers conducted a total of 44 interviews: 33 individual interviews and 11 family interviews. The family interviews were aimed at engaging participants in joint discussions about their experiences.

Life Histories

Life histories are narrative self-disclosures about individual life experiences. Ethnographers frequently use individual life histories to learn about cultural patterns. A famous example of this is Oscar Lewis' (1959, 1961) life history of poor families in Mexico, which gave rise to the controversial concept of *culture of poverty*.

With a life history approach, researchers ask respondents to provide, often in chronologic sequence, a narration of their ideas and experiences, either orally or in writing. Life histories may take months, or even years, to record, with researchers providing only gentle guidance in the telling of the story. Narrated life histories are often backed up by intensive observation of the person, interviews with friends or family members, or a scrutiny of letters, photographs, or other materials.

Leininger (1985) noted that comparative life histories are especially valuable for the study of the patterns and meanings of health and health care, especially among elderly people. Her highly regarded essay provides a protocol for obtaining a life health care history.

Example of life histories:
Abrums (2000) studied the meaning of death and the experience of grieving among deeply religious members of a store-front church. Life history interviews were used to explore these concepts.

Oral Histories

Researchers use the technique known as **oral history** to gather personal recollections of events and their perceived causes and consequences. Oral histories, unlike life histories, typically focus on describing important themes rather than individuals. Oral histories are a method for connecting individual experiences with broader social and cultural contexts.

Oral histories are an important method for historical researchers when the topic under study is the not-too-distant past, and people who experienced the event can still be asked about those experiences. Oral histories are also a tool used by feminist researchers and other researchers with an ideological perspective because oral histories are a way to reach groups that have been ignored or oppressed.

Depending on the focus of the oral history, researchers can conduct interviews with a number of persons or concentrate on multiple interviews with one individual. Researchers usually use unstructured interviews to collect oral history data.

Example of oral histories:
Rafael (2000) collected contemporary oral history data on public health nursing in southwestern Ontario. Rafael interviewed 14 public nurses and asked them about the period of 1980 to 1996, when dramatic changes in public nursing were tak-

ing place. The findings debunked the myth that public health nurses were resistant to change.

Critical Incidents

The **critical incidents technique** is a method of gathering information about people's behaviors by examining specific incidents relating to the behavior under investigation (Flanagan, 1954). The technique, as the name suggests, focuses on a factual incident, which may be defined as an observable and integral episode of human behavior. The word *critical* means that the incident must have had a discernible impact on some outcome; it must make either a positive or negative contribution to the accomplishment of some activity of interest. For example, if we were interested in understanding the use of humor in clinical practice, we might ask a sample of nurses the following questions: "Think of the last time you used humor in your interactions with a hospital patient. What led up to the situation? Exactly what did you do? How did the patient react? Why did you feel it would be all right to use a humorous approach? What happened next?"

The technique differs from other self-report approaches in that it focuses on something specific about which respondents can be expected to testify as expert witnesses. Usually, data on 100 or more critical incidents are collected, but this typically involves interviews with a much smaller number of people because each participant can often describe multiple incidents. The critical incident technique has been used in both individual and focus group interviews.

Example of a critical incident study:
Mårtensson, Dracup, and Fridlund (2001) used the critical incident technique to explore decisive situations influencing spouses' support of patients with heart failure. Interviews with 23 spouses yielded 193 critical incidents. An example of questions used to elicit the data is: "Describe an incident in which you were an asset and/or not an asset to your spouse with regard to his/her heart failure" (p. 343).

Diaries and Journals

Personal **diaries** have long been used as a source of data in historical research. It is also possible to generate new data for a nonhistorical study by asking study participants to maintain a diary or journal over a specified period. Diaries can be useful in providing an intimate description of a person's everyday life.

The diaries may be completely unstructured; for example, individuals who have undergone an organ transplantation could be asked simply to spend 10 to 15 minutes a day jotting down their thoughts and feelings. Frequently, however, subjects are requested to make entries into a diary regarding some specific aspect of their experience, sometimes in a semistructured format. For example, studies of the effect of nutrition during pregnancy on fetal outcomes frequently require subjects to maintain a complete diary of everything they ate over a 1- to 2-week period. Nurse researchers have used health diaries to collect information about how people prevent illness, maintain health, experience morbidity, and treat health problems.

Although diaries are very useful means of learning about ongoing experiences, one limitation is that they can be used only by people with adequate literacy skills, although there are examples of studies in which diary entries were audiotaped rather than written out. Diaries also depend on a high level of participant cooperation.

Example of diaries:
Kaunonen, Aalto, Tarkka, and Paunonen (2000) used diaries in a study of a new oncology nursing intervention—a supportive telephone call to a significant other after the death of a patient. Each nurse involved in the intervention was asked to maintain a diary after every call. The data were analyzed with regard to both the family members' experiences and the nurse's interactions.

The Think-Aloud Method

The **think-aloud method** is a qualitative method that has been used to collect data about cognitive processes, such as thinking, problem-solving, and decision-making. This method involves having people use audio-recording devices to talk about decisions as they are being made or while problems are being solved, over an extended period (e.g., throughout a shift). The method produces an inventory of decisions as they occur in a naturalistic context, and allows researchers to examine sequences

of decisions or thoughts, as well as the context in which they occur (Fonteyn, Kuipers, & Grober, 1993). Think-aloud procedures have been used in a number of studies of clinical nurses' decision-making.

The think-aloud method has been used in both naturalistic and simulated settings. Although simulated settings offer the opportunity of controlling the context of the thought process (e.g., presenting people with a common problem to be solved), naturalistic settings offer the best opportunity for understanding clinical processes.

Think-aloud sessions are sometimes followed up with personal interviews or focus group interviews in which the tape may be played (or excerpts from the transcript quoted). Participants are then questioned about aspects of their reasoning and decision-making.

Example of the think-aloud method:
Aitken and Mardegan (2000) described two studies in which they used the think-aloud method to examine the decision-making of expert critical care practitioners. In the first study they explored critical care nurses' hemodynamic assessment and management during 2-hour periods of care for critically ill patients. The second study focused on expert nurses' clinical judgments while managing pain in postoperative patients.

Photo Elicitation Interviews

Photo elicitation involves an interview stimulated and guided by photographic images. This procedure, most often used in ethnographics, has been described as a method that can break down barriers between researchers and study participants, and promote a more collaborative discussion (Harper, 1994). The photographs typically are ones that researchers or associates have made of the participants' world, through which researchers can gain insights into a new culture. Participants may need to be continually reassured that their taken-for-granted explanations of the photos are providing new and useful information.

Photo elicitation can also be used with photos that participants have in their homes, although in such case researchers have less time to frame useful questions, and no opportunity to select the photos that will be the stimulus for discussion. Researchers have also used the technique of asking participants to take photographs themselves and interpret them.

Example of photo elicitation:
Bender, Harbour, Thorp, and Morris (2001) studied perceptions of quality of prenatal care among immigrant Latina women attending two prenatal clinics. They conducted in-depth interviews using seven "photo prompts" designed to portray stages of the prenatal care appointment. The interview guide asked women to describe the photograph, including how the women portrayed were feeling. Then the women were asked if the photograph reminded them of an experience they had had, and if so, they were asked to tell the story of that experience.

Self-Report Narratives on the Internet

A potentially rich data source for qualitative researchers involves narrative self-reports available on or through the Internet. Data can be solicited directly from a large audience of Internet users. For example, researchers can post a web page requesting that people with particular experiences describe them. They can also enter into long conversations with other users in a chat room, or solicit information through an e-mail listserv that distributes messages to users participating in a network. In some cases data that can be analyzed qualitatively are simply "out there," as when a researcher enters a chat room or goes to a bulletin board and analyzes the content of the existing, unsolicited messages.

Using the Internet to access narrative data has obvious advantages. This approach is economical and allows researchers to obtain information from geographically dispersed and perhaps remote Internet users. However, a number of ethical concerns have been raised, and issues of authenticity need to be considered (Robinson, 2001).

Example of Internet data use:
Dickerson, Flaig, and Kennedy (2000) did a study to understand common themes of help-seeking on the Internet for people with implantable cardioverter defibrillators (ICDs). Data were

collected on-line from a public electronic bulletin board for people with ICDs. A total of 469 postings by 75 users over a 5-month period was analyzed.

Gathering Qualitative Self-Report Data

The purpose of gathering narrative self-report data is to enable researchers to construct reality in ways that are consistent with the constructions of the people being studied. This goal requires researchers to take steps to overcome communication barriers and to enhance the flow of meaning. Asking good questions and eliciting good narrative data are far more difficult than appears. This section offers some suggestions about gathering qualitative self-report data through in-depth interviews. Further suggestions are offered by Weiss (1995) and Seidman (1998).

Preparing for the Interview

Although qualitative interviews are conversational, this does not mean that they are entered into casually. The conversations are purposeful ones that require advance thought and preparation. For example, careful thought should be given to the wording of questions. To the extent possible, the wording should make sense to respondents and reflect their world view.

An important issue is that researchers and respondents should have a common vocabulary. If the researcher is studying a different culture or a subgroup that uses distinctive terms or slang, efforts should be made even before data collection to understand those terms and their nuances.

Researchers usually prepare for the interview by developing (mentally or in writing) the broad questions to be asked (or at least the initial questions, in unstructured interviews). Sometimes it is useful to do a practice interview with a stand-in respondent. If there are questions that are especially sensitive, it is a good idea to ask such questions late in the interview when rapport has been established.

TIP: Memorize the central questions if you have written them out, so that you will be able to maintain eye contact with participants.

It is also important to decide in advance how to present oneself—as a researcher, as a nurse, as an ordinary person as much like participants as possible, as a humble "learner," and so on (Fontana & Frey, 1994). One advantage of assuming the nurse role is that people often trust nurses. On the other hand, people frequently defer to those who are viewed as having more education or more expertise. Moreover, participants may use the interview as an opportunity to ask numerous health questions, or to solicit opinions about particular health practitioners.

Another part of the preparation involves decisions about places where the interviews can be conducted. Morse and Field (1995) advocate letting participants chose the setting. It is, however, important to give thought in advance about possibilities to suggest to them. In-home interviews are often preferred because interviewers then have the opportunity to observe the participants' world, and to take observational notes. When in-home interviews are not desired by participants (e.g., if they are worried that the interview would be overheard by household members and prefer more privacy), it is wise to have alternative suggestions, such as in an office, in a coffee shop, and so on. The important thing is to select places that offer some privacy, that protect insofar as possible against interruptions, and that are adequate for recording the interview. (Of course, in some cases the setting will be dictated by circumstances, as when interviews take place while participants are hospitalized.)

For interviews done in the field, researchers must anticipate the equipment and supplies that will be needed. Preparing a checklist of all such items is helpful. The checklist typically would include audiotape-recording equipment, batteries, tapes, consent forms, forms for obtaining demographic information, notepads, and pens. Other possibilities include laptop computers, incentive payments, cookies or donuts to help break the ice, and distracting toys or picture books if it is likely that children will be home. It may be necessary to bring forms of identification to assure participants of the legitimacy of the visit. And, if the topic under study is likely to elicit emotional narratives, tissues should be readily at hand.

 TIP: Use high-quality tapes for audio-recording interviews. Make sure that the size of the tape corresponds to the size used in the transcription equipment.

Conducting the Interview

Qualitative interviews are typically long—sometimes lasting up to several hours. Researchers often find that the respondents' construction of their experience only begins to emerge after lengthy, in-depth dialogues. Interviewers must prepare respondents for the interview by putting them at ease. Part of this process involves sharing pertinent information about the study (e.g., about the study aims and protection of confidentiality). Another part of this process is using the first few minutes for pleasantries and ice-breaking exchanges of conversation before actual questioning begins. Up-front "small talk" can help to overcome stage fright, which can occur for both interviewers and respondents. Participants may be particularly nervous when the interviews are being tape-recorded, which is the preferred method of recording information. They typically forget about the tape recorder after the interview is underway, so the first few minutes should be used to help both parties "settle in."

 TIP: If possible, place the actual tape recording equipment on the floor or somewhere out of sight.

Respondents will not share much information with interviewers if they do not trust them. Close rapport with respondents provides access to richer information and to personal, intimate details of their stories. Interviewer personality plays a role in developing rapport: Good interviewers are usually congenial, friendly people who have the capacity to see the situation from the respondent's perspective. Nonverbal communication can be critical in conveying concern and interest. Facial expressions, postures, nods, and so on, help to set the tone for the interview.

The most critical interviewing skill for in-depth interviews is being a good listener. A central issue is not how to *talk* to respondents, but how to *listen* to them. It is especially important not to interrupt respondents, to "lead" them, to offer advice or opinions, to counsel them, or to share personal experiences. The interviewer's job is to listen intently to the respondents' stories, a task that is often exhausting. Only by attending carefully to what respondents are saying can in-depth interviewers develop appropriate follow-up questions. Even when a topic guide is used, interviewers must not let the flow of dialogue be bound by those questions. In semistructured interviews, many questions that appear on a topic guide are answered spontaneously over the course of the interview, usually out of sequence.

TIP: In-depth interviewers must be comfortable with pauses and silences, and should let the pace be determined by respondents. Interviewers can encourage respondents with nods and nonspecific prompts, such as "Mmhm."

In-depth interviewers need to be prepared for strong emotions, such as anger, fear, or grief, to surface. Narrative disclosures can "bring it all back" for respondents, which can be a cathartic or therapeutic experience if interviewers create an atmosphere of concern and caring—but it can also be stressful for them.

Interviewers may need to manage a number of potential crises during the interviews. One that happens at least once in most qualitative studies is the failed or improper recording of the interview. Thus, even when interviews are tape recorded, notes should be taken during or immediately after the interview to ensure the highest possible reliability of data and to prevent a total information loss. Interruptions (usually the telephone) and other distractions are another common problem. If respondents are willing, telephones can be controlled by unplugging them or taking the receiver off the hook. Interruptions by personal intrusions of friends or family members may be more difficult to manage. In some cases, the interview may need to be terminated and rescheduled—for example, when a woman is discussing domestic violence and the perpetrator enters and stays in the room.

Interviewers should strive for a positive closure to the interview. The last questions in in-depth interviews should usually be along these lines: "Is there anything else you would like to tell me?" or "Are there any other questions that you think I should have asked you?" Such probes can often elicit a wealth of important information. In closing, interviewers normally ask respondents whether they would mind being contacted again, in the event that additional questions come to mind after reflecting on the information, or in case interpretations of the information need to be verified.

TIP: It is usually unwise to schedule back-to-back interviews. For one thing, it is important not to rush or cut short the first interview to be on time for the next one. It is also important to have an opportunity to write out notes, impressions, and analytic ideas, and it is best to do this when an interview is fresh in your mind.

Postinterview Procedures

Tape-recorded interviews should be listened to and checked for audibility and completeness soon after the interview is over. If there have been problems with the recording, the interview should be reconstructed in as much detail as possible. Listening to the interview may also suggest possible follow-up questions that could be asked if respondents are recontacted. Morse and Field (1995) recommend that interviewers listen to the tapes objectively and critique their own interviewing style, so that improvements can be made in subsequent interviews.

Steps also need to be taken to ensure that the transcription of interviews is done with rigor (Poland, 1995). It is prudent to hire experienced transcribers, to check the quality of initial transcriptions, and to give the transcribers feedback. Transcribers can sometimes unwittingly change the meaning of data by misspelling words, by omitting words, or by not adequately entering information about pauses, laughter, crying, or volume of the respondents' speech (e.g., shouting).

TIP: If transcribers need to be hired, transcriptions can be the most expensive part of a study. It generally takes about 3 hours of transcription time for every hour of interviewing. New, improved voice recognition computer software is available to help with transcribing interviews.

Evaluation of Qualitative Approaches

In-depth interviews are an extremely flexible approach to gathering data and, in many research contexts, offer distinct advantages. In clinical situations, for example, it is often appropriate to let people talk freely about their problems and concerns, allowing them to take much of the initiative in directing the flow of information. In general, qualitative interviews are of greatest utility when a new area of research is being explored. In such situations, an unstructured approach may allow investigators to ascertain what the basic issues or problems are, how sensitive or controversial the topic is, how easy it is to secure respondents' cooperation in discussing the issues, how individuals conceptualize and talk about the problems, and what range of opinions or behaviors exist relevant to the topic. In-depth interviews may also help elucidate the underlying meaning of a pattern or relationship repeatedly observed in more structured research.

On the other hand, qualitative methods are extremely time-consuming and demanding of researchers' skills in analyzing and interpreting the resulting data. Samples tend to be small because of the quantity of information produced, so it may be difficult to know whether findings are idiosyncratic. Qualitative methods do not lend themselves to the rigorous testing of hypotheses about cause-and-effect relationships.

QUANTITATIVE SELF-REPORT INSTRUMENTS

A researcher collecting structured self-report data for a quantitative study almost always uses a formal, written instrument. The instrument is an **interview schedule** when the questions are asked orally in either face-to-face or telephone interviews. It is called a **questionnaire** or an **SAQ** (self-administered questionnaire) when respondents complete the instrument themselves, usually in a paper-and-pencil format but occasionally directly onto a computer. Some studies embed an SAQ into an interview schedule, with interviewers asking some questions orally but respondents answering others in writing.

Structured instruments consist of a set of questions (also known as **items**) in which the wording of both the questions and, in most cases, response alternatives is predetermined. When structured interviews or questionnaires are used, subjects are asked to respond to the same questions, in the same order, and with the same set of response options. In developing structured instruments, much effort is usually devoted to the content, form, and wording of questions.

Open and Closed Questions

Structured instruments vary in *degree* of structure through different combinations of open-ended and closed-ended questions. **Open-ended questions** allow respondents to respond in their own words, in narrative fashion. The question, "What was the biggest problem you faced after your surgery?" is an example of an open-ended question (such as would be used in qualitative studies). In questionnaires, respondents are asked to give a written reply to open-ended items and, therefore, adequate space must be provided to permit a full response. Interviewers are expected to quote responses verbatim or as closely as possible, as would be the case in qualitative interviews that are not tape recorded.

Closed-ended (or **fixed-alternative**) **questions** offer respondents alternative replies, from which subjects must choose the one that most closely matches the appropriate answer. The alternatives may range from the simple "yes" or "no" variety ("Have you smoked a cigarette within the past 24 hours?") to complex expressions of opinion or behavior.

Both open- and closed-ended questions have certain strengths and weaknesses. Good closed-ended items are often difficult to construct but easy to administer and, especially, to analyze. With closed-ended questions, researchers need only tabulate the number of responses to each alternative to gain some understanding about what the sample as a whole thinks about an issue. The analysis of open-ended items, on the other hand, is more difficult and time-consuming. The usual procedure is to develop categories and assign open-ended responses to them. That is, researchers essentially transform open-ended responses to fixed categories in a post hoc fashion so that tabulations can be made.

Closed-ended items are more efficient than open-ended questions because respondents can complete more closed- than open-ended questions in a given amount of time. In questionnaires, subjects may be less willing to compose written responses than to check off or circle appropriate alternatives. Closed-ended items are also preferred with respondents who are unable to express themselves well verbally. Furthermore, some questions are less objectionable in closed form than in open form. Take the following example:

1. What was your family's total annual income last year?
2. In what range was your family's total annual income last year:
   ( ) Under $25,000,
   ( ) $25,000 to $49,999,
   ( ) $50,000 to $74,999,
   ( ) $75,000 to $99,999,
   ( ) or $100,000 or more?

The second question is more likely to be answered because the range of options gives respondents a greater measure of privacy than the blunter open-ended question.

These various advantages of closed-ended questions are offset by some shortcomings. The major drawback is the possibility that researchers may have neglected or overlooked potentially important responses. The omission of possible alternatives can lead to inadequate understanding of the issues or to outright bias if respondents choose an alternative that misrepresents their position. When the area of research is relatively new, open-ended questions may be better than closed-ended ones for avoiding bias.

Another objection to closed-ended items is that they can be superficial. Open-ended questions allow

for a richer and fuller perspective on the topic of interest, if respondents are verbally expressive and cooperative. Some of this richness may be lost when researchers tabulate answers by developing a system of classification, but excerpts taken directly from the open-ended responses can be valuable in imparting the flavor of the replies in a report.

Finally, some respondents may object to being forced into choosing from response options that do not reflect their opinions precisely. Open-ended questions give freedom to respondents and, therefore, offer the possibility of spontaneity and elaboration.

The decision to use open- and closed-ended questions is based on a number of considerations, such as the sensitivity of the topic, the verbal ability of respondents, the amount of time available, and so forth. Combinations of both types are recommended to offset the strengths and weaknesses of each. Questionnaires typically use closed-ended questions predominantly, to minimize respondents' writing burden. Interview schedules, on the other hand, are more variable in their mixture of these two question types.

Questionnaires Versus Interviews

Before developing questions, researchers need to decide whether to collect data through interviews or questionnaires. Each method has advantages and disadvantages.

Advantages of Questionnaires

Self-administered questionnaires, which can be distributed in person, by mail, or over the Internet, offer some advantages. The strengths of questionnaires include the following:

- *Cost.* Questionnaires, relative to interviews, are in general much less costly and require less time and energy to administer. Distributing questionnaires to groups (e.g., to students in a classroom) is clearly an inexpensive and expedient approach. And, with a fixed amount of funds or time, a larger and more geographically diverse sample can be obtained with mailed or web-based questionnaires than with interviews.
- *Anonymity.* Unlike interviews, questionnaires offer the possibility of complete anonymity. A

guarantee of anonymity can be crucial in obtaining candid responses, particularly if the questions are personal or sensitive. Anonymous questionnaires often result in a higher proportion of socially unacceptable responses (i.e., responses that place respondents in an unfavorable light) than interviews.

- *Interviewer bias.* The absence of an interviewer ensures that there will be no interviewer bias. Interviewers ideally are neutral agents through whom questions and answers are passed. Studies have shown, however, that this ideal is difficult to achieve. Respondents and interviewers interact as humans, and this interaction can affect responses.

Web-based surveys are especially economical, and can yield a data set directly amenable to analysis, without having to have staff entering data (the same is also true for CAPI and CATI interviews). Internet surveys also provide opportunities for interactively providing participants with customized feedback, and for prompts that can minimize missing responses.

Advantages of Interviews

The strengths of interviews far outweigh those of questionnaires. It is true that interviews are costly, prevent respondent anonymity, and bear the risk of interviewer bias. Nevertheless, interviews are considered superior to questionnaires for most research purposes because of the following advantages:

- *Response rates.* Response rates tend to be high in face-to-face interviews. People are more reluctant to refuse to talk to an interviewer who directly solicits their cooperation than to discard or ignore a questionnaire. A well-designed and properly conducted interview study normally achieves response rates in the vicinity of 80% to 90%, whereas mailed and web-based questionnaires typically achieve response rates of 50% or lower. Because nonresponse is not random, low response rates can introduce serious biases. (However, if questionnaires are personally distributed to people in a particular setting— e.g., maternity patients about to be discharged from the hospital—reasonably good response rates can be achieved.)

Examples of response rates: Stranahan (2001), who sent mailed questionnaires to all nurse practitioners in Indiana to learn about their attitudes about spiritual care, achieved a response rate of 40%. Resnick (2000) conducted face-to-face interviews with residents of a life care community; 97% of those invited to participate did so.

- *Audience.* Many people simply cannot fill out a questionnaire. Examples include young children and blind, elderly, illiterate, or uneducated individuals. Interviews, on the other hand, are feasible with most people. For web-based questionnaires, a particularly important drawback is that not everyone has access to computers or uses them regularly even if they do.
- *Clarity.* Interviews offer some protection against ambiguous or confusing questions. Interviewers can determine whether questions have been misunderstood and can clarify matters. In questionnaires, misinterpreted questions can go undetected by researchers, and thus responses may lead to erroneous conclusions.
- *Depth of questioning.* The information obtained from questionnaires tends to be more superficial than interview data, largely because questionnaires typically contain mostly closed-ended items. Open-ended questions are avoided in questionnaires because most people dislike having to compose and write out a reply. Much of the richness and complexity of respondents' experiences are lost if closed-ended items are used exclusively. Furthermore, interviewers can enhance the quality of self-report data through probing.
- *Missing information.* Respondents are less likely to give "don't know" responses or to leave a question unanswered in an interview than on questionnaires.
- *Order of questions.* In an interview, researchers have control over question ordering. Questionnaire respondents are at liberty to skip around from one section of the instrument to another. It is possible that a different ordering of questions from the one originally intended could bias responses.

- *Sample control.* Interviews permit greater control over the sample. Interviewers know whether the people being interviewed are the intended respondents. People who receive questionnaires, by contrast, can pass the instrument on to a friend, relative, and so forth, and this can change the sample composition. Web-based surveys are especially vulnerable to the risk that people not targeted by researchers will respond, unless there are password protections.
- *Supplementary data.* Finally, face-to-face interviews can result in additional data through observation. Interviewers are in a position to observe or judge the respondents' level of understanding, degree of cooperativeness, social class, lifestyle, and so forth. Such information can be useful in interpreting responses.

Many advantages of face-to-face interviews also apply to telephone interviews. Long or detailed interviews or ones with sensitive questions usually are not well suited for telephone administration, but for relatively brief instruments, telephone interviews are more economical than personal interviews and tend to yield a higher response rate than mailed questionnaires.

USING AND PREPARING STRUCTURED SELF-REPORT INSTRUMENTS

Assembling a high-quality structured self-report instrument is a challenging task. This section discusses components of such instruments and offers some guidance in constructing them.

Specific Types of Closed-Ended Questions

It is especially challenging to create good-quality closed-ended questions. Researchers must pay careful attention to the wording of questions and to the content, wording, and formatting of response options. Nevertheless, the analytic advantages of closed-ended questions are compelling. Various types of closed-ended questions, many of which are illustrated in Table 15-1, are discussed here.

- **Dichotomous questions** require respondents to make a choice between two response alternatives, such as yes/no or male/female. Dichotomous questions are considered most appropriate for gathering factual information.
- **Multiple-choice questions** offer more than two response alternatives. Dichotomous items often are considered too restrictive by respondents, who may resent being forced to see an issue as either "yes" or "no." Graded alternatives are preferable for opinion or attitude questions because they give researchers more information (intensity as well as direction of opinion) and because they give respondents a chance to express a range of views. Multiple-choice questions most commonly offer three to seven alternatives.
- **Cafeteria questions** are a special type of multiple-choice question that asks respondents to select a response that most closely corresponds to their view. The response options are usually full expressions of a position on the topic.
- **Rank-order questions** ask respondents to rank target concepts along a continuum, such as most to least important. Respondents are asked to assign a 1 to the concept that is most important, a 2 to the concept that is second in importance, and so on. Rank-order questions can be useful but need to be handled carefully because respondents sometimes misunderstand them. Rank-order questions should involve 10 or fewer rankings.
- **Forced-choice questions** require respondents to choose between two statements that represent polar positions or characteristics. Several personality tests use a forced-choice format.
- **Rating questions** ask respondents to evaluate something along an ordered dimension. Rating questions are typically **bipolar**, with the end points specifying opposite extremes on a continuum. The end points and sometimes intermediary points along the scale are verbally labeled. The number of gradations or points along the scale can vary but should always be an odd number, such as 7, 9, or 11, to allow for a neutral midpoint. (In the example in Table 15-1, the rating question has 11 points, numbered 0 to 10.)

TABLE 15.1 Examples of Closed-Ended Questions

QUESTION TYPE	EXAMPLE
1. Dichotomous question	Have you ever been hospitalized? 1. Yes 2. No
2. Multiple-choice question	How important is it to you to avoid a pregnancy at this time? 1. Extremely important 2. Very important 3. Somewhat important 4. Not important
3. Cafeteria question	People have different opinions about the use of estrogen replacement therapy for women at menopause. Which of the following statements best represents your point of view? 1. Estrogen replacement is dangerous and should be banned. 2. Estrogen replacement has undesirable side effects that suggest the need for caution in its use. 3. I am undecided about my views on estrogen replacement. 4. Estrogen replacement has many beneficial effects that merits its use. 5. Estrogen replacement is a wonder treatment that should be administered routinely to most menopausal women.
4. Rank-order question	People value different things in life. Below is a list of things that many people value. Please indicate their order of importance to you by placing a "1" beside the most important, "2" beside the second-most important, and so on. _____ Career achievement/work _____ Family relationships _____ Friendships, social interactions _____ Health _____ Money _____ Religion
5. Forced-choice question	Which statement most closely represents your point of view? 1. What happens to me is my own doing. 2. Sometimes I feel I don't have enough control over my life.
6. Rating question	On a scale from 0 to 10, where 0 means "extremely dissatisfied" and 10 means "extremely satisfied," how satisfied were you with the nursing care you received during your hospitalization? 0 1 2 3 4 5 6 8 9 10 Extremely dissatisfied Extremely satisfied

The next question is about things that may have happened to you personally. Please indicate how recently, if ever, these things happened to you:

	Yes, within past 12 months	Yes, 2-3 years ago	Yes, more than 3 years ago	No,never
a. Has someone ever yelled at you all the time or put you down on purpose?	1	2	3	4
b. Has someone ever tried to control your every move?	1	2	3	4
c. Has someone ever threatened you with physical harm?	1	2	3	4
d. Has someone ever hit, slapped, kicked, or physically harmed you?	1	2	3	4

FIGURE 15.1 Example of a checklist.

• **Checklists** encompass several questions that have the same response format. A checklist is a two-dimensional arrangement in which a series of questions is listed along one dimension (usually vertically) and response alternatives are listed along the other. This two-dimensional character of checklists has led some people to call these **matrix questions**. Checklists are relatively efficient and easy for respondents to understand, but because they are difficult to read orally, they are used more frequently in SAQs than in interviews. Figure 15-1 presents an example of a checklist.

• **Calendar questions** are used to obtain retrospective information about the chronology of different events and activities in people's lives. Questions about start dates and stop dates of events are asked and recorded on a calendar grid, such as the one shown in Figure 15-2. Respondents can often better reconstruct the dates of events when several events are recorded in juxtaposition.

• **Visual analogue scales** (VAS) are used to measure subjective experiences, such as pain, fatigue, nausea, and dyspnea. The VAS is a straight line, the end anchors of which are labeled as the extreme limits of the sensation or feeling being measured. Subjects are asked to mark a point on the line corresponding to the amount of sensation experienced. Traditionally, the VAS line is 100 mm in length, which facilitates the deriva-

tion of a score from 0 to 100 through simple measurement of the distance from one end of the scale to the subject's mark on the line. An example of a VAS is presented in Figure 15-3.

Composite Scales

A **scale** provides a numeric score to place respondents on a continuum with respect to an attribute being measured, like a scale for measuring people's weight. Many studies that collect data through self-report use a psychosocial scale, which is used to discriminate quantitatively among people with different attitudes, fears, motives, perceptions, personality traits, and needs. Scales are usually created by combining several closed-ended items (such as those described in the previous section) into a single composite score. Many sophisticated scaling techniques have been developed, only two of which are discussed here.*

---

*One early type of psychosocial scale was the **Thurstone scale**, named after the psychologist L. L. Thurstone. Thurstone's approach to scaling is elaborate and time-consuming and has fallen into relative disuse. Another scaling method, developed by Louis Guttman in the 1940s, is known as the **Guttman** or **cumulative scales**. Advanced scaling procedures include **ratio scaling**, **magnitude estimation scaling**, **multidimensional scaling**, and **multiple scalogram analysis**. Textbooks on psychological scaling and psychometric procedures should be consulted for more information about these scaling strategies.

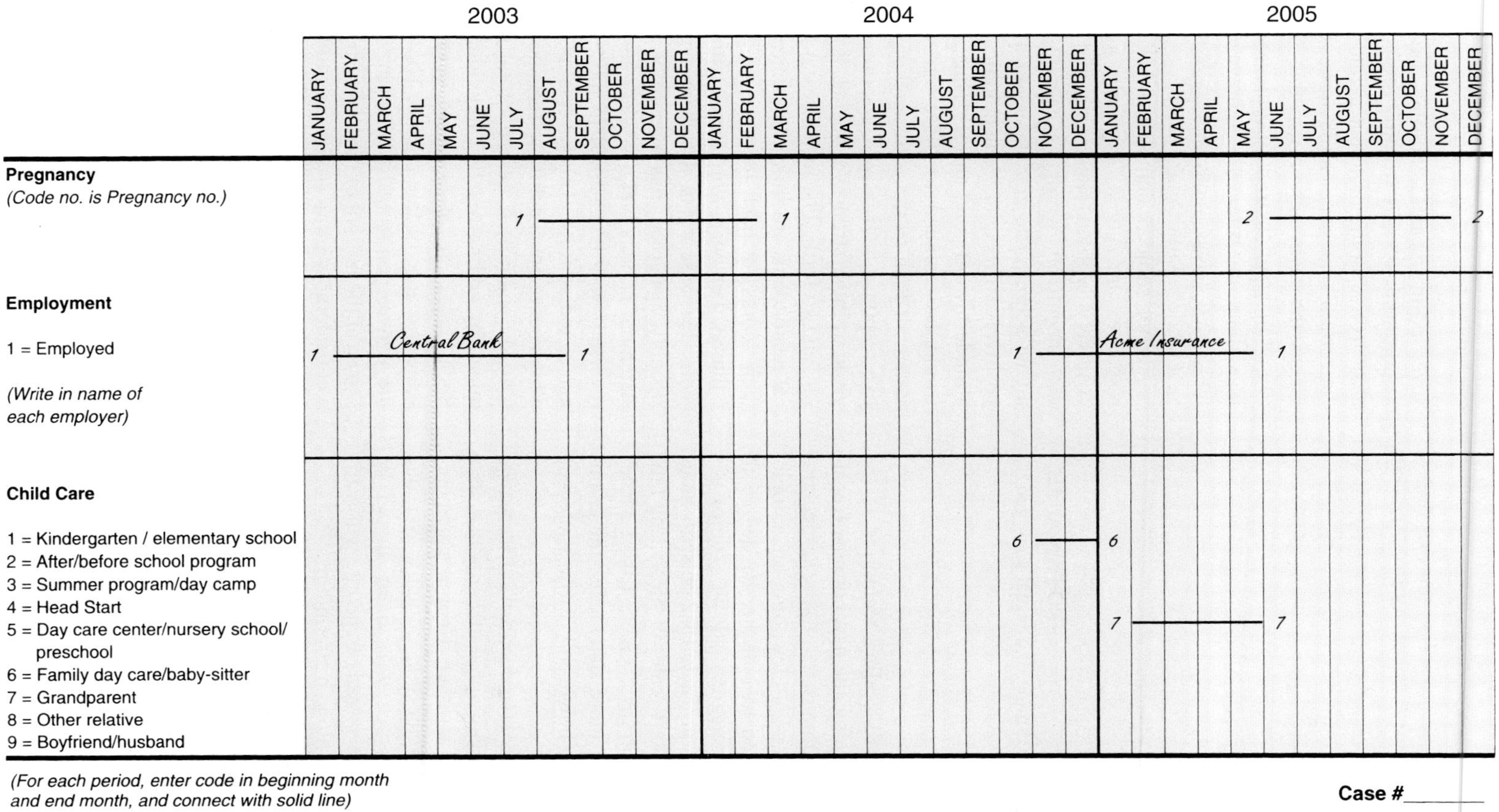

FIGURE 15.2 Example of a calendar grid (completed).

Calendar grid

2003

Category	JAN	FEB	MAR	APR	MAY	JUN	JUL	AUG	SEP	OCT	NOV	DEC
Pregnancy (Code no. is Pregnancy no.)							1					
Employment (1 = Employed) — *Central Bank*	1								1			
Child Care												

2004

Category	JAN	FEB	MAR	APR	MAY	JUN	JUL	AUG	SEP	OCT	NOV	DEC
Pregnancy			1									
Employment — *Acme Insurance*										1		
Child Care										6		

2005

Category	JAN	FEB	MAR	APR	MAY	JUN	JUL	AUG	SEP	OCT	NOV	DEC
Pregnancy					2							2
Employment — *Acme Insurance*	1					1						
Child Care	6											
Child Care	7				7							

Pregnancy
(Code no. is Pregnancy no.)

Employment

1 = Employed

(Write in name of each employer)

Child Care

1 = Kindergarten / elementary school
2 = After/before school program
3 = Summer program/day camp
4 = Head Start
5 = Day care center/nursery school/ preschool
6 = Family day care/baby-sitter
7 = Grandparent
8 = Other relative
9 = Boyfriend/husband

(For each period, enter code in beginning month and end month, and connect with solid line)

Case # _____

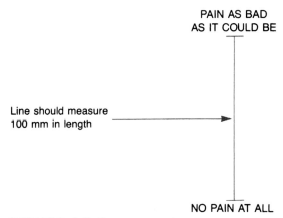

PAIN AS BAD
AS IT COULD BE

Line should measure
100 mm in length

NO PAIN AT ALL

FIGURE 15.3 Example of a visual analogue scale.

Likert Scales

The most widely used scaling technique is the **Likert scale**, named after the psychologist Rensis Likert. A Likert scale consists of several declarative items that express a viewpoint on a topic. Respondents are asked to indicate the degree to which they agree or disagree with the opinion expressed by the statement. Table 15-2 presents an illustrative six-item Likert scale for measuring attitudes toward condom use. Good Likert scales usually include 10 or more statements; the example in Table 15-2 is shown only to illustrate key features.

The first step in constructing a Likert-type scale is to develop a large pool of items that state different positions on an issue. Neutral statements or statements so extreme that virtually everyone would agree or disagree with them should be avoided. The aim is to spread out people with various attitudes or traits along a continuum.*

There are differences of opinion about the number of response alternatives to use. Likert used five categories of agreement/disagreement, such as are shown in Table 15-2. Some researchers prefer

seven-point scales, adding the alternatives "slightly agree" and "slightly disagree." There are also diverse opinions about including an explicit "uncertain" category. Some argue that this option makes the task more acceptable to people who cannot make up their minds or have no strong feelings about an issue. Others, however, feel that an undecided category encourages *fence-sitting*, that is, a tendency not to take sides.

After subjects complete a Likert scale, their responses are scored. Typically, agreement with positively worded statements and disagreement with negatively worded statements are assigned higher scores. The first statement in Table 15-2 is positively worded; agreement indicates a favorable attitude toward condom use. Thus, a higher score would be assigned to those agreeing with this statement than to those disagreeing with it. With five response alternatives, a score of 5 would be given to those strongly agreeing, 4 to those agreeing, and so forth. The responses of two hypothetical respondents are shown by a check or an X, and their scores for each item are shown in far right columns. Person 1, who agreed with the first statement, has a score of 4, whereas person 2, who strongly disagreed, has a score of 1. The second statement is negatively worded, and so scoring is reversed—a 1 is assigned to those who strongly agree, and so forth. This reversal is needed so that a high score consistently reflects positive attitudes toward condoms. A person's total score is determined by adding together individual item scores. Such scales are often called **summated rating scales** because of this feature. The total scores of the two respondents to items in Table 15-2 are shown at the bottom of the table. The scores reflect a considerably more positive attitude toward condoms on the part of person 1 than person 2.

TIP: Investigators who do not include an explicit "uncertain" option proceed in principle as though they were working with a 5- or 7-point scale, even though only four or six alternatives are given: nonresponse to a given item is *scored* as though a neutral response had been chosen (e.g., a "3" on a 5-point scale).

---

*Advanced students developing a Likert scale for widespread use should consult a reference on psychometric procedures, such as *Psychometric Theory* by Nunnally and Bernstein (1994).

TABLE 15.2 Example of a Likert Scale to Measure Attitudes Toward Condoms

DIRECTION OF SCORING*	ITEM	RESPONSES†					SCORE	
		SA	A	?	D	SD	Person 1 (✔)	Person 2 (✕)
+	1. Using a condom shows you care about your partner.		✔			✕	4	1
–	2. My partner would be angry if I talked about using condoms.			✕		✔	5	3
–	3. I wouldn't enjoy sex as much if my partner and I used condoms.			✕	✔		4	2
+	4. Condoms are a good protection against AIDS and other sexually transmitted diseases.				✔	✕	3	2
+	5. My partner would respect me if I insisted on using condoms.	✔				✕	5	1
–	6. I would be too embarrassed to ask my partner about using a condom.			✕		✔	5	2
	Total score						26	11

*Researchers would not indicate the direction of scoring on a Likert scale administered to subjects. The scoring direction is indicated in this table for illustrative purposes only.

†SA, strongly agree; A, agree; ?, uncertain; D, disagree; SD, strongly disagree.

The summation feature of such scales makes it possible to make fine discriminations among people with different points of view. A single question allows people to be put into only five categories. A six-item scale, such as the one in Table 15-2, permits finer gradation—from a minimum possible score of 6 (6 × 1) to a maximum possible score of 30 (6 × 5).

Although traditional Likert scales were used to measure attitudes, summated rating scales can be used to measure a wide array of attributes. In such cases, the bipolar scale would not be agree/disagree but might be always true/never true, extremely likely/extremely unlikely, and so on.

Example of a summated rating scale:
Aiken and Patrician (2000) created a summated rating scale to measure organizational aspects of environments in which nurses practice, the Nursing Work Index, Revised. The measure, comprising 4 subscales, includes 57 items. Examples of items (attributes present in a current job) include "Opportunities for advancement," and "A supervisory staff that is supportive of nurses."

Semantic Differential Scales

Another technique for measuring psychosocial traits is the **semantic differential (SD)**. With the SD, respondents are asked to rate a concept (e.g., primary nursing, team nursing) on a series of bipolar adjectives, such as effective/ineffective, good/bad, important/unimportant, or strong/weak. Respondents place a check at the appropriate point on seven-point rating scales extending from one extreme of the dimension to the other. Figure 15-4 shows an example of the format for an SD for rating the concept *nurse practitioner*.

Semantic differentials are flexible and easy to construct. The concept being rated can be virtually anything—a person, place, situation, abstract idea, controversial issue, and so forth. The concept can be presented as a word, as a phrase, or even as visual material (e.g. photos, drawings). Typically, several concepts are included on an SD so that comparisons can be made across concepts (e.g., male nurse, female nurse, male physician, female physician).

Researchers also have leeway in selecting the scales, but two considerations should guide the selection. First, the adjective pairs should be appropriate for the concepts being used and for the information being sought. The addition of the adjective pair tall/short in Figure 15-4 would add little understanding of how people react to nurse practitioners.

The second consideration in selecting adjective pairs is the extent to which the adjectives measure the same dimension of the concept. Osgood, Suci, and Tannenbaum (1957), through extensive research with SD scales, found that adjective pairs tend to cluster along three independent dimensions: evaluation, potency, and activity. The most important group of adjectives are evaluative ones, such as effective/ineffective, valuable/worthless, good/bad, fair/unfair, and so forth. Potency adjectives include strong/weak and large/small, and examples of activity adjectives are active/passive and fast/slow. These three dimensions need to be considered separately because subjects' evaluative ratings of a concept are independent of their activity or potency ratings. For example, two people who associate high levels of activity with the concept *nurse practitioner* might have divergent views about how to evaluate nurse practitioners. Researchers must decide whether to represent all three dimensions or whether only one or two are needed. Each dimension must be scored separately.

Scoring of SD responses is essentially the same as for Likert scales. Scores from 1 to 7 are

NURSE PRACTITIONERS

competent	7*	6	5	4	3	2	1	incompetent
worthless	1	2	3	4	5	6	7	valuable
important								unimportant
pleasant								unpleasant
bad								good
cold								warm
responsible								irresponsible
successful								unsuccessful

*The score values would not be printed on the form administered to actual subjects. The numbers are presented here solely for the purpose of illustrating how semantic differentials are scored.

FIGURE 15.4 Example of a semantic differential.

assigned to each bipolar scale response, with higher scores usually associated with the positively worded adjective. Responses are then summed across the bipolar scales to yield a total score.

Example of a study using an SD:
Phillips, Brewer, and deArdon (2001) developed the Elder Image Scale, an SD instrument that measures a caregiver's mental image of an elder derived from past associations and present observations. Examples of adjective pairs include reasonable/unreasonable, even-tempered/hot-tempered, and considerate/abusive.

Existing Self-Report Scales and Psychological Measures

Clinical nurse researchers have studied many psychosocial traits, and numerous self-report scales have been developed to measure them, often using a summated rating scale format. Table 15-3 illustrates a number of important constructs that nurse researchers have measured using existing composite scales. Note that many scales and test instruments must be purchased from the publisher, or require the author's permission to use them.

A special reference section at the end of this chapter provides citations for locating existing self-report scales, and Box 15-1 lists some helpful websites. In addition, both the nursing and non-nursing indexes and abstracting services should be consulted for references to studies that have developed scales. The CINAHL database includes information on the scales used in research studies. Information on standardized tests and psychological measures can be retrieved through a computerized literature search of the database called *Mental Measurement Yearbook*, produced by the Buros Institute of Mental Measurements, or through *Health and Psychosocial Instruments Online*.

Response Biases

Although self-reports represent a powerful mechanism for obtaining data, researchers who use this approach should always be aware of the risk of **response biases**—that is, the tendency of respon-

dents to distort their responses. Perhaps the most pervasive problem is people's tendency to present a favorable image of themselves. **Social desirability response bias** refers to the tendency of some individuals to misrepresent their responses consistently by giving answers that are congruent with prevailing social values. This problem is often difficult to combat. Subtle, indirect, and delicately worded questioning sometimes can help to alleviate this response bias. The creation of a permissive atmosphere and provisions for respondent anonymity also encourage frankness.

TIP: If you are collecting self-report data about a socially unacceptable characteristic or behavior, you might want to consider administering a special scale such as the Marlowe-Crowne Social Desirability Scale to determine whether respondents have a systematic tendency to give responses biased in the direction of "looking good."

Some response biases are most commonly observed in composite scales. These biases are sometimes referred to as **response sets**. Scale scores are seldom entirely accurate and pure measures of the critical variable. A number of irrelevant factors are also being measured at the same time. Because response set factors can influence or bias responses to a considerable degree, investigators who construct scales must attempt to eliminate or minimize them.

Extreme responses are an example of a response set that introduces biases when some individuals consistently select extreme alternatives (e.g., "strongly agree"). These extreme responses distort the findings because they do not necessarily signify the most intense feelings about the phenomenon under study. There is little a researcher can do to counteract this bias, but there are procedures for detecting it.

Some people have been found to agree with statements regardless of content. Such people are called **yea-sayers**, and the bias is known as the **acquiescence response set**. A less common problem is the opposite tendency for other individuals, called **nay-sayers**, to disagree with statements independently of question content.

The effects of response biases should not be exaggerated, but it is important that researchers

TABLE 15.3 Examples of Concepts Frequently Measured With Composite Scales in Nursing Studies

CONCEPT	RESEARCH EXAMPLE REFERENCE	INSTRUMENT USED
Anxiety	Brady, Henry, Luth, & Casper-Bruett, 2001	State-Trait Anxiety Inventory (STAI)
Caregiver reactions	Teel, Duncan, & Lai, 2001	Caregiver Reaction Assessment (CRA)
Coping	Myors, Johnson, & Langdon, 2001	Revised Jalowiec Coping Scale
Depression	Lyon & Munro, 2001 Vines Ng, Breggia, & Mahoney, 2000	Center for Epidemiological Studies Depression Scale (CESD) Beck Depression Inventory
Fatigue	Meek et al., 2000 Clark, 2002	Multidimensional Assessment of Fatigue, Lee Fatigue Scale Piper Fatigue Scale (PFS)
Health behaviors	Vines et al., 2000 Acton, 2002	Personal Lifestyle Questionnaire (PLQ) Health-Promoting Lifestyle Profile II (HPLP)
Health status	Ross & Ostrow, 2001	Short-Form Health Survey (SF-36)
Hope	Johnson & Pearson, 2000 Hendricks et al., 2000	Herth Hope Scale (HHS) Miller Hope Scale (MHS)
Mood states	Ross & Ostrow, 2001	Profile of Mood States (POMS)
Pain	LeFort, 2000 Vines et al., 2000	McGill Pain Questionnaire (MPQ) McGill Pain Questionnaire—Short Form
Quality of life	Ross & Ostrow, 2001 Acton, 2002	Quality of Life Index (QLI) Index of Well-Being (IWB)
Self-esteem	Pedro, 2001; Anderson, 2000 Dirksen, 2000	Rosenberg Self-Esteem Scale (RSE) Coopersmith Self-Esteem Inventory
Social support	Dirksen, 2000 Pedro, 2001	Personal Resources Questionnaire (PRQ) Norbeck Social Support Questionnaire (SSQ)
Spirituality	Teel et al., 2001	Spiritual Perspectives Scale (SPS)
Stress	Teel et al., 2001 Gaffney, 2000	Perceived Stress Scale (PSS) Difficult Life Circumstances (DLC)
Symptoms of distress	Flaskerud & Lee, 2001 Berger & Walker, 2001	Symptom Checklist-90 (SCL-90) Modified Symptom Distress Scale (M-SDS)
Uncertainty in illness	Dirksen, 2000	Mishel's Uncertainty in Illness Scale (MUIS)

BOX 15.1 Websites for Locating Scales and Measures

- http://www.nyu.edu/library/bobst/research/sci/health/tests.html (V. G. Rankow's "Selected resources for medical, nursing, and psychological tests, surveys, and research instruments")
- http://www.fiu.edu/~library/assistance/psyched.html (Florida International University's "Psychological, Educational, and Health Tests and Measurements: Selected Sources")
- http://www.med.yale.edu/library/reference/publications/tests.html (Yale Medical Library's "Bibliographic Resource Guide/Behavioral Tests and Measures in the Health Sciences")
- http://www.biomed.lib.umn.edu/tsq.html (University of Minnesota Bio-Medical Library's "Finding Tests, Surveys and Questionnaires")

who are using self-reports give these issues some thought. If an instrument or scale is being developed for general use by others, evidence should be gathered to demonstrate that the scale is sufficiently free from response biases to measure the critical variable.

Developing Structured Self-Report Instruments

A well-developed interview schedule or questionnaire cannot be prepared in minutes or even in hours. To design useful, accurate instruments, researchers must carefully analyze the research requirements and attend to minute details. The steps for developing structured self-report instruments follow closely those outlined in Chapter 14. However, a few additional considerations should be mentioned.

Once data needs have been identified, related constructs should be clustered into separate **modules** or areas of questioning. For example, an interview schedule may consist of a module on demographic information, another on health symptoms, a third on stressful life events, and a fourth on health-promoting activities.

Some thought needs to be given to sequencing modules, and questions within modules, to arrive at an order that is psychologically meaningful and encourages candor and cooperation. The schedule should begin with questions that are interesting, motivating, and not too sensitive. The instrument also needs to be arranged to minimize bias. The

possibility that earlier questions might influence responses to subsequent questions should be kept in mind. Whenever both general and specific questions about a topic are included, general questions should be placed first to avoid "coaching."

Every instrument should be prefaced by introductory comments about the nature and purpose of the study. In interviews, the introductory comments would be read to respondents by the interviewer, and often incorporated into an informed consent form. In SAQs, the introduction usually takes the form of a **cover letter** that accompanies the questionnaire. The introduction should be carefully constructed because it represents the first point of contact with potential respondents. An example of a cover letter for a mailed questionnaire is presented in Figure 15-5.

When a first draft of the instrument is in reasonably good order, it should be discussed critically with people who are knowledgeable about questionnaire construction and with experts on the instrument's substantive content. The instrument also should be reviewed by someone capable of detecting technical problems, such as spelling mistakes, grammatical errors, and so forth. When these various people have provided feedback, a revised version of the instrument can be pretested. The pretest should be administered to individuals who are similar to actual participants. Ordinarily, 10 to 20 pretests are sufficient.*

---

*If a new summated rating scale is being developed, a much larger pretest sample is advisable.

Dear _____ :

We are conducting a study to examine how women who are approaching retirement age (age 55 to 65) feel about various issues relating to health and health care. This study, which is sponsored by the State Department of Health, will enable health-care providers to better meet the needs of women in your age group. Would you please assist us in this study by completing the enclosed questionnaire? Your opinions and experiences are very important to us and are needed to give an accurate picture of the health-related needs of women in the greater Middletown area.

Your name was selected at random from a list of residents in your community. The questionnaire is completely anonymous, so you are not asked to put your name on it or to identify yourself in any way. We therefore hope that you will feel comfortable about giving your honest opinions. If you prefer not to answer any particular question, please feel perfectly free to leave it blank. Please do answer the questions if you can, though, and if you have any comments or concerns about any question just write your comments in the margin.

A postage-paid return envelope has been provided for your convenience. We hope that you will take a few minutes to complete and return the questionnaire to us—it should take only about 15 minutes of your time. To analyze the information in a timely fashion, we ask that you return the questionnaire to us by May 12.

Thank you very much for your cooperation and assistance in this endeavor. If you would like a copy of the summary of the results of this study, please check the box at the bottom of page 10.

FIGURE 15.5 Fictitious example of a cover letter for a mailed questionnaire.

Tips for Developing Structured Self-Report Instruments

Although we all are accustomed to asking questions, the proper phrasing of questions for a study is an arduous task. In this section, we provide some tips on wording questions and response options for self-report instruments. Although most advice is specific to structured self-reports, some suggestions are equally appropriate for qualitative interviews.

Tips for Wording Questions

In wording questions for self-reports, researchers should keep four important considerations in mind.

1. *Clarity.* Questions should be worded clearly and unambiguously. This is usually easier said than done. Respondents do not necessarily understand what information is needed and do not always have the same mind-set as the researchers.

2. *Ability of respondents to give information.* Researchers need to consider whether respondents can be expected to understand the ques-

tion or are qualified to provide meaningful information.

3. *Bias.* Questions should be worded in a manner that will minimize the risk of response biases.

4. *Sensitive information.* Researchers should strive to be courteous, considerate, and sensitive to the needs and rights of respondents, especially when asking questions of a private nature.

Here are some specific suggestions with regard to these four considerations:

TIP: • Clarify in your own mind the information you are trying to obtain. The question, "When do you usually eat your evening meal?" might elicit such responses as "around 6 PM," or "when my son gets home from soccer practice," or "when I feel like cooking." The question itself contains no words that are difficult, but the question is unclear because the researcher's intent is not apparent.

• State questions in the affirmative rather than the negative, and particularly avoid sentences with double negatives.

- Avoid long sentences or phrases, and avoid technical terms (e.g., parity) if more common terms (e.g., number of children) are equally appropriate. Use words that are simple enough for the *least* educated respondents in your sample. Don't assume that even nurses have extensive knowledge on all aspects of nursing and medical terminology.
- Avoid "double-barreled" questions that contain two distinct ideas. The statement, "The mentally ill are incapable of caring for themselves and should be denied responsibilities and rights," might lead to conflicts of opinion in a single person if he or she agrees with only one part of the statement.
- Do not assume that respondents will be aware of, or informed about, issues or questions in which you are interested. Furthermore, avoid giving the impression that they *ought* to be informed. Questions on complex or specialized issues sometimes can be worded in such a way that respondents will be comfortable admitting ignorance (e.g., "Many people have not had a chance to learn much about factors that increase the risk of asthma. Do you happen to know of any contributing factors?"). Another approach is to preface a question by a short statement of explanation about terminology or issues.
- Avoid leading questions that suggest a particular kind of answer. A question such as, "Do you agree that nurse—midwives play an indispensable role in the health team?" is not neutral.
- State a range of alternatives within the question itself when possible. For instance, the question, "Do you normally prefer to get up early in the morning on weekends?" is more suggestive of the "right" answer than "Do you normally prefer to get up early in the morning or to sleep late on weekends?"
- For questions that deal with controversial opinions or socially unacceptable behavior (e.g., excessive drinking habits, noncompliance with medical instructions), closed-ended questions may be preferred. It is easier to check off having engaged in socially disapproved actions than to verbalize those actions in response to open-ended questions. Moreover, when unac-

ceptable behaviors are presented as options, respondents are more likely to realize that they are not alone in their behavior, and admissions of such behavior becomes less difficult.
- Impersonal wording of a question is sometimes useful in minimizing embarrassment and encouraging honesty. To illustrate this point, compare these two statements with which respondents would be asked to agree or disagree: (1) "I am personally dissatisfied with the nursing care I received during my hospitalization," (2) "The quality of nursing care in this hospital is unsatisfactory." A respondent might feel more comfortable admitting dissatisfaction with nursing care in the less personally worded second question.
- Researchers concerned about possible respondent confusion or misinterpretation sometimes conduct **cognitive questioning** during the pretest. Cognitive questioning invites respondents to think aloud about the meaning of the question and what comes to mind when they hear it. For example, if we wanted to ask, "Are you exempt from the hospital's requirement to be fingerprinted?" but we weren't sure if respondents understood the concept of an exemption, we might in the pretest ask, "Please tell me in your own words what an exemption is," and "What came to mind when I asked if you were exempt from fingerprinting?"

Tips for Preparing Response Alternatives

If closed-ended questions are used, researchers also need to develop response alternatives. Below are some suggestions for preparing them.

TIP: • Responses options should cover all significant alternatives. If respondents are forced to choose a response from options provided by researchers, they should feel reasonably comfortable with the available options. As a precaution, researchers often have as one response option a phrase such as "other—please specify."
- Alternatives should be mutually exclusive. The following categories for a question on a person's age are *not* mutually exclusive: 30 years or younger, 30–40 years, 40–50, or 50 years or

older. People who are exactly 30, 40, or 50 would qualify for two of the four categories.

- There should be an underlying rationale for ordering alternatives. Options often can be placed in order of decreasing or increasing favorability, agreement, or intensity. When options have no "natural" order, alphabetic ordering of the alternatives is less likely to lead respondents to a particular response (e.g., see question 4 in Table 15-1).
- Response alternatives should not be too lengthy. One sentence or phrase for each alternative should almost always be sufficient to express a concept. Response alternatives should be about equal in length.

Tips for Formatting an Instrument

The appearance and layout of an instrument may seem a matter of minor administrative importance. However, a poorly designed format can have substantive consequences if respondents (or interviewers) become confused, miss questions, or answer questions they should have omitted. The format is especially important in questionnaires because respondents typically do not have a chance to seek assistance. The following suggestions may be helpful in laying out an instrument:

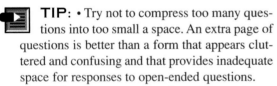 **TIP:** • Try not to compress too many questions into too small a space. An extra page of questions is better than a form that appears cluttered and confusing and that provides inadequate space for responses to open-ended questions.

- Set off the response options from the question or stem itself. Response alternative are usually aligned vertically (Box 15-2). In questionnaires, respondents can be asked either to circle their answer or to place a check in the appropriate box.
- Give special care to formatting **filter questions**, which are designed to route respondents through different sets of questions depending on their responses. In interview schedules, the typical procedure is to use **skip patterns** that instruct interviewers to skip to a specific question (e.g., SKIP TO Q10). In SAQs, skip instructions may be confusing. It is usually better to put

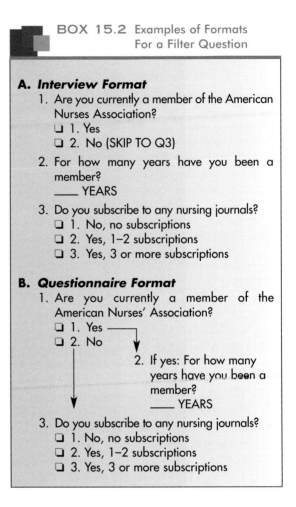

BOX 15.2 Examples of Formats For a Filter Question

A. Interview Format

1. Are you currently a member of the American Nurses Association?
   ❏ 1. Yes
   ❏ 2. No (SKIP TO Q3)

2. For how many years have you been a member?
   ____ YEARS

3. Do you subscribe to any nursing journals?
   ❏ 1. No, no subscriptions
   ❏ 2. Yes, 1–2 subscriptions
   ❏ 3. Yes, 3 or more subscriptions

B. Questionnaire Format

1. Are you currently a member of the American Nurses' Association?
   ❏ 1. Yes
   ❏ 2. No

   2. If yes: For how many years have you been a member?
      ____ YEARS

3. Do you subscribe to any nursing journals?
   ❏ 1. No, no subscriptions
   ❏ 2. Yes, 1–2 subscriptions
   ❏ 3. Yes, 3 or more subscriptions

questions appropriate to a subset of respondents apart from the main series of questions, as illustrated in Box 15-2, part B. An important advantage of CAPI, CATI, and audio-CASI is that skip patterns are built into the computer program, leaving no room for human error.

- Avoid forcing all respondents to go through inapplicable questions in an SAQ. That is, question 2 in Box 15-2 part B could have been worded as follows: "If you are a member of the American Nurses Association, for how long have you been a member?" Nonmembers may not be sure how to handle this question and may be annoyed at having to read through irrelevant material.

ADMINISTERING STRUCTURED SELF-REPORT INSTRUMENTS

Administering interview schedules and questionnaires requires different skills and involves different considerations. In this section, we examine issues in the administration of structured instruments, and ways of handling difficulties.

Collecting Interview Data

The quality of interview data depends heavily on interviewer proficiency. Interviewers for large survey organizations receive extensive general training in addition to specific training for individual studies. Although we cannot in this introductory book cover all the principles of good interviewing, we can identify some major issues.

A primary task of interviewers is to put respondents at ease so that they will feel comfortable in expressing opinions honestly. Respondents' personal reactions to interviewers can affect their willingness to participate. Interviewers, therefore, should always be punctual (if an appointment has been made), courteous, and friendly. Interviewers should strive to appear unbiased and to create a permissive atmosphere that encourages candor. All opinions of respondents should be accepted as natural; interviewers should not express surprise, disapproval, or even approval.

When a structured interview schedule is being used, interviewers should follow question wording precisely. Similarly, interviewers should not offer spontaneous explanations of what questions mean. Repetitions of the questions are usually adequate to dispel misunderstandings, particularly if the instrument has been properly pretested. Interviewers should not read questions mechanically. A natural, conversational tone is essential in building rapport with respondents, and this tone is impossible to achieve if interviewers are not thoroughly familiar with the questions.

When closed-ended questions have lengthy or complicated response alternatives, or when a series of questions has the same response alternatives, interviewers should hand subjects a **show card** that lists response options. People cannot be expected to remember detailed unfamiliar material and may choose the last alternative if they cannot recall earlier ones. Closed-ended items are recorded by checking or circling the appropriate alternative, but responses to open-ended questions must be recorded in full. Interviewers should not paraphrase or summarize respondents' replies.

Obtaining complete, relevant responses to open-ended questions is not always an easy matter. Respondents may reply to seemingly straightforward questions with irrelevant remarks or partial answers. Some may say, "I don't know" to avoid giving their opinions on sensitive topics, or to stall while they think over the question. In such cases, the interviewers' job is to probe. The purpose of a probe is to elicit more useful information than respondents volunteered during their initial reply. A probe can take many forms: Sometimes it involves a repetition of the original question, and sometimes it is a long pause intended to communicate to respondents that they should continue. Frequently, it is necessary to encourage a more complete response by a nondirective supplementary question, such as, "How is that?" Interviewers must be careful to use only *neutral* probes that do not influence the content of a response. Box 15-3 gives some examples of

BOX 15.3 Examples of Neutral, Nondirective Probes

Is there anything else?
Go on.
Are there any other reasons?
How do you mean?
Could you tell me more about that?
Why do you feel that way?
Would you tell me what you have in mind?
There are no right or wrong answers; I'd just like to get your thinking.
Could you please explain that?
Could you give me an example?

neutral, nondirective probes used by professional interviewers to get more complete responses to questions. The ability to probe well is perhaps the greatest test of an interviewer's skill. To know when to probe and how to select the best probes, interviewers must comprehend fully the purpose of each question and the type of information being sought.

Guidelines for telephone interviews are essentially the same as those for face-to-face interviews, but additional effort usually is required to build rapport over the telephone. In both cases, interviewers should strive to make the interview a pleasant and satisfying experience in which respondents are made to understand that the information they are providing is important.

Collecting Questionnaire Data

Questionnaires can be distributed in various ways, including personal distribution, through the mail, and over the Internet. The most convenient procedure is to distribute questionnaires to a group of people who complete the instrument together at the same time. This approach has the obvious advantages of maximizing the number of completed questionnaires and allowing researchers to clarify any possible misunderstandings. Group administrations are often possible in educational settings and may be feasible in some clinical situations.

Personal presentation of questionnaires to individual respondents is another alternative. Personal contact with respondents has a positive effect on response rates for SAQs. Furthermore, researchers can help explain or clarify particular items or the study purpose. Personal involvement may be relatively time-consuming and expensive if questionnaires have to be delivered and picked up at respondents' homes. The distribution of questionnaires in clinical settings, on the other hand, is often inexpensive and efficient and likely to yield a high rate of completed questionnaires.

Questionnaires are often mailed to respondents, but this approach tends to yield low response rates. When only a subsample of respondents return their questionnaires, it may be unreasonable to assume that those who responded were typical of the overall sample. That is, researchers are faced with the possibility that people who did not complete a questionnaire would have answered questions differently from those who did return it.

If the response rate is high, the risk of nonresponse bias may be negligible. A response rate greater than 65% is probably sufficient for most purposes, but lower response rates are common. Researchers should attempt to discover how representative respondents are, relative to the selected sample, in terms of basic demographic characteristics, such as age, gender, and marital status. This comparison may lead researchers to conclude that respondents and nonrespondents are sufficiently similar. When demographic differences are found, investigators can make inferences about the direction of the biases.

Response rates can be affected by the manner in which the questionnaires are designed and mailed. The physical appearance of the questionnaire can influence its appeal, so some thought should be given to the layout, quality and color of paper, method of reproduction, and typographic quality of the instrument. The standard procedure for distributing mailed questionnaires is to include a stamped, addressed return envelope. Failure to enclose a return envelope can have a serious effect on response rates.

TIP: People are more likely to complete a mailed questionnaire if they are encouraged to do so by someone whose name (or position) they recognize. If possible, include a letter of endorsement from someone visible (e.g., a hospital or government official), or write the cover letter on the stationery of a well-respected organization.

The use of **follow-up reminders** is effective in achieving higher response rates for mailed (and Internet) questionnaires. This procedure involves additional mailings urging nonrespondents to complete and return their forms. Follow-up reminders are typically sent about 10 to 14 days after the initial mailing. Sometimes reminders simply involve a letter of encouragement to nonrespondents. It is preferable, however, to enclose a second copy of the questionnaire with the reminder letter because many nonrespondents will have misplaced the original or thrown it away. Telephone follow-ups can be even more successful, but are costly and time-consuming. With anonymous questionnaires, researchers may be unable to distinguish between respondents and nonrespondents for the purpose of sending follow-up letters. In such a situation, the simplest procedure is to send out a follow-up letter to the entire sample, thanking those who have already answered and asking others to cooperate.

Example of response rate improvement: Charles, Piper, Mailey, Davis, and Baigis (2000) mailed questionnaires to hospitals and other employers of nurses in the District of Columbia to determine nurse supply and nurse salaries. Their initial response rate was only 34%, but telephone and in-person follow-up raised the rate to 81%.

As questionnaires are returned, researchers should keep a log of incoming receipts daily. Each questionnaire should be opened, checked for usability, and assigned an identification number. Such record-keeping assists in assembling results, monitoring response rates, and making decisions about the timing of follow-up mailings and cutoff dates.

TIP: The problems associated with mailed questionnaires cannot be handled with interpersonal skills. Building "rapport" into a questionnaire often depends on attention to details. Even though procedural matters may seem trivial, the success of the project may depend on their careful execution.

The Internet is increasingly being used to collect structured self-report data. Web-based surveys appear to be an especially promising approach for accessing groups of people interested in very specific topic domains. Using the Internet to distribute questionnaires requires appropriate equipment and some technical skills, but there are a growing number of aids for doing such surveys.

Web-based surveys can be administered in different ways. One method is to design a questionnaire in a word processing program (e.g., Microsoft Word, WordPerfect, WordPro), as would usually be the case for mailed questionnaires. The file containing the questionnaire would be attached to e-mail messages and distributed to a list of potential respondents. Respondents then complete the questionnaire and return it as an e-mail attachment (or they can print it and return it by mail or fax). This method may be problematic if respondents have trouble opening attachments or if they use a different word processing program. It is also possible to create files containing the survey in executable format (.exe), using a database program such as Paradox or Access.

Internet surveys are increasingly being administered using web-based forms. This approach requires researchers to have their own website on which the survey form is placed. Respondents typically access the website by a hypertext link (i.e., by clicking on the hypertext, which sends the user to another website). For example, respondents may be invited to participate in the survey through an e-mail message that includes the hyperlink to the survey, or they may be invited to participate when they enter a website related in content to the survey (e.g., the website of a cancer support organization). There are also mechanisms for having the survey website included on search engines. However, it is important to weigh the tradeoffs between having a broad population and receiving survey data from inappropriate respondents.

Web-based forms are designed for online response, and may in some cases be programmed to include interactive features. By having dynamic features, respondents can receive as well as give information—a feature that increases people's motivation to participate. For example, respondents can be given information about their own responses (e.g., how they scored on a scale) or about responses of other participants. A major advantage of web-based forms are that the entered data are directly amenable to analysis.

Several reference books are available to help researchers who wish to launch an Internet survey. For example, the books by Nesbary (2000) and Birnbaum (2001) provide useful information. There are also commercial vendors that can help with programming requirements, such as WWW Survey Assistant (http://or.psychology.dal.ca/~wcs/-hidden/home.html) or Opinion Search, Inc. (http://www.opinionsearch.com).

Example of an Internet survey:
Thomas and colleagues (2000) designed and administered a survey about women's perceptions of breast health education and screening to an international population of women. The survey website was linked to other websites frequented by women.

RESEARCH EXAMPLES

This section provides examples of both qualitative and quantitative studies that relied on self-reports.

Research Example of Qualitative Self-Reports

Norton and Bowers (2001) conducted a grounded theory study of end-of-life decision-making. The research focused on clinicians' strategies to change patients' treatment decisions from unrealistic ones (curative) to more realistic choices (palliative). The sample consisted of 10 nurses, 5 physicians, and 5 family members. Interviews were conducted at a time and place convenient to participants over a 16-month period. All interviews were tape recorded and later transcribed and checked for accuracy. The researchers conducted all interviews themselves.

Interviewing changed over the course of the study as the theory emerged. For the first four interviews, which lasted 60 to 90 minutes, Norton and Bowers used broad, open-ended questions, such as "How do patient care decisions get made here?" and "How do decisions get made when it doesn't look like the patient is going to recover?" (p. 261).

Interviews conducted later in the study were shorter, lasting 30 to 60 minutes. The questions used to guide these later interviews became more focused as categories were generated from the analysis. The following questions illustrate interview questions used toward the end of this grounded theory study: "How do you figure out whether a treatment decision is realistic?", What difference does it make if everyone involved (patient, family, and providers) agree on how to proceed?", and "What do you do when that is not the case?" (p. 261). Memos and matrices were used to track the evolving theory and document the researchers' methodologic choices.

Results revealed that the shifting of patients' and families' choices from curative to palliative was accomplished by changing their understanding of the "big picture" of the patient's condition. The strategies clinicians used to make this shift included laying the groundwork, shifting the picture, and accepting the new picture.

Research Example of Structured Self-Reports

Friedman and Griffin (2001) used a structured self-report method to study the relationship of physical symptoms and physical functioning to depression among patients with heart failure. Participants were interviewed twice by trained nursing research assistants. The first interview was a personal interview during the subjects' hospitalization for heart failure. The second interview, conducted 4 to 6 weeks after discharge, was completed with participants in their homes by telephone. Interviewers read the questions slowly over the telephone, and repeated to clarify questions and response options.

A total of 247 patients were determined to be eligible for the study. Most of the eligibles (86%) agreed to participate in the first interview. Those who refused expressed lack of interest or fatigue as their reason. Some 80% of those interviewed in the hospital completed the follow-up interview. The final study sample included 170 subjects (average age of 73 years) with two rounds of interview data.

The interview schedule consisted of four modules. One module focused on sociodemographic data (age, race, martial status, education, and living arrangements). This module was not included in the follow-up interview. Another module consisted of a symptom checklist developed by the researchers. The checklist included 13 symptoms derived from a list of heart failure symptoms contained in the Agency for Health Care Policy Research's practice guidelines on heart failure. In the third module, the researchers included the 10-item physical functioning subscale from the widely used Medical Outcomes Study Short Form Health Survey (SF-36). Finally, the researchers measured depression using the short form (10-item) Center for Epidemiological Studies Depression scale (the CES-D). Friedman and Griffin noted that their selection of the CES-D as the measure of depression in this study was based in part on the fact that this scale "is brief, understandable, and does not confound somatic symptoms that normally accompany aging, thereby making it a useful tool to measure depression in the elderly–even those with a physical illness" (p. 100).

The results indicated that increased physical symptoms and reduced physical functioning over time was associated with greater depressive symptoms in this sample.

SUMMARY POINTS

- Self-report data usually are collected by an oral **interview** or written **questionnaire**. Self-reports vary widely in their degree of structure or standardization.
- Unstructured and loosely structured self reports, which provide respondents and interviewers latitude in formulating questions and answers, yield rich narrative data for qualitative analysis.
- Methods of collecting qualitative self-report data include the following: (1) **unstructured interviews**, which are conversational discussions on the topic of interest; (2) **semistructured interviews**, in which interviewers are guided by a **topic guide** of questions to be asked; (3) **focus group interviews**, which involve discussions with small, homogeneous groups about topics covered in a topic guide; (4) **joint interviews**, which involve simultaneously talking with members of a dyad (e.g., two spouses); (5) **life histories**, which encourage respondents to narrate, in chronologic sequence, their life experiences; (6) **oral histories**, which arc used to gather personal recollections of events and their perceived causes and consequences; (7) **critical incidents interviews**, which involve probes about the circumstances surrounding a behavior or incident that is critical to an outcome of interest; (8) **diaries** and journals, in which respondents are asked to maintain daily records about some aspects of their lives; (9) the **think-aloud method,** which involves having people use audio-recording devices to talk about decisions as they are making them; (10) **photo elicitation interviews**, which are stimulated and guided by photographic images; and

(11) solicited or unsolicited narrative communications on the Internet.
- In preparing for in-depth interviews, researchers learn about the language and customs of participants, formulate broad questions, make decisions about how to present themselves, develop ideas about interview settings, and take stock of equipment needs.
- Conducting good in-depth interviews requires considerable interviewer skill in putting people at ease, developing trust, listening intently, and managing possible crises in the field.
- In-depth self-report methods tend to yield data of considerable richness and are useful in gaining an understanding about little-researched phenomena, but they are time-consuming and yield a wealth of data that are challenging to analyze.
- Structured self-report instruments may include open- or closed-ended questions. **Open-ended questions** permit respondents to reply in narrative fashion, whereas **closed-ended** (or **fixed-alternative**) **questions** offer response options from which respondents must choose.
- Questionnaires are less costly and time-consuming than interviews, offer the possibility of anonymity, and run no risk of interviewer bias; however, interviews tend to yield higher response rates, to be suitable for a wider variety of people, and to yield richer data than questionnaires.
- Types of closed-ended questions include (1) **dichotomous questions**, which require a choice between two options (e.g., yes/no); (2) **multiple-choice questions**, which offer a range of alternatives; (3) **cafeteria questions**, in which respondents are asked to select a statement best representing their view; (4) **rank-order questions**, in which respondents are asked to rank a list of alternatives along a continuum; (5) **forced-choice questions**, which require respondents to choose between two competing positions; (6) **rating questions**, which ask respondents to make judgments along an ordered, bipolar dimension; (7) **checklists** or **matrix questions** in which several questions requiring the same response format are

listed; (8) **calendar questions**, which ask the stop and start dates of various events, recorded on a calendar grid; and (9) **visual analogue scales** (VAS), which are continua used to measure subjective experiences such as pain.

- Composite psychosocial **scales** are multiple-item self-report tools for measuring the degree to which individuals possess or are characterized by target traits or attributes.
- **Likert scales** comprise a series of statements worded favorably or unfavorably toward a phenomenon. Respondents indicate degree of agreement or disagreement with each statement; a total score is computed by the summing item scores, each of which is scored for the intensity and direction of favorability expressed. Likert scales are also called **summated rating scales**.
- **Semantic differentials** (SDs) consist of a series of bipolar rating scales on which respondents indicate their reaction toward some phenomenon; scales can measure an evaluative (e.g., good/bad), activity (e.g., active/passive), or potency (e.g., strong/weak) dimension.
- Self-reports are vulnerable to the risk of reporting biases, which are often called **response set biases**; this problem concerns the tendency of some people to respond to items in characteristic ways, independently of the item's content.
- The **social desirability response bias** stems from a person's desire to appear in a favorable light. The **extreme response set** results when a person characteristically endorses extreme response alternatives. Another response bias is known as **acquiescence**, which is a **yea-sayer's** tendency to agree with statements regardless of their content. A converse problem arises when people (**nay-sayers**) disagree with most statements.
- Data quality in interviews depends heavily on interviewers' interpersonal skills. Interviewers must put respondents at ease and build rapport with them, and need to be skillful at **probing** for additional information when respondents give incomplete or irrelevant responses.
- Group administration is the most convenient and economical way to distribute questionnaires. Another approach is to mail them, but this

method is plagued with the risk of low **response rates**, which can result in a biased sample.
- A number of techniques, such as the use of **follow-up reminders** and good **cover letters**, are designed to increase response rates.

STUDY ACTIVITIES

Chapter 15 of the *Study Guide to Accompany Nursing Research*: *Principles and Methods*, 7th edition, offers various exercises and study suggestions for reinforcing concepts presented in this chapter. In addition, the following study questions can be addressed:

1. Identify which qualitative self-report methods might be appropriate for the following research problems:
   a. What are the coping strategies of parents who have lost a child through sudden infant death syndrome?
   b. How do nurses in emergency departments make decisions about their activities?
   c. What are the health beliefs and practices of Haitian immigrants in the United States?
   d. What is it like to experience having a family member undergo open heart surgery?
2. Voluntary nonemployment of nurses contributes to nursing shortages. Suppose you were planning to conduct a statewide study of the plans and intentions of nonemployed registered nurses in your state. Would you collect structured or unstructured data? Would you adopt an interview or questionnaire approach? If a questionnaire, how would you distribute it?
3. Suppose that the study of nonemployed nurses were done by a mailed questionnaire. Draft a cover letter to accompany it.
4. Suppose you were interested in studying pregnant women's attitudes toward breast-feeding. Develop five positively worded and five negatively worded statements that could be used in constructing a Likert scale for such a study.
5. List 10 pairs of bipolar adjectives that would be appropriate for rating *all* the following concepts

for an SD scale: cigarettes, alcohol, marijuana, heroin, cocaine.

6. Suggest ways of improving the following questions:
    a. When do you usually administer your injection of insulin?
    b. Would you disagree with the statement that nurses should not unionize?
    c. Do you agree or disagree with the following statement? Alcoholics deserve more pity than scorn and should be encouraged to seek medical rather than spiritual assistance.
    d. What is your opinion about the new health reform bill?
    e. Don't you think that the role of nurses ought to be expanded?

SUGGESTED READINGS

Methodologic References

General References on Self-Reports

Alreck, P. L., & Settle, R. B. (1994). *The survey research handbook*. New York: McGraw-Hill.

Birnbaum, M. H. (2001). *Introduction to behavioral research on the Internet*. Upper Saddle River, NJ: Prentice-Hall.

Collins, C., Given, B., Given, C. W., & King, S. (1988). Interviewer training and supervision. *Nursing Research, 37*, 122–124.

Côté-Arsenault, D., & Morrison-Beedy, D. (1999). Practical advice for planning and conducting focus groups. *Nursing Research, 48*, 280–283.

DeVellis, R. F. (1991). *Scale development: Theory and applications*. Newbury Park, CA: Sage.

Dillman, D. (1999). *Mail and internet surveys: The tailored design method* (2nd ed.). New York: John Wiley & Sons.

Flanagan, J. C. (1954). The critical-incident technique. *Psychological Bulletin, 51*, 327–358.

Fontana, A., & Frey, J. H. (1994). Interviewing: The art of the science. In N. K. Denzin & Y. S. Lincoln (Eds.), *Handbook of qualitative research* (pp. 361–376). Thousand Oaks, CA: Sage.

Fonteyn, M. E., Kuipers, B., & Grober, S. J. (1993). A description of the think aloud method and protocol analysis. *Qualitative Health Research, 3*, 430–441.

Fowler, F. J. (1995). *Improving survey questions*. Thousand Oaks, CA: Sage.

Fowler, F. J., & Mangione, T. W. (1990). *Standardized survey interviewing*. Thousand Oaks, CA: Sage.

Gable, R. K., & Wolf, M. B. (1993). *Instrument development in the affective domain* (2nd ed.). Norwell, MA: Kluwer Academic Publishers.

Gift, A. G. (1989). Visual analogue scales: Measurement of subjective phenomena. *Nursing Research, 38*, 286–288.

Glaser, B. G., & Strauss, A. (1967). *The discovery of grounded theory: Strategies for qualitative research*. New York: Aldine de Gruyter.

Gubrium, J. F., & Holstein, J. A. (Eds.), (2001). *Handbook of interview research: Context and method*. Thousand Oaks, CA: Sage.

Harper, D. (1994). On the authority of the image: Visual methods at the crossroads. In N. K. Denzin & Y. S. Lincoln (Eds.), *Handbook of qualitative research* (pp. 403–412). Thousand Oaks, CA: Sage.

Jones, R. K. (2000). The unsolicited diary as a qualitative research tool for advanced research capacity in the field of health and illness. *Qualitative Health Research, 10*, 555–567.

Kahn, D. L. (2000). How to conduct research. In M. Z. Cohen, D. L. Kahn, & R. H. Steeves (Eds.), *Hermeneutic phenomenological research* (pp. 57–70). Thousand Oaks, CA: Sage.

Kidd, P. S., & Parshall, M. B. (2000). Getting the focus and the group: Enhancing analytic rigor in focus group research. *Qualitative Health Research, 10*, 293–308.

Kingry, M. J., Fiedje, L. B., & Friedman, L. L. (1990). Focus groups: A research technique for nursing. *Nursing Research, 39*, 124–125.

Krueger, R. A., & Casey, M. A. (2000). *Focus groups: A practical guide for applied research* (3rd ed.). Thousand Oaks, CA: Sage.

Lee, K. A., & Kieckhefer, G. M. (1989). Measuring human responses using visual analogue scales. *Western Journal of Nursing Research, 11*, 128–132.

Leininger, M. M. (1985). Life-health-care history: Purposes, methods and techniques. In M. M. Leininger (Ed.), *Qualitative research methods in nursing* (pp. 119–132). New York: Grune & Stratton.

Morgan, D. L. (1997). *Focus groups as qualitative research* (2nd ed.). Thousand Oaks, CA: Sage.

Morris, S. M. (2001). Joint and individual interviewing in the context of cancer. *Qualitative Health Research, 11*, 553–567.

Morrison-Beedy, D., Côté-Arsenault, D., & Feinstein, N. F. (2001). Maximizing results with focus groups:

Moderator and analysis issues. *Applied Nursing Research, 14*, 48–53.

Morse, J. M., & Field, P. A. (1995). *Qualitative research methods for health professionals* (2nd ed.). Thousand Oaks, CA: Sage.

Nesbary, D. (1999). *Survey research and the world wide web*. Bostan, MA: Allyn & Bacon.

Nunnally, J. C., & Bernstein, I. H. (1994). *Psychometric theory* (3rd ed.) New York: McGraw-Hill.

Osgood, C. E., Suci, G. J., & Tannenbaum, P. H. (1957). *The measurements of meaning*. Urbana, IL: University of Illinois Press.

Paterson, B., & Bramadat, I. J. (1992). Use of the preinterview in oral history. *Qualitative Health Research, 2*, 99–115.

Poland, B. D. (1995). Transcription quality as an aspect of rigor in qualitative research. *Qualitative Inquiry, 1*, 190–310.

Reiskin, H. (1992). Focus groups: A useful technique for research and practice in nursing. *Applied Nursing Research, 5*, 197–201.

Robinson, K. M. (2001). Unsolicited narratives from the Internet: A rich source of qualitative data. *Qualitative Health Research, 11*, 706–714.

Seidman, I. (1998). *Interviewing as qualitative research: A guide for researchers in education and the social sciences* (2nd ed.). New York: Teachers College Press.

Spradley, J. (1979). *The ethnographic interview*. New York: Holt Rinehart & Winston.

Van Manen, M. (1990). *Researching lived experience*. New York: State University of New York Press.

Waltz, C. F., Strickland, O. L., & Lenz, E. R. (1991). *Measurement in nursing research* (2nd ed.). Philadelphia: F. A. Davis.

Weiss, R. S. (1995). *Learning from strangers: The art and method of qualitative interview studies*. New York: The Free Press.

Woods, N. F. (1981). The health diary as an instrument for nursing research. *Western Journal of Nursing Research, 3*, 76–92.

Wykle, M. L., & Morris, D. L. (1988). The health diary. *Applied Nursing Research, 1*, 47–48.

References for Scales and Psychological Measures

Aiken, L. R., & Aiken, L. A. (1996). *Rating scales and checklists: Evaluating behavior, personality, and attitudes*. New York: John Wiley & Sons.

Anastasi, A., & Urbina, S. (1997). *Psychological testing* (7th ed.). Englewood Cliffs, NJ: Prentice-Hall.

Fischer, J., & Corcoran, K. (2000). *Measures for clinical practice* (3rd ed.). New York: The Free Press.

Frank-Stromberg, M., & Olsen, S. (1997). *Instruments for clinical health care research*. Boston: Jones and Bartlett.

Impara, J. C., & Plake, B. S. (Eds.). (1998). *The 13th mental measurements yearbook*. Lincoln, NE: The Buros Institute.

McDowell, I., & Newell, C. (1996). *Measuring health: A guide to rating scales and questionnaires* (2nd ed.). New York: Oxford University Press.

Murphy, L. L., Impara, J. C., & Plake, B. S. (Eds.). (1999). *Tests in print V*. Lincoln, NE: The Buros Institute.

Robinson, J. P., Shaver, P. R., & Wrightsman, L. S. (Eds.). (1991). *Measures of personality and social psychological attitudes* (3rd ed.). New York: Academic Press.

Strickland, O. L., & Waltz, C. (1988). *Measurement of nursing outcomes: Vol. II. Measuring nursing performance*. New York: Springer.

Waltz, C. F. (2000). *Measurement of nursing outcomes: Measuring nursing performance in practice, education, and reason* (2nd ed.). New York: Springer.

Waltz, C. F., & Strickland, O. L. (1988). *Measurement of nursing outcomes: Vol. I. Measuring client outcomes*. New York: Springer.

Studies Cited in Chapter 15

Abrums, M. (2000). Death and meaning in a storefront church. *Public Health Nursing, 17*, 132–142.

Acton, G. J. (2002). Health-promoting self care in family caregivers. *Western Journal of Nursing Research, 24*, 73–86,

Aiken, L. H., & Patrician, P. A. (2000). Measuring organizational traits of hospital: The Revised Nursing Work Index. *Nursing Research, 49*, 146–153.

Aitken, L. M., & Mardegan, K. J. (2000). "Thinking aloud": Data collection in the natural setting. *Western Journal of Nursing Research, 22*, 841–853.

Anderson, E. H. (2000). Self-esteem and optimism in men and women infected with HIV. *Nursing Research, 49*, 262–271.

Åsbring, P., & Närvänen, A. (2002). Women's experiences of stigma in relation to chronic fatigue syndrome and fibromyalgia. *Qualitative Health Research, 12*, 148–160.

Bannister, E. M. (1999). Women's midlife experience of their changing bodies. *Qualitative Health Research, 9*, 520–537.

Bender, D. E., Harbour, C., Thorp, J., & Morris, P. (2001). Tell me what you mean by "Si": Perceptions of quality of prenatal care among immigrant Latina women. *Qualitative Health Research, 11*, 780–794.

Brady, L. H., Henry, K., Luth, J. F., & Casper-Bruett, K. K. (2001). The effects of shiatsu on lower back pain. *Journal of Holistic Nursing, 19*, 57–70.

Charles, J. P., Piper, S., Mailey, S. K., Davis, P., & Baigis, J. (2000). Nurse salaries in Washington DC and nationally. *Nursing Economics, 18*, 243–249.

Clark, P. C. (2002). Effects of individual and family hardiness on caregiver depression and fatigue. *Research in Nursing & Health, 25*, 37–48.

Cohen, M. Z., Ley, C., & Tarzian, A. J. (2001). Isolation in blood and marrow transplantation. *Western Journal of Nursing Research, 23*, 592–609.

Dickerson, S. S., Flaig, D. M., & Kennedy, M. C. (2000). Therapeutic connection: Help seeking on the Internet for persons with implantable cardioverter defibrillators. *Heart & Lung, 29*, 248–255.

Dirksen, S. R. (2000). Predicting well-being among breast cancer survivors. *Journal of Advanced Nursing, 32*, 937–943.

Flaskerud, J. H., & Lee, P. (2001). Vulnerability to health problems in female informal caregivers of persons with HIV/AIDS and age-related dementias. *Journal of Advanced Nursing, 33*, 60–68.

Freeman, K., O'Dell, C., & Meola, C. (2000). Issues in families of children with brain tumors. *Oncology Nursing Forum, 27*, 843–848.

Friedman, M. M., & Griffin, J. A. (2001). Relationship of physical symptoms and physical functioning to depression in patients with heart failure. *Heart & Lung, 30*, 98–104.

Gaffney, K. F. (2000). Prenatal risk factors among foreign-born Central American women. *Public Health Nursing, 17*, 415–422.

Gibson, C. (1998). Semi-structured and unstructured interviewing: A comparison of methodologies in research with patients following discharge from an acute psychiatric hospital. *Journal of Psychiatric & Mental Health Nursing, 5*, 469–477.

Hendricks, C. S., Hoffman, H. P., Robertson-Laxton, L., Tavakoli, A., Mathis, D., Hackett, D., & Byrd, L. (2000). Hope as a predictor of health promoting behavior among rural southern early adolescents. *Journal of Multicultural Nursing & Health, 6*, 6–11.

Johnson, J., & Pearson, V. (2000). The effects of a structured education course on stroke survivors living in the community. *Rehabilitation Nursing, 25*, 59–65, 79–80.

Kalischuk, R. G., & Davies, B. (2001). A theory of healing in the aftermath of youth suicide. *Journal of Holistic Nursing, 19*, 163–186.

Kaunonen, M., Aalto, P., Tarkka, M., & Paunonen, M. (2000). Oncology ward nurses' perspectives of family grief and a supportive telephone call after the death of the significant other. *Cancer Nursing, 23*, 3144–324.

LeFort, S. M. (2000). A test of Braden's Self-Help Model in adults with chronic pain. *Image: The Journal of Nursing Scholarship, 32*, 153–160.

Lewis, O. (1959). *Five families.* New York: Basic Books.

Lewis, O. (1961). *The children of Sanchez.* New York: Random House.

Lyon, D. E., & Munro, C. (2001). Disease severity and symptoms of depression in black Americans infected with HIV. *Applied Nursing Research, 14*, 3–10.

Mårtensson, J., Dracup, K., & Fridlund, B. (2001). Decisive situations influencing spouses' support of patients with heart failure: A critical incident technique analysis. *Heart & Lung, 30*, 341–350.

Meek, P. M., Nail, L. M., Barsevik, A., Schwartz, A., Stephen, S., Whitmer, K., Beck, S., Jones, L., & Walker, B. (2000). Psychometric testing of fatigue instruments for use with cancer patients. *Nursing Research, 49*, 181–190.

Myors, K., Johnson, M., & Langdon, R. (2001). Coping styles of pregnant adolescents. *Public Health Nursing, 18*, 24–32.

Norton, S. A., & Bowers, B. J. (2001). Working toward consensus: Providers' strategies to shift patients from curative to palliative treatment choices. *Research in Nursing & Health, 24*, 258–269.

Pedro, L. W. (2001). Quality of life for long-term survivors of cancer. *Cancer Nursing, 24*, 1–11.

Phillips, L. R., Brewer, B. B., & deArdon, E. T. (2001). The Elder Image Scale: A method for indexing history and emotion in family caregiving. *Journal of Nursing Measurement, 9*, 23–47.

Rafael, A. R. F. (2000). Nurses' orientations to change: Debunking the "resistant to change" myth. *Journal of Professional Nursing, 16*, 336–344.

Resnick, M. (2000). Health promotion practices of the older adult. *Public Health Nursing, 17*, 160–168.

Ross, A. C., & Ostrow, L. (2001). Subjectively perceived quality of life after coronary artery bypass surgery. *American Journal of Critical Care, 10*, 11–16.

Stranahan, S. (2001). Spiritual perception, attitudes about spiritual care, and spiritual care practices among nurse practitioners. *Western Journal of Nursing Research, 23*, 90–104.

Teel, C. S., Duncan, P., & Lai, S. M. (2001). Caregiving experiences after stroke. *Nursing Research, 50,* 53–60.

Thomas, B., Stamler, L. L., Lafreniere, K., & Dumala R. (2000). The Internet: An effective tool for nursing research with women. *Computers in Nursing, 18,* 13–8.

Vines, S. W., Ng, A., Breggia, A., & Mahoney, R. (2000). Multimodal chronic pain rehabilitation program: Its effect on immune function, depression, and health behaviors. *Rehabilitation Nursing, 25,* 185–191.

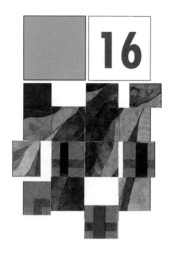

16

Collecting Observational Data

Research observation involves the systematic selection, observation, and recording of behaviors, events, and settings relevant to a problem under study. Like self-report methods, observational methods include both unstructured methods that primarily yield qualitative data and structured approaches that yield mostly quantitative data. Both approaches are discussed in this chapter. First, however, we present an overview of some general issues.

OBSERVATIONAL ISSUES

When nurse researchers observe an event—such as a nurse interacting with a patient—they have to know (at least broadly) what to observe. Researchers cannot absorb and record an infinite number of details; they need guidelines about how to focus the observations. In this section, we describe the versatility of observational methods and note some considerations for observing phenomena.

Phenomena Amenable to Observations

Nurse researchers make observations of human behaviors or the characteristics of individuals, events, environments, or objects. The following list of observable phenomena is suggestive rather than exhaustive:

1. *Characteristics and conditions of individuals.* A lot of information about people's attributes and states can be gathered by direct observation, including both enduring traits such as physical appearance and more temporary conditions such as rashes. (Physiologic conditions can be observed either directly through the senses, or with the aid of observational apparatus, such as a radiograph.) Examples of this class of observable phenomena include patients' sleep—wake state, the presence of edema in congestive heart failure, alopecia during cancer chemotherapy, or symptoms of infusion phlebitis in hospitalized patients.

 Example of observing personal characteristics:
Whittington, Patrick, and Roberts (2000) reported on a national study of pressure ulcer prevalence and incidence in acute care hospitals. Some 17,560 patients in 116 hospitals were observed and assessed by RNs for stage I to stage IV pressure ulcers.

2. *Activities and behavior.* Many actions are amenable to observation and constitute valuable data for nurse researchers. Activities and behavior that indicate health status or physical and emotional functioning are particularly important. The following kinds of activities or behaviors lend themselves to observational

study: patients' eating habits, length and number of visits by friends and relatives to hospitalized patients, and aggressive actions among children in the hospital playroom.

Example of observing behavior:
Twomey, Bevis, and McGibbon (2001) observed bicycle riders' risk-taking behavior regarding the use of bicycle helmets.

3. *Skill attainment and performance.* Nurses are routinely called on to develop skills among clients. Skill attainment is often demonstrated behaviorally, and is therefore amenable to observation. As examples, nurse researchers might want to observe the following kinds of behavior: the ability of stroke patients to scan a food tray if homonymous hemianopia is present, diabetic patients' skill in testing their urine for sugar and acetone, or infants' ability to suck when positioned for breastfeeding. Nurses' on-the-job performance and decision-making behaviors are also of interest to researchers.

Example of observing performance:
Gerdtz and Bucknall (2001) studied the decision tasks performed by Australian triage nurses when making acuity assessments, through observation of 26 nurses performing 404 occasions of triage.

4. *Verbal communication.* The content and structure of people's conversations are readily observable, easy to record, and, thus, a potential data source. Among the kinds of verbal communications that a nurse researcher may be interested in observing are information given by nurses to patients, exchange of information among nurses at change-of-shift report, and conversations among nursing home residents.

Example of observing verbal communication:
Payne, Hardey, and Coleman (2000) conducted an ethnographic study in which they observed the interactions between nurses caring for acutely ill elderly patients during handovers at change-of-shift.

5. *Nonverbal communication.* People communicate their attitudes and emotions in many ways

other than just with words. The kinds of nonverbal behavior amenable to observational methods include facial expressions, touch, posture, gestures and other body movements, crying or laughing, and extralinguistic behavior (i.e., the manner in which people speak, aside from the content, such as the intonation, loudness, and continuity of the speech).

Example of observing nonverbal communication:
Butt and Kisilevsky (2000) studied the behavioral effect of music on preterm infants' recovery from heel lance. Infant pain was assessed based on observations of such nonverbal behavior as facial expressions.

6. *Environmental characteristics.* People's surroundings can affect their behavior, and numerous studies have explored the relationship between observable environmental attributes on the one hand and human actions and characteristics on the other. Examples of observable environmental attributes include hospital noise levels, nursing home decor, safety hazards in an elementary school classroom, or the cleanliness of the homes in a community.

Example of observing environmental characteristics:
Kisida, Holditch-Davis, Miles, and Carlson (2001) observed unsafe environmental hazards and unsafe caregiving practices in the homes of premature children at 3 years of age.

Units of Observation

In selecting behaviors, attributes, or situations to be observed, researchers must decide what constitutes a unit. There are two basic approaches, which actually are end points of a continuum. The **molar approach** entails observing large units of behavior and treating them as a whole. For example, psychiatric nurse researchers might study patient mood swings. An entire constellation of verbal and nonverbal behaviors might be construed as signaling aggressive behaviors, for example. Most qualitative observational studies rely on observations that are reasonably molar. At the other extreme, the **molecular approach** uses small, highly specific behaviors as observational units. Each movement, action, gesture, or phrase is treated as a separate entity. The choice of approaches depends mostly on the nature of the research problem. The molar approach is more susceptible to observer errors because of greater ambiguity in what is being observed. On the other hand, in reducing observations to concrete, specific elements, investigators may fail to understand how small elements work in concert in a behavior pattern.

The Observer–Observed Relationship

Researchers can interact with individuals in an observational setting to varying degrees. The issue of the relationship between observers and those observed is important and has stirred much controversy. Two important aspects of this issue concern *intervention* and *concealment*. The decisions researchers make in establishing a strategy for these considerations should be based on an understanding of ethical and methodologic implications.

Observational studies may involve an experimental intervention of the type described in Chapter 8, which deals with experimental design. For example, a nurse researcher may observe patients' postoperative behaviors after an intervention designed to improve the patients' ability to cough and breathe after surgery. Sometimes, however, observational researchers intervene to structure research settings (called **directed settings**) without introducing an experimental treatment (i.e., without manipulating the independent variable). For instance, researchers sometimes stage a situation to provoke behaviors. Certain activities are rare in naturalistic settings, making it inexpedient to wait for them to happen. For example, several studies have examined the behavior of bystanders in crises. Because crises are unpredictable and infrequent, investigators have staged emergencies to observe helping behavior (or lack of it) among onlookers. Such studies, which are high on the intervention dimension, may be practical when there is little

opportunity to observe activities or events as they unfold naturally; however, such studies may lack external validity.

The second dimension that concerns the observer–observed relationship is the degree to which participants are aware of the observation and their role in a study. In naturalistic settings, researchers are sometimes concerned that their presence, if known, would alter behaviors under observation. Therefore, observers sometimes adopt a completely passive role, attempting insofar as possible to become unobtrusive bystanders. Behavioral distortions that result from the known presence of observers are **reactive measurement effects** or, more simply, **reactivity**. Reactivity can be eliminated if the observations are made without people's knowledge, through some type of concealment. In some directed settings, concealed observations can be accomplished through the use of one-way mirrors.

Concealment offers another distinct advantage, even beyond the elimination of reactivity. Some people might deny researchers the opportunity to observe them altogether, so that the alternative to concealed observation is no observation at all. Total concealment, however, is difficult to attain except in formal or highly active observational settings. Furthermore, concealed observation, without the knowledge and consent of those observed, is ethically problematic (see Chapter 7).

Sometimes participants are aware of the presence of observers, but not of their underlying motives, which gives researchers access to more in-depth information than is usually possible with total concealment. Because the researcher is not totally concealed, there also may be fewer ethical problems. Nevertheless, the issues of subject deception and failure to obtain informed voluntary consent remain thorny ones. Furthermore, a serious drawback of this second approach is the possibility that the interaction between observers and the observed will alter participants' behavior. Even when the observed individuals are unaware of being study participants, there is always a risk that researchers' presence will alter their normal activities or conversations.

Researchers doing observational research will be confronted with methodologic, substantive, or ethical issues all along the concealment and intervention dimensions.

QUALITATIVE OBSERVATIONAL METHODS: PARTICIPANT OBSERVATION

Qualitative researchers collect unstructured or loosely structured observational data for some studies, often as an important supplement to self-report data. The aim of their research is to understand the behaviors and experiences of people as they actually occur in naturalistic settings. Qualitative researchers seek to observe people and their environments with a minimum of structure and interference.

Unstructured observational data are most often gathered in field settings through a process known as **participant observation**. Participant observers participate in the functioning of the social group under investigation and strive to observe, ask questions, and record information within the contexts, structures, and symbols that are relevant to group members. Bogdan (1972) defines participant observation as " ... research characterized by a prolonged period of intense social interaction between the researcher and the subjects, in the milieu of the latter, during which time data ... are unobtrusively and systematically collected" (p. 3).

 Example of a participant observation study:

Pierce (2001) conducted a study focusing on expressions of spirituality by African-American family caregivers of stroke patients. Pierce interviewed 8 key informants on 3 occasions and 16 secondary informants once, and in all cases made observations. In addition, she conducted several participatory observation sessions of 4 to 6 hours each, during which time she assisted in the caregiving process.

Not all qualitative observational research is *participant* observation (i.e., with observations occurring from *within* the group under study). Some unstructured observations involve watching and recording unfolding behaviors without the observers

interacting with participants in activities. If a key research objective, however, is to learn how group interactions and activities give meaning to human behaviors and experiences, then participant observation is the appropriate method. The members of any group or culture are influenced by assumptions they take for granted, and observers can, through active participation as members, gain access to these assumptions. Participant observation is used by grounded theory researchers, ethnographers, and researchers with ideological perspectives.

 Example of a qualitative nonparticipant observation study:

Lotzkar and Bottorff (2001) used ethologic analysis to study the development of a nurse–patient relationship. Eight patients were observed by videotape (continuous videotaping for 72 hours); their interactions with nurses were then analyzed qualitatively.

The Observer—Participant Role in Participant Observation

The role that observers play in the groups under study is important because the observers' social position determines what they are likely to see. That is, the behaviors that are likely to be available for observation depend on observers' position in a network of relations.

Leininger (1985) describes a participant observer's role as evolving through a four-phase sequence:

1. Primarily observation
2. Primarily observation with some participation
3. Primarily participation with some observation
4. Reflective observation

In the initial phase, researchers observe and listen to those under study to obtain a broad view of the situation. This phase allows both observers and the observed to "size up" each other, to become acquainted, and to become more comfortable interacting. This first phase is sometimes referred to as "learning the ropes." In the next phase, observation is enhanced by a modest degree of participation. By participating in the group's activities, researchers can study not only people's behaviors, but also people's reactions to them. In phase 3, researchers strive to become more active participants, learning by the actual experience of doing rather than just by watching and listening. In phase 4, researchers reflect on the total process of what transpired and how people interacted with and reacted to them.

Junker (1960) described a somewhat different continuum that does not assume an evolving process: complete participant, participant as observer, observer as participant, and complete observer. Complete participants conceal their identity as researchers, entering the group ostensibly as regular members. For example, a nurse researcher might accept a job as a clinical nurse with the express intent of studying, in a concealed fashion, some aspect of the clinical environment. At the other extreme, complete observers do not attempt participation in the group's activities, but rather make observations as outsiders. At both extremes, observers may have difficulty asking probing questions—albeit for different reasons. Complete participants may arouse suspicion if they make inquiries not congruent with a total participant role, and complete observers may not have personal access to, or the trust of, those being observed.

Most observational field work lies in between these two extremes and shifts over time in emphasis between observation and participation, as noted by Leininger. Junker described participants as observers as marked by "subjectivity and sympathy"; observers as participants adopt a somewhat more detached stance characterized by "objectivity and sympathy."

TIP: Being a fully participating member of a group does not *necessarily* offer the best perspective for studying a phenomenon—just as being an actor in a play does not offer the most advantageous view of the performance.

Getting Started

Observers must overcome at least two initial hurdles: gaining entrée into the social group or culture under study, and establishing rapport and developing trust within the social group. Without gaining entrée, the study cannot proceed; but without the group's

trust, researchers could be restricted to what Leininger (1985) refers to as "front stage" knowledge, that is, information distorted by the group's protective facades. The observer's goal is to "get back stage"—to learn about the realities of the group's experiences and behaviors. This section discusses some practical and interpersonal aspects of getting started in the field.

Gaining an Overview

Before fieldwork begins, or in the very earliest stage of fieldwork, it is usually useful to gather some written or pictorial descriptive information that provides an overview of the setting. In an institutional setting, for example, it is helpful to obtain a floor plan, an organizational chart, an annual report, and so on. Then, a preliminary personal tour of the setting should be undertaken to gain familiarity with its ambiance and to note major activities, social groupings, transactions, and events.

In community studies, ethnographers sometimes conduct what is referred to as a **windshield survey**, which involves an intensive tour (usually in an automobile, and hence the name) to "map" important features of the community under study. Such community mapping can include documenting community resources (e.g., churches, businesses, public transportation, community centers), community liabilities (e.g., vacant lots, empty stores, public housing units), and social and environmental characteristics (e.g., condition of streets and buildings, traffic patterns, types of signs, children playing in public places).

Example of a windshield survey:
Carruth, Gilbert, and Lewis (1997) studied environmental health hazards in a southern community, and conducted a windshield survey to assess the residential community, analyze drainage pathways away from the site, and get an overview of outdoor activity patterns.

Gaining Entrée

In many cases, researchers need permission to conduct the study, or need access to people who can make important introductions. Gaining entrée typically requires strong interpersonal skills, and knowledge about who to approach as the "gate-keepers" to the community or group. Wilson (1985) noted that successful participant observation research may require researchers to "go through channels, cultivate relationships, contour [their] appearances, withhold evaluative judgments, and be as unobtrusive and charming as possible" (p. 376). Participant observers must learn to take full advantage of anyone who can help in gaining entrée. Evaneshko (1985) offers excellent advice on strategies for gaining entrée in qualitative nursing studies.

TIP: Bear in mind that no matter how enthusiastic and persuasive you are about your project, no matter how sincere and credible you appear, gatekeepers may express numerous concerns because you are asking permission to participate in private and possibly hidden activities and events. Prepare in advance by rehearsing how to respond to the many questions gatekeepers are likely to ask. You will almost always need to be prepared for the question, "What's in it for us?"

Establishing Rapport

After researchers obtain permissions or information about contacts to make from gatekeepers, the next step is to enter the field. In some cases it may be possible just to "blend in" or ease into a social group, but often researchers walk into a "head-turning" situation in which there is considerable curiosity because they stand out as strangers. Participant observers often find that, for their own comfort level and also for that of participants, it is best to have a brief, simple explanation about their presence. Except in rare cases, deception is neither necessary nor recommended, but vagueness has many advantages. People rarely want to know *exactly* what researchers are studying, they simply want an introduction and enough information to satisfy their curiosity and erase any suspicions they may have about the researchers' ulterior motives.

After initial introductions with members of the group, it is usually best to keep a fairly low profile. At the beginning, researchers are not yet familiar with the customs, language, and norms of the group, and it

is critical to learn these things. Politeness and friendliness are, of course, essential, but effusive socializing is not appropriate at the early stages of field work.

TIP: At this point, your job is to listen intently and learn what it is going to take to fit into the group, that is, what you need to do to become accepted as a member. To the extent possible, you should downplay any expertise you might have, because you do not want to distance yourself from participants. Your overall goal is to gain people's trust and to move relationships to a deeper level.

As rapport is developed and trust is established, researchers can begin to play a more active participatory role and to collect observational data in earnest.

Gathering Unstructured Observational Data

Participant observers typically place few restrictions on the nature of the data collected, in keeping with the goal of minimizing observer-imposed meanings and structure. Nevertheless, participant observers often have a broad plan for the types of information to be gathered. Among the aspects likely to be considered relevant are the following:

1. *The physical setting.* What are the main features of the physical setting? What is the context within which human behavior unfolds? What types of behaviors and characteristics are promoted (or constrained) by the physical environment? How does the environment contribute to what is happening?

2. *The participants.* What are the characteristics of the people being observed? How many people are there? What are their roles? Who is given free access to the setting—who "belongs"? What brings these people together?

3. *Activities and interactions.* What is going on—what are people doing and saying, and how are they behaving? Is there a discernible progression of activities? How do people interact with one another? What methods do they use to communicate, and how frequently do they do so? What is the tone of their communications? What type

of emotions do they show during their interactions? How are participants interconnected to one another or to activities underway?

4. *Frequency and duration.* When did the activity or event begin, and when is it scheduled to end? How much time has elapsed? Is the activity a recurring one, and if so, how regularly does it recur? How typical of such activities is the one that is under observation?

5. *Precipitating factors.* Why is the event or interaction happening? What contributes to how the event or interaction unfolds?

6. *Organization.* How is the event or interaction organized? How are relationships structured? What norms or rules are in operation?

7. *Intangible factors.* What did *not* happen (especially if it ought to have happened)? Are participants saying one thing verbally but communicating other messages nonverbally? What types of things were disruptive to the activity or situation?

Clearly, this is far more information than can be absorbed in a single session (and not all categories may be relevant to the research question). However, this framework provides a starting point for thinking about observational possibilities while in the field.

TIP: When we enter a social setting in our everyday lives, we unconsciously process many of the questions on this list. Usually, however, we do not consciously *attend* to our observations and impressions in any systematic way, and are not careful about making note of the details that contribute to our impressions. This is precisely what participant observers must learn to do.

Spradley (1980) distinguishes three levels of observation that typically occur during fieldwork. The first level is **descriptive observation**, which tends to be broad and is used to help observers figure out what is going on. During these descriptive observations, researchers make every attempt to observe as much as possible. Later in the inquiry, observers do **focused observations** on more carefully selected events and interactions. Based on the research aims and on what has been learned from

the descriptive observations, participant observers begin to focus more sharply on key aspects of the setting. From these focused observations, they may develop a system for organizing observations, such as a taxonomy or category system. Finally, **selective observations** are the most highly focused, and are undertaken to facilitate comparisons between categories or activities. Spradley describes these levels as analogous to a funnel, with an increasingly narrow and more systematic focus.

While in the field, participant observers have to make decisions about how to sample observations and to select observational locations. **Single positioning** means staying in a single location for a period to observe behaviors and transactions in that location. **Multiple positioning** involves moving around the site to observe behaviors from different locations. **Mobile positioning** involves following a person throughout a given activity or period. It is usually useful to use a combination of positioning approaches in selecting observational locations.

Because participant observers cannot spend a lifetime in one site and because they cannot be in more than one place at a time, observation is almost always supplemented with information obtained in unstructured interviews or conversations. For example, informants may be asked to describe what went on in a meeting that the observer was unable to attend, or to describe events that occurred before the observer entered the field. In such a case, the informant functions as the observer's observer.

Recording Observations

Participant observers may find it tempting to put more emphasis on the *participation* and *observation* parts of their research than on the recording of those activities. Without systematic daily recording of the observational data, however, the project will flounder. Observational information cannot be trusted to memory; it must be diligently recorded as soon after the observations as possible.

Types of Observational Records

The most common forms of record-keeping in participant observation are logs and field notes, but photographs and videotapes may also be used. A **log** (or **field diary**) is a daily record of events and conversations in the field. A log is a historical listing of how researchers have spent their time and can be used for planning purposes, for keeping track of expenses, and for reviewing what work has already been completed. Box 16-1 presents an example of a log entry from Beck's (2002) study of mothers of multiples.

Field notes are much broader, more analytic, and more interpretive than a simple listing of occurrences. Field notes represent the participant observer's efforts to record information and also to synthesize and understand the data. The next sections discuss the content of field notes and the process of writing them.

The Content of Field Notes

Participant observers' field notes contain a narrative account of what is happening in the field; they serve as the data for analysis. Most "field" notes are not written while observers are literally in the field but rather are written after an observational session in the field has been completed.

Field notes are usually lengthy and time-consuming to prepare. Observers need to discipline themselves to provide a wealth of detail, the meaning and importance of which may not emerge for weeks. Descriptions of what has transpired must include enough contextual information about time, place, and actors to portray the situation fully. The term **thick description** is often used to characterize the goal of participation observers' field notes.

 TIP: Especially in the early stages of fieldwork, a general rule of thumb is this: When in doubt, write it down.

Field notes are both descriptive and reflective. **Descriptive notes** (or **observational notes**) are objective descriptions of observed events and conversations; information about actions, dialogue, and context are recorded as completely and objectively as possible.

Reflective notes, which document the researcher's personal experiences, reflections, and progress while in the field, can serve a number of different purposes:

- **Methodologic notes** are reflections about the strategies and methods used in the observations. Sometimes participant observers do things that do not "work," and methodologic notes document their thoughts about new strategies and reasons why they might be needed—or thoughts about why a strategy that was used was

 BOX 16.1 Example of a Log Entry

Log entry for Mothers of Multiples Support Group Meeting (Beck, 2002)
July 15, 1999 10–11:30 AM

This is my fourth meeting that I have attended. Nine mothers came this morning with their twins. One other woman attended. She was pregnant with twins. She came to the support group for advice from the other mothers regarding such issues as what type of stroller to buy, etc. All the moms sat on the floor with their infants placed on blankets on the floor next to them. Toddlers and older children played together off to the side with a box of toys. I sat next to a mom new to the group with her twin 4-month-old girls. I helped her hold and feed one of the twins. On my other side was a mom who had signed up at the last meeting to participate in my study. I hadn't called her yet to set up an appointment. She asked how my research was going. We then set up an appointment for next Thursday at 10 AM at her home for me to interview her. The new mother that I sat next to also was eager to participate in the study. In fact she said we could do the interview right after the meeting ends today but I couldn't, due to another meeting. We scheduled an interview appointment for next Thursday at 1 PM. I also set up a third appointment for an interview for next week with I.K. for Monday at 1 PM. She had participated in an earlier study of mine. She came right over to me this morning at the support group meeting.

especially effective. Methodologic notes also can provide instructions or reminders about how subsequent observations will be made.

- **Theoretical notes** (or **analytical notes**) document researchers' thoughts about how to make sense of what is going on. These notes are the researchers' efforts to attach meaning to observations while in the field, and serve as a starting point for subsequent analysis.
- **Personal notes** are comments about researchers' own feelings while in the field. Almost inevitably, field experiences give rise to personal emotions,

and challenge researchers' assumptions. It is essential to reflect on such feelings because there is no other way to determine whether the feelings are influencing what is being observed or what is being done in the participant role. Personal notes can also contain reflections relating to ethical dilemmas and possible conflicts.

Box 16-2 presents examples of various types of field notes from Beck's (2002) study of mothering multiples.

Reflective notes are typically not integrated into the descriptive notes, but are kept separately as

BOX 16.2 Example of Field Notes: Mothering Multiples Grounded Theory Study

Observational Notes: O.L. attended the mothers of multiples support group again this month but she looked worn out today. She wasn't as bubbly as she had been at the March meeting. She explained why she wasn't doing as well this month. She and her husband had just found out that their house has lead-based paint in it. Both twins do have increased lead levels. She and her husband are in the process of buying a new home.

Theoretical Notes: So far all the mothers have stressed the need for routine in order to survive the first year of caring for twins. Mothers, however, have varying definitions of routine. I.R. had the firmest routine with her twins. B.L. is more flexible with her routine, i.e., the twins are always fed at the same time but aren't put down for naps or bed at night at the same time. Whenever one of the twins wants to go to sleep is fine with her. B.L. does have a daily routine in regards to housework. For example, when the twins are down in the morning for a nap, she makes their bottles up for the day (14 bottles total).

Methodologic Notes: The first sign-up sheet I passed around at the Mothers of Multiples Support Group for women to sign up to participate in interviews for my grounded theory study only consisted of 2 columns: one for the mother's name and one for her telephone number. I need to revise this sign-up sheet to include extra columns for the age of the multiples, the town where the mother lives, and for older siblings and their ages. My plan is to start interviewing mothers with multiples around one year of age so that the moms can reflect back over the process of mothering their infants for the first 12 months of their lives.

Right now I have no idea of the ages of the infants of the mothers who signed up to be interviewed. I will need to call the nurse in charge of this support group to find out the ages.

Personal Notes: Today was an especially challenging interview. The mom had picked the early afternoon for me to come to her home to interview her because that is the time her 2-year-old son would be napping. When I arrived at her house her 2-year-old ran up to me and said hi. The mom explained that he had taken an earlier nap that day and that he would be up during the interview. So in the living room with us during our interview were her 2 twin daughters (3 months old) swinging in the swings and her 2-year-old son. One of the twins was quite cranky for the first half hour of the interview. During the interview the 2-year-old sat on my lap and looked at the two books I had brought as a little present. If I didn't keep him occupied with the books, he would keep trying to reach for the microphone of the tape recorder.

From Beck, C.T. (2002). Releasing the pause button: Mothering twins during the first year of life. Qualitative Health Research, 12, 593–608.

parallel notes; they may be maintained in a journal or series of self-memos. Strauss and Corbin (1990) argue that these reflective memos or journals help researchers to achieve analytic distance from the actual data, and therefore play a critical role in the project's success.

> **TIP:** Personal notes should begin even before entering the field. By writing down your feelings, assumptions, and expectations, you will have a baseline against which to compare feelings and experiences that emerge in the field.

The Process of Writing Field Notes

The success of any participant observation study depends heavily on the quality of the field notes. This section describes some techniques for enhancing their quality.

A fundamental issue concerns the timing of field note preparation: They should be written as soon as possible after an observation is made because memory is bound to fail if there is too long a delay. The longer the interval between an observation and field note preparation, the greater the risk of losing or distorting the data. If the delay is long, intricate details will be forgotten; moreover, memory of what was observed may be biased by things that happen subsequently.

> **TIP:** Be sure not to talk to anyone about your observation before you have had a chance to write up the observational notes. Such discussions could color what you record.

Participant observers cannot usually write their field notes while they are in the field observing, in part because this would distract them from their job of being keen observers, and also because it would undermine their role as ordinary group participants. Researchers must develop the skill of making detailed mental notes that can later be committed to a permanent record. In addition, observers usually try to jot down unobtrusively a phrase or sentence that will later serve as a reminder of an event, conversation, or impression. Many experienced field workers use the tactic of frequent trips to the bathroom to record these **jottings**, either in a small notebook or

perhaps into a recording device. With the widespread use of cell phones, researchers can also excuse themselves to make a call, and "phone in" their jottings to an answering machine. Observers use the jottings and mental recordings to develop more extensive field notes.

It is important to schedule enough time for properly recording field notes after an observation. An hour of observation can take 3 or 4 hours to record, so advance planning is essential. This also means that observation sessions must be relatively brief.

> **TIP:** Try to find a quiet place for recording field notes, preferably a location where you can work undisturbed for several hours. Because most researchers now record field notes on computers, the place will ideally be able to accommodate computer equipment.

Observational field notes obviously need to be as complete and detailed as possible. This in turn means that hundreds of pages of field notes typically will be created, and so systems need to be developed for recording and managing them. For example, each entry should have the date and time the observation was made, the location, and the name of the observer (if several are working together as a team). It is useful to give observational sessions a name that will trigger a memory (e.g., "Emotional Outburst by a Patient With Ovarian Cancer").

Thought also needs to be given to how to record participants' dialogue. The goal is to record conversations as accurately as possible, but it is not always possible to maintain verbatim records because tape recordings are seldom made if researchers are trying to maintain a stance as regular participants. Systems need to be developed to distinguish different levels of accuracy in recording dialogue (e.g., by using quotation marks and italics for true verbatim recordings, and a different designation for paraphrasings).

Observation, participation, and record-keeping are exhausting, labor-intensive activities. It is important to establish the proper pace of these activities to ensure the highest possible quality notes for analysis.

Evaluation of Participant Observation

Participant observation can provide a deeper and richer understanding of human behaviors and social situations than is possible with more structured procedures. Participant observation is particularly valuable for its ability to "get inside" a particular situation and lead to a more complete understanding of its complexities. Furthermore, this approach is inherently flexible and therefore gives observers the freedom to reconceptualize problems after becoming more familiar with the situation. Participant observation is the preferred method for answering questions about intangible phenomena that are difficult for insiders to explain or articulate because these phenomena are taken for granted (e.g., group norms, cultural patterns, approaches to problem-solving).

However, like all research methods, there are potential problems with the approach that need to be considered. The risk of observer bias and observer influence are prominent difficulties. Observers may lose objectivity in viewing and recording actual observations; they may also inappropriately sample events and situations to be observed. Once researchers begin to participate in a group's activities, the possibility of emotional involvement becomes a salient concern. Researchers in their member role may fail to attend to many scientifically relevant aspects of the situation or may develop a myopic view on issues of importance to the group. Participant observation may thus be an unsuitable approach when the risk of identification is strong. Another important issue concerns the ethical dilemmas that often emerge in participant observation studies. Finally, participant observation depends more on the observational and interpersonal skills of the observer than do highly structured techniques—skills that may be difficult to cultivate.

On the whole, participant observation and other unstructured observational methods are extremely profitable for in-depth research in which researchers wish to develop a comprehensive conceptualization of phenomena within a social setting or culture. The more structured observational methods discussed next are better suited to the formal testing of research hypotheses.

OBSERVATIONAL METHODS: STRUCTURED OBSERVATIONS

Researchers using structured observational methods specify in advance the behaviors or events to be observed and use record-keeping forms that yield numeric information. Observers using structured observation are still required to make some inferences and exercise judgment, but they are restrained with regard to the kinds of phenomena that will be watched and recorded. The creativity of structured observation lies not in the observation itself but rather in the formulation of a system for accurately categorizing, recording, and encoding the observations. Because structured techniques depend on plans developed before the actual observation, they are not appropriate when researchers have limited knowledge about the phenomena under investigation.

Categories and Checklists

The most common approach to making structured observations consists of constructing a category system for classifying observed phenomena. A **category system** represents an attempt to designate in a systematic or quantitative fashion the qualitative behaviors and events transpiring in the observational setting.

Considerations in Using Category Systems

A critical requirement for a good category system is the careful and explicit definition of behaviors and characteristics to be observed. Each category must be explained in detail with an operational definition so that observers have relatively clearcut criteria for determining the occurrence of a specified phenomenon. Virtually all category systems do, however, require observers to make some inferences, although there is considerable variability on this dimension.

Example of low observer inference: Holditch-Davis, Miles, and Belyea (2000) studied the interactions between mothers and their premature infants during periods of feeding and nonfeeding in relation to infant behaviors, such as sleep—wake states. Observers categorized sleep—wake states into four mutually exclusive categories: Sleep, Drowse/Transition, Alert, and Active Waking. The "Alert" category, for example, was defined as follows: "The infant's eyes are open and scanning. Motor activity is typically low, particularly during the first two weeks, but the infant may be active" (p. 325).

In this system, assuming that observers were properly trained, relatively little inference would be required to allocate the infant's state to the proper category. Other category systems, however, require considerable inference.

Example of high observer inference:

The Abnormal Involuntary Movement Scale (AIMS), which was developed by the National Institute for Mental Health, has been used by several nurse researchers for studying tardive dyskinetic movements. For example, Herman (1997) evaluated the clinical response of chronic schizophrenic patients to clozapine treatment using AIMS. This scale contains such broad categories as "incapacitation due to abnormal movements."

In scales like the AIMS, even when categories are defined in detail, a heavy inferential burden is placed on observers. The decision concerning how much observer inference is appropriate depends on a number of factors, including the research purposes and the observers' skills. Beginning researchers are advised to construct or use category systems that require only a moderate degree of inference.

Another consideration in structured category systems concerns the exhaustiveness of what is to be observed. Some category systems are constructed to classify *all* observed behaviors of a certain type (e.g., all body movements) into mutually exclusive categories.

A contrasting technique is to develop a nonexhaustive system in which only *particular* types of behavior are categorized. For example, if we were observing children's aggressive behavior, we might develop such categories as "strikes another child," "calls other children names," "throws objects around the room," and so forth. In this category system,

many behaviors (all those that are nonaggressive) would not be classified. Such nonexhaustive systems are adequate for many research purposes, but they run the risk of providing data that are difficult to interpret. When a large number of observed behaviors are unclassified, investigators may have difficulty placing categorized behaviors into a proper context.

When observers use an exhaustive system— that is, when all behaviors of a certain type, such as verbal interaction, are observed and recorded— researchers must be careful to define categories so that observers know when one behavior ends and a new one begins. Another essential feature is that referent behaviors should be mutually exclusive. If overlapping categories are not eliminated, observers will have difficulty deciding how to classify a particular observation. The underlying assumption in the use of such a category system is that behaviors, events, or attributes that are allocated to a particular category are equivalent to every other behavior, event, or attribute in that same category.

Checklists for Exhaustive Systems

A category system is the basis for constructing a **checklist**, which is the instrument observers use to record observed phenomena. The checklist is usually formatted with the list of behaviors or events from the category system on the left and space for tallying the frequency or duration of occurrence of behaviors on the right. In complex social situations with multiple actors, the right-hand portion may be divided into panels according to characteristics of the actors (e.g., nurse/physician; male patients/ female patients) or by individual subjects' names or identification numbers.

The observers' task with an exhaustive checklist is to place all behaviors in only one category for each element. By **element**, we refer to either a unit of behavior, such as a sentence in a conversation, or to a time interval. To illustrate, suppose we were studying the problem-solving behavior of a group of public health workers discussing a new intervention for the homeless. Our category system involves eight categories: (1) seeks information, (2) gives information, (3) describes problem, (4) offers suggestion, (5) opposes suggestion, (6) supports suggestion, (7) summarizes, and (8) miscellaneous. Observers would be required to classify every group member's contribution—using, for example, each sentence as the element—in terms of one of these eight categories.

Another approach with exhaustive systems is to categorize relevant behaviors at regular time intervals. For example, in a category system for infants' motor activities, the researcher might use 15-second time intervals as the element; observers would categorize infant movements within 15-second periods. Checklists based on exhaustive category systems are demanding because the recording task is continuous.

Checklists for Nonexhaustive Systems

The second approach, which is sometimes referred to as a **sign system**, begins with a list of behaviors (or symptoms) that subjects may or may not manifest. The observer's task is to watch for instances of the behaviors on the list. When a behavior occurs, observers either place a checkmark beside the behavior category to designate its occurrence or make a cumulative tally of the number of times the behavior occurred. The resulting product is a kind of demography of events transpiring in the observational period. With this type of checklist, the observer does not classify *all* behaviors or characteristics of those being observed, but rather identifies the occurrence of particular ones.

Example of a nonexhaustive checklist: Feldt (2000) created a checklist to capture the occurrence of nonverbal pain indicators. Observers indicate whether, during an observational session, subjects demonstrate such pain-related behaviors as nonverbal vocal complaints (e.g., moans, grunts, sighs); facial grimaces (e.g., furrowed brow, clenched teeth); and bracing (clutching onto side rails). Behaviors unrelated to pain are not captured.

Rating Scales

The major alternative to a checklist for recording structured observations is a **rating scale** that requires observers to rate a phenomenon along a descriptive continuum that is typically bipolar. The ratings are quantified for subsequent statistical analysis.

Observers may be required to rate behaviors or events at specified intervals throughout the observational period (e.g., every 15 minutes), in much the same way that a checklist would be used. Alternatively, observers may rate entire events or transactions after observations are completed. Postobservation ratings require observers to integrate a number of activities and to judge which point on a scale most closely fits their interpretation of the overall situation. For example, suppose we were comparing the behaviors of nurses working in intensive care units with those of nurses in other units. After each 15-minute observation session, observers are asked to rate the perceived degree of tension of nurses in each unit. The rating scale might take the form of a graphic rating scale:

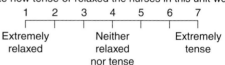

Rate how tense or relaxed the nurses in this unit were:

1 2 3 4 5 6 7

Extremely relaxed — Neither relaxed nor tense — Extremely tense

Global observational rating scales are often included at the end of structured interviews. For example, in a study of the health problems of nearly 4000 welfare mothers, interviewers were asked to observe and rate the safety of the home environment with regard to structural or potential health hazards to the children on five-point scales, from completely safe to extremely unsafe (Polit, London, & Martinez, 2001).

Rating scales can also be used as an extension of checklists, in which observers not only record the occurrence of a behavior but also rate some qualitative aspect of it, such as its magnitude or intensity. A particularly good example is Weiss's (1992) Tactile Interaction Index (TII) for observing patterns of interpersonal touch. The TII comprises four dimensions: location (part of body touched, such as arm, abdomen); action (the specific gesture or movement used, such as grabbing, hitting, patting); duration (temporal length of the touch); and intensity. Observers using the index must both classify the nature and duration of the touch *and* rate the intensity on a four-point scale: light, moderate, strong, and deep. When rating scales are coupled with a category scheme in this fashion, considerable information about a phenomenon can be obtained, but it places an immense burden on observers, particularly if there is extensive activity.

TIP: It is usually useful to spend a period of time with study participants before the actual observations and recording of data. Having a warm-up period helps to relax people (especially if audio or video equipment is being used) and can be helpful to observers (e.g., if participants have a linguistic style to which observers must adjust, such as a strong regional accent).

Constructing Versus Borrowing Structured Observational Instruments

The development, testing, and refinement of a new observational instrument may require weeks or months of effort, particularly if the system is intended for use by other researchers or clinicians. In some cases, researchers have no alternative but to design new observational instruments if existing ones are inappropriate. As with self-report instruments, however, we encourage researchers to explore the literature fully for potentially usable observational instruments. The use of an existing system not only saves considerable work but also facilitates comparisons among investigations.

A few source books describe available observational instruments for certain research applications. For example, the reference books by Frank-Stromberg and Olsen (1997) and Strickland and Waltz (1988), which describe instruments for measuring variables of relevance to nursing, include some observational instruments. The best source for such instruments, however, is recent research literature on the study topic. For example, if you wanted to conduct an observational study of infant pain, a good place to begin would be recent research on this or similar topics to obtain information on how infant pain was operationalized.

Table 16-1 provides examples of some concepts for which observational instruments have been developed and lists a recent nursing study that used these instruments. Note that many of these instruments focus on phenomena for which self-reports are not an option, such as behaviors and characteristics of infants, young children, and the very old.

Sampling for Structured Observations

Researchers must decide how and when structured observational instruments will be used. Observational sampling is sometimes needed to obtain representative examples of behaviors without having to observe for prolonged periods. Note that observational sampling concerns the selection of *behaviors* to be observed, not the selection of study participants.

One method is **time sampling**, which involves the selection of time periods during which observations will occur. The time frames may be systematically selected (e.g., 30 seconds at 2-minute intervals), selected at random, or selected by a quota system. As an example, suppose we were studying mothers' interactions with their handicapped children. Experimental group mothers have received instruction for addressing their conflict over their children's dependence—independence needs, whereas control group mothers have not. To examine program effects, mother—child interactions are observed in a playground setting. During a 1-hour observation period, we sample moments to observe, rather than observing the entire session. Let us say that observations are made in 3-minute intervals. If we used a systematic sampling approach, we would observe for 3 minutes, then cease observing for a prespecified period, say 3 minutes. With this scheme, a total of ten 3-minute observations would be made. A second approach is to sample randomly 3-minute periods from the total of 20 such periods in an hour; a third is to use all 20 periods. The decision with regard to the length and number of periods for creating a suitable sample must be made in accordance with research aims. In

TABLE 16.1 Examples of Observational Instruments Used by Nurse Researchers

CONCEPT	RESEARCH EXAMPLE	INSTRUMENT
Aggression in elders	Rateau, 2000	Ryden Aggression Scale (RAS-2)
Confusion in elders	Cacchione, 2002 Rateau, 2000	NEECHAM Confusion Scale Clinical Assessment of Confusion-A
Competence in elders	Mallick & Whipple, 2000	Multidimensional Observation Scale for Elderly Subjects (MOSES)
Functional ability	Roberts et al., 1999	Barthel Index for Functional Status
Home environment quality for children	Gaffney, Barndt-Maglio, Myers, & Kollar, 2002	Home Observation for Measurement of the Environment (HOME)
Infant behavior organization/state	Harrison, Williams, Berbaum, Stern, & Leeper, 2000 Medoff-Cooper McGrath, & Bilker, 2000 Neu, Browne, & Vojir, 2000	Brazelton Neonatal Behavioral Assessment Scale Anderson Behavioral State Scale (ABSS) Assessment Behavioral Systems Organization Scale (ABSO)
Infant development	Holditch-Davis, Docherty, Miles, & Burchinal, 2001	Bayley Scales of Infant Development (BSID)
Mother–infant interaction	Macke, 2001 Gaffney et al., 2002	Nursing Child Assessment Feeding Scale (NCAFS) NCAST Teaching Total Parent Scale
Pain in children	LaMontagne, Wells, Hepworth, Johnson, & Manes, 1999	Observational Scale of Behavioral Distress
Quality of nursing care	Archibong, 1999	Quality of Patient Care Scale (QualPacs)
Sleep–wake patterns	Thomas, 2000	Nursing Child Assessment Sleep Activity Record (NCASA)

establishing time units, a key consideration is determining a psychologically meaningful time frame. A good deal of pretesting and experimentation with different sampling plans may be necessary.

Example of time sampling:
Kolanowski, Litaker, and Catalano (2002) conducted a case study of the emotional well-being of a man with dementia. Observers rated his affect

and his mood over a 35-day period. Observations were made in 20-minute sessions, sampling behaviors in three time periods: morning (10 AM), afternoon (2 PM), and evening (6 PM).

Event sampling is a second system for obtaining observations. This approach uses integral behaviors or events for observation. Event sampling requires that the investigator either have some knowledge about the occurrence of events, or be in a position to await (or arrange) their occurrence. Examples of integral events suitable for event sampling include shift changes of nurses in a hospital, cast removals of pediatric patients, and cardiac arrests in the emergency department. This approach is preferable to time sampling when the events of interest are infrequent and are at risk of being missed if time sampling is used. Event sampling also has the advantage that situations are observed in their entirety rather than being fragmented into segments. Still, when behaviors and events are frequent, time sampling has the virtue of enhancing the representativeness of observed behaviors.

Example of event sampling:
Neu, Browne, and Vojir (2000) made observations of infants' behavior during two different types of transfer techniques used in skin-to-skin care: nurse transfer and parent transfer.

Structured Observations by Nonresearch Observers

The research discussed thus far involves observations made and recorded by researchers or observer assistants. Sometimes, however, researchers ask others not connected with the research team to provide structured observational data, based on their observations of the characteristics, activities, and behaviors of others. This method has much in common (in terms of format and scoring) with the self-report scales described in Chapter 15; the primary difference is that the person completing the scale is asked to describe the attributes and behaviors of another person, based on their observations of that person. For example, a mother might be asked to describe the behavior problems of her preschool child or staff

nurses might be asked to evaluate the functional capacity of nursing home residents.

Obtaining observational data from nonresearchers has practical advantages: It is economical compared with using trained observers. For example, observers might have to watch children for hours or days to describe the nature and intensity of behavior problems, whereas parents or teachers could do this readily. Some behaviors might never lend themselves to outsider observation because of reactivity, occurrence in private situations, or infrequency (e.g., sleepwalking).

On the other hand, such methods may have the same problems as self-report scales (e.g., response-set bias) in addition to observer bias. Observer bias may in some cases be extreme, such as often happens when parents are asked to provide information about their children. Nonresearch observers are typically not trained, and interobserver agreement usually cannot be determined. Thus, this approach has some problems but will inevitably continue to be used because, in many cases, there are no alternatives.

Example of observations by nonresearch personnel:
Hawranik and Strain (2001) studied the link between disruptive behaviors by elders with cognitive impairment and use of home care services. Disruptive behaviors were measured by having caregivers complete the Dementia Behavior Disturbance Scale, based on their observations of the elders.

MECHANICAL AIDS IN OBSERVATIONS

Our discussion has focused on observations made by observers directly through their visual and auditory senses. In this section, we look at mechanical aids that can be used to extend the human senses and secure permanent records of observational data.

The health care field has a rich array of observational equipment that makes available conditions or attributes that are ordinarily imperceptible. Nasal specula, stethoscopes, bronchoscopes, radiographic and imaging equipment, ultrasound technology, and a myriad of other medical instruments make it possible to gather observational information about people's health status and functioning for both clinical and research purposes.

In addition to equipment for enhancing physiologic observations, mechanical devices are available for recording behaviors and events, making analysis or categorization at a later time possible. When the behavior of interest is primarily auditory, tape recordings can be obtained and used as a permanent observational record. Transcripts from such recordings can then be prepared to facilitate the coding or classification process. Such equipment may not be feasible in participant observation studies, unless recordings can be done unobtrusively or unless events being recorded are public, such as lectures or speeches. Other technologic instruments to aid auditory observation have been developed, such as laser devices that are capable of recording sounds by being directed on a window to a room, and voice tremor detectors that are sensitive to stress. Auditory recordings can also be subjected to computerized speech software analysis to obtain objective quantitative measures of certain features of the recordings (e.g., volume, pitch).

When visual records are desired, videotapes can be used. In addition to being permanent, videotapes can capture complex behaviors that might elude notice by on-the-spot observers. Visual records are also more capable than the naked eye of capturing fine units of behavior, such as micromomentary facial expressions. Videotapes offer the possibility of checking the accuracy of coders or the recording skills of participant observers and so are useful as a training aid. Finally, it is often easier to conceal a camera than a human observer. Video records also have a number of drawbacks, some of which are fairly technical, such as lighting requirements, lens limitations, and so forth. Other problems result from the fact that the camera angle adopted could present a lopsided view of an event or situation. Also, some participants may be more self-conscious in front of a video camera than they would otherwise be. Still, for many applications, permanent visual records offer unparalleled opportunities to expand the range and scope of observational studies.

Ethnographers sometimes create videotapes and photographs, particularly to document physical settings and other visually relevant aspects of a culture (e.g., modes of dress). Harper (1994), who has written about visual methods as research tools, has discussed the importance of learning to see through the lenses of the culture under study, and to take photographs reflecting that viewpoint.

Also of interest is the growing technology for assisting with the encoding and recording of observations made directly by on-the-spot observers. For example, there is equipment that permits observers to enter observational data directly into a computer as the observation occurs, and in some cases, the equipment can record physiologic data concurrently. Such a system was used in an interesting nursing study by White, Williams, Alexander, Powell-Cope, and Conlon (1990), who tested whether a taped bedtime story read to hospitalized children by their parents would help to ease separation anxiety.

Example of the use of equipment:
Fuller (2000) studied infant behaviors in relation to levels of infant pain, and used a number of mechanical aids to measure key variables. The analyses were based on 3-minute videotaped segments of 64 infants categorized as being in no pain, mild pain, moderate pain, and severe pain. The videotapes were coded for the infants' behavioral state (e.g., consolability in response to comfort efforts) using behavioral analysis software. Four cry measures (e.g., mean cry energy) were derived from the sound tracks of the videotapes, which were analyzed using speech laboratory software and hardware.

OBSERVER BIASES

Although observation is an important method of data collection, both unstructured and structured observations are vulnerable to biases. Human perceptual errors and inadequacies are a continuous threat to the quality of obtained information. Observation and interpretation are demanding tasks, requiring attention, sensation, perception, and conception. To accomplish these activities in a completely objective fashion is challenging and perhaps impossible.

Several types of observational bias are especially common. One bias is the **enhancement of contrast effect**, in which observers distort observations in the direction of dividing content into clearcut entities. The converse effect—a bias toward **central tendency**—occurs when extreme events are distorted toward a middle ground. A series of biases are called **assimilatory**, in which observers distort observations in the direction of identity with previous inputs. This bias would have the effect of miscategorizing information in the direction of regularity and orderliness. Assimilation to the observer's expectations and attitudes also occurs.

Rating scales and other evaluative observations are also susceptible to bias. The **halo effect** is the tendency of observers to be influenced by one characteristic in judging other, unrelated characteristics. For example, if we formed a positive general impression of a person, we would probably be likely to rate that person as intelligent, loyal, and dependable simply because these traits are positively valued. Rating scales may reflect observers' personality. The **error of leniency** is the tendency for observers to rate everything positively, and the **error of severity** is the contrasting tendency to rate too harshly.

Biases are especially likely to operate when a high degree of observer inference is required. Although the degree of observer bias is not a function of the degree of structure imposed on observations, it is usually more difficult to assess the extent of bias when using unstructured methods.

The careful construction and pretesting of checklists and rating scales (with structured observation) and the proper training and preparation of observers are techniques that can play an important role in minimizing or estimating biases. If people are to become good instruments for collecting observational data, then they must be trained to observe in such a way that accuracy is maximized and biases are minimized. Even when the principal investigator is the primary observer, self-training and dry runs are essential. The setting during the trial period should resemble as closely as possible the settings that will be the focus of actual observations.

Ideally, training should include practice sessions during which the comparability of the observers' recordings is assessed. That is, two or more observers should watch a trial event or situation, and observational notes or coding should then be compared. Procedures for establishing the **interrater reliability** of structured observational instruments are described in Chapter 18.

TIP: Observers should observe behaviors and events in a neutral and nonjudgmental manner. People being observed are more likely to mask their emotions or behave atypically if they think they are being critically appraised. Even positive cues (such as nodding approval) should be withheld because approval may induce repetition of a behavior that might not otherwise have occurred. (Positive cues may be impossible to withhold in participant observation studies, which makes it all the more important for observers to be reflective and to keep personal notes.)

RESEARCH EXAMPLES

Two examples that illustrate observational research follow. The first is an example of a study in which participant observation was used, and the second is a quantitative study that used structured instruments.

Research Example of Participant Observation

Holt and Reeves (2001) conducted an ethnonursing study of caring practices designed to nurture hope in a rural village in the Dominican Republic. Participant observation and interviews with key informants were conducted over a 5-week period when the primary researcher was fully immersed in the culture of the Dominican Republic. One week was spent living with the nurses in this country and learning about the health care system. The remaining 4 weeks were spent in a mountain village living with one of the Dominican families.

Leininger's Observation–Participation–Reflection model was used to transition into different research roles. The first 2 weeks of the study were devoted primarily to pure observation, and to questioning villagers about their lives and medical care. However, some participation began in the first week of living in the village. The researcher observed all the activities she could, ranging from haircuts to preparing a spaghetti dinner. The researcher participated in a wide variety of social and religious events in the village, such as attending the Catholic Church at the center of the village.

A total of 13 small-group interviews were conducted with 45 villagers, who were identified as potential informants by a village leader who was also a health care worker. The researcher wrote field notes after each interview. Field notes were also used to capture and remember the events and conversations that occurred during the 5 weeks of participant observation.

The results of the study revealed five themes related to hope in this village in the foothills of the Dominican Republic. Holt and Reeves combined these five themes into a definition of hope for this group of Dominicans: "Hope is an essential but dynamic life force that grows out of faith in God; is supported by relationships, resources, and work; and results in the energy necessary to work for a desired future. Hope gives meaning and happiness" (pp. 128–129).

Research Example of Structured Observation

Holditch-Davis, Docherty, Miles, and Burchinal (2001) compared developmental outcomes and mother–infant interactions of infants with bronchopulmonary dysplasia (BPD) with those of other medically fragile infants. A wide variety of observational data were collected for 23 infants with BDP and 39 medically fragile infants without BDP.

Mother–infant interactions were observed in 1-hour observational sessions at multiple points in time: at the point of enrollment into the study, every 2 months during the infant's hospitalization, 1 month after discharge, and at 6 months and 12 months of age, corrected for prematurity. During the observations, the presence or absence of five maternal and five infant behaviors was recorded during each 10-second interval. The maternal behavior categories were medicalized caregiving, interaction, talk, positive affect, and negative affect; the infant categories were child alert, child vocalize, child negative affect, child talk, and child locomotion. Mothers' *positive*

affect, for example, was operationally defined as "The mother directs positive affect to the child (e.g., smiling, praising, or affectionate touching)" (p. 185). The behavior categories were not mutually exclusive; if a particular behavior occurred more than once in a 10-second interval, its incidence was counted, rather than its frequency. The final 10 variables were expressed as percentages of the total observation. That is, percentages were calculated as the number of 10-second periods in which a specified behavior occurred, divided by the number of 10-second periods in the observational session.

Holditch-Davis and her colleagues also collected other types of observational data. For example, the Bayley Scales of Infant Development, which depends on the test administrator's observations of the child, was used to measure infants' mental development. The research team had been trained by a psychologist in the administration of the Bayley Scales. The sessions were videotaped to ensure standard administration and proper scoring.

Finally, observers completed an instrument known as the Home Observation for Measurement of the Environment (HOME) scale. This widely used 45-item instrument relies on a semistructured interview with the mother, observation of mother–child interactions, and observations of cognitively stimulating material available in the home.

The results of the study indicated that there were no differences between the two groups of infants in any developmental outcomes or interactive behaviors. However, the mother's positive attention and higher-quality home environments were predictive of better developmental outcomes in both groups.

SUMMARY POINTS

- **Observational methods** are techniques for acquiring research data through the direct observation and recording of phenomena.
- Researchers focus on different **units of observation**. The **molar approach** entails observations of large segments of behaviors as integral units; the **molecular approach** treats small, specific actions as separate entities.
- Concealed observation, with people unaware that they are being observed or participating in a study, is done to reduce **reactivity** (i.e., behavioral distortions due to the presence of an observer).

- Observational **intervention** refers to the degree to which observers structure the observational setting in line with research demands, as opposed to being passive observers.
- Qualitative researchers collect unstructured observational data, often through **participant observation**. Participant observers obtain information about the dynamics of social groups or cultures within members' own frame of reference.
- In the initial phase of participant observation studies, researchers are primarily observers getting a preliminary understanding of the site. As time passes, researchers becomes more active participants.
- Observations tend to become more focused over time, ranging from **descriptive observation** (broad observations) to **focused observation** of more carefully selected events or interactions, and then to **selective observations** designed to facilitate comparisons.
- Participant observers usually select events to be observed through a combination of **single positioning** (observing from a fixed location), **multiple positioning** (moving around the site to observe in different locations), and **mobile positioning** (following a person around a site).
- **Logs** of daily events and **field notes** are the major methods of recording unstructured observational data. Field notes are both descriptive and reflective.
- Descriptive notes (sometimes called **observational notes**) are detailed, objective accounts of what transpired in an observational session. Observers strive for detailed, **thick description**.
- **Reflective notes** include **methodologic notes** that document observers' thoughts about their strategies; **theoretical notes** (or **analytic notes**) that represent ongoing efforts to make sense of the data; and **personal notes** that document observers' feelings and experiences.
- Structured observational methods impose constraints on observers to enhance the accuracy and objectivity of the observations and to obtain an adequate representation of the phenomena of interest.
- **Checklists** are tools for recording the occurrence or frequency of predesignated behaviors, events, or characteristics. Checklists are based on **category systems** for encoding observed phenomena into discrete, mutually exclusive categories.
- Some checklists categorize exhaustively all behaviors of a particular type (e.g., body movements) in an ongoing fashion, whereas others use a **sign system** to record particular behaviors while ignoring others.
- With **rating scales**, another record-keeping device for structured observations, observers are required to rate phenomena along a dimension that is typically bipolar (e.g., passive/aggressive or excellent health/poor health); ratings are made either at specific intervals during the observations (e.g., every 15 minutes) or after observations are completed.
- Some structured observations use sampling to select behaviors or events to be observed. **Time sampling** involves the specification of the duration and frequency of both observational periods and intersession intervals. **Event sampling** selects integral behaviors or events of a special type for observation.
- Technologic advances have greatly augmented researchers' capacity to collect, record, and preserve observational data. Such devices as audiotape recorders and videotape cameras permit behaviors and events to be described or categorized after their occurrence.
- Observational methods are subject to various biases. The greater the degree of observer inference and judgment, the more likely that perceptual errors and distortions will occur. The most prevalent observer biases include the **enhancement of contrast effect**, **central tendency bias**, the **halo effect**, **assimilatory biases**, **errors of leniency**, and **errors of severity**.

STUDY ACTIVITIES

Chapter 16 of the *Study Guide to Accompany Nursing Research: Principles and Methods, 7th edition*, offers various exercises and study suggestions for reinforcing concepts presented in this chapter. In addition, the following study questions can be addressed:

1. Suppose you were interested in observing fathers' behavior in the delivery room during the

birth of their first child. Identify the observer–observed relationship or the concealment and intervention dimensions that you would recommend adopting for such a study, and defend your recommendation. What are the possible drawbacks of your approach, and how might you deal with them?

2. Would a psychiatric nurse researcher be well suited to conduct a participant observation study of the interactions between psychiatric nurses and their clients? Why or why not?

3. A nurse researcher is planning to study temper tantrums displayed by hospitalized children. Would you recommend using a time sampling approach? Why or why not?

4. The following is a list of research questions. Indicate which of these problems could be studied by using an observational method. For each problem that is amenable to observation, indicate whether you think a structured or unstructured approach would be preferable.

a. Does team nursing versus primary nursing affect the type of communication patterns between nurses and patients?

b. Is there a relationship between prenatal instruction and delivery room behaviors of primiparas?

c. Is the number of hours of direct clinical practice for nursing students related to their performance on the licensure examination?

d. Do the attitudes of nurses toward abortion affect the quality of care given to patients undergoing abortion?

e. Do industrial alcohol programs have a positive impact on on-the-job accident rates?

f. Is the touching behavior of nurses related to their ethnic or cultural background?

SUGGESTED READINGS

Methodologic References

Aiken, L. R., & Aiken, L. A. (1996). *Rating scales and checklists: Evaluating behavior, personality, and attitudes.* New York: John Wiley.

Bogdan, R. C. (1972). *Participant observation in organizational settings.* Syracuse, NY: Syracuse University Press.

Bogdewic, S. P. (1992). Participant observation. In B. F. Crabtree & W. L. Miller (Eds.), *Doing qualitative research* (pp. 47–69). Newbury Park, CA: Sage.

Dowrick, P., & Biggs, S. J. (Eds.). (1983). *Using video: Psychological and social applications.* New York: John Wiley & Sons.

Evaneshko, V. (1985). Entrée strategies for nursing field research studies. In M. M. Leininger (Ed.), *Qualitative research methods in nursing* (pp. 133–147). Orlando, FL: Grune & Stratton.

Frank-Stromberg, M., & Olsen, S. J. (1997). *Instruments for clinical health-care research.* Sudbury, MA: Jones and Bartlett.

Hammersley, M., & Atkinson, P. (1995). *Ethnography: Principles and practice* (2nd ed.). New York: Routledge.

Harper, D. (1994). On the authority of the image: Visual methods at the crossroads. In N. K. Denzin & Y. S. Lincoln (Eds.), *Handbook of qualitative research* (pp. 403–412). Thousand Oaks, CA: Sage.

Junker, B. H. (1960). *Field work: An introduction to the social sciences.* Chicago: University of Chicago Press.

Kerlinger, F. N., & Lee, H. B. (2000). *Foundations of behavioral research* (4th ed.). Orlando, FL: Harcourt College Publishers.

Leininger, M. (1985). Ethnography and ethnonursing: Models and modes of qualitative data analysis. In M. M. Leininger (Ed.), *Qualitative research methods in nursing* (pp. 33–71). New York: Grune & Stratton.

Lobo, M. L. (1992). Observation: A valuable data collection strategy for research with children. *Journal of Pediatric Nursing, 7,* 320–328.

Lofland, J., & Lofland, L. (1995). *Analyzing social settings: A guide to qualitative observation and analysis* (3rd ed.). Belmont, CA: Wadsworth.

Morrison, E. F., Phillips, L. R., & Chal, Y. M. (1990). The development and use of observational measurement scales. *Applied Nursing Research, 3,* 73–86.

Savage, J. (2000). Participant observation: Standing in the shoes of others? *Qualitative Health Research, 10,* 324–339.

Schatzman, L., & Strauss, A. (1982). *Field research: Strategies for a natural sociology* (2nd ed.). Englewood Cliffs, NJ: Prentice-Hall.

Scisney-Matlock, M., Algase, D., Boehm, S., Coleman-Burns, P., Oakley, D., Rogers, A. E., Yeo, S., Young, E., & Yu, M. (2001). Measuring behavior: Electronic devises in nursing studies. *Applied Nursing Research, 13,* 97–102.

Spradley, J. P. (1980). *Participant observation.* New York: Holt, Rinehart & Wilson.

Strauss, A., & Corbin, J. (1990). *Basics of qualitative research: Grounded theory procedures and techniques.* Newbury Park, CA: Sage.

Strickland, O. L., & Waltz, C. (Eds.). (1988). *Measurement of nursing outcomes.* New York: Springer.

Wilson, H. S. (1985). *Research in nursing.* Menlo Park, CA: Addison-Wesley.

Studies Cited in Chapter 16

Archibong, U. E. (1999). Evaluating the impact of primary nursing practice on the quality of nursing care: A Nigerian study. *Journal of Advanced Nursing, 29,* 680–689.

Beck, C. T. (2002). Releasing the pause button: Mothering twins during the first year of life. *Qualitative Health Research, 12,* 593–608.

Butt, M. L., & Kisilevsky, B. S. (2000). Music modulates behaviour of premature infants following heel lance. *Canadian Journal of Nursing Research, 31,* 17–39.

Cacchione, P. Z. (2002). Four acute confusion assessment instruments: Reliability and validity for use in long-term care facilities. *Journal of Gerontological Nursing, 28,* 12–19.

Carruth, A. K., Gilbert, K., & Lewis, B. (1997). Environmental health hazards: The impact on a southern community. *Public Health Nursing, 14,* 259–267.

Feldt, K. S. (2001). Checklist of Nonverbal Pain Indicators. *Pain Management Nursing, 1,* 13–21.

Fuller, B. G. (2000). Fluctuations in established infant pain behaviors. *Clinical Nursing Research, 9,* 298–316.

Gaffney, K. F., Barndt-Maglio, B., Myers, S., & Kollar, S. J. (2002). Early clinical assessment for harsh child discipline strategies. *MCN: American Journal of Maternal Child Nursing, 27,* 34–40.

Gerdtz, M. F., & Bucknall, T. K. (2001). Triage nurses' clinical decision making: An observational study of urgency assessment. *Journal of Advanced Nursing, 35,* 550–561.

Harrison, L. L., Williams, A. K., Berbaum, M. L., Stern, J. T., & Leeper, J. (2000). Physiologic and behavioral effects of gentle human touch on preterm infants. *Research in Nursing & Health, 23,* 435–446.

Hawranik, P. G., & Strain, L. A. (2001). Cognitive impairment, disruptive behaviors, and home care utilization. *Western Journal of Nursing Research, 23,* 148–162.

Herman, M. (1997). Clinical response to clozapine treatment of 11 chronic patients in a state psychiatric ward. *Australia-New Zealand Journal of Mental Health Nursing, 6,* 129–133.

Holditch-Davis, D., Docherty, S., Miles, M. S., & Burchinal, M. (2001), Developmental outcomes of infants with bronchopulmonary dysplasia: Comparison with other medically fragile infants. *Research in Nursing & Health, 24,* 181–193.

Holditch-Davis, D., Miles, M. S., & Belyea, M. (2000). Feeding and nonfeeding interactions of mothers and prematures. *Western Journal of Nursing Research, 22,* 320–334.

Holt, J., & Reeves, J. S. (2001). The meaning of hope and generic caring practices to nurture hope in a rural village in the Dominican Republic. *Journal of Transcultural Nursing, 12,* 123–131.

Kisida, N., Holditch-Davis, D., Miles, M. S., & Carlson, J. (2001). Unsafe caregiving practices experienced by 3-year-old-children born prematurely. *Pediatric Nursing, 27,* 13–18.

Kolanowski, A. M., Litaker, M. S., & Catalano, P. A. (2002). Emotional well-being in a person with dementia. *Western Journal of Nursing Research, 24,* 28–48.

LaMontagne, L. L., Wells, N., Hepworth, J. T., Johnson, B. D., & Manes, R. (1999). Parent coping and child distress behaviors during invasive procedures for childhood cancer. *Journal of Pediatric Oncology Nursing, 16,* 3–12.

Lotzkar, M., & Bottorff, J. L. (2001). An observational study of the development of a nurse-patient relationship. *Clinical Nursing Research, 10,* 275–294.

Macke, J. K. (2001). Analgesia for circumcision: Effects on newborn behavior and mother/infant interaction. *Journal of Obstetric, Gynecologic, and Neonatal Nursing, 30,* 507–514.

Mallick, M. J., & Whipple, T. W. (2000). Validity of the nursing diagnosis of relocation stress syndrome. *Nursing Research, 49,* 97–100.

Medoff-Cooper, B., McGrath, J. M., & Bilker, W. (2000). Nutritive sucking and neurobehavioral development in preterm infants from 34 weeks PCA to term. *MCN: American Journal of Maternal-Child Nursing, 25,* 64–70.

Neu, M., Browne, J. V., & Vojir, C. (2000). The impact of two transfer techniques used during skin-to-skin care on the physiologic and behavioral responses of preterm infants. *Nursing Research, 49,* 215–223.

Payne, S., Hardey, M., & Coleman, P. (2000). Interactions between nurses during handovers in elderly care. *Journal of Advanced Nursing, 32,* 277–285.

Pierce, L. L. (2001). Caring and expressions of spirituality by urban caregivers of people with stroke in

African American families. *Qualitative Health Research, 11*, 339–352.

Polit, D. F., London, A. S., & Martinez, J. M. (2001). *The health of poor urban women.* New York: MDRC.

Rateau, M. R. (2000). Confusion and aggression in restrained elderly persons undergoing hip repair surgery. *Applied Nursing Research, 13*, 50–54.

Roberts, J., Browne, G., Milne, C., Spooner, L., Gafni, A., Drummond-Young, M., LeGris, J., Watt, S., LeClair, K., Beaumont, L., & Roberts J. (1999). Problem-solving counseling for caregivers of the cognitively impaired: Effective for whom? *Nursing Research, 48*, 162–172.

Thomas, K. A. (2000). Differential effects of breast- and formula-feeding on preterm infants sleep-wake patterns. *Journal of Obstetric, Gynecologic, and Neonatal Nursing, 29*, 145–152.

Twomey, J. G., Bevis, M. C., & McGibbon, C. A. (2001). Associations between adult and child bicycle helmet use. *MCN: American Journal of Maternal Child Nursing, 26*, 272–277.

Weiss, S. J. (1992). Measurement of the sensory qualities in tactile interaction. *Nursing Research, 41*, 82–86.

White, M. A., Williams, P. D., Alexander, D. J., Powell-Cope, G. M., & Conlon, M. (1990). Sleep onset latency and distress in hospitalized children. *Nursing Research, 39*, 134–139.

Whittington, K., Patrick, M., & Roberts, J. (2000). A national study of pressure sore prevalence and incidence in acute care hospitals. *Journal of Wound, Ostomy, and Continence Nursing, 27*, 209–215.

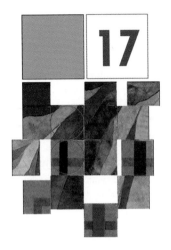

17

Collecting Biophysiologic and Other Data

Most nursing research studies involve the collection of data through self-reports or observations. However, there are other methods of collecting data, several of which are reviewed in this chapter. The most important alternative method is biophysiologic measures, which are used primarily in quantitative studies.

BIOPHYSIOLOGIC MEASURES

The trend in nursing research has been toward increased use of measures to assess the physiologic status of study participants, and to evaluate clinical outcomes. Indeed, the National Institute for Nursing Research has emphasized the need for more physiologically based nursing research. Bond and Heitkemper (2001) note that enormous advances in basic physiologic science (e.g., the human genome project) in the past decade offer new opportunities for the evolving physiologic nursing science.

Many clinically relevant variables do not require biophysiologic instrumentation for their measurement. Data on physiologic activity or dysfunction can often be gathered through direct observation (e.g., vomiting, cyanosis, edema, wound status). Other biophysiologic data can be gathered by asking people directly (e.g., ratings of

pain, fatigue, or nausea). This section focuses on biophysiologic phenomena that are measured through specialized technical equipment.

Settings in which nurses operate are typically filled with a wide variety of technical instruments for measuring physiologic functions. It is beyond the scope of this book to describe the many kinds of biophysiologic measures available to nurse researchers. Our goals are to present an overview of biophysiologic measures, to illustrate their use in research, and to note considerations in decisions to use them.

Purposes of Biophysiologic Measures

Clinical nursing studies may involve specialized equipment and instruments both for creating independent variables (e.g., an intervention using biofeedback equipment) and for measuring dependent variables. For the most part, our discussion focuses on the use of biophysiologic measures as outcome or dependent variables. Most nursing studies in which biophysiologic measures have been used fall into one of six classes.

1. *Basic physiologic processes.* Some studies investigate basic physiologic processes that are relevant to nursing care. Such studies often involve subjects who are healthy and normal, or some subhuman animal species.

Example of a study of basic physiologic processes:
Nantais-Smith and her colleagues (2001) studied plasma and nipple aspirate levels in lactating and postwean women to explore whether the transport of carotenoid from the blood to the breast is enhanced by lactation.

2. *Physiologic outcomes of nursing care.* Nurse researchers are increasingly interested in exploring and documenting the ways in which nursing actions affect patients' biophysiologic outcomes. Some of these studies are undertaken when there is concern that standard procedures are not having the intended beneficial effects.

Example of a study of physiologic outcomes:
Jellema and colleagues (2000) investigated the hemodynamic changes induced by manual lung hyperinflation (MLH) in patients with septic shock. Their intent was to assess if the changes were sufficiently adverse to warrant prohibition of MLH as a routine procedure in caring for these patients.

3. *Evaluations of nursing interventions.* These evaluation studies differ from those in the second category in that they involve the testing of a new intervention, usually in comparison with standard methods of care or with alternative interventions. Typically, these studies involve a hypothesis stating that the innovative nursing procedure will result in improved biophysiologic outcomes among patients.

Example of an evaluation:
Wong, Lopez-Nahas, and Molassiotis (2001) evaluated the effectiveness of music therapy in decreasing anxiety in ventilator-dependent patients. Mean blood pressure and respiratory rate were used to assess anxiety.

4. *Product assessments.* A number of nursing studies are designed to evaluate alternative products designed to enhance patient health or comfort, rather than to evaluate nursing interventions.

Example of a product assessment study:
Cohen, Hayes, Tordella, and Puente (2002) used an experimental design to evaluate the thermal efficiency of three heat-loss prevention products (prewarmed cotton, reflective, and forced-warm-air inflatable blankets) in trauma patients undergoing resuscitation in the emergency department. Body temperatures were recorded every 15 minutes for the first hour, and then hourly.

5. *Measurement and diagnosis improvement.* Nurse researchers sometimes undertake studies to improve the measurement and recording of biophysiologic information regularly gathered by nurses. Similarly, some researchers investigate methods to improve clinical diagnosis.

Example of a study on measurement/diagnosis:
Gray, McClain, Peruggia, Patrie, and Steers (2001) conducted a study to construct an optimal model for diagnosing motor urge incontinence. Urodynamic testing was used to diagnose type of urinary incontinence. A voiding pressure study was used to evaluate bladder outlet obstruction.

6. *Studies of physiologic correlates.* Nurse researchers have also studied biophysiologic outcomes in relation to social or psychological characteristics. In some cases, the studies are prospective and are designed to identify antecedents to physiologic problems. In other cases, the researcher is trying to describe concurrently the psychological status of people with different physiologic conditions.

Example of a study of physiologic correlates:
Belza, Steele, Hunziker, Lakshminaryan, Holt, and Buchner (2001) examined relationships between functional performance (physical activity), functional capacity (e.g., forced expiratory volume during spirometry), and symptom experiences in people with chronic obstructive pulmonary disease.

The physiologic phenomena that interest nurse researchers run the full gamut of available measures, some of which are discussed next.

Types of Biophysiologic Measures

Physiologic measurements can be classified in one of two major categories. **In vivo measurements** are those performed directly in or on living organisms. Examples include measures of oxygen saturation, blood pressure, and body temperature. An **in vitro measure**, by contrast, is performed outside the organism's body, as in the case of measuring serum potassium concentration in the blood.

In Vivo Measures

In vivo measures often involve the use of highly complex instrumentation systems. An **instrumentation system** is the apparatus and equipment used to measure one or more attributes of a subject and the presentation of that measurement data in a manner that humans can interpret. Organism—instrument systems involve up to six major components:

1. A stimulus
2. A subject
3. Sensing equipment (e.g., transducers)
4. Signal-conditioning equipment (to reduce interference signals)
5. Display equipment
6. Recording, data processing, and transmission equipment

Not all instrumentation systems involve all six components. Some systems, such as an electronic thermometer, are simple; others are extremely complex. For example, some electronic monitors yield simultaneous measures of such physiologic variables as cardiac responsivity, respiratory rate and rhythm, core temperature, and muscular activity.

In vivo instruments have been developed to measure all bodily functions, and technologic improvements continue to advance our ability to measure biophysiologic phenomena more accurately, more conveniently, and more rapidly than ever before. The uses to which such instruments have been put by nurse researchers are richly diverse and impressive.

Example of an in vivo study:
Wipke-Tevis, Stotts, Williams, Froelicher, and Hunt (2001) conducted a study to compare the partial pressure of transcutaneous tissue oxygen ($TcPO_2$) in people with venous ulcers in four body positions, both with and without inspired oxygen. Tissue perfusion was measured with a Novametrix 840 PrO_2 and $PtcO_2$ Monitor. Arterial oxygen saturation (SaO_2) was measured by an Oximax 100 pulse oximeter.

In Vitro Measures

With in vitro measures, data are gathered by extracting physiologic material from subjects and submitting it for laboratory analysis. Nurse researchers may or may not be involved in the extraction of the material; however, the analysis is normally done by specialized laboratory technicians. Usually, each laboratory establishes a range of normal values for each measurement, and this information is critical for interpreting the results.

Several classes of laboratory analysis have been used in studies by nurse researchers, including the following:

- *Chemical measurements*, such as the measure of hormone levels, sugar levels, or potassium levels
- *Microbiologic measures*, such as bacterial counts and identification
- *Cytologic or histologic measures*, such as tissue biopsies

It is impossible, of course, to catalog the thousands of laboratory tests available. Laboratory analyses of blood and urine samples are the most frequently used in vitro measures in nursing investigations.

Example of an in vitro study:
Bliss and her colleagues (2001) compared the effects of a fiber supplement in community-living adults who were incontinent of loose or liquid stools. Stool specimens from before and after the intervention were subjected to laboratory analysis.

Selecting a Biophysiologic Measure

For nurses unfamiliar with the hundreds of biophysiologic measures available in institutional settings, the selection of appropriate research measures may pose a challenge. There are, unfortunately, no comprehensive handbooks to guide interested researchers to the measures, instruments, and interpretations that may be required in collecting physiologic data. Probably the best approach is to consult knowledgeable colleagues or experts at a local institution. It also may be possible to obtain useful information on biophysiologic measures from research articles on a problem similar to your own, a review article on the central phenomenon under investigation, manufacturers' catalogs, and exhibits of manufacturers at professional conferences.

Obviously, the most basic issue to address in selecting a physiologic measure is whether it will yield good information about the research variable. In some cases, researchers need to consider whether the variable should be measured by observation or self-report instead of (or in addition to) using biophysiologic equipment. For example, stress could be measured by asking people questions (e.g., using the State–Trait Anxiety Inventory); by observing their behavior during exposure to stressful stimuli; or by measuring heart rate, blood pressure, or levels of adrenocorticotropic hormone in urine samples.

Several other considerations should be kept in mind in selecting a biophysiologic measure. Some key questions include the following:

- Is the equipment or laboratory analysis you need readily available to you? If not, can it be borrowed, rented, or purchased?
- If equipment must be purchased, is it affordable? Can funding be acquired to cover the purchase (or rental) price?
- Can you operate the required equipment and interpret its results, or do you need training? Are there resources available to help you with operation and interpretation?
- Will you have difficulty obtaining permission to use the equipment from an Institutional Review Board or other institutional authority?
- Does the measure need to be direct (e.g., a direct measure of blood pressure by way of an arterial line), or is an indirect measure (e.g., blood pressure measurement by way of a sphygmomanometer) sufficient?

- Is continuous monitoring necessary (e.g., electrocardiogram readings), or is a point-in-time measure adequate?
- Do your activities during data collection permit you to record data simultaneously, or do you need an instrument system with recording equipment (or a research assistant)?
- Is a mechanical stimulus needed to get meaningful measurements? Does available equipment include the required stimulus?
- Is a single measure of your dependent variable sufficient, or are multiple measures preferable? If multiple measures are better, what burden does this place on you and on subjects?
- Are your measures likely to be influenced by reactivity (i.e., subjects' awareness of their subject status)? If so, can alternative or supplementary nonreactive measures be identified, or can the extent of reactivity bias be assessed?
- Can your research variable be measured using a noninvasive procedure, or is an invasive procedure required?
- Is the measure you plan to use sufficiently accurate and sensitive to variation?
- Are you thoroughly familiar with rules and safety precautions, such as grounding procedures, especially when using electrical equipment?

Evaluation of Biophysiologic Measures

Biophysiologic measures offer the following advantages to nurse researchers:

- Biophysiologic measures are relatively accurate and precise, especially compared with psychological measures (e.g., self-report measures of anxiety).
- Biophysiologic measures are objective. Two nurses reading from the same spirometer output are likely to record the same tidal volume measurements, and two different spirometers are likely to produce identical readouts. Patients cannot easily distort measurements of biophysiologic functioning deliberately.
- Biophysiologic instrumentation provides valid measures of the targeted variables: thermometers

can be depended on to measure temperature and not blood volume, and so forth. For nonbiophysiologic measures, the question of whether an instrument is really measuring the target concept is an ongoing concern.

- Because equipment for obtaining biophysiologic measurements is available in hospital settings, the cost of collecting biophysiologic data may be low or nonexistent.

Biophysiologic measures also have a few disadvantages:

- The measuring tool may affect the variables it is attempting to measure. The presence of a sensing device, such as a transducer, located in a blood vessel partially blocks that vessel and, hence, alters the pressure–flow characteristics being measured.
- There are normally interferences that create artifacts in biophysiologic measures. For example, noise generated in a measuring instrument interferes with the signal being produced.
- Energy must often be applied to the organism when taking the biophysiologic measurements; extreme caution must continually be exercised to avoid the risk of damaging cells by high-energy concentrations.

The difficulty in choosing biophysiologic measures for nursing research investigations lies not in their shortage, nor in their questionable utility, nor in their inferiority to other methods. Indeed, they are plentiful, often highly reliable and valid, and extremely useful in clinical nursing studies. However, care must be exercised in selecting appropriate instruments or laboratory analyses with regard to practical, ethical, medical, and technical considerations.

RECORDS, DOCUMENTS, AND AVAILABLE DATA

Thus far, we have examined data collection strategies that require researchers to collect their own data and, in some cases, to develop data collection instruments. However, data that are gathered for

nonresearch purposes can often be used to answer research questions of both qualitative and quantitative researchers.

Data Sources

The places where nurse researchers can find useful records and documents are too numerous to list, but a few suggestions may be helpful. In hospitals and other health care settings, excellent records are kept routinely. For example, patient charts, physicians' and nurses' orders, care plan statements, and shift reports constitute rich data sources. In addition to medical and nursing records, hospitals maintain financial records, personnel records, nutrition records, and so forth.

Example of a hospital records study:
Sobie, Gaves, and Tringali (2000) examined the medical records of 104 emergency department (ED) patients to determine if "ED-hold" patients and "ED-direct admit" patients differed with respect to the timeliness and type of nursing assessments.

Educational institutions maintain various records. For example, most schools of nursing have permanent files on their students. Public school systems also keep records, including both academic and health-related information. Industries and businesses normally maintain a variety of records that may interest industrial nurse researchers, such as information on employees' absenteeism, health status, on-the-job accidents, job performance ratings, and alcoholism or drug problems. Governments also maintain records of potential interest, such as birth or death records.

Example of a school records study:
Hammond, Ali, Fendler, Dolan, and Donovan (2000) studied the effect of using an alcohol gel hand sanitizer in elementary school settings on student and teacher absenteeism. Analysis of the absence records from 16 schools (some of which got the handwash product) revealed a substantial drop in absenteeism due to infection in the product schools.

In addition to quantified institutional records, narrative documents are potential data sources for qualitative researchers. Personal documents such as diaries and letters are sometimes available. Ethnographers frequently collect and analyze a range of personal documents and institutional records, including minutes of meetings, organizational bylaws or policy statements, and promotional literature, to name only a few. Such materials can provide useful insight into lived experiences.

Example of a study using documents:
Powers (2001) conducted an ethnographic study of everyday ethics in the care of nursing home residents with dementia. For a 2-year period, Powers used participant observation and in-depth interviewing in a 147-bed nursing home. The researcher supplemented these data with various documents, including newsletters, activity calendars, daily care worksheets, in-service education calendars and teaching tools, annual reports, and documents associated with the work of the ethics committee.

Advantages and Disadvantages of Using Records

Research data obtained from records and documents are advantageous for several reasons. The most salient advantage of records is that they are economical; the collection of original data is often time-consuming and costly. Preexisting records also permit an examination of trends over time, if the information is collected repeatedly. Problems of reactivity and response bias may be completely absent when researchers obtain data from records. Furthermore, investigators do not have to rely on participants' cooperation.

On the other hand, when researchers are not responsible for collecting and recording data, they may be unaware of the records' limitations and biases. Two major sources of bias in records are **selective deposit** and **selective survival**. If the available records are not the entire set of all possible such records, researchers must address the question of how representative existing records are. Many record keepers *intend* to maintain an entire universe of records but may fail to adhere to this

ideal. Lapses from the ideal may be the result of systematic biases, and careful researchers should attempt to learn just what those biases may be.

Another problem confronting researchers is the increasing reluctance of institutions to make their records available for study. The Privacy Act, a federal regulation enacted to protect individuals against possible misuse of records, has made hospitals, agencies, schools, and businesses sensitive to the possibility of legal action from people who think their right to privacy has been violated. The major issue is divulgence of individual identities. If records are maintained with an identifying number rather than a name, permission to use the records may be easy to secure. Most institutions *do* maintain records by their clients' names, however. In such situations, researchers may need the help of staff at the institution to maintain client anonymity, and some organizations may be unwilling to use their staff for such purposes.

Other difficulties also may be relevant. Sometimes records have to be verified for their authenticity, authorship, or accuracy, a task that may be difficult if the records are old. Researchers using records must be prepared to deal with forms and file systems they do not understand. Codes and symbols that had meaning to the record keeper may have to be translated to be usable. In using records to study trends, researchers should be alert to possible changes in record-keeping procedures. For example, does a dramatic increase or decrease in the incidence of sudden infant death syndrome reflect changes in the causes or cures of this problem, or does it reflect a change in diagnosis or record-keeping?

Thus, although existing records may be plentiful, inexpensive, and accessible, they should not be used without paying attention to potential problems.

Q METHODOLOGY

Q methodology (Stephenson, 1975) refers to a constellation of substantive, statistical, and psychometric concepts for research on individuals. Q methodology uses a **Q-sort** procedure, which involves sorting a deck of cards according to specified criteria.

Q-Sort Procedures

In a Q-sort study, participants are presented with a set of cards on which words, statements, or other messages are written. Participants are asked to sort the cards along a particular dimension, such as approve/disapprove, most like me/least like me, or highest priority/lowest priority. The number of cards is typically between 60 and 100. Usually, cards are sorted into 9 or 11 piles, with researchers designating the number of cards to be placed in each pile. Subjects typically are asked to place fewer cards at either of the two extremes and more cards toward the middle. Table 17-1 shows a hypothetical distribution of 60 cards in 9 piles.

Q sorts have many possible applications. Attitudes can be studied by asking people to sort statements on a agree/disagree continuum. Researchers can study personality by describing personality characteristics on the cards (e.g., *friendly*, *aggressive*); people can then be requested to sort the cards on a "very much like me" to "not at all like me" continuum. Self-concept can be explored by comparing responses to this "like me" dimension with people's responses elicited when the instructions are to sort cards according to what they consider ideal personality traits.

Q sorts can be used to study individuals in depth. For example, participants could be asked to sort traits as they apply to themselves in different roles, such as employee, parent, spouse, and friend. The technique can be used to gain information about how individuals see themselves, how they perceive others seeing them, how they believe others would like them to be, and so forth. Other applications include asking patients to rate nursing behaviors on a continuum of most helpful to least helpful or asking cancer patients to rate aspects of their treatment on a most distressing to least distressing dimension.

The number of cards in a Q sort varies, but it is best to use at least 50 because it is difficult to achieve stable and reliable results with a smaller number. On the other hand, the task is tedious and difficult with more than 100 cards.

Q sorts have sometimes been used by qualitative researchers (Brown, 1996), but more often are analyzed statistically. The statistical analysis of Q-sort data is a somewhat controversial matter. Options range from the most elementary, descriptive statistical procedures, such as rank ordering, averages, and percentages, to highly complex procedures, such as factor analysis. Factor analysis, a procedure designed to reveal the underlying dimensions or common elements in a set of items, is described in Chapter 21. Some researchers insist that factor analysis is essential in the analysis of Q-sort data. Specific computer software (Qmethod) has been designed for analyzing Q-sort data (Brown, 1996).

Q sorts can be constructed by researchers and tailored to the needs of specific studies, but there are also existing Q sorts. The advantages of using a previously developed Q sort are that it is time-saving, provides opportunities for comparisons with other studies, and usually includes established information about data quality. An example of a widely

TABLE 17.1 Example of a Distribution of Q-Sort Cards									
	APPROVE OF LEAST								**APPROVE OF MOST**
Category	1	2	3	4	5	6	7	8	9
Number of cards	2	4	7	10	14	10	7	4	2

used Q sort is the Child-Rearing Practices Report (CRPR), a 91-item Q sort that provides information about parenting behavior.

Example of using an existing Q sort:
Hillman (1997) used the CRPR to compare the child-rearing practices of parents of children with cancer and parents of healthy children. The two groups of parents differed in terms of discipline and protectiveness.

Evaluation of Q Methodology

Q methodology can be a powerful tool but, like other data collection techniques, has drawbacks as well. On the plus side, Q sorts are versatile and can be applied to a wide variety of problems. Q sorts can be an objective and reliable procedure for the intensive study of an individual. They have been used effectively to study the progress of people during different phases of therapy, particularly psychotherapy. The requirement that individuals place a predetermined number of cards in each pile virtually eliminates response-set biases. Furthermore, sorting cards may be a more agreeable task to some people than completing a paper-and-pencil instrument.

On the other hand, it is difficult and time-consuming to administer Q sorts to large samples. The sampling problem is compounded by the fact that Q sorts cannot normally be administered through the mail, thereby making it difficult to obtain a geographically diverse sample. Some critics argue that the forced procedure of distributing cards according to researchers' specifications is artificial and excludes information about how people would ordinarily distribute their opinions.

Another criticism of Q-sort data relates to permissible statistical operations. Most statistical tests assume that item responses are independent of one another. In a Likert scale, for example, a person's response to one item does not restrict responses to other items. Techniques of this type yield **normative measures**, with which individual scores can be compared with average group scores. Q sorts are a forced-choice procedure: A person's response to one item depends on, and is restricted by, responses

to other items. Referring to Table 17-1, a respondent who has placed two cards in category 1 ("approve of least") is not free to place another card in this category.* Such an approach produces **ipsative measures**. With ipsative measures, a group average is an irrelevant point of comparison because the average is identical for everyone. With the nine-category Q sort shown in Table 17-1, the average value of the sorted cards will always be five. (The average of a *particular item* can be meaningfully computed and compared among individuals or groups, however.) Strictly speaking, ordinary statistical tests are inappropriate with non-independent ipsative measures. In practice, many researchers feel that the violation of assumptions in applying standard statistical procedures to Q-sort data is not a serious transgression, particularly if the number of cards is large.

Example of a Q-sort study:
Snethen and Broome (2001) used a Q sort to explore the perceptions of adolescents living with end-stage renal disease. Statements describing how subjects might view themselves and their disease were placed on cards (e.g., "I guess at my age, knowing about all of this stuff going on with my kidneys, I'm just kind of depressed a little," p. 161). Adolescents sorted the 48 cards into 11 piles on a "most like me" to "most unlike me" continuum.

PROJECTIVE TECHNIQUES

Self-report methods normally depend on respondents' willingness to share personal information, but projective techniques obtain psychological data with a minimum of cooperation. **Projective techniques** present participants with a stimulus of low structure, permitting them to "read in" their own interpretations and in this way provide researchers with information about their way of thinking. The rationale underlying these techniques is that the

---

* People are usually told, however, that they can move cards around from one pile to another until the desired distribution is obtained.

manner in which people react to unstructured stimuli is a reflection of their needs, motives, values, or personality traits. Projective methods give free play to participants' imagination by providing them with tasks that permit an almost unlimited variety of responses—responses that are typically in narrative form but that are sometimes quantified.

Types of Projective Techniques

Projective techniques are flexible because virtually any unstructured stimuli can be used to induce projections. One class of projective methods uses pictorial materials. The Rorschach ink blot test is an example of a **pictorial projective device**. Another example is the Thematic Apperception Test (TAT). The TAT materials consist of 20 cards that contain pictures. People are asked to make up a story for each picture, inventing an explanation of what led up to the event shown, what is happening at the moment, what the characters are feeling and thinking, and what kind of outcome will result. Examples of variables that have been derived from TAT-type pictures include need for affiliation, parent–child relationships, creativity, attitude toward authority, and fear of success.

Example of a study using the TAT:
Krulik and Florian (1995) used the TAT to study social isolation experienced by school-aged children with chronic illnesses. Themes of isolation in response to the TAT were compared for 57 children with chronic health problems and 91 healthy children.

Verbal projective techniques present participants with an ambiguous verbal stimulus. Verbal methods include association techniques and completion techniques. An example of an association technique is the **word-association method**, which presents participants with a series of words, to which they respond with the first thing that comes to mind. The word list often combines both neutral and emotionally tinged words, which are included for the purpose of detecting impaired thought processes or internal conflicts. The word-association technique has also been used to study creativity,

interests, and attitudes. The most common completion technique is **sentence completion**. The person is given a set of incomplete sentences and asked to complete them in any desired manner. This approach is frequently used as a method of measuring attitudes or some aspect of personality. Some examples of incomplete sentences include the following:

When I think of a nurse, I feel ....
The thing I most admire about nurses is ....
A good nurse should always ....

The sentence stems are designed to elicit responses toward some attitudinal object or event in which the investigator is interested. Responses are typically categorized or rated according to a prespecified plan.

A third class of projective measures is known as **expressive methods**. These techniques encourage self-expression, in most cases, through the construction of some product out of raw materials. The major expressive methods are play techniques, drawing and painting, and role-playing. The assumption is that people express their needs, motives, and emotions by working with or manipulating materials.

Example of a study using expressive methods:
Instone (2000) conducted a grounded theory study of children with human immunodeficiency virus infection. The study included projective drawings, which were analyzed for themes of emotional distress, disturbed self-image, and social isolation.

Evaluation of Projective Measures

Projective measures are fairly controversial. Critics point out that it is difficult to evaluate information from projective techniques objectively. A high degree of inference is required in gleaning data from projective tests, and data quality depends heavily on researchers' sensitivity and interpretive skill. Critics suggest that researchers' interpretations of responses are almost as projective as participants' reactions to original stimuli.

Another problem with projective techniques is that it is difficult to demonstrate that they are, in fact, measuring the variables they purport to measure. If a pictorial device is scored for aggressive expressions, can researchers be confident that individual differences in aggressive responses really reflect underlying differences in aggressiveness?

Projective techniques also have supporters. Advocates argue that the techniques probe the unconscious mind, encompass the whole personality, and provide data of a breadth and depth unattainable by more traditional methods. Projective instruments are less susceptible to faking than self-report measures. Also, it is often easier to build rapport and gain people's trust with projective measures than with a questionnaire or scale. Finally, some projective techniques are particularly useful with special groups, especially children.

TIP: If you decide to use an alternative method such as a projective technique or a Q sort, a good strategy might be to supplement it with a more traditional measure of the construct, as a means of assessing the validity of the alternative approach.

VIGNETTES

Another data collection alternative is called *vignettes*. Vignettes rely on self-reports by participants, but involve a stimulus.

Uses of Vignettes

Vignettes are brief descriptions of events or situations to which respondents are asked to react. The descriptions, which can either be fictitious or based on fact, are structured to elicit information about respondents' perceptions, opinions, or knowledge about some phenomenon. The vignettes are usually written narrative descriptions, but researchers have also used videotaped vignettes. The questions posed to respondents after the vignettes may be either open-ended (e.g., How would you recommend handling this situation?) or closed-ended (e.g., On the scale below, rate how well you believe the nurse handled the situation). The number of vignettes included in a study normally ranges from 4 to 10.

Sometimes the underlying purpose of vignette studies is not revealed to participants, especially if the technique is used as an indirect measure of attitudes, prejudices, and stereotypes using embedded descriptors. For example, a researcher interested in exploring stereotypes of male nurses could present people with a series of vignettes describing fictitious nurses' actions. For each vignette, the nurse would be described as a male half the time (at random) and as a female the other half. Participants could then be asked to describe the fictitious nurses in terms of likableness, effectiveness, and so forth. Any differences presumably result from attitudes toward male and female nurses.

Example of a study using vignettes: Arslanian-Engoren (2001) studied emergency department nurses' triage decisions in relation to patients' age and gender. She distributed vignettes for cases that contained identical cues for myocardial infarction, but that differed in patient gender and age. Nurses perceived middle-aged men as needing more urgent triage than same-aged women with the same symptoms.

Evaluation of Vignettes

Vignettes are an economical means of eliciting information about how people might behave in situations that would be difficult to observe in daily life. For example, we might want to assess how patients feel about nurses with different personal styles of interaction. In clinical settings, it would be difficult to expose patients to different nurses who have been evaluated as having different personal styles. Another advantage of vignettes is that the stimuli (the vignettes) can be manipulated experimentally by randomly assigning vignettes to groups, as in the study of nurses' triage decisions. Furthermore, vignettes often represent an interesting task for subjects. Finally, vignettes can be incorporated into questionnaires distributed by mail or over the Internet, and are therefore an inexpensive data collection strategy.

The principal problem with vignettes concerns the validity of responses. If respondents describe how they would react in a situation portrayed in the vignette, how accurate is that description of their actual behavior? Thus, although the use of vignettes can be profitable, the possibility of response biases should be recognized.

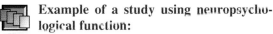 **TIP:** Sometimes the methods described in this chapter are attractive because they are unusual and may therefore seem like a more creative approach to collecting data than self-report and observational methods. However, the prime considerations in selecting a data collection method should always be the conceptual congruence between the constructs of interest and the method, and the quality of data that the method yields.

COGNITIVE AND NEUROPSYCHOLOGICAL TESTS

Nurse researchers sometimes are interested in assessing the cognitive skills of study participants. There are several different types of **cognitive tests**.

Intelligence tests are attempts to evaluate a person's global ability to perceive relationships and solve problems. *Aptitude tests* are designed to measure a person's potential for achievement, usually achievement of an academic nature. In practice, the terms *aptitude, intelligence,* and *general mental ability* are often used interchangeably. Of the many such tests available, some have been developed for individual (one-on-one) administration, whereas others have been developed for group use. Individual tests, such as the Stanford-Binet or Wechsler I.Q. tests, must be administered by a person who has received training as a tester. Group tests of ability, such as the Scholastic Assessment Test (SAT)**,** can be administered with little training. Intelligence or aptitude tests give scores for global ability and, usually, subscores for different areas, such as quantitative, verbal, and spatial ability. Nurse researchers have been particularly likely to use ability tests in studies of high-risk groups, such as low-birth-weight children. Good sources for learning more about ability tests

are the books by Anastasi and Urbina (1997) and Walsh and Betz (1995).

Example of a study using cognitive tests: Bender and colleagues (2000) described a pilot study of changes in cognitive function among patients with melanoma receiving interferon alfa-2b. The Wechsler Adult Intelligence Scale (WAIS) and other cognitive tests were administered before treatment and at several points during and after treatment.

Some cognitive tests are specially designed to assess neuropsychological functioning among those with potential cognitive impairments, such as the Mini-Mental Status Examination (MMSE). These tests capture varying types of competence, such as the ability to concentrate and the ability to remember. Nurses have used such tests extensively in studies of elderly patients and patients with Alzheimer's disease.

Example of a study using neuropsychological function: Souder and O'Sullivan (2000) examined the extent to which nurses document the cognitive status of hospitalized individuals. Participants were administered the MMSE and Neurobehavioral Cognitive Status Examination. A chart review revealed no mention of cognitive impairment for the 42 subjects, but the tests revealed considerable impairment.

Nurse researchers sometimes use achievement tests designed to measure a person's present level of proficiency in a knowledge area. Because both practicing nurses and nurse educators engage in teaching, measuring instructional effectiveness is of interest to some nurse researchers. Achievement tests may be standardized for use by thousands, or specially constructed to assess specific knowledge. Standardized tests are carefully developed and tested, and normally cover broad achievement objectives. The constructors of such tests establish **norms**, which permit comparisons between study participants and a reference group. The NLN Achievement Test is an example of a standardized test. For specific learning objectives, researchers may be required to construct new tests. The development of an achievement test that is objective, accurate, and valid is a challenging task; Ebel's (1991) book, *Essentials of Educational Measurement* (5th ed.), is a useful reference.

■ **TIP:** As with other methods of data collection, the importance of adequate training of data collectors for the alternative methods described in this chapter cannot be overemphasized. Even when using existing records, data collectors need to be trained with respect to the extraction of relevant data and the recording of that data in an appropriate manner.

RESEARCH EXAMPLES OF STUDIES USING ALTERNATIVE DATA COLLECTION METHODS

This section presents descriptions of two studies that used some of the data collection methods described in this chapter.

Research Example of Biophysiologic Measures and Records

Brooks-Brunn (2000) conducted a study to identify risk factors for the development of postoperative pulmonary complications (PPCs) after total abdominal hysterectomy. Her data sources included physiologic measures, self-reports, and medical records. In her multisite study, 120 patients undergoing a total abdominal hysterectomy were included in the sample. The design was prospective: Women were recruited into the sample before surgery and their PPC status was subsequently determined after surgery.

Brooks-Brunn collected data on a wide range of risk factors that had previously been identified in the literature and that were accessible to the health care team. These included preoperative, intraoperative, and postoperative risk factors. Preoperative factors included information on the subjects' health habits, demographic characteristics, and medical history. This information was obtained through a structured interview and review of medical charts. Information about intraoperative risk factors (e.g., duration of anesthesia and location, direction, and length of the incision) was obtained from charts as well. Postoperative risk factors included the presence of a nasogastric tube and the initial method of pain management. After surgery, subjects underwent a daily interview and chest examination. The dependent variable, presence of absence of PPCs, was based on a combination of biophysiologic measures, such as body temperature, abnormal breath sounds, and cough/sputum production.

In the research sample, some 11% developed a PPC. Brooks-Brunn's results indicated that patients most likely to develop a PPC were older, had a history of smoking, and had a history of cancer or congestive heart failure. Also, women at highest risk were ones who had an upper (vs. lower) abdominal surgical location, and had a vertical incision.

Research Example of Records, Documents, and Available Data

D'Antonio (2001) conducted a historical study of the relationship between families and health care institutions in early 19th century Philadelphia. The research focused on the Friends Asylum for the Insane and the historical roots of these kinds of relationships in a Quaker community. The Friends Asylum was the first institution created by families, not professionals, to provide temporary respite for families from the daily stress of caring for their insane relatives.

D'Antonio's data sources included diaries, letters, and religious writings of the founders of the Friends Asylum and relatives that had family members as patients there. Other sources of data were the Annual Reports (1817–1850) and committee minutes of the Friends Asylum managers. These reports/minutes provided data on the creation and maintenance of this institution. D'Antonio identified two additional data sources as deserving particular attention: the Necrology File (NF) in the Haverford College Quaker Collection and the daily diaries of the Friends Asylum's lay superintendents. In the NF were archival and bibliographic references that helped to explain the social and class context of early 19th century. The lay superintendents' diaries revealed detailed descriptions of the patterns of use of the Asylum and also the relationships among families, the Asylum's staff, and the institution.

Review of these various data sources revealed that families in the early 19th century presented health care professionals not only with dilemmas but also with solutions. This historical study reminds nurses that it may not be nurses who empower patients, but at times it may be the patients who empower nurses.

SUMMARY POINTS

- For certain research problems, alternatives to self-report and observation—especially **biophysiologic measures**—may be appropriate data collection techniques.
- **Biophysiologic measures** can be classified as either **in vivo measurements** (those performed within or on living organisms, like blood pressure measurement) or **in vitro measurements** (those performed outside the organism's body, such as blood tests).
- In vivo measures often rely on complex **instrumentation systems**, the components of which include the stimulus, subject, sensing equipment, signal-conditioning equipment, display equipment, and recording equipment.
- Biophysiologic measures have the advantage of being objective, accurate, and precise, but care must be taken in using such measures with regard to practical, technical, and ethical considerations.
- Existing **records** and documents provide an economical source of research data. Two major potential sources of bias in records are **selective deposit** and **selective survival**.
- **Q sorts**, in which people sort a set of card statements into piles according to specified criteria, can be used to measure attitudes, personality, and other psychological traits.
- One limitation of Q sorts is that they yield **ipsative measures**; the average across cards is an irrelevant basis of comparison because the forced-choice approach produces the same average for all subjects. This differs from other techniques that produce **normative measures** (e.g., Likert scales) because each choice is independent of other choices.
- **Projective techniques** are data collection methods that rely on people's projection of psychological traits in response to vaguely structured stimuli. **Pictorial methods** present pictures or cartoons and ask participants for their reactions.

Verbal methods present people with an ambiguous verbal stimulus rather than a picture; two types of verbal methods are **word association** and **sentence completion**. **Expressive methods** take the form of play, drawing, or role playing.
- **Vignettes** are brief descriptions of an event or situation to which respondents are asked to react. They are used to assess respondents' hypothetical behaviors, opinions, and perceptions.
- Various aspects of cognitive functioning can be measured by **cognitive tests**, including intelligence or aptitude, neuropsychological functioning, and achievement.

STUDY ACTIVITIES

Chapter 17 of the *Study Guide to Accompany Nursing Research: Principles and Methods, 7th edition*, offers various exercises and study suggestions for reinforcing concepts presented in this chapter. In addition, the following study questions can be addressed:

1. Formulate a research question for which each of the following could be used as measures of the dependent variable:
   a. Blood pressure
   b. Electromyograms
   c. Tidal volume
   d. Blood sugar levels
2. Identify some of the in vivo or in vitro measures you might use to address the following research questions:
   a. Does clapping the lungs before suctioning result in better patient outcomes than suctioning without clapping?
   b. What is the effect of various bed positions on the development of respiratory acidosis or alkalosis?
   c. What are the cardiovascular effects of administering liquid potassium chloride in three different solutions (orange juice, fruit punch, cranberry juice)?
   d. What is the rate of respiratory increase for designated decreases in the pH level of cerebrospinal fluid?

3. Suppose that you were interested in studying the following variables: fear of death in patients, fathers' reactions to their newborn infants, caretakers' stress, and patients' spirituality. Describe at least two ways of collecting data relating to these concepts, using the following approaches:

a. Vignettes
b. Verbal projective techniques
c. Pictorial projective techniques
d. Records
e. Q sorts

SUGGESTED READINGS

Methodologic References

Biophysiologic References

Abbey, J. (Guest Ed.). (1978). Symposium on bioinstrumentation for nurses. *Nursing Clinics of North America, 13*, 561–640.

Bauer, J. D., Ackermann, P. G., & Toro, G. (1982). *Clinical laboratory methods* (9th ed.). St. Louis: C. V. Mosby.

Chernecky, C., & Berger, B. J. (2001). *Laboratory tests and diagnostic procedures* (3rd ed.). Philadelphia: W. B. Saunders.

Fischbach, F. T. (1999). *A manual of laboratory diagnostic tests* (6th ed.). Philadelphia: Lippincott Williams & Wilkins.

Kraemer, H. C. (1992). *Evaluating medical tests: Objective and quantitative guidelines*. Newbury Park, CA: Sage.

Pagana, K. D., & Pagana, T. J. (1998). *Mosby's manual of diagnostic and laboratory tests*. St. Louis: C. V. Mosby.

Pugh, L. C., & DeKeyser, F. G. (1995). Use of physiologic variables in nursing research. *Image: The Journal of Nursing Scholarship, 27*, 273–276.

Tietz, N. E. (Ed.). (1995). *Clinical guide to laboratory tests* (3rd ed.). Washington, DC: AACC Press.

Webster, J. G. (1988). *Encyclopedia of medical devices and instrumentation*. New York: John Wiley & Sons.

References for Other Data Collection Methods

Aaronson, L. S., & Burman, M. E. (1994). Use of health records in research: Reliability and validity issues. *Research in Nursing and Health, 17*, 67–74.

Anastasi, A., & Urbina, S. (1996). *Psychological testing* (7th ed.). Englewood Cliffs, NJ: Prentice-Hall.

Angell, R. C., & Freedman, R. (1953). The use of documents, records, census materials, and indices. In L. Festinger & D. Katz (Eds.), *Research methods in the behavioral sciences* (pp. 300–326). New York: Holt, Rinehart & Winston.

Block, J. (1978). *The Q-Sort method in personality assessment and psychiatric research* (2nd ed.). Springfield, IL: Charles C Thomas.

Bond, E. F., & Heitkemper, M. M. (2001). Physiological nursing science: Emerging directions. *Research in Nursing & Health, 24*, 345–348.

Brown, S. R. (1996). Q methodology and qualitative research. *Qualitative Health Research, 6*, 561–567.

Cordingley, L., Webb, C., & Hillier V. (1997). Q methodology. *Nurse Researcher, 4*, 31–45.

Crumbaugh, J. C. (1989). *A primer of projective techniques of psychological assessment*. San Diego, CA: Libra.

Ebel, R. (1991). *Essentials of educational measurement* (5th ed.) Englewood Cliffs, NJ: Prentice-Hall.

Flaskerud, J. H. (1979). Use of vignettes to elicit responses toward broad concepts. *Nursing Research, 28*, 210–212.

Groth-Marnet, G. (1997). *Handbook of psychological assessment* (3rd ed.) New York: John Wiley & Sons.

Lanza, M. L. (1988). Development of a vignette. *Western Journal of Nursing Research, 10*, 346–351.

Lezak, M. D. (1995). *Neuropsychological assessment*. New York: Oxford University Press.

Ludwick, R., & Zeller, R. A. (2001). The factorial survey: An experimental method to replicate real world problems. *Nursing Research, 50*, 129–133.

Semeomoff, B. (1976). *Projective techniques*. New York: John Wiley & Sons.

Simpson, S. H. (1989). Use of Q-sort methodology in cross-cultural nutrition and health research. *Nursing Research, 38*, 289–290.

Stephenson, W. (1975). *The study of behavior: Q technique and its methodology*. Chicago: University of Chicago Press.

Tetting, D. W. (1988). Q-sort update. *Western Journal of Nursing Research, 10*, 757–765.

Walsh, W. B., & Betz, N. E. (1995). *Tests and assessments* (3rd ed.) Englewood Cliffs, NJ: Prentice-Hall

Waltz, C. F., Strickland, O. L., & Lenz, E. R. (1991). *Measurement in nursing research* (2nd ed.). Philadelphia: F. A. Davis.

Studies Cited in Chapter 17

Arslanian-Engoren, C. (2001). Gender and age differences in nurses' triage decisions using vignette patients. *Nursing Research, 50,* 61–66.

Belza, B., Steele, B. G., Hunziker, J., Lakshminaryan, S., Holt, L., & Buchner, D. (2001). Correlates of physical activity in chronic obstructive pulmonary disease. *Nursing Research, 50,* 195–202.

Bender, C. M., Yasko, J., Kirkwood, J., Ryan, C., Dunbar-Jacob, J., Zullo, T. (2000). Cognitive function and quality of life in interferon therapy for melanoma. *Clinical Nursing Research, 9,* 352–63.

Bliss, D. Z., Jung, H., Savik, K., Lowry, A., MeMoine, M., Jensen, L., Werner, C., & Schaffer, K. (2001). Supplementation with dietary fiber improves fecal incontinence. *Nursing Research, 50,* 203–213.

Brooks-Brunn, J. A. (2000). Risk factors associated with postoperative pulmonary complications following total abdominal hysterectomy. *Clinical Nursing Research, 9,* 27–46.

Cohen, S., Hayes, J., Tordella, T., & Puente I. (2002). Thermal efficiency of prewarmed cotton, reflective, and forced-warm-air inflatable blankets in trauma patients. *International Journal of Trauma Nursing, 8,* 4–8.

D'Antonio, P. (2001). Founding friends: Families and institution building in early 19th century Philadelphia. *Nursing Research, 50,* 260–266.

Gray, M., McClain, R., Peruggia, M., Patrie, J., & Steers, W. D. (2001). A model for predicting motor urge urinary incontinence. *Nursing Research, 50,* 116–122.

Hammond, B., Ali, Y., Fendler, E., Dolan, M., & Donovan, S. (2000). Effect of hand sanitizer use on elementary school absenteeism. *American Journal of Infection Control, 28,* 340–346.

Hillman, K. A. (1997). Comparing child-rearing practices in parents of children with cancer and parents of healthy children. *Journal of Pediatric Oncology Nursing, 14,* 53–67.

Instone, S. L. (2000). Perceptions of children with HIV infection when not told for so long. *Journal of Pediatric Health Care, 14,* 235–243.

Jellema, W. T., Groeneveld, J., van Goudoever, J., Wesseling, K. H., Westerhof, N., Lubbers, M. J., Kesecioglu, J., & van Lieshout, J. J. (2000). Hemodynamic effects of intermittent manual lung hyperinflation in patients with septic shock. *Heart & Lung, 29,* 356–366.

Krulik, T., & Florian, V. (1995) Social isolation of school-age children with chronic illnesses. *Social Sciences in Health: International Journal of Research & Practice, 1,* 164–174.

Nantais-Smith, L. M., Covington, C., Nordstrom-Klee, B., Grubbs, C., Eto, I., Lawson, D., Pieper, B., & Northouse, L. (2001). Differences in plasma and nipple aspirate carotenoid by lactation status. *Nursing Research, 50,* 172–177.

Powers, B. A. (2001). Ethnographic analysis of everyday ethics in the care of nursing home residents with dementia. *Nursing Research, 50,* 332–339.

Snethen, J. A., & Broome, M. E. (2001). Adolescents' perception of living with end stage renal disease. *Pediatric Nursing, 27,* 159–167.

Sobie, J. M., Gaves, D., & Tringali, A. (2000). ED "hold" patients: Is their care also being held? *Journal of Emergency Nursing, 26,* 549–553.

Souder, E., & O'Sullivan, P. (2000). Nursing documentation versus standardized assessment of cognitive status in hospitalized medical patients. *Applied Nursing Research, 13,* 29–36.

Wipke-Tevis, D. D., Stotts, N. A., Williams, D. A., Froelicher, E. S., & Hunt, T. K. (2001). Tissue oxygenation, perfusion, and position in patients with venous leg ulcers. *Nursing Research, 50,* 24–32.

Wong, H. L., Lopez-Nahas, V., & Molassiotis, A. (2001). Effects of music therapy on anxiety in ventilator-dependent patients. *Heart & Lung, 30,* 376–387.

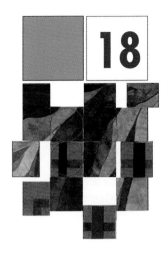

18

Assessing Data Quality

An ideal data collection procedure is one that captures a construct in a way that is relevant, credible, accurate, truthful, and sensitive. For most concepts of interest to nurse researchers, there are few data collection procedures that match this ideal. Biophysiologic methods have a higher chance of success in attaining these goals than self-report or observational methods, but no method is flawless. In this chapter, we discuss criteria for evaluating the quality of data obtained in a study. We begin by discussing principles of measurement and assessments of quantitative data. Later in this chapter, we discuss assessments of qualitative data.

MEASUREMENT

Quantitative studies derive data through the measurement of variables. **Measurement** involves the assignment of numbers to represent the amount of an attribute present in an object or person, using a specified set of rules. As this definition implies, quantification and measurement go hand in hand. An often-quoted statement by early American psychologist L. L. Thurstone advances a fundamental position: "Whatever exists, exists in some amount and can be measured." Attributes are not constant: They vary from day to day, from situation to situation, or from one person to another. This variability is presumed to be capable of a numeric expression that signifies *how much* of an attribute is present.

The purpose of assigning numbers is to differentiate between people or objects that possess varying degrees of the critical attribute.

Rules and Measurement

Measurement involves assigning numbers to objects according to rules, rather than haphazardly. Rules for measuring temperature, weight, blood pressure, and other physical attributes are familiar to us. Rules for measuring many variables for nursing research studies, however, have to be invented. Whether the data are collected by observation, self-report,. or some other method, researchers must specify under what conditions and according to what criteria the numeric values are to be assigned to the characteristic of interest.

As an example, suppose we were studying attitudes toward distributing condoms in school-based clinics and asked parents to express their extent of agreement with the following statement:

Teenagers should have access to contraceptives in school clinics.
  { } Strongly agree
  { } Agree
  { } Slightly agree
  { } Neither agree nor disagree
  { } Slightly disagree
  { } Disagree
  { } Strongly disagree

Responses to this question can be quantified by developing a system for assigning numbers to them. Note that *any* rule would satisfy the definition of measurement. We could assign the value of 30 to "strongly agree," 27 to "agree," 20 to "slightly agree," and so on, but there is no justification for doing so. In measuring attributes, researchers strive to use good, meaningful rules. Without any *a priori* information about the "distance" between the seven options, the most defensible procedure is to assign a 1 to "strongly agree" and a 7 to "strongly disagree." This rule would quantitatively differentiate, in increments of one point, among people with seven different reactions to the statement. With a new instrument, researchers seldom know in advance if their rules are the best possible. New measurement rules reflect researchers' hypotheses about how attributes function and vary. The adequacy of the hypotheses—that is, the worth of the instruments—needs to be assessed empirically.

Researchers endeavor to link numeric values to reality. To state this goal more technically, measurement procedures must be isomorphic to reality. The term **isomorphism** signifies equivalence or similarity between two phenomena. An instrument cannot be useful unless the measures resulting from it correspond with the real world.

To illustrate the concept of isomorphism, suppose the Scholastic Assessment Test (SAT) were administered to 10 students, who obtained the following scores: 345, 395, 430, 435, 490, 505, 550, 570, 620, and 640. These values are shown at the top of Figure 18-1. Now suppose that in reality the true scores of these same students on a hypothetically perfect test were as follows: 360, 375, 430, 465, 470, 500, 550, 610, 590, and 670, as shown at the bottom of Figure 18-1. This figure shows that, although not perfect, the test came fairly close to representing true scores; only two people (H and I) were improperly ordered in the actual test. This example illustrates a measure whose isomorphism with reality is high, but improvable.

Researchers almost always work with fallible measures. Instruments that measure psychological phenomena are less likely to correspond to reality than physical measures, but few instruments are error free.

Advantages of Measurement

What exactly does measurement accomplish? Consider how handicapped health care professionals—and researchers—would be in the absence of measurement. What would happen, for example, if there were no measures of body temperature or blood pressure? Subjective evaluations of clinical outcomes would have to be used. A principal strength of measurement is that it removes subjectivity and guesswork. Because measurement is

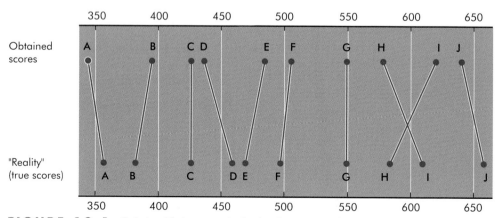

FIGURE 18.1 Relationship between obtained and true scores for a hypothetical set of test scores.

based on explicit rules, resulting information tends to be objective, that is, it can be independently verified. Two people measuring the weight of a person using the same scale would likely get identical results. Not all measures are completely objective, but most incorporate mechanisms for minimizing subjectivity.

Measurement also makes it possible to obtain reasonably precise information. Instead of describing Nathan as "rather tall," we can depict him as being 6 feet 2 inches tall. If we chose, we could obtain even greater precision. With precise measures, researchers can more readily differentiate among people with different degrees of an attribute.

Finally, measurement is a language of communication. Numbers are less vague than words and therefore can communicate information more accurately. If a researcher reported that the average oral temperature of a sample of patients was "somewhat high," different readers might develop different conceptions about the sample's physiologic state. However, if the researcher reported an average temperature of 99.6°F, there would be no ambiguity.

Errors of Measurement

Both the procedures involved in applying measurements and the objects being measured are susceptible to influences that can alter the resulting data. Some influences can be controlled to a certain degree, and attempts should always be made to do so, but such efforts are rarely completely successful.

Instruments that are not perfectly accurate yield measurements containing some error. Conceptually, an **observed** (or **obtained**) **score** can be decomposed into two parts—an error component and a true component. This can be written symbolically as follows:

$$\text{Obtained score} = \text{True score} \pm \text{Error}$$

or

$$X_O = X_T \pm X_E$$

The first term in the equation is an observed score—for example, a systolic blood pressure reading or a score on an anxiety scale. X_T is the value that would be obtained with an infallible measure. The **true score** is hypothetical—it can never be known because measures are *not* infallible. The final term in the equation is the **error of measurement**. The difference between true and obtained scores is the result of factors that distort the measurement.

Decomposing obtained scores in this fashion highlights an important point. When researchers measure an attribute, they are also *measuring* attributes that are not of interest. The true score component is what they hope to isolate; the error component is a composite of other factors that are also being measured, contrary to their wishes. This concept can be illustrated with an exaggerated example. Suppose a researcher measured the weight of 10 people on a spring scale. As subjects step on the scale, the researcher places a hand on their shoulders and applies some pressure. The resulting measures (the X_Os) will be biased upward because the scores reflect both actual weight (X_T) and the researcher's pressure (X_E). Errors of measurement are problematic because their value is unknown and also because they are variable. In this example, the amount of pressure applied likely would vary from one subject to the next. In other words, the proportion of true score component in an obtained score varies from one person to the next.

Many factors contribute to errors of measurement. The most common are the following:

1. *Situational contaminants.* Scores can be affected by the conditions under which they are produced. A participant's awareness of an observer's presence (reactivity) is one source of bias. The anonymity of the response situation, the friendliness of researchers, or the location of the data gathering can affect subjects' responses. Other environmental factors, such as temperature, lighting, and time of day, can represent sources of measurement error.
2. *Transitory personal factors.* A person's score can be influenced by such temporary personal states as fatigue, hunger, anxiety, or mood. In some cases, such factors directly affect the measurement, as when anxiety affects a pulse

rate measurement. In other cases, personal factors can alter scores by influencing people's motivation to cooperate, act naturally, or do their best.

3. *Response-set biases.* Relatively enduring characteristics of respondents can interfere with accurate measures. Response sets such as social desirability, acquiescence, and extreme responses are potential problems in self-report measures, particularly in psychological scales (see Chapter 15).

4. *Administration variations.* Alterations in the methods of collecting data from one person to the next can result in score variations unrelated to variations in the target attribute. If observers alter their coding categories, if interviewers improvise question wording, if test administrators change the test instructions, or if some physiologic measures are taken before a feeding and others are taken after a feeding, then measurement errors can potentially occur.

5. *Instrument clarity.* If the directions for obtaining measures are poorly understood, then scores may be affected by misunderstanding. For example, questions in a self-report instrument may be interpreted differently by different respondents, leading to a distorted measure of the variable. Observers may miscategorize observations if the classification scheme is unclear.

6. *Item sampling.* Errors can be introduced as a result of the sampling of items used in the measure. For example, a nursing student's score on a 100-item test of nursing knowledge will be influenced somewhat by *which* 100 questions are included. A person might get 95 questions correct on one test but only 92 right on another similar test.

7. *Instrument format.* Technical characteristics of an instrument can influence measurements. Open-ended questions may yield different information than closed-ended ones. Oral responses to a question may be at odds with written responses to the same question. The ordering of questions in an instrument may also influence responses.

RELIABILITY OF MEASURING INSTRUMENTS

The reliability* of a quantitative instrument is a major criterion for assessing its quality and adequacy. An instrument's **reliability** is the consistency with which it measures the target attribute. If a scale weighed a person at 120 pounds one minute and 150 pounds the next, we would consider it unreliable. The less variation an instrument produces in repeated measurements, the higher its reliability. Thus, reliability can be equated with a measure's stability, consistency, or dependability.

Reliability also concerns a measure's accuracy. An instrument is reliable to the extent that its measures reflect true scores—that is, to the extent that errors of measurement are absent from obtained scores. A reliable measure maximizes the true score component and minimizes the error component.

These two ways of explaining reliability (consistency and accuracy) are not so different as they might appear. Errors of measurement that impinge on an instrument's accuracy also affect its consistency. The example of the scale with variable weight readings illustrates this point. Suppose that the true weight of a person is 125 pounds, but that two independent measurements yielded 120 and 150 pounds. In terms of the equation presented in the previous section, we could express the measurements as follows:

$$120 = 125 - 5$$
$$150 = 125 + 25$$

The errors of measurement for the two trials (-5 and $+25$, respectively) resulted in scores that are inconsistent *and* inaccurate.

The reliability of an instrument can be assessed in various ways. The method chosen depends on the nature of the instrument and on the aspect of reliability of greatest concern. Three key aspects are stability, internal consistency, and equivalence.

---

*The discussion of reliability presented here is based on classic measurement theory. Readers concerned with assessing the reliability of instructional measures that can be classified as mastery-type or criterion-referenced should consult Thorndike (1996).

Stability

The **stability** of an instrument is the extent to which similar results are obtained on two separate administrations. The reliability estimate focuses on the instrument's susceptibility to extraneous factors over time, such as subject fatigue or environmental conditions.

Assessments of an instrument's stability involve procedures that evaluate **test–retest reliability**. Researchers administer the same measure to a sample on two occasions and then compare the scores. The comparison is performed objectively by computing a **reliability coefficient**, which is a numeric index of the magnitude of the test's reliability.

To explain a reliability coefficient, we must briefly discuss a statistic known as the **correlation coefficient**.* We have pointed out repeatedly that researchers strive to detect and explain relationships among phenomena: Is there a relationship between patients' gastric acidity levels and exposure to stress? Is there a relationship between body temperature and physical exertion? The correlation coefficient is a tool for quantitatively describing the magnitude and direction of a relationship between two variables. The computation of this index does not concern us here. It is more important to understand how to read a correlation coefficient.

Two variables that are obviously related are people's height and weight. Tall people tend to be heavier than short people. We would say that there was a **perfect relationship** if the tallest person in a population were the heaviest, the second tallest person were the second heaviest, and so forth. Correlation coefficients summarize how perfect relationships are. The possible values for a correlation coefficient range from −1.00 through .00 to +1.00. If height and weight were perfectly correlated, the correlation coefficient expressing this relationship would be 1.00. Because the relationship does exist but is not perfect, the correlation coefficient is typically in the vicinity of .50 or .60. The relationship between height and

weight can be described as a **positive relationship** because increases in height tend to be associated with increases in weight.

When two variables are totally unrelated, the correlation coefficient equals zero. One might expect that women's dress sizes are unrelated to their intelligence. Large women are as likely to perform well on IQ tests as small women. The correlation coefficient summarizing such a relationship would presumably be in the vicinity of .00.

Correlation coefficients running from .00 to −1.00 express **inverse** or **negative relationships**. When two variables are inversely related, increases in one variable are associated with *decreases* in the second variable. Suppose that there is an inverse relationship between people's age and the amount of sleep they get. This means that, on average, the older the person, the fewer the hours of sleep. If the relationship were perfect (e.g., if the oldest person in a population got the least sleep, and so on), the correlation coefficient would be −1.00. In actuality, the relationship between age and sleep is probably modest—in the vicinity of −.15 or −.20. A correlation coefficient of this magnitude describes a weak relationship wherein older people tend to sleep fewer hours and younger people tend to sleep more, but a "crossing of lines" is common. That is, many young people sleep few hours, and many older people sleep a lot.

Now we can discuss the use of correlation coefficients to compute reliability estimates. With test–retest reliability, an instrument is administered twice to the same sample. Suppose we wanted to assess the stability of a self-esteem scale. Self-esteem is a fairly stable attribute that does not fluctuate much from day to day, so we would expect a reliable measure of it to yield consistent scores on two occasions. To check the instrument's stability, we administer the scale 3 weeks apart to a sample of 10 people. Fictitious data for this example are presented in Table 18-1. It can be seen that, in general, differences in scores on the two testings are not large. The reliability coefficient for test–retest estimates is the correlation coefficient between the two sets of scores. In this example, the computed reliability coefficient is .95, which is high.

---

*Computational procedures and additional information concerning correlation coefficients (Pearson's *r*) are presented in Chapter 19.

TABLE 18.1 Fictitious Data for Test–Retest Reliability of Self-Esteem Scale

SUBJECT NUMBER	TIME 1	TIME 2
1	55	57
2	49	46
3	78	74
4	37	35
5	44	46
6	50	56
7	58	55
8	62	66
9	48	50
10	67	63 $r = .95$

The value of the reliability coefficient theoretically can range between −1.00 and +1.00, like other correlation coefficients. A negative coefficient would have been obtained in our example if those with high self-esteem scores at time 1 had low scores at time 2. In practice, reliability coefficients normally range between .00 and 1.00. The higher the coefficient, the more stable the measure. Reliability coefficients above .70 usually are considered satisfactory. In some situations, a higher coefficient may be required, or a lower one may be acceptable.

The test–retest method is a relatively easy approach to estimating reliability, and can be used with self-report, observational, and physiologic measures.* The test–retest approach has certain disadvantages, however. One issue is that many traits *do* change over time, independently of the measure's stability. Attitudes, behaviors, knowledge, physical condition, and so forth can be

modified by experiences between testings. Test–retest procedures confound changes from measurement error and those from true changes in the attribute being measured. Still, there are many relatively enduring attributes for which a test–retest approach is suitable.

Stability estimates suffer from other problems, however. One possibility is that subjects' responses or observers' coding on the second administration will be influenced by their memory of initial responses or coding, regardless of the actual values the second day. Such memory interference results in spuriously high reliability coefficients. Another difficulty is that subjects may actually change *as a result of* the first administration. Finally, people may not be as careful using the same instrument a second time. If they find the process boring on the second occasion, then responses could be haphazard, resulting in a spuriously low estimate of stability.

On the whole, reliability coefficients tend to be higher for short-term retests than for long-term retests (i.e., those greater than 1 or 2 months) because of actual changes in the attribute being measured. Stability indexes are most appropriate for relatively enduring characteristics such as personality, abilities, or certain physical attributes such as adult height.

Example of test–retest reliability:
Gauthier and Froman (2001) developed an instrument called the Preferences for Care near the End of Life (PCEOL) scale. The scale's reliability assessment included administering the scale to 38 adults 2 weeks apart. The test–retest reliability coefficients for subscales of the PCEOL ranged from .80 to .94.

Internal Consistency

Scales and tests that involve summing items are often evaluated for their internal consistency. Scales designed to measure an attribute ideally are composed of items that measure that attribute and nothing else. On a scale to measure nurses' empathy, it would be inappropriate to include an item that measures diagnostic competence. An instrument may be

---

*There are more sophisticated methods of assessing test–retest reliability, as described by Yen and Lo (2002).

said to be **internally consistent** or **homogeneous** to the extent that its items measure the same trait.

Internal consistency reliability is the most widely used reliability approach among nurse researchers. Its popularity reflects the fact that it is economical (it requires only one test administration) and is the best means of assessing an especially important source of measurement error in psychosocial instruments, the sampling of items.

TIP: Many scales and tests contain multiple **subscales** or subtests, each of which tap distinct, but related, concepts (e.g., a measure of independent functioning might include subscales for motor activities, communication, and socializing). The internal consistency of the subscales is typically assessed and, if subscale scores are summed for an overall score, the scale's internal consistency would also be assessed.

One of the oldest methods for assessing internal consistency is the **split-half technique**. For this approach, items on a scale are split into two groups and scored independently. Scores on the two half-tests then are used to compute a correlation coefficient. To illustrate, the 10 fictitious scores from the first administration of the self-esteem scale are reproduced in the second column of Table 18-2. Let us say that the total instrument consists of 20 questions, and so the items must be divided into two groups of 10. Although many splits are possible, the usual procedure is to use odd items versus even items. One half-test, therefore, consists of items 1, 3, 5, 7, 9, 11, 13, 15, 17, and 19, and the even-numbered items compose the second half-test. Scores on the two halves are shown in the third and fourth columns of Table 18-2. The correlation coefficient for scores on the two half-tests gives an estimate of the scale's internal consistency. If the odd items are measuring the same attribute as the even items, then the reliability coefficient should be high. The correlation coefficient computed on these fictitious data is .67.

The correlation coefficient computed on split-halves tends to underestimate the reliability of the entire scale. Other things being equal, longer scales are more reliable than shorter ones. The correlation coefficient for the data in Table 18-2 is the estimated reliability for a 10-item, not a 20-item, instrument. A correction formula has been developed to give a reliability estimate for the entire test. The equation,

TABLE 18.2 Fictitious Data for Split-Half Reliability of the Self-Esteem Scale

SUBJECT NUMBER	TOTAL SCORE	ODD-NUMBERS SCORE	EVEN-NUMBERS SCORE
1	55	28	27
2	49	26	23
3	78	36	42
4	37	18	19
5	44	23	21
6	50	30	20
7	58	30	28
8	62	33	29
9	48	23	25
10	67	28	39 $r = .80$

known as the **Spearman-Brown prophecy formula**, is as follows for this situation:

$$r^1 = \frac{2r}{1 + r}$$

where r = the correlation coefficient computed on the split halves

r^1 = the estimated reliability of the entire test

Using the formula, the reliability for our hypothetical 20-item measure of self-esteem would be:

$$r^1 = \frac{(2)(.67)}{1 + .67} = .80$$

The split-half technique is easy to use, but is handicapped by the fact that different reliability estimates can be obtained with different splits. That is, it makes a difference whether one uses an odd—even split, a first-half—second-half split, or some other method of dividing items into two groups.

The most widely used method for evaluating internal consistency is **coefficient alpha** (or **Cronbach's alpha**). Coefficient alpha can be interpreted like other reliability coefficients described here; the normal range of values is between .00 and +1.00, and higher values reflect a higher internal consistency. Coefficient alpha is preferable to the split-half procedure because it gives an estimate of the split-half correlation for *all possible* ways of dividing the measure into two halves. It is beyond the scope of this text to explain this method in detail, but more information is available in textbooks on psychometrics (e.g., Cronbach, 1990; Nunnally & Bernstein, 1994).*

---

*The coefficient alpha equation, for the advanced student, is as follows:

$$r = \frac{k}{k - 1} \left[1 - \frac{\Sigma \sigma_i^2}{\sigma y^2} \right]$$

where r = the estimated reliability

k = the total number of items in the test

σ_i^2 = the variance of each individual item

σy^2 = the variance of the total test scores

Σ = the sum of

In summary, indices of homogeneity or internal consistency estimate the extent to which different subparts of an instrument are equivalent in measuring the critical attribute. The split-half technique has been used to estimate homogeneity, but coefficient alpha is preferable. Neither approach considers fluctuations over time as a source of unreliability.

Example of internal consistency reliability: Brown, Becker, Garcia, Barton, and Hanis (2002) adapted a measure of health beliefs for use with Spanish-speaking Mexican Americans with type 2 diabetes. The adapted instrument, administered to 326 Mexican Americans, was found to have 5 subscales, with alpha coefficients ranging from .56 to .90.

Equivalence

Nurse researchers estimate a measure's reliability by way of the **equivalence** approach primarily with observational measures. In Chapter 16, we pointed out that a potential weakness of observational methods is observer error. The accuracy of observer ratings and classifications can be enhanced by careful training, the specification of clearly defined, nonoverlapping categories, and the use of a small number of categories. Even when such care is taken, researchers should assess the reliability of observational instruments. In this case, "instrument" includes both the category or rating system *and* the observers making the measurements.

Interrater (or **interobserver**) **reliability** is estimated by having two or more trained observers watching an event simultaneously, and independently recording data according to the instrument's instructions. The data can then be used to compute an index of equivalence or agreement between observers. For certain types of observational data (e.g., ratings), correlation techniques are suitable. That is, a correlation coefficient is computed to demonstrate the strength of the relationship between one observer's ratings and another's.

Another procedure is to compute reliability as a function of agreements, using the following equation:

$$\frac{\text{Number of agreements}}{\text{Number of agreements} + \text{disagreements}}$$

This simple formula unfortunately tends to overestimate observer agreements. If the behavior under investigation is one that observers code for absence or presence every, say, 10 seconds, the observers will agree 50% of the time by chance alone. Other approaches to estimating interrater reliability may be of interest to advanced students. Techniques such as Cohen's kappa, analysis of variance, intraclass correlations, and rank-order correlations have been used to assess interobserver reliability.

Example of interrater reliability: Kovach and Wells (2002) observed the behaviors of older people with dementia over 30-minute observation sessions. Interrater reliability, calculated as percentage agreement between two raters, was .74 for the variable *activity*, .92 for *noxiousness*, and .84 for *agitation*.

Interpretation of Reliability Coefficients

Reliability coefficients are important indicators of an instrument's quality. Unreliable measures do not provide adequate tests of researchers' hypotheses. If data fail to confirm a prediction, one possibility is that the instruments were unreliable—not necessarily that the expected relationships do not exist. Knowledge about an instrument's reliability thus is critical in interpreting research results, especially if research hypotheses are not supported.

For group-level comparisons, coefficients in the vicinity of .70 are usually adequate, although coefficients of .80 or greater are highly desirable. By group-level comparisons, we mean that researchers compare scores of groups, such as male versus female or experimental versus control subjects. If measures are used for making decisions about individuals, then reliability coefficients ideally should be .90 or better. For instance, if a test score was used as a criterion for admission to a graduate nursing program, then the accuracy of the test would be of critical importance to both individual applicants and the school of nursing.

Reliability coefficients have a special interpretation that should be briefly explained without elaborating on technical details. This interpretation relates to the earlier discussion of decomposing observed scores into error components and true components. Suppose we administered a scale that measures hope to 50 cancer patients. It would be expected that the scores would vary from one person to another—that is, some people would be more hopeful than others. Some variability in scores is true variability, reflecting real individual differences in hopefulness; some variability, however, is error. Thus,

$$V_O = V_T + V_E$$

where V_O = observed total variability in scores

V_T = true variability

V_E = variability owing to random errors

A reliability coefficient is directly associated with this equation. *Reliability is the proportion of true variability to the total obtained variability*, or

$$r = \frac{V_T}{V_O}$$

If, for example, the reliability coefficient were .85, then 85% of the variability in obtained scores would represent true individual differences, and 15% of the variability would reflect random, extraneous fluctuations. Looked at in this way, it should be clearer why instruments with reliability lower than .70 are risky to use.

Factors Affecting Reliability

Researchers who develop or adapt instruments for their own use or for use by others must undertake reliability assessments. The availability of computer programs to calculate coefficient alphas has made this task convenient and economical. There are also things that instrument developers should keep in mind during the development process that can enhance reliability.

First, as previously noted, the reliability of composite self-report and observational scales is partly a function of their length (i.e., number of items). To improve reliability, more items tapping the same concept should be added. Items that have no discriminating power (i.e., that elicit similar responses from everyone) should, however, be removed. Scale developers can assess whether items are tapping the same construct and are sufficiently discriminating by doing an **item analysis**. In general, items that elicit a 50/50 split (e.g., agree/disagree or correct/incorrect) have the best discriminating power. As a general guideline, if the split is 80/20 or worse, the item should probably be replaced. Another aspect of an item analysis is an inspection of the correlations between individual items and the overall scale score. Item-to-total correlations below .30 are usually considered unacceptably low.

With observational scales, reliability can usually be improved by greater precision in defining categories, or greater clarity in explaining the underlying dimension for rating scales. The most effective means of enhancing reliability in observational studies, however, is thorough training of observers.

The reliability of an instrument is related in part to the heterogeneity of the sample with which it is used. The more homogeneous the sample (i.e., the more similar their scores), the lower the reliability coefficient will be. This is because instruments are designed to measure differences among those being measured. If the sample is homogeneous, then it is more difficult for the instrument to discriminate reliably among those who possess varying degrees of the attribute being measured. For example, a depression scale will be less reliable when administered to a homeless sample than when it is used with a general population.

Choosing an instrument previously demonstrated to be reliable is no guarantee of its high quality in a new study. An instrument's reliability is not a fixed entity. *The reliability of an instrument is a property not of the instrument but rather of the instrument when administered to a certain sample under certain conditions.* A scale that reliably measures dependence in hospitalized adults may be unreliable with nursing homes residents. This means that in selecting an instrument, it is important to know the characteristics of the group with whom it was developed. If the group is similar to the population for a new study, then the reliability estimate provided by the scale developer is probably a reasonably good index of the instrument's accuracy in the new study.

TIP: You should not be satisfied with an instrument that will *probably* be reliable in your study. The recommended procedure is to compute estimates of reliability whenever research data are collected. For physiologic measures that are relatively impervious to fluctuations from personal or situational factors, this procedure may be unnecessary. However, observational tools, self-report measures, tests of knowledge or ability, and projective tests—all of which are highly susceptible to errors of measurement—should be subjected to a reliability check as a routine step in the research process.

Finally, reliability estimates vary according to the procedures used to obtain them. A scale's test–retest reliability is rarely the same value as its internal consistency reliability. In selecting an instrument, researchers need to determine which aspect of reliability (stability, internal consistency, or equivalence) is most relevant.

Example of different reliability estimates: Chaiyawat and Brown (2000) did a psychometric assessment of the Thai version of the State-Trait Anxiety Inventory for Children. The test–retest reliability was .68 for the Trait subscale and .63 for the State subscale. Cronbach alphas for both subscales at both administrations exceeded .80.

VALIDITY

The second important criterion for evaluating a quantitative instrument is its validity. **Validity** is the degree to which an instrument measures what it is supposed to measure. When researchers develop an instrument to measure hopelessness, how can they be sure that resulting scores validly reflect this construct and not something else, like depression?

Reliability and validity are not independent qualities of an instrument. *A measuring device that is unreliable cannot possibly be valid.* An instrument cannot validly measure an attribute if it is inconsistent and inaccurate. An unreliable instrument contains too much error to be a valid indicator of the target variable. An instrument can, however, be reliable without being valid. Suppose we had the idea to assess patients' anxiety by measuring the circumference of their wrists. We could obtain highly accurate, consistent, and precise measurements of wrist circumferences, but such measures would not be valid indicators of anxiety. Thus, the high reliability of an instrument provides no evidence of its validity; low reliability of a measure *is* evidence of low validity.

Like reliability, validity has different aspects and assessment approaches. Unlike reliability, however, an instrument's validity is difficult to establish. There are no equations that can easily be applied to the scores of a hopelessness scale to estimate how good a job the scale is doing in measuring the critical variable.

Face Validity

Face validity refers to whether the instrument *looks* as though it is measuring the appropriate construct. Although face validity should not be considered primary evidence for an instrument's validity, it is helpful for a measure to have face validity if other types of validity have also been demonstrated. For example, it might be easier to persuade people to participate in an evaluation if the instruments being used have face validity.

Example of face validity:
Shin and Colling (2000) undertook a cultural verification of the Profile of Mood States (POMS) scale for Korean elders. One part of the study involved an assessment of the translated scale's face validity, using a panel of Korean experts.

Content Validity

Content validity concerns the degree to which an instrument has an appropriate sample of items for the construct being measured. Content validity is relevant for both affective measures (i.e., measures relating to feelings, emotions, and psychological traits) and cognitive measures.

For cognitive measures, the content validity question is, How representative are the questions on this test of the universe of questions on this topic? For example, suppose we were testing students'

knowledge about major nursing theories. The test would not be content valid if it omitted questions about, for example, Orem's self-care theory.

Content validity is also relevant in the development of affective measures. Researchers designing a new instrument should begin with a thorough conceptualization of the construct so the instrument can capture the entire content domain. Such a conceptualization might come from rich first-hand knowledge, an exhaustive literature review, or findings from a qualitative inquiry.

Example of using qualitative data for content validity:
Holley (2000) developed a self-report scale to measure distress from fatigue in cancer patients. Items for the scale were drawn from 23 in-depth interviews with patients experiencing cancer-related fatigue.

An instrument's content validity is necessarily based on judgment. There are no completely objective methods of ensuring the adequate content coverage of an instrument. However, it is becoming increasingly common to use a panel of substantive experts to evaluate and document the content validity of new instruments. The panel typically consists of at least three experts, but a larger number may be advisable if the construct is complex. The experts are asked to evaluate individual items on the new measure as well as the entire instrument. Two key issues in such an evaluation are whether individual items are relevant and appropriate in terms of the construct, and whether the items adequately measure all dimensions of the construct. With regard to item relevance, some researchers compute interrater agreement indexes and a formal **content validity index** (CVI) across the experts' ratings of each item's relevance. One procedure is to have experts rate items on a four-point scale (from $1 =$ not relevant to $4 =$ very relevant). The CVI for the total instrument is the proportion of items rated as either 3 or 4. A CVI score of .80 or better indicates good content validity.

Example of using a content validity index:
Rew (2000) developed a scale to tap nurses' acknowledgment of using intuition in clinical

decision making. In the first phase of the study, scale items were generated from published literature and a CVI of .96 was computed on responses from a panel of five experts.

Criterion-Related Validity

Establishing **criterion-related validity** involves determining the relationship between an instrument and an external criterion. The instrument is said to be valid if its scores correlate highly with scores on the criterion. For example, if a measure of attitudes toward premarital sex correlates highly with subsequent loss of virginity in a sample of teenagers, then the attitude scale would have good validity. For criterion-related validity, the key issue is whether the instrument is a useful predictor of other behaviors, experiences, or conditions.

One requirement of this approach is the availability of a reliable and valid criterion with which measures on the instrument can be compared. This is, unfortunately, seldom easy. If we were developing an instrument to measure the nursing effectiveness of nursing students, we might use supervisory ratings as our criterion—but can we be sure that these ratings are valid and reliable? The ratings might themselves need validation. Criterion-related validity is most appropriate when there is a concrete, well-accepted criterion. For example, a scale to measure smokers' motivation to quit smoking has a clearcut, objective criterion (subsequent smoking).

Once a criterion is selected, criterion validity can be assessed easily. A correlation coefficient is computed between scores on the instrument and the criterion. The magnitude of the coefficient is a direct estimate of how valid the instrument is, according to this validation method. To illustrate, suppose researchers developed a scale to measure nurses' professionalism. They administer the instrument to a sample of nurses and also ask the nurses to indicate how many articles they have published. The publications variable was chosen as one of many potential objective criteria of professionalism. Fictitious data are presented in Table 18-3. The correlation coefficient of .83 indicates that the professionalism scale correlates fairly well with the number of published articles. Whether the scale is really measuring professionalism is a different issue—an issue that is the concern of construct validation discussed in the next section.

TABLE 18.3 Fictitious Data for Criterion-Related Validity Example

SUBJECT	SCORE ON PROFESSIONALISM SCALE	NUMBER OF PUBLICATIONS
1	25	2
2	30	4
3	17	0
4	20	1
5	22	0
6	27	2
7	29	5
8	19	1
9	28	3
10	15	1 $r = .83$

A distinction is sometimes made between two types of criterion-related validity. **Predictive validity** refers to the adequacy of an instrument in differentiating between people's performance on some future criterion. When a school of nursing correlates incoming students' SAT scores with subsequent grade-point averages, the predictive validity of the SATs for nursing school performance is being evaluated.

Example of predictive validity:
Marsh, Prochada, Pritchett, and Vojir (2000) used a predictive validity approach in their assessment of their Alzheimer's Hospice Placement Evaluation Scale (AHOPE), a scale designed to measure the appropriateness of hospice care. The criterion used was survival status 6 months after the scale was administered.

Concurrent validity refers to an instrument's ability to distinguish individuals who differ on a present criterion. For example, a psychological test to differentiate between those patients in a mental institution who can and cannot be released could be correlated with current behavioral ratings of health care personnel. The difference between predictive and concurrent validity, then, is the difference in the timing of obtaining measurements on a criterion.

Example of concurrent validity:
Resnick and Jenkins (2000) developed the Self-Efficacy for Exercise Scale (SEE). As one of their methods of validating the scale, they correlated SEE scores with whether participants engaged in regular exercise activity, defined as 20 minutes of aerobic activity three times a week.

Validation by means of the criterion-related approach is most often used in applied or practically oriented research. Criterion-related validity is helpful in assisting decision makers by giving them some assurance that their decisions will be effective, fair, and, in short, valid.

Construct Validity

Validating an instrument in terms of **construct validity** is a challenging task. The key construct validity questions are: What is this instrument really measuring? Does it adequately measure the abstract concept of interest? Unfortunately, the more abstract the concept, the more difficult it is to establish construct validity; at the same time, the more abstract the concept, the less suitable it is to rely on criterion-related validity. Actually, it is really not just a question of suitability: What objective criterion is there for such concepts as empathy, role conflict, or separation anxiety? Despite the difficulty of construct validation, it is an activity vital to the development of a strong evidence base. The constructs in which nurse researchers are interested must be validly measured.

Construct validity is inextricably linked with theoretical factors. In validating a measure of death anxiety, we would be less concerned with the adequate sampling of items or with its relationship to a criterion than with its correspondence to a cogent conceptualization of death anxiety. Construct validation can be approached in several ways, but it always involves logical analysis and tests predicted by theoretical considerations. Constructs are explicated in terms of other abstract concepts; researchers make predictions about the manner in which the target construct will function in relation to other constructs.

One construct validation approach is the **known-groups technique**. In this procedure, the instrument is administered to groups expected to differ on the critical attribute because of some known characteristic. For instance, in validating a measure of fear of the labor experience, we could contrast the scores of primiparas and multiparas. We would expect that women who had never given birth would be more anxious than women who had done so, and so we might question the instrument's validity if such differences did not emerge. We would not necessarily expect large differences; some primiparas would feel little anxiety, and some multiparas would express some fears. On the whole, however, we would anticipate differences in average group scores.

Example of the known-groups technique:
Davies and Hodnett (2002) developed a scale to measure nurses' self-efficacy in providing

support to women in labor. To validate the scale, they compared the scores of labor and delivery nurses with those of nurses who worked in postpartum care and found significantly higher scores among the first group, as predicted.

Another method of construct validation involves an examination of relationships based on theoretical predictions, which is really a variant of the known-groups approach. A researcher might reason as follows:

- According to theory, construct X is positively related to construct Y.
- Instrument A is a measure of construct X; instrument B is a measure of construct Y.
- Scores on A and B are correlated positively, as predicted by theory.
- Therefore, it is inferred that A and B are valid measures of X and Y.

This logical analysis is fallible and does not constitute proof of construct validity, but yields important evidence. Construct validation is essentially an evidence-building enterprise.

Example of testing relationships: Ryden and her colleagues (2000) created a Satisfaction with the Nursing Home Instrument (SNHI). Their approach to construct validation included a scrutiny of the correlation between SNHI scores with scores on two affective measures. As predicted, SNHI scores were negatively associated with depression and positively associated with morale.

A significant construct validation tool is a procedure known as the **multitrait–multimethod matrix method** (**MTMM**) (Campbell & Fiske, 1959). This procedure involves the concepts of convergence and discriminability. **Convergence** is evidence that different methods of measuring a construct yield similar results. Different measurement approaches should converge on the construct. **Discriminability** is the ability to differentiate the construct from other similar constructs. Campbell and Fiske argued that evidence of both convergence and discriminability should be brought to bear in the construct validity question.

To help explain the MTMM approach, fictitious data from a study to validate a "need for autonomy" measure are presented in Table 18-4. In using this approach, researchers must measure the critical concept by two or more methods. Suppose we measured need for autonomy in nursing home residents by (1) giving a sample of residents a self-report summated rating scale (the measure we are attempting to validate); (2) asking nurses to rate residents after observing them in a task designed to elicit autonomy or dependence; and (3) having residents respond to a pictorial (projective) stimulus depicting an autonomy-relevant situation.

TABLE 18.4 Multitrait–Multimethod Matrix

METHOD	TRAITS	SELF-REPORT (1)		OBSERVATION (2)		PROJECTIVE (3)	
		AUT_1	AFF_1	AUT_2	AFF_2	AUT_3	AFF_3
Self-report (1)	AUT_1	(.88)					
	AFF_1	−.38	(.86)				
Observation (2)	AUT_2	.60	−.19	(.79)			
	AFF_2	−.21	.58	−.39	(.80)		
Projective (3)	AUT_3	.51	−.18	.55	−.12	(.74)	
	AFF_3	−.14	.49	−.17	.54	−.32	(.72)

AUT, need for autonomy trait; AFF, need for affiliation trait.

A second requirement of the full MTMM is to measure a differentiating construct, using the same measuring methods. In the current example, suppose we wanted to differentiate "need for autonomy" from "need for affiliation." The discriminant concept must be similar to the focal concept, as in our example: We would expect that people with high need for autonomy would tend to be relatively low on need for affiliation. The point of including both concepts in a single validation study is to gather evidence that the two concepts are distinct, rather than two different labels for the same underlying attribute.

The numbers in Table 18-4 represent the correlation coefficients between the scores on six different measures (two traits $\times$ three methods). For instance, the coefficient of $-.38$ at the intersection of AUT_1–AFF_1 expresses the relationship between self-report scores on the need for autonomy and need for affiliation measures. Recall that a minus sign before the correlation coefficient signifies an inverse relationship. In this case, the $-.38$ tells us that there was a slight tendency for people scoring high on the need for autonomy scale to score low on the need for affiliation scale. (The numbers in parentheses along the diagonal of this matrix are the reliability coefficients.)

Various aspects of the MTMM matrix have a bearing on construct validity. The most direct evidence (**convergent validity**) comes from the correlations between two different methods measuring the same trait. In the case of AUT_1–AUT_2, the coefficient is .60, which is reasonably high. Convergent validity should be large enough to encourage further scrutiny of the matrix. Second, the convergent validity entries should be higher, in absolute magnitude,* than correlations between measures that have neither method nor trait in common. That is, AUT_1–AUT_2 (.60) should be greater than AUT_2–AFF_1 ($-.21$) or AUT_1–AFF_2 ($-.19$), as it is in fact. This requirement is a minimum one that, if failed, should cause re-searchers to have serious doubts about the measures. Third, convergent validity coefficients should be greater than coefficients between measures of different traits by a single method. Once again, the matrix in Table 18-4 fulfills this criterion: AUT_1–AUT_2 (.60) and AUT_2–AUT_3 (.55) are higher in absolute value than AUT_1–AFF_1 ($-.38$), AUT_2–AFF_2 ($-.39$), and AUT_3–AFF_3 ($-.32$). The last two requirements provide evidence for **discriminant validity**.

The evidence is seldom as clearcut as in this contrived example. Indeed, a common problem with the MTMM is interpreting the pattern of coefficients. Another issue is that there are no clearcut criteria for determining whether MTMM requirements have been met—that is, there are no objective means of assessing the magnitude of similarities and differences within the matrix. The MTMM is nevertheless a valuable tool for exploring construct validity. Researchers sometimes decide to use MMTM concepts even when the full model is not feasible, as in focusing only on convergent validity. Executing any part of the model is better than no effort at construct validation.

Example of convergent validity:
Garvin and Kim (2000) evaluated the reliability and validity of three instruments measuring patients' preference for information. Convergent validity between two of the three measures was fair in both a Korean and U.S. sample (.30 and .51, respectively), but the third instrument had inadequate convergent validity.

Example of divergent validity:
Cacchione (2002) compared four acute confusion assessment instruments. She found that only one of them (the Visual Analog Scale for Acute Confusion) demonstrated divergent validity with a measure of geriatric depression.

Another approach to construct validation uses a statistical procedure known as factor analysis.*

---

*The **absolute magnitude** refers to the value without a plus or minus sign. A value of $-.50$ is of a higher absolute magnitude than $+.40$.

---

*Another sophisticated and complex approach to construct validation is based on **item response theory**. For an explanation, see Chapter 10 of Nunnally and Bernstein (1994). See also Hambleton, Swaminathan, and Rogers (1991).

Although factor analysis, which is discussed in Chapter 21, is computationally complex, it is conceptually rather simple. **Factor analysis** is a method for identifying clusters of related variables. Each cluster, called a **factor**, represents a relatively unitary attribute. The procedure is used to identify and group together different items measuring an underlying attribute. In effect, factor analysis constitutes another means of looking at the convergent and discriminant validity of a large set of items. Indeed, a procedure known as **confirmatory factor analysis** is sometimes used as a method for analyzing MTMM data (Ferketich, Figueredo, & Knapp, 1991; Lowe & Ryan-Wenger, 1992).

Construct validation is the most important type of validity for a quantitative instrument. Instrument developers should use one or more of the techniques described here in their effort to assess the instrument's worth.

Interpretation of Validity

Like reliability, validity is not an all-or-nothing characteristic of an instrument. An instrument does not possess or lack validity; it is a question of degree. An instrument's validity is not proved, established, or verified but rather is supported to a greater or lesser extent by evidence.

Strictly speaking, researchers do not validate an instrument but rather an application of it. A measure of anxiety may be valid for presurgical patients on the day of an operation but may not be valid for nursing students on the day of a test. Of course, some instruments may be valid for a wide range of uses with different types of samples, but each use requires new supporting evidence. The more evidence that can be gathered that an instrument is measuring what it is supposed to be measuring, the more confidence researchers will have in its validity.

TIP: Instrument developers usually gather evidence of the validity and reliability of their instruments in a thorough **psychometric assessment** before making them available for general use. If you use an existing instrument, choose one with demonstrated high reliability and validity. If you select an instrument for which there is no published psychometric information, try contacting the instrument developer and ask about evidence of data quality.

OTHER CRITERIA FOR ASSESSING QUANTITATIVE MEASURES

Reliability and validity are the two most important criteria for evaluating quantitative instruments. High reliability and validity are a necessary, although not sufficient, condition for good quantitative research. Researchers sometimes need to consider other qualities of an instrument, as discussed in this section.

Sensitivity and Specificity

Sensitivity and specificity are criteria that are important in evaluating instruments designed as screening instruments or diagnostic aids. For example, a researcher might develop a new scale to measure risk of osteoporosis. Such screening/diagnostic instruments could be self-report, observational, or biophysiologic measures.

Sensitivity is the ability of an instrument to identify a "case" correctly, that is, to screen in or diagnosis a condition correctly. An instrument's sensitivity is its rate of yielding "true positives." **Specificity** is the instrument's ability to identify noncases correctly, that is, to screen *out* those without the condition correctly. Specificity is an instrument's rate of yielding "true negatives." To determine an instrument's sensitivity and specificity, researchers need a reliable and valid criterion of "caseness" against which scores on the instrument can be assessed.

There is, unfortunately, a tradeoff between the sensitivity and specificity of an instrument. When sensitivity is increased to include more true positives, the number of true negatives declines. Therefore, a critical task is to develop the appropriate **cutoff point**, that is, the score value used to distinguish cases and noncases. To determine the best cutoff point, researchers often use what is called a **receiver operating characteristic curve** (**ROC curve**). To construct an ROC curve, the sensitivity of an instrument (i.e., the rate of correctly identifying a case vis-à-vis a criterion) is plotted against the false-positive rate (i.e., the rate of incorrectly diagnosing someone as a case, which is the inverse of its specificity) over a range of different cutoff points. The cutoff point that yields the best balance between sensitivity and specificity can then be determined. The optimum cutoff is at or near the shoulder of the ROC curve. The example at the end of this chapter illustrates the use of ROC curves. Fletcher, Fletcher, and Wagner (1996) is a good source for further information about these procedures.

Example of sensitivity and specificity: Bergquist and Frantz (2001) studied the use of the Braden scale for predicting pressure ulcers in a sample of community-based adults receiving home health care. The sensitivity and specificity of the scale at cutoff scores between 16 and 22 were assessed against actual pressure ulcer development. The cutoff score of 19 yielded the best balance between sensitivity (61%) and specificity (68%) for stage I to IV pressure ulcers.

Efficiency

Instruments of comparable reliability and validity may differ in their efficiency. A depression scale that requires 10 minutes of people's time is efficient compared with a depression scale that requires 30 minutes to complete. One aspect of efficiency is the number of items incorporated in an instrument. Long instruments tend to be more reliable than shorter ones. There is, however, a point of diminishing returns. As an example, consider a 40-item scale to measure social support that has an internal consistency reliability of .94. Using the Spearman-Brown formula, we can estimate how reliable the scale would be with only 30 items:

$$r^1 = \frac{kr}{1+[(k-1)r]} = \frac{.75(.94)}{1+[(-.25)(.94)]} = .92$$

where k = the factor by which the instrument is being incremented or decreased; in this case, $k = 30 \div 40 = .75$

r^1 = reliability estimate for shorter (longer) scale

As this calculation shows, a 25% reduction in the instrument's length resulted in a negligible decrease in reliability, from .94 to .92. Most researchers likely would sacrifice a modest amount of reliability in exchange for reducing subjects' response burden and data collection costs.

Efficiency is more characteristic of certain types of data collection procedures than others. In self-reports, closed-ended questions are more efficient than open-ended ones. Self-report scales tend to be less time-consuming than projective instruments for a comparable amount of information. Of course, a researcher may decide that other advantages (such as depth of information) offset a certain degree of inefficiency. Other things being equal, however, it is desirable to select as efficient an instrument as possible.

Other Criteria

A few remaining qualities that sometimes are considered in assessing a quantitative instrument can be noted. Most of the following six criteria are actually aspects of the reliability and validity issues:

1. *Comprehensibility.* Subjects and researchers should be able to comprehend the behaviors required to secure accurate and valid measures.
2. *Precision.* An instrument should discriminate between people with different amounts of an attribute as precisely as possible.
3. *Speededness.* For most instruments, researchers should allow adequate time to obtain complete measurements without rushing the measuring process.
4. *Range.* The instrument should be capable of achieving a meaningful measure from the smallest expected value of the variable to the largest.
5. *Linearity.* A researcher normally strives to construct measures that are equally accurate and sensitive over the entire range of values.
6. *Reactivity.* The instrument should, insofar as possible, avoid affecting the attribute being measured.

ASSESSMENT OF QUALITATIVE DATA AND THEIR INTERPRETATION

The criteria and methods of assessment described thus far apply to quantitative data collection instruments. The procedures cannot be meaningfully applied to such qualitative materials as narrative interview data or descriptions from a participant observer's field notes, but qualitative researchers are also concerned with data quality. The central question underlying the concepts of reliability and validity is: Do the data reflect the truth? Qualitative researchers are as eager as quantitative researchers to have data reflecting the true state of human experience.

Nevertheless, there has been considerable controversy about the criteria to use for assessing the "truth value" of qualitative research. Whittemore, Chase, and Mandle (2001), who listed different criteria recommended by 10 influential authorities, noted that the difficulty in achieving universally accepted criteria (or even universally accepted labels for those criteria) stems in part from various tensions, such as the tension between the desire for rigor and the desire for creativity.

The criteria currently thought of as the gold standard for qualitative researchers are those outlined by Lincoln and Guba (1985). As noted in Chapter 2, these researchers have suggested four criteria for establishing the **trustworthiness** of qualitative data: credibility, dependability, confirmability, and transferability. These criteria go beyond an assessment of qualitative *data* alone, but rather are concerned with evaluations of interpretations and conclusions as well. These standards are often used by qualitative researchers in all major traditions, but some exceptions are noted.

Credibility

Credibility is viewed by Lincoln and Guba as an overriding goal of qualitative research, and is considered in the Whittemore et al. (2001) synthesis as a primary validity criterion. **Credibility** refers to confidence in the truth of the data and interpreta-

tions of them. Lincoln and Guba point out that credibility involves two aspects: first, carrying out the study in a way that enhances the believability of the findings, and second, taking steps to *demonstrate* credibility to consumers. They suggest a variety of techniques for improving and documenting the credibility of qualitative research.

Prolonged Engagement and Persistent Observation

Lincoln and Guba recommend several activities that make it more likely to produce credible data and interpretations. A first and very important step is **prolonged engagement**—the investment of sufficient time collecting data to have an in-depth understanding of the culture, language, or views of the group under study and to test for misinformation and distortions. Prolonged engagement is also essential for building trust and rapport with informants, which in turn makes it more likely that useful, accurate, and rich information will be obtained.

Example of prolonged engagement:
Albertín-Carbó, Domingo-Salvany, and Hartnoll (2001) studied the meaning that injecting drug users attribute to risk behaviors linked to HIV transmission. They gathered participant observation data (e.g., accompanying people to look for drugs, walking the streets) during 10 months of fieldwork in a district of Barcelona that had a high prevalence of opiate use.

Credible data collection in naturalistic inquiries also involves **persistent observation**, which concerns the salience of the data being gathered and recorded. Persistent observation refers to the researchers' focus on the characteristics or aspects of a situation or a conversation that are relevant to the phenomena being studied. As Lincoln and Guba (1985) note, "If prolonged engagement provides scope, persistent observation provides depth" (p. 304).

Example of persistent observation:
Beck (2002) conducted a grounded theory study of mothering twins during the first year of

life. In addition to prolonged engagement for 10 months of fieldwork, she engaged in persistent observation. After interviewing mothers in their homes, Beck often stayed and helped them with their twins, using the time for persistent observation of the mothers caretaking (e.g., details of what and how the mothers talked to their twins).

Triangulation

Triangulation can also enhance credibility. As previously noted, triangulation refers to the use of multiple referents to draw conclusions about what constitutes truth, and has been compared with convergent validation. The aim of triangulation is to "overcome the intrinsic bias that comes from single-method, single-observer, and single-theory studies" (Denzin, 1989, p. 313). It has also been argued that triangulation helps to capture a more complete and contextualized portrait of the phenomenon under study—a goal shared by researchers in all qualitative traditions. Denzin (1989) identified four types of triangulation: data triangulation, investigator triangulation, method triangulation, and theory triangulation.

Data triangulation involves the use of multiple data sources for the purpose of validating conclusions. There are three basic types of data triangulation: time, space, and person. **Time triangulation** involves collecting data on the same phenomenon or about the same people at different points in time. Time triangulation can involve gathering data at different times of the day, or at different times in the year. This concept is similar to test–retest reliability assessment; that is, the point is not to study the phenomenon longitudinally to determine how it changes, but to determine the congruence of the phenomenon across time. **Space triangulation** involves collecting data on the same phenomenon in multiple sites. The aim is to validate the data by testing for cross-site consistency. Finally, **person triangulation** involves collecting data from different levels of persons: individuals, groups (e.g., dyads, triads, families), and collectives (e.g., organizations, communities, institutions), with the aim of validating data through multiple perspectives on the phenomenon.

 Example of data (person/space) triangulation:

Lipson (2001) studied the experience of living with multiple chemical sensitivity (MCS). She collected data in four sites (Dallas, San Francisco, Vancouver, and Halifax). Participant observation included two treatment centers, a support organization, and an Internet chat room; Lipson conducted interviews with MCS sufferers, activists, and educators.

The second major type of triangulation is **investigator triangulation**, which refers to the use of two or more researchers to analyze and interpret a data set. Through collaboration, investigators can reduce the possibility of a biased interpretation of the data. Moreover, if the investigators bring to the analysis task a complementary blend of skills and expertise, the analysis and interpretation can benefit from divergent perspectives. Blending diverse methodologic, disciplinary, and clinical skills also can contribute to other types of triangulation. Investigator triangulation is conceptually somewhat similar to interrater reliability in quantitative studies.

Example of investigator triangulation:

Woodhouse, Sayre, and Livingood (2001), who evaluated youth tobacco prevention policies in Florida, did an ethnography of tobacco possession enforcement. Interview data were analyzed simultaneously and separately by two researchers. The two analyses were compared and contrasted "to perfect the definition of themes and provide triangulation of findings" (p. 687).

With **theory triangulation,** researchers use competing theories or hypotheses in the analysis and interpretation of their data. Qualitative researchers who develop alternative hypotheses while still in the field can test the validity of each because the flexible design of qualitative studies provides ongoing opportunities to direct the inquiry. Theory triangulation can help researchers to rule out rival hypotheses and to prevent premature conceptualizations. The quantitative analogue for theory triangulation is construct validation.

Method triangulation involves the use of multiple methods of data collection about the same phenomenon. In qualitative studies,* researchers often use a rich blend of unstructured data collection methods (e.g., interviews, observations, documents) to develop a comprehensive understanding of a phenomenon. Multiple data collection methods provide an opportunity to evaluate the extent to which an internally consistent picture of the phenomenon emerges.

Example of method triangulation:
Carter (2002) studied the experiences of chronic pain in children and their families. Data were collected by means of journals (in which study participants reflected on what it was like to live with chronic pain) and in-depth interviews.

Although Denzin's (1989) seminal work discussed these four types of triangulation as a method of converging on valid understandings about a phenomenon, other types have been suggested. For example, Kimchi, Polivka, and Stephenson (1991) have described **analysis triangulation** (i.e., using two or more analytic techniques to analyze the same set of data). This approach offers another opportunity to validate the meanings inherent in a qualitative data set. Analysis triangulation can also involve using multiple units of analysis (e.g., individuals, dyads, families). Finally, **multiple triangulation** is used when more than one of these types of triangulation is used in the collection and analysis of the same data set.

In summary, the purpose of using triangulation is to provide a basis for convergence on the truth. By using multiple methods and perspectives, researchers strive to sort out "true" information from "error" information, thereby enhancing the credibility of the findings.

Peer Debriefing

Another technique for establishing credibility involves external validation. **Peer debriefing** involves

sessions with peers to review and explore various aspects of the inquiry. Peer debriefing exposes researchers to the searching questions of others who are experienced in either the methods of naturalistic inquiry, the phenomenon being studied, or both.

In a peer debriefing session, researchers might present written or oral summaries of the data that have been gathered, categories and themes that are emerging, and researchers' interpretations of the data. In some cases, taped interviews might be played. Among the questions that peer debriefers might address are the following:

- Is there evidence of researcher bias?
- Have the researchers been sufficiently reflexive?
- Do the gathered data adequately portray the phenomenon?
- If there are important omissions, what strategies might remedy this problem?
- Are there any apparent errors of fact?
- Are there possible errors of interpretation?
- Are there competing interpretations? More comprehensive or parsimonious interpretations?
- Have all important themes been identified?
- Are the themes and interpretations knit together into a cogent, useful, and creative conceptualization of the phenomenon?

Example of peer debriefing:
Phillips, Cohen, and Tarzian (2001) conducted a phenomenological study of the experience of breast cancer screening for African-American women. The researchers interviewed 23 low- and middle-income women; then another objective researcher reviewed each interview, including the questions and techniques used. This peer reviewer debriefed with the three researchers before the next interview was conducted.

Member Checking

Lincoln and Guba consider member checking the most important technique for establishing the credibility of qualitative data. In a **member check**, researchers provide feedback to study participants regarding the emerging data and interpretations, and obtain participants' reactions. If researchers purport

---

*We have already discussed method triangulation involving a combination of qualitative and quantitative approaches (see Chapter 12).

that their interpretations are good representations of participants' realities, participants should be given an opportunity to react to them. Member checking with participants can be carried out both informally in an ongoing way as data are being collected, and more formally after data have been fully analyzed.

TIP: Not all qualitative researchers use member checking to ensure credibility. For example, member checking is not a component of Giorgi's method of descriptive phenomenology. Giorgi (1989) argued that asking participants to evaluate the researcher's psychological interpretation of their own descriptions exceeds the role of participants.

Member checking is sometimes done in writing. For example, researchers can ask participants to review and comment on case summaries, interpretive notes, thematic summaries, or drafts of the research report. Member checks are more typically done in face-to-face discussions with individual participants or small groups of participants. Many of the questions relevant for peer debriefings are also appropriate in the context of member checks.

Despite the role that member checking can play in enhancing credibility and demonstrating it to consumers, several issues need to be kept in mind. One is that some participants may be unwilling to participate in this process. Some—especially if the research topic is emotionally charged—may feel they have attained closure once they have shared their concerns, feelings, and experiences. Further discussion might not be welcomed. Others may decline being involved in member checking because they are afraid it might arouse suspicions of their families. Choudhry (2001) encountered this in her study of the challenges faced by elderly women from India who had immigrated to Canada. When Choudhry asked participants for a second interview to examine the transcripts of their first interviews, the participants refused. They feared that a second visit to their homes might arouse suspicions among their family members and increase their sense of loss and regret.

A second issue is that member checks can lead to misleading conclusions of credibility if partici-

pants "share some common myth or front, or conspire to mislead or cover up" (Lincoln & Guba, p. 315). At the other extreme, some participants might express agreement (or fail to express disagreement) with researchers' interpretations either out of politeness or in the belief that researchers are "smarter" or more knowledgeable than they themselves are.

TIP: It is important to explain to participants the helpful role that member checking plays in establishing trustworthiness. Participants should be given every encouragement to provide critical feedback about factual or interpretive errors or inadequacies.

Example of member checking:
King, Cathers, Polgar, MacKinnon, and Havens (2000) interviewed 10 adolescents with cerebral palsy to determine how they defined success in life. After the researchers' original thematic analysis, major themes and text segments representing themes were presented to a subgroup of participants in a member-checking focus group. Participants were asked to appraise critically the researchers' interpretations, and the importance of honest feedback was emphasized. Major themes were confirmed, but focus group members provided additional information elaborating on the themes.

Searching for Disconfirming Evidence

The credibility of a data set can be enhanced by the researcher's systematic search for data that will challenge an emerging categorization or descriptive theory. The search for disconfirming evidence occurs through purposive sampling methods but is facilitated through other processes already described here, such as prolonged engagement and peer debriefings. As noted in Chapter 13, the purposive sampling of individuals who can offer conflicting accounts or points of view can greatly strengthen a comprehensive description of a phenomenon.

Lincoln and Guba (1985) refer to a similar activity of **negative case analysis**—a process by which researchers revise their interpretations by including cases that appear to disconfirm earlier hypotheses. The goal of this procedure is to continuously refine a hypothesis or theory until it accounts for *all* cases.

Example of negative case analysis:

Beck (1995) developed three different versions describing the experience of burnout in nursing students, with refinements stemming from negative cases. The original formulation was: "Burnout occurs in nursing students as they become engulfed with competing demands from school, work, and family. Fatigue is all encompassing. Students gain weight from overeating due to stress. Social activities and physical exercise are outlets for this stress." This description had to be revised when other nursing students revealed that they had lost weight because of a lack of appetite and not having enough time to eat. The second version was: "Burnout occurs in nursing students as they become engulfed with competing demands from school, work, and family. Fatigue is all encompassing. Stress affects students' weight but not in a uniform direction. Some nursing students gain weight while others lose weight. Social activities and physical exercise are outlets for this stress." A third revision became necessary as subsequent interviews revealed that other students noted their lack of outlets for their stress because they did not have free time to socialize or exercise. Based on these negative cases, the latest version was as follows: "Burnout occurs in nursing students as they become engulfed with competing demands from school, work, and family. Fatigue is all encompassing. Stress affects students' weight but not in a uniform direction. Some nursing students gain weight while others lose weight. Outlets such as physical exercise and social activities are life savers but not for all nursing students. Due to time pressures, some could not indulge in these stress relieving activities."

Researcher Credibility

Another aspect of credibility discussed by Patton (2002) is **researcher credibility**, that is, the faith that can be put in the researcher. In qualitative studies, researchers *are* the data collecting instruments—as well as creators of the analytic process.

Therefore, researcher qualifications, experience, and reflexivity are important in establishing confidence in the data.

It is sometimes argued that, for readers to have confidence in the validity of a qualitative study's findings, the research report should contain information about the researchers, including information about credentials. In addition, the report may need to make clear the personal connections they had to the people, topic, or community under study. For example, it is relevant for a reader of a report on the coping mechanisms of AIDS patients to know that the researcher is HIV positive. Patton argues that researchers should report "any personal and professional information that may have affected data collection, analysis and interpretation—either negatively or positively..." (p. 566).

Example of researcher credibility:

Mohr (2000) studied how families with children under care in mental health care settings experience that care. In a section of her report labeled "Reflexive Notes," Mohr presented her credentials as a nurse (various nursing roles in psychiatric hospitals), her personal background (her mother was schizophrenic), and her strong advocacy activities (involvement with the National Alliance for the Mentally Ill). In addition, a brief biography establishing her credentials was included at the end of the report, a common feature in the journal *Qualitative Health Research*.

Dependability

The second criterion used to assess trustworthiness in qualitative research is dependability. The **dependability** of qualitative data refers to the stability of data over time and over conditions. This is similar conceptually to the stability and equivalence aspects of reliability assessments in quantitative studies (and similar also to time triangulation).

One approach to assessing the dependability of data is to undertake a procedure referred to as **stepwise replication**. This approach involves having a research team that can be divided into two groups. These groups deal with data sources separately and conduct, essentially, independent inquiries through which data can be compared. Ongoing, regular communication between the groups is essential for the success of this procedure.

Another technique relating to dependability is the **inquiry audit**. An inquiry audit involves a scrutiny of the data and relevant supporting documents by an external reviewer, an approach that also has a bearing on the confirmability of the data, a topic we discuss next.

Example of dependability:
Williams, Schutte, Evers, and Holkup (2000) used a stepwise replication and inquiry audit in their study of coping with normal results from predictive gene testing for neurodegenerative disorders. Ten participants were interviewed three times. Three researchers read through transcripts of the first set of interviews and made marginal notes for coding. The three researchers compared their codes and revised them until agreement was reached. All transcripts from the remaining interviews were coded independently, and the researchers met periodically to compare codes and reach a consensus. Once coding was completed, a qualitative nurse researcher reviewed the entire set of transcribed interviews and validated the findings with the three researchers.

Confirmability

Confirmability refers to the objectivity or neutrality of the data, that is, the potential for congruence between two or more independent people about the data's accuracy, relevance, or meaning. Bracketing (in phenomenological studies) and maintaining a reflexive journal are methods that can enhance confirmability, although these strategies do not actually document that it has been achieved.

Inquiry audits can be used to establish both the dependability and confirmability of the data. For an inquiry audit, researchers develop an **audit trail**, that is, a systematic collection of materials and documentation that allows an independent auditor to come to conclusions about the data. There are six classes of records that are of special interest in creating an adequate audit trail: (1) the raw data

(e.g., field notes, interview transcripts); (2) data reduction and analysis products (e.g., theoretical notes, documentation on working hypotheses); (3) process notes (e.g., methodologic notes, notes from member check sessions); (4) materials relating to researchers' intentions and dispositions (e.g., reflexive notes); (5) instrument development information (e.g., pilot forms); and (6) data reconstruction products (e.g., drafts of the final report).

Once the audit trail materials are assembled, the inquiry auditor proceeds to audit, in a fashion analogous to a financial audit, the trustworthiness of the data and the meanings attached to them. Although the auditing task is complex, it can serve as an invaluable tool for persuading others that qualitative data are worthy of confidence. Relatively few comprehensive inquiry audits have been reported in the literature, but some studies report partial audits or the assembling of auditable materials. Rodgers and Cowles (1993) present useful information about inquiry audits.

Example of confirmability:
In her research on mothering twins, Beck (2002) developed a four-phased grounded theory entitled, "life on hold: releasing the pause button." In her report, Beck provided a partial audit trail for phase three, which she called "striving to reset."

Transferability

In Lincoln and Guba's (1985) framework, **transferability** refers essentially to the generalizability of the data, that is, the extent to which the findings can be transferred to other settings or groups. This is, to some extent, a sampling and design issue rather than an issue relating to the soundness of the data per se. However, as Lincoln and Guba note, the responsibility of the investigator is to provide sufficient descriptive data in the research report so that consumers can evaluate the applicability of the data to other contexts: "Thus the naturalist cannot specify the external validity of an inquiry; he or she can provide only the thick description necessary to enable someone interested in making a transfer to reach a conclusion about whether transfer can be contemplated as a possibility" (p. 316). Thick description, as noted earlier, refers to a rich and thorough description of the research setting or context and of the transactions and processes observed during the inquiry. Thus, if there is to be transferability, the burden of proof rests with the investigator to provide sufficient information to permit judgments about contextual similarity.

Example of transferability:
In their phenomenological study of homeless patients' experience of satisfaction with health care, McCabe, Macnee, and Anderson (2001) interviewed 17 homeless people at a nurse-managed primary health care clinic for the homeless, at three shelters, and at a night-time soup kitchen. To assess the transferability of their themes, the researchers checked their findings with a group of homeless people who had not participated in the study and who lived in a shelter in a neighboring city.

TIP: Establishing the trustworthiness of focus group data poses special challenges to researchers. Morrison-Beedy, Côté-Arsenault, and Feinstein (2001) include many excellent suggestions.

Other Criteria for Assessing Quality in Qualitative Research

Qualitative researchers who take steps to enhance, assess, and document quality are most likely to use Lincoln and Guba's criteria. However, as noted previously, other criteria have been proposed, and new ways of thinking about quality assessments for qualitative studies are emerging.

Whittemore, Chase, and Mandle (2001), in their synthesis of qualitative criteria, use the term *validity* as the overarching goal. Although this term has been eschewed by many qualitative researchers as a "translation" from quantitative perspectives, Whittemore and her colleagues argue that validity is the most appropriate term. According to their view, the dictionary definition of validity as "the state or quality of being sound, just, and well-founded" lends itself equally to qualitative and quantitative research.

In their synthesis of criteria that can be used to develop evidence of validity in qualitative studies, Whittemore and associates proposed four primary criteria and six secondary criteria. In their view, the primary criteria are essential to all qualitative inquiry, whereas secondary criteria provide supplementary benchmarks of validity and are not relevant to every study. They argue that judgment is needed to determine the optimal weight given to each of the 10 criteria in specific studies. The primary criteria include credibility (as discussed earlier), authenticity, criticality, and integrity. The six secondary criteria include explicitness, vividness, creativity, thoroughness, and congruence. Table 18-5 lists these 10 criteria and the assessment questions relevant to achieving each. The questions are ones that can be used by qualitative researchers in their efforts to enhance the rigor of their studies and by consumers to evaluate the quality of the evidence studies yield.

A scrutiny of Table 18-5 reveals that the list contains many of the same concerns as those encompassed in Guba and Lincoln's four criteria. This overlap is further illustrated by considering techniques that can be used to contribute evidence of study validity according to these 10 criteria. As shown in Table 18-6, many of the techniques previously described in this chapter, as well as some methods discussed in earlier chapters, are important strategies for developing evidence of validity. These techniques can be used throughout the data collection and analysis process, and in preparing research reports.

Meadows and Morse (2001) discuss the components of rigor in qualitative studies and, similar to Whittemore and colleagues, conclude that the traditional terms of validity and reliability are appropriate in qualitative studies. Meadows and Morse argued that by not using traditional quantitative terminology, qualitative research has not yet taken its rightful place in the world of evidence and science. They call for the use of three components of rigor: verification, validation, and validity. Verification refers to strategies researchers use to enhance validity in the process of conducting a high-quality study. Verification strategies include the

TABLE 18.5 Primary and Secondary Qualitative Validity Criteria*

CRITERIA	ASSESSMENT QUESTIONS
Primary Criteria	
Credibility	Do the research results reflect participants' experiences and their context in a believable way?
Authenticity	Has the researcher adequately represented the multiple realities of those being studied? Has an emic perspective been accurately portrayed?
Criticality	Has the inquiry involved critical appraisal and reflexivity?
Integrity	Does the research reflect ongoing checks on the many aspects of validity? Are the findings humbly presented?
Secondary Criteria	
Explicitness	Have methodologic decisions been explained and justified? Have biases been identified? Is evidence presented in support of conclusions and interpretations?
Vividness	Have rich, evocative, and compelling descriptions been presented?
Creativity	Do the findings illuminate in an insightful and original way? Are new perspectives and rich imagination brought to bear on the inquiry?
Thoroughness	Has sufficient attention been paid to sampling adequacy, information richness, data saturation, and contextual completeness?
Congruence	Is there congruity between the questions and the methods, the methods and the participants, the data and categories? Do themes fit together in a coherent way?
Sensitivity	Has the research been undertaken in a way that is sensitive to the cultural, social, and political contexts of those being studied?

*Criteria are from Whittemore and colleagues' (2001) synthesis of qualitative validity criteria. The assessment questions are adapted from Whittemore and colleagues and other sources.

conduct of a thorough literature review, bracketing, theoretical sampling, and data saturation. Validation deals with the researcher's efforts to *assess* validity, apart from efforts to enhance it. Validation techniques include those discussed earlier, such as member checking, inquiry audits, triangulation, and so on. The final step in achieving validity involves the use of external judges to assess whether the project as a whole is trustworthy and valid.

 TIP: Unfortunately, most qualitative reports do *not* provide information about validity

efforts and assessments. With increasing emphasis on developing evidence for practice, nurses should expect such information when they read reports, and include it in the reports they prepare.

RESEARCH EXAMPLES

In this section, we describe the efforts of researchers to develop and evaluate a structured self-report instrument, and of another researcher to evaluate her qualitative data.

(text continues on page 440)

TABLE 18.6 Techniques for Addressing Criteria for Qualitative Validity

| | | | | | CRITERIA | | | | | |
TECHNIQUE	Credibility	Authenticity	Criticality	Integrity	Explicitness	Vividness	Creativity	Thoroughness	Congruence	Sensitivity
Data Generation										
Persistent observation	X	X		X						X
Prolonged engagement	X	X								X
Bracketing			X							
Reflexive journaling		X	X							
Comprehensive field notes				X		X				
Theoretical sampling	X							X		
Disconfirming evidence	X		X					X		
Triangulation (data, method)	X	X						X		
Verbatim recording	X	X			X	X				
Stepwise replication					X			X		
Data saturation								X		
Data Management										
Transcription rigor	X		X							
Maintenance of audit trail				X	X				X	

Data Analysis

Investigator triangulation	X					X	
Theory triangulation	X	X				X	
Analysis triangulation		X				X	
Peer debriefing	X					X	
Member checking						X	
Negative case analysis		X				X	

Report Preparation

Thick description		X				X	
Researcher credibility			X				
Evidence supporting interpretation			X	X	X		
Demonstrating reflexivity				X			
Humble presentation					X		

Research Example Involving Assessment of a Structured Scale

Beck studied the phenomenon of postpartum depression (PPD) in a series of qualitative studies, using both a phenomenological approach (1992, 1996) and a grounded theory approach (1993). Based on her in-depth understanding of PPD, she began in the late 1990s to develop a scale that could be used to screen for PPD, the Postpartum Depression Screening Scale (PDSS). Working with an expert psychometrician, Beck refined and evaluated the PDSS, as documented in two reports (Beck & Gable, 2000, 2001).

The PDSS is a Likert scale designed to tap seven dimensions, such as sleeping/eating disturbances and cognitive impairment. A 56-item pilot form of the PDSS was developed (8 per dimension), using direct quotes from women interviewed in Beck's studies of PPD (e.g., "I felt like I was losing my mind"). The reading level of the PDSS was assessed as at the seventh grade level. The pilot form was subjected to two content validation procedures, including ratings by a panel of five content experts. Feedback from these procedures led to several changes (e.g., removal and addition of some items).

The revised PDSS was then subjected to rigorous psychometric testing. Eight health care facilities in 6 states and a PPD support group distributed the PDSS to a sample of 525 new mothers. Item analysis procedures were used to streamline the scale while maintaining adequate reliability. That is, Beck and Gable determined that three items could be deleted from each subscale without sacrificing internal consistency; they examined the correlations between individual items and subscale scores to select which items to delete.

Figure 18-2 shows a portion of the computer printout for the reliability analysis of the five selected items for the cognitive impairment subscale. Some information in this table is difficult to explain to those without statistical backgrounds, but we will point out a few salient pieces of information. In the panel labeled "Item-total Statistics," the first column identifies the items in the subscale by number: I11, I18, and so on (I11 is the "I felt like I was losing my mind" item). In the fourth column are correlation coefficients indicating the strength of the relationship between a woman's score on an item and her score on the total five-item subscale. I11 has an item-total correlation of nearly .80, which is very high; all five items have excellent correlations with the total score. The sixth and

final column indicates what the internal consistency reliability would be if an item were deleted. If I11 were removed from the subscale and only the four other items remained, the reliability coefficient would be .8876; in the panel below, we see that the reliability for the 5-item scale is even higher: alpha − .9120. Deleting any of the five items on the scale would reduce the internal consistency of the scale, albeit by a rather small amount. On the seven subscales of the PDSS, each now with five items, the reliability coefficients ranged from .83 to .94, demonstrating high internal consistency across all dimensions.

Beck and Gable (2000) used confirmatory factor analysis to evaluate the construct validity of the PDSS. Essentially, this procedure involves a validation of Beck's hypotheses about how individual items map onto underlying constructs, like cognitive impairment. Item response theory was also used, and both techniques provided evidence of the scale's construct validity.

Beck and Gable (2001) administered the PDSS to a second sample of 150 new mothers in a further effort to validate the scale, and to establish the best possible cutoff points for diagnostic assessment. In this new study, reliability coefficients were also strong, ranging from .80 to .91 for the seven subscales.

A convergent validity approach was used to examine construct validity of the overall scale. Women in the sample completed two measures of PPD and one measure of general depression. Correlations among the three were high. Validity was further established by having each study participant interviewed by a nurse psychotherapist, who used a rigorous interviewing process to confirm and document a suspected diagnosis for major or minor depression with postpartum onset. The correlation between this expert diagnosis and scores on the PDSS was .70, which was higher than the correlations between the diagnosis and scores on the other two depression scales, indicating its superiority as a screening instrument.

ROC curves were then constructed to examine the sensitivity and specificity of the PDSS at different cutoff points, using the expert diagnosis to establish true positives and true negatives. Figure 18-3 presents the ROC curve for a diagnosis of major or minor depression (46 of the 150 mothers had this diagnosis). Sensitivity, the rate of true positives, is plotted on the vertical axis. The rate of false positives (the inverse of the true-negative rate, or specificity) is plotted on the horizontal axis. To illustrate how to read ROC information, let us suppose we used a cutoff score of 95 on

****** Method 2 (covariance matrix) will be used for this analysis ******

R E L I A B I L I T Y   A N A L Y S I S   -   S C A L E   (A L P H A)

1. I11
2. I18
3. I25
4. I39
5. I53

		Mean	Std Dev	Cases
1.	I11	2.3640	1.4243	522.0
2.	I18	2.2146	1.2697	522.0
3.	I25	2.2050	1.3736	522.0
4.	I39	2.3985	1.3511	522.0
5.	I53	2.2759	1.3491	522.0

Correlation Matrix

	I11	I18	I25	I39	I53
I11	1.0000				
I18	.6540	1.0000			
I25	.8143	.6031	1.0000		
I39	.6456	.6594	.6519	1.0000	
I53	.6469	.7508	.6012	.7240	1.0000

N of Cases = 522.0

Item Means	Mean	Minimum	Maximum	Range	Max/Min	Variance
	2.2916	2.2050	2.3985	.1935	1.0877	.0076

Item Variances	Mean	Minimum	Maximum	Range	Max/Min	Variance
	1.8347	1.6122	2.0285	.4163	1.2582	.0225

Item-total Statistics

	Scale Mean if Item Deleted	Scale Variance if Item Deleted	Corrected Item-Total Correlation	Squared Multiple Correlation	Alpha if Item Deleted
I11	9.0939	21.3712	.7991	.7145	.8876
I18	9.2433	23.0060	.7639	.6231	.8951
I25	9.2529	22.0972	.7696	.6912	.8937
I39	9.0594	22.2901	.7687	.6097	.8938
I53	9.1820	22.1760	.7812	.6662	.8912

R E L I A B I L I T Y   A N A L Y S I S   -   S C A L E   (A L P H A)

Reliability Coefficients   5 items

Alpha =   .9120 Standardized item alpha =   .9122

FIGURE 18.2   Reliability analysis for the Postpartum Depression Screening Scale.

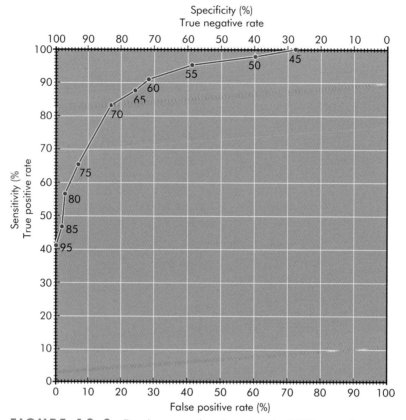

FIGURE 18.3 Receiver operating characteristic (ROC) curve for Postpartum Depression Screening Scale (PDSS): major or minor postpartum depression. Area = 0.91 (SD = 0.03). Used with permission from Beck, C. T., & Gable, R. K. (2001). Further validation of the Postpartum Depression Screening Scale. *Nursing Research, 50,* 161.

the PDSS to screen in PPD cases. With this score, the sensitivity is 41%, meaning that only 41% of the women actually diagnosed with PPD would be identified. A score of 95 has a specificity of 100%, meaning that all cases without an actual PPD diagnosis would be accurately screened out as based on the scale. At the other extreme, a cutoff score of 45 would have 100% sensitivity but only 28% specificity (i.e., 62% false positive), an unacceptable rate of overdiagnosis. Screening instruments that perform well have ROC curves that crowd into the upper left corner, and whose area under the curve is a high proportion of overall space. The area under the curve in Figure 18-3 is .91, which is excellent. Based on these results, Beck and Gable recommended a cutoff score of 60,

which would accurately screen in 91% of PPD cases, and would mistakenly screen in 28% who do not have this mood disorder. In a further analysis, they determined that using this cutoff point would have correctly classified 85% of their sample.

Research Example Involving Assessment of Qualitative Data

Stubblefield and Murray (2001) examined how parents whose children have undergone lung transplantation perceive their relationships with others before, during, and after the transplantation. Fifteen parents of 12 children who had undergone lung transplantation were interviewed. Interviews ranged in length from 45 minutes to 2½ hours. The researchers used several strategies to help ensure credibility, including prolonged engagement. The researchers were in contact with the parents over a 9-month period, facilitating their understanding of what it was like to live with a lung transplant.

Investigator triangulation and peer debriefings were additional techniques used to increase credibility. The investigators discussed their descriptive categories as they were developing them each other and with a peer who was an expert in qualitative research. The peer debriefings had two purposes: (1) data analysis decisions were supported and credibility was thereby enhanced, and (2) discussions with the peer provided the researchers with an opportunity for much-needed catharsis after conducting the emotionally difficult interviews. Member checks were done by returning to the parents for a final validating step. Parents were asked how the findings compared with their experiences with the transplantation situation. Data saturation (i.e., obtaining redundant information) was yet another method used to enhance credibility.

With respect to dependability and confirmability, Stubblefield and Murray maintained an audit trail that identified the analytical decisions made during data collection and data analysis. Transferability was facilitated through rich description of the parents' experiences with their children's lung transplantation. Also, the report included information about the demographic characteristics of the parents and children, which can be used to determine transferability of the study findings.

According to Stubblefield and Murray's report, some parents perceived a sense of diminished support from family and friends as they coped with living with the transplant. Parents felt misunderstood and labeled.

SUMMARY POINTS

- **Measurement** involves the assignment of numbers to objects to represent the amount of an attribute, using a specified set of rules. Researchers strive to develop or use measurements whose rules are **isomorphic** with reality.
- Few quantitative measuring instruments are infallible. Sources of measurement error include situational contaminants, response-set biases, and transitory personal factors, such as fatigue.
- **Obtained scores** from an instrument consist of

a **true score** component (the value that would be obtained for a hypothetical perfect measure of the attribute) and an error component, or **error of measurement**, that represents measurement inaccuracies.

- **Reliability**, one of two primary criteria for assessing a quantitative instrument, is the degree of consistency or accuracy with which an instrument measures an attribute. The higher the reliability of an instrument, the lower the amount of error in obtained scores.
- There are different methods for assessing an instrument's reliability and for computing a **reliability coefficient**. A reliability coefficient typically is based on the computation of a **correlation coefficient** that indicates the magnitude and direction of a relationship between two variables.
- Correlation coefficients can range from -1.00 (a **perfect negative relationship**) through zero to $+1.00$ (a **perfect positive relationship**). Reliability coefficients usually range from .00 to 1.00, with higher values reflecting greater reliability.
- The **stability** aspect of reliability, which concerns the extent to which an instrument yields the same results on repeated administrations, is evaluated by **test–retest procedures.**
- The **internal consistency** aspect of reliability, which refers to the extent to which all the instrument's items are measuring the same attribute, is assessed using either the **split-half reliability technique** or, more likely, **Cronbach's alpha method**.
- When the reliability assessment focuses on **equivalence** between observers in rating or coding behaviors, estimates of **interrater** (or **interobserver**) **reliability** are obtained.
- Reliability coefficients reflect the proportion of true variability in a set of scores to the total obtained variability.
- **Validity** is the degree to which an instrument measures what it is supposed to be measuring.
- **Face validity** refers to whether the instrument appears, on the face of it, to be measuring the appropriate construct.

- **Content validity** is concerned with the sampling adequacy of the content being measured. Expert judgments can be used to compute a **content validity index** (**CVI**), which provides ratings across experts of the relevance of items on a scale.
- **Criterion-related validity** (which includes both **predictive validity** and **concurrent validity**) focuses on the correlation between the instrument and an outside criterion.
- **Construct validity** is an instrument's adequacy in measuring the focal construct. One construct validation method is the **known-groups technique**, which contrasts scores of groups presumed to differ on the attribute; another is **factor analysis**, a statistical procedure for identifying unitary clusters of items or measures.
- Another construct validity approach is the **multitrait–multimethod matrix technique**, which is based on the concepts of convergence and discriminability. **Convergence** refers to evidence that different methods of measuring the same attribute yield similar results. **Discriminability** refers to the ability to differentiate the construct being measured from other, similar concepts.
- Sensitivity and specificity are important criteria for screening and diagnostic instruments. **Sensitivity** is the instrument's ability to identify a case correctly (i.e., its rate of yielding true positives). **Specificity** is the instrument's ability to identify noncases correctly (i.e., its rate of yielding true negatives).
- Sensitivity is sometimes plotted against specificity in a **receiver operating characteristic curve** (**ROC curve**) to determine the optimum **cutoff point** for caseness.
- A **psychometric assessment** of a new instrument is usually undertaken to gather evidence about validity, reliability, and other assessment criteria.
- There is less agreement among qualitative researchers about criteria to use in enhancing and documenting data quality. The most widely used approach is Lincoln and Guba's method of evaluating the **trustworthiness** of data and interpretations, using the criteria of credibility, dependability, confirmability, and transferability.

- **Credibility** refers to the believability of the data. Techniques to improve the credibility include **prolonged engagement**, which strives for adequate scope of data coverage, and **persistent observation**, which is aimed at achieving adequate depth.
- **Triangulation** is the process of using multiple referents to draw conclusions about what constitutes the truth. The four major forms are **data triangulation**, **investigator triangulation**, **theoretical triangulation**, and **method triangulation**.
- Two important tools for establishing credibility are **peer debriefings**, wherein the researcher obtains feedback about data quality and interpretive issues from peers, and **member checks**, wherein informants are asked to comment on the data and interpretations.
- Credibility can also be enhanced through a systematic search for disconfirming evidence (including a **negative case analysis**), and by having investigators whose credibility is evident through their training and experience.
- **Dependability** of qualitative data refers to the stability of data over time and over conditions, and is somewhat analogous to the concept of reliability in quantitative studies.
- **Confirmability** refers to the objectivity or neutrality of the data. Independent **inquiry audits** by external auditors can be used to assess and document dependability and confirmability.
- **Transferability** is the extent to which findings from the data can be transferred to other settings or groups. Transferability can be enhanced through thick descriptions of the context of the data collection.
- Criteria that have been proposed in a recent synthesis of qualitative validity approaches include credibility, authenticity, criticality, and integrity (primary criteria), and explicitness, vividness, creativity, thoroughness, and congruence (secondary criteria).

STUDY ACTIVITIES

Chapter 18 of the accompanying *Study Guide for Nursing Research: Principles and Methods, 7th ed.*, offers various exercises and study suggestions for reinforcing the concepts presented in this chapter. In addition, the following study questions can be addressed:

1. Explain in your own words the meaning of the following correlation coefficients:
   a. The relationship between intelligence and grade-point average was found to be .72.
   b. The correlation coefficient between age and gregariousness was −.20.
   c. It was revealed that patients' compliance with nursing instructions was related to their length of stay in the hospital ($r = -.50$).
2. Suppose the split-half reliability of an instrument to measure attitudes toward contraception was .70. Calculate the reliability of the full scale by using the Spearman-Brown formula.
3. If a researcher had a 20-item scale whose reliability was .60, about how many items would have to be added to achieve a reliability of .80?
4. An instructor has developed an instrument to measure knowledge of research terminology. Would you say that more reliable measurements would be yielded before or after a year of instruction on research methodology, using the exact same test, or would there be no difference? Why?
5. In Figure 18-2, if Beck had wanted a four-item subscale rather than a five-item subscale, which item would she have eliminated?
6. What types of groups do you feel might be useful for a known-groups approach to validating a measures of the following: emotional maturity, attitudes toward alcoholics, territorial aggressiveness, job motivation, and subjective pain?
7. Suppose you were interested in doing an in-depth study of people's struggles with obesity. Outline a data collection plan that would include opportunities for various types of triangulation.
8. Suppose you were going to conduct a grounded theory study investigating parenting of children with attention-deficit/hyperactivity disorder (ADHD). What measures could you take to enhance the credibility of your study?
9. You have been asked to be a peer debriefer for two nurse researchers who are conducting a phenomenological study on the experiences of women who have been physically abused during pregnancy. What are some questions you could ask these researchers during the debriefing sessions?

SUGGESTED READINGS

Methodologic References

Banik, B. J. (1993). Applying triangulation in nursing research. *Applied Nursing Research, 6,* 47–52.

Beck, C. T. (1993). Qualitative research: The evaluation of its credibility, fittingness, and auditability. *Western Journal of Nursing Research, 15,* 263–266.

Beck, C. T. (1994). Reliability and validity issues in phenomenological research. *Western Journal of Nursing Research, 16,* 254–267.

Berk, R. A. (1990). Importance of expert judgment in content-related validity evidence. *Western Journal of Nursing Research, 12,* 659–670.

Campbell, D. T., & Fiske, D. W. (1959). Convergent and discriminant validation by the multitrait-multimethod matrix. *Psychological Bulletin, 56,* 81–105.

Cronbach, L. J. (1990). *Essentials of psychological testing* (5th ed.). New York: Harper & Row.

Davis, L. L., & Grant, J. S. (1993). Guidelines for using psychometric consultants in nursing studies. *Research in Nursing & Health, 16,* 151–155.

DeKeyser, F. G., & Pugh, L. C. (1990). Assessment of the reliability and validity of biochemical measures. *Nursing Research, 39,* 314–317.

Denzin, N. K. (1989). *The research act* (3rd ed.). New York: McGraw-Hill.

Ferketich, S. L., Figueredo, A., & Knapp, T. R. (1991). The multitrait-multimethod approach to construct validity. *Research in Nursing & Health, 14,* 315–319.

Fletcher, R. H., Fletcher, S. W., & Wagner, E. H. (1996). *Clinical epidemiology: The essentials.* Baltimore: Williams & Wilkins.

Giorgi, A. (1989). Some theoretical and practical issues regarding the psychological and phenomenological method. *Saybrook Review, 7,* 71–85.

Goodwin, L. D., & Goodwin, W. L. (1991). Estimating construct validity. *Research in Nursing & Health, 14,* 235–243.

Grant, J. S., & Davis, L. L. (1997). Selection and use of content experts for instrument development. *Research in Nursing & Health, 20,* 269–274.

Hambleton, R., Swaminathan, H., & Rogers, H. J. (1991). *Fundamentals of item response theory.* Newbury Park, CA: Sage.

Hoffart, N. (1991). A member check procedure to enhance rigor in naturalistic research. *Western Journal of Nursing Research, 13,* 522–534.

Hopkins, K. D. (1997). *Educational and psychological measurement and evaluation* (8th ed.). Boston: Allyn Bacon.

Hutchinson, S., & Wilson, H. S. (1992). Validity threats in scheduled semistructured research interviews. *Nursing Research, 41,* 117–119.

Kimchi, J., Polivka, B., & Stevenson, J. S. (1991). Triangulation: Operational definitions. *Nursing Research, 40,* 364–366.

Lincoln, Y. S., & Guba, E. G. (1985). *Naturalistic inquiry.* Newbury Park, CA: Sage.

Lowe, N. K. & Ryan-Wenger, N. M. (1992). Beyond Campbell and Fiske: Assessment of convergent and discriminant validity. *Research in Nursing & Health, 15,* 67–75.

Lynn, M. R. (1986). Determination and quantification of content validity. *Nursing Research, 35,* 382–385.

Meadows, L. M., & Morse, J. M. (2001). Constructing evidence within the qualitative project. In J. M. Morse, J. M. Swanson, & A. J. Kuzel (Eds.), *The nature of qualitative evidence* (pp. 187–200). Thousand Oaks, CA: Sage.

Morrison-Beedy, D., Côté-Arsenault, D., & Feinstein, N. F. (2001). Maximizing results with focus groups: Moderator and analysis issues. *Applied Nursing Research, 14,* 48–53.

Morse, J. M. (1999). Myth # 93: Reliability and validity are not relevant to qualitative inquiry. *Qualitative Health Research, 9,* 717–718.

Nunnally, J., & Bernstein, I. H. (1994). *Psychometric theory* (3rd ed.). New York: McGraw-Hill.

Patton, M. Q. (2002). *Qualitative evaluation and research methods* (3rd ed.). Thousand Oaks, CA: Sage.

Rodgers, B. L., & Cowles, K. V. (1993). The qualitative research audit trail: A complex collection of documentation. *Research in Nursing and Health, 16,* 219–226.

Sim J., & Sharp, K. (1998). A critical appraisal of the role of triangulation in nursing research. *International Journal of Nursing Studies, 35,* 23–31

Slocumb, E. M., & Cole, F. L. (1991). A practical approach to content validation. *Applied Nursing Research, 4,* 192–195.

Thorndike, R. L. (1996). *Measurement and evaluation in psychology and education* (6th ed.). Columbus, OH: Prentice-Hall.

Tilden, V. P., Nelson, C. A., & May, B. A. (1990). Use of qualitative methods to enhance content validity. *Nursing Research, 39,* 172–175.

Whittemore, R., Chase, S. K., & Mandle, C. L. (2001). Validity in qualitative research. *Qualitative Health Research, 11,* 522–537.

Wright, B., & Masters, G. (1982). *Rating scale analysis.* Chicago: Mesa Press.

Yen, M., & Lo, L. (2002). Examining test–retest reliability: An intraclass correlation approach. *Nursing Research, 51,* 59–62.

Studies Cited in Chapter 18

Albertín-Carbó, P., Domingo-Salvany, A., & Hartnoll, R. L. (2001). Psychosocial consideration for the prevention of HIV prevention of HIV infection of injecting drug users. *Qualitative Health Research, 11,* 26–39.

Beck, C. T. (1992). The lived experience of postpartum depression: A phenomenological study. *Nursing Research, 41,* 166–170.

Beck, C. T. (1993). Teetering on the edge: A substantive theory of postpartum depression. *Nursing Research, 42,* 42–48.

Beck, C. T. (1995). Burnout in undergraduate nursing students. *Nurse Educator, 20,* 19–23.

Beck, C. T. (1996). Postpartum depressed mothers interacting with their children. *Nursing Research, 45,* 98–104.

Beck, C. T. (2002). Releasing the pause button: Mothering twins during the first year of life. *Qualitative Health Research, 12,* 593–608.

Beck, C. T., & Gable, R. K. (2000). Postpartum Depression Screening Scale: Development and psychometric testing. *Nursing Research, 49,* 272–282.

Beck, C. T., & Gable, R. K. (2001). Further validation of the Postpartum Depression Screening Scale. *Nursing Research, 50,* 155–164.

Bergquist, S., & Frantz, R. (2001). Braden Scale: Validity in community-based older adults receiving home health care. *Applied Nursing Research, 14,* 36–43.

Brown, S. A., Becker, H. A., Garcia, A. A., Barton, S. A., & Hanis, C. L. (2002). Measuring health beliefs in Spanish-speaking Mexican Americans with type 2 diabetes: Adapting an existing instrument. *Research in Nursing & Health, 25,* 145–158.

Cacchione, P. Z. (2002). Four acute confusion assessment instruments: Reliability and validity for use in long-term care facilities. *Journal of Gerontological Nursing, 28,* 12–19.

Carter, B. (2002).Chronic pain in childhood and the medical encounter: Professional ventriloquism and hidden voices. *Qualitative Health Research, 12*, 28–41.

Chaiyawat, W., & Brown, J. K. (2000). Psychometric properties of the Thai versions of State-Trait Anxiety Inventory for Children and Child Medical Fear Scale. *Research in Nursing & Health, 23*, 406–414.

Choudhry, U. K. (2001). Uprooting and resettlement experiences of South Asian immigrant women. *Western Journal of Nursing Research, 23*, 376–393.

Davies, B. L., & Hodnett, E. (2002). Labor support: Nurses' self-efficacy and views about factors influencing implementation. *Journal of Obstetric, Gynecologic, and Neonatal Nursing, 31*, 48–56.

Garvin, B., & Kim, C. (2000). Measurement of preference for information in U.S. and Korean cardiac catheterization patients. *Research in Nursing & Health, 23*, 310–318.

Gauthier, D. M., & Froman, R. D. (2001). Preferences for care near the end of life: Scale development and validation. *Research in Nursing & Health, 24*, 298–306.

Holley, S. K. (2000) Evaluating patient distress from cancer-related fatigue: An instrument development study. *Oncology Nursing Forum, 27*, 1425–1431.

King, G. A., Cathers, T., Polgar, J. M., MacKinnon, E., & Havens, S. (2000). Success in life for older adolescents with cerebral palsy. *Qualitative Health Research, 10*, 734–749.

Kovach, C. R., & Wells, T. (2002). Pacing of activity as a predictor of agitation. *Journal of Gerontological Nursing, 28*, 28–35.

Lipson, J. (2001). We are the canaries: Self-care in multiple chemical sensitivity sufferers. *Qualitative Health Research, 11*, 103–116.

Marsh, G., Prochada, K., Pritchett, E., & Vojir, C. (2000). Predicting hospice appropriateness for patients with dementia of the Alzheimer's type. *Applied Nursing Research, 13*, 187–196.

McCabe, S., Macnee, C. L., & Anderson, M. K. (2001). Homeless patients' experience of satisfaction with care. *Archives of Psychiatric Nursing, 15*, 78–85.

Mohr, W. K. (2000). Rethinking professional attitudes in mental health settings. *Qualitative Health Research, 10*, 595–611.

Phillips, J. M., Cohen, M. Z., & Tarzian, A. J. (2001). African American women's experiences with breast cancer screening. *Journal of Nursing Scholarship, 33*, 135–140.

Resnick, B., & Jenkins, L. S. (2000). Testing the reliability and validity of the Self-Efficacy for Exercise Scale. *Nursing Research, 49*, 154–159.

Rew, L. (2000). Acknowledging intuition in clinical decision making. *Journal of Holistic Nursing, 18*, 94–113.

Ryden, M., Gross, C., Savik, K. Snyder, M., Oh, H., Jang, Y., Wang, J., & Krichbaum, K. (2000). Development of a measure of resident satisfaction with the nursing home. *Research in Nursing & Health, 23*, 237–245.

Shin, Y., & Colling, K. B. (2000). Cultural verification and application of the Profile of Mood States (POMS) with Korean elders. *Western Journal of Nursing Research, 22*, 68–83.

Stubblefield, C., & Murray, R. L. (2001). Pediatric lung transplantation: Families' need for understanding. *Qualitative Health Research, 11*, 58–68.

Williams, J. K., Schutte, D. L., Evers, C., & Holkup, P. A. (2000). Redefinition: Coping with normal results from predictive gene testing for neurodegenerative disorders. *Research in Nursing & Health, 23*, 260–269.

Woodhouse, L. D., Sayre, J. J., & Livingood, W. C. (2001). Tobacco policy and the role of law enforcement in prevention. *Qualitative Health Research, 11*, 682–692.

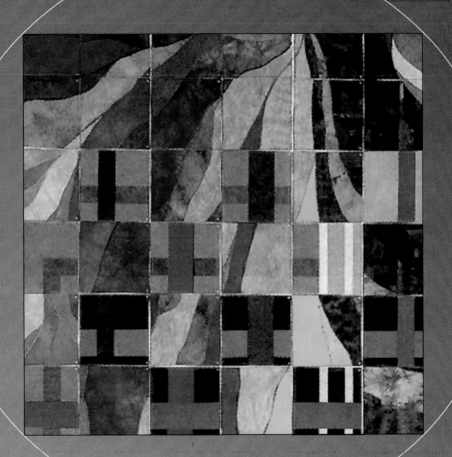

The Analysis of
Research Data

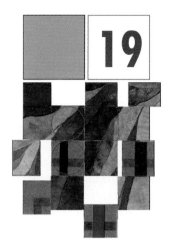

Analyzing Quantitative Data: Descriptive Statistics

tatistical analysis helps researchers make sense of quantitative information. Without statistics, quantitative data would be a chaotic mass of numbers. Statistical procedures enable researchers to summarize, organize, evaluate, interpret, and communicate numeric information.

This textbook does not emphasize the theory or mathematic basis of statistics. Even computation is underplayed because this is not a statistics textbook and because statistics are seldom calculated by hand. We focus on how to use statistics appropriately in different situations, and how to understand what they mean once they have been applied. Mathematic talent is not required to use or understand statistical analysis—only logical thinking ability is needed.

Statistics are either descriptive or inferential. **Descriptive statistics** are used to describe and synthesize data. Averages and percentages are examples of descriptive statistics. Actually, when such indexes are calculated on data from a population, they are called **parameters**. A descriptive index from a sample is called a **statistic**. Research questions are about parameters, but researchers calculate sample statistics to estimate them, using **inferential statistics** to make inferences about the population. This chapter discusses descriptive statistics, and Chapter 20 focuses on inferential statistics. First, however, we discuss the concept of levels of measurement.

LEVELS OF MEASUREMENT

Scientists have developed a system for categorizing measures. This system is important because the analyses that can be performed on data depend on their measurement level. The four major classes, or levels, of measurement are nominal, ordinal, interval, and ratio.

Nominal Measurement

The lowest level of measurement is **nominal measurement**, which involves assigning numbers to classify characteristics into categories. Examples of variables amenable to nominal measurement include gender, blood type, and marital status.

The numeric codes assigned in nominal measurement do not convey quantitative information. If we classify males as 1 and females as 2, the numbers have no inherent meaning. The number 2 clearly does not mean "more than" 1. It would be perfectly acceptable to reverse the code and use 1 for females and 2 for males. The numbers are merely symbols that represent two different values of the gender attribute. Indeed, instead of numeric codes, we could have used alphabetical symbols, such as M and F. We recommend, however, thinking in terms of numeric codes if data analysis is done by computer.

Nominal measurement provides no information about an attribute except equivalence and nonequivalence. If we were to "measure" the gender of Jon, Michael, James, Sheila, and Helen, we would—according to our rule—assign them the codes 1, 1, 1, 2, and 2, respectively. Jon, Michael, and James are considered equivalent on the gender attribute but are not equivalent to Sheila and Helen.

Nominal measures must have categories that are mutually exclusive and collectively exhaustive. For example, if we were measuring ethnicity, we might use the following codes: 1 = whites, 2 = African Americans, 3 = Hispanics. Each subject must be classifiable into one and only one category. The requirement for collective exhaustiveness would not be met if, for example, there were individuals of Asian descent in the sample.

The numbers used in nominal measurement cannot be treated mathematically. It is, for example, nonsensical to calculate the average gender of a sample. We can, however, count elements in the categories, and make statements about frequency of occurrence. In a sample of 50 patients, if there are 30 men and 20 women, we could say that 60% of the subjects are male and 40% are female. No further mathematic operations would be meaningful with nominal data.

It may strike you as odd to think of nominal classification as measurement. Nominal measurement does, however, involve assigning numbers to attributes according to rules. The rules are not sophisticated, to be sure, but they are rules nonetheless.

Example of nominal measures:
Wong, Ho, Chiu, Lui, Chan, and Lee (2002) studied factors contributing to hospital readmission in a Hong Kong hospital. Their dependent variable (readmission versus not) and several independent variables (e.g., working versus not working, gender, and receives financial assistance or not) were nominal-level variables.

Ordinal Measurement

Next in the measurement hierarchy is **ordinal measurement**, which involves sorting objects on the basis of their relative standing on an attribute.

This level of measurement goes beyond mere categorization: The attributes are *ordered* according to some criterion. If a researcher rank-orders subjects from heaviest to lightest, ordinal measurement has been used.

With ordinal measurement, unlike nominal measurement, information concerning not only equivalence but relative standing among objects is captured. When we assign numbers to classify a mother's method of delivery (vaginal versus cesarean), the numbers are not meaningful. Now, consider this scheme for coding a client's ability to perform activities of daily living: (1) completely dependent, (2) needs another person's assistance, (3) needs mechanical assistance, (4) completely independent. In this case, the measurement is ordinal. The numbers are not arbitrary—they signify incremental ability to perform activities of daily living. Individuals assigned a value of four are equivalent to each other with regard to functional ability *and*, relative to those in the other categories, have more of that attribute.

Ordinal measurement does not, however, tell us anything about how much greater one level is than another. We do not know if being completely independent is twice as good as needing mechanical assistance. Nor do we know if the difference between needing another person's assistance and needing mechanical assistance is the same as that between needing mechanical assistance and being completely independent. Ordinal measurement tells us only the relative ranking of the attribute's levels.

As with nominal scales, the types of mathematic operation permissible with ordinal-level data are restricted. Averages are usually meaningless with rank-order measures. Frequency counts, percentages, and several other statistical procedures to be discussed later are appropriate for analyzing ordinal-level data.

Example of ordinal measures:
Bours, Halfens, Abu-Saad, and Grot (2002) studied the prevalence of pressure ulcers in 89 health care institutions in the Netherlands. Over 15,000 patients were assessed for pressure ulcer severity, using the 4-stage classification of the

American and European Pressure Ulcer Advisory Panel. This classification is on an ordinal scale.

Interval Measurement

Interval measurement occurs when researchers can specify the rank-ordering of objects on an attribute and can assume equivalent distance between them. Most psychological and educational tests are based on interval scales. The Scholastic Assessment Test (SAT) is an example of this level of measurement. A score of 550 on the SAT is higher than a score of 500, which in turn is higher than 450. In addition, a difference between 550 and 500 on the test is presumably equivalent to the difference between 500 and 450.

Interval measures are more informative than ordinal measures, but interval measures do not give information about absolute magnitude. The Fahrenheit temperature scale illustrates this point. A temperature of 60°F is 10°F warmer than 50°F. A 10°F difference similarly separates 40°F and 30°F, and the two differences in temperature are equivalent. However, it cannot be said that 60°F is twice as hot as 30°F, or three times as hot as 20°F. The Fahrenheit scale involves an arbitrary zero point. Zero on the thermometer does not signify a total absence of heat. In interval scales, there is no real or rational zero point.

Interval scales greatly expand analytic possibilities. The intervals between numbers can be meaningfully added and subtracted: The interval between 10°F and 5°F is 5°F, or $10 - 5 - 5$. This same operation could not be performed with ordinal measures. Because of this feature, interval-level data can be averaged. It is reasonable, for example, to compute an average daily temperature for hospital patients from whom four temperature readings were taken. Many widely used statistical procedures require measurements on at least an interval scale.

Example of interval measures:
Cheng and Boey (2002) studied the effectiveness of a cardiac rehabilitation program on self-efficacy. An interval level measure, the Exercise Tolerance Self-Efficacy Expectation Scale, was used as one of the dependent variables.

Ratio Measurement

The highest level of measurement is **ratio measurement**. Ratio scales have a rational, meaningful zero. Measures on a ratio scale provide information concerning the rank-ordering of objects on the critical attribute, the intervals between objects, *and* the absolute magnitude of the attribute. Many physical measures provide ratio-level data. A person's weight, for example, is measured on a ratio scale because zero weight is an actual possibility. It is perfectly acceptable to say that someone who weighs 200 pounds is twice as heavy as someone who weighs 100 pounds.

Because ratio scales have an absolute zero, all arithmetic operations are permissible. One can meaningfully add, subtract, multiply, and divide numbers on a ratio scale. All the statistical procedures suitable for interval-level data are also appropriate for ratio-level data.

Example of ratio measures:
Lindeke, Stanley, Else, and Mills (2002) studied academic performance and the need for special services among school-aged children who had been in a level 3 neonatal intensive care unit (NICU). Numerous ratio-level measures of neonatal characteristics (e.g., birth weight, length at birth, head circumference, and number of days in the NICU) were used to describe the sample and to predict outcomes.

Comparison of the Levels

The four levels of measurement constitute a hierarchy, with ratio scales at the top and nominal measurement at the base. Moving from a higher to a lower level of measurement results in an information loss. Let us demonstrate this with an example of people's weight. Table 19-1 presents fictitious data for 10 subjects. The second column shows ratio-level data (i.e., actual weight in pounds).

In the third column, the ratio data have been converted to interval measures by assigning a score of 0 to the lightest individual (Heather), a score of 5 to the person 5 pounds heavier than the lightest person (Amy), and so forth. Note that the resulting

TABLE 19.1 Fictitious Data for Four Levels of Measurement

SUBJECTS	RATIO-LEVEL	INTERVAL-LEVEL	ORDINAL-LEVEL	NOMINAL
Nathan	180	70	10	2
Heather	110	0	1	1
Colby	165	55	8	2
Amanda	130	20	5	1
Trevor	175	65	9	2
Amy	115	5	2	1
Haley	125	15	4	1
Chance	150	40	7	1
Gabriel	145	35	6	1
Erin	120	10	3	1

scores are still amenable to addition and subtraction; differences in pounds are equally far apart, even though they are at different parts of the scale. The data no longer tell us, however, anything about the subjects' weights. Heather, the lightest individual, might be a 10-pound infant or a 120-pound adult.

In the fourth column of Table 19-1, ordinal measurements were assigned by rank-ordering the sample from the lightest (assigned the score of 1), to the heaviest (assigned the score of 10). Now even more information is missing. The data provide no indication of how much heavier Nathan is than Heather. The difference separating them might be 5 pounds or 150 pounds.

Finally, the fifth column presents nominal measurements in which subjects were classified as either *heavy* or *light*. The criterion applied in categorizing individuals was arbitrarily set at a weight greater than 150 pounds (2), or less than or equal to 150 pounds (1). These nominal data are very limited. Within a category, there are no clues as to who is heavier than whom. With this level of measurement, Nathan, Colby, and Trevor are equivalent with regard to the attribute heavy/light, as defined by the classification criterion.

This example illustrates that at every successive level in the measurement hierarchy, there is a loss of information. It also illustrates another point: With information at one level, it is possible to convert data to a lower level, but the converse is not true. If we were given only the nominal measurements, it would be impossible to reconstruct actual weights.

It is not always a straightforward task to identify the level of measurement for a variable. Nominal and ratio measures usually are discernible with little difficulty, but the distinction between ordinal and interval measures is more problematic. Some methodologists argue that most psychological measures that are treated as interval measures are really only ordinal measures. Although instruments such as Likert scales produce data that are, strictly speaking, ordinal, most analysts believe that treating them as interval measures results in too few errors to warrant using less powerful statistical procedures.

TIP: In operationalizing research variables, it is usually best to use the highest level of measurement possible. Higher levels of measurement yield more information and are amenable to more powerful analyses than lower levels. There are, however, exceptions to this guideline, as when researchers use people's scores on interval- or ratio-level measures to create groups. Sometimes group membership is more meaningful than continuous scores. For example, for some research and clinical purposes, it may be more relevant to designate infants as being of low versus normal birth weight (nominal level) than to use actual birth weight values (ratio level).

FREQUENCY DISTRIBUTIONS

Unanalyzed quantitative data are overwhelming. It is not even possible to discern general trends until some order is imposed on the data. Consider the 60 numbers presented in Table 19-2. Let us say these are the scores of 60 high school students on a 30-item test of knowledge about AIDS—scores that are ratio level because there is a rational zero point (no correct answers). Visual inspection of the numbers does not help us understand how students performed.

A set of data can be completely described in terms of three characteristics: the shape of the distribution of values, central tendency, and variability. Central tendency and variability are dealt with in subsequent sections.

Constructing Frequency Distributions

Frequency distributions are a method of organizing numeric data. A **frequency distribution** is a systematic arrangement of values from lowest to highest, together with a count of the number of times each value was obtained. The 60 fictitious test scores are presented as a frequency distribution in Table 19-3. This organized scheme makes it possible to see at a glance what the highest and lowest scores were, what the most common score was, where the bulk of scores clustered, and how many students were in the sample (total sample size is typically depicted as N in research reports). None of this was apparent before the data were organized.

Constructing frequency distributions is simple. They consist of two parts: observed values or measurements (the Xs) and the frequency of cases at each value (the fs). Values are listed in numeric order in one column, and corresponding frequencies are listed in another. Table 19-3 shows the intermediary step of tallying by the familiar method of four vertical bars and then a slash for the fifth observation. In frequency distributions, the categories or score values must be mutually exclusive and collectively exhaustive. The sum of numbers appearing in the frequency column must equal the sample size. In less verbal terms, $\Sigma f = N$, which translates as the sum of (signified by the Greek letter sigma, Σ) the frequencies (f) equals the sample size (N).

It is usually useful to display not only frequency counts but percentages for each score value, as shown in the fourth column of Table 19-3. Percentages are calculated by the simple formula: $\% = (f \div N) \times 100$. Just as the sum of all frequencies should equal N, the sum of all percentages should equal 100.

Some researchers display frequency data graphically. Graphs have the advantage of communicating a lot of information almost instantly. The most widely used graphs for displaying interval- and ratio-level data are **histograms** and **frequency**

TABLE 19.2	AIDS Knowledge Test Scores								
22	27	25	19	24	25	23	29	24	20
26	16	20	26	17	22	24	18	26	28
15	24	23	22	21	24	20	25	18	27
24	23	16	25	30	29	27	21	23	24
26	18	30	21	17	25	22	24	29	28
20	25	26	24	23	19	27	28	25	26

TABLE 19.3 Frequency Distribution of Test Scores

SCORE (X)	TALLIES	FREQUENCY (f)	PERCENTAGE (%)
15	I	1	1.7
16	II	2	3.3
17	II	2	3.3
18	III	3	5.0
19	II	2	3.3
20	IIII	4	6.7
21	III	3	5.0
22	IIII	4	6.7
23	IIHI	5	8.3
24	IHI IIII	9	15.0
25	IHI II	7	11.7
26	IHI I	6	10.0
27	IIII	4	6.7
28	III	3	5.0
29	III	3	5.0
30	II	2	3.3
		$N = 60 = \Sigma f$	$\Sigma\% = 100.0\%$

polygons, which are constructed in a similar fashion. First, score classes are placed on a horizontal dimension, with the lowest value on the left, ascending to the highest value on the right. Frequencies or percentages are displayed vertically, with values usually starting at zero. A histogram is constructed by drawing bars above the score classes to the height corresponding to the frequency for that score class. Figure 19-1 shows a histogram constructed using the AIDS knowledge test scores.

Instead of vertical bars, frequency polygons use dots connected by straight lines to show frequencies. A dot corresponding to the frequency is placed above each score, as shown in Figure 19-2. It is customary to connect the line to the base at the score below the minimum value obtained and above

the maximum value obtained. In this example, however, the graph is terminated at 30 and brought down to the base at that point with a dotted line because a score of 31 was not possible.

Shapes of Distributions

Data displayed in a frequency polygon can assume many shapes. A distribution is **symmetric** in shape if, when folded over, the two halves are superimposed on one another. Symmetric distributions thus consist of two halves that are mirror images of one another. All the distributions in Figure 19-3 are symmetric. With real data sets, distributions are rarely perfectly symmetric, but minor discrepancies are ignored in characterizing a distribution's shape.

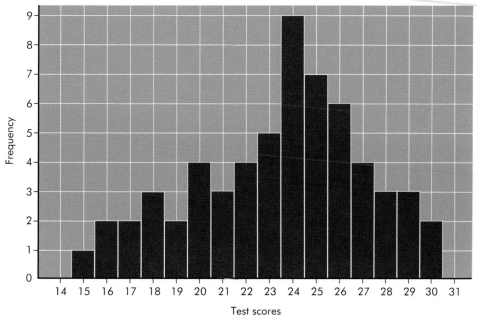

FIGURE 19.1   Histogram of test scores.

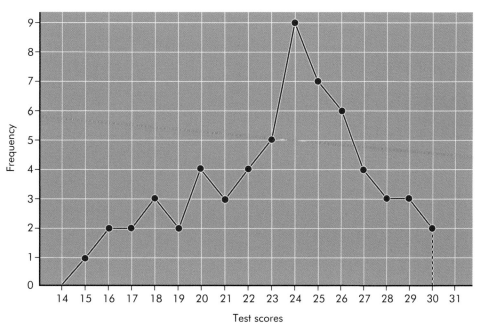

FIGURE 19.2   Frequency polygon of test scores.

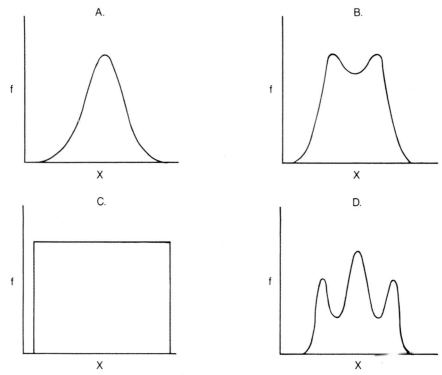

FIGURE 19.3 Examples of symmetric distributions.

In **asymmetric** or **skewed distributions**, the peak is off center and one tail is longer than the other. When the longer tail points to the right, the distribution is **positively skewed**. Figure 19-4A shows a positively skewed distribution. Personal in-come, for example, is positively skewed. Most peo-ple have low to moderate incomes, with relatively few people in high-income brackets in the tail. If the tail points to the left, the distribution is **negatively skewed**, as illustrated in Figure 19-4B. An example

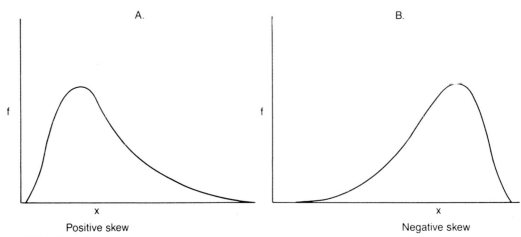

FIGURE 19.4 Examples of skewed distributions.

of a negatively skewed attribute is age at death. Here, most people are at the upper end of the distribution, with relatively few dying at an early age.

A second aspect of a distribution's shape is modality. A **unimodal distribution** has only one peak or high point (i.e., a value with high frequency), whereas a **multimodal distribution** has two or more peaks (i.e., values of high frequency). The most common multimodal distribution is one with two peaks, which is called **bimodal**. Figure 19-3A is unimodal, whereas multimodal distributions are illustrated in Figure 19-3B and D. Symmetry and modality are completely independent aspects of a distribution. Knowledge of skewness does not tell you anything about how many peaks the distribution has.

Some distributions are encountered so frequently that they have special names. Of particular importance is the **normal distribution** (sometimes called a **bell-shaped curve**). A normal distribution is symmetric, unimodal, and not too peaked, as illustrated in Figure 19-3A. Many physical and psychological attributes of humans approximate a normal distribution. Examples include height and intelligence. As we discuss in Chapter 20, the normal distribution plays a central role in inferential statistics.

CENTRAL TENDENCY

Frequency distributions are a good way to organize data and clarify patterns. Often, however, a pattern is of less interest than an overall summary. Researchers usually ask such questions as, "What is the average oxygen consumption of myocardial infarction patients during bathing?" or "What is the average stress level of AIDS patients?" Such questions seek a single number that best represents a distribution of data values. Because an index of typicalness is more likely to come from the center of a distribution than from either extreme, such indexes are called measures of **central tendency**. Lay people use the term *average* to designate central tendency. Researchers avoid this ambiguous term because there are three kinds of averages, or indexes of central tendency: the mode, the median, and the mean.

The Mode

The **mode** is the most frequently occurring score value in a distribution. The mode is simple to determine; it is not computed but rather is established by inspecting a frequency distribution. In the following distribution of numbers, we can readily see that the mode is 53:

50 51 51 52 53 53 53 53 54 55 56

The score of 53 occurred four times, a higher frequency than for any other number. In the example of AIDS knowledge test scores (Table 19-3), the mode is 24. In multimodal distributions, of course, there is more than one score value that has high frequencies.

The mode is seldom used in research reports as the only index of central tendency. Modes are a quick way to determine the most popular score, but cannot be used for further computation and are rather unstable. By unstable, we mean that modes tend to fluctuate widely from sample to sample drawn from the same population. The mode is used primarily to describe typical values on nominal-level measures. For instance, researchers often characterize their samples by providing modal information on nominal-level demographic variables, as in the following example: "The typical (modal) subject was an unmarried white woman, living in an urban area, with no prior history of sexually transmitted diseases."

The Median

The **median** is the point in a distribution above which and below which 50% of cases fall. As an example, consider the following set of values:

2 2 3 3 4 5 6 7 8 9

The value that divides the cases exactly in half is 4.5, which is the median for this set of numbers. The point that has 50% of the cases above and below it is halfway between 4 and 5.

An important characteristic of the median is that it does not take into account the quantitative values of scores. The median is an index of average *position* in a distribution. It is insensitive to extreme values. Consider making one change to the previous set of numbers:

2 2 3 3 4 5 6 7 8 99

Although the last value was increased from 9 to 99, the median is still 4.5. Because of this property, the median is often the preferred index of central tendency when a distribution is skewed. In research reports, the median may be abbreviated as **Md** or **Mdn**.

The Mean

The **mean** is equal to the sum of all scores divided by the total number of scores. The mean is the index usually referred to as an *average*. The computational formula for a mean is

$$\overline{X} = \frac{\Sigma X}{N}$$

where $\overline{X}$ = the mean
Σ = the sum of
X = each individual raw score
N = the number of cases

Let us apply this formula to compute the mean weight of eight subjects with the following weights:

85 109 120 135 158 177 181 195

$$\overline{X} = \frac{85+109+120+135+158+177+181+195}{8} = 145$$

Unlike the median, the mean is affected by each and every score. If we were to exchange the 195-pound subject in this example for one weighing 275 pounds, the mean would increase from 145 to 155. Such a substitution would leave the median unchanged.

The mean is the most widely used measure of central tendency. Many important tests of statistical significance, described in Chapter 20, are based on the mean. When researchers work with interval-level or ratio-level measurements, the mean, rather than the median or mode, is usually the statistic reported. In research reports, the mean is often symbolized as M or $\overline{X}$.

Comparison of the Mode, Median, and Mean

The mean is the most stable index of central tendency. If repeated samples were drawn from a population, means would fluctuate less than modes or medians. Because of its stability, the mean is the most useful estimate of central tendency. Sometimes, however, the primary concern is to understand what is typical, in which case a median might be preferred. If we wanted to know about the economic well-being of U.S. citizens, for example, we would get a distorted impression by considering mean income. The mean in this case would be inflated by the wealth of a minority. The median would better reflect how a typical person fares financially.

When a distribution of scores is symmetric and unimodal, the three indexes of central tendency coincide. In skewed distributions, the values of the mode, median, and mean differ. The mean is always pulled in the direction of the long tail, as shown in Figure 19-5.

A variable's level of measurement plays a role in determining the appropriate index of central tendency to use. In general, the mode is most suitable for nominal measures, the median is appropriate for ordinal measures, and the mean is appropriate for interval and ratio measures.

VARIABILITY

Measures of central tendency do not totally summarize a distribution. Two sets of data with identical means could differ in several respects. For instance, two distributions with the same mean could have different shapes. The characteristic of concern in this section is the **variability** of a distribution, that is, how spread out or dispersed the data are.

Consider the two distributions in Figure 19-6, which represent hypothetical SAT scores of students at two nursing schools. Both distributions have a mean of 500, but the score patterns are clearly different. School A has a wide range of scores, with some below 300 and some above 700. This school has many students who performed

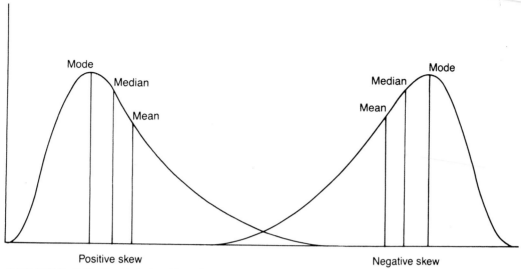

FIGURE 19.5 Relationships of central tendency indexes in skewed distributions.

among the best possible, but also has many students who scored well below average. In school B, on the other hand, there are few students at either extreme. School A is more **heterogeneous** than school B, and school B is more **homogeneous** than school A.

There are indexes of variability that express the extent to which scores deviate from one an-

other. The most common indexes are the range, semiquartile range, and standard deviation.

The Range

The **range** is simply the highest score minus the lowest score in a distribution. In the examples shown in Figure 19-6, the range for school A is

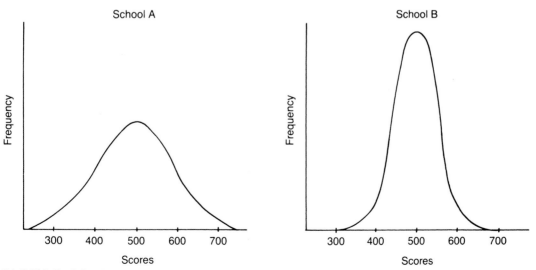

FIGURE 19.6 Two distributions of different variability.

approximately 500 (750 − 250), and the range for school B is approximately 300 (650 − 350).

The chief virtue of the range is its computational ease, but its shortcomings outweigh this modest advantage. The range, being based on only two scores, is highly unstable. From sample to sample drawn from the same population, the range tends to fluctuate considerably. Another limitation is that the range ignores variations in scores between the two extremes. In school B of Figure 19-6, suppose one student obtained a score of 250 and one other student obtained a score of 750. The range of both schools would then be 500, despite obvious differences in the heterogeneity of scores. For these reasons, the range is used largely as a gross descriptive index and is typically reported in conjunction with, not instead of, other measures of variability.

Semiquartile Range*

As previously discussed, the median is the point below which 50% of the cases fall. It is possible to compute the point below which any percentage of scores fall. The **semiquartile range** is calculated based on quartiles of a distribution. The upper quartile (Q_3) is the point below which 75% of the cases fall, and the lower quartile (Q_1) is the point below which 25% of the scores lie.† The semiquartile range (SQR) is half the distance between Q_1 and Q_3, or

$$SQR = \frac{Q_3 - Q_1}{2}$$

Because this index is based on middle cases rather than extreme scores, it is more stable than the range. In Figure 19-6, the semiquartile range of schools A and B is approximately 125 and 75, respectively. The addition of one deviant case at each extreme for school B would leave the semiquartile range virtually untouched.

----

*Some statistical texts use the term *semiquartile range,* whereas others refer to this statistic as the *semi-interquartile range* or the *quartile deviation.*

†The computational formulas for percentiles are not presented here. Most standard statistics texts contain this information.

Standard Deviation

With interval- or ratio-level data, the most widely used measure of variability is the standard deviation. The **standard deviation** indicates the average amount of deviation of values from the mean. Like the mean, the standard deviation is calculated using every score.

A variability index needs to capture the degree to which scores deviate from one another. This concept of deviation is represented in both the range and the semiquartile range by the presence of a minus sign, which produces an index of deviation, or difference, between two score points. The standard deviation is similarly based on score differences. In fact, the first step in calculating a standard deviation is to compute deviation scores for each subject. A **deviation score** (symbolized as x) is the difference between an individual score and the mean. If a person weighed 150 pounds and the sample mean were 140, then the person's deviation score would be +10. The formula for a deviation score is

$$x = X - \overline{X}$$

Because what one is essentially looking for is an *average* deviation, one might think that a good variability index could be arrived at by summing deviation scores and then dividing by the number of cases. This gets us close to a good solution, but the difficulty is that the sum of a set of deviation scores is always zero. Table 19-4 presents an example of deviation scores computed for nine numbers. As shown in the second column, the sum of the xs is zero. Deviations above the mean always balance exactly deviations below the mean.

The standard deviation overcomes this problem by squaring each deviation score before summing. After dividing by the number of cases, the square root is taken to bring the index back to the original unit of measurement. The formula for the standard deviation (often abbreviated as **s** or **SD**)* is

$$SD = \sqrt{\frac{\Sigma x^2}{N}}$$

A standard deviation has been completely worked out for the data in Table 19-4. First, a deviation score is calculated for each of the nine raw scores by subtracting the mean ($\overline{X} = 7$) from them.

TABLE 19.4 Computation of a Standard Deviation

X	$x = X - \bar{X}$	$x^2 = (X - \bar{X})^2$
4	-3	9
5	-2	4
6	-1	1
7	0	0
7	0	0
7	0	0
8	1	1
9	2	4
10	3	9
$\Sigma X = 63$	$\Sigma x = 0$	$\Sigma x^2 = 28$
$\bar{X} = 7$		

$$SD = \sqrt{\frac{28}{9}} = \sqrt{3.11} = 1.76$$

The third column shows that each deviation score is squared, thereby converting all values to positive numbers. The squared deviation scores are summed ($\Sigma x^2 = 28$), divided by 9 (N), and a square root taken to yield an SD of 1.76.

Most researchers routinely report the means and standard deviation of key variables. Sometimes, however, one finds a reference to an index of variability known as the *variance*. The **variance** is simply the value of the standard deviation before a square root has been taken. In other words,

$$\text{Variance} = \frac{\Sigma x^2}{N} = SD^2$$

---

*Some statistical texts indicate that the formula for an unbiased estimate of the population standard deviation is

$$SD = \sqrt{\frac{\Sigma x^2}{N - 1}}$$

Knapp (1970) clarifies when N or $N - 1$ should be used in the denominator. He indicates that N is appropriate when the researcher is interested in *describing* variation in sample data.

In the preceding example, the variance is 1.76^2, or 3.11. The variance is rarely reported because it is not in the same unit of measurement as the original data, but it is an important component in inferential statistical tests that we discuss later.

A standard deviation is typically more difficult for students to interpret than other statistics, such as the mean or range. In our example, we calculated an SD of 1.76. One might well ask, 1.76 *what*? What does the number mean? First, as we already know, the standard deviation is a variability index for a set of scores. If two distributions had a mean of 25.0, but one had an SD of 7.0 and the other had an SD of 3.0, we would immediately know that the second sample was more homogeneous.

A second way to conceptualize the standard deviation is to think of it as an average of deviations from the mean. The mean tells us the single best value for summarizing a distribution; a standard deviation tells us how much, on average, scores deviate from that mean. A standard deviation might thus be interpreted as indicating our degree of error when we use a mean to describe the entire sample.

The standard deviation can also be used in interpreting individual scores in a distribution. Suppose we had weight measures from a sample whose mean weight was 125 pounds and whose SD was 10 pounds. The standard deviation provides a *standard* of variability. Weights greater than 1 SD away from the mean (i.e., greater than 135 or less than 115 pounds) are greater than the average variability for that distribution. Weights within 1 SD of the mean, by consequence, are less than the average variability for that sample.

When distributions are normal or nearly normal, it is possible to say more about the standard deviation. There are about 3 SDs above and 3 SDs below the mean in a normal distribution. To illustrate, suppose we had normally distributed scores with a mean of 50 and an SD of 10, as shown in Figure 19-7. In a normal distribution, a fixed percentage of cases falls within certain distances from the mean. Sixty-eight percent of all cases fall within 1 SD of the mean (34% above and 34% below the mean). In this example, nearly 7 of every 10 scores fall between 40 and 60. Ninety-five percent of the

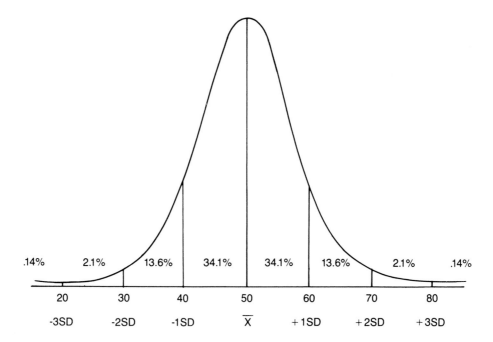

.14%   2.1%   13.6%   34.1%   34.1%   13.6%   2.1%   .14%

20	30	40	50	60	70	80
-3SD	-2SD	-1SD	$\overline{X}$	+1SD	+2SD	+3SD

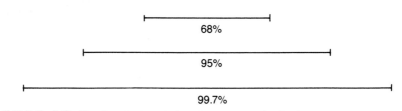

68%

95%

99.7%

FIGURE 19.7   Standard deviations in a normal distribution.

scores in a normal distribution fall within 2 SDs from the mean. Only a handful of cases—approximately 2% at each extreme—lie more than 2 SDs from the mean. Using this figure, we can see that a person with a score of 70 got a higher score than approximately 98% of the sample.

In summary, the standard deviation is a useful variability index for describing a distribution and interpreting individual scores in relation to other scores in the sample. Like the mean, the standard deviation is a stable estimate of a parameter and is the preferred index of a distribution's variability. Standard deviations are appropriate only for variables measured on the interval or ratio scale.

TIP: Descriptive statistics (percentages, means, standard deviations, and so on) are used for various purposes. They may be used to answer research questions, but inferential statistics (see Chapter 20) are much more likely to be used for this purpose. Descriptive statistics are most often used to summarize sample characteristics, describe key research variables, and document methodological features (e.g., the response rate or attrition rate).

Example of descriptive statistics:
Table 19-5 presents descriptive statistics based on data from a nursing study that examined predictors of physical functioning among elderly

TABLE 19.5 Example of Descriptive Statistics: Physical Functioning Scores (SF-36) of Elderly Cancer Patients*

	BEFORE DIAGNOSIS		6–8 WEEKS AFTER DIAGNOSIS	
	Mean (SD)	Median	Mean (SD)	Median
Patients with breast cancer	80 (24)	90	68 (24)	70
Patients with colon cancer	85 (27)	95	61 (27)	65
Patients with lung cancer	72 (28)	85	44 (28)	35
Patients with prostate cancer	88 (19)	100	76 (26)	85

*Adapted from Given, B., Given, C., Azzouzz, F., & Stommel, M. (2001). Physical functioning of elderly cancer patients prior to diagnosis and following initial treatment. *Nursing Research, 50,* 222–232.

cancer patients (Given, Given, Azzouzz, & Stommel, 2001). The table shows the means, standard deviations, and medians of physical functioning scores, using the SF-36 scale, for four groups of cancer patients before diagnosis and then 6 to 8 weeks after diagnosis. According to these data, physical functioning deteriorated in all groups, but especially among lung cancer patients. Variability was constant over time except for prostate cancer patients, who became more heterogeneous after diagnosis. Differences between the medians and means indicate that the distributions were skewed, mostly negatively.

BIVARIATE DESCRIPTIVE STATISTICS: CONTINGENCY TABLES AND CORRELATION

So far we have focused on descriptions of single variables. The mean, mode, standard deviation, and so forth are **univariate** (one-variable) **descriptive statistics** that describe one variable at a time. Most research is about relationships between variables, and **bivariate** (two-variable) **descriptive statistics** describe such relationships.

Contingency Tables

A **contingency table** is a two-dimensional frequency distribution in which the frequencies of two variables are **cross-tabulated**. Suppose we had data on patients' gender and whether they were nonsmokers, light smokers (<1 pack of cigarettes a day), or heavy smokers (≥ 1 pack a day). The question is whether there is a tendency for men to smoke more heavily than women, or vice versa (i.e., whether there is a relationship between smoking and gender). Fictitious data on these two variables are shown in a contingency table in Table 19-6. Six **cells** are created by placing one variable (gender) along the vertical dimension and the other variable (smoking status) along the horizontal dimension. After subjects' data are allocated to the appropriate cells, percentages are computed. This procedure allows us to see at a glance that, in this sample, women were more likely than men to be nonsmokers (45.4% versus 27.3%) and less likely to be heavy smokers (18.2% versus 36.4%). Contingency tables usually are used with nominal data or ordinal data that have few levels or ranks. In the present example, gender is a nominal measure, and smoking status, as defined, is an ordinal measure.

Example of a contingency table:
Table 19-7 shows a cross-tabulation table from a study that examined dyspnea in emergency department visits among patients with chronic cardiorespiratory diseases (Parshall, 1999). The table shows whether there was a dyspnea complaint for patients with different diseases. Overall, 76.3% of

TABLE 19.6 Contingency Table for Gender and Smoking Status Relationship

| SMOKING STATUS | GENDER | | | | | |
| | Women | | Men | | Total | |
	n	%	*n*	%	*n*	%
Nonsmoker	10	45.4	6	27.3	16	36.4
Light smoker	8	36.4	8	36.4	16	36.4
Heavy smoker	4	18.2	8	36.4	12	27.3
TOTAL	22	100.0	22	100.0	44	100.0

the sample reported dyspnea. Asthmatic patients were especially likely to report dyspnea: 87.6% of asthmatic patients, compared with 61.6% of those with congestive heart failure, reported it.

A comparison of Tables 19-6 and 19-7 illustrates that cross-tabulated data can be presented in two ways: Cell percentages can be computed based on either row totals or column totals. In Table 19-6,

the number 10 in the first cell (nonsmoking women) was divided by the *column* total (i.e., total number of women—22) to arrive at the percentage of women who were nonsmokers (45.4%). The table *could* have shown 62.5% in this cell—the percentage of nonsmokers who were women. In Table 19-7, the number 187 in the first cell (patients with chronic obstructive pulmonary disease [COPD] with dyspnea) was divided by the *row* total

TABLE 19.7 Example of a Contingency Table: Study of Dyspnea in Relation to Diagnoses and Dispositions

| DIAGNOSIS | DYSPNEA | | NO DYSPNEA | | Total *N* |
	n	%	*n*	%	
COPD	187	78.2	52	21.8	239
Asthma	346	87.6	49	12.4	395
Mixed COPD and asthma	12	66.7	6	33.3	18
Restrictive	10	71.4	4	28.6	14
Congestive heart failure	197	61.6	123	38.4	320
TOTAL	752	76.3	234	23.7	986

COPD, chronic obstructive pulmonary disease.
Adapted from Parshall, M.D. (1999). Adult emergency visits for chronic cardio respiratory disease: Does dyspnea matter? *Nursing Research, 48,* 62–70, Table 2.

(i.e., total number of patients with COPD —239) to yield the percentage of 78.2%. Computed the other way, the percentage of patients with dyspnea who had a COPD diagnosis would be 24.9%. Either approach is acceptable, but the former is often preferred because then the column percentages add up to 100%.

Correlation

Relationships between two variables are usually described through **correlation** procedures. Correlation coefficients can be computed with two variables measured on either the ordinal, interval, or ratio scale. Correlation coefficients were briefly described in Chapter 18, and this section extends that discussion.

The correlation question is: To what extent are two variables related to each other? For example, to what degree are anxiety test scores and blood pressure readings related? This question can be answered graphically or, more commonly, by calculating an index that describes the *magnitude* and *direction* of the relationship.

Correlations between two variables can be graphed on a **scatter plot** or **scatter diagram**. Constructing a scatter plot involves making a rec-

tangular coordinate graph with the two variables laid out at right angles. Values for one variable (*X*) are scaled along the horizontal axis, and values for the second variable (*Y*) are scaled vertically, as shown in Figure 19-8. This graph presents data for 10 subjects (a–j) for variables *X* and *Y*. For subject a, the values for *X* and *Y* are 2 and 1, respectively. To graph subject a's position, we go two units to the right along the *X* axis, and one unit up on the *Y* axis. This procedure is followed for all subjects. The letters on the plot are shown to help identify subjects, but normally only dots appear.

In a scatter plot, the direction of the slope of points indicates the direction of the correlation. As noted in Chapter 18, a positive correlation occurs when high values on one variable are associated with high values on a second variable. If the slope of points begins at the lower left corner and extends to the upper right corner, the relationship is positive. In the current example, we would say that *X* and *Y* are positively related. People with high scores on variable *X* tend to have high scores on variable *Y*, and low scorers on *X* tend to score low on *Y*.

A negative (or inverse) relationship is one in which high values on one variable are related to low values on the other. Negative relationships on a

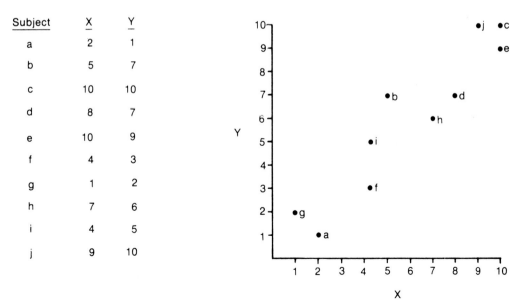

FIGURE 19.8 Construction of a scatter plot.

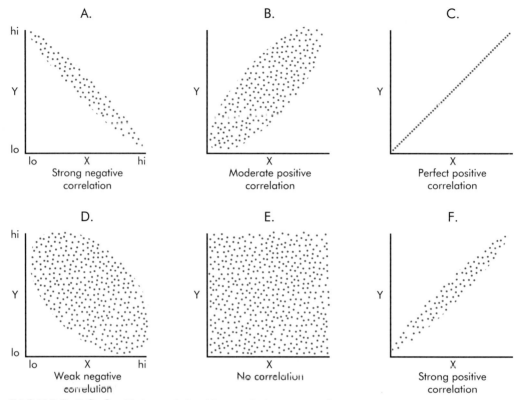

FIGURE 19.9 Various relationships graphed on scatter plots.

scatter plot are depicted by points that slope from the upper left corner to the lower right corner. A negative correlation is shown in Figure 19-9A and D.

When relationships are perfect, it is possible to predict perfectly the value of one variable by knowing the value of the second. For instance, if all people who were 6 feet 2 inches tall weighed 180 pounds, and all people who were 6 feet 1 inch tall weighed 175 pounds, and so on, then we could say that weight and height were perfectly, positively related. In such a situation, we would only need to know a person's height to know his or her weight, or vice versa. On a scatter plot, a perfect relationship is represented by a sloped straight line, as shown in Figure 19-9C. When a relationship is not perfect, as is usually the case, one can interpret the *degree* of correlation from a scatter plot by seeing how closely the points cluster around a straight line. The more closely packed the points are around a diagonal

slope, the stronger the correlation. When the points are scattered all over the graph, the relationship is low or nonexistent. Various degrees and directions of relationships are presented in Figure 19-9.

It is more efficient to express relationships between variables by computing a correlation coefficient. As noted earlier, the correlation coefficient is an index with values ranging from −1.00 for a perfect negative correlation, through zero for no relationship, to +1.00 for a perfect positive correlation. All correlations that fall between .00 and −1.00 are negative, and ones that fall between .00 and +1.00 are positive. The higher the absolute value of the coefficient (i.e., the value disregarding the sign), the stronger the relationship. A correlation of −.80, for instance, is much stronger than a correlation of +.20.

The most commonly used correlation index is the **product–moment correlation coefficient**, also referred to as **Pearson's r**. This coefficient is computed with variables measured on either an interval or ratio scale. (The correlation index usually used for ordinal-level measures is **Spearman's rho**, discussed in Chapter 20). The calculation of the *r* statistic is laborious and seldom performed by hand.*

It is difficult to offer guidelines on what to interpret as strong or weak relationships because it depends on the variables in question. If we measured patients' body temperatures orally and rectally, a correlation (*r*) of .70 between the two measurements would be low. For most psychosocial variables (e.g., stress and severity of illness), an *r* of .70 is high; correlations between such variables are typically in the .10 to .40 range. Perfect correlations (+1.00 and −1.00) are rare.

Correlation coefficients are often reported in tables displaying a two-dimensional **correlation matrix**, in which every variable is displayed in both a row and a column and coefficients are displayed at the intersections. An example of a correlation matrix is presented at the end of this chapter.

THE COMPUTER AND DESCRIPTIVE STATISTICS

Researchers usually use a computer to calculate statistics. This section aims to familiarize you with printouts from a widely used computer program called Statistical Package for the Social Sciences (SPSS).

Suppose we were evaluating the effectiveness of an intervention for low-income pregnant adolescents. The intervention is a program of intensive health care, nutrition education, and contraceptive counseling. Thirty pregnant young women are randomly assigned to either the special program or routine care. Two key outcomes are infant birth weight and repeat pregnancy within 18 months of delivery. Fictitious data are presented in Table 19-8.

Figure 19-10 presents information from a frequency distribution printout for infant birth weight. Several descriptive statistics are shown first. The *Mean* is 104.7, the *Median* is 102.5, and the *Mode* is 99, suggesting a modestly skewed distribution. The SD (*Std Deviation*) is 10.9549, and the *Variance* is 120.0103 (10.9549²). The *Range* is 52, which is equal to the *Maximum* of 128 minus the *Minimum* of 76. Quartile values are then shown; for example, 25% of the birth weight values were below 98.75.

The frequency distribution is shown in the second panel. Each birth weight is listed in ascending order in the first column, from the low value of 76 to the high value of 128. The next column, *Frequency*, shows the number of occurrences of each birth weight. There was one 76-ounce baby, two 89-ounce babies, and so on. The next column, *Percent*, indicates the percentage of infants in each birth weight category: 3.3% weighed 76 ounces, 6.7% weighed 89 ounces, and so on. The next column, *Valid Percent*, indicates the percentage in each category after removing any missing values. In this example, birth weights were obtained for all 30 infants, but if one birth weight had been missing, the **adjusted frequency** for the 76-ounce baby would have been 3.4% (1 ÷ 29 rather than 30). The last column, *Cumulative Percent*, adds the percentage for a given birth weight value to the percentage for all preceding values. Thus, we can tell by looking at the row for 99 ounces that, cumulatively, 33.3% of the babies weighed *under* 100 ounces.

Many computer programs also produce graphs. Figure 19-11 shows a histogram for maternal age. The age values (ranging from 13 to 21) are on the horizontal axis, and frequencies are on the vertical axis. The histogram shows at a glance that the modal age is 19 (*f* = 7) and that age is negatively skewed (i.e., there are fewer younger than older mothers). Descriptive statistics above the histogram indicate that the mean age for this group is 18.1667, with an SD of 2.0858.

---

*For those who may wish to understand how a correlation coefficient is computed, we offer the following formula:

$$r_{xy} = \frac{\Sigma(X - \overline{X})(Y - \overline{Y})}{\sqrt{[\Sigma(X - \overline{X})^2][\Sigma(Y - \overline{Y})^2]}}$$

where r_{xy} = the correlation coefficient for variable X and Y
  X = an individual score for variable X
  $\overline{X}$ = the mean score for variable X
  Y = an individual score for variable Y
  $\overline{Y}$ = the mean score for variable Y
  Σ = the sum of

TABLE 19.8 Fictitious Data on Low-Income Pregnant Adolescents

GROUP*	INFANT BIRTH WEIGHT	REPEAT PREGNANCY†	MOTHER'S AGE (YEARS)	NO. OF PRIOR PREGNANCIES	SMOKING STATUS‡
1	107	1	17	1	1
1	101	0	14	0	0
1	119	0	21	3	0
1	128	1	20	2	0
1	89	0	15	1	1
1	99	0	19	0	1
1	111	0	19	1	0
1	117	1	18	1	1
1	102	1	17	0	0
1	120	0	20	0	0
1	76	0	13	0	1
1	116	0	18	0	1
1	100	1	16	0	0
1	115	0	18	0	0
1	113	0	21	2	1
2	111	1	19	0	0
2	108	0	21	1	0
2	95	0	19	2	1
2	99	0	17	0	1
2	103	1	19	0	0
2	94	0	15	0	1
2	101	1	17	1	0
2	114	0	21	2	0
2	97	0	20	1	0
2	99	1	18	0	1
2	113	0	18	0	1
2	89	0	19	1	0
2	98	0	20	0	0
2	102	0	17	0	0
2	105	0	19	1	1

*Group: 1 = experimental; 2 = control.
†Repeat pregnancy: 1 = yes; 0 = no.
‡Smoking status: 1 = smokes; 0 = does not smoke.

Frequencies

Statistics

Infant birth weight in ounces

N	Valid	30
	Missing	0
Mean		104.7000
Median		102.5000
Mode		99.00
Std. Deviation		10.9549
Variance		120.0103
Range		52.00
Minimum		76.00
Maximum		128.00
Percentiles	25	98.7500
	50	102.5000
	75	113.2500

Infant birth weight in ounces

	Frequency	Percent	Valid Percent	Cumulative Percent
Valid 76.00	1	3.3	3.3	3.3
89.00	2	6.7	6.7	10.0
94.00	1	3.3	3.3	13.3
95.00	1	3.3	3.3	16.7
97.00	1	3.3	3.3	20.0
98.00	1	3.3	3.3	23.3
99.00	3	10.0	10.0	33.3
100.00	1	3.3	3.3	36.7
101.00	2	6.7	6.7	43.3
102.00	2	6.7	6.7	50.0
103.00	1	3.3	3.3	53.3
105.00	1	3.3	3.3	56.7
107.00	1	3.3	3.3	60.0
108.00	1	3.3	3.3	63.3
111.00	2	6.7	6.7	70.0
113.00	2	6.7	6.7	76.7
114.00	1	3.3	3.3	80.0
115.00	1	3.3	3.3	83.3
116.00	1	3.3	3.3	86.7
117.00	1	3.3	3.3	90.0
119.00	1	3.3	3.3	93.3
120.00	1	3.3	3.3	96.7
128.00	1	3.3	3.3	100.0
Total	30	100.0	100.0	

FIGURE 19.10 Frequency distribution printout for infant birth weight.

Frequencies

Statistics

Mother's age

N	Valid	30
	Missing	0
Mean		18.1667
Median		18.5000
Mode		19.00
Std. Deviation		2.0858
Variance		4.3506
Range		8.00
Minimum		13.00
Maximum		21.00

Mother's age

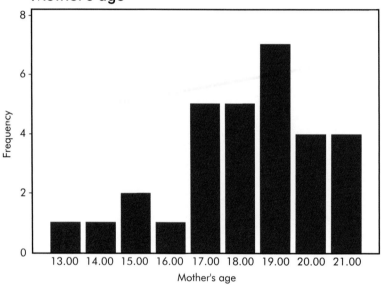

FIGURE 19.11

Histogram for maternal age.

If we wanted to compare the repeat-pregnancy rate of experimental versus control group mothers, we would instruct the computer to cross-tabulate the two variables, as shown in the contingency table in Figure 19-12. This cross-tabulation resulted in four key cells: (1) experimental subjects with no repeat pregnancy (upper left cell); (2) control subjects with no repeat pregnancy; (3) experimental subjects with a repeat pregnancy; and (4)

control subjects with a repeat pregnancy. Each of these cells contains four pieces of information. The first is number of subjects in the cell (*Count*). In the first cell, 10 experimental subjects did not have a repeat pregnancy within 18 months of delivery. Below the 10 is the *row* percentage or *% within Repeat pregnancy*: 47.6% of the women who did not become pregnant again were experimentals (10 ÷ 21). The next entry is the *column* percentage or

			GROUP		
			Experimental	Control	Total
Repeat pregnancy	No	Count	10	11	21
		% within Repeat pregnancy	47.6%	52.4%	100.0%
		% within GROUP	66.7%	73.3%	70.0%
		% of Total	33.3%	36.7%	70.0%
	Yes	Count	5	4	9
		% within Repeat pregnancy	55.6%	44.4%	100.0%
		% within GROUP	33.3%	26.7%	30.0%
		% of Total	16.7%	13.3%	30.0%
Total		Count	15	15	30
		% within Repeat pregnancy	50.0%	50.0%	100.0%
		% within GROUP	100.0%	100.0%	100.0%
		% of Total	50.0%	50.0%	100.0%

FIGURE 19.12 Repeat pregnancy* GROUP cross-tabulation.

% within GROUP: 66.7% of the experimental subjects did not become pregnant (10 ÷ 15). Last is the *overall* percentage of the sample who were in that cell (10 ÷ 30 = 33.3%). Thus, Figure 19-12 indicates that a somewhat higher percentage of experimental (33.3%) than control subjects (26.7%) had an early repeat pregnancy. The row totals on the far right indicate that, overall, 30.0% of the sample (N = 9) had a subsequent pregnancy. The column totals at the bottom indicate that 50.0% of the subjects were in the experimental group, and 50.0% were in the control group.

RESEARCH EXAMPLE

Dwyer, Coty, Smith, Dulemba, and Wallston (2001) undertook a study to compare two methods of assessing disease activity in the joints of people with rheumatoid arthritis (RA). The two methods were (1) clinician joint count, including clinician's ratings of joint tenderness, joint swelling, and joint range of motion; and (2) a self-reported assessment of pain and tenderness using an instrument called the Rapid Assessment of Disease Activity in Rheumatology (RADAR). Dwyer and her colleagues examined the relationship of these two methods to one another, and the relationship of both to self-reported pain and scores on an objective functional performance index.

A sample of 207 persons diagnosed with RA were recruited into the study, and data were gathered in the homes of 185 subjects (89.4% response rate). The mean age of subjects was 54 years, and the median time elapsed since diagnosis was 2 years.

The research report for this study contained a variety of descriptive statistics. The means, standard deviations, and ranges of key study variables were displayed in the first table. The value of these indexes for the three clinician assessments were as follows:

1. Joint tenderness: $\overline{X} = 10.8$, SD = 8.0, range = 0–28
2. Joint swelling: $\overline{X} = 5.4$, SD = 4.9, range = 0–21
3. Joint limited range of motion: $\overline{X} = 4.3$, SD = 4.8, range = 0–23

All three clinician ratings were based on assessments of 28 joints, and each joint was scored as normal or abnormal. Total scores reflect the total number of abnormal joints. Thus, the *theoretical* range of scores for each indicator is 0 to 28, a range

TABLE 19.9 Correlation Matrix for Key Study Variables: Disease Activity in the Joints

VARIABLE	1	2	3	4	5	6
1 Joint tenderness, clinician's rating	1.00					
2 Joint swelling, clinician's rating	.55	1.00				
3 Joint limited range of motion, clinician rating	.36	.35	1.00			
4 RADAR score (self-assessment)	.54	.31	.35	1.00		
5 Pain index	.40	.24	.32	.67	1.00	
6 Performance index	−.46	−.35	−.44	−.42	−.36	1.00

Adapted from Dwyer, K. A., Coty, M., Smith, C., Dulemba, S., & Wallston, K. A. (2001). A comparison of two methods of assessing disease activity in the joints. *Nursing Research, 50*, 214–221.

that in fact occurred for the joint tenderness assessment. Smaller ranges were observed for swelling and range of motion. The descriptive statistics also tell us that joint tenderness ($\overline{X} = 10.8$) was assessed to be far more prevalent than swelling ($\overline{X} = 5.4$) or limited range of motion ($\overline{X} = 4.3$). The values of the standard deviations are quite large, relative to the value of the means. This tells us that the clinician's ratings were not normally distributed, but rather were positively skewed. If joint tenderness, for example, were normally distributed, we would have expected a mean of about 14 and an SD of about 4.7, given that ratings ranged from 0 to 28. With a positively skewed distribution, the bulk of ratings would be less than the mean of 10.8, with the mean being inflated by the scores of the minority of subjects with very high ratings.

Table 19-9, adapted from Table 2 of the research report, presents the correlation matrix for key study variables.* This table lists, on the left, six variables: the three clinician ratings (variables 1, 2, and 3), self-reported RADAR scores (4), pain index scores (5), and subject performance, based on clinician's observations of performance in both upper and lower extremities. The numbers in the top row, from 1 to 6, correspond to the six variables: 1 is the clinician's ratings of joint tenderness, and so on. The correlation matrix shows, in the first column, the correlation coefficient between joint tenderness ratings with all six variables. At the intersection of row 1 and column 1, we find the value 1.00, which simply indicates that joint tenderness ratings are perfectly correlated with themselves. The next entry in the first column is the correlation between joint tenderness and joint swelling. The value of .55 (which can be read as +.55) indicates a moderate and positive relationship between these two variables: people rated with abnormal joint tenderness tended to have ratings of abnormal swelling. Looking down at the last row in this table, we see that subjects' scores on the performance index were negatively correlated with all other variables. In other words, the greater the tenderness, swelling, and limited range of motion, the lower the performance.

Several correlations deserve special mention. First, we see that the RADAR scores (variable 4) were moderately and positively correlated with the clinician's ratings. The correlation between RADAR scores and the clinician's rating of joint tenderness was .54, for example. The table also shows us that the RADAR scores were nearly as well correlated with performance scores (−.42) as were the clinician's ratings of tenderness (−.46). Finally, RADAR scores were even *more* strongly correlated with self-reported pain (.67) than were the clinician's rating of tenderness (.40). Dwyer and her colleagues concluded that self-reported joint counts have sufficient validity for research purposes to be used in place of more costly clinician assessments.

---

*Although we present only descriptive information, Dwyer and her colleagues also applied inferential statistics.

SUMMARY POINTS

- There are four **levels of measurement:** (1) **nominal measurement**—the classification of characteristics into mutually exclusive categories; (2) **ordinal measurement**—the ranking of objects based on their relative standing to each other on an attribute; (3) **interval measurement**—indicating not only the ranking of objects but the amount of distance between them; and (4) **ratio measurement**—distinguished from interval measurement by having a rational zero point.
- **Descriptive statistics** enable researchers to summarize and describe quantitative data.
- In **frequency distributions,** which impose order on raw data, numeric values are ordered from lowest to highest, accompanied by a count of the number (or percentage) of times each value was obtained.
- **Histograms** and **frequency polygons** are two common methods of displaying frequency information graphically.
- Data for a variable can be completely described in terms of the shape of the distribution, central tendency, and variability.
- A distribution is **symmetric** if its two halves are mirror images of each other. A **skewed distribution**, by contrast, is asymmetric, with one tail longer than the other.
- In a **positively skewed distribution** the long tail points to the right (e.g., personal income); in a **negatively skewed distribution** the long tail points to the left (e.g., age at death).
- The modality of a distribution refers to the number of peaks present: A **unimodal distribution** has one peak, and a **multimodal distribution** has more than one peak.
- A **normal distribution** (bell-shaped curve) is symmetric, unimodal, and not too peaked.
- Measures of **central tendency** are indexes, expressed as a single number, that represent the average or typical value of a set of scores. The **mode** is the value that occurs most frequently in the distribution; the **median** is the point above which and below which 50% of the cases fall; and the **mean** is the arithmetic average of all

scores. The mean is usually the preferred measure of central tendency because of its stability.
- Measures of **variability**—how spread out the data are—include the range, semiquartile range, and standard deviation. The **range** is the distance between the highest and lowest scores; the **semiquartile range** indicates one half of the range of scores within which the middle 50% of scores lie; and the **standard deviation** indicates how much, on average, scores deviate from the mean.
- The standard deviation (SD) is calculated by first computing **deviation scores**, which represent the degree to which each person's score deviates from the mean. The **variance** is equal to the standard deviation squared.
- **Bivariate descriptive statistics** describe relationships between two variables.
- A **contingency table** is a two-dimensional frequency distribution in which the frequencies of two nominal- or ordinal-level variables are **cross-tabulated.**
- **Correlation coefficients** describe the direction and magnitude of a relationship between two variables, and range from -1.00 (perfect negative correlation) through .00 to $+1.00$ (perfect positive correlation).
- The most frequently used correlation coefficient is the **product–moment correlation coefficient** (**Pearson's r**), used with interval- or ratio-level variables.
- Graphically, the relationship between two variables is displayed on a **scatter plot** or **scatter diagram**.

STUDY ACTIVITIES

Chapter 19 of the accompanying *Study Guide for Nursing Research: Principles and Methods, 7th ed.,* offers various exercises and study suggestions for reinforcing concepts presented in this chapter. In addition, the following study questions can be addressed:

1. Construct a frequency distribution for the following set of scores:

   32 20 33 22 16 19 25 26 25 18 22 30 24 26 27
   23 28 26 21 24 31 29 25 28 22 27 26 30 17 24

2. Construct a frequency polygon or histogram with the preceding data. Describe the resulting distribution of scores in terms of symmetry and modality. How closely does the distribution approach a normal distribution?

3. What are the mean, median, and mode for the following set of data?

    13 12 9 15 7 10 16 8 6 1

    Compute the range and standard deviation.

4. Two hospitals are interested in comparing the tenure rates of their nursing staff. Hospital A finds that the current staff has been employed for a mean of 4.3 years, with an SD of 1.5. Hospital B, on the other hand, finds that the nurses have worked there for a mean of 6.4 years, with an SD of 4.2 years. Discuss what these results signify.

SUGGESTED READINGS

Methodologic References

Jaccard, J., & Becker, M. A. (2001). *Statistics for the behavioral sciences* (4th ed.). Belmont, CA: Wadsworth.

Knapp, T. R. (1970). N vs. N − 1. *American Educational Research Journal, 7,* 625–626.

McCall, R. B. (2000). *Fundamental statistics for behavioral sciences* (8th ed.). Belmont, CA: Wadsworth.

Munro, B. H. (Ed.). (2001). *Statistical methods for health-care research* (4th ed.). Philadelphia: Lippincott Williams & Wilkins.

Polit, D. F. (1996). *Data analysis and statistics for nursing research.* Stamford, CT: Appleton & Lange.

Triola, M. (2000). *Elementary statistics* (8th ed.). Menlo Park, CA: Addison-Wesley.

Studies Cited in Chapter 19

Bours, G., Halfens, R., Abu-Saad, H., & Grot, R. (2002). Prevalence, prevention, and treatment of pressure ulcers: Descriptive study in 89 institutions in The Netherlands. *Research in Nursing & Health, 25,* 99–110.

Cheng, T. Y. L., & Boey, K. W. (2002). The effectiveness of a cardiac rehabilitation program on self-efficacy and exercise tolerance. *Clinical Nursing Research, 11,* 10–21.

Dwyer, K. A., Coty, M., Smith, C., Dulemba, S., & Wallston, K. A. (2001). A comparison of two methods of assessing disease activity in the joints. *Nursing Research, 50,* 214–221.

Given, B., Given, C., Azzouzz, F., & Stommel, M. (2001). Physical functioning of elderly cancer patients prior to diagnosis and following initial treatment. *Nursing Research, 50,* 222–232.

Lindeke, L. L., Stanley, J. R., Else, B. S., & Mills, M. M. (2002). Neonatal predictors of school-based services used by NICU graduates at school age. *MCN: Journal of Maternal—Child Nursing, 27,* 41–46.

Parshall, M. B. (1999). Adult emergency visits for chronic cardiorespiratory disease: Does dyspnea matter? *Nursing Research, 48,* 62–70.

Wong, F., Ho, M., Chiu, I., Lui, W., Chan, C., & Lee, K. (2002). Factors contributing to hospital readmission in a Hong Kong regional hospital. *Nursing Research, 51,* 40–49.

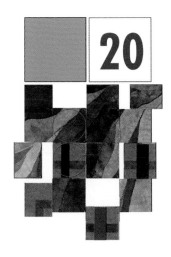

20

Analyzing Quantitative Data: Inferential Statistics

Researchers usually want to do more than *describe* their data. **Inferential statistics**, which are based on the **laws of probability**, provide a means for drawing conclusions about a population, given data from a sample. Inferential statistics would help us with such questions as, "What do I know about 3-minute Apgar scores of premature babies (the population) after learning that the mean Apgar score in a sample of 100 premature babies was 7.5?" or "What can I conclude about an intervention to promote breast self-examination among women older than 25 years (the population) after finding in a sample of 200 women that 50% of experimental subjects and 30% of controls practiced breast self-examination 3 months later?"

With inferential statistics, researchers estimate population parameters from sample statistics. These probabilistic estimates involve some error, but inferential statistics provide a framework for making judgments about their reliability in a systematic, objective fashion. Different researchers applying inferential statistics to the same data would likely draw identical conclusions.

SAMPLING DISTRIBUTIONS

To estimate population parameters, it is clearly advisable to use representative samples. As we saw in Chapter 13, probability samples are the best way to get representative samples. Inferential statistics are based on the assumption of random sampling from populations—although this assumption is widely violated.

Even when random sampling is used, however, sample characteristics are seldom identical to population characteristics. Suppose we had a population of 25,000 nursing school applicants whose mean score on the Scholastic Assessment Test (SAT) was 500 with a standard deviation (SD) of 100. Suppose we do not know these parameters but must estimate them from the scores of a random sample of 25 students. Should we expect a mean of *exactly* 500 and an SD of 100 for this sample? Obtaining the exact population value would be improbable. Let us say the sample mean is 505. If a new sample were drawn and another mean computed, we might obtain a value such as 497. The tendency for statistics to fluctuate from one sample to another is known as **sampling error**. The challenge for researchers is to determine whether sample values are good estimates of population parameters.

Researchers work with only *one* sample on which statistics are computed and inferences made. To understand inferential statistics, however, we must perform a mental exercise. Consider drawing a sample of 25 students from the population of 25,000, calculating a mean, replacing the students,

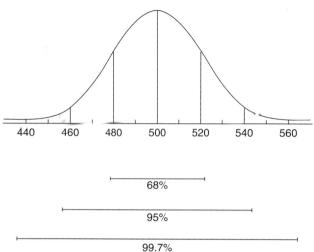

FIGURE 20.1 Sampling distribution.

and drawing a new sample. Each mean is considered a separate datum. If we drew 5000 such samples, we would have 5000 means (data points) that could be used to construct a frequency polygon, as shown in Figure 20-1. This distribution is a **sampling distribution of the mean**. A sampling distribution is a theoretical rather than actual distribution because in practice no one draws consecutive samples from a population and plots their means. Theoretical distributions of sample values are the basis of inferential statistics.

Characteristics of Sampling Distributions

When an infinite number of samples is drawn from an infinite population, the sampling distribution of the mean has certain characteristics. Our example of a population of 25,000 applicants, and 5000 samples with 25 students each, deals with finite quantities, but the numbers are large enough to approximate these characteristics.

Statisticians have demonstrated that sampling distributions of means are normally distributed. Furthermore, the mean of a sampling distribution with an infinite number of sample means always equals the population mean. In the example shown

in Figure 20-1, the mean of the sampling distribution is 500, the same as the population mean.

As discussed in Chapter 19, 68% of the cases fall between ±1 SD from the mean when data are normally distributed. Because a sampling distribution of means *is* normally distributed, we can say that 68 out of 100 sample means will lie between +1 SD and −1 SD of the sampling distribution (and population) mean. Thus, if we could estimate the value of the sampling distribution's standard deviation, we could interpret the accuracy of any sample mean.

Standard Error of the Mean

The standard deviation of a sampling distribution of the mean is called the **standard error of the mean** (**SEM**). The word *error* signifies that the various means in the sampling distribution have some error as estimates of the population mean. The smaller the SEM—that is, the less variable the sample means—the more accurate are the means as estimates of the population value.

But no one actually constructs a sampling distribution, so how can its standard deviation be computed? Fortunately, there is a formula for estimating the SEM from a single sample, using two pieces of information: the sample's SD and sample size. The equation for the SEM (symbolized as $s_{\bar{x}}$) is:

$$s_{\bar{x}} = \frac{SD}{\sqrt{N}}$$

where SD = the standard deviation of the sample
  N = sample size
  $s_{\bar{x}}$ = standard error of the mean

If we use this formula to calculate the SEM for an SD of 100 with a sample of 25 students we obtain

$$s_{\bar{x}} = \frac{100}{\sqrt{25}} = 20.0$$

The standard deviation of the sampling distribution is 20, as shown in Figure 20-1. This SEM is an estimate of how much sampling error there is from one sample mean to another when samples of 25 are randomly drawn.

Given that a sampling distribution of means follows a normal curve, we can estimate the probability of drawing a sample with a certain mean. With a sample size of 25, the chances are about 95 out of 100 that any sample mean will fall between 460 and 540 (i.e., 2 SDs above and below the mean of 500). Only 5 times out of 100 would the mean of a randomly selected sample exceed 540 or be less than 460. In other words, only 5 times out of 100 would we get a sample whose mean deviated from the population mean by more than 40 points.

Because the SEM is partly a function of sample size, we need only increase sample size to increase the accuracy of our estimate. Suppose that instead of using a sample of 25 applicants, we used a sample of 100. With this many students, the SEM would be 10:

$$s_{\bar{x}} = \frac{100}{\sqrt{100}} = 10.0$$

In this situation, the chances are about 95 out of 100 that a sample mean will be between 480 and 520. The chances of drawing a sample with a mean very different from the population mean is reduced as sample size increases because large numbers promote the likelihood that extreme cases will cancel each other out.

ESTIMATION OF PARAMETERS

Statistical inference consists of two techniques: estimation of parameters and hypothesis testing. Hypothesis testing is more common in research reports, but estimation is also important.

Parameter estimation is used to estimate a single parameter, like a mean. Estimation can take two forms: point estimation or interval estimation. **Point estimation** involves calculating a single statistic to estimate the population parameter. To continue with the SAT example, if we calculated the mean SAT score for a sample of 25 applicants and found that it was 510, then this number would be the point estimate of the population mean.

Point estimates convey no information about accuracy. **Interval estimation** of a parameter is more useful because it indicates a range of values within which the parameter has a specified probability of lying. With interval estimation, researchers construct a **confidence interval (CI)** around the estimate; the upper and lower limits are called **confidence limits**. Constructing a confidence interval around a sample mean establishes a range of values for the population mean as well as the probability of being right—the estimate is made with a certain degree of confidence. Researchers conventionally use either a 95% or a 99% confidence interval.

Calculating confidence limits involves the use of the SEM. As shown in Figure 20-1, 95% of the scores in a normal distribution lie within about 2 SDs (more precisely, 1.96 SDs) from the mean. In our example, suppose the point estimate for mean SAT scores is 510, and the SD is 100. The SEM for a sample of 25 would be 20. We can build a 95% confidence interval with the following formula:

$$\text{Conf. } (\overline{X} \pm 1.96 \, s_{\bar{x}}) = 95\%$$

That is, the confidence is 95% that the population mean lies between the values equal to 1.96 times the standard error, above and below the sample mean. In the example at hand, we would obtain the following:

$$\text{Conf. } (510 \pm (1.96 \times 20.0)) = 95\%$$

$$\text{Conf. } (510 \pm (39.2)) = 95\%$$

$$\text{Conf. } (470.0 \leq \mu \leq 549.2) = 95\%$$

The final statement may be read as follows: the confidence is 95% that the population mean (symbolized by the Greek letter mu [μ] by convention) is between 470.8 and 549.2.

Confidence intervals reflect the degree of risk researchers are willing to take of being wrong. With a 95% confidence interval, researchers accept the probability that they will be wrong five times out of 100. A 99% confidence interval sets the risk at only 1% by allowing a wider range of possible values. The formula is as follows:

$$\text{Conf. } (\overline{X} \pm 2.58 \ s_{\overline{x}}) = 99\%$$

The 2.58 reflects the fact that 99% of all cases in a normal distribution lie within ± 2.58 SD units from the mean. In the example, the 99% confidence interval would be:

$$\text{Conf. } (510 \pm (2.58 \times 20.0)) = 99\%$$

$$\text{Conf. } (510 \pm (51.6)) = 99\%$$

$$\text{Conf. } (458.4 \leq \mu \leq 561.6) = 99\%$$

In samples with 25 subjects, 99 out of 100 confidence intervals so constructed would contain the population mean. One accepts a reduced risk of being wrong at the price of reduced specificity. With a 95% interval, the range between confidence limits was only about 80 points; here, the range is more than 100 points. The acceptable risk of error depends on the nature of the problem. In research that could affect human health, a stringent 99% confidence interval might be used; for most studies, a 95% confidence interval is sufficient.

Example of confidence intervals:
Pieper and Templin (2001) studied the prevalence of chronic venous insufficiency in people with a history of injection drug use. They reported the percentages of cases in seven disease severity classes, with a 95% confidence interval around each.

HYPOTHESIS TESTING

Statistical hypothesis testing provides objective criteria for deciding whether hypotheses are supported by empirical evidence. Suppose we hypothesized that participation of cancer patients in a stress management program would lower anxiety levels. The sample is 25 patients in a control group who do not participate in the program and 25 experimental subjects who do. All 50 subjects complete a post-treatment scale of anxiety, and the mean anxiety score for experimentals is 15.8 and that for controls is 17.9. Should we conclude that the hypothesis was correct? True, group differences are in the predicted direction, but the results might simply be due to sampling fluctuations. The two groups might *happen* to be different by chance, regardless of the intervention. Perhaps with a new sample the group means would be nearly identical. Statistical hypothesis testing allows researchers to make objective decisions about study results. Researchers need such a mechanism for deciding which results likely reflect chance sample differences and which reflect true population differences.

The Null Hypothesis

The procedures used in testing hypotheses are based on rules of negative inference. In the stress management program example, we found that those participating in the intervention had lower mean anxiety scores than subjects in the control group. There are two possible explanations for this result: (1) the intervention was successful in reducing patients' anxiety; or (2) the differences resulted from chance factors, such as group differences in anxiety even before the treatment. The first explanation is our research hypothesis, and the second is the null hypothesis. The **null hypothesis**, it may be recalled, states that there is no relationship between variables. Statistical hypothesis testing is basically a process of disproof or rejection. It cannot be demonstrated directly that the research hypothesis is correct, but it is possible to show, using theoretical sampling distributions, that the null hypothesis has a high probability of being incorrect. Researchers seek to reject the null hypothesis through various **statistical tests**.

The null hypothesis in our example can be stated formally as follows:

$$H_0: \mu_E = \mu_C$$

The null hypothesis (H_0) claims that the mean population anxiety score for experimental subjects (μ_E) is the same as that for controls (μ_C). The **alternative**, or research, **hypothesis** (H_A) claims the means are *not* the same:

$$H_A: \mu_E \neq \mu_C$$

Although null hypotheses are accepted or rejected based on sample data, the hypothesis is about population values. Hypothesis testing uses samples to draw conclusions about relationships within the population.

Type I and Type II Errors

Researchers decide whether to accept or reject a null hypothesis by determining how probable it is that observed group differences are due to chance. Because researchers lack information about the population, they cannot flatly assert that a null hypothesis is or is not true. Researchers must be content to conclude that hypotheses are either *probably* true or *probably* false. Statistical inferences are based on incomplete information, so there is always a risk of error.

Researchers can make two types of error: rejecting a true null hypothesis or accepting a false null hypothesis. Figure 20-2 summarizes possible outcomes of researchers' decisions. Researchers make a **Type I error** by rejecting the null hypothesis when it is, in fact, true. For instance, if we concluded that the experimental treatment was more effective than the control condition in alleviating patients' anxiety, when in fact observed differences in anxiety scores resulted from sampling fluctuations, we would be making a Type I error. Conversely, if we concluded that group differences in anxiety scores resulted by chance, when in fact the intervention *did* reduce anxiety, we would be committing a **Type II error** by accepting a false null hypothesis.

Level of Significance

Researchers do not know when an error in statistical decision making has been made. The validity of a null hypothesis could be ascertained only by collecting data from the population, in which case there would be no need for statistical inference. Researchers do, however, control the *risk* of a Type I error by selecting a **level of significance**, which signifies the probability of rejecting a true null hypothesis.

The two most frequently used significance levels (referred to as **alpha** or α) are .05 and .01.

The actual situation is that the null hypothesis is:

		True	False
The researcher calculates a test statistic and decides that the null hypothesis is:	**True** (Null accepted)	Correct decision	Type II error
	False (Null rejected)	Type I error	Correct decision

FIGURE 20.2 Outcomes of statistical decision making.

With a .05 significance level, we are accepting the risk that out of 100 samples drawn from a population, a true null hypothesis would be rejected only 5 times. With a .01 significance level, the risk of a Type I error is *lower*: in only 1 sample out of 100 would we erroneously reject the null hypothesis. The minimum acceptable level for α usually is .05. A stricter level (e.g., .01 or .001) may be needed when the decision has important consequences.

Naturally, researchers want to reduce the risk of committing both types of error, but unfortunately lowering the risk of a Type I error increases the risk of a Type II error. The stricter the criterion for rejecting a null hypothesis, the greater the probability of accepting a false null hypothesis. Researchers must deal with tradeoffs in establishing criteria for statistical decision making, but the simplest way of reducing the risk of a Type II error is to increase sample size. Procedures for addressing Type II errors are discussed later in this chapter.

Example of significance levels:
Stark (2001) studied the relationship between the psychosocial tasks of pregnancy (e.g., preparation for labor) and pregnant women's capacity to focus attention. Stark stated the following with regard to significance levels: "For all tests an alpha of .05 was designated a priori for significance. Because this is a new area of study, tests with an alpha of <.10 were examined for trends" (p. 197).

Critical Regions

Researchers establish a decision rule by selecting a significance level. The decision rule is to reject the null hypothesis if the test statistic falls at or beyond a **critical region** on the applicable theoretical distribution, and to accept the null hypothesis otherwise. The critical region, defined by the significance level, indicates whether the null hypothesis is *improbable*, given the results.

A simple example illustrates the statistical decision-making process. Suppose we measured attitudes toward in vitro fertilization (IVF) among infertile couples. We ask a sample of 100 patients with infertility to express their attitude toward IVF on a scale ranging from 0 (extremely negative) to 10 (extremely positive). We want to determine whether the mean rating for the population of patients with infertility is different from 5.0, the score that represents a neutral attitude. The null hypothesis is H_0: $\mu = 5.0$, and the alternate hypothesis is H_A: $\mu \neq 5.0$.

Now suppose that data from the 100 patients result in a mean rating of 5.5 with an SD of 2.0. This mean is consistent with the alternative hypothesis that patients are not neutral, but can we reject the null hypothesis? Because of sampling fluctuation, there is a possibility that the mean of 5.5 occurred simply by chance and not because the population in general is somewhat favorable toward IVF.

In hypothesis testing, researchers *assume* the null hypothesis is true and then gather evidence to disprove it. In this example, we would assume the population mean is 5.0 and then estimate the standard deviation of the sampling distribution (i.e., the SEM) by dividing the actual standard deviation (2.0) by the square root of the sample size (100). In this example, the SEM is 0.2 ($s_{\bar{x}} = 2.0 \div \sqrt{100}$).

The resulting sampling distribution is shown in Figure 20-3. Based on knowledge of normal distributions, we can determine probable and improbable values of sample means drawn from the infertility patient population. If, as assumed, the population mean is 5.0, then 95% of all sample means would fall roughly between 4.6 and 5.4—that is, about 2 SDs above and below the mean. Only 5% of sample means would be less than 4.6 or greater than 5.4 if the null hypothesis of population neutrality were true. The obtained sample mean of 5.5 is improbable using a significance level of .05 as our criterion of improbability. We can reject the null hypothesis that the population mean equals 5.0. We cannot say we have *proved* the alternative hypothesis: There is a 5% possibility that we made a Type I error. But we can *accept* the alternative hypothesis that patients with infertility are not, on average, neutral about IVF.

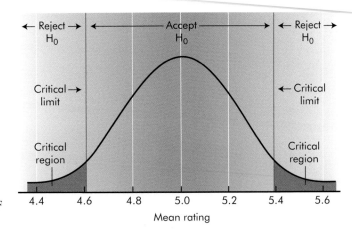

FIGURE 20.3 Critical regions in the sampling distribution for a two-tailed test, IVF attitudes example.

Statistical Tests

In practice, researchers do not construct sampling distributions and calculate critical regions. Research data are used to compute **test statistics**, using appropriate formulas. For every test statistic, there is a related theoretical distribution. Researchers compare the value of the computed test statistic to values in a table that specify **critical limits** for the applicable distribution.

When researchers calculate a test statistic that is beyond the critical limit, the results are said to be **statistically significant**. The word *significant* should not be read as *important* or *clinically relevant*. In statistics, *significant* means that obtained results are not likely to have been the result of chance, at a specified level of probability. A **nonsignificant result** means that any observed difference or relationship could have resulted from chance fluctuations.

> **TIP:** When a statistical test indicates that the null hypothesis should be retained (i.e., when the results are nonsignificant), this is sometimes referred to as a **negative result**. Negative results are often disappointing to researchers and sometimes leads to rejection of a manuscript by a journal editor. Research reports with negative results are not rejected because editors are prejudiced against certain types of outcomes; they are rejected because negative results are usually inconclusive

and difficult to interpret. A nonsignificant result indicates that the result *could* have occurred as a result of chance, but offers no evidence that the research hypothesis is *not* correct.

One-Tailed and Two-Tailed Tests

In most hypothesis-testing situations, researchers use **two-tailed tests**. This means that both ends, or tails, of the sampling distribution are used to determine improbable values. In Figure 20-3, for example, the critical region that contains 5% of the sampling distribution's area involves $2\frac{1}{2}\%$ at one end of the distribution and $2\frac{1}{2}\%$ at the other. If the level of significance were .01, the critical regions would involve $\frac{1}{2}\%$ of the distribution in each tail.

When researchers have a strong basis for a directional hypothesis (see Chapter 4), they sometimes use a **one-tailed test**. For example, if we instituted an outreach program to improve the prenatal practices of low-income rural women, we would expect that birth outcomes for the two groups would not just be *different*; we would expect experimental subjects to have an *advantage*. It might make little sense to use the tail of the distribution signifying *worse* outcomes among experimental group mothers.

In one-tailed tests, the critical region of improbable values is entirely in one tail of the distribution—the tail corresponding to the direction of the hypothesis,

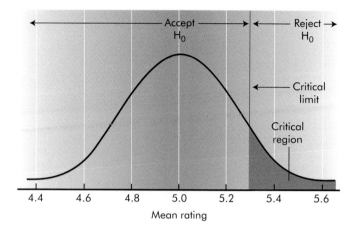

FIGURE 20.4 Critical region in the sampling distribution for a one-tailed test, IVF attitudes example.

as illustrated in Figure 20-4. The alternative hypothesis being tested is not just that the population mean is different from 5.0; it is testing the hypothesis that the population mean is greater than 5.0, that is, that patients with infertility are somewhat positive toward IVF, on average. When a one-tailed test is used, the critical 5% area of "improbability" covers a bigger region of the specified tail, and so one-tailed tests are less conservative. This means it is easier to reject the null hypothesis with a one-tailed test than with a two-tailed test. In our example, any sample mean of 5.3 or greater would result in the rejection of the null hypothesis at the .05 level for a one-tailed test, rather than 5.4 for a two-tailed test.

The use of one-tailed tests is somewhat controversial. Most researchers use a two-tailed test even if they have a directional hypothesis. In reading research reports, one can assume two-tailed tests were used unless one-tailed tests are specifically mentioned. However, when there is a strong logical or theoretical reason for a directional hypothesis and for assuming that findings in the opposite direction are virtually impossible, a one-tailed test may be warranted. In the remainder of this chapter, the examples are for two-tailed tests.

Parametric and Nonparametric Tests

There are two broad classes of statistical tests. Researchers more often use **parametric tests**, which are characterized by three attributes: (1) they involve the estimation of a parameter; (2) they require measurements on at least an interval scale; and (3) they involve several assumptions, such as the assumption that the variables are normally distributed in the population.

Nonparametric tests, by contrast, do not estimate parameters. They are usually applied when data have been measured on a nominal or ordinal scale. Nonparametric methods involve less restrictive assumptions about the shape of the variables' distribution than do parametric tests. For this reason, nonparametric tests are sometimes called **distribution-free statistics**.

Parametric tests are more powerful than nonparametric tests and are usually preferred, but there is some disagreement about the use of nonparametric tests. Purists insist that if the requirements of parametric tests are not met, these tests are inappropriate. Many statistical studies have shown, however, that statistical decision making is not affected when the assumptions for parametric tests are violated. The more moderate position in this debate, and one that we think is reasonable, is that nonparametric tests are most useful when data cannot in any manner be construed as interval-level or when the distribution is markedly non-normal.

Between-Subjects Tests and Within-Subjects Tests

Another distinction in statistical tests concerns the nature of the comparisons. When comparisons involve different people (e.g., men versus women), the study uses a between-subjects design, and the statistical test is a **between-subjects test** (or **test for independent groups**).

Other research designs involve one group of subjects (e.g., with a repeated-measures design, subjects are exposed to two or more treatments). In this situation, comparisons across treatments are not independent because the same subjects are used in all conditions. The appropriate statistical tests for such designs are **within-subjects tests** (or **tests for dependent groups**).

Overview of Hypothesis-Testing Procedures

This chapter presents several statistical tests. The discussion emphasizes applications rather than computations. One computational example is worked out to show that test values are not just pulled out of a hat, but computers have virtually eliminated manual calculations. Those of you who will be doing statistical analyses are urged to consult other references for a fuller explanation of statistical methods. In this research methods textbook, our main interest is to provide an overview of the use and interpretation of some common statistical tests.

Each statistical test described in this chapter has a particular application, but the overall process of testing hypotheses is basically the same. The steps are as follows:

1. *Select a test statistic.* Table 20-10, presented later in this chapter, offers assistance in selecting appropriate tests. Researchers consider such factors as whether a parametric test is justified, which levels of measurement were used, whether a between-groups test is needed, and how many groups are being compared.
2. *Establish the level of significance.* Researchers establish the criterion for accepting or rejecting the null hypothesis before analyses are undertaken. An α level of .05 is usually acceptable.
3. *Select a one-tailed or two-tailed test.* In most cases, a two-tailed test should be used, but in some cases a one-tailed test may be warranted.

4. *Compute a test statistic.* Using collected data, researchers calculate a test statistic using appropriate computational formulas, or instruct a computer to calculate the statistic.
5. *Calculate the degrees of freedom* (symbolized as *df*). **Degrees of freedom** is a concept that refers to the number of observations free to vary about a parameter. The concept is too complex for full elaboration here, but fortunately *df* is easy to compute.
6. *Obtain a tabled value for the statistical test.* There are theoretical distributions for all test statistics. These distributions enable researchers to determine whether obtained values of the test statistic are beyond the range of what is probable if the null hypothesis were true. Researchers examine a table for the appropriate test statistic and obtain the critical value corresponding to the degrees of freedom and significance level.
7. *Compare the test statistic with the tabled value.* In the final step, researchers compare the value in the table with the value of the computed test statistic. If the absolute value of the test statistic is *larger* than the tabled value, the results are statistically significant. If the computed value is *smaller,* the results are nonsignificant.

When a computer is used to analyze data, researchers follow only the first two steps, and then give commands to the computer. The computer calculates the test statistic, the degrees of freedom, and the *actual* probability that the null hypothesis is true. For example, the computer may show that the probability (*p*) of an experimental group doing better than a control group on a measure of anxiety by chance alone is .025. This means that only 25 times out of 1000 would a difference between the two groups as large as the one obtained reflect haphazard differences rather than true differences resulting from an intervention. The computed probability level can then be compared with the desired level of significance. If the significance level desired were .05, then the results would be significant, because .025 is more stringent than .05. If .01

were the significance level, then the results would be nonsignificant (sometimes abbreviated *NS*). By convention, any computed probability greater than .05 (e.g., .20) indicates a nonsignificant relationship—that is, one that could have occurred by chance in more than 5 out of 100 samples.

In the sections that follow, several specific statistical tests and their applications are described. Examples of hypothesis testing using the computer are provided at the end of the chapter.

TESTING DIFFERENCES BETWEEN TWO GROUP MEANS

A common research situation involves comparing two groups of subjects on a dependent variable. For instance, we might compare an experimental and control group of patients on a physiologic measure such as blood pressure. Or, we might contrast the average number of school days missed among children who had been born preterm versus full-term. This section describes methods for testing the statistical significance of differences between two group means.

The parametric procedure for testing differences in group means is the **t-test** (sometimes referred to as **Student's** t). The t-test can be used when there are two independent groups (e.g., experimental versus control, male versus female), and when the sample is paired or dependent (e.g., when pretreatment and post-treatment scores are compared for a single group).

t-Tests for Independent Groups

Suppose we wanted to test the effect of early discharge of maternity patients on perceived maternal competence. We administer a scale of perceived maternal competence at discharge to 10 primiparas who remained in the hospital 48 to 72 hours (group A, regular discharge) and to 10 primiparas discharged less than 48 hours after delivery (group B, early discharge). The mean scale scores for these two groups are 25.0 and 19.0, respectively. Are these differences *real* (i.e., would they be found in the population of early-discharge and later-

discharge mothers?), or are group differences the result of chance fluctuations? The hypotheses are

$$H_0: \mu_A = \mu_B \qquad H_A: \mu_A \neq \mu_B$$

To test these hypotheses, a t-statistic is computed. With independent samples such as in the current example, the formula is

$$t = \frac{\overline{X}_A - \overline{X}_B}{\sqrt{\dfrac{\Sigma_{x_A^2} + \Sigma_{x_B^2}}{n_A + n_B - 2}\left(\dfrac{1}{n_A} + \dfrac{1}{n_B}\right)}}$$

This formula looks complex, but it boils down to components that can be calculated with simple arithmetic. Let us work through an example with data shown in Table 20-1.

The first column presents the scores of the regular-discharge group, whose mean score of 25.0 is shown at the bottom of column 1. In column 4, scores are shown for the early-discharge group, whose mean is 19.0. The 20 scores vary from one person to another. Some variability reflects individual differences in perceived maternal competence, some may be due to measurement error (i.e., low reliability of the scale), some may be the result of subjects' moods on that particular day, and so forth. The research question is: Can a significant part of the six-point mean group difference be attributed to the independent variable, time of hospital discharge? Calculating a t-statistic allows us to answer this question objectively.

After calculating the group means, deviation scores then are computed for each subject, as shown in columns 2 and 5: 25.0 is subtracted from each score in group A, and 19.0 is subtracted from each score in group B. Then, deviation scores are squared (columns 3 and 6), and the squared deviation scores are added. We now have all the components for the t-test formula, as follows:

$$\overline{X}_A = 25.0 \text{ mean of group A}$$
$$\overline{X}_B = 19.0 \text{ mean of group B}$$
$$\Sigma_{x_A^2} = 242 \text{ sum of group A squared}$$
$$\text{deviation scores}$$
$$\Sigma_{x_B^2} = 154 \text{ sum of group B squared}$$
$$\text{deviation scores}$$

TABLE 20.1 Computation of the t-Statistic for Independent Samples

GROUP A (REGULAR-DISCHARGE GROUP)			GROUP B (EARLY-DISCHARGE GROUP)			
(1)	(2)	(3)	(4)	(5)	(6)	
X_A	x_A	x_A^2	X_B	x_B	x_B^2	
30	5	25	23	4	16	
27	2	4	17	-2	4	$t = \dfrac{25 - 19}{\sqrt{\dfrac{242 + 154}{(10 + 10 - 20)}\left(\dfrac{1}{10} + \dfrac{1}{10}\right)}} =$
25	0	0	22	3	9	
20	-5	25	18	-1	1	
24	-1	1	20	1	1	
32	7	49	26	7	49	$t = \dfrac{6}{\sqrt{(22)(.2)}} =$
17	-8	64	16	-3	9	
18	-7	49	13	-6	36	
28	3	9	21	2	4	$t = \dfrac{6}{\sqrt{4.4}} =$
29	4	16	14	-5	25	
$\Sigma X_A = 250$		$\Sigma x_A^2 = 242$	$\Sigma X_B = 190$		$\Sigma x_B^2 = 154$	
$\bar{X}_A = 25.0$			$\bar{X}_B = 19.0$			$t = \dfrac{6}{2.1} = 2.86$

$n_A =$ 10 number of subjects in group A
$n_B =$ 10 number of subjects in group B

When these numbers are used in the t-equation, the value of the t-statistic is computed to be 2.86. To determine whether this t-value is statistically significant, we consult a table for the t-statistic. To use such a table, we need two pieces of information: (1) the α level sought, that is, the risk of a Type I error we are willing to accept; and (2) degrees of freedom. For a t-test with independent samples, the formula for degrees of freedom is

$$df = n_A + n_B - 2$$

That is, df equals the number of subjects in the two groups, minus 2. In the current example, df equals 18 [(10 + 10) − 2].

A table of t-values is presented in Table A-1, Appendix A. The left column lists various degrees of freedom, and the top row specifies different α values. Using a two-tailed probability (p) level of .05, we find that with 18 df, the tabled value of t is 2.10. This value is the upper limit to what is probable, if the null hypothesis were true; values greater than 2.10 are considered improbable. Thus, our calculated t of 2.86* is improbable, that is, statistically significant. We can now say that primiparas discharged early had significantly lower perceptions of maternal competence than those who were not discharged early. The probability that the mean difference of 6 points was the result of chance factors rather than early discharge is less than 5 in 100 ($p < .05$). The null hypothesis is rejected and the alternative hypothesis is accepted.

---

*The tabled t-value should be compared with the absolute value of the calculated t. Thus, if the calculated t-value had been −2.86, then the results would still be significant.

Example of independent *t*-tests:
Schultz, Drew, and Hewitt (2002) used a double-blind experiment to compare normal saline and heparinized saline for patency of intravenous locks in patients in the neonatal intensive care unit. The mean duration of patency for angiocatheters flushed with heparinized solution was 38.5 hours (SD = 33.3), compared with 34.4 hours (SD = 27.3) for those flushed with normal saline. With $t = .457$ and $df = 45$, the group difference was not significant ($p = .65$).

Paired *t*-Tests

Researchers sometimes obtain two measures from the same subjects, or measures from paired sets of subjects (e.g., two siblings). Whenever two sets of scores are not independent, researchers must use a **paired *t*-test**—a *t*-test for dependent groups.

Suppose we were studying the effect of a special diet on the cholesterol level of elderly men. A sample of 50 men is randomly selected, and their cholesterol levels are measured before the intervention and again after 2 months on the special diet. The hypotheses being tested are

$$H_0: \mu_x = \mu_y \qquad H_A: \mu_x \neq \mu_y$$

where X = pretreatment cholesterol levels
Y = postreatment cholesterol levels

A *t*-statistic then would be computed from pretest and posttest data (using a different formula).* The obtained *t* would be compared with the *t*-values in Table A-1, Appendix A. For this type

---

*The paired *t*-statistic is computed according to the following formula:

$$t = \frac{\overline{D}_{x-y}}{\sqrt{\dfrac{\Sigma d^2}{N(N-1)}}}$$

where D_{x-y} = the difference between two paired scores
$\overline{D}_{x-\bar{y}}$ = the mean difference between the paired scores
d = the deviation scores for the difference measure
Σd^2 = the sum of the squared deviation scores
N = number of pairs

of *t*-test, degrees of freedom equals the number of paired observations minus one ($df = N - 1$).

Example of paired *t*-tests:
Damato (2000) studied whether maternal attachment to twin fetuses differed between twins. A sample of 214 pregnant women completed a maternal—fetal attachment scale for twin A (typically, the presenting fetus) and twin B (the nonpresenting fetus). A paired *t*-test was used to compare mean scores for the twins. Women reported significantly greater attachment to twin B than to twin A; with a *t* of -3.08 and $df = 201$, the difference was significant beyond the .01 level ($p = .002$).

Other Two-Group Tests

In certain two-group situations, *t*-tests may not be appropriate. If the dependent variable is on an ordinal scale, or if the distribution is markedly nonnormal, then a nonparametric test may be needed. We mention a few such tests here without actually working out examples.

The **median test** involves comparing two independent groups based on deviations from the median rather than the mean. In the median test, scores for both groups are combined and an overall median is calculated. Then, the number of cases above and below this median is counted separately for each group, resulting in a 2×2 contingency table; (above/below median) $\times$ (group A/group B). From such a contingency table, a chi-square statistic (described in a subsequent section) can be computed to test the null hypothesis that the medians are the same for the two populations.

The **Mann-Whitney *U* test** is another nonparametric procedure for testing the difference between two independent groups when the dependent variable is measured on an ordinal scale. The test involves assigning ranks to the two groups of measures. The sum of the ranks for the two groups can be compared by calculating the *U* statistic. The Mann-Whitney *U* test throws away less information than a median test and so is more powerful.

When ordinal-level data are paired (dependent), either the sign test or the Wilcoxon signed-rank test can be used. The **sign test** is a simple procedure involving the assignment of a "+" or "−" to the differences between a pair of scores, depending on whether X is larger than Y, or vice versa. The **Wilcoxon signed-rank test** involves taking the difference between paired scores and ranking the absolute difference.

Compared with t-tests, all these nonparametric tests are computationally easy. However, the ease of computation should not be the basis for selecting a statistic, especially if a computer is being used to analyze the data.

Example of the Mann-Whitney U test: Connelly, Gunzerath, and Knebel (2000) compared mood states in mechanically ventilated patients who either did ($n = 8$) or did not ($n = 11$) successfully wean. The difference in mean mood scores for the two groups was tested using the Mann-Whitney U-test, and was not significant ($U = 38.5$, $p > .05$).

TESTING DIFFERENCES BETWEEN THREE OR MORE GROUP MEANS

Analysis of variance (**ANOVA**) is another commonly used parametric procedure for testing differences between means where there are three or more groups. The statistic computed in an ANOVA is the **F-ratio** statistic. ANOVA decomposes total variability in a dependent variable into two parts: (1) variability attributable to the independent variable; and (2) all other variability, such as individual differences, measurement error, and so on. Variation *between* groups is contrasted to variation *within* groups to get an F-ratio. When differences between groups are large relative to fluctuations within groups, the probability is high that the independent variable is related to, or has resulted in, group differences.

One-Way ANOVA

Suppose we were comparing the effectiveness of different interventions to help people stop smoking. One group of smokers receives intensive nurse

counseling (group A); a second group is treated by a nicotine patch (group B); and a third control group receives no special treatment (group C). The dependent variable is cigarette consumption the week after the intervention. Thirty smokers who wish to quit smoking are randomly assigned to one of the three conditions. ANOVA tests the following hypotheses:

$$H_0: \mu_A = \mu_B = \mu_C \qquad H_A: \mu_A \neq \mu_B \neq \mu_C$$

The null hypothesis states that the population means for post-treatment cigarette smoking is the same for all three groups, and the alternative (research) hypothesis predicts inequality of means. Table 20-2 presents fictitious data for each subject, and group means for the three groups. The mean numbers of post-treatment cigarettes consumed are 20, 25, and 33 for groups A, B, and C, respectively. These means are different, but are they significantly different—or do differences reflect random fluctuations?

In calculating an F-statistic, total variability in the data is broken down into two sources. The portion of the variance resulting from group membership (i.e., exposure to different treatments) is determined by calculating the **sum of squares between groups**, or SS_B. The SS_B represents the

TABLE 20.2 Fictitious Data for a One-Way ANOVA

GROUP A	GROUP B	GROUP C
28	22	33
0	31	44
17	26	29
20	30	40
35	34	33
19	37	25
24	0	22
0	19	43
41	24	29
16	27	32
$\Sigma X_A = 200$	$\Sigma X_B = 250$	$\Sigma X_C = 330$
$\bar{X}_A = 20.0$	$\bar{X}_A = 25.0$	$\bar{X}_C = 33.0$

TABLE 20.3 ANOVA Summary Table

SOURCE OF VARIANCE	SS	df	MEAN SQUARE	F	p
Between groups	860.0	2	430.00	3.84	<.05
Within groups	3,022.0	27	111.93		
TOTAL	3,882.0	29			

sum of squared deviations of individual group means from the overall mean for all subjects (often referred to as the **grand mean**). SS_B reflects variability in scores attributable to group membership.

The second component is the **sum of squares within groups**, or SS_W. This index is the sum of the squared deviations of each individual score from its *own* group mean. SS_W indicates variability attributable to individual differences, measurement error, and so on.

Recall from Chapter 19 that the formula for calculating a variance is $\Sigma x^2 \div N$.* The two sums of squares are like the numerator of this variance equation: both SS_B and SS_W are sums of squared deviations from means. So, to compute variance within and variance between groups, we must divide the sums of squares by something similar to N: the degrees of freedom for each sum of squares. For between groups, $df_B = G - 1$ (i.e., number of groups minus 1). For within groups, $df_W = (n_A - 1) + (n_B - 1) + \ldots (n_G - 1)$. That is, degrees of freedom within groups is the sum of the number of subjects less 1, for each group.

In an ANOVA context, the variance is conventionally referred to as the **mean square** (MS). The formulas for the mean square between groups and the mean square within groups are

$$MS_B = \frac{SS_B}{df_B} \qquad MS_W = \frac{SS_W}{df_W}$$

---

*When the population variance is being estimated, the denominator is $N - 1$, rather than just N.

The F-ratio statistic is the ratio of these mean squares, or

$$F = \frac{MS_B}{MS_W}$$

Computations for the data in Table 20-2 are presented in an ANOVA summary table (Table 20-3), which shows that the calculated F-statistic for this example is 3.84. Next, we must compare 3.84 with the value from a theoretical F distribution. Table A-2, Appendix A, contains the upper limits of probable values for distributions with varying degrees of freedom. The first part of the table lists values for a significance level of .05, and the second and third parts list those for .01 and .001 significance levels. Let us say that we have chosen the .05 probability level. To enter the table, we find the column headed by df_B (2), and go down this column until we reach the row corresponding to df_W (27). The tabled value of F with 2 and 27 df is 3.35. Because our obtained F-value of 3.84 exceeds 3.35, we reject the null hypothesis that the population means are equal. Group differences in post-treatment cigarette smoking are beyond chance expectations. In fewer than 5 samples out of 100 would differences this great be obtained by chance alone.

The data support the hypothesis that the interventions affected cigarette smoking, but we cannot tell from these results if treatment A was significantly more effective than treatment B. Statistical analyses known as **multiple comparison procedures** (or **post hoc tests**) are needed. Their function is to isolate the differences between group means that are responsible for rejecting the overall ANOVA null hypothesis. Note that it is *not* appropriate to use a series of *t*-tests (group A versus B, A versus C, and B versus C) because this would increase the risk of a Type I error. Multiple comparison methods are described in most intermediate statistical textbooks, such as that by Polit (1996).

Example of a one-way ANOVA:
Logsdon and Usui (2001) compared levels of postpartum depression in three groups of women: middle-class white mothers of term infants (group 1), middle-class white mothers of preterm infants (group 2), and low-income African-American mothers of term infants (group 3). Mean depression scores for these groups were 14.5, 20.7, and 20.5, respectively, and the differences were significant ($F = 6.81$, $p = .001$). Post hoc tests indicated that white mothers of term infants were significantly less depressed that mothers in groups 2 or 3, but that mothers in groups 2 and 3 were not significantly different from each other.

Multifactor ANOVA

One-way ANOVA, as just described, is used to test the effect of one independent variable (e.g., different interventions) on a dependent variable. Data from studies with multiple independent variables are sometimes analyzed by a **multifactor ANOVA**. In this section, we describe some principles underlying a **two-way ANOVA** without working out computations.

Suppose we wanted to determine whether the two smoking cessation treatments (intensive nurse counseling and a nicotine patch) were equally effective in helping men and women stop smoking, with no control group in the study. We use a randomized block design, with four groups: women and men are randomly assigned, separately, to the two treatment conditions. After the intervention, subjects report the number of cigarettes they smoked. Fictitious data for this example are shown in Table 20-4.

With two independent variables, three hypotheses are tested. First, we are testing the effectiveness, for both men and women, of intensive

nurse counseling versus the nicotine patch. Second, we are testing whether postintervention smoking differs for men and women, regardless of treatment. These are the tests for **main effects**. Third, we are testing for **interaction effects** (i.e., differential treatment effects on men and women). Interaction concerns whether the effect of one independent variable is consistent for all levels of a second independent variable.

The data in Table 20-4 reveal that, overall, subjects in treatment 1 smoked less than those in treatment 2 (19.0 versus 25.0); that women smoked less than men after treatment (21.0 versus 23.0); and that men smoked less when exposed to treatment 1, but women smoked less when exposed to treatment 2. By performing a two-way ANOVA on these data, it would be possible to learn whether these differences were statistically significant.

Multifactor ANOVA is not restricted to two-way analyses. In theory, any number of independent variables is possible, but in practice studies with more than three factors are rare. Other statistical techniques typically are used with three or more independent variables, as we discuss in Chapter 21.

Example of a three-way ANOVA:
Hojat and colleagues (2001) conducted a cross-cultural study of attitudes toward physician–nurse collaboration. An attitude scale was administered to 639 male and female physicians and nurses in the United States and Mexico. A three-way ANOVA was used to test attitude differences by profession, country, and gender. Attitudes were significantly more positive among U.S. than Mexican respondents, and among nurses than physicians. There were no significant main effects for gender. The interaction between country and profession was also significant: U.S. nurses had especially favorable attitudes.

Repeated-Measures ANOVA

Repeated-measures ANOVA (or **within-subjects ANOVA**) is used when there are three or more measures of the same dependent variable for each subject. As discussed in Chapter 8, a repeated-measures

TABLE 20.4 Fictitious Data for a Two-Way (2 × 2) ANOVA

FACTOR B—GENDER	FACTOR A—TREATMENT		
	Nurse Counseling (1)	Nicotine Patch (2)	
Female (1)	24 28 22 19 27 25 $\bar{X}_{A1B1} = 22.0$ 18 21 0 36	27 0 45 19 22 23 $\bar{X}_{A2B1} = 20.0$ 18 20 12 14	Female $\bar{X}_{B1} = 21.0$
Male (2)	10 21 17 0 33 16 $\bar{X}_{A1B2} - 16.0$ 18 13 15 17	36 31 28 32 25 22 $\bar{X}_{A2B2} = 30.0$ 19 30 35 42	Male $\bar{X}_{B2} = 23.0$
	Treatment 1 $\bar{X}_{A1} = 19.0$	Treatment 2 $\bar{X}_{A2} = 25.0$	$\bar{X}_T = 22.0$

experimental design is sometimes used to expose subjects to two or more treatment conditions, with subjects acting as their own controls. When there are only two such conditions—that is, when subjects are exposed to treatment A and treatment B, with order of exposure determined at random—then a paired *t*-test can be used. However, when there are three or more treatment conditions, a repeated-measures ANOVA is required. Repeated-measures ANOVA can also be used when multiple measures of the same dependent variable are collected longitudinally. For instance, in some studies, physiologic measures such as blood pressure or heart rate might be collected before, during, and after a medical procedure.

In some applications of repeated-measures ANOVA, there are multiple measures of the dependent variables for subjects in two or more groups. For example, suppose we collected heart rate data at 2 hours (T1), 4 hours (T2), and 6 hours (T3) postsurgery for subjects in an experimental and control group. Structurally, the ANOVA for analyzing these data would look similar to a multifactor ANOVA, but calculations would differ. An *F*-statistic would be computed to test for a **between-subjects effect** (i.e., differences between experimental and control subjects). This statistic indicates whether, across all time periods, the mean heart rate differed in the two treatment groups. Another *F*-statistic is computed to test for a **within-subjects effect** (i.e., differences at T1, T2, and T3). This statistic indicates whether, across both groups, mean heart rates differed over time. Finally, an interaction effect would be tested to determine whether group differences varied across time. Given the many situations in which nurse researchers collect data from subjects at multiple time points, repeated-measures ANOVA is an important analytic tool.

Example of repeated-measures ANOVA: Cimprich and Ronis (2001) examined ability to direct attention over time among older women who either had or had not undergone surgery for breast cancer. The main effect for time on a measure of attention was not significant ($F = 0.93, p = .34$), and the time by group interaction narrowly missed significance ($F = 3.28, p = .07$). Scores did, however, differ significantly between the breast cancer and healthy groups ($F = 8.23, p < .01$).

Nonparametric "Analysis of Variance"

Nonparametric tests do not, strictly speaking, analyze variance. There are, however, nonparametric analogs to ANOVA for use with ordinal-level data or when a markedly non-normal distribution makes parametric tests inadvisable. The **Kruskal-Wallis test** is a generalized version of the Mann-Whitney U test, based on assigning ranks to the scores of various groups. This test is used when the number of groups is greater than two and a one-way test for independent samples is desired. When multiple measures are obtained from the same subjects, the **Friedman test** for "analysis of variance" by ranks can be used. Both tests are described in Polit (1996).

TESTING DIFFERENCES IN PROPORTIONS

Tests discussed thus far involve dependent variables measured on an interval or ratio scale, when group means are being compared. In this section, we examine tests of group differences when the dependent variable is on a nominal scale.

The Chi-Square Test

The **chi-square** (χ^2) **test** is a nonparametric procedure used to test hypotheses about the proportion of cases that fall into different categories, as when a contingency table has been created. Suppose we were studying the effect of nursing instruction on patients' compliance with a self-medication regimen. Nurses implement a new instructional approach with 100 experimental group patients, while 100 control group patients are cared for by nurses using the usual mode of instruction. The hypothesis is that a higher proportion of experimental subjects than control subjects report self-medication compliance.

The chi-square statistic is computed by comparing observed frequencies (i.e., those observed in the data) and expected frequencies. **Observed frequencies** for our example are shown in Table 20-5. As this table shows, 60 experimental subjects

TABLE 20.5 Observed Frequencies for Chi-Square Example

PATIENT COMPLIANCE	EXPERIMENTAL GROUP	CONTROL GROUP	TOTAL
Compliant	60	40	100
Noncompliant	40	60	100
TOTAL	100	100	200

$\chi^2 = 8.00, df = 1, p < .01$

(60%), but only 40 controls (40%), reported self-medication compliance. The chi-square test enables us to decide whether a difference in proportions of this magnitude is likely to reflect a real experimental effect or only chance fluctuations. **Expected frequencies**, which are the cell frequencies that would be found if there were *no* relationship between the two variables, are calculated on the basis of row totals and column totals. In this example, if there were no relationship between compliance and treatment group, the expected frequency would be 50 subjects per cell because overall exactly half the subjects complied.

The chi-square statistic is computed* by summarizing differences between observed and expected frequencies for each cell. In our example, there are four cells, and thus χ^2 is the sum of four numbers. In this example, $\chi^2 = 8.00$. Then we need to compare the test statistic with the value from a theoretical chi-square distribution. Table A-3 (Appendix A) presents chi-square values for various degrees of freedom and significance levels. For the chi-square statistic, degrees of freedom are equal to the number of rows minus 1 times the number of columns minus 1 [$(R - 1) \times (C - 1)$]. In the current case, $df = 1 \times 1 = 1$. With 1 df, the value that must be exceeded to establish significance at the .05 level is 3.84. The obtained value of 8.00 is substantially larger than would be expected by chance. We can conclude that a significantly larger proportion of experimental patients than control patients were compliant.

Example of chi-square test:
Parker, Bliwise, and Rye (2000) studied the relationship between the timing of hemodialysis (HD) and levels of daytime sleepiness. A sample of 92 patients receiving HD who received treatment either on shift 1 (6 to 10 AM), shift 2 (10 AM to 2 PM), or shift 3 (2 to 6 PM) were categorized as having either average or above-average sleepiness. Patients on shift 2 were significantly less sleepy than those on the other shifts ($\chi^2 = 6.20$, df = 2, $p = .04$).

Other Tests of Proportions

In some situations it is not appropriate to calculate a chi-square statistic. When the total sample size is small (total N of 30 or less) or when there are cells with 0 frequencies, **Fisher's exact test** can be used to test the significance of differences in proportions. When the proportions being compared are from two paired groups (e.g., when a pretest—posttest design is used to compare changes in proportions on a dichotomous variable), the appropriate test is the **McNemar test**.

Example of Fisher's exact test:
Elpern and her colleagues (2000) studied instances of aspiration with a sample of 15 adults with tracheostomies. Using Fisher's exact test, the researchers determined that there were no significant differences between those who aspirated material on presentation of thin liquid and those who did not, in terms of gender and feeding access (gastrostomy tube versus nasogastric tube).

TESTING RELATIONSHIPS BETWEEN TWO VARIABLES

The tests discussed thus far are used to test differences between *groups*; that is, they involve situations in which the independent variable is a nominal-level variable. In this section, we consider statistical tests used when the independent variable is on a higher level of measurement.

Pearson's *r*

In Chapter 19, we explained the interpretation of the Pearson product—moment correlation coefficient. Pearson's *r*, which is calculated when two variables

---

*The formula for the chi-square statistic is

$$\chi^2 = \sum \frac{(f_O - f_E)^2}{f_E}$$

where f_O = observed frequency for a cell
f_E = expected frequency for a cell
$\sum$ = sum of the $(f_O - f_E)^2/f_E$ ratios for all cells

$$f_E = \frac{f_R f_C}{N}$$

where f_R = observed frequency for the given row
f_C = observed frequency for the given column
N = total number or subjects

are measured on at least the interval scale, is both descriptive and inferential. As a descriptive statistic, the correlation coefficient summarizes the magnitude and direction of a relationship between two variables. As an inferential statistic, r is used to test hypotheses about population correlations, which are symbolized by the Greek letter rho, or ρ. A frequently tested null hypothesis is that there is no relationship between two variables. Stated formally,

$$H_0: \rho = 0 \qquad H_A: \rho \neq 0$$

For instance, suppose we were testing the relationship between patients' self-reported level of stress and the pH level of their saliva. With a sample of 50 subjects, we find that $r = -.29$. This value indicates that there was a modest tendency for people with higher stress scores to have lower pH levels than those with lower stress scores. But can we generalize this finding to the population? Does the coefficient of $-.29$ reflect a random fluctuation, observable only for the particular subjects sampled, or is the relationship *real*? Table A-4 (Appendix A) allows us to make the determination. Degrees of freedom for correlation coefficients are equal to the number of subjects minus 2, or $(N - 2)$. With $df = 48$, the critical value for r (for a two-tailed test with $\alpha = .05$) lies between .2732 and .2875, or about .2803. Because the absolute value of the calculated r is .29, the null hypothesis can be rejected. We accept the alternative hypothesis that, in the population, the correlation between stress and saliva acidity is not equal to zero.

Pearson's r can be used in both within-group and between-group situations. The example about the relationship between stress scores and the pH levels is a between-group situation: The question is whether people with high stress scores tend to have significantly lower pH levels than *different* people with low stress scores. If stress scores were obtained both before and after surgery, however, the correlation between the two scores would be a within-group situation.

Example of Pearson's *r*:
Steward and Pridham (2002) examined the growth patterns of extremely low-birth-weight preterm infants. They found a significant negative correlation between the infants' birth weight and number of days of ventilator support ($r = -.44$, $p < .05$) and a positive correlation between birth weight and growth velocity ($r = .60, p < .05$).

Other Tests of Bivariate Relationships

Pearson's r is a parametric statistic. When the assumptions for a parametric test are violated, or when the data are ordinal-level, then the appropriate coefficient of correlation is either **Spearman's rho** (r_S) or **Kendall's tau**. The values of these statistics range from -1.00 to $+1.00$, and their interpretation is similar to that of Pearson's r.

Measures of the magnitude of relationships can also be computed with nominal-level data. For example, the **phi coefficient** (ϕ) is an index describing the relationship between two dichotomous variables. **Cramér's *V*** is an index of relationship applied to contingency tables larger than 2×2. Both of these statistics are based on the chi-square statistic and yield values that range between .00 and 1.00, with higher values indicating a stronger association between variables.

Example of Spearman's rho:
Parshall, Welsh, Brockopp, Heiser, Schooler, and Cassidy (2001) studied dyspnea distress (measured on an ordinal scale, from 0 to 4) among patients with heart failure who presented to the emergency department (ED). The correlation between distress at decision (coming into the ED) and remembered distress the week before was $r_S = .31$, $p < .03$, a modest but significant correlation.

POWER ANALYSIS

Many published nursing studies (and even more *un*published ones) result in nonsignificant findings. Although statistical textbooks pay considerable attention to the problem of Type I errors, less attention has been paid to Type II errors

As indicated earlier in this chapter, the probability of committing a Type I error (wrongly rejecting a *true* null hypothesis) is established by researchers as the level of significance, or alpha (α). The probability of a Type II error (wrongly accepting a *false* null hypothesis) is **beta** (β). The complement of beta ($1 - \beta$) is the *probability of obtaining a significant result* and is referred to as the **power** of a statistical test. Polit and Sherman (1990) found that many published nursing studies have insufficient power, placing them at risk for Type II errors.

Power analysis is a method of reducing the risk of Type II errors and for estimating their occurrence. There are four components in a power analysis, three of which must be known or estimated; power analysis solves for the fourth. The four components are as follows:

1. *The significance criterion*, α. Other things being equal, the more stringent this criterion, the lower the power.
2. *The sample size, N*. As sample size increases, power increases.
3. *The population effect size, gamma* (γ). Gamma is a measure of how wrong the null hypothesis is, that is, how strong the effect of the independent variable is on the dependent variable in the population.
4. *Power, or $1 - \beta$*. This is the probability of rejecting the null hypothesis.

Researchers typically use power analysis before a study is undertaken, to estimate the sample size needed to obtain significant results. (Power analysis can also be used to determine the power of a statistical test after it has been applied, in which case the N is known.) To estimate needed sample size, researchers must specify α, γ, and $1 - \beta$. Researchers usually establish the risk of a Type I error (α) as .05. Just as .05 is used as the standard for α, the conventional standard for $1 - \beta$ is .80. With power equal to .80, there is a 20% risk of committing a Type II error. Although this risk may seem high, a stricter criterion requires sample sizes much larger than most researchers could afford; power is usually well below .80.

With α and $1 - \beta$ specified, the information needed to solve for N is γ, the population effect size. The **effect size** is the magnitude of the relationship between the research variables. When relationships (effects) are strong, they can be detected at statistically significant levels even with small research samples. When relationships are modest, large sample sizes are needed to avoid Type II errors.

Population effect size is never *known*; if it were known, there would be no need for a new study. Effect size must be estimated using available evidence. Sometimes evidence comes from a pilot study, an excellent approach when the main study is costly. More often, an effect size is calculated (through procedures that follow) based on findings from earlier studies on a similar problem.* When there are *no* relevant earlier findings, researchers use conventions based on expectations of a *small, medium,* or *large* effect. Most nursing studies have modest effects.

Procedures for estimating effects and sample size needs vary from one statistical situation to another. We discuss a few here; Cohen (1988) and Jaccard and Becker (2001) discuss power analysis in the context of many other situations.†

Sample Size Estimates for Test of Difference Between Two Means

Suppose we were testing the hypothesis that cranberry juice reduces the urinary pH of diet-controlled patients. We plan to assign some subjects randomly to a control condition (no cranberry juice) and others to an experimental condition in which they will be given 200 mL of cranberry juice with each meal for 5 days. How large a sample is needed for this study, given an α of .05 and power equal to .80?

---

*Researchers can usually find more than one study from which the effect size can be estimated. In such a case, the estimate should be based on the study with the most reliable results or whose design most closely approximates that of the new study. Researchers can also estimate effect size by combining information from multiple high-quality studies through averaging or weighted averaging.

†Computer software for performing power analyses is available for personal computers (Borenstein & Cohen, 1988).

To answer this, we must first estimate γ. In a two-group situation in which the difference of means is of interest, the formula for the effect size is

$$\gamma = \frac{\mu_1 - \mu_2}{\sigma}$$

That is, γ is the difference between the two population means, divided by the population standard deviation. These values are not known in advance, but must be estimated based on available information. For example, suppose we found an earlier non-experimental study that compared the urinary pH of subjects who had or had not ingested cranberry juice in the previous 24 hours. The earlier and current studies are different. In the nonexperimental study,

the diets are uncontrolled, there likely are selection biases in who drinks or does not drink cranberry juice, the length of ingestion is only 1 day, and so on. This study is, however, a reasonable starting point. Suppose the results were as follows:

$\overline{X}_1$ (no cranberry juice) = 5.70
$\overline{X}_2$ (cranberry juice) = 5.50
SD = .50

Thus, the estimated value of γ would be .40:

$$\gamma = \frac{5.70 - 5.50}{.50} = .40$$

Table 20-6 presents approximate sample size requirements for various effect sizes and powers,

TABLE 20.6 Approximate Sample Sizes* Necessary To Achieve Selected Levels of Power as a Function of Estimated Effect Size for Test of Difference of Two Means

	ESTIMATED EFFECT†									
POWER	**.10**	**.15**	**.20**	**.25**	**.30**	**.40**	**.50**	**.60**	**.70**	**.80**
PART A: $\alpha = .05$										
.60	977	434	244	156	109	61	39	27	20	15
.70	1230	547	308	197	137	77	49	34	25	19
.80	1568	697	392	251	174	98	63	44	32	25
.90	2100	933	525	336	233	131	84	58	43	33
.95	2592	1152	648	415	288	162	104	72	53	41
.99	3680	1636	920	589	409	230	147	102	75	58
PART B: $\alpha = .01$										
.60	1602	712	400	256	178	100	64	44	33	25
.70	1922	854	481	308	214	120	77	53	39	30
.80	2339	1040	585	374	260	146	94	65	48	37
.90	2957	1324	745	477	331	186	119	83	61	47
.95	3562	1583	890	570	396	223	142	99	73	56
.99	4802	2137	1201	769	534	300	192	133	98	65

*Sample size requirements for *each* group; total sample size would be twice the number shown.
†Estimated effect (γ) is the estimated population mean group difference divided by the estimated population standard deviation, or:

$$\gamma = \frac{\mu_1 - \mu_2}{\sigma}$$

for two values of α (for two-tailed tests), in a two-group mean-difference situation. In part A of the table for $\alpha = .05$, we find that the estimated n (number per group) to detect an effect size of .40 with power equal to .80 is 98 subjects. That is, assuming that the earlier study provided a good estimate of the population effect size, the total number of subjects needed in the new study would be about 200, with half assigned to the control group (no cranberry juice) and the other half assigned to the experimental group. A sample size smaller than 200 would have a greater than 20% chance of resulting in a Type II error. For example, a sample size of 100 (50 per group) would have almost a 50% chance of incorrect nonsignificant results.

If there is *no* prior relevant research, the researcher can, as a last resort, estimate whether the expected effect is small, medium, or large. By a convention developed by Cohen (1988), the value of γ in a two-group test of mean differences is estimated at .20 for small effects, .50 for medium effects, and .80 for large effects. With an α value of .05 and power of .80, the n (number of subjects per group) for studies with expected small, medium, and large effects would be 392, 63, and 25, respectively. Most nursing studies cannot expect effect sizes in excess of .50; those in the range of .20 to .40 are most common. In Polit and Sherman's (1990) analysis of effect sizes for all studies published in *Nursing Research* and *Research in Nursing & Health* in 1989, the average effect size for *t*-test situations was .35. Cohen (1988) noted that in new areas of research inquiry, effect sizes are likely to be small. A medium effect should be estimated only when the effect is so substantial that it can be detected by the naked eye (i.e., without formal research procedures).

Sample Size Estimates for Test of Difference Between Three or More Means

Suppose we were testing the effectiveness of three different modes of stimulation—auditory, visual, and tactile—on preterm infants' sensorimotor development. The dependent variable is a standardized scale of infant development, such as the Bayley Scale.

With an α of .05 and power of .80, how many infants should be randomly assigned to the three groups?

There are alternative approaches to doing a power analysis in an ANOVA context. The simplest approach is to estimate **eta-squared** (η^2), the index indicating the proportion of variance explained in ANOVA. Eta-squared, which equals the sum of squares between (SS_B) divided by the total sum of squares (SS_T), can be used directly as the estimate of effect size.

In our example of infant stimulation, suppose we found an earlier study that tested a similar hypothesis, and the study resulted in an η^2 of .05. Table 20-7 presents approximate sample size requirements for various ANOVA situations. For the sake of economy, this table presents information only for powers ranging from .70 to .95, for an α of .05, and for the most common group sizes (3, 4, and 5). Jaccard and Becker (2001) provide expanded tables for different αs, powers, and group sizes.

With a power of .80, an α of .05, and an estimated η^2 of .05, Table 20-7 tells us that the number of infants needed in each of the three stimulation groups is 62. If the study were undertaken with only 50 infants per group, there would be a 30% chance (power = .70) of finding nonsignificant results, even when the null hypothesis is false.

When eta-squared cannot be estimated, researchers can predict whether effects are likely to be small, medium, or large. For ANOVA situations, the conventional estimates for small, medium, and large effects would be values of η^2 equal to .01, .06, and .14, respectively. This corresponds to sample size requirements of about 319, 53, or 22 subjects *per group* in a three-group study, assuming an α of .05 and power of .80.*

Sample Size Estimates for Bivariate Correlation Tests

Suppose we were studying the relationship between primiparas' acceptance of the motherhood

---

*When analysis of covariance is used in lieu of *t*-tests or ANOVA, sample size requirements are smaller—sometimes appreciably so—because of reduced error variance.

TABLE 20.7 Approximate Sample Sizes* Necessary To Achieve Selected Levels of Power for $\alpha = .05$ as a Function of Estimated Population Values of Eta-Squared

POWER	.01	.03	.05	.07	.10	.15	.20	.25	.30	.35
POPULATION ETA-SQUARED										
GROUPS = 3										
.70	255	84	50	35	24	16	11	9	7	6
.80	319	105	62	44	30	19	14	11	9	7
.90	417	137	81	57	39	25	18	14	11	9
.95	511	168	99	69	47	30	22	16	13	11
GROUPS = 4										
.70	219	72	43	30	21	13	10	8	6	5
.80	272	90	53	37	26	17	12	9	7	6
.90	351	115	68	48	33	21	15	12	9	8
.95	426	140	83	58	40	25	18	14	11	9
GROUPS = 5										
.70	193	64	38	27	18	12	9	7	6	4
.80	238	78	46	33	23	15	10	8	7	5
.90	306	101	59	42	29	18	13	10	8	7
.95	369	121	72	50	34	22	16	12	10	8

*The values are the number of subjects *per group.*

role and their social support. The hypothesis is that women with greater social support are more accepting of the role transition to motherhood. Both variables are measured by scales that yield interval measures. How many women should be included in the study, given an α of .05 and power of .80?

In this example, the relationship between the two variables will be tested using Pearson's *r*. The estimated value of γ in this situation is ρ, that is, the expected population correlation coefficient.

Suppose we found an earlier study that correlated a measure of social support (the number of people subjects felt they could count on) with an observational measure of maternal warmth. The resulting correlation coefficient was .18, which we use as our estimate of ρ and hence of γ. Table 20-8 shows sample size requirements for various powers and effect sizes in situations in which Pearson's *r* is used. With an α of .05 and power of .80, the sample size needed in the study lies between 197 (effect size = .20) and 349 (effect size = .15). Extrapolating for an effect size of .18, we would need a sample of about 250 subjects. With a sample this size, we would wrongly reject the null hypothesis only 5 times out of 100 and wrongly retain the null hypothesis 20 times out of 100. To increase power to .95 (wrongly retaining the null hypothesis only 5 times out of 100), we would need a sample of about 400 women.

TABLE 20.8 Approximate Sample Sizes Necessary To Achieve Selected Levels of Power as a Function of Estimated Population Value of ρ

POWER	POPULATION CORRELATION COEFFICIENT									
	.10	.15	.20	.25	.30	.40	.50	.60	.70	.80
PART A: α = .05										
.60	489	218	123	79	55	32	21	15	11	9
.70	616	274	155	99	69	39	26	18	14	11
.80	785	349	197	126	88	50	32	23	17	13
.90	1050	468	263	169	118	67	43	30	22	17
.95	1297	577	325	208	145	82	53	37	27	21
.99	1841	819	461	296	205	116	75	52	39	30
PART B: α = .01										
.60	802	357	201	129	90	51	33	23	17	14
.70	962	428	241	155	108	61	39	28	21	16
.80	1171	521	293	188	131	74	48	33	25	19
.90	1491	663	373	239	167	94	61	42	31	24
.95	1782	792	446	286	199	112	72	50	37	28
.99	2402	1068	601	385	267	151	97	67	50	39

When prior estimates of effect size are unavailable, the conventional values of small, medium, and large effect sizes in a bivariate correlation situation are .10, .30, and .50, respectively (i.e., samples of 785, 88, and 32 for a power of .80 and a significance level of .05). In Polit and Sherman's (1990) study, the average correlation found in nursing studies was in the vicinity of .20.

Sample Size Estimates for Testing Differences in Proportions

Estimating sample size requirements for testing differences in proportions between groups is complex and so we restrict our discussion to 2×2 contingency tables. Other references, such as Cohen (1988) or Jaccard and Becker (2001), should be consulted for other situations.

Suppose we were comparing breastfeeding rates for two groups of women: those receiving a special intervention (home visits by nurses in which the advantages of breastfeeding are described), and those in a control group not receiving home visits. How many subjects should be randomly assigned to the two groups to minimize the risk of a Type II error?

The effect size for contingency tables is influenced not only by expected differences in proportions (e.g., 60% in one group versus 40% in another, a 20–percentage point difference), but by the absolute values of the proportions. The effect size for 60% versus 40% is *not* the same as that for 30% versus 10%. In general, the effect size is *larger* (and consequently, sample size needs are *smaller*) at the extremes than near the midpoint. A 20–percentage point difference is easier to detect if the percentages are 10% and 30% than if they are near the middle, such as 40% and 60%.

Computing the effect size index involves a complex transformation that we do not explain here. Rather than present sample size estimates based on effect size, Table 20-9 presents approximate sample size requirements for detecting differences in various proportions, assuming an α of .05 and a power of .80. To use this table, we need estimates of the proportions for both groups. Then we would find the proportion for one group in the first column and the proportion for the second group in the top row. The approximate sample size requirement *for each group* is found at the intersection. In our example, if we estimated (based on a pilot study, say) that 20% of the control group mothers and 40% of the experimental group mothers breastfed their infants, the sample

size needed to keep the risk of a Type II error down to 20% is 80 subjects per group.

Because we have not presented information on the computationally complex effect size for contingency tables, we cannot conveniently identify Cohen's convention for small, medium, and large effects. We can, however, give *examples* of differences in proportions (i.e., the proportions in group 1 versus group 2) that conform to the conventions:

Small: .05 versus .10, .20 versus .29, .40 versus .50, .60 versus .70, .80 versus .87
Medium: .05 versus .21, .20 versus .43, .40 versus .65, .60 versus .82, .80 versus .96
Large: .05 versus .34, .20 versus .58, .40 versus .78, .60 versus .92, .80 versus .96

Thus, if the researcher expected a medium effect in which the proportion for group 1 was expected to be about .40, the number of subjects in

TABLE 20.9 Approximate Sample Sizes* Necessary To Achieve a Power of .80 for α = .05 for Estimated Population Difference Between Two Proportions

GROUP II PROPORTIONS	GROUP I PROPORTIONS														
	.10	.15	.20	.25	.30	.35	.40	.45	.50	.55	.60	.70	.80	.90	1.00
.05	421	133	69	44	31	24	19	15	13	11	9	7	5	4	2
.10		689	196	97	59	41	30	23	18	15	12	9	6	5	3
.15			901	247	118	71	48	34	26	21	16	11	8	5	3
.20				1090	292	137	80	53	38	28	22	14	10	6	3
.25					1252	327	151	87	57	40	30	18	12	8	4
.30						1371	356	161	93	60	42	23	14	9	4
.35							1480	374	169	96	61	31	18	10	5
.40								1510	385	172	97	42	22	12	5
.45									1570	393	173	60	28	15	6
.50										1570	389	93	38	18	6
.55											1539	162	53	23	7
.60												356	80	30	8
.70													292	59	12
.80														195	18
.90															38

*The values are the number of subjects *per group*.

each of the two groups would need to be about 70 to 75 to achieve adequate power. As in other situations, researchers are encouraged to avoid using the conventions, if possible, in favor of more precise estimates from prior empirical evidence. If the conventions cannot be avoided, conservative estimates should be used to minimize the risk of finding nonsignificant results.

Example of a power analysis:

Wang and Laffrey (2001) studied well-being in relation to self-care among rural elderly women in Taiwan. They reported that in prior studies "the average correlation coefficient ... between self-care and well-being was .25" (p. 125). To estimate needed N, they used an even more conservative value of $r = .20$; this called for a sample of about 200 for $\alpha = .05$ and power $= .80$. A total of 300 women were invited to participate in the study, and 284 agreed to do so.

THE COMPUTER AND INFERENTIAL STATISTICS

We have stressed the logic and uses of various statistical tests rather than computational formulas.* Because computers are almost always used for hypothesis testing, and because it is important to know how to read a computer printout, we include examples of computer analyses for two statistical tests.

We return to the example described in Chapter 19, which involved an experiment to test the effects of a special prenatal program for young low-income women. The raw data for the 30 subjects in this example were presented in Table 19-8 in Chapter 19. Given these data, let us test some hypotheses.

Hypothesis One: *t*-Test

Our first research hypothesis is that the babies of experimental subjects have higher birth weights than babies of control subjects. The *t*-test for independent samples is used to test the hypothesis of mean group differences. The null and alternative hypotheses are:

H_0: μ experimental $=$ μ control
H_A: μ experimental $\neq$ μ control

Figure 20-5 presents the computer printout for the *t*-test. The top panel presents some descriptive statistics (mean, standard deviation, and standard error of the mean) for the birth weight variable, separately for the two groups. The mean birth weight of the babies in the experimental group is 107.5333 ounces, compared with 101.8667 ounces for those in the control group. The data are consistent with the research hypothesis, that is, the average weight of babies in the experimental group is higher than that of controls. But is the difference attributable to the intervention, or does it reflect random fluctuations?

The second panel of Figure 20-5 presents results of Levene's test for equality of variances. An assumption underlying use of the *t*-test is that the population variances for the two groups are equal. The top panel shows that the standard deviations (and thus the variances) are quite different, with substantially more variability among experimentals than controls. Levene's test tells us that the two variances are, in fact, significantly different (Sig. $= .046$).

The third panel has two rows of information. The top row is for the **pooled variance *t*-test,** which is used when equality of variances can be assumed. Given the significantly different variances in this sample, however, we need to use information in the second row, which uses a **separate variance *t*-test** formula. The value of the *t* statistic is 1.443, and the two-tailed probability (Sig.) for the differences in group means is .163. This means that in about 16 samples out of 100, we could expect a mean difference in weights this large as a result of chance alone. Therefore, because $p > .05$ (a nonsignificant result), we cannot conclude that the special intervention was effective in improving the birth weights of experimental group infants.

---

*Note that this introduction to inferential statistics has necessarily been superficial. We urge readers to undertake further exploration of statistical principles.

Group Statistics

	GROUP	N	Mean	Std. Deviation	Std. Error Mean
Infant birth weight in ounces	Experimental	15	107.5333	13.3784	3.4543
	Control	15	101.8667	7.2394	1.8692

Independent Samples Test

		Levene's Test for Equality of Variances	
		F	Sig.
Infant birth weight in ounces	Equal variances assumed	4.370	.046
	Equal variances not assumed		

		t-test for Equality of Means						
							95% Confidence Interval of the Difference	
		t	df	Sig. (2-tailed)	Mean Difference	Std. Error Difference	Lower	Upper
Infant birth weight in ounces	Equal variances assumed	1.443	28	.160	5.6667	3.9276	−2.3787	13.7120
	Equal variances not assumed	1.443	21.552	.163	5.6667	3.9276	−2.4885	13.8218

FIGURE 20.5 *t*-Test printout.

Early in this chapter we discussed the use of confidence intervals to determine the probable range of values within which the mean of a single population is expected to lie. Confidence intervals can also be developed for the difference between two population means (as well as for other parameters). The last two columns of the bottom panel of Figure 20-5 show the 95% confidence intervals for the population mean difference. We can conclude with 95% confidence that the mean difference in birth weights for the population of young mothers exposed and not exposed to the intervention lies between −2.4885 ounces and +13.8218 ounces. Zero is within this interval, indicating the possibility that there are no group differences in the population. This is consistent with the fact that we could not reject the null hypothesis of equality of means on the basis of the *t*-test.

TIP: Nurse researchers, like researchers in many social/behavioral science disciplines, typically report the results of test statistics rather than confidence intervals. Medical researchers, however, typically include confidence interval

Correlations

		Infant birth weight in ounces	Mother's age
Infant birth weight in ounces	Pearson Correlation	1.000	.594**
	Sig. (2-tailed)	.	.001
	N	30	30
Mother's age	Pearson Correlation	.594**	1.000
	Sig. (2-tailed)	.001	.
	N	30	30

**Correlation is significant at the 0.01 level (2-tailed)

FIGURE 20.6 Correlation matrix printout for the hypothesis test.

information. Rothstein and Tonges (2000) argue that statistical significance testing should be supplemented, if not replaced, by effect size estimation and confidence interval analysis because they offer richer information that is more amenable to accumulating evidence in nursing.

It was noted earlier than power analysis can be used to estimate both sample size needs *and* power. In our example, the effect size estimate is as follows:

$$\gamma = (107.5333 - 101.8667) \div 10.955 = .52$$

The estimated effect size is the experimental mean minus the control mean, divided by the overall (pooled) standard deviation, which is 10.955. The obtained effect size of .52 is moderate, but an examination of Table 20-6 indicates that with a sample size of only 15 per group, our power to detect a true population difference is less (actually *far* less) than .60. This means that we had a very large probability of incorrectly retaining the null hypothesis. We can also see that with an effect size of .52, we would need about 60 subjects in each group to achieve a power of .80.

Hypothesis Two: Pearson Correlation

Our second research hypothesis is as follows: Older mothers have babies of higher birth weight than younger mothers. In this case, both birth weight and age are measured on the ratio scale and the appropriate test statistic is the Pearson product-moment correlation. The hypotheses are

H_0: ρ birth weight—age $= 0$

H_A: ρ birth weight—age $\neq 0$

The printout for the hypothesis test is presented in Figure 20-6. The correlation matrix shows, in row one, the correlation of infant birth weight with infant birth weight and of birth weight with mother's age; and in row two, the correlation of mother's age with infant birth weight and of age with age. In the cell created at the intersection of age and birth weight, we find three numbers. The first is the correlation coefficient ($r = .594$), which indicates a moderately strong positive relationship: the older the mother, the higher the baby's weight tends to be, consistent with the research hypothesis. The second number in the cell shows the probability that the correlation occurred by chance: Sig. (for significance level) $= .001$ for a two-tailed test. In other words, a relationship this strong would be found by chance in fewer than 1 out of 1000 samples of 30 young mothers. Therefore, the research hypothesis is accepted. The final number in the cell is 30, the total sample size (*N*).

We can determine power for this test by referring back to Table 20-8. The effect size is .594, the same as *r*. With this effect size and a sample size of 30, power is about .90 when α is .05. For an effect size this large, we would have needed only 23 subjects in total to achieve a power $= .80$.

GUIDE TO BIVARIATE STATISTICAL TESTS

The selection and use of a statistical test depends on several factors, such as the number of groups and the levels of measurement of the research variables. To aid you in selecting a test statistic (or evaluating statistics used by other researchers), a chart summarizing the major features of several commonly used tests is presented in Table 20-10. This table does not include every test you may need, but it does include the bivariate statistical tests most often used by nurse researchers.

You may also find it helpful to consult the glossary of symbols in the inside back cover of this book to determine the meaning of statistical symbols that might be used in research reports. Note that not all symbols in this glossary are described in this book; therefore, it may be necessary to refer to a statistics textbook, such as that of Polit (1996), for further information.

RESEARCH EXAMPLE

Guided by the Health Belief Model (HBM), Welch (2001) conducted a study to determine whether beliefs differed among patients undergoing hemodialysis at different stages of adherence to fluid limitations. Based on responses to a series of interview questions, 148 patients were categorized into one of three groups: *Precontemplation*, not currently limiting fluids to 1 kg per day, and no plans to do so; *Contemplation*, not yet limiting fluids, but thinking about doing so; and *Action/Maintenance*, limiting fluids, with the intention of continuing.

The three groups were compared in terms of several variables from the HBM. These included perceived benefits of adhering to fluid limitations, perceived barriers to fluid adherence, perceived seriousness of the consequences of fluid nonadherence, perceived susceptibility to those consequences, and self-efficacy (i.e., the belief that one has the capability of executing a given course of action). Five one-way ANOVAs were performed to test the null hypothesis that the three populations of patients had comparable means on these measures.

Most of the means were in a direction consistent with predictions from the HBM. The analyses revealed, however, that differences among the three groups were not statistically significant at the .05 level for three dependent

variables: perceived barriers, perceived seriousness, and self-efficacy. For example, the mean self-efficacy scores were 26.5, 26.0, and 27.3 for the Precontemplation, Contemplation, and Action groups, respectively. The resulting F of 1.53 $(df = 2, 147)$ was not significant. The groups did, however, differ in terms of perceived benefits and perceived susceptibility. For example, mean scores on the perceived benefit scale were 28.8, 30.4, and 31.5, respectively. For this ANOVA, the F was 6.76, which was significant beyond the .01 level. To isolate which group difference contributed to the value of F, post hoc tests were performed. These tests indicated that the Precontemplation and Action groups were significantly different from each other. In other words, patients who were adhering to fluid limitations perceived significantly more benefits than patients in the precontemplation stage.

Welch also presented interesting information about the power of her analyses. For each statistical test, she computed an effect size and observed power, based on her own data. The power was greater than .80 for only one test, the ANOVA for perceived benefits $(1 - \beta = .91)$. Power was especially low in the test for differences in perceived seriousness $(1 - \beta = .11)$.

Welch concluded that some beliefs vary across the stages of adherence and that stage-appropriate interventions may be needed to target specific beliefs about adherence.

SUMMARY POINTS

- **Inferential statistics,** which are based on the **laws of probability,** allow researchers to make inferences about a population based on data from a sample; they offer a framework for deciding whether the **sampling error** that results from sampling fluctuation is too high to provide reliable population estimates.
- The **sampling distribution of the mean** is a theoretical distribution of the means of an infinite number of samples drawn from a population. Because the sampling distribution of means follows a normal curve, it is possible to indicate the probability that a specified sample value will be obtained.
- The **standard error of the mean (SEM)**—the standard deviation of this theoretical distribution — indicates the degree of average error of a sample mean; the smaller the SEM, the more accurate are the estimates of the population mean based on a sample mean.

- Statistical inference consists of two major types of approaches: estimating parameters and testing hypotheses. **Parameter estimation** is used to estimate a single parameter, like a mean.
- **Point estimation** provides a single numeric value. **Interval estimation** provides the upper and lower limits of a range of values—the **confidence interval**—between which the population value is expected to fall, at a specified probability level. Researchers establish the degree of confidence that the population value lies within this range.
- **Hypothesis testing** through statistical procedures enables researchers to make objective decisions about the validity of their hypotheses.

TABLE 20.10 Guide to Widely Used Bivariate Statistical Tests

TEST NAME	TEST STATISTIC	BETWEEN OR WITHIN	PURPOSE	MEASUREMENT LEVEL* IV	DV
Parametric Tests					
t-test for independent groups	*t*	Between	To test the difference between two independent group means	Nominal	Interval, ratio
Paired *t*-test	*t*	Within	To test the difference between two related group means	Nominal	Interval, ratio
Analysis of variance (ANOVA)	F	Between	To test the difference among the means of 3+ independent groups, or of 2+ independent variables	Nominal	Interval, ratio
Repeated-measures ANOVA	F	Within	To test the difference among the means of 3+ related groups or sets of scores	Nominal	Interval, ratio
Pearson's product–moment correlation	*r*	Between, within	To test that a correlation is different from zero (that a relationship exists)	Interval, ratio	Interval, ratio
Nonparametric Tests					
Mann–Whitney *U*-test	*U*	Between	To test the difference in ranks of scores of two independent groups	Nominal	Ordinal
Median test	χ^2	Between	To test the difference between the medians of two independent groups	Nominal	Ordinal

(continued)

TABLE 20.10 Guide to Widely Used Bivariate Statistical Tests (*continued*)

TEST NAME	TEST STATISTIC	BETWEEN OR WITHIN	PURPOSE	MEASUREMENT LEVEL*	
				IV	DV
Nonparametric Tests					
Kruskal–Wallis test	H	Between	To test the difference in ranks of scores of 3+ independent groups	Nominal	Ordinal
Wicoxon signed–rank test	Z	Within	To test the difference in ranks of scores of two related groups	Nominal	Ordinal
Friedman test	χ^2	Within	To test the difference in ranks of scores of 3+ related groups	Nominal	Ordinal
Chi–square test	χ^2	Between	To test the difference in proportions in 2+ independent groups	Nominal	Nominal
McNemar's test	χ^2	Within	To test the difference in proportions for paired samples (2×2)	Nominal	Nominal
Fisher's exact test	—	Between	To test the difference in proportions in a 2×2 contingency table when $N < 30$	Nominal	Nominal
Spearman's rho	ρ	Between, within	To test that a correlation is different from zero (that a relationship exists)	Ordinal	Ordinal
Kendall's tau	τ	Between, within	To test that a correlation is different from zero (that a relationship exists)	Ordinal	Ordinal
Phi coefficient	ϕ	Between	To examine the magnitude of a relationship between two dichotomous variables	Nominal	Nominal
Cramér's V	V	Between	To examine the magnitude of a relationship between variables in a contingency table (not restricted to 2×2)	Nominal	Nominal

*IV, independent variable, DV, dependent variable.

- The **null hypothesis** states that no relationship exists between research variables, and that any observed relationship is due to chance. Rejection of the null hypothesis lends support to the research hypothesis; failure to reject it indicates that observed differences may be due to chance.
- If a null hypothesis is incorrectly rejected, this is a **Type I error**. A **Type II error** occurs when a null hypothesis that should be rejected is accepted.
- Researchers control the risk of making a Type I error by establishing a **level of significance** (or **alpha** level), which specifies the probability that such an error will occur. The .05 level means that in only 5 out of 100 samples would the null hypothesis be rejected when it should have been accepted.
- In testing hypotheses, researchers compute a **test statistic** and then determine whether the statistic falls at or beyond the **critical region** on the relevant theoretical distribution. If the value of the test statistic indicates that the null hypothesis is "improbable," the result is **statistically significant** (i.e., obtained results are not likely to result from chance fluctuations at the specified level of probability).
- Most hypothesis testing involves **two-tailed tests**, in which both ends of the sampling distribution are used to define the region of improbable values, but a **one-tailed test** may be appropriate if there is a strong rationale for a directional hypothesis.
- **Parametric tests** involve the estimation of at least one parameter, the use of interval- or ratio-level data, and assumptions of normally distributed variables; **nonparametric tests** are used when the data are nominal or ordinal or when a normal distribution cannot be assumed.
- There are **between-subjects tests** (or **tests for independent groups**) for comparing separate groups of subjects, and **within-subjects tests** (or **tests for dependent groups**) for comparing the same group of subjects over time or conditions.
- Two common statistical tests are the **t-test** and **analysis of variance** (**ANOVA**), both of which are used to test the significance of the difference between group means; ANOVA is used when there are three or more groups (**one-way ANOVA**) or when there is more than one independent variable (e.g., **two-way ANOVA**).
- Nonparametric analogues of t-tests and ANOVA include the **median test**, the **Mann-Whitney U test**, the **sign test** and the **Wilcoxon signed-rank test** (two-group situations), and the **Kruskal-Wallis** and **Friedman tests** (three-group or more situations).
- The most frequently used nonparametric test is the **chi-square test**, which is used to test hypotheses relating to differences in proportions.
- Statistical tests to measure the magnitude of bivariate relationships and to test whether the relationship is significantly different from zero include Pearson's *r* for interval-level data, **Spearman's rho** and **Kendall's tau** for ordinal-level data, and the **phi coefficient** and **Cramér's V** for nominal-level data.
- **Power analysis** is a method of estimating either the likelihood of committing a Type II error or sample size requirements. Power analysis involves four components: desired significance level (α), **power** ($1 - \beta$), sample size (N), and estimated **effect size** (γ).

STUDY ACTIVITIES

Chapter 20 of the accompanying *Study Guide for Nursing Research: Principles and Methods, 7th ed.*, offers various exercises and study suggestions for reinforcing the concepts presented in this chapter. In addition, the following study questions can be addressed:

1. A researcher has administered a Job Satisfaction Scale to a sample of 50 primary nurses and 50 team nurses. The mean score on this scale was found to be 35.2 for primary nurses and 33.6 for team nurses. The computed t-statistic is 1.89. Interpret this result, using the table for t-values in Appendix B.
2. Given that:
   a. There are three groups of cancer patients (breast, ovarian, and lung), with 50 in each group

b. Mean scores on a scale to measure anxiety: 25.8, 29.3, and 23.4 for groups A, B, and C, respectively

c. Level of significance = .05

d. Value of test statistic = 4.43

Specify:

a. What test statistic was used

b. How many degrees of freedom there are

c. Whether the test statistic is statistically significant

d. What the test statistic means

3. What inferential statistic would you choose for the following sets of variables? Explain your answers (refer to Table 20-10.)

a. Variable 1 represents the weights of 100 patients; variable 2 is the patients' resting heart rate.

b. Variable 1 is the patients' marital status; variable 2 is the patient's level of preoperative stress.

c. Variable 1 is whether an amputee has a leg removed above or below the knee; variable 2 is whether the amputee shows signs of aggressive behavior during rehabilitation.

4. Estimate the required total sample sizes for the following situations:

a. Comparison of two group means: $\alpha = .01$; power = .90; $\gamma = .35$.

b. Comparison of three group means: $\alpha = .05$; power = .80; $\eta^2 = .07$.

c. Correlation of two variables: $\alpha = .01$; power = .85; $\rho = .27$.

d. Comparison of two proportions: $\alpha = .05$; power = .80, $P_1 = .35$; $P_2 = .50$.

5. What was the power of the t-test in the Schultz et al. (2002) study, described in this chapter?

SUGGESTED READINGS

Methodologic References

Borenstein, M., & Cohen, J. (1988). *Statistical power analysis: A computer program.* Hillsdale, NJ: Lawrence Erlbaum Associates.

Cohen, J. (1988). *Statistical power analysis for the behavioral sciences* (2nd ed.) Hillsdale, NJ: Lawrence Erlbaum Associates.

Holm, K., & Christman, N. J. (1985). Post hoc tests following analysis of variance. *Research in Nursing & Health, 8,* 207–210.

Jaccard, J., & Becker, M. A. (2001). *Statistics for the behavioral sciences* (4th ed.). Belmont, CA: Wadsworth.

Jacobsen, B. S., Tulman, L., & Lowery, B. J. (1991). Three sides of the same coin: The analysis of paired data from dyads. *Nursing Research, 40,* 359–363.

McCall, R. B. (2000). *Fundamental statistics for behavioral sciences* (8th ed.). Belmont, CA: Wadsworth.

Munro, B. H. (Ed.). (2001). *Statistical methods for health-care research* (4th ed.). Philadelphia: Lippincott Williams & Wilkins.

Polit, D. F. (1996). *Data analysis and statistics for nursing research.* Stamford, CT: Appleton & Lange.

Polit, D. F., & Sherman, R. (1990). Statistical power in nursing research. *Nursing Research, 39,* 365–369.

Rothstein, H., & Tonges, M. C. (2000). Beyond the significance test in administrative research and policy decisions. *Image: The Journal of Nursing Scholarship, 32,* 65–70.

Sidani, S., & Lynn, M. R. (1993). Examining amount and pattern of change: Comparing repeated measures ANOVA and individual regression analysis. *Nursing Research, 42,* 283–286.

Triola, M. (2000). *Elementary statistics* (8th ed.). Menlo Park, CA: Addison-Wesley.

Welkowitz, J., Ewen, R. B., & Cohen, J. (2000). *Introductory statistics for the behavioral sciences* (5th ed.). New York: Harcourt College Publishers.

Studies Cited in Chapter 20

Cimprich, B., & Ronis, D. L. (2001). Attention and symptom distress in women with and without breast cancer. *Nursing Research, 50,* 86–94.

Connelly, B., Gunzerath, L., & Knebel, A. (2000). A pilot study exploring mood state and dyspnea in mechanically ventilated patients. *Heart & Lung, 29,* 173–179.

Damato, E. G. (2000). Maternal-fetal attachment in twin pregnancies. *Journal of Obstetric, Gynecologic, and Neonatal Nursing, 29,* 598–605.

Elpern, E., Okonek, M., Bacon, B., Gerstung, C., & Skrzynski, M. (2000). Effect of the Passy-Muir tracheostomy speaking valve on pulmonary aspiration in adults. *Heart & Lung, 29,* 287–293.

Hojat, M., Masca, T., Cohen, M., Fields, S., Rattner, S., Griffits, M., Ibarra, D., deGonzales, A., Torres-Ruiz,

A., Ibarra, G., & Garcia, A. (2001). Attitudes toward physician-nurse collaboration: A cross-cultural study of male and female physicians and nurses in the United States and Mexico. *Nursing Research, 50,* 1230–128.

Logsdon, M. C., & Usui, W. (2001). Psychosocial predictors of postpartum depression in diverse groups of women. *Western Journal of Nursing Research, 23,* 563–574.

Parker, K. P., Bliwise, D., & Rye, D. (2000). Hemodialysis disrupts basic sleep regulatory mechanisms: Building hypotheses. *Nursing Research, 49,* 327–331.

Parshall, M., Welsh, J. D., Brockopp, D., Heiser, R., Schooler, M., & Cassidy, K. (2001). Dyspnea duration, distress, and intensity in emergency department visits for heart failure. *Heart & Lung, 30,* 47–56.

Pieper, B., & Templin, T. (2001). Chronic venous insufficiency in persons with a history of injection drug use. *Research in Nursing & Health, 24,* 423–432.

Schultz, A. A., Drew, D., & Hewitt, H. (2002). Comparison of normal saline and heparinized saline for patency of IV locks in neonates. *Applied Nursing Research, 15,* 28–34.

Stark, M. (2001). Relationship of psychosocial tasks of pregnancy and attentional functioning in the third trimester. *Research in Nursing & Health, 24,* 194–202.

Steward, D. K., & Pridham, K. F. (2002). Growth patterns of extremely low-birthweight hospitalized preterm infants. *Journal of Obstetric, Neonatal, and Gynecologic Nursing, 31,* 57–65.

Wang, H., & Laffrey, S. C. (2001). A predictive model of well-being and self-care for rural elderly women in Taiwan. *Research in Nursing & Health, 24,* 122–132.

Welch, J. L. (2001). Hemodialysis patient beliefs by stage of fluid adherence. *Research in Nursing & Health, 24,* 105–112.

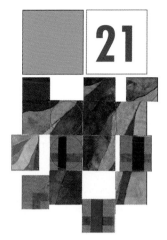

21

Analyzing Quantitative Data: Multivariate Statistics

The phenomena of interest to nurse researchers usually are complex. Patients' spirituality, nurses' effectiveness, or abrupt elevations of patients' temperature are phenomena with multiple facets and multiple determinants. Scientists, in attempting to explain or predict phenomena, have recognized that two-variable studies are often inadequate for these purposes. The classic approach to data analysis and research design, which involved studying the effect of a single independent variable on a single dependent variable, is being replaced by more sophisticated **multivariate* procedures**. Regardless of whether a study is designed for multivariate analysis, the fact remains that the determinants of most nursing outcomes are fundamentally multivariate.

Unlike the statistical methods reviewed in Chapters 19 and 20, multivariate statistics are computationally formidable. Our purpose is to provide a general understanding of how, when, and why multivariate statistics are used, without working out computations. Those needing more comprehensive coverage should consult the references at the end of this chapter.

The mostly widely used multivariate procedure (and therefore the one we describe in greatest

depth) is multiple regression analysis, which is used to understand the effects of two or more independent variables on a dependent variable. The terms **multiple correlation** and **multiple regression** will be used almost interchangeably in reference to this technique, consistent with the strong bond between correlation and regression. To comprehend the nature of this bond, we first explain simple (that is, bivariate) regression.

SIMPLE LINEAR REGRESSION

Regression analysis is used to make predictions about phenomena. In simple (bivariate) regression, one independent variable (X) is used to predict a dependent variable (Y). For instance, we could use simple regression to predict weight from height, nursing school achievement from Scholastic Assessment Test (SAT) scores, or stress from noise levels. An important feature of regression is that the higher the correlation between two variables, the more accurate the prediction. If the correlation between diastolic and systolic blood pressure were perfect (i.e., if $r = 1.00$), we would need to measure only one to know the value of the other. Because most variables are not perfectly correlated, predictions made through regression analysis usually are imperfect.

---

*We use the term *multivariate* in this chapter to refer to analyses with at least three variables. Some statisticians reserve the term for problems involving more than one dependent variable.

The basic linear regression equation is

$$Y' = a + bX$$

where Y' = prediced value of variable Y
a = intercept constant
b = regression coefficient (slope of the line)
X = actual value of variable X

Regression analysis solves for a and b, so for any value of X, a prediction about Y can be made. You may remember from high school algebra that the preceding equation is the algebraic equation for a straight line. **Linear regression** is used to determine a straight-line fit to the data that minimizes deviations from the line.

As an illustration, consider the data for five subjects on two variables (X and Y) shown in columns 1 and 2 of Table 21-1. These two variables are strongly related ($r = .90$). We use the five pairs of X and Y values to solve for a and b in a regression equation, which will allow us to predict Y values for a *new* group of people about whom we will have information on variable X only.

The formulas for these two components are as follows:

$$b = \frac{\Sigma xy}{\Sigma x^2} \qquad a = \bar{Y} - b\bar{X}$$

where b = regression coefficient
a = intercept constant
$\bar{Y}$ = mean of variable Y
$\bar{X}$ = mean of variable X
x = deviation scores from $\bar{X}$
y = deviation scores from $\bar{Y}$

Calculations for the current example are presented in columns 3 through 7 of Table 21-1. As shown at the bottom of the table, the solution to the regression equation is $Y' = 1.5 + .9X$. Now suppose for the moment that the X values in column 1 are the only data we have, and we want to predict values for Y. For the first subject, $X = 1$; we would predict that $Y' = 1.5 + (.9)(1)$, or 2.4. Column 8 shows Y' values for each X. These numbers show that Y' does not exactly equal the actual values obtained for Y (column 2). Most **errors of**

TABLE 21.1 Computations for Simple Linear Regression

(1) X	(2) Y	(3) x	(4) x²	(5) y	(6) y²	(7) xy	(8) Y'	(9) e	(10) e²
1	2	−4	16	−4	16	16	2.4	−.4	.16
3	6	−2	4	0	0	0	4.2	1.8	3.24
5	4	0	0	−2	4	0	6.0	−2.0	4.00
7	8	2	4	2	4	4	7.8	.2	.04
9	10	4	16	4	16	16	9.6	.4	.16
$\Sigma X = 25$	$\Sigma Y = 30$		40		40	36		0.0	$\Sigma e^2 = 7.60$

$\bar{X} = 5.0$ $\bar{Y} = 6.0$
$r = .90$

$$b = \frac{\Sigma xy}{\Sigma x^2} = \frac{36}{40} = .9$$

$$a = \bar{Y} - b\bar{X} = 6.0 - (.9)(5.0) = 1.5$$

$$Y' = a + b\bar{X} = 1.5 + .9X$$

prediction (*e*) are small, as shown in column 9. Errors of prediction occur because the correlation between X and Y is not perfect. Only when $r = 1.00$ or -1.00 does $Y' = Y$. The regression equation solves for a and b in a way that minimizes such errors. More precisely, the solution minimizes the sums of squares of prediction errors, which is why standard regression analysis is said to use a **least-squares** criterion. Indeed, standard regression is sometimes referred to as **ordinary least squares**, or **OLS**, regression. In column 10 of Table 21-1, the error terms—referred to as the **residuals**—have been squared and summed to yield a value of 7.60. Any values of a and b other than 1.5 and .9 would have yielded a larger sum of squared residuals.

Figure 21-1 displays the solution to this regression analysis graphically. The actual X and Y values are plotted on the graph with circles. The line running through these points represents the regression solution. The intercept (*a*) is the point at which the line crosses the Y axis, which in this case is 1.5. The slope (*b*) is the angle of the line. With $b = .90$, the line slopes so that for every 4 units on

the X axis, we must go up 3.6 units (.9 × 4) on the Y axis. The line, then, embodies the regression equation. To predict a value for Y, we would go to the point on the X axis for an obtained X value, go up to vertically to the point on the regression line directly above the X score, and then read the predicted Y' value horizontally on the Y axis. For example, for an X value of 5, we would predict a Y' of 6, indicated by the star.

The correlation coefficient, it may be recalled, is an index of the degree to which variables are related. From a statistical point of view, relationships are concerned with how variation in one variable is associated with variation in another. The square of r (r^2) tells us the proportion of variance in Y that can be accounted for by X. In our example, $r = .90$, so $r^2 = .81$. This means that 81% of the variability in Y values can be understood in terms of variability in X values. The remaining 19% is variability resulting from other sources.

In the regression problem, the sum of the squared residuals (*es*) is 7.6. Column 6 of Table 21-1 also tells us that the sum of the squared

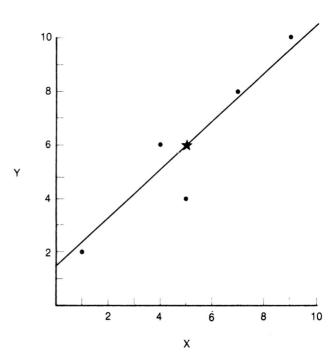

FIGURE 21.1   Example of simple linear regression.

deviations of Y values from the mean of Y (Σy^2) is 40, which represents variability in Y. To demonstrate that the residuals are 19% of the unexplained variability in Y, we compute the following ratio:

$$\frac{7.6}{40} = .19 = 1 - r^2$$

Although the computations are not shown, the sum of the squared deviations of the Y' values from the mean of Y' ($\Sigma y'^2$) equals 32.4. As a proportion of the variability in the *actual* Y values, this would equal

$$\frac{32.4}{40} = .81 = r^2$$

These calculations reinforce a point made earlier: The stronger the correlation, the better the prediction; the stronger the correlation, the greater the percentage of variance explained.

MULTIPLE LINEAR REGRESSION

Because the correlation between two variables is rarely perfect, researchers often try to improve predictions of Y by including more than one independent (predictor) variable. Multiple regression is used for this purpose.

Basic Concepts for Multiple Regression

Suppose we wanted to predict graduate nursing students' grade-point averages (GPA). Only a limited number of students can be accepted, so we want to select applicants with the greatest chance of success. Suppose we had previously found that students with high scores on the verbal portion of the Graduate Record Examination (GRE) tended to get better grades than those with lower GRE scores. The correlation between GRE verbal scores (GRE-V) and graduate GPAs has been calculated as .50. With only 25% ($.50^2$) of the variance of graduate GPA accounted for, there will be many errors of prediction: Many admitted students will not perform as well as expected, and many rejected

applicants would have made successful students. It may be possible, by using additional information, to make more accurate predictions through multiple regression. The basic multiple regression equation is

$$Y' = a + b_1 X_1 + b_2 X_2 + \ldots b_k X_k$$

where Y' = predicted value for variable Y
a = intercept constant
k = number of predictor (independent) variables
b_1 to b_k = regression coefficients for the k variables
X_1 to X_k = scores or values on the k independent variables

When the number of predictor variables exceeds two, computations to solve this equation are very complex and so we restrict our discussion to hypothetical rather than worked-out examples.

In our example of predicting graduate nursing students' GPAs, suppose we hypothesized that information on undergraduate GPA (GPA U) and scores on the quantitative portion of the GRE (GRE-Q) would improve our ability to predict graduate GPA. The resulting equation might be

$$Y' = .4 + .05(\text{GPA-U}) + .003(\text{GRE-Q}) + .002(\text{GRE-V})$$

For instance, suppose an applicant had a GRE-V score of 600, a GRE-Q score of 550, and a GPA-U of 3.2. The predicted graduate GPA would be

$$Y' = .4 + (.05)(3.2) + .003(550) + .002(600) = 3.41$$

We can assess the degree to which adding two independent variables improves our ability to predict graduate school performance through the multiple correlation coefficient. In bivariate correlation, the index is Pearson's r. With two or more independent variables, the correlation index is the **multiple correlation coefficient**, or R. Unlike r, R does not have negative values. R varies only from .00 to 1.00, showing the *strength* of the relationship between several independent variables and a dependent variable but not *direction*. Direction cannot be shown because X_1 might be positively related to Y, while X_2 might be negatively related. The R statistic, when squared (R^2), indicates the proportion of variance in Y accounted for by the combined, simultaneous influence of the independent variables.

R^2 provides a way to evaluate the accuracy of a prediction equation. Suppose that with the three predictor variables in the current example, the value of $R = .71$. This means that 50% ($.71^2$) of the variability in graduate students' grades can be explained by their verbal and quantitative GRE scores and undergraduate grades. The addition of two predictors doubled the variance accounted for by the single independent variable (GRE-V), from .25 to .50.

The multiple correlation coefficient cannot be less than the highest bivariate correlation between an independent variable and the dependent variable. Table 21-2 presents a correlation matrix with the correlation coefficients for all pairs of variables in this example. The independent variable most strongly correlated with graduate performance is (GPA-U), $r = .60$. The value of R could not have been less than .60.

Another important point is that R can be more readily increased when the independent variables have relatively low correlations among themselves. In the current case, the lowest correlation coefficient is between GRE-Q and GPA-U ($r = .40$), and the highest is between GRE-Q and GRE-V ($r = .70$). All correlations are fairly substantial, a fact that helps to explain why R is not much higher than the r between the dependent variable and undergraduate grades alone (.71 compared with .60). This somewhat puzzling phenomenon results from redundancy of information among predictors. When correlations among independent variables are high, they tend to add little predictive power to each other. With low correlations among predictor variables, each one can contribute something unique to the prediction of the dependent variable.

Figure 21-2 illustrates this concept. Each circle represents total variability in a variable. The circle on the left (Y) is the dependent variable (graduate GPA). The overlap between this circle and the other circles represents variability that the variables have in common. If the overlap were complete—if the entire Y circle were covered by the other circles—R^2 would be 1.00. As it is, only half the circle is covered, because $R^2 = .50$. The hatched area designates the independent contribution of undergraduate GPA in explaining graduate grades. This contribution amounts to 36% of Y's variance ($.60^2$). The remaining two independent variables do not contribute as much as we would expect by considering their bivariate correlation with graduate GPA (r for GRE-V = .50; r for GRE-Q = .55). In fact, their *combined* additional contribution is only 14% ($.50 - .36 = .14$), designated by the dotted area on the figure. The contribution is small because the two

	GPA-GRAD	GPA-U	GRE-Q	GRE-V
TABLE 21.2 Correlation Matrix				
GPA-GRAD	1.00			
GPA-U	.60	1.00		
GRE-Q	.55	.40	1.00	
GRE-V	.50	.50	.70	1.00

GPA, grade point average; GRE, Graduate Record Examination; GPA-GRAD, graduate GPA; GPA-U, undergraduate GPA; GRE-Q, GRE quantitative score; GRE-V, GRE verbal score.

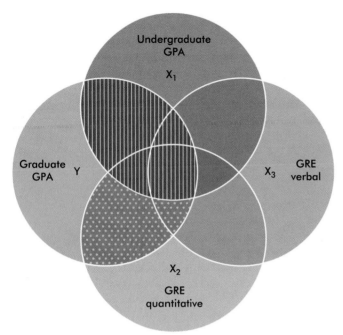

FIGURE 21.2 Visual representation of multiple regression example.

GRE scores have redundant information with undergraduate grades.

A related point is that, as more independent variables are added to the regression equation, increments to R tend to decrease. It is rare to find predictor variables that correlate well with a criterion but modestly with one another. Redundancy is difficult to avoid as more and more variables are added to the equation. The inclusion of independent variables beyond the first four or five typically does little to improve the proportion of variance accounted for or the accuracy of prediction.

The dependent variable in multiple regression analysis, as in analysis of variance (ANOVA), should be measured on an interval or ratio scale. Independent variables, on the other hand, can either be interval- or ratio-level variables *or* dichotomous variables. A text such as that by Polit (1996) should be consulted for information on how to use and interpret dichotomous **dummy variables**.

Tests of Significance

Multiple regression analysis is not used solely (or even primarily) to develop prediction equations. Researchers almost always ask inferential questions about relationships in the regression analysis (e.g., Is the calculated R the result of chance fluctuations, or is does it reflect true relationships in the population?) There are several relevant significance tests, each used to address different questions.

Tests of the Overall Equation and R

The most basic test in multiple regression concerns the null hypothesis that the population multiple correlation coefficient equals zero. The test for the significance of R is based on principles analogous to those for ANOVA. We stated in Chapter 20 that the general form for calculating an F-ratio is as follows:

$$F = \frac{SS_{between}/df_{between}}{SS_{within}/df_{within}}$$

In the case of multiple regression, the form is similar:

$$F = \frac{SS_{\text{due to regression}}/df_{\text{regression}}}{SS_{\text{of residuals}}/df_{\text{residuals}}}$$

The basic principle is the same in both cases: Variance resulting from independent variables is contrasted with variance attributable to other factors, or error. To calculate the F-statistic for regression, we can use the following alternative formula:

$$F = \frac{R^2/k}{(1 - R^2)/(N - k - 1)}$$

where k = number of predictor variables

N = total sample size

In the example of predicting graduate GPAs, suppose a multiple correlation coefficient of .71 (R^2 = .50) has been calculated for a sample of 100 graduate students. The value of the F-statistic is

$$F = \frac{.50/3}{.50/96} = 32.05$$

The tabled value of F with 3 and 96 degrees of freedom for a significance level of .01 is about 4.0; thus, the probability that R = .71 resulted from chance fluctuations is considerably less than .01.

Example of multiple regression:
Badr (2001) examined predictors of development among low-birth-weight infants of Latino background. The two dependent variables were the motor and mental development subscales scores of the Bayley Scales of Infant Development. There were 11 independent variables measuring primarily maternal factors such as maternal confidence, maternal depression, and family income. The value of R^2 was .40 for motor development and .60 for mental development scores, both $p < .01$.

Tests for Adding Predictors

Another question researchers may want to answer is: Does *adding* X_k to the regression equation significantly improve the prediction of Y over that achieved with X_{k-1}? For example, does a third predictor increase our ability to predict Y after two predictors have been used? An F-statistic can be computed to answer this question.

Let us number each independent variable in the current example: X_1 = GPA-U; X_2 = GRE-Q; and X_3 = GRE-V. We can then symbolize various correlation coefficients as follows:

$R_{y.1}$ = the correlation of Y with GPA-U

$R_{y.12}$ = the correlation of Y with GPA-U *and* GRE-Q

$R_{y.123}$ = the correlation of Y with all three predictors

The values of these Rs are as follows:

$R_{y.1}$ = .60 $\qquad$ $R^2_{y.1}$ = .36
$R_{y.12}$ = .71 $\qquad$ $R^2_{y.12}$ = .50
$R_{y.123}$ = .71 $\qquad$ $R^2_{y.123}$ = .50

These figures indicate that GRE-V scores made no independent contribution to the multiple correlation coefficient. The value of $R_{y.12}$ is identical to the value of $R_{y.123}$. Figure 21-2 illustrates this point: If the circle for GRE-V were completely removed, the area of the Y circle covered by X_1 and X_2 would remain the same.

We cannot tell at a glance, however, whether adding X_2 to X_1 *significantly* increased the prediction of Y. What we want to know is whether X_2 would improve predictions in the population, or if its added predictive power in this sample resulted from chance. The F-statistic formula to test the significance of variables added to the regression equation is

$$F = \frac{(R^2_{Y.12...k_1} - R^2_{Y.12 \; k_2})/(k_1 - k_2)}{(1 - R^2_{Y.12...k_1})/(N - k_1 - 1)}$$

where $R^2_{y.12...k_1}$ = squared multiple correlation coefficient for Y correlated with k_1 predictor variables

k_1 = the number of predictors for the larger of the two sets of predictors

$R^2_{y.12...k_2}$ = squared R for Y correlated with k_2 predictor variables

k_2 = the number of predictors for the smaller of the two sets of predictors

In the current example, the F-statistic for testing whether adding GRE-Q scores significantly improves our prediction of Y is

$$F = \frac{(.50 - .36)/1}{.50/97} = 27.16$$

Consulting Table A-2 in Appendix A, we find that with $df = 1$ and 97 and a significance level of .01, the critical value is about 6.90. Therefore, adding GRE-Q to the regression equation significantly improved the accuracy of predicting graduate GPA, beyond the .01 level.

 Example of adding predictors in multiple regression:

McCarter-Spaulding and Kearney (2001) studied mothers' perceptions of insufficient milk. They first examined demographic predictors of these perceptions (age, education, and parity), which yielded a nonsignificant R^2 of .02. They then added a fourth predictor, scores on a parenting self-efficacy scale. R^2 increased to .25; the .23 increment was statistically significant.

Tests of the Regression Coefficients

Researchers often want to know the significance of individual predictors in the regression equation, which can be done by calculating t statistics that test the unique contribution of each independent variable. A significant t indicates that the regression coefficient (b) is significantly different from zero.

Regression coefficients in multiple regression must be interpreted differently than coefficients in bivariate regression. In simple regression, the value of b indicates the amount of change in predicted values of Y, for a specified rate of change in X. In multiple regression, the coefficients represent the number of units the dependent variable is predicted to change for each unit change in a given independent variable *when the effects of other predictors are held constant.* This "holding constant" of other variables means that they are statistically controlled, a very important feature that can enhance a study's internal validity. If a regression coefficient is significant and extraneous variables are included in the regression equation, it means that the variable associated with the coefficient contributes significantly to the regression, even after extraneous variables are taken into account.

Strategies for Handling Predictors in Multiple Regression

There are various strategies for entering predictor variables into regression equations. The three most common are simultaneous, hierarchical, and stepwise regressions.

Simultaneous Multiple Regression

The most basic strategy, **simultaneous multiple regression**, enters all predictor variables into the regression equation at the same time. A single regression equation is developed, and statistical tests indicate the significance of R and of individual regression coefficients. The study about predicting infant development cited earlier (Badr, 2001) used a simultaneous approach: All 11 independent variables were put into the regression equation at the same time. This strategy is most appropriate when there is no basis for considering any particular predictor as causally prior to another, and when the predictors are of comparable importance to the research problem.

Hierarchical Multiple Regression

Many researchers use **hierarchical multiple regression**, which involves entering predictors into the equation in a series of steps. Researchers control the order of entry, with the order typically based on logical or theoretical considerations. For example, some predictors may be thought of as causally or temporally prior to others, in which case they could be entered in an early step. Another common reason for using hierarchical regression is to examine the effect of a key independent variable after first removing the effect of extraneous variables. The study by McCarter-Spaulding and Kearney (2001) exemplifies this strategy. Demographic characteristics were entered in step 1, and then parenting self-efficacy

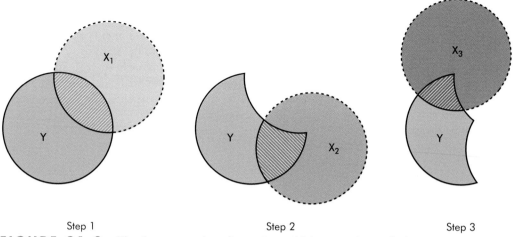

| Step 1 | Step 2 | Step 3 |

FIGURE 21.3   Visual representation of stepwise multiple regression analysis.

was entered in step 2. The findings indicated that, even after taking age, parity, and education into account, parenting self-efficacy was a significant predictor of the mothers' perceptions about insufficient milk supply.

With hierarchical regression, researchers determine the number of steps as well as the number of predictors included in each step. When several variables are added as a block, as in the McCarter-Spaulding and Kearney example, the analysis is a simultaneous regression for those variables at that stage. Thus, hierarchical regression can be considered a controlled sequence of simultaneous regressions.

Stepwise Multiple Regression

Stepwise multiple regression is a method of empirically selecting the combination of independent variables with the most predictive power. In stepwise multiple regression, predictors enter the regression equation in the order that produces the greatest increments to R^2. The first step selects the single best predictor of the dependent variable, that is, the independent variable with the highest bivariate correlation with Y. The second variable to enter the equation is the one that produces the largest increase to R^2 when used simultaneously with the variable selected in the first step. The pro-

cedure continues until no additional predictor significantly increases the value of R^2.

Figure 21-3 illustrates stepwise multiple regression. The first variable (X_1), has a correlation of .60 with Y ($r^2 = .36$); no other predictor variable is correlated more strongly with the dependent variable. The variable X_1 accounts for the portion of the variability of Y represented by the hatched area in step 1 of the figure. This hatched area is, in effect, removed from further consideration, because this portion of Y's variability is explained or accounted for. Thus, the variable chosen in step 2 is not necessarily the X variable with the second largest correlation with Y. The selected predictor is the one that explains the largest portion of what *remains* of Y's variability after X_1 has been taken into account. Variable X_2, in turn, removes a second part of Y so that the independent variable selected in step 3 is the one that accounts for the most variability in Y after *both* X_1 and X_2 are removed.

TIP: Stepwise regression is a somewhat controversial procedure because variables are entered into the regression equation based solely on statistical rather than theoretical criteria. Pure stepwise regression is best suited to exploratory work, but cross-validation is essential. If a sample is sufficiently large, we recommend that it be split in half to determine if similar equations result with both subsets of data.

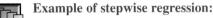

Example of stepwise regression:
Tarkka, Paunonen, and Laippala (2000) explored factors associated with first-time mothers' ability to cope with their child care responsibilities, using stepwise regression with seven predictors (perceived maternal competence, maternal attachment to the child, self-concept, relationship with her spouse, breastfeeding status, decision-making support, and activity level of the child). All were significant predictors, and the cumulative R^2 was .55. Perceived competence entered the equation first.

Relative Contribution of Predictors

Scientists want not only to predict phenomena, but to explain them. Predictions can be made in the absence of understanding. For instance, in our graduate school example, we could predict performance moderately well without understanding the factors contributing to students' success. For practical applications, it may be sufficient to make accurate predictions, but scientists typically want to understand phenomena and contribute to knowledge.

In multiple regression, one approach to understanding a phenomenon is to explore the relative importance of independent variables. Unfortunately, the determination of the relative contributions of independent variables in predicting a dependent variable is one of the thorniest issues in regression analysis. When independent variables are correlated, as they usually are, there is no ideal way to disentangle the effects of variables in the equation.

It may appear that the solution is to compare the contributions of the Xs to R^2. In our graduate school example, GPA-U accounted for 36% of Y's variance; GRE-Q explained an additional 14%. Should we conclude that undergraduate grades are more than twice as important as GRE-Q scores in explaining graduate school grades? This conclusion would be inaccurate because the order of entry of variables in a regression equation affects their apparent contribution. If these two predictor variables were entered in reverse order (i.e., GRE-Q first), R^2 would remain unchanged at .50; however, GRE-Q's contribution would be .30 ($.55^2$), and

GPA-U's contribution would be .20 (.50 − .30). This is because whatever variance the independent variables have in common is attributed to the first variable entered in the analysis.

Another approach to assessing the relative importance of the predictors is to compare regression coefficients. Earlier, the regression equation was given as

$$Y' = a + b_1X_1 + b_2X_2 + \ldots b_kX_k$$

where b_1 to b_k = regression coefficients

These b values cannot be directly compared because they are in the units of original scores, which differ from one X to another. X_1 might be in milliliters, X_2 in degrees Fahrenheit, and so forth. The use of **standard scores** (or z scores) eliminates this problem by transforming all variables to scores with a mean of 0.0 and a standard deviation (SD) of 1.00. The formula for converting raw scores to standard scores* is

$$z_X = \frac{X - \overline{X}}{SD_X}$$

In standard score form, the regression equation is

$$z_{Y'} = \beta_1 z_{X_1} + \beta_2 z_{X_2} + \ldots \beta_k z_{X_k}$$

where $z_{Y'}$ = predicted value of the standard score for Y

β_1 to β_k = standardized regression weights for k independent variables

z_{X_1} to z_{X_k} = standard scores for the k predictors

With all the βs (referred to as **beta [β] weights**) in the same measurement units, can their relative size shed light on how much importance to attach to predictor variables? Many researchers have interpreted beta weights in this fashion, but there are problems in doing so. These regression coefficients will be the same no matter what the order of entry of the variables. The difficulty, however, is that regression weights are unstable. The values of β tend to fluctuate from sample to sample. Moreover, when a variable is added to or

---

*Consult a standard statistical textbook for a complete discussion of standard scores.

subtracted from the regression equation, the beta weights change. Because there is nothing absolute about the values of the regression coefficients, it is difficult to attach theoretical importance to them.

Another method of disentangling relationships is through causal modeling, which represents an important tool in testing theoretical expectations about relationships. Causal modeling is described later in this chapter.

Sample Size for Multiple Regression

Small samples are especially problematic in multiple regression and other multivariate procedures. Inadequate sample size can lead to Type II errors, and can also yield erratic and misleading regression coefficients.

There are two approaches to estimating sample size needs. One concerns the ratio of predictor variables to total number of cases. Tabachnick and Fidell (2000) indicate that the barest minimum is to include five times as many cases as there are predictors in the regression equation. They *recommend*, however, a ratio of 20 to 1 for simultaneous and hierarchical regression and a ratio of 40 to 1 for stepwise. More cases are needed for stepwise regression because this procedure capitalizes on the idiosyncrasies of a specific data set.

A better way to estimate sample size needs is to perform a power analysis. The number of subjects needed to reject the null hypothesis that R equals zero is estimated as a function of effect size, number of predictors, desired power, and the significance criterion. For multiple regression, the estimated population effect size is:

$$\gamma = \frac{R^2}{1 - R^2}$$

Researchers must either predict the value of R^2 on the basis of earlier research, or use the convention that the effect size will be small ($R^2 = .02$), moderate ($R^2 = .13$), or large ($R^2 = .30$). Next, the following formula is applied:

$$N = \frac{L}{\gamma} + k + 1$$

where N = estimated number of subjects needed
L = tabled value for the desired α and power
k = number of predictors
γ = estimated effect size

Table 21-3 presents values for L when $\alpha = .05$ and power is .50 to .95, in situations in which there are up to 20 predictor variables.

As an example, suppose we were planning a study to predict functional ability in nursing home residents using five predictor variables. We estimate a moderate effect size ($R^2 = .13$) and want to achieve a power of .80 and $\alpha = .05$. With $R^2 = .13$, the estimated population effect size (γ) is .149 (.13 ÷ .87). From Table 21-3, we find that the value of $L = 12.83$. Thus:

$$N = \frac{12.83}{.149} + 5 + 1 = 92.1$$

Thus, a sample of about 92 nursing home residents is needed to detect a population R^2 of .13 with five predictors, with a 5% chance of a Type I error and a 20% chance of a Type II error.

TIP: If you are testing hypotheses and analyzing data by computer, you should definitely consider using multivariate procedures in lieu of bivariate ones because the commands to the computer are not appreciably more complicated. Researchers can come to the wrong conclusions about their hypotheses (i.e., commit Type I errors) when extraneous variables are not controlled, and multivariate procedures offer a way to control them.

ANALYSIS OF COVARIANCE

Analysis of covariance (**ANCOVA**) has much in common with multiple regression, but it also has features of ANOVA. Like ANOVA, ANCOVA is used to compare the means of two or more groups, and the central question for both is the same: Are mean group differences likely to be *real*, or do they reflect chance fluctuations? Like multiple regression, however,

TABLE 21.3 Power Analysis Table for Multiple Regression: Values of L for α = .05

	Power (1 − β)					
k	.50	.70	.80	.95	.90	.95
1	3.84	6.17	7.85	8.98	10.51	13.00
2	4.96	7.70	9.84	10.92	12.65	15.44
3	5.76	8.79	10.90	12.30	14.17	17.17
4	6.42	9.68	11.94	13.42	15.41	18.57
5	6.99	10.45	12.83	14.39	16.47	19.78
6	7.50	11.14	13.62	15.26	17.42	20.86
7	7.97	11.77	14.35	16.04	18.28	21.84
8	8.41	12.35	15.02	16.77	19.08	22.74
9	8.81	12.89	15.65	17.45	19.83	23.59
10	9.19	13.40	16.24	18.09	20.53	24.39
15	10.86	15.63	18.81	20.87	23.58	27.84
20	12.26	17.50	20.96	23.20	26.13	30.72

k = number of predictor variables.

ANCOVA permits researchers statistically to control extraneous variables.

Uses of Analysis of Covariance

ANCOVA is especially useful in certain situations. For example, if a nonequivalent control group design is used, researchers must consider whether obtained results are influenced by preexisting group differences. When experimental control through randomization is lacking, ANCOVA offers post hoc statistical control. Even in true experiments, ANCOVA can result in more precise estimates of group differences because, even with randomization, there are typically slight differences between groups. ANCOVA adjusts for initial differences so that the results more precisely reflect the effect of an intervention.

Strictly speaking, ANCOVA should not be used with preexisting groups because randomization is an underlying assumption of ANCOVA. This assumption is often violated, however. Random assignment should be done whenever possible, but when randomization is not feasible ANCOVA can make an important contribution to the internal validity of a study.

Analysis of Covariance Procedures

Suppose we were testing the effectiveness of biofeedback therapy on patients' anxiety. An experimental group in one hospital is exposed to the treatment, and a comparison group in another hospital is not. Subjects' anxiety levels are measured both before and after the intervention and so pretest anxiety scores can be statistically controlled through ANCOVA. In such a situation, the dependent variable is the posttest anxiety scores, the independent variable is experimental/comparison group status, and the **covariate** is pretest anxiety

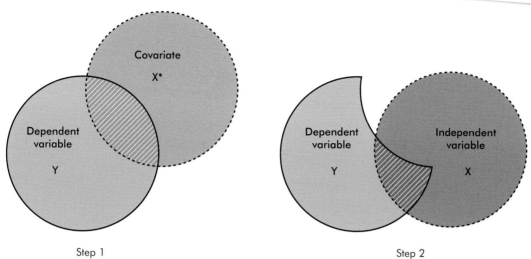

FIGURE 21.4 Visual respresentation of analysis of covariance.

scores. Covariates can either be continuous variables (e.g., anxiety test scores) or dichotomous variables (male/female); the independent variable is always a nominal-level variable.

ANCOVA tests the significance of differences between group means after first adjusting scores on the dependent variable to remove the effect of the covariate. The adjustment uses regression procedures. In essence, the first step in ANCOVA is the same as the first step in hierarchical multiple regression. Variability in the dependent measure that can be explained by the covariate is removed from further consideration. ANOVA is performed on what remains of Y's variability to see whether, once the covariate is controlled, significant differences between group means exist. Figure 21-4 illustrates this two-step process: Y is patients' posttest anxiety scores, the covariate X^* is pretest anxiety scores, and the independent variable X designates whether patients were exposed to the biofeedback therapy.

Let us consider another example to explore further aspects of ANCOVA. Suppose we were testing the effectiveness of three weight-loss diets, and we randomly assign 30 subjects to 1 of 3 groups. An ANCOVA, using pretreatment weight as the covariate, permits a more sensitive analysis

of weight change than simple ANOVA. Some hypothetical data for such a study are displayed in Table 21-4.

Two aspects of the weight values in this table are discernible. First, despite random assignment to treatment groups, initial group means are different. Subjects in diet B differ from those in diet C by an average of 10 pounds (175 versus 185 pounds). This difference is not significant*; it reflects chance sampling fluctuations. Second, post-treatment means are also different by a maximum of only 10 pounds (160 to 170). However, the mean number of pounds *lost* ranged from 10 pounds for diets A and B to 25 pounds for diet C.

A summary table for ordinary ANOVA is presented in part A of Table 21-5. According to the results, group differences in post-treatment means result in a nonsignificant F-value. Based on ANOVA, we would conclude that all three diets had equal effects on weight loss.

Part B of Table 21-5 presents the summary table for ANCOVA. The first step of the analysis breaks total variability in post-treatment weights into two components: (1) variability explained by

*Calculations demonstrating nonsignificance are not shown. The calculated $F = .45$. With 2 and 27 df, $p > .05$.

TABLE 21.4 Fictitious Data for ANCOVA Example

DIET A (X_A)		DIET B (X_B)		DIET C (X_C)	
X_A^*	Y_A	X_B^*	Y_B	X_C^*	Y_C
195	185	205	200	175	160
180	170	150	140	210	165
160	150	145	135	150	130
215	200	210	190	185	170
155	145	185	185	205	180
205	195	160	150	190	165
175	165	190	175	160	135
180	170	165	150	165	140
140	135	180	165	180	160
195	185	160	160	230	195
1800	1700	1750	1650	1850	1600
$\bar{X}_A^* = 180.0$	$\bar{Y}_A = 170.0$	$\bar{X}_B^* = 175.0$	$\bar{Y}_B = 165.0$	$\bar{X}_C^* - 185.0$	$\bar{Y}_C = 160.0$

X, independent variable (diet); X*, covariate (pretreatment weight); Y, dependent variable (posttreatment weight).

the covariate, pretreatment weights; and (2) residual variability. The table shows that the covariate accounted for a significant amount of variance, which is not surprising given the strong relationship between pretreatment and post-treatment weights ($r = .91$). This merely indicates that people who started out especially heavy tended to stay that way, relative to others in the sample. In the second phase of the analysis, residual variance is broken down to reflect between-group and within-group contributions. With 2 and 26 degrees of freedom, the F of 17.54 is significant beyond the .01 level. The conclusion is that, after controlling for initial weight, there is a significant difference in weight loss attributable to exposure to different diets.

This fictitious example was contrived so that the ANOVA result of "no difference" would be altered by adding a covariate. Most actual results are less dramatic than this example. Nonetheless, ANCOVA yields a more sensitive statistical test than ANOVA

if appropriate covariates are used. The increase in sensitivity results from the fact that the covariate reduces the error term (within-group variability), against which treatment effects are compared. In part A of Table 21-5, it can be seen that the within-group term is extremely large (12,300), masking the contribution of the experimental treatments.

Theoretically, it is possible to use any number of covariates. It is probably unwise, however, to use more than five or six. For one thing, including more covariates is often unnecessary because of the typically high degree of redundancy beyond the first few variables. Moreover, it is unwise to add covariates that do not explain a significant amount of variability in a dependent variable. Each covariate uses up a degree of freedom, and fewer degrees of freedom means that a higher computed F is required for significance. For instance, with 2 and 26 df, an F of 5.53 is required for significance at the .01 level, but with 2 and 23 df (i.e., adding three covariates), an F of 5.66 is needed.

TABLE 21.5 Comparison of ANOVA and ANCOVA Results

SOURCE OF VARIATION		SUM OF SQUARES	df	MEAN SQUARE	f	p
A. Summary Table for Anova						
Between groups		500.0	2	250.0	0.55	>.05
Within groups		12,300.0	27	455.6		
TOTAL		12,800.0	29			
B. Summary Table for Ancova						
Step 1	Covariate	10,563.1	1	10,563.1	132.23	<.01
	Residual	2236.9	28	79.9		
	TOTAL	12,800.0	29			
Step 2	Between groups	1284.8	2	642.4	17.54	<.01
	Within groups	952.1	26	36.6		
	TOTAL	2236.9	28			

TIP: ANCOVA is almost always preferable to ANOVA or t-tests, and is relatively easy to run on the computer. Covariates are usually available: At a minimum, you can use key background characteristics, such as age, gender, and so on. Covariates should be variables that you suspect are correlated with the dependent variable, and demographic characteristics usually are related to many other attributes. A pretest measure (i.e., a measure of the dependent variable before the occurrence of the independent variable) is an excellent choice for a covariate.

Adjusted Means

As shown in part B of Table 21-5, an ANCOVA summary table provides information about significance tests. The table indicates that at least one of the three groups had a post-treatment weight that is significantly different from the overall grand mean, after adjusting for pretreatment weights. It sometimes is useful to examine **adjusted means**, that is, group means on the dependent variable after adjusting for (i.e., removing the effect of) covariates. Means can be adjusted through a process sometimes referred to as **multiple classification analysis** (MCA). Adjusted means allow researchers to determine **net effects** (i.e., group differences on the dependent variable that are *net* of the effect of the covariate.) A subsequent section of this chapter, which presents computer examples of multivariate statistics, provides an illustration of adjusted means.

Example of ANCOVA:
Badger and Collins-Joyce (2000) studied depression in relation to functional ability in older adults. The sample was divided into two groups (depressed or not depressed). After statistically controlling for scores on a physical health impairment measure, they found that those in the

depressed group had significantly lower functional ability scores than those in the nondepressed group ($F = 7.22$, $df = 1{,}76$, $p < .01$).

FACTOR ANALYSIS

The major purpose of **factor analysis** is to reduce a large set of variables into a smaller, more manageable set. Factor analysis disentangles complex interrelationships among variables and identifies variables that "go together" as unified concepts. This section deals with a type of factor analysis known as **exploratory factor analysis**. Another type—**confirmatory factor analysis**—uses more complex modeling and estimation procedures and more sophisticated computer programs, as described later.

Suppose we developed 100 Likert-type items measuring women's attitudes toward menopause. Our goal is to compare the attitudes of urban versus rural women. If we do not combine items to form a scale, we would have to perform 100 separate statistical tests (such as chi-square tests) to compare the two groups of women on the 100 items. We could form a scale by adding together scores from several individual items, but which items should be combined? Would it be reasonable to combine all 100 items? Probably not, because the 100 items are not all tapping exactly the same thing. There are various aspects to women's attitude toward menopause. One aspect may relate to aging, and another to loss of reproductive ability. Other questions may involve sexuality, and yet others may concern avoidance of monthly aggravation. There are, in short, multiple dimensions to women's attitudes toward menopause, and each dimension should be captured on a separate scale. Women's attitude on one dimension may be independent of their attitude on another. The identification of dimensions can be made *a priori* by researchers, but different researchers may read different concepts into the items. Factor analysis offers an empirical method of clarifying the underlying dimensionality of a large set of measures. Underlying dimensions thus identified are called **factors**.

Mathematically, a factor is a linear combination of variables in a **data matrix**, which contains the scores of N people on k different measures. For instance, a factor might be defined by the following equation:

$$F = b_1X_1 + b_2X_2 + b_3X_3 + \ldots b_kX_k$$

where

$$F = \text{a factor score}$$
$$X_1 \text{ to } X_k = \text{values on the } k \text{ original variables}$$
$$b_1 \text{ to } b_k = \text{weights}$$

The development of such equations allows us to reduce the X_k scores to one or more factor scores.

Factor Extraction

Most factor analyses involve two phases. The first phase (**factor extraction**) condenses variables in the data matrix into a smaller number of factors. The general goal is to extract clusters of highly interrelated variables from a correlation matrix. There are various methods of performing the first step, each of which uses different criteria for assigning weights to variables. The most widely used factor extraction method is called **principal components** (or principal factor or principal axes), but other methods include the image, alpha, centroid, maximum likelihood, and canonical techniques.

Factor extraction results in an **unrotated factor matrix**, which contains coefficients or weights for all original variables on each extracted factor. (Because unrotated factor matrixes are difficult to interpret, we postpone a detailed discussion of factor matrixes until the second factor analysis phase is described.) In the principal components method, weights for the first factor are defined such that the average squared weight is maximized, permitting a maximum amount of variance to be extracted by the first factor. The second factor, or linear combination, is formed so that the highest possible amount of variance is extracted from what *remains* after the first factor has been taken into account. The factors thus represent independent sources of variation in the data matrix.

TABLE 21.6 Summary of Factor Extraction Results

FACTOR	EIGENVALUE	PERCENTAGE OF VARIANCE EXPLAINED	CUMULATIVE PERCENTAGE OF VARIANCE EXPLAINED
1	12.32	29.2	29.2
2	8.57	23.3	52.5
3	6.91	15.6	68.1
4	2.02	8.4	76.5
5	1.09	6.2	82.7
6	.98	5.8	88.5
7	.80	4.5	93.0
8	.62	3.1	96.1
9	.47	2.2	98.3
10	.25	1.7	100.0

Factoring should continue until there is no further meaningful variance left, and so a criterion must be applied to determine when to stop extraction and move on to the second phase. There are several possible criteria, a fact that makes factor analysis a semisubjective process. Several of the most commonly used criteria can be described by illustrating information generated in a factor analysis. Table 21-6 presents fictitious values for eigenvalues, percentages of variance accounted for, and cumulative percentages of variance accounted for, for 10 factors. **Eigenvalues** are equal to the sum of the squared weights for the factor. Many researchers establish as their cutoff point for factor extraction eigenvalues greater than 1.00. In our example, the first five factors meet this criterion. Another cutoff rule is factors with a minimum of 5% explained variance, in which case six factors would qualify in this example. Yet another criterion is based on a principle of discontinuity: A sharp drop in the percentage of explained variance indicates the appropriate termination point. In Table 21-6, we might argue that there is considerable discontinuity between the third and fourth factors. The general consensus is that it is better to extract too many factors than too few.

Factor Rotation

The second phase of factor analysis (**factor rotation**) is performed on factors that have met the extraction criteria. The concept of rotation can be best explained graphically. Figure 21-5 shows two coordinate systems, marked by axes A1 and A2 and B1 and B2. The primary axes (A1 and A2) represent factors I and II, respectively, as defined before rotation. The points 1 through 6 represent six variables in this two-dimensional space. The weights associated with each variable can be determined in reference to these axes. For instance, before rotation, variable 1 has a weight of .80 on factor I and .85 on factor II, and variable 6 has a weight of −.45 on factor I and .90 on factor II. Unrotated axes account for a maximum amount of variance but rarely provide a structure with conceptual meaning. Interpretability is enhanced by rotating the axes so that clusters of variables are distinctly associated with a factor. In the figure, B1 and B2 represent rotated factors. The rotation has been done in such a way that variables 1, 2, and 3 have large weights on factor I and small weights on factor II, and the reverse is true for variables 4, 5, and 6.

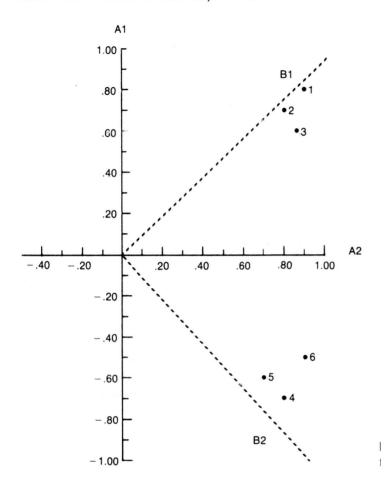

FIGURE 21.5 Illustration of factor rotation.

Researchers choose from two classes of rotation. Figure 21-5 illustrates **orthogonal rotation**, in which factors are kept at right angles to one another. Orthogonal rotations maintain the independence of factors—that is, orthogonal factors are uncorrelated with one another. **Oblique rotations**, on the other hand, permit rotated axes to depart from a 90-degree angle. In our figure, an oblique rotation would have put axis B1 between variables 2 and 3 and axis B2 between variables 5 and 6. This placement strengthens the clustering of variables around an associated factor, but results in correlated factors. Some researchers insist that orthogonal rotation leads to greater theoretical clarity; others claim that it is unrealistic. Those advo-

cating oblique rotation point out that if the concepts *are* correlated, then the analysis should reflect this fact. In practice, similar conclusions are often reached by both rotation procedures.

Researchers work with a **rotated factor matrix** in interpreting the factor analysis. An example of such a matrix is displayed in Table 21-7. To make the discussion less abstract, let us say that the 10 variables listed in the table are the first 10 of the 100 items measuring attitudes toward menopause, and that 3 factors have been extracted and rotated. The entries under each factor are the weights, called **factor loadings**. For orthogonally rotated factors, factor loadings can range from −1.00 to +1.00 and can be interpreted like correlation coefficients—they

TABLE 21.7 Rotated Factor Matrix

VARIABLE	FACTOR I	FACTOR II	FACTOR III
1	.75	.15	.23
2	−.02	.61	.18
3	−.59	−.11	.03
4	.05	.08	.48
5	.21	.79	.02
6	−.07	−.52	−.29
7	.08	.19	.80
8	.68	.12	−.01
9	−.04	.08	−.61
10	−.43	−.13	.06

express the correlations between individual variables and factors (underlying dimensions). In this example, variable 1 is fairly highly correlated with factor 1, .75. By examining factor loadings, it is possible to find which variables "belong" to a factor. Variables 1, 3, 8, and 10 have fairly sizable loadings on factor I. (Loadings with an absolute value of about .40 or .30 normally are used as cutoff values.) The underlying dimensionality of the data can then be interpreted. By inspecting items 1, 3, 8, and 10, we would search for a common theme that makes the variables go together. Perhaps these four questions have to do with the link between menopause and infertility, and perhaps items 2, 5, and 6 (items with high loadings on factor II) are related to sexuality. The naming of factors is a process of identifying underlying constructs.

Factor Scores

When the main purpose of factor analysis is to delineate the conceptual makeup of a set of measures, the analysis may end at this point. Frequently, however, researchers want to develop **factor scores** to use in subsequent analyses. For instance, the factor analysis of the 100 menopause items might indicate 5 underlying dimensions. By reducing 100 variables to 5 new variables, the analysis of differences between urban and rural women using t-tests or ANCOVA would be greatly simplified.

Several methods can be used to form factor scores, one of which is to weight variables according to their factor loading on each factor. For example, a factor score for the first factor in Table 21-7 could be computed for each subject by the following formula:

$$F_1 = .75X_1 - .02X_2 - .59X_3 + .05X_4 \\ + .21X_5 - .07X_6 + .08X_7 + .68X_8 - .04X_9 \\ - .43X_{10} \ldots b_{100}X_{100}$$

where the X values* = subjects' scores on the 100 items

Most factor analysis computer programs can directly compute this type of factor score.

A second method of obtaining factor scores is to select variables to represent the factor and to combine them with unit weighting. This method

---

*Standardized (z) scores are often used in lieu of raw scores in computing factor scores when the means and standard deviations of the variables differ substantially.

would produce the following factor score on the first factor of our example:

$$F_1 = X_1 - X_3 + X_8 - X_{10} \pm \cdots$$

The variables are those with high loadings on factor I (the "? . . ." indicates that some of the other 90 items with high loadings would be included). This procedure is computationally and conceptually simpler than the first approach, and yields similar results.

To illustrate more concretely, consider the rotated factor matrix in Table 21-7 and assume that factor scores are being computed on the basis of this 10-item analysis, omitting for the sake of simplicity the remaining 90 items on the menopause scale. Suppose two respondents had the following scores on the first 10 items:

Subject 1: 7, 1, 1, 5, 1, 6, 7, 6, 3, 2
Subject 2: 2, 5, 6, 3, 7, 3, 2, 3, 4, 4

Factor I has high loadings on variables 1, 3, 8, and 10. Thus, the two subjects' factor scores on factor 1 would be

$$7 - 1 + 6 - 2 = 10$$
$$2 - 6 + 3 - 4 = -5$$

The minus signs reflect the negative loadings on variables 3 and 10.* The same procedure would be performed for all three factors, yielding the following factor scores:

Subject 1: 10, −3, 9
Subject 2: −5, 9, 1

Factor scores would be computed for all respondents, and these scores could be used in subsequent analyses as measures of different dimensions of attitudes toward menopause.

Example of factor analysis:
Misener and Cox (2001) developed a scale to measure nurse practitioner job satisfaction. They administered 77 items to a sample of 342 nurse practitioners, whose responses were factor analyzed. An eigenvalue of 1.00 was used as the extraction criterion; 33 items with factor loadings less than .35 were discarded. The remaining items formed six factors: collegiality; autonomy; interactions; professional growth; and benefits.

OTHER LEAST-SQUARES MULTIVARIATE TECHNIQUES

In this section, the methods known as discriminant function analysis, canonical correlation, and multivariate analysis of variance are introduced. The introduction is brief, and computations are entirely omitted because these procedures are very complex. The intent is to acquaint you with the types of research situations for which these methods are appropriate. Advanced statistical texts such as the ones listed in the references may be consulted for more information.

Discriminant Analysis

In multiple regression, the dependent variable is normally a measure on either the interval or ratio scale. The regression equation makes predictions about scores that take on a range of values, such as heart rate, weight, or scores on a depression scale. **Discriminant analysis**, in contrast, makes predictions about membership in categories or groups. The purpose of the analysis is to distinguish groups from one another on the basis of available independent variables. For instance, we may wish to predict membership in such groups as complying versus noncomplying cancer patients, graduating nursing students versus dropouts, or normal pregnancies versus those terminating in a miscarriage.

Discriminant analysis develops a regression equation—called a **discriminant function**—for a categorical dependent variable, with independent variables that are either dichotomous or continuous. Researchers begin with data from subjects whose group membership is known, and develop an equation to predict membership when only measures of the independent variables are available. The discriminant function indicates to which group each subject will probably belong.

---

*Researchers forming scale scores with Likert items often reverse the direction of the scoring on negatively loaded items before forming factor scores. Direction of an item can be reversed by subtracting the raw score from the sum of 1 + the maximum item value. For example, in a five-point scale, a score of 2 would be reversed to 4 [(1 + 5) − 2]. When such reversals have been done, all raw scores can be added to compute factor scores.

Discriminant analysis for predicting membership into only two groups (e.g., nursing school dropouts versus graduates) is relatively simple and can be interpreted in much the same way as multiple regression. When there are more than two groups, the calculations and interpretations are more complex. With three or more groups (e.g., very—low-birth-weight, low-birth-weight, and normal-birth-weight infants), the number of discriminant functions is either the number of groups minus 1 or the number of independent variables, whichever is smaller. The first discriminant function is the linear combination of predictors that maximizes the ratio of between-group to within-group variance. The second function is the linear combination that maximizes this ratio, after the effect of the first function is removed. Because independent variables have different weights on the various functions, it is possible to develop theoretical interpretations based on the knowledge of which predictors are important in discriminating among different groups.

As with multiple regression analysis, it is possible to use a stepwise approach to enter predictors into a discriminant analysis equation. Discriminant analysis also produces an index designating the proportion of variance in the dependent variable accounted for by predictor variables. The index is **Wilks' lambda** (λ), which actually indicates the proportion of variance *unaccounted for* by predictors, or $\lambda = 1 - R^2$.

Example of discriminant analysis:
Aminzadeh and Edwards (2000) examined predictors of cane use among community-dwelling older adults. Using a stepwise discriminant analysis, they determined that age, subjective norms, and attitudes predicted cane use. The discriminant function accounted for 67% of the variance in cane use ($\lambda = .33$), and correctly categorized 91% of the cases.

Canonical Correlation

Canonical correlation analyzes the relationship between two or more independent variables *and* two or more dependent variables. Conceptually, one can think of this technique as an extension of multiple regression to more than one dependent variable. Mathematically and interpretatively, the gap between multiple regression and canonical correlation is greater than this statement suggests.

Like other techniques described thus far, canonical correlation uses the least-squares principle to partition and analyze variance. Basically, two linear composites are developed, one of which is associated with the dependent variables, the other of which is for the independent variables. The relationship between the two linear composites is expressed by the **canonical correlation coefficient**, R_C, which, when squared, indicates the proportion of variance accounted for in the analysis. When there is more than one dimension of covariation in the two sets of variables, more than one canonical correlation can be found.

Examples of research using canonical correlation are not common, perhaps because of its complexity and perhaps because it is problematic as a hypothesis-testing technique.

Example of canonical correlation:
Lucas, Orshan, and Cook (2000) used canonical correlation to explore various components of Pender's Health Promotion Model. They studied the role of cognitive-perceptual factors (e.g., self-esteem, perceived health) and modifying factors (e.g., age, income) in various health-promoting behaviors (e.g., stress management) among community-dwelling older women. Two dimensions of covariation were identified; the value of R_C for the first canonical variate was .74.

Multivariate Analysis of Variance

Multivariate analysis of variance (**MANOVA**) is the extension of ANOVA to more than one dependent variable. MANOVA is used to test the significance of differences in group means for two or more dependent variables, considered simultaneously. For instance, if we wanted to examine the effect of two methods of exercise on both diastolic and systolic blood pressure, MANOVA would be appropriate. Researchers often analyze such data by performing two separate univariate ANOVAs. Strictly speaking, this practice is incorrect. Separate ANOVAs imply that the dependent variables have been obtained independently of one another when, in fact, they have been obtained from the same subjects and are correlated. MANOVA takes the intercorrelations of dependent variables into account in computing the test statistics. However, ANOVA is a more widely understood procedure than MANOVA, and thus its results may be more easily communicated to a broad audience.

MANOVA can be readily extended in ways analogous to ANOVA. For example, it is possible to perform **multivariate analysis of covariance (MANCOVA)**, which allows for the control of extraneous variables (covariates) when there are two or more dependent variables. MANOVA can also be used when there are repeated measures of the dependent variables.

TIP: One problem with using multivariate procedures is that the findings are less accessible to statistically unsophisticated readers, such as practicing nurses. You may thus opt to use simpler analyses to enhance the utilizability of the findings (e.g., three separate ANOVAs rather than a MANOVA). If the primary reason for *not* using appropriate multivariate procedures is for communication purposes, you should consider running the analyses both ways. You could present bivariate results (e.g., from an ANOVA) in the report, but then note whether a more complex test (e.g. MANOVA) changed the conclusions.

Example of MANOVA:
Fuller (2000) studied infant behaviors in relation to infant age, distress, and level of pain using a three-factor ($2 \times 2 \times 4$) MANOVA. The dependent variables included several measures of infants' behavioral state (e.g., body movements) and four cry measures (e.g., pitch, cry energy). There were numerous significant main effects for all three factors, as well as interaction effects. For example, mean differences in least distressed versus most distressed infants with regard to "arching back," "arm waving," and "knitted brows" were all significant at the .01 level.

Links Among Least-Squares Multivariate Techniques

We could state an analogy that canonical correlation is to multiple regression what MANOVA is to ANOVA. This analogy, although correct, obscures a point that astute readers have perhaps suspected, and that is the close affinity between multiple regression and ANOVA.

In fact, ANOVA and multiple regression are virtually identical. Both techniques analyze total variability in a dependent measure and contrast variability attributable to independent variables with that attributable to random error. Both multiple regression and ANOVA boil down to an F-ratio. By tradition, experimental data typically are analyzed by ANOVA, and correlational data are analyzed by regression. Nevertheless, *any data for which ANOVA is appropriate can also be analyzed by multiple regression*, although the reverse is not true. Multiple regression often is preferable because it is more flexible and provides more information, such as a prediction equation and an index of association, R. (However, most ANOVA programs also indicate the value eta-squared, which also summarizes the strength of association between variables.)

CAUSAL MODELING

Causal modeling involves the development and testing of a hypothesized causal explanation of a phenomenon, typically with data from nonexperimental studies. In a causal model, researchers posit explanatory linkages among three or more variables, and then test whether hypothesized pathways from the causes to the effect are consistent with the data. We briefly describe some features of two approaches to causal modeling without discussing analytic procedures.

Path Analysis

Path analysis, which relies on multiple regression, is a method for studying causal patterns among variables. Path analysis is not a method for discovering causes; rather, it is a method applied to a pre-specified model formulated on the basis of prior knowledge and theory.

Path analytic reports often display results in a **path diagram**; we use such a diagram (Figure 21-6) to illustrate key concepts. This model postulates that the dependent variable, patients' length of hospitalization (V4), is the result of their capacity for self-care (V3); this, in turn, is affected by nursing actions (V1) and the severity of their illness (V2). This model is a **recursive model**, which means that the causal flow is unidirectional and without feedback loops. In other words, it is assumed that variable 2 is a cause of variable 3, and that variable 3 is *not* a cause of variable 2.

In path analysis, a distinction is made between exogenous and endogenous variables. An **exogenous variable** is a variable whose determinants lie outside the model. In Figure 21-6, nursing actions (V1) and illness severity (V2) are exogenous; no attempt is made in the model to elucidate what causes different nursing actions or different degrees of illness. An **endogenous variable**, by contrast, is one whose variation is determined by other variables in the model. In our example, self-care capacity (V3) and length of hospitalization (V4) are endogenous.

Causal linkages are shown on a path diagram by arrows drawn from presumed causes to presumed effects. In our illustration, severity of illness is hypothesized to affect length of hospitalization both directly (path p_{42}) and indirectly through the **mediating variable** self-care capacity (paths p_{32} and p_{43}). Correlated exogenous variables are indicated by curved lines, as shown by the curved line between nursing actions and illness severity.

Ideally, the model would totally explain the outcome of interest (i.e., length of hospitalization).

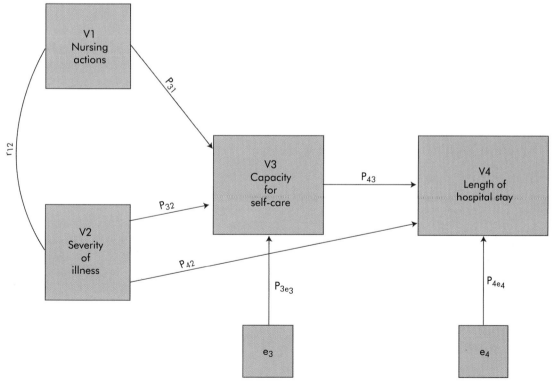

FIGURE 21.6 Path diagram.

In practice, this almost never happens because there are other determinants of the outcome, referred to as **residual variables**. In Figure 21-6, there are two boxes labeled *e*, which denote a composite of all determinants of self-care capacity and hospital stay that are not in the model. If we can identify and measure additional causal forces and incorporate them into the theory, they should be in the model.

Path analysis solves for **path coefficients**, which are the weights representing the effect of one variable on another. In Figure 21-6, causal paths indicate that one variable (e.g., V3) is caused by another (e.g., V2), yielding a path labeled p_{32}. In research reports, path symbols would be replaced by actual path coefficients, which are derived through regression procedures. Path coefficients are standardized partial regression slopes. For example, path p_{32} is equal to $\beta_{32.1}$—the beta weight between variables 2 and 3, holding variable 1 constant. Because path coefficients are in standard form, they indicate the proportion of a standard deviation difference in the caused variable that is directly attributable to a 1.00 SD difference in the specified causal variable. Thus, the path coefficients give us indication about the relative importance of various determinants.

Path analysis estimates path coefficients through the use of **structural equations**. The structural equations for Figure 21-6 are as follows:

$$z_1 = e_1$$
$$z_2 = e_2$$
$$z_3 = p_{31}z_1 + p_{32}z_2 + e_3; \text{ and}$$
$$z_4 = p_{43}z_3 + p_{42}z_2 + e_4$$

These equations indicate that z_1 and z_2 (standard scores for variables 1 and 2) are determined by outside variables (*e*s); that z_3 depends directly on z_1 and z_2 plus outside variables; and that z_4 depends directly on z_2, z_3, and outside variables. These structural equations could be solved to yield path coefficients by performing two multiple regressions: by regressing variable 3 on variables 1 and 2; and by regressing variable 4 on variables 2 and 3.

Path analysis involves a number of procedures for testing causal models and for determining effects. Polit (1996) and Pedhazur (1997) provide an overview of path analytic techniques, and advanced students should refer to books such as the classic text by Blalock (1972).

Example of path analysis:
Berger and Walker (2001) tested an explanatory model of fatigue in women receiving adjuvant breast cancer chemotherapy. The predictor variables in the model included health and functional status, type of chemotherapy protocol, health-promoting lifestyle behaviors, nutritional status, interpersonal relations, symptom distress, and initial reaction to the diagnosis of cancer. In the final model, symptom distress had the strongest direct path to perceived fatigue 48 hours after treatment.

Linear Structural Relations Analysis—LISREL

A drawback of path analysis using ordinary least-squares regression is that the method's validity is based on a set of restrictive assumptions, most of which are virtually impossible to meet. First, it is assumed that variables are measured without error, but (as discussed in Chapter 18) most measures contain some error. Second, it is assumed that residuals (error terms) in the different regression equations are uncorrelated. This assumption is seldom tenable because error terms often represent unmeasured individual differences—differences that are not entirely random. Third, traditional path analysis assumes that the causal flow is unidirectional or recursive. In reality, causes and effects are often reciprocal or iterative.

Linear structural relations analysis, usually abbreviated as **LISREL**,* is a more general and powerful approach that avoids these problems. Unlike path analysis, LISREL can accommodate measurement errors, correlated residuals, and

---

*LISREL is actually the name of a specific computer program for analyzing covariance structures and for performing structural equations modeling, but the software has come to be almost synonymous with the approach.

nonrecursive models that allow for reciprocal causation. Another attractive feature of LISREL is that it can be used to analyze causal models involving latent variables. A **latent variable** is an unmeasured variable corresponding to an abstract construct. For example, factor analysis yields information about underlying, latent dimensions that are not measured directly. In LISREL, latent variables are captured by two or more measured variables (**manifest variables**) that are indicators of the underlying construct.

Path analysis uses least-squares estimation with its associated assumptions and restrictions. LISREL uses a different estimation procedure known as **maximum likelihood estimation**. Maximum likelihood estimators are ones that estimate the parameters most likely to have generated the observed measurements.

LISREL proceeds in two phases. In the first phase, which corresponds to a confirmatory factor analysis (CFA), a measurement model is tested. When there is evidence of an adequate fit of the data to the hypothesized measurement model, the causal model is tested by structural equation modeling.

The Measurement Model Phase

The **measurement model** stipulates the hypothesized relationships among latent and manifest variables. In path analysis, it is assumed—unrealistically—that underlying constructs on the one hand and the scales used to measure them on the other are identical. In LISREL, constructs are treated as unobserved variables measured by two or more fallible indicators. Thus, a major strength of LISREL is that it enables researchers to separate latent variables from errors, and then to study causal relationships among latent variables. The process depends on the judicious selection of indicators. A faulty selection of measured variables to represent a latent variable leads to questions about whether the theory's constructs are really embedded in the causal model.

During the measurement model phase, LISREL tests three things: (1) causal relationships between measured and latent variables, (2) correlations between pairs of latent variables, and (3) correlations among the errors associated with the measured variables. The measurement model is essentially a factor analytic model that seeks to confirm a hypothesized factor structure. Thus, loadings on the factors (the latent variables) provide a method for evaluating relationships between observed and unobserved variables.

We illustrate with a simplified example involving the relationship between two latent variables: a student's cognitive ability and academic success. In our example, depicted in Figure 21-7, cognitive ability is captured by two indicators: scores on the verbal and quantitative portions of the GRE. According to the model, people's test scores are *caused by* their cognitive ability (and thus the arrows indicating a hypothesized causal path), and are also affected by error (e_1 and e_2). Moreover, it is hypothesized that the error terms are correlated, as indicated by the curved line connecting e_1 and e_2. Correlated measurement errors on the GRE might arise as a result of the person's test anxiety or level of fatigue—factors that would systematically depress test scores on both parts of the examination. The second latent variable is academic success, which is captured by undergraduate and graduate GPAs. The error terms associated with these two manifest variables are presumed not to be correlated but, within the measurement model, the two latent variables *are* hypothesized to be correlated.

The hypothesized measurement model then would be tested against actual data using LISREL. The analysis would provide loadings of the observed variables on the latent variables, the correlation between the two latent variables, and the correlation between e_1 and e_2. The analysis would also indicate whether the overall model fit is good, based on a **goodness-of-fit statistic**. If the hypothesized model is not a good fit to the study data, the measurement model could be respecified and retested.

The Structural Equations Model Phase

After an adequate measurement model has been found, the second phase of LISREL can proceed. As in path analysis, researchers specify the theoretical causal model to be tested. As an example, we could use LISREL to test a model in which we hypothesized that the latent variable cognitive ability

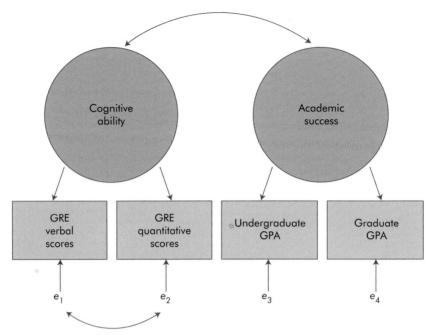

FIGURE 21.7 Example of a measurement model.

caused the latent variable academic success. The model being tested would look similar to the one in Figure 21-7, except that there would be a straight line and an arrow (i.e., a path) from cognitive ability to academic success. There would also be an arrow leading to academic success from a residual term.

In this part of the analysis, LISREL yields information about the hypothesized causal parameters—that is, the path coefficients, which are presented as beta weights. The coefficients indicate the expected amount of change in the latent endogenous variable that is caused by a change in the latent causal variable. The LISREL program provides information on the significance of individual paths. The residual terms—the amount of unexplained variance for the latent endogenous variables—can also be calculated from the LISREL analysis. The overall fit of the causal model to the research data can be tested by means of several alternative statistics. Two such statistics are the **goodness-of-fit index (GFI)** and the **adjusted goodness-of-fit index (AGFI)**. For both indexes, a value of .90 or greater indicates a good fit of the model to the data.

LISREL has gained considerable popularity among nurse researchers, but is a highly complex procedure. Readers interested in further information on LISREL are urged to consult Jöreskog and Sörbom (1997), Kelloway (1998), or Bollen and Bollen (1989).

Example of LISREL:
Mahon and Yarcheski (2001) used LISREL to test two models predicting health outcomes and interpersonal outcomes in relation to depression among early adolescents. In both models, depressed mood contributed fairly strongly to depressive symptoms, which in turn affected health and interpersonal outcomes.

OTHER MULTIVARIATE STATISTICAL PROCEDURES

The statistical procedures described in this and the previous two chapters cover most of the techniques for analyzing quantitative data used by nurse researchers today. However, the widespread use of computers and new developments in statistical analysis have combined to give researchers more options for analyzing their data than in the past. Although a full exposition of other sophisticated statistical procedures is beyond the scope of this book, we briefly describe a few advanced techniques and provide references for those interested in fuller discussion.

Survival and Event History Analysis

Survival analysis (or **life table analysis**) is widely used by epidemiologists and medical researchers when the dependent variable is a time interval between an initial event and a terminal event (e.g., when the initial event is disease onset or initiation of treatment, and death is the end event). Survival analysis calculates a survival score, which compares survival time for one subject with that for other subjects. When researchers are interested in group comparisons—for example, comparing the survival function of subjects in an experimental group versus a control group—a statistic can be computed to test the null hypothesis that the groups are samples from the same survival distribution.

Survival analysis can be applied to many situations unrelated to mortality. For example, survival analysis could be used to analyze such time-related phenomena as length of time in labor, length of time elapsed between release from a psychiatric hospital and reinstitutionalization, and length of time between the termination of a first pregnancy and the onset of a second one. Further information about survival analysis can be found in Harrell (2001) and Lee (1992).

More recently, extensions of survival analysis have been developed that allow researchers to examine determinants of survival-type transitions in a multivariate framework. In these analyses, independent variables are used to model the risk (or hazard) of experiencing an event at a given point in time, given that one has not experienced the event before that time. The most common specification of the hazard is known as the **Cox proportional hazards model**. Further information may be found in Therneau and Grambsh (2000) and Hougaard (2000).

Example of a hazards model:
Cowan, Pike, and Budzynski (2001) used Cox proportional hazards regression to assess the impact of psychosocial nursing therapy after sudden cardiac arrest on 2-year survival. The risk of cardiovascular death was significantly reduced by the intervention, even after controlling for such factors as depression, prior myocardial infarction, and decreased heart rate variability.

Logistic Regression

Logistic regression (sometimes referred to as **logit analysis**) uses maximum likelihood estimation for analyzing relationships between multiple independent variables and a categorical dependent variable. Logistic regression transforms the probability of an event occurring (e.g., that a woman will practice breast self-examination) into its odds. The **odds** of an event is the ratio of two probabilities: the probability of an event occurring to the probability that it will not occur. Probabilities that range between zero and one in actuality are transformed into continuous variables that range between zero and infinity. Because this range is still restricted, a further transformation is performed, namely calculating the logarithm of the odds. The range of this new variable (known as the **logit**) is from minus to plus infinity. Using the logit as the dependent variable, a maximum likelihood procedure estimates the coefficients of the independent variables.

Logistic regression is based on the assumption that the underlying relationships among variables is an S-shaped probabilistic function—an assumption that is usually more tenable than the least-squares assumption of linearity and multivariate normality. Logistic regression thus is often more technically appropriate than discriminant analysis, which also has categorical dependent variables. In practice, logistic regression and discriminant analysis often yield the same results. Logistic regression, however, is better suited to many research questions because it models the probability of an outcome rather than predicting group membership. Also, logistic regression enables the researcher to generate odds ratios that can be meaningfully interpreted and graphically displayed. An **odds ratio** (OR) is the ratio of one odds to another odds, and thus is an index of relative risk—that is, the risk of an event occurring given one condition, versus the risk of it occurring given a different condition. Logistic regression was rarely used 20 years ago because of the lack of convenient computer programs, but that is no longer the case.

Example of logistic regression:
Nyamathi, Leake, Longshore, and Gelberg (2001) examined the congruity between homeless women's self-reports of cocaine use and hair assays for the presence of cocaine. They used logistic regression analysis to predict underreporting of cocaine use. Being Latina, younger, and living primarily in shelters were significant predictors of underreporting. For example, the odds of underreporting were twice as high among women whose usual living place in the prior month was shelters than among other women (OR = 2.01, $p < .05$).

THE COMPUTER AND MULTIVARIATE STATISTICS

Multivariate analyses are invariably done by computer because computations are complex. To illustrate computer analyses for two multivariate techniques, we return to the example described in Chapters 19 and 20, involving the implementation of a special prenatal intervention for low-income young women. Data for these examples were presented in Table 19-8.

Example of Multiple Regression

In Chapter 20, we tested the hypothesis that older mothers in the sample had infants with higher birth weights than younger mothers, using Pearson's r. The calculated value of r was .594, which was highly significant, thereby supporting the research hypothesis.

Suppose now that we want to test whether we can significantly *improve* our ability to predict infant birth weight by adding two predictor variables in a multiple regression analysis: whether the mother smoked while pregnant, and number of

prior pregnancies. Figure 21-8 presents part of the Statistical Package for the Social Sciences (SPSS) printout for a stepwise multiple regression in which infant birth weight is the dependent variable and maternal age, smoking status, and number of prior pregnancies are predictor variables. We will explain some of the most noteworthy aspects of this printout.

The top panel of Figure 21-8 shows that the first variable to enter the regression equation is mother's age. The second panel (Model Summary) indicates that $R = .594$–the same value shown in Figure 20-6 as the bivariate correlation. The value of R^2 is .353 ($.594^2$), which represents the proportion of variance in birth weight accounted for by mother's age.* Maternal age was the first of the three predictor variables stepped into the equation because it had the highest bivariate correlation with birth weight. (The r between birth weight and number of pregnancies is .32, and the r between birth weight and smoking status is $-.24$.)

The next panel (ANOVA) shows the calculation of the F-ratio in which variability due to regression (i.e., to the relationship between birth weight and maternal age) is contrasted with residual variability. The value of F (15.252) with 1 and 28 df is significant at the .001 level, consistent with information from Figure 20-6.

The actual regression equation is presented in the next panel (Coefficients). If we wanted to predict new values of birth weight based on maternal age at birth, the equation would be:

Birth weight' = (3.119 × age) + 48.040

That is, predicted birth weight values would be equal to the regression coefficient ($b = 3.119$) times values of maternal age (X), plus the value of the intercept constant ($a = 48.040$).

In regression, a statistical test can be performed for each regression coefficient by dividing b by the standard error for b; this is shown here

---

*The adjusted R^2 of .330 is the R^2 after it has been adjusted to reflect more closely the goodness of fit of the regression model in the population, through a formula that involves sample size and number of independent variables.

Regression

Variables Entered/Removed[a]

Model	Variables Entered	Variables Removed	Method
1	Mother's age		Stepwise (Criteria: Probability-of-F-to-enter <= .050, Probability-of-F-to-remove >= .100)

a. Dependent Variable: Infant birth weight in ounces

Model Summary

Model	R	R Square	Adjusted R Square	Std. Error of the Estimate
1	.594[a]	.353	.330	8.9702

a. Predictors: (Constant), Mother's age

ANOVA[b]

Model		Sum of Squares	df	Mean Square	F	Sig.
1	Regression	1227.283	1	1227.283	15.252	.001[a]
	Residual	2253.017	28	80.465		
	Total	3480.300	29			

a. Predictors: (Constant), Mother's age
b. Dependent Variable: Infant birth weight in ounces

Coefficients[a]

Model		Unstandardized Coefficients		Standardized Coefficients	t	Sig.
		B	Std. Error	Beta		
1	(Constant)	48.040	14.600		3.290	.003
	Mother's age	3.119	.799	.594	3.905	.001

a. Dependent Variable: Infant birth weight in ounces

Excluded Variables[b]

Model		Beta In	t	Sig.	Partial Correlation	Colinearity Statistics Tolerance
1	No. of prior pregnancies	.020[a]	.108	.915	.021	.727
	Smoking status	−.072[a]	−.446	.659	−.086	.910

a. Predictor: in the model (Constant), Mother's age
b. Dependent Variable: infact birth weight in ounces

FIGURE 21.8 Statistical Package for the Social Sciences (SPSS) printout for a stepwise multiple regression.

under the columns *t* and Sig. The value of *t* for the age coefficient is 3.905, which is significant at the .001 level.

The final panel (Excluded Variables) shows the two predictors not yet in the equation, number of prior pregnancies and smoking status. The figure shows that the *t* values associated with the regression coefficients for the two predictors are both nonsignificant (*p* = .915 and .659, respectively), once variation due to maternal age is taken into account. Because of this fact, the stepwise regression ends at this point, without adding new predictors. Given the significance criterion of .05 (shown in the top panel of "probability of *F* to enter = .050"), neither of the two predictor variables would have significantly added to the prediction of birth weight, over and above what was already achieved with maternal age.

It is, of course, possible to *force* the two additional predictors into the regression equation by doing a simultaneous regression. When this is done (not shown in the table), the value of *R* increases from .594 to .598, a negligible and nonsignificant increase. Thus, we conclude that we cannot improve our ability to predict infant birth weight with the two additional predictors available.

Example of Analysis of Covariance

In Chapter 20, we tested the hypothesis that infants in the experimental group have higher birth weights than infants in the control group, using a *t*-test. The computer calculated *t* to be 1.44, which was nonsignificant with 28 *df*. The research hypothesis was therefore rejected.

Through ANCOVA, we can test the same hypothesis controlling for maternal age, which, as we have just seen, is significantly correlated with birth weight. Figure 21-9 presents the printout for ANCOVA for this analysis, with birth weight as the dependent variable, maternal age (AGE) as the covariate, and GROUP (experimental versus control) as the independent variable. The first panel shows that the group variable involves 15 experimentals and 15 controls. In

the next panel (Tests of between-subjects effects), we see that the *F*-value for the covariate AGE is 24.358, significant at the .000 level (i.e., beyond the .001 level). After controlling for AGE, the *F*-value for the independent variable GROUP is 8.719, which is significant at the .006 level. In other words, once AGE is controlled, the research hypothesis about experimental versus control differences is supported rather than rejected. The total amount of variability explained with the two variables (1777.228), when contrasted with residual variability (1703.072), is also significant (*F* = 14.088, *p* < .000). The multiple R^2 for predicting birth weight, based on both AGE and GROUP, is .511—substantially more than the R^2 between maternal age and birth weight alone (.352).

The next panel shows the overall mean (104.70) for the sample; the standard error (1.45); and the 95% confidence interval for estimating the population mean (CI = 101.725 to 107.675). The bottom panel shows the group means after they are adjusted for maternal age (i.e., the results of an MCA). The original, unadjusted means for the experimental and control groups were 107.53 and 101.87, respectively (Figure 20-5). After adjusting for maternal age, however, the experimental mean is 109.08, and the control mean is 100.32, a much more sizable difference.

GUIDE TO MULTIVARIATE STATISTICAL TESTS

With the widespread availability of computers and user-friendly programs for performing statistical analysis, multivariate statistics have become increasingly common in nursing studies. As with bivariate statistical tests, the selection of a multivariate procedure depends on several factors, including the nature of the research question and the measurement level of the variables. Table 21-8 summarizes some of the major features of several of the multivariate statistics discussed in this chapter and thus serves as an aid to the selection of an appropriate procedure.

Univariate Analysis of Variance

Between-Subjects Factors

		Value	Label	N
Treatment group	1	Experimenta l	15
	2	Control	15

Test of Between-Subjects Effects

Dependent Variable: Infant birth weight in ounces

Source	Type III Sum of Squares	df	Mean Square	F	Sig.
Corrected Model	1777.228[a]	2	888.614	14.088	.000
Intercept	572.734	1	572.734	9.080	.006
AGE	1536.395	1	1536.395	24.358	.000
GROUP	549.945	1	549.945	8.719	.006
Error	1703.072	27	63.077		
Total	332343.000	30			
Corrected Total	3480.300	29			

a. R Squared = .511 (Adjusted R Squared = .474)

Estimated Marginal Means

1. Grand Mean

Dependent Variable: Infant birth weight in ounces

Mean	Std. Error	95% Confidence Interval	
		Lower Bound	Upper Bound
104.700[a]	1.450	101.725	107.675

a. Evaluated at covariates appeared in the model: Mother's age = 18.1667.

2. Treatment group

Dependent Variable: Infant birth weight in ounces

Treatment group	Mean	Std. Error	95% Confidence Interval	
			Lower Bound	Upper Bound
Experimental	109.080[a]	2.074	104.824	113.337
Control	100.320[a]	2.074	96.063	104.576

a. Evaluated at covariates appeared in the model: Mother's age = 18.1667.

FIGURE 21.9 Printout for ANCOVA analysis.

TABLE 21.8 Guide to Selected Multivariate Analyses

TEST NAME	PURPOSE	MEASUREMENT LEVEL OF VARIABLES*			NUMBER OF VARIABLES†		
		IV	DV	Cov	IVs	DVs	Cov
Multiple regression/ correlation	To test the relationship between 2+ IVs and 1 DV; to predict a DV from 2+ IVs	N, I, R	I, R	—	2+	1	—
Analysis of covariance (ANCOVA)	To test the difference between the means of 2+ groups, while controlling for 1+ covariate	N	I, R	N, I, R	1+	1	1+
Multivariate analysis of variance (MANOVA)	To test the difference between the means of 2+groups for 2+ DVs simultaneously	N	I, R	—	1+	2+	—
Multivariate analysis of covariance (MANCOVA)	To test the difference between the means of 2+ groups for 2+ DVs simul-taneously, while controlling for 1+ covariate	N	I, R	N, I, R	1+	2+	1+
Discriminant analysis	To test the relationship between 2+ IVs and 1 DV; to predict group membership; to classify cases into groups	N, I, R	N	—	2+	1	—
Canonical correlation	To test the relationship between 2 sets of variables	N, I, R	N, I, R	—	2+	2+	—
Factor analysis	To determine the dimen-sionality and structure of a set of variables	—	—	—	—	—	—
Logistic regression	To test the relationship between 2+ IVs and 1 DV; to predict the probability of on event; to estimate relative risk	N, I, R	N	—	2+	1	—

*Variables: IV, independent variable; DV, dependent variable; Cov, covariate.

†Measurement levels: N, nominal; I, interval; R, ratio.

RESEARCH EXAMPLE

Johnson and her colleagues (1999) conducted an evaluation of a nurse-delivered smoking cessation intervention for hospitalized cardiac disease patients and used many multivariate procedures. They used a nonequivalent control group before—after design, using smokers admitted to two inpatient cardiac units in a large Canadian hospital. Patients in one unit received the intervention, which involved two in-hospital contacts followed by 3 months of telephone support. Patients in the other unit received no special intervention.

The main outcome measures in the study were (1) self-reported smoking status 6 months after enrollment, and (2) self-reported smoking cessation self-efficacy, measured using the Smoking Abstinence Self-Efficacy Scale. When factor analyzed, this 20-item Likert scale revealed three stable factors, which were used to form three subscales: a positive/social subscale, a negative/affective subscale, and a habit/addictive subscale.

Using bivariate tests (*t*-tests and chi-squared tests), the researchers compared baseline characteristics of the experimental and comparison group in terms of age, gender, marital status, education, and other demographic characteristics. The two groups were found to be comparable in most respects, but the experimental group was significantly more affluent and significantly less likely to have been admitted for cardiac surgery. The groups had similar smoking histories.

Six months after enrollment in the study, 30.8% of control subjects and 46.0% of experimental subjects reported they were not smoking. A chi-squared test indicated that, although sizable, this difference was not statistically significant. The researchers then conducted a logistic regression to predict smoking abstinence based on group assignment, while controlling for important covariates (e.g., income, surgical status, prior smoking history). They found that those in the control group were about three times as likely as those in the experimental group to resume smoking, net of background factors (OR = 3.18), which was significant at the .05 level.

Multiple regression was used to predict scores on the three subscales of the self-efficacy scale. These analyses revealed that, with background variables controlled, being in the treatment group was a significant predictor of scores on the positive/social and habit/addictive subscales. The total amount of variance accounted for in these two regression analyses was 33% and 39%, respectively. Although the researchers used a quasi-

experimental design, their strategy of statistically controlling a number of background characteristics strengthened the internal validity of the study.

SUMMARY POINTS

- **Multivariate statistical procedures** are increasingly being used in nursing research to untangle complex relationships among three or more variables.
- Simple **linear regression** makes predictions about the values of one variable based on values of a second variable. **Multiple regression** is a method of predicting a continuous dependent variable on the basis of two or more independent variables.
- The **multiple correlation coefficient** (R) can be squared (R^2) to estimate the proportion of variability in the dependent variable accounted for by the independent variables.
- **Simultaneous multiple regression** enters all predictor variables into the regression equation at the same time. **Hierarchical multiple regression** enters predictors into the equation in a series of steps controlled by researchers. **Stepwise multiple regression** enters predictors in steps using a statistical criterion for order of entry.
- **Analysis of covariance** (ANCOVA) extends ANOVA by removing the effect of extraneous variables (**covariates**) before testing whether mean group differences are statistically significant.
- **Multiple classification analysis** (MCA) is a supplement to ANCOVA that yields information about the **adjusted means** of groups on a dependent variable, after removing the effect of covariates.
- **Factor analysis** is used to reduce a large set of variables into a smaller set of underlying dimensions, called **factors**. Mathematically, each factor is a linear combination of variables in a data matrix.
- The first phase of factor analysis (**factor extraction**) identifies clusters of variables with a high degree of communality and condenses a larger set of variables into a smaller number of factors.

- The second phase of factor analysis involves **factor rotation**, which enhances the interpretability of the factors by aligning variables more distinctly with a particular factor.
- **Factor loadings** shown in a rotated factor matrix can be examined to identify and name the underlying dimensionality of the original set of variables and to compute **factor scores**.
- **Discriminant analysis** is used to make predictions about dependent variables that are categorical (i.e., predictions about membership in groups) on the basis of two or more predictor variables.
- **Canonical correlation** analyzes the relationship between two or more independent *and* two or more dependent variables; it yields a canonical correlation coefficient, R_C.
- **Multivariate analysis of variance** (**MANOVA**) is the extension of ANOVA to situations in which there is more than one dependent variable.
- **Causal modeling** involves the development and testing of a hypothesized causal explanation of a phenomenon.
- **Path analysis**, a regression-based method for testing causal models, involves the preparation of a **path diagram** that stipulates hypothesized causal links among variables. Path analysis tests **recursive models**, that is, ones in which causation is presumed to be unidirectional.
- Path analysis applies **ordinary least-squares regression** to a series of **structural equations**, resulting in a series of **path coefficients**. The path coefficients represent weights associated with a causal path, in standard deviation units.
- **Linear structural relations analysis** (**LISREL**), another approach to causal modeling, does not have as many assumptions and restrictions as path analysis. LISREL can accommodate measurement errors, **nonrecursive models** that allow for reciprocal causal paths, and correlated errors.
- LISREL can analyze causal models involving **latent variables**, which are not directly measured but which are captured by two or more **manifest variables** (i.e., measured variables).
- LISREL proceeds in two sequential phases: the measurement model phase and the structural equations modeling phase. The **measurement model** stipulates the hypothesized relationship between latent variables and manifest variables; if the measurement model fits the data, the hypothesized causal model is then tested.
- Most multivariate procedures described in the chapter are based on least-squares estimation, but LISREL is based on a different estimation procedure known as **maximum likelihood**; maximum likelihood estimates the parameters most likely to have generated observed data.
- **Logistic regression,** another multivariate procedure based on maximum likelihood estimation, is used to predict categorical dependent variables. A useful feature of this technique is that it yields an **odds ratio** that is an index of relative risk, that is, the risk of an outcome occurring given one condition, versus the risk of it occurring given a different condition.
- **Survival analysis** and other related event history methods are used when the dependent variable of interest is a time interval (e.g., time from onset of a disease to death).

STUDY ACTIVITIES

Chapter 21 of the accompanying *Study Guide for Nursing Research: Principles and Methods, 7th ed.*, offers various exercises and study suggestions for reinforcing the concepts presented in this chapter. In addition, the following study questions can be addressed:

1. Refer to Figure 21-1. What would the value of Y' be for the following X values: 8, 1, 3, 6?
2. A researcher has examined the relationship between preventive health care attitudes on the one hand and the person's educational level, age, and gender on the other. The multiple correlation coefficient is .62. Explain the meaning of this statistic. How much variation in attitudinal scores is explained by the three predictors? How much is *unexplained*? What other variables might improve the power of the prediction?

3. Using power analysis, determine the sample size needed to achieve power = .80 for α = .05, when:
   a. estimated R^2 = .15, k = 5
   b. estimated R^2 = .33, k = 10
4. Which multivariate statistical procedures would you recommend using in the following situations:
   a. A researcher wants to test the effectiveness of a nursing intervention for reducing stress levels among surgical patients, using an experimental group of patients from one hospital and a control group from another hospital.
   b. A researcher wants to predict which college students are at risk of a sexually transmitted disease using background information such as gender, academic grades, socioeconomic status, religion, and attitudes toward sexual activity.
   c. A researcher wants to test the effects of three different diets on blood sugar levels and blood pH.

SUGGESTED READINGS

Methodologic References

Aaronson, L. S. (1989). A cautionary note on the use of stepwise regression. *Nursing Research, 38,* 309–311.

Aaronson, L. S., Frey, M., & Boyd, C. J. (1988). Structural equation models and nursing research: Part II. *Nursing Research, 37,* 315–318.

Blalock, H. M., Jr. (1972). *Causal inferences in nonexperimental research.* New York: W. W. Norton.

Bollen, K., & Bollen, W. (1989). *Structural equations with latent variables.* New York: John Wiley.

Boyd, C. J., Frey, M. A., & Aaronson, L. S. (1988). Structural equation models and nursing research: Part I. *Nursing Research, 37,* 249–253.

Cohen, J., & Cohen, P. (1984). *Applied multiple regression: Correlation analysis for behavioral sciences* (2nd ed.). Hillsdale, NJ: Lawrence Erlbaum.

Goodwin, L. D. (1984). Increasing efficiency and precision of data analysis: Multivariate vs. univariate statistical techniques. *Nursing Research, 33,* 247–249.

Hair, J. F., Anderson, R. E., Tatham, R. L., & Black, W. (1998). *Multivariate data analysis* (5th ed.). Upper Saddle River, NJ: Prentice-Hall.

Harrell, F. E. (2001). *Regression modeling strategies: With applications to linear models, logistic regression, and survival analysis.* New York: Springer-Verlag.

Holt, F., Merwin, E., & Stern S. (1996). Alternative statistical methods to use with survival data. *Nursing Research, 45,* 345–349.

Hougaard, P. (2000). *Analysis of multivariate survival data.* New York: Springer-Verlag.

Jaccard, J., & Becker, M. A. (2001). *Statistics for the behavioral sciences* (4th ed.). Belmont, CA: Wadsworth.

Jöreskog, K. G., & Sörbom, D. (1997). *LISREL 8: User's reference guide.* Mooresville, IN: Scientific Software International.

Kelloway, E. K. (1998). *Using LISREL for structural equation modeling: A researcher's guide.* Thousand Oaks, CA: Sage.

Kim, J., Kaye, J., & Wright L. K. (2001). Moderating and mediating effects in causal models. *Issues in Mental Health Nursing, 22,* 63–75.

Knapp, T. R. (1994). Regression analysis: What to report. *Nursing Research, 43,* 187–189.

Knapp, T. R., & Campbell-Heider, N. (1989). Numbers of observations and variables in multivariate analyses. *Western Journal of Nursing Research, 11,* 634–641.

Lee, E. T. (1992). *Statistical methods for survival data analysis* (2nd ed.). New York: John Wiley & Sons.

Mason-Hawkes, J. & Holm, K. (1989). Causal modeling: A comparison of path analysis and LISREL. *Nursing Research, 38,* 312–314.

Musil, C. M., Jones, S. L., & Warner, C. D. (1998). Structural equation modeling and its relationship to multiple regression and factor analysis. *Research in Nursing & Health, 21,* 271–281.

Pedhazur, E. J. (1997). *Multiple regression in behavioral research* (3rd ed.). New York: Harcourt College Publishers.

Polit, D. F. (1996). *Data analysis and statistics for nursing research.* Stamford, CT: Appleton & Lange.

Tabachnick, B. G., & Fidell, L. S. (2000). *Using multivariate statistics* (4th ed.). New York: HarperCollins College Publishers.

Weisberg, S. (1985). *Applied linear regression* (2nd ed.). New York: John Wiley & Sons.

Welkowitz, J., Ewen, R. B., & Cohen, J. (2000). *Introductory statistics for the behavioral sciences* (5th ed.). New York: Harcourt College Publishers.

Wu, Y. B., & Slakter, M. J. (1989). Analysis of covariance in nursing research. *Nursing Research, 38*, 306–308.

Studies Cited in Chapter 21

Aminzadeh, F., & Edwards, N. (2000). Factors associated with cane use among community dwelling older adults. *Public Health Nursing, 17*, 474–483.

Badger, T. A., & Collins-Joyce, P. (2000). Depression, psychosocial resources, and functional ability in older adults. *Clinical Nursing Research, 9*, 238–255.

Badr (Zahr), L. K. (2001). Quantitative and qualitative predictors of development for low birth-weight infants of Latino background. *Applied Nursing Research, 14*, 125–135.

Berger, A. M., & Walker, S. N. (2001). An explanatory model of fatigue in women receiving adjuvant breast cancer chemotherapy. *Nursing Research, 50*, 42–52.

Cowan, M. J., Pike, K., & Budzynski, H. K. (2001). Psychosocial nursing therapy following sudden cardiac arrest: Impact on two-year survival. *Nursing Research, 50*, 68–76.

Fuller, B. F., (2000). Fluctuations in established infant pain behaviors. *Clinical Nursing Research, 9*, 298–316.

Johnson, J. L., Budz, B., Mackay, M., & Miller, C. (1999). Evaluation of a nurse-delivered smoking cessation intervention for hospitalized patients with cardiac disease. *Heart & Lung, 28*, 55–64.

Lucas, J. A., Orshan, S. A., & Cook, F. (2000). Determinants of health-promoting behavior among women ages 65 and above living in the community. *Scholarly Inquiry for Nursing Practice, 14*, 77–100.

Mahon, N. E., & Yarcheski, A. (2001). Outcomes of depression in early adolescents. *Western Journal of Nursing Research, 23*, 360–375.

McCarter-Spaulding, D. E. & Kearney, M. H. (2001). Parenting self-efficacy and perception of insufficient breast milk. *Journal of Obstetric, Gynecologic, and Neonatal Nursing, 30*, 515–522.

Misener, T. R., & Cox, D. L. (2001). Development of the Misener Nurse Practitioner Job Satisfaction Scale. *Journal of Nursing Measurement, 9*, 91–108.

Nyamathi, A., Leake, B., Longshore, D., & Gelberg, L. (2001). Reliability of homeless women's reports: Concordance between hair assay and self report of cocaine use. *Nursing Research, 50*, 165–171

Tarkka, M. T., Paunonen, M., & Laippala, P. (2000). First-time mothers and child care when the child is 8 months old. *Journal of Advanced Nursing, 31*, 20–26.

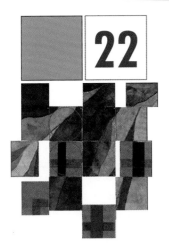

22

Designing and Implementing a Quantitative Analysis Strategy

The successful analysis of quantitative data requires careful planning and attention to detail. This chapter provides an overview of steps that are normally taken in designing and implementing a **data analysis plan**. The final phase of data analysis, interpreting the results, also is discussed.

PHASES IN THE ANALYSIS OF QUANTITATIVE DATA

The data analysis process varies from one project to another. With small, simple sets of data, researchers may be able to proceed quickly from data collection to data analysis. In most cases, however, intermediary steps are necessary. Figure 22-1 shows what the flow of tasks might look like, organized in a series of phases. Progress in analyzing quantitative data is not always as linear as this figure suggests, but the figure provides a framework for discussing various steps in the analytic process.

PREANALYSIS PHASE

The first set of steps, shown in Figure 22-1 as the Preanalysis Phase, involves various clerical and administrative tasks. These might include logging

data in and maintaining appropriate administrative records, reviewing data forms for completeness and legibility, taking steps to retrieve pieces of missing information, and assigning identification (ID) numbers. Another task involves selecting a statistical ssoftware package for doing the data analyses. Once these tasks have been performed, researchers typically must code the data and enter them onto computer files to create a **data set** (the total collection of data for all sample members) for analysis.

TIP: The most widely used statistical software packages are the Statistical Package for the Social Sciences (SPSS) and the Statistical Analysis System (SAS). Both packages contain programs for a variety of descriptive, bivariate, and multivariate analyses.

Coding Quantitative Data

Computers usually cannot process data in the form they are collected. **Coding** is the process of transforming data into symbols compatible with computer analysis.

Coding Inherently Quantitative Variables

Certain variables are inherently quantitative (e.g., age, body temperature) and do not normally require

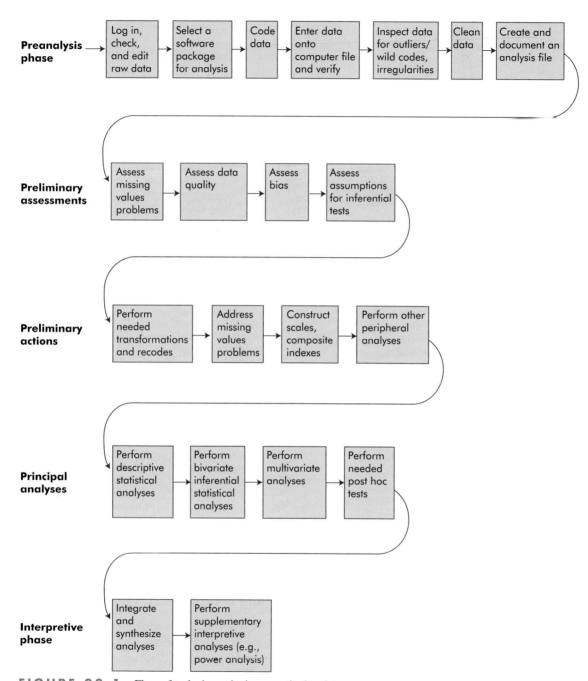

FIGURE 22.1 Flow of tasks in analyzing quantitative data.

coding. Researchers may, however, ask for information of this type in a way that *does* call for some coding. If a researcher asks respondents to indicate whether they are younger than 30 years of age, between the ages of 30 and 49 years, or 50 years or older, then responses would have to be coded. When responses to questions such as age, height, and so forth are obtained in their full form, the information should not be reduced to coded categories for data entry purposes; this can be accomplished later, if desired.

Even with "naturally" quantitative data, researchers should inspect and edit their data. All responses should be of the same form and precision. For example, in entering a person's height onto a computer file, researchers would need to decide whether to use feet and inches or to convert the information entirely to inches. Whichever method is adopted, it must be used consistently for all subjects. There must also be consistency in the method of handling information reported with different degrees of precision (e.g., coding a response such as 5 feet 2½ inches).

Precoded Data

Most data from structured instruments can be precoded (i.e., codes assigned even before data are collected). For example, closed-ended questions with fixed response alternatives can be preassigned a numeric code, as in the following:

> From what type of program did you receive your basic nursing preparation?
> 1. Diploma school
> 2. Associate degree program
> 3. Baccalaureate degree program

Nurses who received their nursing preparation from a diploma school would be coded 1 for this variable, and so on.

Codes are often arbitrary, as in the case of a variable such as gender. Whether a female subject is coded 1 or 2 has no bearing on subsequent analyses as long as female subjects are consistently assigned one code and male subjects another. Other variables,

such as ordinal-level variables, have a less arbitrary coding scheme, as in the following example:

> How often do you take a nap?
> 1. Almost never
> 2. Once or twice a year
> 3. Three to 11 times a year
> 4. Once a month or more often

Respondents sometimes can check off more than one response to a question, as in the following:

> To which of the following journals do you subscribe?
> ( ) *Applied Nursing Research*
> ( ) *Canadian Journal of Nursing Research*
> ( ) *Clinical Nursing Research*
> ( ) *Nursing Research*
> ( ) *Qualitative Health Research*
> ( ) *Research in Nursing & Health*
> ( ) *Western Journal of Nursing Research*

With questions of this type, it is not appropriate to adopt a 1-2-3-4-5-6-7 code because respondents may check several, or none, of the responses. The correct procedure for such questions is to treat each journal separately. In other words, researchers would code responses as though the item were seven separate questions, that is, "Do you subscribe to *Applied Nursing Research*? Do you subscribe to the *Canadian Journal of Nursing Research*?" and so on. A check mark beside a journal would be treated as a "yes." The question would yield seven dichotomous variables, with one code (e.g., 1) signifying "yes" and another code (e.g., 2) signifying "no."

Coding Uncategorized Data

Qualitative data from open-ended questions, unstructured observations, and other narrative forms must be coded if they are going to be used in quantitative analysis. Sometimes researchers can develop codes for such variables ahead of time. For instance, a question might ask, "What is your occupation?" In this case, it might be possible to predict major job categories (e.g., professional, managerial, clerical).

Usually, however, unstructured data are collected specifically because it is difficult to anticipate the kind of information that will be obtained. In such situations, codes are developed after the data are collected. Researchers typically begin by reviewing a sizable portion of the data to get a feel for the content, and then develop a category scheme. The scheme should reflect both theoretical and analytic goals as well as the substance of the information. The amount of detail in the category scheme can vary, but too much detail usually is better than too little detail. In developing such a coding scheme, the only rule is that the categories should be both mutually exclusive and collectively exhaustive.

Precise coding instructions should developed and documented in a coding manual. Coders, like observers and interviewers, must be properly trained. Intercoder reliability checks are strongly recommended.

Coding Missing Values

A code should be assigned to each variable for every sample member, even if no response is available. **Missing values** can be of various types. A person responding to an interview question may be undecided, refuse to answer, or say, "Don't know." When skip patterns are used, there is missing information for those questions that are irrelevant to some sample members. In observational studies, an observer may get distracted during a 10-second sampling frame, may be undecided about an appropriate categorization, or may observe behavior not listed on the observation schedule. It is sometimes important to distinguish between various types of missing data with different codes (e.g., distinguishing refusals and "don't knows"). In other cases, a single missing values code may suffice. This decision must be made with the conceptual aims of the research in mind.

Researchers often strive to code missing data in a similar fashion for all or most variables. If a nonresponse is coded as a 4 on variable 1, a 6 on variable 2, a 5 on variable 3, and so forth, there is a greater risk of error than if a uniform code is adopted. The choice of what code to use for missing data is fairly arbitrary, but numeric codes must be ones that have not been used for actual pieces of information. Many researchers follow the convention of coding missing data as 9 because this value is out of the range of real codes for most variables. Others use blanks, periods, or negative values to indicate missing information.

TIP: Some statistical software specifies how missing data should be coded, so you should decide what software to use before finalizing coding decisions.

Entering, Verifying, and Cleaning Data

Coded data must be entered onto a computer file for analysis, and then verified and cleaned. This section provides an overview of these procedures, but technological advances make it inevitable that the information we provide will need to be updated.

Data Entry

Coded data typically are transferred onto a data file through a keyboard or computer terminal. Various computer programs can be used for data entry, including spreadsheets or databases. Major software packages for statistical analysis also have data editors that make data entry fairly easy.

Figure 22-2 presents a portion of a data file for the Statistical Package for the Social Sciences (SPSS), for data that we used in analytic examples in the preceding three chapters and that were displayed in Table 19-8. The entire data file is a 30-by-10 matrix, with 30 rows (1 for each subject) and 10 columns (1 to 3 for each variable); this figure displays data for only the first 15 subjects (all experimental group subjects) to conserve space. Each variable had to be given a brief name (id, bweight, etc.). The computer also had to be told whether each variable was categorical or continuous; for example, group (experimental versus control) is categorical with only two values, 1 or 2. Birth weight (bweight), however, is continuous, ranging from 76 on up. Researchers have to specify the maximum "width" of continuous variables (e.g., could the variable *priors*, number of prior pregnancies, equal 10 or more, which would

	id	group	bweight	repeat	age	priors	smokstat
1	1	1	107	1	17	1	1
2	2	1	101	0	14	0	0
3	3	1	119	0	21	3	0
4	4	1	128	1	20	2	0
5	5	1	89	0	15	1	1
6	6	1	99	0	19	0	1
7	7	1	111	0	19	1	0
8	8	1	117	1	18	1	1
9	9	1	102	1	17	0	0
10	10	1	120	0	20	0	0
11	11	1	76	0	13	0	1
12	12	1	116	0	18	0	1
13	13	1	100	1	16	0	0
14	14	1	115	0	18	0	0
15	15	1	113	0	21	2	1

FIGURE 22.2 Portion of an SPSS data file.

require two columns?). It is sometimes necessary to indicate how many places to the right of the decimal point are required (two places is the typical default). Once this information is specified, coded data can be typed in, one subject at a time.

Each subject should be assigned a unique ID number, and this number should be entered along with actual data. This allows researchers to go back to the original source if there are any difficulties with the data file. Usually, a consecutive numbering scheme is used, running from number 1 to the number of actual cases. The ID number normally is entered as the first variable of the record, as was the case in Figure 22-2.

Data Verification and Cleaning

Data entry is a tedious and error-prone task and so it is necessary to verify the entries and correct any mistakes. Several methods of verification exist. The first is to compare visually the numbers printed on a printout of the data file with codes on the original source. A second possibility is to enter all the data twice and to compare the two sets of records, either visually or by computer. Finally, there are special verifying programs designed to perform comparisons during direct data entry.

Even verified data usually contain some errors. Such errors could result from data entry mistakes, coding problems, or misreporting of information. Data are not ready for analysis until they have been cleaned. **Data cleaning** involves two types of checks. The first is a check for outliers and wild codes. **Outliers** are values that lie outside the normal range of values for other cases. Outliers can be found by inspecting frequency distributions, paying special attention to the lowest and highest values. In some cases, the outliers are true, legitimate values (e.g., an annual income of $2 million in a distribution where all other incomes are below $200,000). In other cases, however, outliers indicate an error in data entry that needs to be corrected, as when the frequency distribution reveals a **wild code**—that is, a code that is not possible. For example, the variable gender might have the following three defined codes: 1 = female, 2 = male, and 9 = not reported. If we discovered a code of 5 in our data file for gender, it would be clear that an error had been made. The computer could be instructed to list the ID number of the culpable record, and the error could be corrected by finding the proper code on the original source. Another procedure is to use a program for data entry that automatically performs range checks.

Editing of this type, of course, will never reveal all errors. If the gender of a male subject is entered incorrectly as a 1, the mistake may never be detected. Because errors can have a big effect on the analysis and interpretation of data, it is naturally important to perform the coding, entering, verifying, and cleaning with great care.

The second data-cleaning procedure involves **consistency checks**, which focus on internal data consistency. In this task, researchers check for errors by testing whether data for different variables are compatible. For example, one question in a survey might ask respondents their current marital status, and another might ask how many times they had been married. If the data were internally consistent, respondents who answered "Single, never married" to the first question should have a zero (or a missing values code) for the second. As another example, if the respondent's gender were entered with the code for male and there was an entry of 2 for the variable "Number of pregnancies," then one of those two fields would contain an error. Researchers should search for opportunities to check the consistency of entered data.

Creating and Documenting the Analysis Files

Once the data set has been created and cleaned, researchers proceed to develop an analysis file, using one of the many available statistical software packages. If the data set was not created within a statistical software package—that is, if it is simply a file of numeric data values—the computer must be told basic information about the data set, such as what the variable names are, where to find values for those variables in the file, and how to determine where one case ends and another one begins.

The decisions that researchers make about coding, variable naming, and so on should be documented in full. Memory should not be trusted; several weeks after coding, researchers may no longer remember if male subjects were coded 1 and female subjects 2, or vice versa. Moreover, colleagues may wish to borrow the data set to perform a secondary analysis. Regardless of whether one anticipates a secondary analysis, documentation should be sufficiently thorough so that a person unfamiliar with the original research project could use the data.

Documentation primarily involves preparing a codebook. A **codebook** is essentially a listing of each variable together with information about placement in the file, codes associated with the values of the variable, and other basic information. Codebooks can be generated by statistical or data entry programs.

Figure 22-3 presents a portion of the SPSS-generated codebook for the first three variables in the data set shown in Figure 22-2. This codebook shows variable names in the left column, variable position in the file in the right column, and then various types of information about the variables (e.g., measurement level, width of the data, coded values) in the middle. We see that the variable GROUP, for example, has an extended label, "Treatment Group." GROUP is specified as a nominal variable occupying only one column (F1). Data for this variable have values coded either 1 for experimental subjects or 2 for controls. No missing data code is specified because all subjects are known to be in either one or the other group. By contrast, the variable BWEIGHT (infant birth weight in ounces) allows for missing data, with a missing values code of 999.

List of variables on the working file

Name		Position
ID	Subject identification number	1
	Measurement Level: Nominal	
	Column Width : Unknown Alignment: Center	
	Print Format : F2	
	Write Format : F2	
GROUP	Treatment group	2
	Measurement Level: Nominal	
	Column Width : Unknown Alignment: Center	
	Print Format : F1	
	Write Format : F1	

Value	Label
1	Experimental
2	Control

Name		Position
BWEIGHT	Infant birth weight in ounces	3
	Measurement Level: Scale	
	Column Width : 6 Alignment: Center	
	Print Format : F3	
	Write Format : F3	
	Missing Values: 999	

FIGURE 22.3   Portion of an SPSS-generated codebook.

PRELIMINARY ASSESSMENTS AND ACTIONS

Researchers typically undertake preliminary assessments of their data and several preanalytic activities before they test their hypotheses. Several preparatory activities are discussed next.

Assessing and Handling Missing Values Problems

Researchers usually find that their data set has some missing values. There are various ways of dealing with missing data. In selecting an approach, researchers should first determine the distribution and patterning of missing data. The appropriate solution depends on such factors as the extent of missing data, the role the variable with missing data plays in the analysis (i.e., whether the missing values are for dependent, independent, or descriptive variables), and the randomness of the missing data (i.e., whether missing values are related in any systematic way to important variables in the study). The magnitude of the problem differs if only 2% of the values for a relatively minor variable are missing, as opposed to 20% of the values for the main dependent variable. Also, if the missing values disproportionately come from people with certain characteristics, there is likely some bias.

The first step, then, is to determine the extent of the problem by examining frequency distributions on a variable-by-variable basis. (Most researchers routinely begin data analysis by running **marginals**—constructing frequency distributions—for all or most variables in their data set.) Another step is to examine the cumulative extent of missing values. Statistical programs can be used to create **flags** to count how many variables are missing for each sample member. Once a missing values flag has been created, a frequency distribution can be computed for this new variable, which would show how many cases had no missing values, one missing value, and so on.

Another task is to evaluate the randomness of missing values. A simple procedure is to divide the sample into two groups—those with missing data on a specified variable and those without missing data. The two groups can then be compared in terms of other variables in the data set to determine if the two groups are comparable (e.g., were men more likely than women to leave certain questions blank?). Similarly, groups can be created based on the missing values flag (e.g., those with no missing data versus those with *any* missing data) and compared on other variables.

Once researchers have assessed the extent and patterning of missing values, decisions must be made about how to address the problem. Solutions include the following:

1. *Delete missing cases.* One simple strategy is to delete a case (i.e., a subject) entirely if there is missing information. When samples are small, it is irksome to throw away an entire case—especially if data are missing for only one or two variables. It is, however, advisable to delete cases for subjects with extensive missing information. This strategy is sometimes referred to as **listwise deletion** of missing values.

2. *Delete the variable.* Another option is to throw out information for particular variables for all subjects. This option is especially suitable when a high percentage of cases have missing values on a specific variable. This may occur if, for example, a question was objectionable and was left blank, or if many respondents did not understand directions and inadvertently skipped it. When missing data on a variable are extensive, there may be systematic biases with regard to those subjects for whom data *are* available. This approach clearly is not attractive if the variable is a critical independent or dependent variable.

3. *Substitute the mean or median value.* When missing values are reasonably random and when the problem is not extensive, it may be useful to substitute real data values for missing value codes. Such a substitution represents a "best guess" about what the value would have been, had data actually been collected. Because of this fact, researchers usually substitute a value that is typical for the sample, and typical values usually come from the center of the distribution. For example, if data for a subject's age were missing and if the average age of subjects in the sample were 45.2 years, we might substitute the value 45 in place of the missing values code for subjects whose age is unknown.

This approach is especially useful when there are missing values for variables that comprise a multiple-item scale, such as a Likert scale. Suppose, for example, we had a 20-item scale that measures anxiety, and that one person answered only 18 of the 20 items. It would not be appropriate to score the scale by adding together responses on the 18 items only, and it would be a waste of information on the 18 answered items to code the entire scale as missing. Thus, for the two missing items, the researcher could substitute the most typical responses (based on either the mean, median, or mode, depending on the distribution of scores), so that a scale score on the full 20 items could be computed. Needless to say, this approach makes sense only when a small proportion of scale items is missing. And, if the scale is a test of knowledge rather than a measure of a psychosocial characteristics, it usually is more appropriate to consider a missing value as a "don't know" and to mark the item as incorrect.

4. *Estimate the missing value.* When researchers substitute a mean value for a missing value, there is a risk that the substitution is erroneous, perhaps dramatically so. For example, if the mean value of 45 is substituted for a missing value on a subject's age, but the range of ages in the sample is 25 to 70 years, then the substituted

value could be wrong by 20 years or more. When only a couple of cases have missing data for the variable age, an error of even this magnitude is unlikely to alter the results. However, if missing values are more widespread, it is sometimes worthwhile to substitute values that have a greater likelihood of being accurate.

Various procedures can be used to derive estimates of what the missing value should be. One simple method is to use the mean for a subgroup that is most like the case with the missing value. For example, suppose the mean age for women in the sample were 42.8 years and the mean age for men were 48.9 years. The researcher could then substitute 43 for women with missing age data and 49 for men with missing age data. This likely would result in improved accuracy, compared with using the overall mean of 45 for all subjects with missing age data.

Another method is to use multiple regression to "predict" the correct value of missing data. To continue with the example used previously, suppose that subjects' age was correlated with gender, education, and marital status in this research sample. Based on data from subjects without missing values, these three variables could be used to develop a regression equation that could predict age for subjects whose age information is missing but whose values for the three other variables are not missing.

Some statistical software packages (such as SPSS) have a special procedure for estimating the value of missing data. These procedures can also be used to examine the relationship between the missing values and other variables in the data set.

5. *Delete cases pairwise*. Perhaps the most widely used (but not necessarily the best) approach is to delete cases selectively, on a variable-by-variable basis. For example, in describing the characteristics of the sample, researchers might use whatever information is available for each characteristic, resulting in a fluctuating number of cases across descriptors. Thus, the mean age might be based on 95 cases, the gender distrib-

ution might be based on 102 cases, and so on. If the number of cases fluctuates widely across characteristics, the information is difficult to interpret because the sample of subjects is essentially a "moving target."

The same strategy is sometimes used to handle missing information for dependent variables. For example, in an evaluation of an intervention to reduce patient anxiety we might have blood pressure, self-reported anxiety, and an observational measure of stress-related behavior as the dependent variables. Suppose that 10 people out of a sample of 100 failed to complete the anxiety scale. We might base the analyses of the anxiety data on the 90 subjects who completed the scale, but use the full sample of 100 subjects in the analyses of the other dependent variables. The problem with this approach is that it can cause interpretive problems, especially if there are inconsistent findings across outcomes. For example, if there were experimental versus control group differences on all outcomes except the anxiety scale, one possible explanation is that the anxiety scale sample is not representative of the full sample. Researchers usually strive for a **rectangular matrix** of data: data values for all subjects on all important variables. In the example just described, we should, at a minimum, perform supplementary analyses using the rectangular matrix—that is, rerun *all* analyses using the 90 subjects for whom complete data are available. If the results are different from when the full sample was used, we would at least be in a better position to interpret results.

In analyses involving a correlation matrix, researchers sometimes use **pairwise deletion** of cases with missing values. Figure 22-4 illustrates a correlation matrix with four variables in which pairwise deletion of missing values was used on a nonrectangular data matrix. As this figure shows, correlations between pairs of variables are based on varying numbers of cases (shown in the row labeled *N*), ranging from 425 subjects for the correlation

Correlations

		Highest school grade completed	Total # people in hh	Total Household Income	CES-D Score (Range 0 to 60)
Highest school grade completed	Pearson Correlation sig. (2 tailed) N	1.000 484	−.127** .005 483	.068 .154 437	−.081 .082 460
Total # people in hh	Pearson Correlation sig. (2 tailed) N	−.127** .005 483	1,000 492	.196** .000 446	−.021 .649 467
Total Household Income	Pearson Correlation sig. (2-tailed) N	.068 .154 437	.196** .000 446	1.000 446	−.178** .000 425
CES-D score (Range 0 to 60)	Pearson Correlation Sig. (2-tailed) N	−.081 .082 460	−.021 .649 467	−.178** .000 425	1.000 468

**Correlation is significant at the 0.01 level (2-tailed).

FIGURE 22.4 Correlation matrix for a nonrectangular data matrix.

between Center for Epidemiological Studies Depression scale (CES-D) scores and total income, to 483 subjects for the correlation between highest grade and total number of people in the household. Pairwise deletion is acceptable for descriptive purposes if data are missing at random and differences in *N*s are small. It is especially imprudent to use this procedure for multivariate analyses such as multiple regression because the criterion correlations (i.e., the correlations between the dependent variable and the various predictors) are based on nonidentical subsets of subjects.

Each of these solutions has accompanying problems, so care should be taken in deciding how missing data are to be handled. Procedures for dealing with missing data are discussed at greater length in Allison (2000), Little and Rubin (1990), and Kneipp and McIntosh (2001).

Example of handling missing values:
Berger and Walker (2001) used path analysis to model fatigue in women receiving adjuvant breast cancer chemotherapy. Many of their variables, including the dependent variable, were measured using composite psychosocial scales. The report noted that "sample median substitutions were performed for missing items on all scales; there were no cases in which more than 10% of the responses were missing" (p. 48).

Assessing Quantitative Data Quality

Steps are often undertaken to assess data quality in the early stage of analysis. For example, when psychosocial scales or composite indexes are used, researchers should usually assess their internal consistency reliability (see Chapter 18). The distribution of data values for key variables also should be examined to determine any anomalies, such as limited variability, extreme skewness, or the presence of ceiling or floor effects. For example, a vocabulary test for 10-year-olds likely would yield a clustering of high scores in a sample of 11-year-olds, creating a **ceiling effect** that would reduce correlations between test scores and other characteristics of the children. Conversely, there likely would be a clustering of low scores on the test with a sample of 9-year-olds, resulting in a **floor effect** with similar consequences. In such situations, data may need to be transformed to meet the requirements for certain statistical tests.

Assessing Bias

Researchers often undertake preliminary analyses to assess the direction and extent of any biases, including the following:

- *Nonresponse bias.* When possible, researchers should determine whether a biased subset of people participated in a study. If there is information about the characteristics of all people who were asked to participate in a study (e.g., demographic information from hospital records), researchers should compare the characteristics of those who did and did not participate to determine the nature and direction of any biases. This means that the data file would have to include both respondents and nonrespondents, and a variable indicating their response status (e.g., a variable could be coded 1 for participants and 2 for those who declined to participate).
- *Selection bias.* When nonequivalent comparison groups are used (in quasi-experimental or nonexperimental studies), researchers should check for selection biases by comparing the groups' background characteristics. It is particularly important to examine possible group differences on extraneous variables that are strongly related to the dependent variable. These variables can (and should, if possible) then be controlled—for example, through analysis of covariance (ANCOVA) or multiple regression. Even when an experimental design has been used, researchers should check the success of randomization. Random assignment does not *guarantee* equivalent groups, so researchers should be aware of characteristics for which the groups are not, in fact, comparable.
- *Attrition bias.* In longitudinal studies, it is always important to check for attrition biases, which involves comparing people who did and

did not continue to participate in the study in later waves of data collection, based on characteristics of these groups at the initial wave.

In performing any of these analyses, significant group differences are an indication of bias, and such bias must be taken into consideration in interpreting and discussing the results. Whenever possible, the biases should be controlled in testing the main hypotheses.

Example of assessing bias: Cimprich and Ronis (2001) studied differences in capacity to direct attention among older women with and without breast cancer. Before undertaking the main analyses, the two groups were compared in terms of background characteristics. Significant group differences were observed for age, marital status, and health problems; these variables were used as covariates in the substantive analyses.

Testing Assumptions for Statistical Tests

Most statistical tests are based on a number of assumptions—conditions that are presumed to be true and, when violated, can lead to misleading or invalid results. For example, parametric tests assume that variables are distributed normally. Frequency distributions, scatter plots, and other assessment procedures provide researchers with information about whether underlying assumptions for statistical tests have been violated.

Frequency distributions can reveal whether the normality assumption is tenable; graphic displays of data values indicate whether the distribution is severely skewed, multimodal, too peaked (**leptokurtic**), or too flat (**platykurtic**). There are also statistical indexes of skewness or peakedness that statistical programs can compute to determine whether the shape of the distribution deviates significantly from normality.

Example of testing assumptions: Gulick (2001) used multiple regression to explore the relationship of emotional distress, social support, and personal attributes vis-à-vis functional status in people with multiple sclerosis. She examined scatter plots and performed other analysis to determine if the assumptions of linearity and normality were met.

Performing Data Transformations

Raw data entered directly onto a computer file often need to be modified or transformed before hypotheses can be tested. Various **data transformations** can easily be handled through commands to the computer. All statistical software packages can create new variables through arithmetic manipulations of variables in the original data set. We present a few examples of such transformations, covering a range of realistic situations.

- *Performing item reversals.* Sometimes response codes to certain variables need to be reversed (i.e., high values becoming low, and vice versa) so that items can be combined in a composite scale. For example, the widely used CES-D scale consists of 20 items, 16 of which are statements indicating negative feelings in the prior week (e.g., item 9 states, "I thought my life had been a failure"), and four of which indicate positive feelings (e.g., item 8 states, "I felt hopeful about the future"). The positively worded items must be reversed before items are added together. CES-D items have four response options, from 1 (rarely felt that way) to 4 (felt that way most days). To reverse an item (i.e., to convert a 4 to a 1, and so on), the raw value of the item is subtracted from the maximum possible value, plus 1. In SPSS, this can be accomplished through the "Compute" command, which could be used to set the value of a new variable to 5 minus the value of the original variable; for example, a new variable CESD8R could be computed as the value of $5 - CESD8$, where CESD8 is the original value of item 8 on the CESD scale.
- *Constructing scales.* Transformations are also used to construct composite scale variables, using responses to individual items. Commands

for creating such scales in statistical software packages are straightforward, using algebraic conventions. In SPSS, the "Compute" command could again be used to create a new variable; for example, a new variable STRESS could be set equal to $Q1 + Q2 + Q3 + Q4 + Q5$.
- *Performing counts.* Sometimes composite indexes are created when researchers want a cumulative tally of the occurrence of some attribute. For example, suppose we asked people to indicate which types of illegal drug they had used in the past month, from a list of 10 options. Use of each drug would be answered independently in a yes (coded 1) or no (coded 2) fashion. We could then create a variable indicating the number of different drugs used. In SPSS, the "Count" command would be used, creating a new variable (e.g., DRUGS) equal to the sum of all the "1" codes for the 10 drug items. Note that counting is the approach used to create missing values flags, described earlier in this chapter.
- *Recoding variables.* Other transformations involve recoding values to change the nature of the original data. For example, in some analyses, an infant's original birth weight (entered on the computer file in grams) might be used as a dependent variable. In other analyses, however, the researcher might be interested in comparing the subsequent morbidity of low-birth-weight versus normal-birth-weight infants. For example, in SPSS, the "Recode Into Different Variable" command could be used to recode the original variable (BWEIGHT) into a new dichotomous variable with a code of 1 for a low-birth-weight infant and a code of 2 for a normal-birth-weight infant, based on whether BWEIGHT was less than 2500 grams.
- *Meeting statistical assumptions.* Transformations also can be undertaken to render data appropriate for statistical tests. For example, if a distribution is markedly non-normal, a transformation can sometimes be done to make parametric procedures appropriate. A logarithmic transformation, for example, tends to normalize distributions. In SPSS, the "Compute" command could be used

to normalize the distribution of values on family income (INCOME), for instance, by computing a new variable (e.g., INCLOG) set equal to the natural log of the values on INCOME. Discussions of the use of transformations for changing the characteristics of a distribution can be found in Dixon and Massey (1983) and Ferketich and Verran (1994).

Example of transforming variables:
Faulkner, Hathaway, Milstead, and Burghen (2001) studied heart rate variability in adolescents and adults with type 1 diabetes, compared with healthy control subjects. Several of their measures of heart beat variability (e.g., changes in heart rate with deep breathing and the Valsalva maneuver) were positively skewed, and so logarithmically transformed variables were used as the dependent variables.

• *Creating dummy variables.* Data transformations may be needed to convert codes for multivariate statistics. For example, for dichotomous variables, researchers most often use a 0-1 code (rather than, say, a 1-2 code) to facilitate interpretation of regression coefficients. Thus, if the original codes for gender were 1 for women and 2 for men, men could be recoded to 0 for a regression analysis.

TIP: Whenever you create transformed variables, it is important to check that the transformations were done correctly by examining a sample of values for the original and transformed variables. This can be done by instructing the computer to list the values of the newly created variables and the original variables used to create them for a sample of cases.

Performing Additional Peripheral Analyses

Depending on the study, additional peripheral analyses may be needed before proceeding to substantive analyses. It is impossible to catalog all such analyses, but a few examples are provided to alert readers to the kinds of issues that need to be given some thought.

• *Data pooling.* Researchers sometimes obtain data from more than one source or from more than one type of subject. For example, to enhance the generalizability of their findings, researchers sometimes draw subjects from multiple sites, or may recruit subjects with different medical conditions. The risk in doing this is that subjects may not really be drawn from the same population, and so it is wise in such situations to determine whether **pooling** of data (combining data for all subjects) is warranted. This involves comparing the different subsets of subjects (i.e., subjects from the different sites, and so on) in terms of key research variables.

Example of testing for pooling:
Kammer (1994) studied the relationship between stress appraisal and coping among people responsible for older adults placed in nursing homes. Subjects from two sites were compared on key variables to determine if the data could be pooled.

• *Cohort effects.* Nurse researchers sometimes need to gather data over an extended period of time to achieve adequate sample sizes. This can result in **cohort effects**, that is, differences in outcomes or subject characteristics over time. This might occur because sample characteristics evolve over time or because of changes in the community, in families, in health care, and so on. If the research involves an experimental treatment, it may also be that the treatment itself is modified—for example, if early program experience is used to improve the treatment or if those administering the treatment simply get better at doing it. Thus, researchers with a long period of sample intake should consider testing for cohort effects because such effects can confound the results or even mask existing relationships. This activity usually involves examining correlations between entry dates and key research variables.

Example of testing for cohort effects:
Polit, London, and Martinez (2001), in their study of health problems among low-income mothers, used survey data that were collected over a 12-month period. They discovered that women interviewed later were significantly more disadvantaged than those interviewed early. In their multivariate analysis, a variable for timing of the interview was statistically controlled.

• *Ordering effects.* When a crossover design is used (i.e., subjects are randomly assigned to different orderings of treatments), researchers should assess whether outcomes are different for people in the different treatment-order groups.

Example of testing for ordering effects:
Keele-Smith and Price-Daniel (2001) tested the hypothesis that blood pressure measurements are higher when people cross their legs. Subjects were randomly assigned to different orderings of the treatment (crossing versus not crossing legs), and blood pressure was measured in both conditions. The researchers found that blood pressure was significantly higher when subjects legs' were crossed; ordering of conditions (crossed first versus uncrossed first) did not affect the outcome.

• *Manipulation checks.* In testing an intervention, the primary research question is whether the treatment was effective in achieving the intended outcome. Researchers sometimes also want to know whether the intended treatment was, in fact, received. Subjects may perceive a treatment, or respond to it, in unanticipated ways, and this can influence treatment effectiveness. Therefore, researchers sometimes build in mechanisms to test whether the treatment was actually in place. For example, suppose we were testing the effect of noise levels on stress, exposing two groups of subjects to two different noise levels in a laboratory setting. As a **manipulation check**, we could ask subjects to rate how noisy they perceived the settings to be. If subjects did not rate the noise levels in the two

settings differently, it would probably affect our interpretation of the results—particularly if stress in the two groups turned out not to be significantly different.

Example of a manipulation check:
Melnyk and co-researchers (2001) did a pilot study to evaluate the effectiveness of an early neonatal intensive care unit intervention. The mothers in the study were administered a brief "test" to ensure that they had processed information they had received.

PRINCIPAL ANALYSES

At this point in the analysis process, researchers have a cleaned data set, with missing data problems resolved and needed transformations completed; they also have some understanding of data quality and the extent of biases. They can now proceed with more substantive data analyses.

The Substantive Data Analysis Plan

In many studies, researchers collect data on dozens, and often hundreds, of variables. They cannot realistically analyze every variable in relation to all others, and so a plan to guide data analysis must be developed. Research hypotheses and questions provide only broad and general direction.

One approach is to prepare a list of the analyses to be undertaken, specifying both the variables and the statistical test to be used. Another approach is to develop table shells. **Table shells** are layouts of how researchers envision presenting the research findings in a report, without any numbers in the table. Once a table shell has been prepared, researchers can undertake analyses to fill in the table entries.

Table 22-1 presents an example of an actual table shell created for an evaluation of an intervention for low-income women. This table guided a series of ANCOVAs that compared experimental and control groups in terms of several indicators of emotional well-being, after controlling for various characteristics measured at random assignment. The

TABLE 22.1 Example of a Table Shell: Program Impacts on Indicators of Emotinal Well-Being at the Time of the Follow-up Interview*

OUTCOME	EXPERIMENTAL GROUP	CONTROL GROUP	DIFFERENCE	p
Mean score on the CES-D (depression) scale				
Percentage at risk of clinical depression (scores of 16 and above on the CES-D)				
Mean score, Mastery (self-efficacy) scale				
Mean score, Difficult Life Circumstances scale				
Percentage who cited no one available as a social support				
Mean number of categories of social support cited as available				
Mean level of satisfaction with available social support				

*Analyses to be performed using ANCOVA, controlling for 15 baseline characteristics.

completed table that eventually appeared in the research report was somewhat different than this table shell (e.g., another outcome variable was added). Researchers do not need to adhere rigidly to table shells, but they provide an excellent mechanism for organizing the analysis of large amounts of data.

Substantive Analyses

The next step is to perform the actual substantive analyses, typically beginning with descriptive analyses. For example, researchers usually develop a descriptive profile of the sample, and often look descriptively at correlations among variables. These initial analyses may suggest further analyses or further data transformations that were not originally envisioned. They also give researchers an opportunity to become familiar with their data.

TIP: When you begin to do analyses to acquaint yourself better with the data, resist the temptation of going on a "fishing expedition,"

that is, hunting for *any* interesting relationships between variables. The facility with which computers can generate statistical information makes it easy to run analyses rather indiscriminately. The risk is that you will serendipitously find significant correlations between variables as a function of chance. For example, in a correlation matrix with 10 variables (which results in 45 nonredundant correlations), there are likely to be two to three *spurious* significant correlations when alpha = .05 (i.e., .05 × 45 = 2.25).

Researchers then perform statistical analyses to test their hypotheses. Researchers whose data analysis plan calls for multivariate analyses (e.g., multivariate analysis of variance [MANOVA]) may proceed directly to their final analyses, but they may begin with various bivariate analyses (e.g., a series of analyses of variance [ANOVAs]). The primary statistical analyses are complete when all the research questions are addressed and, if relevant, when all table shells have the applicable numbers in them.

INTERPRETATION OF RESULTS

The analysis of research data provides the **results** of the study. These results need to be evaluated and interpreted, giving consideration to the aims of the project, its theoretical basis, the existing body of related research knowledge, and limitations of the adopted research methods. The interpretive task involves a consideration of five aspects of the results: (1) their credibility, (2) their meaning, (3) their importance, (4) the extent to which they can be generalized, and (5) their implications.

Credibility of the Results

One of the first interpretive tasks is assessing whether the results are accurate. This assessment, in turn, requires a careful analysis of the study's methodologic and conceptual limitations. Regardless of whether one's hypotheses are supported, the validity and meaning of the results depend on a full understanding of the study's strengths and shortcomings.

Such an assessment relies heavily on researchers' critical thinking skills and on their ability to be reasonably objective. Researchers should carefully evaluate (e.g., using criteria such as those presented in Chapter 26) the major methodologic decisions they made in planning and executing the study and consider whether different decisions might have yielded different results.

In assessing the credibility of results, researchers seek to assemble different types of evidence. One type of evidence comes from prior research on the topic. Investigators should examine whether their results are consistent with those of other studies; if there are discrepancies, a careful analysis of the reasons for any differences should be undertaken. Evidence can often be developed through peripheral data analyses, some of which were discussed earlier in this chapter. For example, researchers can have greater confidence in the accuracy of their findings if they have established that their measures are reliable and have ruled out biases.

Another recommended strategy is to conduct a power analysis. In Chapters 20 and 21, we de-scribed how power analysis can be used before a study is undertaken to estimate sample size needs. Researchers can also determine the *actual* power of their analyses, to determine the probability of having committed a Type II error. It is especially useful to perform a power analysis when the results of statistical tests are not statistically significant.

For example, suppose we were testing the effectiveness of an intervention to reduce patients' pain. The sample of 200 subjects (100 subjects each in an experimental and a control group) are compared in terms of pain scores, using a *t*-test. Suppose further that the mean pain score for the experimental group was 7.90 (standard deviation [SD] = 1.3), whereas the mean for the control group was 8.29 (SD = 1.3), indicating lower pain among experimental subjects. Although the results are in the hypothesized direction, the *t*-test was nonsignificant. We can provide a context for interpreting the accuracy of the nonsignificant results by performing a power analysis. First, we must estimate the effect size, using the formula presented in Chapter 20:

$$\gamma = \frac{8.29 - 7.90}{1.3} = .30$$

Table 20-6 in Chapter 20 shows us that, with an effect size of .30, $\alpha = .05$, and a sample size of 100 per group, the power of the statistical test is less than .60. This means that we had more than a 40% risk of committing a Type II error—that is, of incorrectly concluding that the groups were not different.

A critical analysis of the research methods and a scrutiny of various types of external and internal evidence almost inevitably indicates some limitations. These limitations must be taken into account in interpreting the results.

Meaning of the Results

In qualitative studies, interpretation and analysis occur virtually simultaneously. In quantitative studies, however, results are in the form of test statistics and probability levels, to which researchers need to attach meaning. This sometimes involves supplementary analyses that were not originally planned. For example, if research findings are contrary to the hypotheses, other information in the data set sometimes can be examined to help researchers understand what the findings mean. In this section, we discuss the interpretation of various research outcomes within a hypothesis testing context.

Interpreting Hypothesized Results

Interpreting results is easiest when hypotheses are supported. Such an interpretation has been partly accomplished beforehand because researchers have already brought together prior findings, a theoretical framework, and logical reasoning in developing the hypotheses. This groundwork forms the context within which more specific interpretations are made.

Naturally, researchers are gratified when the results of many hours of effort support their predictions. There is a decided preference on the part of individual researchers, advisers, and journal reviewers for studies whose hypotheses have been supported. This preference is understandable, but it is important not to let personal preferences interfere with the critical appraisal appropriate to all interpretive situations. A few caveats should be kept in mind.

First, it is best to be conservative in drawing conclusions from the data. It may be tempting to go beyond the data in developing explanations for what results mean, but this should be avoided. An example might help to explain what we mean by "going beyond" the data. Suppose we hypothesized that pregnant women's anxiety level about labor and delivery is correlated with the number of children they have already borne. The data reveal that a significant negative relationship between anxiety levels and parity ($r = -.40$) exists. We conclude that increased experience with childbirth results in decreased anxiety. Is this conclusion supported by the data? The conclusion appears to be logical, but in fact, there is nothing in the data that leads directly to this interpretation. An important, indeed critical, research precept is: *correlation does not prove causation*. The finding that two

variables are related offers no evidence suggesting which of the two variables—if either—caused the other. In our example, perhaps causality runs in the opposite direction, that is, that a woman's anxiety level influences how many children she bears. Or perhaps a third variable not examined in the study, such as the woman's relationship with her husband, causes or influences both anxiety and number of children.

Alternative explanations for the findings should always be considered and, if possible, tested directly. If competing interpretations can be ruled out, so much the better, but every angle should be examined to see if one's own explanation has been given adequate competition.

Empirical evidence supporting research hypotheses never constitutes *proof* of their veracity. Hypothesis testing is probabilistic. There is always a possibility that observed relationships resulted from chance. Researchers must be tentative about their results and about interpretations of them. In summary, even when the results are in line with expectations, researchers should draw conclusions with restraint and should give due consideration to limitations identified in assessing the accuracy of the results.

 Example of hypothesized significant results:

Steele, French, Gatherer-Boyles, Newman, and Leclaire (2001) tested four hypotheses about the effect of acupressure by Sea-Bands on nausea and vomiting during pregnancy. All four hypotheses were supported.

Interpreting Nonsignificant Results

Failure to reject a null hypothesis is problematic from an interpretative point of view. Statistical procedures are geared toward disconfirmation of the null hypothesis. Failure to reject a null hypothesis can occur for many reasons, and researchers do not know which one applies. The null hypothesis *could* actually be true, for example. The nonsignificant result, in this case, accurately reflects the absence of a relationship among research variables. On the other hand, the null hypothesis could be false, in which case a Type II error has been committed.

Retaining a false null hypothesis can result from such problems as poor internal validity, an anomalous sample, a weak statistical procedure, unreliable measures, or too small a sample. Unless the researcher has special justification for attributing the nonsignificant findings to one of these factors, interpreting such results is tricky. We suspect that failure to reject null hypotheses is often a consequence of insufficient power, usually reflecting too small a sample size. For this reason, conducting a power analysis can help researchers in interpreting nonsignificant results, as indicated earlier.

In any event, researchers are never justified in interpreting a retained null hypothesis as proof of the *absence* of relationships among variables. *Nonsignificant results provide no evidence of the truth or the falsity of the hypothesis.* Thus, if the research hypothesis is that there are no group differences or no relationships, traditional hypothesis testing procedures will *not* permit the required inferences.

When significant results are not obtained, there may be a tendency to be overcritical of the research methods and undercritical of the theory or reasoning on which hypotheses were based. This is understandable: It is easier to say, "My ideas were sound, I just didn't use the right approach," than to admit to faulty reasoning. It is important to look for and identify flaws in the research methods, but it is equally important to search for theoretical shortcomings. The result of such endeavors should be recommendations for how the methods, the theory, or an experimental intervention could be improved.

Example of nonsignificant results:
Vines, Ng, Breggia, and Mahoney (2000) did a pilot study to test the effect of a multimodal pain rehabilitation program on the immune function, pain and depression levels, and health behaviors of patients with chronic back pain. Changes in these measures between baseline and the last week of the treatment program were not significant,

which the researchers speculated might reflect the small sample size ($N = 23$).

Interpreting Unhypothesized Significant Results

Unhypothesized significant results can occur in two situations. The first involves finding relationships that were not considered while designing the study. For example, in examining correlations among variables in the data set, we might notice that two variables that were not central to our research questions were nevertheless significantly correlated—and interesting. To interpret this finding, we would need to evaluate whether the relationship is real or spurious. There may be information in the data set that sheds light on this issue, but we might also need to consult the literature to determine if other investigators have observed similar relationships.

The second situation is more perplexing: obtaining results *opposite* to those hypothesized. For instance, we might hypothesize that individualized teaching about AIDS risks is more effective than group instruction, but the results might indicate that the group method was better. Or a positive relationship might be predicted between a nurse's age and level of job satisfaction, but a negative relationship might be found.

It is, of course, unethical to alter a hypothesis after the results are "in." Some researchers view such situations as awkward or embarrassing, but there is little basis for such feelings. The purpose of research is not to corroborate researchers' notions, but to arrive at truth and enhance understanding. There is no such thing as a study whose results "came out the wrong way," if the "wrong way" is the truth.

When significant findings are opposite to what was hypothesized, it is less likely that the methods are flawed than that the reasoning or theory is incorrect. As always, the interpretation of the findings should involve comparisons with other research, a consideration of alternate theories, and a critical scrutiny of data collection and analysis procedures. The result of such an examination should be a tentative explanation for the unexpected findings, together with suggestions for how such explanations could be tested in other research projects.

Example of unhypothesized significant results:

Pellino (1997) tested the Theory of Planned Behavior to predict postoperative analgesic use after elective orthopedic surgery. The theory predicted that patients with high levels of perceived control would be more likely to intend to use analgesics than those with low levels of perceived control. Just the opposite was found to be true, however, leading Pellino to conclude that the findings "raise issues for research in the use of medications" (p. 104).

Interpreting Mixed Results

Interpretation is often complicated by **mixed results**: Some hypotheses are supported by the data, whereas others are not. Or a hypothesis may be accepted when one measure of the dependent variable is used but rejected with a different measure. When only some results run counter to a theoretical position or conceptual scheme, the research methods are the first aspect of the study deserving critical scrutiny. Differences in the validity and reliability of the various measures may account for such discrepancies, for example. On the other hand, mixed results may suggest that a theory needs to be qualified, or that certain constructs within the theory need to be reconceptualized. Mixed results sometimes present opportunities for making conceptual advances because efforts to make sense of disparate pieces of evidence may lead to key breakthroughs.

Example of mixed results:

Neitzel, Miller, Shepherd, and Belgrade (1999) tested the effects of implementing evidence-based postoperative pain management strategies on patient, provider, and fiscal outcomes. As hypothesized, there were significant effects on provider behavior (e.g., decreased use of meperidine) and nurses' knowledge, as well as on costs. However, patient outcomes (e.g., decreased pain intensity, increased satisfaction) were not affected by the intervention.

In summary, interpreting research results is a demanding task, but it offers the possibility of unique intellectual rewards. Researchers must in essence play the role of scientific detectives, trying to make pieces of the puzzle fit together so that a coherent picture emerges.

TIP: In interpreting your data, remember that others will be reviewing your interpretation with a critical and perhaps even a skeptical eye. Part of your job is to convince others of your interpretation, in a fashion similar to convincing a jury in a judicial proceeding. Your hypotheses and interpretations are, essentially, on trial—and the null hypothesis is considered "innocent" until proven "guilty." Look for opportunities to gather and present supplementary evidence in support of your conclusion. This includes evidence from other studies as well as internal evidence from your own study. Scrutinize your data set to see if there are further analyses that could lend support to your explanation of the findings.

Importance of the Results

In quantitative studies, results that support the researcher's hypotheses are described as significant. A careful analysis of study results involves an evaluation of whether, in addition to being statistically significant, they are important.

Attaining statistical significance does not necessarily mean that the results are meaningful to nurses and their clients. Statistical significance indicates that the results were unlikely to be a function of chance. This means that observed group differences or relationships were probably real, but not necessarily important. With large samples, even modest relationships are statistically significant. For instance, with a sample of 500, a correlation coefficient of .10 is significant at the .05 level, but a relationship this weak may have little practical value. Researchers must pay attention to the numeric values obtained in an analysis in addition to significance levels when assessing the importance of the findings.

Conversely, the absence of statistically significant results does not mean that the results are unimportant—although because of the difficulty in interpreting nonsignificant results, the case is more complex. Suppose we compared two alternative procedures for making a clinical assessment (e.g., body temperature). Suppose further that we retained the null hypothesis, that is, found no statistically significant differences between the two methods. If a power analysis revealed an extremely low probability of a Type II error (e.g., power = .99, a 1% risk of a Type II error), we might be justified in concluding that the two procedures yield equally accurate assessments. If one of these procedures is more efficient or less painful than the other, nonsignificant findings could indeed be clinically important.

Generalizability of the Results

Researchers also should assess the generalizability of their results. Researchers are rarely interested in discovering relationships among variables for a specific group of people at a specific point in time. The aim of research is typically to reveal relationships for broad groups of people. If a new nursing intervention is found to be successful, others will want to adopt it. Therefore, an important interpretive question is whether the intervention will "work" or whether the relationships will "hold" in other settings, with other people. Part of the interpretive process involves asking the question, "To what groups, environments, and conditions can the results of the study reasonably be applied?"

Implications of the Results

Once researchers have drawn conclusions about the credibility, meaning, importance, and generalizability of the results, they are in a good position to make recommendations for using and building on the study findings. They should consider the implications with respect to future research, theory development, and nursing practice.

Study results are often used as a springboard for additional research, and researchers themselves often can readily recommend "next steps." Armed with an understanding of the study's limitations and strengths, researchers can pave the way for new studies that would avoid known pitfalls or capitalize on known strengths. Moreover, researchers are in a

good position to assess how a new study might move a topic area forward. Is a replication needed, and, if so, with what groups? If observed relationships are significant, what do we need to know next for the information to be maximally useful?

For studies based on a theoretical or conceptual model, researchers should also consider the study's theoretical implications. Research results should be used to document support for the theory, suggest ways in which the theory ought to be modified, or discredit the theory as a useful approach for studying the topic under investigation.

Finally, researchers should carefully consider the implications of the findings for nursing practice and nursing education. How do the results contribute to a base of evidence to improve nursing? Specific suggestions for implementing the results of the study in a real nursing context are extremely valuable in the utilization process, as we discuss in Chapter 27.

RESEARCH EXAMPLE

Researchers typically undertake many of the steps depicted in Figure 22-1 without describing them in their research reports. Thus, the research literature does not offer many examples that fully explain the design and implementation of an analysis plan.

Considerable analytic detail, however, was provided in a study by Davis, Maguire, Haraphongse, and Schaumberger (1994), who examined whether the type of preparatory information provided to patients receiving cardiac catheterization (CC) was equally effective in reducing anxiety for patients with different coping styles. The coping styles of the 145 patients who served as subjects in this study were first assessed, and patients were then categorized as either "monitors" (people who coped through information-seeking strategies) or "blunters" (people who coped through an information-avoiding strategy). Using a randomized block design, the two coping-style groups were then randomly assigned to one of three preparatory information treatment conditions: (1) procedural information presented on videotape, (2) procedural–sensory information presented on videotape, and (3) procedural–sensory information presented in a booklet. Anxiety was measured at four points in time: preintervention, postintervention, pre-CC procedure, and post-CC procedure.

The central hypothesis regarding effects on patient anxiety was tested with a 2 × 3 × 4 ANOVA (coping style × preparatory treatment × time period). In addition, the researchers undertook the following analyses:

- The six treatment groups (two coping styles 3 three treatment groups) were compared in terms of basic demographic characteristics (age and education) and preintervention anxiety—an analysis aimed at assessing potential selection effects. One significant difference emerged: Monitors reported more preintervention anxiety than blunters.
- The researchers then wondered whether gender might be implicated in the observed preintervention anxiety differences. A 2 × 3 × 2 ANOVA (coping style × treatment group × gender) yielded a significant gender effect on preintervention anxiety scores (women were significantly more anxious than men). The researchers concluded that gender should be taken into account in their analyses but realized that they had too few women in the sample to analyze results for women separately.
- A subgroup analysis was, however, undertaken with the 107 men in the sample. This analysis revealed a significant coping style × treatment interaction for the preintervention anxiety measure. Male blunters randomly assigned to the three treatment groups were found to be comparable in terms of pretreatment anxiety, but male monitors were not. This analysis, then, indicated that the random assignment did not result in the sought-after anxiety equivalency among the subgroup of male monitors. (A further analysis was performed to determine whether the nonequivalence among groups was the result of only one or two extreme scores on the preintervention anxiety measure, but this proved not to be the case).
- The investigators then explored whether to use preintervention anxiety as a covariate in subsequent analyses, which would allow them to control statistically differences in preintervention anxiety among male blunters. They found that the correlations between preintervention anxiety and postintervention anxiety varied across time and across groups, which discouraged them from using preintervention anxiety as a covariate. The researchers used ANOVA (rather than ANCOVA) for the main analyses, but their knowledge of pretreatment differences was taken into consideration in interpreting the results.

- The researchers calculated effect sizes to draw conclusions about effects that were both statistically and clinically significant. They determined that any mean difference on the anxiety scale of 3 points or greater constituted an effect size of .30, which they established as their criterion for clinical significance.
- The researchers found that, as hypothesized, there was a significant three-way ANOVA interaction. The results indicated that the procedural–sensory videotape treatment was especially beneficial for monitors; the procedural modeling video was the best treatment for blunters. Over time, monitors and blunters in each treatment group had decreased anxiety scores.

The researchers' results included both expected and unexpected findings, which they addressed in the Discussion section of their report. The finding that coping styles moderated the effects of the preparation strategies was predicted from theory and prior research. The finding that women were significantly more anxious than their male counterparts in both coping-style groups led the researchers to recommend that gender be considered as a primary rather than an incidental variable in CC preparatory intervention research.

The unexpected nonequivalence among male monitors led the researchers to consider the following:

> From a theoretic standpoint, it was determined that the observed nonequivalence in state anxiety among the male monitor groups might reflect an important and heretofore unexamined aspect of coping style: the relationship between subjects' monitoring and blunting repertoires and their procedural anxiety levels (p. 136).

The researchers pursued the implications of this suggestion with several supplementary analyses.

In summary, the researchers implemented a thorough and thoughtful analysis plan that took unexpected findings and design quality issues into account in their interpretation.

SUMMARY POINTS

- Researchers who collect quantitative data typically progress through a series of steps in the analysis and interpretation of their data. The careful researcher lays out a **data analysis plan** in advance to guide that progress.

- Quantitative data must be converted to a form amenable to computer analysis through **coding**, which typically transforms all research data into numbers. Special codes need to be developed to code **missing values**.

- Researchers typically document decisions about coding, variable naming, and variable location in a **codebook.**

- **Data entry** is an error-prone process that requires **verification** and **cleaning**. Cleaning involves (1) a check for **outliers** (values that lie outside the normal range of values) and **wild codes** (codes that are not legitimate), and (2) **consistency checks**.

- An important early task in analyzing data involves taking steps to evaluate and address missing data problems. These steps include deleting cases with missing values (i.e., **listwise deletion**), deleting variables with missing values, substitution of mean values, estimation of missing values, and selective **pairwise deletion** of cases. Researchers strive to achieve a **rectangular matrix** of data (valid information on all variables for all cases), and these strategies help researchers to attain this goal.

- Raw data entered directly onto a computer file often need to be transformed for analysis. Examples of **data transformations** include reversing of the coding of items, combining individual variables to form composite scales, recoding the values of a variable, altering data for the purpose of meeting statistical assumptions, and creating dichotomous dummy variables for multivariate analyses.

- Before the main analyses can proceed, researchers usually undertake additional steps to assess data quality and to maximize the value of the data. These steps include evaluating the reliability of measures, examining the distribution of values on key variables for any anomalies, and analyzing the magnitude and direction of any biases.

- Sometimes peripheral analyses involve tests to determine whether **pooling** of subjects is warranted, tests for **cohort effects** or **ordering effects**, and **manipulation checks**.

- Once the data are fully prepared for substantive analysis, researchers should develop a formal analysis plan, to reduce the temptation to go on a "fishing expedition." One approach is to develop **table shells**, that is, fully laid-out tables without any numbers in them.

- The interpretation of research findings typically involves five subtasks: (1) analyzing the credibility of the results, (2) searching for underlying meaning, (3) considering the importance of the results, (4) analyzing the generalizability of the findings, and (5) assessing the implications of the study regarding future research, theory development, and nursing practice.

STUDY ACTIVITIES

Chapter 22 of the accompanying *Study Guide for Nursing Research: Principles and Methods, 7th ed.*, offers various exercises and study suggestions for reinforcing the concepts presented in this chapter. In addition, the following study questions can be addressed:

1. Read the study by Coffman, Levitt, and Brown (1994) entitled "Effects of clarification of support expectations in prenatal couples" (*Nursing Research, 43*, 111–116). Indicate which steps in the process shown in Figure 21-1 are described in this report.
2. Suppose you were studying gender differences in physical health 6 months after loss of a spouse. Create a fictitious table shell for such a study.
3. Read an article in a recent nursing research journal. Write out a brief interpretation of the results based on the reports "Results" section and then compare your interpretation with that of the researchers.

SUGGESTED READINGS

Methodologic References

Allison, P. D. (2000). *Missing data*. Thousand Oaks, CA: Sage.

Dixon, W. J., & Massey, F. J. (1983). *Introduction to statistical analysis* (4th ed.). New York: McGraw-Hill.

Ferketich, S., & Verran, J. (1994). An overview of data transformation. *Research in Nursing & Health, 17,* 393–396.

Harris, M. L. (1991). *Introduction to data processing* (3rd ed.). New York: John Wiley & Sons.

Jacobsen, B. S. (1981). Know thy data. *Nursing Research, 30,* 254–255.

Kniepp, S. M., & McIntosh, M. (2001). Handling missing data in nursing research with multiple imputation. *Nursing Research, 50,* 384–389.

Little, R. J. A., & Rubin, D. B. (1990). The analysis of social science data with missing values. In J. Fox & J. S. Long (Eds.), *Modern methods of data analysis.* Newbury Park, CA: Sage.

Patrician, P. A. (2002). Multiple imputation for missing data. *Research in Nursing & Health, 25,* 76–84.

Polit, D. F. (1996). *Data analysis & statistics for nursing research.* Stamford, CT: Appleton & Lange.

Tabachnick, B. G., & Fidell, L. S. (2000). *Using multivariate statistics* (4th ed.). Boston: Allyn Bacon.

Studies Cited in Chapter 22

Berger, A. M., & Walker, S. N. (2001). An explanatory model of fatigue in women receiving adjuvant breast cancer chemotherapy. *Nursing Research, 50,* 42–52.

Cimprich, B., & Ronis, D. L. (2001). Attention and symptom distress in women with and without breast cancer. *Nursing Research, 50,* 86–94.

Davis, T. M. A., Maguire, T. O., Haraphongse, M., & Schaumberger, M. R. (1994). Preparing adult patients for cardiac catheterization: Informational treatment and coping style interactions. *Heart & Lung, 23,* 130–139.

Faulkner, M. S., Hathaway, D. K., Milstead, E. J., & Burghen, G.A. (2001). Heart rate variability in adolescents and adults with type I diabetes. *Nursing Research, 50,* 95–104.

Gulick, E. E. (2001). Emotional distress and activities of daily living functioning in persons with multiple sclerosis. *Nursing Research, 50,* 147–154.

Kammer, C. H. (1994). Stress and coping of family members responsible for nursing home placement. *Research in Nursing & Health, 17,* 89–98.

Keele-Smith, R., & Price-Daniel, C. (2001). Effects of crossing legs on blood pressure measurements. *Clinical Nursing Research, 10,* 202–213.

Melnyk, B. M., Alpert-Gillis, L., Feinstein, N. F., Fairbanks, E., Schutz-Czarniak, J., Hust, D., Sherman, L., LeMoine, C., Moldenhauser, Z., Small, L., Bender, N., & Sinkin, R. (2001). Improving cognitive development of low-birth-weight premature infants with the COPE program: A pilot study of the benefit of early NICU intervention with mothers. *Research in Nursing & Health, 24,* 373–389.

Neitzel, J. J., Miller, E. H., Shepherd, M. F., & Belgrade, M. (1999). Improving pain management after total joint replacement surgery. *Orthopaedic Nursing, 18,* 37–45.

Pellino, T. A. (1997), Relationships between patient attitudes, subjective norms, perceived control, and analgesic use following elective orthopedic surgery. *Research in Nursing & Health, 20,* 97–105.

Polit, D. F., London, A. S., & Martinez, J. M. (2001). *The health of poor urban women.* New York: MDRC (available at www.mdrc.org).

Steele, N. M., French, J., Gatherer-Boyles, J., Newman, S., & Leclaire, S. (2001) Effect of acupressure by Sea-Bands on nausea and vomiting of pregnancy. *Journal of Obstetric, Gynecologic, and Neonatal Nursing, 30,* 61–70.

Vines, S. W., Ng, A., Breggia, A., & Mahoney R. (2000). Multimodal chronic pain rehabilitation program: its effect on immune function, depression, and health behaviors. *Rehabilitation Nursing, 25,* 185–91.

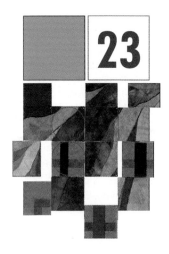

23

Analyzing Qualitative Data

As we have seen, qualitative data take the form of loosely structured, narrative materials, such as verbatim dialogue between an interviewer and a respondent in a phenomenological study, the field notes of a participant observer in an ethnographic study, or diaries used by historical researchers. This chapter describes methods for analyzing such qualitative data.

INTRODUCTION TO QUALITATIVE ANALYSIS

Qualitative analysis is a labor-intensive activity that requires creativity, conceptual sensitivity, and sheer hard work. Qualitative analysis is more complex and arduous than quantitative analysis, in part because it is less formulaic. In this section, we discuss some general considerations relating to qualitative analysis.

Qualitative Analysis: General Considerations

The purpose of both qualitative and quantitative data analysis is to organize, provide structure to, and elicit meaning from research data. In qualitative studies, however, data collection and data analysis usually occur simultaneously, rather than after all data are collected. The search for important themes and concepts begins from the moment data collection begins.

Qualitative data analysis is a particularly challenging enterprise, for three major reasons. First, there are no universal rules for analyzing and presenting qualitative data. The absence of standard analytic procedures makes it difficult to explain how to do such analyses, how to present findings in such a way that their validity is apparent, and how to replicate studies. Some of the procedures described in Chapter 18 (e.g., member checking and investigator triangulation) are important tools for enhancing the trustworthiness of not only the data themselves but also of the analyses and interpretation of those data.

The second challenge of qualitative analysis is the enormous amount of work required. Qualitative analysts must organize and make sense of pages and pages of narrative materials. In a recent multimethod study by one of us (Polit), the qualitative data consisted of transcribed, unstructured interviews with over 100 low-income women discussing life stressors and health problems. The transcriptions ranged from 30 to 50 pages in length, resulting in more than 3000 pages that had to be read, reread, and then organized, integrated, and interpreted.

The final challenge comes in reducing data for reporting purposes. Quantitative results can often be summarized in two or three tables. Qualitative researchers, by contrast, must balance the need to be concise with the need to maintain the richness and evidentiary value of their data.

TIP: Qualitative analyses are more difficult to *do* than quantitative ones, but qualitative findings are usually easier to understand than quantitative ones because the stories are often told in everyday language. The readability of the qualitative reports is usually enhanced by the inclusion of verbatim excerpts taken directly from the narrative data. Qualitative analyses are often harder to evaluate critically than quantitative analyses, however, because readers cannot know first-hand if researchers adequately captured thematic patterns in the data.

Analysis Styles

Crabtree and Miller (1999) observed that there are nearly as many qualitative analysis strategies as there are qualitative researchers, but they identified three major analysis styles that fall along a continuum. At one end is a style that is more systematic and standardized, and at the other is a style that is more intuitive, subjective, and interpretive. The three prototypical styles are as follows:

- *Template analysis style*. In this style, researchers develop a **template** or analysis guide to which the narrative data are applied. The units for the template are typically behaviors, events, and linguistic expressions (e.g., words or phrases). Although researchers begin with a rudimentary template before collecting data, the template undergoes constant revision as more data are gathered. The analysis of the resulting data, once sorted according to the template, is interpretive and not statistical. This style is most likely to be adopted by researchers whose research tradition is ethnography, ethology, discourse analysis, and ethnoscience.
- *Editing analysis style*. Researchers using an editing style act as interpreters who read through the data in search of meaningful segments and units. Once segments are identified and reviewed, they

develop a **categorization scheme** and corresponding codes that can be used to sort and organize the data. The researchers then search for the patterns and structure that connect the thematic categories. Researchers whose research traditions are grounded theory, phenomenology, hermeneutics, and ethnomethodology use procedures that fall within the editing analysis style.

- *Immersion/crystallization style*. This style involves the analyst's total immersion in and reflection of the text materials, resulting in an intuitive crystallization of the data. This highly interpretive and subjective style is exemplified in personal case reports of a semianecdotal nature, and is less frequently encountered in the nursing research literature than the other two styles.

Researchers seldom use terms like *template analysis style* or *editing style* in research reports. These terms are primarily post hoc characterizations of styles adopted by qualitative researchers. However, King (1998) has described the process of undertaking a template analysis, and his approach has been used in qualitative studies.

Example of a template analysis: King, Carroll, Newton, and Dornan (2002) used a template analysis process to analyze transcripts of 22 in-depth interviews in their study of the experience of adaptation to diabetic renal disease. Their template, developed in draft at the outset, included four main categories (immediate reactions to diagnosis; explanations of renal disease; living with renal disease; and hopes, fears, and expectations for the future). Each category and their subcategories in the template were refined in the course of the analysis.

The Qualitative Analysis Process

The analysis of qualitative data is an active and interactive process, especially at the interpretive end of the analysis style continuum. Qualitative researchers typically scrutinize their data carefully and deliberatively, often reading the data over and over again in a search for meaning and deeper understanding. Insights and theories cannot emerge until researchers become completely familiar with their data. Morse and Field (1995) note that qualitative analysis is a "process of fitting data together, of making the invisible obvious, of linking and attributing consequences to antecedents. It is a process of conjecture and verification, of correction and modification, of suggestion and defense" (p. 126).

Several intellectual processes play a role in qualitative analysis. Morse and Field (1995) have identified four such processes:

1. *Comprehending.* Early in the analytic process, qualitative researchers strive to make sense of the data and to learn "what is going on." When comprehension is achieved, they are able to prepare a thorough, rich description of the phenomenon under study, and new data do not add much to that description. Thus, comprehension is completed when saturation has been attained.
2. *Synthesizing.* Synthesizing involves a "sifting" of the data and putting pieces together. At this stage, researchers get a sense of what is typical with regard to the phenomenon, and what variation is like. At the end of the synthesis, researchers can make some generalized statements about the phenomenon and about study participants.
3. *Theorizing.* Theorizing involves a systematic sorting of the data. During this process, researchers develop alternative explanations of the phenomenon, and then hold these explanations up to determine their fit with the data. Theorizing continues to evolve until the best and most parsimonious explanation is obtained.
4. *Recontextualizing.* The process of **recontextualization** involves further development of the theory to explore its applicability to other settings or groups. In qualitative inquiries whose ultimate goal is theory development, it is the theory that must be recontextualized and generalized.

Although the intellectual processes in qualitative analysis are not linear in the same sense that quantitative analysis is, these four processes follow a rough progression over the course of the study.

Comprehension occurs primarily while in the field. Synthesis begins in the field but may continue well after the field work is done. Theorizing and recontextualizing are processes that are difficult to undertake before synthesis has been completed.

QUALITATIVE DATA MANAGEMENT AND ORGANIZATION

Qualitative analysis is supported and facilitated by several tasks that help to organize and manage the mass of narrative data, as described next.

Transcribing Qualitative Data

In qualitative studies, audiotaped interviews and field notes are major data sources. Most researchers have their tapes transcribed for analysis. Verbatim transcription is a critical step in preparing for data analysis, and researchers need to ensure that transcriptions are accurate, that they validly reflect the totality of the interview experience, and that they facilitate analysis.

With regard to the last two points, it is useful to develop transcription conventions or use existing ones. For example, transcribers have to indicate through symbols in the written text who is speaking (e.g., "I" for interviewer, "P" for participant), overlaps in speaking turns, time elapsed between utterances when there are gaps, nonlinguistic utterances (e.g., sighs, sobs, laughter), emphasis of words, and so on. Silverman (1993) offers some guidance with regard to transcription conventions.

Transcription errors are almost inevitable, which means that researchers need to check the accuracy of transcribed data. Poland (1995) notes that there are three categories of error:

1. *Deliberate alterations of the data.* Transcribers may intentionally try to "fix" data to make the transcriptions look more like what they "should" look like. Such alterations are not done out of malice, but rather reflect a desire to be helpful. For example, transcribers may alter profanities, omit extraneous sounds

such as phones ringing, or "tidy up" the text by deleting "ums" and "uhs." It is crucial to impress on transcribers the importance of verbatim accounts.

2. *Accidental alterations of the data.* Inadvertent transcription errors are far more common. One pervasive problem concerns proper punctuation. The insertion or omission of commas, periods, or question marks can alter the interpretation of the text. The most common error in this category is misinterpretation of actual words and substituting words that change the meaning of the dialogue. For example, the actual words might be, "this was totally moot," whereas the transcription might read, "this was totally mute." Researchers should thus never assume that transcriptions are accurate, and should take steps to verify accuracy before analysis gets underway.

3. *Unavoidable alterations.* Data are unavoidably altered by the fact that transcriptions capture only a portion of an interview experience. For example, transcriptions will inevitably miss many nonverbal cues, such as body language, intonation, and so on.

TIP: When checking the accuracy of transcribed data, it is critical to listen to the taped interview while doing the cross-check. This is also a good time to insert in the transcription any nonverbal behavior you captured in your field notes.

Researchers should begin the process of analyzing data with the best-possible quality data, and this requires careful training of transcribers, ongoing feedback, and continuous efforts to verify accuracy.

Developing a Categorization Scheme

Another early step in analyzing qualitative data is to organize them by classifying and indexing them. Researchers must design a mechanism for gaining access to parts of the data, without having repeatedly to reread the data set in its entirety. This phase of data analysis is essentially a reductionistic activity—data must be converted to smaller, more manageable units that can be retrieved and reviewed.

The most widely used procedure is to develop a categorization scheme and then to code data according to the categories. A preliminary categorization system is sometimes prepared before data collection, but in most cases qualitative analysts develop categories based on a scrutiny of actual data. There are, unfortunately, no straightforward or easy guidelines for this task. The development of a high-quality categorization scheme involves a careful reading of the data, with an eye to identifying underlying concepts and clusters of concepts. The nature of the categories may vary in level of detail or specificity, as well as in level of abstraction.

Researchers whose aims are primarily descriptive tend to use categories that are fairly concrete. For example, the category scheme may focus on differentiating various types of actions or events, or different phases in a chronologic unfolding of an experience. In developing a category scheme, related concepts are often grouped together to facilitate the coding process.

Example of a descriptive category scheme: The coding scheme used by Polit, London, and Martinez (2000) to categorize data relating to food insecurity and hunger in low-income families (Fig. 23-1) is an example of a category system that is fairly concrete and descriptive. For example, there are codes for the use of specific resources and food assistance programs. The coding system involved four major category clusters, each with subcodes. An excerpt describing a mother's purchase of day-old bread, for example, would be coded under category C.4.

Studies designed to develop a theory are more likely to involve abstract, conceptual categories. In designing conceptual categories, researchers must break the data into segments, closely examine them, and compare them to other segments for similarities and dissimilarities to determine what type of phenomena are reflected in them, and what the meaning of those phenomena are. (This is part of the process referred to as **constant comparison** by grounded theory researchers.) The researcher asks

A. Use of Food Services/Programs
   1. Food stamps
   2. WIC
   3. Food pantries
   4. Soup kitchens
   5. Free school lunch programs

B. Food Inadequacy Experiences
   1. Problems feeding family, having enough food
   2. Having to eat undesirable food
   3. Hunger

C. Strategies to Avoid Hunger
   1. Bargain shopping
   2. Borrowing money
   3. Getting food from friends, relatives
   4. Eating old or unsafe food
   5. Doubling up to share food costs
   6. Stretching food, smaller portions
   7. Smoking in lieu of eating
   8. Illegal activities, fraud

D. Special Issues
   1. Mothers sacrificing for children
   2. Effects of welfare reform on hunger
   3. Stigma

FIGURE 23.1 Polit et al.'s (2000) coding scheme for food insecurity and hunger in low-income families.

questions such as the following about discrete events, incidents, or statements:

What is this?
What is going on?
What does it stand for?
What else is like this?
What is this distinct from?

Important concepts that emerge from close examination of the data are then given a label that forms the basis for a categorization scheme. These category names are necessarily abstractions, but the labels are usually sufficiently graphic that the nature of the material to which they refer is clear—and often provocative. Strauss and Corbin (1998) advise qualitative researchers as follows: "This is very important—that the conceptual name or label should be suggested by the context in which an event is located" (p. 106).

Example of a conceptual category scheme: Chiu (2000) investigated the experience of spirituality in Taiwanese women with breast cancer through in-depth interviews with 15 women. A review of the interview transcripts led to the development of a fairly abstract coding scheme with four main categories (Living Reality; Creating Meaning; Connectedness; and Transcendence). Each of these had several subcategories. For example, the subthemes of "Living Reality" were "Living with encounter," "Taking full res-

ponsibility," and "Appreciation of life, people, and beloved things."

TIP: A good category scheme is critical to the analysis of qualitative data and so a substantial sample of the data should be carefully read before the scheme is finalized. To the extent possible, you should read materials that vary along important dimensions, to capture a wide range of content. The dimensions might be informant characteristics (e.g., transcripts of men versus women) or aspects of the data collection experience (e.g., data from different sites). Investigator triangulation or peer reviewers can be used to enhance the quality of a category system.

Coding Qualitative Data

Once a categorization scheme has been developed, the data are reviewed and coded for correspondence to or exemplification of identified categories. Coding qualitative material is seldom easy, for several reasons. First, researchers may have difficulty deciding the most appropriate code, or may not fully comprehend the underlying meaning of some aspect of the data. It may take a second or third reading of the material to grasp its nuances.

Second, researchers often discover in going through the data that the initial category system was incomplete or inadequate. It is common for themes to emerge that were not initially identified. When this happens, it is risky to assume that the theme failed to appear in materials that have already been coded. A concept might not be identified as salient until it has emerged three or four times. In such a case, it would be necessary to reread all previously coded material to have a truly complete grasp of that category.

TIP: Even when a category system is "finalized," you should be prepared to amend or even totally revise it. Even simple changes may mean rereading all previously coded material. Making changes midway is often painful and frustrating, but without an effective category system, you will not be able to identify and integrate important themes adequately.

Another issue is that narrative materials usually are not linear. For example, paragraphs from transcribed interviews may contain elements relating to three or four different categories, embedded in a complex fashion.

Example of a multitopic segment: Figure 23-2 shows a multitopic segment of an interview from Polit and colleagues' (2000) study of hunger in low-income families. The six codes in the margins represent codes from the category scheme presented in Figure 23-1.

It is sometimes recommended that a single member of the research team code the entire data set, to ensure the highest possible coding consistency across interviews or observations. Nevertheless, at least a portion of the interviews should be coded by two or more people early in the coding process, to evaluate and ensure intercoder reliability.

Manual Methods of Organizing Qualitative Data

Qualitative data traditionally have been organized manually through a variety of techniques. Although manual methods have a long and respected history, they are becoming increasingly outmoded as a result of the widespread availability of personal computers that can be used to perform the filing and indexing of qualitative material. Here, we briefly describe some manual methods of data organization and management, and the next section describes computer methods.

When the amount of data is small, or when a category system is simple, researchers sometimes use colored paper clips or colored Post-It Notes to code the content of the narrative materials. For example, if we were analyzing responses to an unstructured question about women's attitudes toward the menopause, we might use blue paper clips for text relating to loss of fertility, red clips for text on menopausal side effects, yellow clips for text relating to aging, and so on. Then we could pull out all responses with a certain color clip to examine one aspect of menopausal attitudes at a time.

TIP: In analyzing data from a phenomenological study, researchers often use file cards. Each significant statement from the interviews is placed on a file card of its own. The file cards are then sorted into piles representing themes. Some researchers use different-colored file cards for each participant's data.

Before the advent of computer programs for managing qualitative data, a typical procedure was to

FIGURE 23.2 Coded excerpt from Polit et al. (2000) study.

	I hate being on welfare, it is a pain in the butt. I
	don't need their cash, but the food stamps, they A1
B1	help a lot because it is hard, it is really hard. I got
	to live day by day for food for my kids. I have to
	call down to the shelter to get them to send you A3
	food, and you hate doing that because it is
	embarrassing, but I have to live day by day. I D3
	have to do things so my kids can eat. I don't
	worry about me, just for my kids because I can go
	a day without eating, but as long as my kids eat.
D1	But I never have to worry about my kids starving
	because I have family. C3

develop **conceptual files.** In this approach, researchers create a physical file for each category in their coding scheme, and insert all material relating to that category into the file. To create conceptual files, researchers must first go through all the data, writing relevant codes in the margins, as in Figure 23-2. Then they cut up a copy of the material by category area, and place the cut-out excerpt into the file for that category. All of the content on a particular topic then can be retrieved by going to the applicable file folder.

Creating such conceptual files is a cumbersome and labor-intensive task. This is particularly true when segments of the narrative materials have multiple codes, as is the case for the excerpt in Figure 23-2. In such a situation, there would need to be six copies of the paragraph—one for each file corresponding to the six codes. Researchers must also be sensitive to the need to provide enough context that the cut-up material can be understood (e.g., including material preceding or following the directly relevant materials). Finally, researchers must usually include pertinent administrative information. For example, if the data were from transcribed interviews, informants would be assigned an ID number. Each excerpt filed in the conceptual file would need to include the appropriate ID number so that researchers could, if necessary, obtain additional information from the master copy.

TIP: It is wise to develop a codebook, that is, written documentation describing the exact definition of the various categories used to code the data. Good qualitative codebooks usually include two or three actual excerpts that typify materials coded in each category.

Example of manual data organization: Manns and Chad (2001) explored components of quality of life among people with a quadriplegic or paraplegic spinal cord injury. Interviews with 15 informants were taped and transcribed. The researchers coded their data and then created conceptual files for each category. Their nine categories were as follows: physical function and independence, accessibility, emotional well-being, stigma, spontaneity, relationships and social function, occupation, financial stability, and physical well-being.

Computer Programs for Managing Qualitative Data

Computer programs remove the drudgery of cutting and pasting pages and pages of narrative material and are fast becoming indispensable research tools. These programs permit the entire data file to be entered onto the computer, each portion of an interview or observational record coded, and then portions of the text corresponding to specified codes retrieved and printed (or shown on a screen) for analysis. The current generation of programs has features that go beyond simple indexing and retrieval—they offer possibilities for actual analysis and integration of data.

The most widely used computer programs for qualitative data have been designed for personal computers, and most are for use with IBM-compatible computers, rather than Macintoshes. Some examples of major software include the following: The Ethnograph, MARTIN, and QUALPRO (all for use with IBM-type PCs), and the HyperQual2 (for use with Macs).

A new generation of programs, which Weitzman and Miles (1995) categorize as "conceptual network builders," have been developed to help users formulate and represent conceptual schemes through a graphic network of links. ATLAS/TI and NUD*IST (*N*onnumerical *U*nstructured *D*ata *I*ndexing, *S*earching, and *T*heorizing) are two of the most serious contenders in the category of coding and theory-building software. Barry (1998) compared these two programs on two dimensions: the structure of the software and the complexity of the research project. Barry views ATLAS/TI's strengths as its visual and spatial qualities, its interlinkages, and its creativity. The ability to create hyperlinks, which is offered by ATLAS/TI, allows for building nonhierarchical networks. On the other hand, NUD*IST's strengths include its project management functions, its structured organization, and its sophisticated level of searching. With NUD*IST, hierarchies of coding categories can be built and developed.

TIP: When first using qualitative data analysis software, choosing a software package that is best for your study can be overwhelming. It can be helpful to contact distributors of such software and ask for free demonstration disks. SCOLARI, for example, distributes The Ethnograph, NUD*IST, and HyperResearch, to name a few. Free demo disks can be requested by contacting this distributor at http://www. scolari.com.

Researchers typically begin by entering qualitative data into a word processing program (e.g., Word or WordPerfect). The data are then imported into the analysis program. A few qualitative data management programs (e.g., QUALPRO, HyperQual2) allow text to be entered directly rather than requiring an import file from a word processor.

Next, the researcher marks the boundaries (i.e., the beginning and end) of a segment of data, and then codes the data according to the developed category system. In some programs, this step can be done directly on the computer screen in a one-step process, but others require two steps. The first step involves the numbering of lines of text and the subsequent printing out of the text with the line numbers appearing in the margins. Then, after coding the paper copy, the researcher tells the computer which codes go with which lines of text. Most programs permit overlapping coding and the nesting of segments with different codes within one another.

All major programs permit editing. That is, codes can be altered, expanded, or deleted, and the boundaries of segments of text can be changed. These programs also provide screen displays or printouts of collated segments—however, some programs do this only on a file-by-file basis (e.g., one interview at a time), rather than allowing researchers to retrieve all segments with a given code across files.

Beyond these basic features, available programs vary in the enhancements they offer. The following is a partial list of features available in some programs:

- Automatic coding according to words or phrases found in the data
- Compilation of a master list of all codes used
- Selective searches (i.e., restricted to cases with certain characteristics, such as searching for a code only in interviews with women)
- Searches for co-occurring codes (i.e., retrieval of data segments to which two or more specific codes are attached)

- Retrieval of information on the sequence of coded segments (i.e., on the order of appearance of certain codes)
- Frequency count of the occurrence of codes
- Calculation of code percentages, in relation to other codes
- Calculation of the average size of data segments
- Listing and frequency count of specific words in the data files
- Searches for relationships among coded categories

Several of these enhancements have led to a blurring in the distinction between qualitative data management and data analysis.

Computer programs offer many advantages for organizing qualitative data, but some people prefer manual indexing because it allows them to get closer to the data. Others have raised concerns about using programs for the analysis of qualitative data, objecting to having a process that is basically cognitive turned into an activity that is mechanical and technical. Seidel (1993), for example, noted that there is a dark side of computer technology in qualitative data analysis. He proposed that these technological advances can lead to research behavior that he calls "analytic madness," which he claimed can disturb qualitative sensibilities. Seidel described three forms of such behavior. First, researchers can become infatuated with the amount of data the computer can deal with, which can lead to sacrificing resolution or insight for scope. Second, in assigning code words to identify portions of text, researchers can mistakenly consider these codes as significant just because they appear in certain quantities. Qualitative researchers may not analyze and critically evaluate the code words they have labeled and counted. Finally, the use of computers can distance or separate researchers from their data.

Agar (1993) also urged qualitative researchers to remember that computer programs represent only a portion of the research process. When that portion is taken for the whole, researchers can get the right answer to the wrong question. Qualitative analysis at times emphasizes the interrelated detail in a small, limited number of cases instead of common properties among a large number of cases. For that, Agar stressed that one needs a small amount of data and a lot of right brain.

Despite these concerns, many qualitative researchers have switched to computerized data management. Proponents insist that it frees up their time and permits them to pay greater attention to more important conceptual issues.

TIP: Even if you have little experience using a computer, the available programs for qualitative data management are relatively easy to learn. In selecting a program, try to discuss the merits of various programs with other researchers who have experience using them.

 Example of computerized data organization:
Jett (2002) studied the process of help seeking and help giving among older rural African Americans. Transcribed interviews with 41 informants were entered into The Ethnograph program for coding and sorting of analytic categories, which included aging, frailty, survival, and help-seeking.

ANALYTIC PROCEDURES

Data *management* in qualitative research is reductionist in nature because it involves converting large masses of data into smaller, more manageable segments. By contrast, qualitative data *analysis* is constructionist: It involves putting segments together into a meaningful conceptual pattern. Qualitative analysis is an inductive process that involves determining the pervasiveness of key ideas. Although there are various approaches to qualitative data analysis, some elements are common to several of them. We provide some general guidelines, followed by a description of the procedures used by grounded theory researchers, phenomenologists, and ethnographic researchers. We also provide information about analyzing data from focus group interviews and briefly note a strategy for analyzing triangulated qualitative and quantitative data.

A General Analytic Overview

The analysis of qualitative materials usually begins with a search for themes. DeSantis and Ugarriza (2000), in their thorough review of the way is which the term *theme* is used among qualitative researchers, offer this definition of **theme**: "A theme is an abstract entity that brings meaning and identity to a current experience and its variant manifestations. As such, a theme captures and unifies the nature or basis of the experience into a meaningful whole" (p. 362). Themes emerge from the data. Themes may develop within categories of data (i.e., within categories of the coding scheme used for indexing materials), but may also cut across them. For example, in Polit and colleagues' (2000) study (see Fig. 23-1), one theme was that these single mothers took great *pride in their own resourcefulness* in accessing food services (A codes) and developing strategies to avoid hunger (C codes) for their families.

The search for themes involves not only discovering commonalities across participants, but also seeking natural variation. Themes are never universal. Researchers must attend not only to what themes arise but also to how they are patterned. Does the theme apply only to certain types of people or in certain communities? In certain contexts? At certain periods? What are the conditions that precede the observed phenomenon, and what are the apparent consequences of it? In other words, the qualitative analyst must be sensitive to *relationships* within the data.

Researchers' search for themes, regularities, and patterns in the data can sometimes be facilitated by charting devices that enable them to summarize the evolution of behaviors, events, and processes. For example, for qualitative studies that focus on dynamic experiences—such as decision-making—it is often useful to develop flow charts or time-lines that highlight time sequences, major decision points and events, and factors affecting the decisions.

Example of a time-line:
In Beck's (2002) grounded theory study of mothering twins during the first year of life, time-lines that highlighted a mother's 24-hour schedule

were helpful. Figure 23-3 presents an example for a 23-year-old mother of 2-month-old twins. This mother's twins had been born premature and were in the neonatal intensive care unit for 2 months. The twins had recently been discharged from the hospital. Until the twins were 3 months old, the mother maintained the twins on the same feeding schedule as they had been on in the hospital— every 3 hours. The time-line in the figure illustrates a typical 24-hour period for this mother during the 4 weeks after hospital discharge.

A further step involves validation of the understandings that the thematic exploration has provided.

In this phase, the concern is whether the themes inferred accurately represent the perspectives of the people interviewed or observed. Several validation procedures can be used, as discussed in Chapter 18. If more than one researcher is working on the study, sessions in which the themes are reviewed and specific cases discussed can be highly productive. Investigator triangulation cannot ensure thematic validity, but it can minimize idiosyncratic biases. Using an iterative approach is almost always necessary. That is, researchers derive themes from the narrative materials, go back to the materials with the themes in mind to see if the materials really do fit, and then refine the themes as

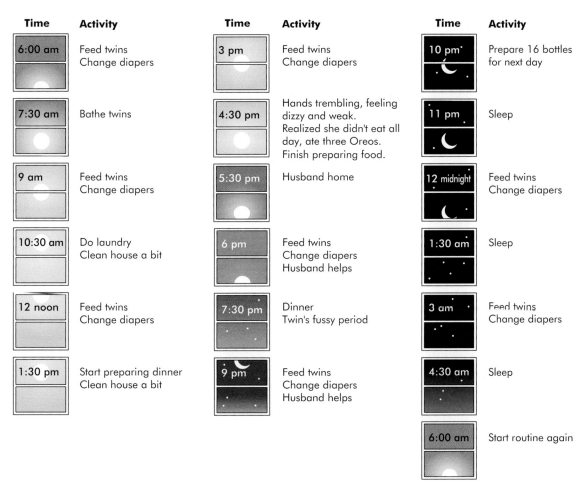

Time	Activity	Time	Activity	Time	Activity
6:00 am	Feed twins Change diapers	3 pm	Feed twins Change diapers	10 pm	Prepare 16 bottles for next day
7:30 am	Bathe twins	4:30 pm	Hands trembling, feeling dizzy and weak. Realized she didn't eat all day, ate three Oreos. Finish preparing food.	11 pm	Sleep
9 am	Feed twins Change diapers	5:30 pm	Husband home	12 midnight	Feed twins Change diapers
10:30 am	Do laundry Clean house a bit	6 pm	Feed twins Change diapers Husband helps	1:30 am	Sleep
12 noon	Feed twins Change diapers	7:30 pm	Dinner Twin's fussy period	3 am	Feed twins Change diapers
1:30 pm	Start preparing dinner Clean house a bit	9 pm	Feed twins Change diapers Husband helps	4:30 am	Sleep
				6:00 am	Start routine again

FIGURE 23.3 Example of a timeline for mothering multiples study.

necessary. It is also useful to undertake member checks—that is, to present the preliminary thematic analysis to some study participants, who can be encouraged to offer comments to support, contradict, or modify the thematic analysis.

At this point some researchers introduce **quasi-statistics**—a tabulation of the frequency with which certain themes, relations, or insights are supported by the data. The frequencies cannot be interpreted in the same way as frequencies generated in survey studies, because of imprecision in the sampling of cases and enumeration of the themes. Nevertheless, as Becker (1970) pointed out,

> Quasi-statistics may allow the investigator to dispose of certain troublesome null hypotheses. A simple frequency count of the number of times a given phenomenon appears may make untenable the null hypothesis that the phenomenon is infrequent. A comparison of the number of such instances with the number of negative cases—instances in which some alternative phenomenon that would not be predicted by his theory appears—may make possible a stronger conclusion, especially if the theory was developed early enough in the observational period to allow a systematic search for negative cases (p. 81).

Sandelowski (2001) believes that numbers are underutilized in qualitative research because of two myths: (1) real qualitative researchers do not count, and (2) qualitative researchers cannot count. Numbers are helpful in highlighting the complexity and work of qualitative research and in generating meaning from the data. Numbers are also useful in documenting and testing interpretations and conclusions and in describing events and experiences. Sandelowski warns, however, of the pitfalls of overcounting.

Example of tabulating data:
Boughn and Holdom (2002) conducted semistructured interviews with 44 women with trichotillomania (a compulsion to pull out one's hair). In analyzing the women's beliefs about the effectiveness of treatments they had used, the researchers quantified their data. They found, for example, that 21 of the women had used Prozac, but that none had found this to have long-term effectiveness.

In the final analysis stage, researchers strive to weave the thematic pieces together into an integrated whole. The various themes need to be interrelated to provide an overall structure (such as a theory or integrated description) to the data. The integration task is a difficult one, because it demands creativity and intellectual rigor if it is to be successful. One strategy that sometimes helps in this task is to cross-tabulate dimensions that have emerged in the thematic analysis.

Example of cross-tabulating dimensions:
Guttman, Nelson, and Zimmerman (2001) explored the perspectives of 26 physicians and nurses working in the emergency departments (EDs) regarding medically nonurgent pediatric ED visits. They identified four orientations toward such visits (restrictive, pragmatic, empowering, and all-inclusive), which represented the intersection of two dimensions: how urgent the medical care was perceived to be (high versus low) and the dominance of the medical model of professional control (high versus low). The "restrictive" orientation, for example, at the intersection of high urgency and high medical model dominance, is exemplified by the stance: "Only true medical emergencies, as defined by medical criteria, should be brought to the ED."

In the remainder of this section, we discuss analytic procedures that have been adopted by grounded theory researchers, phenomenologists, and ethnographers. It should be noted, however, that qualitative researchers who conduct studies that are not based in a formal research tradition may simply say that a content analysis was performed. **Qualitative content analysis** is the analysis of the content of narrative data to identify prominent themes, and patterns among the themes—primarily using an analysis style that can be characterized as either template analysis or editing analysis.

Grounded Theory Analysis

The general analytic procedures just described provide an overview of how qualitative researchers make sense of their data and distill from them insights into processes and behaviors operating in naturalistic settings. However, variations in the goals and philosophies of qualitative researchers also lead to variations in analytic strategies. This section describes data analysis in grounded theory studies. As noted in Chapter 11, one grounded theory approach was developed by Strauss and Corbin (1998), and another is Glaser and Strauss' (1967) grounded theory method of generating theories from data.

Glaser and Strauss' Grounded Theory Method

Grounded theory uses the constant comparative method of data analysis. This method involves a comparison of elements present in one data source (e.g., in one interview) with those identified in another. The process is continued until the content of each source has been compared with the content in all sources. In this fashion, commonalities are identified. The concept of fit is an important element in grounded theory analysis. **Fit** is the process of identifying characteristics of one piece of data and comparing them with the characteristics of another datum to determine if they are similar (Morse & Singleton, 2001). In the analytic process, fit is used to sort and reduce data. Fit enables the researcher to determine if data can be placed in the same category or if they can be related to one another. Glaser (1992) warns qualitative researchers not to force an analytic fit when it is not present in the data. He stated that "if you torture data enough it will give up!" (p. 123). Forcing a fit hinders the development of a relevant theory.

Coding in Glaser and Strauss' grounded theory approach is used to conceptualize data into patterns or concepts. The empirical substance of the topic being studied is conceptualized by **substantive codes**, whereas **theoretical codes** conceptualize how the substantive codes relate to each other.

In the Glaser and Strauss approach, there are two types of substantive codes: open and selective. **Open coding**, used in the first stage of the constant comparative analysis, captures what is going on in the data. Open codes may be the actual words used by the participants. Through open coding, data are broken down into incidents and their similarities and differences are examined. During open coding, researchers ask "What category or property of a category does this incident indicate?" (Glaser,

1978, p. 57). There are three different levels of open coding, depending on the level of abstraction. **Level I codes** (sometimes called **in vivo codes**) are derived directly from the language of the substantive area. They have vivid imagery and "grab." As researchers constantly compare new level I codes with previously identified ones, they condense them into broader categories (**level II codes**). Theoretical constructs, also called **level III codes**, are the most abstract level of codes. These constructs "add scope beyond local meanings" (Glaser, 1978, p. 70) to the generated theory. Collapsing of level II codes aids in identifying constructs.

Open coding ends when the core category is discovered, and then selective coding begins. The **core category** is a pattern of behavior that is relevant or problematic for study participants. In **selective coding**, researchers code only those data that are related to the core variable. One kind of core variable can be a **basic social process (BSP)** that evolves over time in two or more phases. All BSPs are core variables, but not all core variables have to be BSPs.

To help researchers decide on a core category, Glaser (1978, pp. 95–96) provided nine criteria:

1. It must be central, meaning that it is related to many categories.
2. It must reoccur frequently in the data.
3. It takes more time to saturate than other categories.
4. It relates meaningfully and easily to other categories.
5. It has clear and grabbing implications for formal theory.
6. It has considerable carry-through.
7. It is completely variable.
8. It is a dimension of the problem.
9. It can be any kind of theoretical code.

Theoretical codes help the grounded theorist to weave the broken pieces of data back together again. Box 23-1 presents the 18 families of theoretical codes that researchers can use to help determine how the substantive codes relate to each other.

Throughout coding and analysis, grounded theory analysts document their ideas about the

---

BOX 23.1 Families of Theoretical Codes for Grounded Theory Analysis

1. The six C's: causes, contexts, contingencies, consequences, covariances, and conditions
2. Process: stages, phases, passages, transitions
3. Degree: intensity, range, grades, continuum
4. Dimension: elements, parts, sections
5. Type: kinds, styles, forms
6. Strategy: tactics, techniques, maneuverings
7. Interaction: mutual effects, interdependence, reciprocity
8. Identity–self: self-image, self-worth, self-concept
9. Cutting point: boundaries, critical junctures, turning points
10. Means–goal: purpose, end, products
11. Cultural: social values, beliefs
12. Consensus: agreements, uniformities, conformity
13. Mainline: socialization, recruiting, social order
14. Theoretical: density, integration, clarity, fit, relevance
15. Ordering/elaboration: structural ordering, temporal ordering, conceptual ordering
16. Unit: group, organization, collective
17. Reading: hypotheses, concepts, problems
18. Models: pictorial models of a theory

Adapted from Glaser, B. G. (1978). *Theoretical sensitivity.* Mill Valley, CA: Sociological Press.

---

data, themes, and emerging conceptual scheme in memos. Memos preserve ideas that may initially not seem productive but may later prove valuable once further developed. Memos also encourage researchers to reflect on and describe patterns in the data, relationships between categories, and emergent conceptualizations.

 TIP: Glaser (1978) offered guidelines for preparing effective memos to generate substantive theory, including the following:

- Keep memos separate from data.
- Stop coding when an idea for a memo occurs, so as not to lose the thought.
- A memo can be brought on by literally forcing it, by beginning to write about a code.
- Memos can be modified as growth and realizations occur.
- When a lot of memos on different codes appear similar, compare the codes for any difference

that may have been missed. If the codes still seem the same, collapse them into one code.
- As memos are written, do not talk about persons but instead talk conceptually about the substantive codes as they are theoretically coded.
- When you have two ideas, write each idea up as a separate memo to prevent confusion.
- Always remain flexible with memoing approaches.

Glaser and Strauss' grounded theory method is concerned with the generation of categories, properties, and hypotheses rather than testing them. The product of the typical grounded theory analysis is a conceptual or theoretical model that endeavors to explain a pattern of behavior that is both relevant and problematic for study participants. Once the basic problem emerges, the grounded theorist then goes on to discover the process these participants experience in coping with or resolving this problem.

Example of Glaser and Strauss grounded theory analysis:

Faulkner and Mansfield (2002) explored young Latinas' experiences and meanings of sexuality, using Glaser and Strauss' grounded theory method to identify the process of sexual talk. *Reconciling messages* emerged as the core category. Young Latinas accepted messages that fit their value system, rejected those that misrepresented their beliefs, and altered messages to accept their own sexuality.

In the process of developing grounded theory, the concept of **emergent fit** can help to prevent individual substantive theories from being "respected little islands of knowledge" (Glaser, 1978, p. 148). As Glaser pointed out, generating grounded theory does not necessarily require discovering all new categories or ignoring ones previously identified in the literature: "The task is, rather, to develop an emergent fit between the data and a pre-existent category that might work. Therefore, as in the refitting of a generated category as data emerge, so must an extant category be carefully fitted as data emerge to be sure it works. In the bargain, like the generated category, it may be modified to fit and work. In this sense the extant category was not merely borrowed but earned its way into the emerging theory" (p. 4).

Emergent fit does not imply relevant existing literature should be disregarded. Through constant comparison, one compares concepts emerging from the data with similar concepts from existing theory or research to determine which parts have emergent fit with the theory being generated.

Example of emergent fit:

Wuest (2000) described how she grappled with reconciling emergent fit with Glaser's warning to avoid reading the literature until a grounded theory is well on its way. She used examples from her grounded theory study on negotiating with helping systems (e.g., health care, education, religion) to illustrate how emergent fit with existing research on relationships in health care was used to support her emerging theory. Constant comparison provided the checks and balances on using preexisting knowledge.

Strauss and Corbin's Approach

The Strauss and Corbin (1998) approach to grounded theory analysis differs from the original Glaser and Strauss method with regard to method and outcomes. Table 23-1 summarizes major analytic differences between these two grounded theory analysis methods.

Glaser (1978) stressed that to generate a grounded theory, the basic problem must emerge

---

TABLE 23.1 Comparison of Glaser's and Strauss/Corbin's Methods

	GLASER	STRAUSS & CORBIN
Initial data analysis	Breaking down and conceptualizing data involves comparison of incident to incident so patterns emerge	Breaking down and conceptualizing data includes taking apart a single sentence, observation, and incident
Types of coding	Open, selective, theoretical	Open, axial, selective
Connections between categories	18 coding families	Paradigm model (conditions, contexts, action/interactional strategies, and consequences)
Outcome	Emergent theory (discovery)	Conceptual description (verification)

from the data—it must be discovered. The theory is, from the very start, grounded in the data, rather than starting with a preconceived problem. Strauss and Corbin, however, state that the research itself is only one of four possible sources of the research problem. Research problems can, for example, come from the literature or a researcher's personal and professional experience.

The Strauss and Corbin method involves three types of coding: open, axial, and selective coding. In **open coding**, data are broken down into parts and compared for similarities and differences. Similar actions, events, and objects are grouped together as more abstract concepts, which are called *categories*. In open coding, the researcher focuses on generating categories and their properties and dimensions. In **axial coding**, the analyst systematically develops categories and links them with subcategories. Strauss and Corbin (1998) term this process of relating categories and their subcategories as "axial because coding occurs around the axis of a category, linking categories at the level of properties and dimensions" (p. 123). What is called the *paradigm* is used to help identify linkages among categories. The basic components of the paradigm include conditions, actions/interactions, and consequences. **Selective coding** is the process in which the findings are integrated and refined. The first step in integrating the findings is to decide on what Strauss and Corbin term the **central category** (sometimes called the *core category*), which is the main theme of the research. Recommended techniques to facilitate identifying the central category are writing the storyline, using diagrams, and reviewing and organizing memos.

The outcome of the Strauss and Corbin approach is, as Glaser (1992) terms it, a full preconceived conceptual description. On the other hand, the original grounded theory method (Glaser & Strauss, 1967) generates a theory that explains how a basic social problem that emerged from the data is processed in a social scene.

 Example of Strauss and Corbin grounded theory analysis:
Using data from focus groups interviews with 34 women, Borrayo and Jenkins (2001) examined how cultural health beliefs about breast cancer influence Mexican-descent women's decision to participate in breast cancer screening. Data analysis started with open coding of every sentence and word to identify as many discrete concepts as possible. An example of their open coding comes from the quote, "When I had that burning sensation, I went to the doctor, specially because I thought that it was cancer" (p. 814). Borrayo and Jenkins labeled "a burning sensation" as a breast cancer symptom. Axial coding was used to identify possible relationships within and among categories. Selective coding was used to help achieve theoretical integration. The analysis revealed that the basic social-psychological problem of Mexican-descent women was "feeling healthy." When the women were feeling healthy, they did not perceive that there was any reason to participate in breast cancer screening.

Phenomenological Analysis

Schools of phenomenology have developed different approaches to data analysis. Three frequently used methods for descriptive phenomenology are the methods of Colaizzi (1978), Giorgi (1985), and Van Kaam (1966), all of whom are from the Duquesne school of phenomenology, based on Husserl's philosophy. Table 23-2 presents a comparison of the steps involved in these three methods of analysis. The basic outcome of all three methods is the description of the meaning of an experience, often through the identification of essential themes. Phenomenologists search for common patterns shared by particular instances. There are, however, some important differences among these three approaches. Colaizzi's method, for example, is the only one that calls for a validation of results by returning to study participants. Giorgi's analysis relies solely on researchers. His view is that it is inappropriate either to return to participants to validate findings or to use external judges to review the analysis. Van Kaam's method requires that intersubjective agreement be reached with other expert judges.

 Example of a study using Colaizzi's method: Bondas and Eriksson (2001) studied the lived experiences of pregnancy among Finnish

TABLE 23.2 Comparison of Three Phenomenologic Methods

COLAIZZI (1978)	GIORGI (1985)	VAN KAAM (1966)
1. Read all protocols to acquire a feeling for them.	1. Read the entire set of protocols to get a sense of the whole.	1. List and group preliminarily the descriptive expressions that must be agreed upon by expert judges. Final listing presents percentages of these categories in that particular sample.
2. Review each protocol and extract significant statements.	2. Discriminate units from participants' description of phenomenon being studied.	2. Reduce the concrete, vague, and overlapping expressions of the participants to more descriptive terms. (Intersubjective agreement among judges needed.)
3. Spell out the meaning of each significant statement (i.e., formulate meanings).	3. Articulate the psychological insight in each of the meaning units.	3. Eliminate elements not inherent in the phenomenon being studied or that represent blending of two related phenomena.

4. Organize the formulated meanings into clusters of themes.
  a. Refer these clusters back to the original protocols to validate them.
  b. Note discrepancies among or between the various clusters, avoiding the temptation of ignoring data or themes that do not fit.
	4. Synthesize all of the transformed meaning units into a consistent statement regarding participants' experiences (referred to as the "structure of the experience"); can be expressed on a specific or general level.	4. Write a hypothetical identification and description of the phenomenon being studied.

5. Integrate results into an exhaustive description of the phenomenon under study.		5. Apply hypothetical description to randomly selected cases from the sample. If necessary, revise the hypothesized description, which must then be tested again on a new random sample.
6. Formulate an exhaustive description of the phenomenon under study in as unequivocal a statement of identification as possible.		6. Consider the hypothesized identification as a valid identification and description once preceding operations have been carried out successfully.
7. Ask participants about the findings thus far as a final validating step.		

women. Eighty interviews with 40 women, together with data from nonparticipant observations, were analyzed according to Colaizzi's method. The researchers extracted significant statements pertaining to the phenomena from transcriptions. Meanings were formulated and organized into 10 themes, which were clustered into 3 comprehensive categories and integrated into an exhaustive description. The three broad categories were the perfect body, an altered mode of being, and striving for family communion.

A second school of phenomenology is the Utrecht School. Phenomenologists using this Dutch approach combine characteristics of descriptive and interpretive phenomenology. Van Manen's (1990) method is an example of this combined approach in which researchers try to grasp the essential meaning of the experience being studied. According to Van Manen, thematic aspects of experience can be uncovered or isolated from participants' descriptions of the experience by three methods: (1) the holistic approach, (2) the selective or highlighting approach, and (3) the detailed or line-by-line approach. In the **holistic approach**, researchers view the text as a whole and try to capture its meanings. In the **selective approach**, researchers highlight or pull out statements or phrases that seem essential to the experience under study. In the **detailed approach**, researchers analyze every sentence. Once themes have been identified, they become the objects of reflection and interpretation through follow-up interviews with participants. Through this process, essential themes are discovered.

In addition to identifying themes from the participants' descriptions, Van Manen also calls for gleaning thematic descriptions from artistic sources. Van Manen urges qualitative researchers to keep in mind that poetry, literature, music, painting, and other art forms can provide a wealth of experiences that can be used to increase insights in the reflection process as the phenomenologist tries to interpret and grasp the essential meaning of the experience being studied. These experiential descriptions in literature and art help challenge and stretch the phenomenologist's interpretive sensibilities.

 Example of a study using Van Manen's method:

Lauterbach (2001) used Van Manen's method to investigate mothers' experiences with the death of a wished-for baby. Poetry, literature, mourning art, and cemeteries were especially helpful in Lauterbach's interpretation of the mothers' experiences. For instance, Robert Frost's poem, "Home Burial," and John Milton's poem, "On the Death of a Fair Infant Dying of a Cough," were used in data analysis. Also, a painting by Charles Wilson Peale called *Rachel Weeping*, depicting a mother mourning the loss of her infant from smallpox in 1772, and memorial art in cemeteries, provided insight.

A third school of phenomenology is an interpretive approach called *Heideggerian hermeneutics*. Diekelmann, Allen, and Tanner (1989) have described a seven-stage process of data analysis, the outcome of which is a description of shared practices and common meanings. Diekelmann and colleagues' stages of data analysis include:

1. All the interviews or texts are read for an overall understanding.
2. Interpretive summaries of each interview are written.
3. A team of researchers analyzes selected transcribed interviews or texts.
4. Any disagreements on interpretation are resolved by going back to the text.
5. Common meanings and shared practices are identified by comparing and contrasting the text.
6. Relationships among themes emerge.
7. A draft of the themes along with exemplars from texts are presented to the team. Responses or suggestions are incorporated into the final draft.

 Example of a Heideggerian hermeneutical analysis:

Foley, Minick, and Kee (2000) explored the experiences of military nurses as they engaged in advocacy during a military operation, and described their shared practices and common meanings. The hermeneutical analysis used the seven stages described by Diekelmann and colleagues. The stories of the 24

interviewed nurses revealed one constitutive pattern—*safeguarding*—and four related themes: advocating as protecting, advocating as attending the whole person, advocating as being the patient's voice, and advocating as preserving personhood.

Pollio, Henley, and Thompson (1997) propose another method for conducting a hermeneutic phenomenological study. Their method begins with bracketing. Their bracketing is not, however, viewed as a subtractive process of removing one's presuppositions, but instead as a positive process, a way of seeing. Instead of suspending preconceived notions, as described by Husserl, Pollio, and colleagues call for researchers to apply a world view.

Pollio and colleagues' method begins with a bracketing interview. The researcher is the first person to be interviewed about the topic under study, which raises his or her awareness of presuppositions. Once interviews have been conducted and transcribed, the hermeneutic circle begins. This is an interpretive process of continuously relating a part of the text (the transcribed interview) to the whole of the text. Pollio and colleagues described three types of interpretation: group, idiographic (particular), and nomothetic (general). In group interpretation, a transcript is read aloud. Meanings and relationships among meanings are discussed. After one transcript is interpreted, the remaining transcripts are usually interpreted by the primary researcher. At certain times the researcher goes back to the group with idiographic descriptions and nomothetic themes. The group provides feedback on whether the descriptions and themes are supported by the data. Each transcript is interpreted in the context of all other interview transcripts. Figure 23-4 provides a

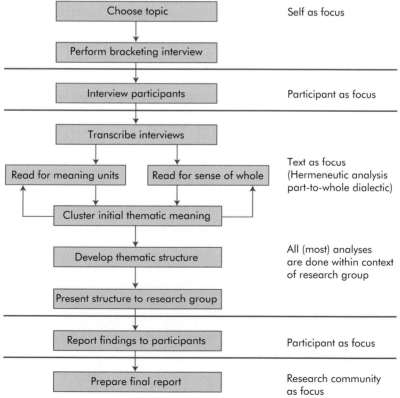

FIGURE 23.4   Schematic summary of Pollio and colleagues' interview process. Used with permission from Pollio, H.R., Henley, T.B., & Thompson, C.J. (1997). *The phenomenology of everyday life.* New York: Cambridge University Press.

schematic summary of Pollio and colleagues' interview process (p. 60).

Example using Pollio and colleagues' method:

Secrest (2000) investigated the quality of life of primary support persons of stroke survivors. Before data collection, the researcher's bracketing interview occurred. Once it was transcribed, the bracketing interview was analyzed by the research group. In-depth interviews were next conducted with 10 participants. Selected transcripts from the 10 interviews were read aloud to members of the research group and were analyzed, comparing the part of a transcript with its whole, and the whole transcript with other transcripts. Through this interpretive process, three themes emerged: fragility, vigilance, and loss/responsibility.

Analysis of Ethnographic Data

Spradley's (1979) developmental research sequence is one method that is often used for data analysis in an ethnographic study. His method is based on the premise that language is the primary mechanism that relates cultural meaning in a culture. The task of an ethnographer is to describe cultural symbols and to identify their coding rules. His sequence of 12 steps, which includes both data collection and data analysis, is as follows:

1. Locating an informant
2. Interviewing an informant
3. Making an ethnographic record
4. Asking descriptive questions
5. Analyzing ethnographic interviews
6. Making a domain analysis
7. Asking structural questions
8. Making a taxonomic analysis
9. Asking contrast questions
10. Making a componential analysis
11. Discovering cultural themes
12. Writing the ethnography

Thus, in Spradley's method there are four levels of data analysis: domain, taxonomic, componential, and theme. **Domain analysis** is the first level of analysis. Domains, which are units of cultural knowledge, are broad categories that encompass smaller categories. There is no preestablished number of domains to be uncovered in an ethnographic study. During this first level of data analysis, ethnographers identify relational patterns among terms in the domains that are used by members of the culture. The ethnographer focuses on the cultural meaning of terms and symbols (objects and events) used in a culture, and their interrelationships.

In **taxonomic analysis**, the second level of data analysis, ethnographers decide how many domains the data analysis will encompass. Will only one or two domains be analyzed in depth, or will a number of domains be studied less intensively? After making this decision, a **taxonomy**—a system of classifying and organizing terms—is developed to illustrate the internal organization of a domain and the relationship among the subcategories of the domain.

In **componential analysis**, multiple relationships among terms in the domains are examined. The ethnographer analyzes data for similarities and differences among cultural terms in a domain. Finally, in **theme analysis**, cultural themes are uncovered. Domains are connected in cultural themes, which help to provide a holistic view of the culture being studied. The discovery of cultural meaning is the outcome.

Example using Spradley's method:

Pierce (2001) conducted an ethnographic study of caring and expressions of spirituality by urban caregivers of people with stroke in African-American families. The study setting was an urban community in northwestern Ohio. Eight key informants (primary caregivers) and 16 general informants (secondary caregivers) participated in this research. Data obtained from interviews were analyzed using Spradley's four levels of analysis. In the theme analysis, eight themes concerning spirituality for all caregivers were discovered: caring was viewed as a filial ethereal value, self-contemplation, motivation for philosophical introspection, filial piety, living in the moment and hope for the future, purpose, motivated by approval from care recipients, and Christian piety.

Analysis of Focus Group Data

Focus group interviews yield rich and complex data that pose special analytic challenges. Indeed, there is little consensus about the analysis of focus group data, despite its use by researchers in several qualitative research traditions.

Unlike data from individual interviews, focus group interviews are very difficult to transcribe, partly because there are often technical problems. For example, it is difficult to place microphones so that the voices of all group members are picked up with equal clarity, particularly because participants tend to speak at different volumes. An additional issue is that, because of the group situation, it is inevitable that several participants will speak at once, making it impossible for transcriptionists to discern everything being said.

A major controversy in the analysis of focus group data is whether the unit of analysis is the group or individual participants. Some writers (e.g., Morrison-Beedy, Côté-Arsenault, and Feinstein, 2001) maintain that the group is the proper unit of analysis. Analysis of group-level data involves a scrutiny of themes, interactions, and sequences within and between groups. Others, however (e.g., Carey and Smith, 1994; Kidd and Parshall, 2000), argue that analysis should occur at both the group level and the individual level. Those who insist that only group-level analysis is appropriate argue that what individuals say in focus groups cannot be treated as personal disclosures because they are inevitably influenced by the dynamics of the group. However, even in personal interviews individual responses are shaped by social processes, and analysis of individual-level data (independent of group) is thought by some analysts to add important insights. Carey and Smith (1994) advocate a third level of analysis—namely, the analysis of individual responses *in relation* to group context (e.g., is a participant's view in accord with or in contrast to majority opinion, and how does that get expressed—or suppressed?).

For those who wish to analyze data from individual participants, it is essential to maintain information about what each person said—a task that is impossible to do if researchers are relying solely on audiotapes. Videotapes, as supplements to audiotapes, are sometimes used to identify who said what in focus group sessions. More frequently, however, researchers have several members of the research team in attendance at the sessions, whose job it is to take detailed field notes about the order of speakers and about significant nonverbal behavior, such as pounding or clenching of fists, crying, aggressive body language, and so on.

Many focus group researchers agree, regardless of their position on the unit of analysis, on the benefit of certain methods of enhancing data quality and analytic rigor. First, it is usually recommended that member checking occur *in situ*. That is, moderators develop a summary of major themes or viewpoints in real time, and present that summary to focus group participants at the end of the session for their feedback. Especially rich data often emerge from participants' reactions to those summaries. Second, postsession debriefings are critical. Team members who were present during the session meet immediately afterward to discuss issues and themes that arose. During these debriefings, which should be tape recorded, team members also share their views about group dynamics, such as coercive group members, censoring of controversial opinions, individual conformity to group viewpoints, and discrepancies between verbal and nonverbal behavior.

Transcription quality is especially important in focus group interviews: Emotional content as well as words must be faithfully recorded because participants are responding not only to the questions being posed but also to the experience of being in a group. Field notes, debriefing notes, and verbatim transcripts ideally must be integrated to yield a more comprehensive transcript for analysis.

Example of integrating focus group data: Morrison-Beedy and her co-authors (2001) provided several examples of integrating data across sources from their own focus group research. For example, one verbatim quote was, "It was no big deal." This was supplemented with data from the field notes that the woman's eyes were cast downward as she said this, and that the words were delivered sarcastically. The complete transcript for this entry, which includes researcher interpretation in brackets, was as follows: "'It was no big deal.' (said sarcastically, with eyes looking downward). [It really was a very big deal to her, but others had not acknowledged that.]" (p. 52).

Because of group dynamics, focus group analysts must be sensitive to both the thematic content of these interviews, and also to how, when, and why themes are developed. Some of the issues that could be central to focus group analysis are the following:

- Does an issue raised in a focus group constitute a *theme* or merely a strongly held viewpoint of one or two members?
- Do the same issues or themes arise in more than one group?
- If there are group differences, why might this be the case—were participants different in background characteristics and experiences, or did group processes affect the discussions?
- Are some issues sufficiently salient that they are discussed not only in direct response to specific questions posed by the moderator, but also spontaneously emerge at multiple points in the session?
- Do group members find certain issues both interesting *and* important?

Some focus group analysts, such as Kidd and Parshall (2000), use quantitative methods as adjuncts to their qualitative analysis. Using NUD*IST, they conduct such analyses as assessing similarities and differences between groups, determining coding frequencies to aid pattern detection, examining codes in relation to participant characteristics, and examining how much individual members contributed. They use such methods not so that interpretation can be based on frequencies, but so that they can better understand context and identify issues that require further critical scrutiny and interpretation. Focus group data are sometimes analyzed according to the procedures of a formal research tradition, such as grounded theory.

Analysis of Triangulated Qualitative–Quantitative Data

Chapter 12 described the growth of multimethod research that triangulates qualitative and quantitative data within the context of a single study or coordinated sequence of studies. Typically, data from such studies are integrated after the fact. That is, quantitative data are analyzed statistically, narrative data are analyzed through qualitative methods, and then researchers interpret overall patterns in light of findings from the two study components.

There is, however, emerging interest in exploring alternative methods of analysis. One such approach is the construction of a **meta-matrix** that permits researchers to recognize important patterns and themes across data sources. This method, which can also be used to integrate multiple types of qualitative data (e.g., interviews and observational field notes), involves the development of a two- or three-dimensional matrix that aligns various types of data (Miles & Huberman, 1994). Typically, one dimension involves a particular study participant. Then, for each participant, a chart is constructed in which data from multiple data sources are entered, so that the analyst can see at a glance such information as scores on psychosocial scales (e.g., scores on the Center for Epidemiological Studies Depression scale), comments from open-ended dialogue with participants (e.g., verbatim narratives relating to depression), hospital record data (e.g., physiologic information), and the researchers' own reflexive comments. A third dimension can be added if there are multiple sources of data relating to multiple constructs (e.g., depression, pain).

The construction of such a meta-matrix allows researchers to explore such issues as whether statistical conclusions are supported by the qualitative data for individual study participants, and vice versa. Patterns of regularities, as well as anomalies, may be easier to see through detailed inspection of such matrices, and can allow for fuller exploration of all sources of data simultaneously.

Example of a meta-matrix:
Wendler (2001) constructed a meta-matrix for her study of the impact of a therapeutic intervention, Tellington touch, on patient anxiety, pain, and physiologic status. She gathered quantitative data on such variables as blood pressure, state anxiety, pain levels, and nicotine and caffeine use. Participants also responded to open-ended questions, and the clinician completed field notes on

impressions and spontaneous participant comments. Participant observers also provided field notes on behaviors. These multiple sources of data were analyzed quantitatively and qualitatively, and then subsequently arrayed in a meta-matrix, which yielded important insights.

INTERPRETATION OF QUALITATIVE FINDINGS

In qualitative studies, interpretation and analysis of the data occur virtually simultaneously. That is, researchers interpret the data as they categorize it, develop a thematic analysis, and integrate the themes into a unified whole. Efforts to validate the qualitative analysis are necessarily efforts to validate interpretations as well. Thus, unlike quantitative analyses, the meaning of the data flows from qualitative analysis.

Nevertheless, prudent qualitative researchers hold their interpretations up for closer scrutiny—self-scrutiny as well as review by peers and outside reviewers. Even when researchers have undertaken member checks and peer debriefings, these procedures do not constitute proof that results and interpretations are credible. For example, in member checks, many participants might be too polite to disagree with researchers' interpretations, or they may become intrigued with a conceptualization that they themselves would never have developed on their own—a conceptualization that is not necessarily accurate. Thus, for qualitative researchers as well as quantitative researchers, it is important to consider possible alternative explanations for the findings and to take into account methodologic or other limitations that could have affected study results.

 Example of seeking alternative explanations:

Cheek and Ballantyne (2001) studied family members' selection process for a long-term care facility for elderly patients being discharged from an acute setting. In describing their methods, they explicitly noted that "attention throughout was paid to looking for rival or competing themes or explanations" (p. 225). In their analysis, they made a conscious effort to weigh alternatives.

In drawing conclusions, qualitative researchers should also consider the transferability of the findings. Although qualitative researchers rarely seek to make generalizations, they often strive to develop an understanding of how the study results can be usefully applied. The central question is: In what other types of settings and contexts could one expect the phenomena under study to be manifested in a similar fashion?

The implications of the findings of qualitative studies, as with quantitative ones, are often multidimensional. First, there are implications for further research: Should the study be replicated? Could the study be expanded (or circumscribed) in meaningful and productive ways? Do the results suggest that an important construct has been identified that merits the development of a more formal instrument? Does the emerging theory suggest hypotheses that could be tested through more controlled, quantitative research? Second, do the findings have implications for nursing practice? For example, could the health care needs of a subculture (e.g., the homeless) be identified and addressed more effectively as a result of the study? Finally, do the findings shed light on the fundamental processes that are incorporated into nursing theory?

RESEARCH EXAMPLES

Example of a Grounded Theory Analysis

Beck (2002) developed a grounded theory study of mothering twins during the first year of life. Figure 23-5 presents her model, which was developed using Glaser and Strauss' constant comparative method. Data for this study consisted of transcripts from 16 in-depth interviews, 14 months of field notes, and participant observation in mothers' homes and during support group meetings for parents of multiples. *Life on hold* was identified as the basic social psychological problem of mothering twins. As one mother expressed, "I would say that my life is on hold since the twins were born. It is a rare occasion when I can undo the pause button."

Coding continued until the basic social psychological process, also the core category, was discovered.

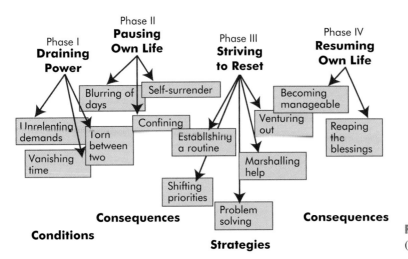

FIGURE 23.5 Beck's (2002) model of mothering twins.

"Releasing the pause button" was the process mothers progressed through as they attempted to resume their lives. Once this core category was discovered, Beck shifted from open coding to selective coding. The core category consisted of the four phases of (1) draining power, (2) pausing own life, (3) striving to reset, and (4) resuming own life.

To help make the wealth of data more manageable, Beck collapsed in vivo (level I) codes into broader, more abstract categories. An example of this process involved collapsing five in vivo codes (enjoying the twins, feeling blessed, getting attention, amazing, and twin bonding) into the level II code of Reaping the Blessings, as shown in Table 23-3. Next, Beck collapsed the codes of Reaping the Blessings and Becoming Manageable into the construct of Resuming Own Life. She used 10 of Glaser's (1978) 18 coding families in her theoretical coding for the process of Releasing the Pause Button. These 10 coding families included the 6 C's, process, degree, strategy, cutting point, dimension, theoretical, ordering or elaboration, means–goals, and model. The family *cutting point* provides an illustration of a theoretical code. Three months seemed to be the cutting or turning point for mothers when life started to become more manageable. The following are a few excerpts from transcripts of interviews that Beck coded as cutting points (the numbers in parentheses refer to the interview number): "I just pushed through the first 3 months, then it got easier and I felt like I would survive" (7). "Three months came around and the twins sort of slept through the night and it made a huge,

huge, difference" (11). "The first 3 months definitely were the hardest. It wasn't very rewarding. It was like being a servant to two demanding people. They really weren't giving anything back" (10).

Example of an Analysis for an Ethnographic Study

Kraatz's (2001) ethnographic study focused on the understanding of health and illness in women living in a Brazilian *favela* (urban slum). The sample consisted of 1 key informant and 10 additional participants. The key informant was one of the original settlers, and she was recognized informally as a leader in the community. Snowball sampling was used to identify other informants. Interviews were usually conducted in the homes. One informant preferred to be interviewed in her grocery store. Data analysis and collection occurred concurrently. At first, Kraatz concentrated on identifying the taxonomy for the two domains of health and illness. Once a tentative taxonomy was developed, additional interviews focused more on componential analysis in which Kraatz explored the similarities and contrasts within the taxonomy.

Data analysis revealed the taxonomy of health and illness, which were seen as playing a contributing role in life. The following six components played a part in both health and illness: going to the doctor, cleanliness, nutrition, spirituality, herbal remedies, and sympathetic magic. An example of

TABLE 23.3 Collapsing Level I Codes Into the Level II Code of *"REAPING THE BLESSINGS"* (Beck, 2002)

QUOTE	LEVEL I CODE
I enjoy just watching the twins interact so much. Especially now that they are mobile. They are not walking yet but they are crawling. I will tell you they are already playing. Like one will go around the corner and kind of peek around and they play hide and seek. They crawl after each other. (3)	Enjoying Twins
With twins it's amazing. She was sick and she had a fever. He was the one acting sick. She didn't seem like she was sick at all. He was. We watched him for like 6–8 hours. We gave her the medicine and he started calming down. Like WOW! That is so weird. Cause you read about it but it's like, Oh come on! You know that doesn't really happen and it does. It's really neat to see. (15)	Amazing
These days it's really neat cause you go to the store or you go out and people are like "Oh, they are twins, how nice". And I say, "Yeah they are. Look, look at my kids". (15)	Getting Attention
I just feel blessed to have two. I just feel like I am twice as lucky as a mom who has one baby. I mean that's the best part. It's just that instead of having one baby to watch grow and change and develop and become a toddler and school age child you have two. (11)	Feeling Blessed
It's very exciting. It's interesting and it's fun to see them and how the twin bond really is. There really is a twin bond. You read about it and you hear about it but until you experience it, you just don't understand. One time they were both crying and they were fed. They were changed and burped. There was nothing wrong. I couldn't figure out what was wrong. So I said to myself, "I am just going to put them together and close the door." I put them in my bed together and they patty caked their hands and put their noses together and just looked at each other and went right to sleep. (15)	Twin Bonding

sympathetic magic playing a part in safeguarding one's health and in curing illness is the cure for warts in the Brazilian *favela*. The following is an excerpt from one of the interviews: "To get rid of a wart you cut the wart; bury it in an anthill. Just that you can't go by there. It's just that you can't even go by there on the road, not even on the road. If you do go by there, then it will come back. That's what they say, you know" (p. 178).

Example of a Phenomenological Analysis

Beck (1998) conducted a descriptive phenomenological study of the experience of panic disorder in new mothers. The purposive sample consisted of six women who had experienced their initial onset of panic disorder in the postpartum period. Each mother participated in an in-depth interview in which she described her experiences living with panic after delivery. All interviews, which lasted from 50 minutes to 2 hours, were audiotaped and transcribed.

Colaizzi's (1978) method was used to analyze verbatim transcripts. After reading the transcripts, Beck extracted significant statements, formulated their meanings, and categorized statements into theme clusters. The findings were then integrated into an exhaustive description of the phenomenon of postpartum panic and validated by two mothers who had participated in the study.

During the early stage of data analysis, Beck initially identified eight themes. After further deliberation she combined two preliminary themes with other themes. Beck concluded that the following six themes described the essence of the experience of postpartum panic:

1. The terrifying physical and emotional components of panic paralyzed women, leaving them feeling totally out of control.
2. During panic attacks, women's cognitive functioning abruptly diminished; between attacks, women experienced a more insidious decrease in cognitive functioning.
3. During the attacks, women feverishly struggled to maintain their composure, leading to exhaustion.
4. Because of the terrifying nature of panic, preventing further attacks was paramount in the lives of the women.
5. As a result of recurring panic attacks, negative changes in women's lifestyles ensued, lowering their self-esteem and leaving them to bear the burden of disappointing both themselves and their families.
6. Mothers were haunted by the prospect that their panic could have residual effects on themselves and their families.

As depicted in these six themes, panic permeated all aspects of a mother's life as she struggled to fulfill her maternal role.

SUMMARY POINTS

- Qualitative analysis is a challenging, labor-intensive activity, guided by few standardized rules.

- Although there are no universal strategies, three prototypical analytic styles have been identified: (1) a **template analysis style** that involves the development of an analysis guide (**template**) to sort the data; (2) an **editing analysis style** that involves an interpretation of the data on which a **categorization scheme** is based; and (3) an **immersion/crystallization style** that is characterized by the analyst's total immersion in and reflection of text materials.
- Qualitative analysis typically involves four intellectual processes: comprehending, synthesizing, theorizing, and **recontextualizing** (exploration of the developed theory vis-à-vis its applicability to other settings or groups).
- In working with audiotaped data that must be transcribed, researchers should use transcription conventions and take steps to ensure that transcription errors are minimized and corrected.
- The first major step in analyzing qualitative data is to organize and index the materials for easy retrieval, typically by coding the content of the data according to a categorization scheme.
- Traditionally, researchers have organized their data by developing **conceptual files**, which are physical files in which coded excerpts of data relevant to specific categories are placed. Now, however, computer programs are widely used to perform basic indexing functions, and to facilitate data analysis.
- The actual analysis of data begins with a search for **themes,** which involves the discovery not only of commonalities across subjects, but also of natural variation and patterns in the data.
- The next analytic step usually involves a validation of the thematic analysis. Some researchers use **quasi-statistics,** which involves a tabulation of the frequency with which certain themes or relations are supported by the data.
- In a final analytic step, the analyst tries to weave the thematic strands together into an integrated picture of the phenomenon under investigation.
- Grounded theory uses the **constant comparative** method of data analysis.

- One approach to grounded theory is the Glaser and Strauss method, in which there are two broad types of codes: **substantive codes** (in which the empirical substance of the topic is conceptualized) and **theoretical codes** (in which the relationships among the substantive codes are conceptualized).
- Substantive coding involves **open coding** to capture what is going on in the data, and then **selective coding**, in which only variables relating to a core category are coded. The **core category**, a behavior pattern that has relevance for participants, is sometimes a **basic social process (BSP)** that involves an evolutionary process of coping or adaptation.
- In the Glaser and Strauss method, open codes begin with **level I (in vivo) codes**, which are collapsed into a higher level of abstraction in **level II codes**. Level II codes are then used to formulate **level III codes**, which are theoretical constructs.
- Through constant comparison, the researcher compares concepts emerging from the data with similar concepts from existing theory or research to determine which parts have **emergent fit** with the theory being generated.
- The Strauss and Corbin method is an alternative grounded theory method whose outcome is a full preconceived conceptual description. This approach to grounded theory analysis involves three types of coding: open (in which categories are generated), **axial coding** (where categories are linked with subcategories), and selective (in which the findings are integrated and refined).
- There are numerous different approaches to phenomenological analysis, including the descriptive methods of Colaizzi, Giorgi, and Van Kaam, in which the goal is to find common patterns of experiences shared by particular instances.
- In Van Manen's approach, which involves efforts to grasp the essential meaning of the experience being studied, researchers search for themes, using either a **holistic approach** (viewing text as a whole); a **selective approach** (pulling out key statements and phrases); or a **detailed approach** (analyzing every sentence).

- One approach to analyzing ethnographic data is Spradley's method, which involves four levels of data analysis: **domain analysis** (identifying categories); **taxonomic analysis** (selecting key domains and constructing taxonomies); **componential analysis** (comparing and contrasting terms in a domain); and **theme analysis** (to uncover cultural themes).
- Some researchers identify neither a specific approach nor a specific research tradition; rather, they might say that they used **qualitative content analysis** as their analytic method.
- A major controversy in the analysis of focus group data is whether the unit of analysis is the group or individual participants.
- One approach to analyzing triangulated data from multiple sources (e.g., qualitative and quantitative data) is the construction of a **meta-matrix** that arrays such data in a table so the analyst can inspect patterns and themes across data sources.

STUDY ACTIVITIES

Chapter 23 of the *Study Guide to Accompany Nursing Research*: *Principles and Methods*, *7th edition*, offers various exercises and study suggestions for reinforcing concepts presented in this chapter. In addition, the following study questions can be addressed:

1. Read a recent qualitative nursing study. If a different investigator had gone into the field to study the same problem, how likely is it that the conclusions would have been the same? How transferable are the researcher's findings? What did the researcher learn that he or she would probably not have learned with a more structured and quantified approach?
2. Ask two people to describe their conception of preventive health care and what it means in their daily lives. Pool descriptions with those of other classmates, and develop a coding scheme to organize responses. What major themes emerged?
3. If possible, listen to an audiotaped interview and transcribe a few minutes of it. Compare your transcription with that of another classmate, or with that of the professional transcriber.

SUGGESTED READINGS

Methodologic References

Agar, M. (1993). The right brain strikes back. In N. G. Fielding, & R. M. Lee (Eds.), *Using computers in qualitative research* (pp. 181–194). Newbury Park, CA: Sage.

Barry, C. A. (1998). Choosing qualitative data analysis software: ATLAS/TI and NUD*IST compared. *Sociological Research Online, 3*(3) [Online.] Available: http://www.socresonline.org.uk/3/3/4.html.

Becker, H. S. (1970). *Sociological work*. Chicago: Aldine.

Boyatzis, R. E. (1998). *Transforming qualitative information: Thematic analysis and code development*. Thousand Oaks, CA: Sage.

Carey, M. A., & Smith, M. W. (1994). Capturing the group effect in focus groups: A special concern in analysis. *Qualitative Health Research, 4*, 123–127.

Colaizzi, P. (1978). Psychological research as the phenomenologist views it. In R. Valle & M. King (Eds.), *Existential phenomenological alternatives for psychology* (pp. 48–71). New York: Oxford University Press.

Crabtree, B. F., & Miller, W. L. (Eds.) (1999). *Doing qualitative research* (2nd ed.). Newbury Park, CA: Sage.

DeSantis, L., & Ugarriza, D. N. (2000). The concept of theme as used in qualitative nursing research. *Western Journal of Nursing Research, 22*, 351–372.

Diekelmann, N. L., Allen, D., & Tanner, C. (1989). *The NLN criteria for appraisal of baccalaureate programs: A critical hermeneutic analysis*. New York: NLN Press.

Gephart, R. P., Jr. (1988). *Ethnostatistics: Qualitative foundations for quantitative research*. Newbury Park, CA: Sage.

Giorgi, A. (1985). *Phenomenology and psychological research*. Pittsburgh, PA: Duquesne University Press.

Glaser, B. G. (1978). *Theoretical sensitivity*. Mill Valley, CA: Sociology Press.

Glaser, B. G. (1992). *Basics of grounded theory analysis*. Mill Valley, CA: Sociology Press.

Glaser, B. G., & Strauss, A. L. (1967). *The discovery of grounded theory: Strategies for qualitative research*. Chicago: Aldine.

Kidd, P. S., & Parshall, M. B. (2000). Getting the focus and the group: Enhancing analytic rigor in focus group research. *Qualitative Health Research, 10*, 293–308.

King, N. (1998). Template analysis. In C. Cassell & G. Symon (Eds.), *Qualitative methods and analysis in organizational research* (pp. 118–134). London: Sage.

Lofland, J., & Lofland, L. H. (1995). *Analyzing social settings: A guide to qualitative observation and analysis* (3rd ed.). Belmont, CA: Wadsworth.

Melia, K. M. (1996). Rediscovering Glaser. *Qualitative Health Research, 6*, 368–378.

Miles, M. B., & Huberman, A. M. (1994). *Qualitative data analysis: An expanded sourcebook* (2nd ed.). Thousand Oaks, CA: Sage.

Morgan, D. L. (1993). Qualitative content analysis: A guide to paths not taken. *Qualitative Health Research, 3*, 112–121.

Morrison-Beedy, D., Côté-Arsenault, D., & Feinstein, N. F. (2001). Maximizing results with focus groups: Moderator and analysis issues. *Applied Nursing Research, 14*, 48–53.

Morse, J. M., & Field, P. A. (1995). *Qualitative research methods for health professionals* (2nd ed.). Thousand Oaks, CA: Sage Publications.

Morse, J. M., & Singleton, J. (2001). Exploring the technical aspects of "fit" in qualitative research. *Qualitative Health Research, 11*, 841–847.

Poland, B. D. (1995). Transcription quality as an aspect of rigor in qualitative research. *Qualitative Inquiry, 1*, 190–310.

Pollio, H. R., Henley, T. B., & Thompson, C. J. (1997). *The phenomenology of everyday life*. New York: Cambridge University Press.

Sandelowski, M. (2001). Real qualitative researchers do not count: The use of numbers in qualitative research. *Research in Nursing & Health, 24*, 230–240.

Seidel, J. (1993). Method and madness in the application of computer technology to qualitative data analysis. In N. G. Fielding & R. M. Lee (Eds.), *Using computers in qualitative research* (pp. 107–116). Newbury Park, CA: Sage.

Silverman, D. (1993). *Interpreting qualitative data: Methods for analyzing talk, text, and interaction*. London: Sage.

Spradley, J. P. (1979). *The ethnographic interview*. New York: Holt, Rinehart, and Winston.

Strauss, A. L., & Corbin, J. M. (1998). *Basics of qualitative research: Techniques and procedures for developing grounded theory* (2nd ed.) Thousand Oaks, CA: Sage.

Van Kaam, A. (1966). *Existential foundations of psychology*. Pittsburgh, PA: Duquesne University Press.

Van Manen, M. (1990). *Researching lived experience*. Albany, NY: State University of New York Press.

Weitzman, E. A., & Miles, M. B. (1995). *Computer programs for qualitative data analysis: A software sourcebook*. Thousand Oaks, CA: Sage.

Substantive References

Beck, C. T. (1998). Postpartum onset of panic disorder. *Image: The Journal of Nursing Scholarship, 30,* 131–135.

Beck, C. T. (2002). Releasing the pause button: Mothering twins during the first year of life. *Qualitative Health Research, 12,* 593–608.

Bondas, T., & Eriksson, K. (2001). Women's lived experiences of pregnancy: A tapestry of joy and suffering. *Qualitative Health Research, 11,* 824–840.

Borrayo, EA., & Jenkins, S. R. (2001). Feeling healthy: So why should Mexican-descent women screen for breast cancer? *Qualitative Health Research, 11,* 812–823.

Boughn, S., & Holdom, J. (2002). Trichotillomania: Women's reports of treatment efficacy. *Research in Nursing & Health, 25,* 135–144.

Cheek, J., & Ballantyne, A. (2001). Moving them on and in: The process of searching for and selecting an aged care facility. *Qualitative Health Research, 11,* 221–237.

Chiu, L. (2000). Lived experience of spirituality in Taiwanese women with breast cancer. *Western Journal of Nursing Research, 22,* 29–53.

Faulkner, S. L., & Mansfield, P. K. (2002). Reconciling messages: The process of sexual talk for Latinas. *Qualitative Health Research, 12,* 310–328.

Foley, B. J., Minick, P., & Kee, C. (2000). Nursing advocacy during a military operation. *Western Journal of Nursing Research, 22,* 492–507.

Guttman, N., Nelson, M. S., & Zimmerman, D. R. (2001). When the visit to the emergency department is medically nonurgent: Provider ideologies and patient advice. *Qualitative Health Research, 11,* 161–178.

Jett, K. (2002). Making the connection: Seeking and receiving help by elderly African Americans. *Qualitative Health Research, 12,* 373–387.

King, N., Carroll, C., Newton, P., & Dornan, T. (2002). "You can't cure it so you have to endure it": The experience of adaptation to diabetic renal disease. *Qualitative Health Research, 12,* 329–346.

Kraatz, E. S. (2001). The structure of health and illness in a Brazilian favela. *Journal of Transcultural Nursing, 12,* 173–179.

Lauterbach, S. S. (2001). Longitudinal phenomenology: An example of "doing" phenomenology over time, phenomenology of maternal mourning: Being-a-mother in another world (1992) and five years later (1997). In P. L. Munhall (Ed.), *Nursing research: A qualitative perspective* (pp. 185–208). Sudbury, MA: Jones & Bartlett.

Manns, P. J., & Chad, K. E. (2001). Components of quality of life for persons with a quadriplegic and paraplegic spinal cord injury. *Qualitative Health Research, 11,* 795–811.

Pierce, L. L. (2001). Caring and expressions of spirituality by urban caregivers of people with stroke in African American families. *Qualitative Health Research, 11,* 339–352.

Polit, D. F., London, A., & Martinez, J. M. (2000). Food security and hunger in poor, mother-headed families in four U.S. cities. New York: MDRC.

Secrest, J. (2000). Transformation of the relationship: The experience of primary support persons of stroke survivors. *Rehabilitation Nursing, 25,* 93–99.

Wendler, M. C. (2001). Triangulation using a metamatrix. *Journal of Advanced Nursing, 35,* 521–525.

Wuest, J. (2000). Negotiating with helping systems: An example of grounded theory evolving through emergent fit. *Qualitative Health Research, 10,* 51–70

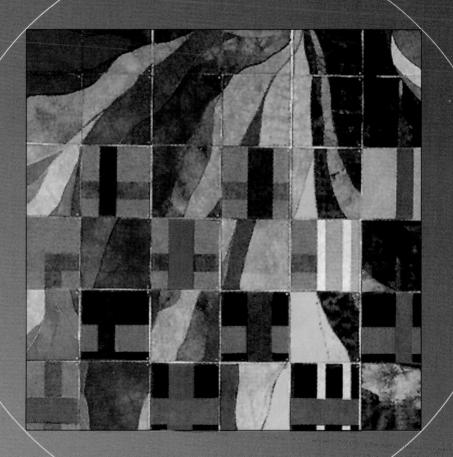

Communicating
Research

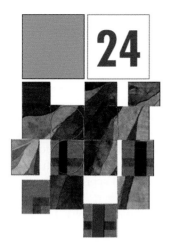

24

Summarizing and Sharing Research Findings

No study is complete until the findings have been shared with others in a research report. Reporting research results contributes to the base of evidence for nursing practice, and is a professional responsibility. This chapter offers guidelines for helping researchers to disseminate their research results.

GETTING STARTED ON DISSEMINATION

Researchers contend with various issues in developing a dissemination plan, as we discuss in this section.

Selecting a Communication Outlet

Research results can be presented in various venues and types of publication. These include student-related outlets (term papers, theses, and dissertations) and professional ones (journal articles, books, reports to funders, conference presentations).

Researchers who want to communicate their findings to other researchers or clinicians can opt to present research findings orally or in writing. Oral presentations (typically at professional conferences) can be a formal talk in front of an audience. Most conferences also give researchers the option of presenting findings in **poster sessions** in which results

are summarized on a poster. Major advantages of oral presentations are that they typically can be done soon after study completion, and offer opportunities for dialogue among people interested in the same topic.

Written reports can take the form of research journal articles published in traditional professional journals, or in a variety of new outlets on the Internet. Written journal articles have the major advantage of being available to a worldwide audience of readers—an important consideration in thinking about how a study can contribute to evidence-based nursing practice.

Research reports for different outlets vary in a number of ways, as we discuss in a subsequent section. Nevertheless, the advice and information in this chapter is generally relevant for most types of dissemination.

Knowing the Audience

Good research communication depends on providing information that can be understood by consumers. Therefore, before researchers develop a dissemination strategy, they should consider the audience they are hoping to reach. Here are some questions to consider:

1. Will the audience include nurses only, or will it include professionals from other disciplines (e.g., physicians, sociologists, anthropologists)?

2. Will the audience be primarily researchers, or will it include other professionals (clinicians, health care administrators, health care policy makers)?
3. Are clients (lay people) a possible audience for the report?
4. Will the audience include people whose native language is not English?
5. Will reviewers, editors, and readers be experts in the field?

These questions underscore an important point, namely, that researchers usually have to write with multiple audiences in mind. This, is turn, means writing clearly and avoiding technical jargon to the extent possible. It is also means that researchers sometimes must develop a multiprong dissemination strategy—for example, publishing a report aimed at other nurse researchers in a journal such *Nursing Research*, and then publishing a short summary of it for clinicians or clients in a hospital newsletter.

Although writing for a broad audience may be an important goal, it is also important to keep in mind the needs of the *main* intended audience. If consumers of a report are mostly clinical nurses (as might be the case at some professional conferences and in specialty journals), it is important to emphasize what the findings mean for the practice of nursing. If the audience is health care administrators or policy makers, explicit information should be included about how the research can be used to improve such outcomes as *cost, efficiency, accessibility*, and so on. Other researchers, if they are the primary targets, need more explicit information about the methods used, study limitations, and implications for future research.

Developing a Plan

Before beginning to prepare research reports, researchers should develop a plan. Part of that plan involves decisions about the communication outlet and the audience for the report. Beyond that, researchers also have to coordinate the actual tasks of preparing a **manuscript** (i.e., an unpublished paper or document).

Deciding on Authorship

When a study has been completed by a team or by several colleagues, one critical part of the plan involves division of labor and authorship. Authorship can be a tricky business. The International Committee of Medical Journal Editors (ICMJE, 1997) advises that authorship credit should be given only to those who have made a substantial contribution to (1) the conception and design of the study, or to data analysis and interpretation; (2) drafting or revising the manuscript; and (3) approving the final version of the manuscript.

The **lead author**, who is usually the first-named author, is the person who has overall responsibility for the report and, usually, for the study. The lead author and co-authors should plan in advance for the roles and responsibilities of each team member in producing the manuscript. To avoid the possibility of subsequent conflicts, they should also plan on the order of authors' names in advance. Ethically, it is most appropriate to order names in the order of authors' contribution to the work, not according to status. When contributions of co-authors are comparable, names are usually listed alphabetically. Issues arising when there are multiple authors are discussed by Erlen, Siminoff, Sereika, and Sutton (1997).

Deciding on Content

Many studies collect far more data than can be reported on in a single journal article, poster, or conference presentation, and thus lend themselves to multiple publications. In such a situation, an early decision involves what aspects of a study to write about in a given paper. If there are multiple and complex research questions or hypotheses, perhaps several papers will be required to communicate important results adequately. Researchers who collect both qualitative and quantitative data often report on each separately. Sometimes there are substantive, theoretical, and methodologic findings, each of which is intended for different audiences and merit separate papers.

It is, however, not appropriate to write several papers when one would suffice. Each paper from a study should independently make a contribution to knowledge. Those who make editorial decisions about manuscripts, as well as readers, expect original work, so unnecessary duplication or overlap should be avoided. It is also considered unethical to submit essentially the same or similar paper to two journals (or two conferences) simultaneously. Oermann (2002) offers excellent guidelines regarding duplicate and redundant publications.

Assembling Materials

The planning process also involves assembling materials needed to begin a draft. One essential ingredient is information about manuscript requirements. Traditional journals, on-line journals, and conferences issue guidelines for authors, and these guidelines should be clearly understood before writing begins. We offer information about acquiring these guidelines and what types of information they contain later in this chapter.

Other materials also need to be pulled together and organized for easy retrieval. This includes notes about the relevant literature and references; instruments used in the study; descriptions of the study sample; output of computer analyses; relevant analytic memos or reflexive notes; figures or photographs that illustrate some aspect of the study; and permissions to use copyrighted materials. If the study needed approvals or obtained funding, the proposals or grant applications that were prepared for those purposes should be on hand. Other important tools are style manuals that provide information about both grammar and language use (e.g., Turabian, 1996; University of Chicago Press, 1993; Strunk, White, & Angell, 2000), as well as more specific information about writing professional and scientific papers (e.g., American Psychological Association, 2001; American Medical Association, 1997; ICMJE, 1997). Finally, there should be an outline and timeline.

Preparing an Outline

Written outlines are extremely useful as an organizing tool. Outlines provide guidance for the content to be covered in a manuscript, and suggest ways in which smooth transitions between sections can be made. Research reports usually follow a fixed flow of content, as we subsequently discuss, but an outline with major headings and subheadings helps researchers to get an overview of the task ahead.

A written outline is essential if there are multiple co-authors who each have responsibility for different sections of the manuscript. The overall outline and individual assignments should be developed collaboratively.

One final advantage of having an outline is that it can be incorporated into a timeline that sets goals or deadlines for completing the manuscript. Having a timeline cannot ensure that a manuscript will be completed in a timely fashion. Without a timeline, the dissemination phase can drag on for months or, worse yet, never reach completion. Authors can use the outline to establish goals for small and relatively manageable tasks.

Writing Effectively

Some researchers are talented writers who do not agonize during this last phase of a study. Many people, however, have a hard time putting their ideas down on paper. It is clearly beyond the scope of this book to teach good writing skills, but we can offer a few suggestions.

One suggestion, quite simply is: *do it*. Get in the habit of writing, even if it is only 10 to 15 minutes a day. "Writer's block" is probably responsible for thousands of unfinished (or never-started) manuscripts each year. So, just begin somewhere, and keep at it regularly. A research report does not have to be written in a linear fashion, from the beginning to the end. Writing can start in the middle (e.g., by describing something you know well, like who the study participants were, or what hypotheses were addressed). The important thing is to get started. Writing is a bit like learning to swim or to play the piano: it gets easier with practice.

Writing *well* is, of course, important, and there are resources that offer suggestions on how to write compelling sentences, select good words, and organize your ideas effectively (e.g., Iles, 1997; Browner, 1999). It is equally important, however, to not get bogged down at the beginning. Writing a first draft is harder than editing and revising. It is usually better to write a draft in its entirety, and then go back later to rewrite awkward sentences, correct spelling and grammatical errors, reorganize sentences or paragraphs, insert more compelling or precise words, smooth the transitions, and generally polish it up.

CONTENT OF RESEARCH REPORTS

As noted, research reports can vary in terms of audience, purpose, and length. Theses or dissertations not only communicate research results, but document students' ability to perform scholarly empirical work; they therefore tend to be long. Journal articles, by contrast, are short because they compete with other reports for limited journal space, and are read by busy professionals. Despite differences in length and amount of detail, the general form and content of research reports are often similar. In this section, we expand on the information presented in Chapter 5 by reviewing in greater depth the type of material covered in qualitative and quantitative research reports. Distinctions among the various kinds of reports are described later in the chapter.

Quantitative Research Reports

Quantitative reports typically follow a conventional format referred to as the **IMRAD format**. This format involves organizing study material into four sections—the **I**ntroduction, **M**ethod, **R**esults, **a**nd **D**iscussion. These sections, respectively, address the following questions:

- Why was the study done? (I)
- How was the study done? (M)
- What was learned? (R)
- What does it mean? (D)

The Introduction
The introduction acquaints readers with the research problem, its significance, and the context in which it was developed. The introduction sets the stage for the study by describing the existing literature, the study's conceptual framework, the problem, research questions, or hypotheses, any underlying assumptions, and the rationale for doing the study. Although the introduction covers various aspects of the study background, it should be concise. Readers are more interested in learning about new findings than about the researcher's breadth of knowledge of prior research or theory. A common critique of research manuscripts by reviewers and editors is that the introduction is too long.

Introductions are often written in a funnel-shaped structure, beginning broadly to establish a framework for understanding the study, and then narrowing to the specifics of what researchers sought to learn. The end point of the introduction should be a concise delineation of the research questions or the study hypotheses, which provides a good transition to the method section.

Some researchers postpone stating the problem until late in the introduction, but readers profit from learning the general problem immediately. An up-front, clearly stated problem statement is of immense value in communicating the study's context. Researchers should explain why the problem is important, in terms of either practical or theoretical significance.

 TIP: The first paragraph should be written with special care, because the goal is to grab the readers' attention. Convey enthusiasm for your topic, and try to present the problem in an imaginative way. For example, sometimes beginning with a provocative question or statement can act as "bait" for a reader.

Example of a first paragraph of an introduction:
Davies and Hodnett (2002), who were interested in nurses' self-efficacy regarding support to women in labor, began their report as follows:

> What are maternity care nurses' views about their experience and ability to provide labor support? To answer this question, a scale was developed to measure nurses' self-efficacy or confidence about providing labor support. Subsequently, the views of practicing labor and delivery nurses were elicited in a survey. The purpose of these two studies was to better understand caregivers'

perspectives for the implementation of clinical practice guideline recommendations (p. 48).

The introduction typically includes a summary of related research to provide a pertinent context. The literature review should be a brief summary rather than an exhaustive review (except for theses or dissertations). The literature review should make clear what is already known, and also gaps or deficiencies in that knowledge. The review thus helps to clarify the contribution that the new study is making to evidence on a topic.

 TIP: Literature reviews are usually done in the early phase of a project, before data collection. When writing your report, be sure to bring your literature review up to date by including new research.

The introduction also should describe the study's theoretical or conceptual framework, if relevant. The theoretical framework should be sufficiently explained so that readers who are unfamiliar with it can nevertheless understand its main thrust and its link to the research problem. The introduction should include definitions of the concepts under investigation. Complete operational definitions are often reserved for the method section, but conceptual definitions belong early in the report.

Introductory materials may not be explicitly grouped under a heading labeled Introduction; many journals articles begin without *any* heading. Some introductory sections, on the other hand, include subheadings such as *Literature Review*, *Conceptual Framework*, or *Hypotheses*. In general, all the material before the method section is considered to be the introduction.

The various background strands need to be convincingly and cogently interwoven to persuade readers that, in fact, the new study holds promise for adding to evidence for nursing.

Example of an ending paragraph of an introduction:

Lampic, Thurfjell, Bergh, Carolsson, and Sjödén (2002), who studied women's life values before and after a breast cancer diagnosis, put this paragraph near the conclusion of their introduction:

In conclusion, some empirical evidence suggests that in the cancer context, an individual may strive to adapt to an illness/loss by changing the perceived importance of life values. With the exception of the study by Nordin et al. (2001), no prospective studies of life value changes in connection with a cancer diagnosis appear to have been performed, despite the limitations of retrospective self-reports. Also, no study has compared the perceptions of life values before versus after a cancer diagnosis (p. 90).

The Method Section

To evaluate the quality of evidence a study offers, readers need to understand exactly what researchers did to address the research problem . The method section ideally provides a sufficiently detailed description of the research methods that another researcher could replicate the study. In theses, this goal should almost always be satisfied. In journal articles and conference presentations, the method section may need to be condensed (e.g., inclusion of a complete interview schedule is rarely possible). The degree of detail should, however, permit readers to evaluate the methods and draw conclusions about the validity of the findings.

TIP: Faulty method sections are the leading cause of manuscript rejection by journals (Byrne, 1998). If readers are not convinced that your methods are sound, they may feel that the remainder of the paper is not worth reading. Your job in writing the method section of a quantitative report is to offer persuasive evidence that your study has internal, external, construct, and statistical conclusion validity. This is not to say, however, that you should gloss over study limitations.

The method section is often subdivided into several parts, which helps readers to locate vital information. As an example, the method section might contain the following subsections in an experimental study:

Research Design
Sample and Setting
Data Collection Instruments
Procedures
Data Analysis

The method section usually begins with the description of the research design and its rationale. The design is often given more detailed coverage in experimental projects than in nonexperimental ones. In experimental and quasi-experimental studies, researchers should indicate what specific design was adopted, what variables were manipulated, how subjects were assigned to groups, and whether "blinding" or "double blinding" was used. Reports for longitudinal studies or studies with multiple points of data collection should indicate the number of times data were collected, and the amount of time elapsed between those points. In all types of quantitative studies, it is important to identify steps taken to control the research situation in general and extraneous variables in particular.

 Example of a description of research design:

Pridham, Brown, Sondel, Clark, and Green (2001) conducted a study of the pattern of growth in premature and full-term infants; they described their research design as follows:

> This longitudinal study was designed to make assessments at 1, 4, 8, and 12 months post-term age. These time points were selected because they precede or are coincident with the occurrence of developmental transformations . . . (p. 286).

Readers also need to know about study participants. This section (which may be labeled *Research Sample*, *Subjects*, or *Study Participants*) normally includes a discussion of the population or community from which the sample was drawn, and a list of inclusion or exclusion criteria, to clarify the group to whom results can be generalized. The method of sample selection and its rationale, recruitment techniques, and sample size should be indicated so readers can understand the strengths and limitations of the sampling plan and determine how representative subjects are of the target population. If a power analysis was undertaken to determine sample size needs, this should be clearly stated. There should also be information about response rates and, if possible, about response bias (or attrition bias, if this is relevant). Finally, the

method section should describe basic characteristics of study participants (e.g., age, gender, medical condition).

 Example of a description of research sample:

Kang and Fox (2001) studied physiologic responses to academic stress in college students, and described their convenience sample as follows:

> The sample consisted of 24 college students, including 13 who reported a history of childhood asthma and 11 students without a history of childhood asthma. . . . There were 13 women and 11 men; the mean age of the sample was 21.8 years ($SD = 3.1$ years). . . . Students were excluded if they smoked, consumed alcohol on a regular basis, or had other significant health problems (p. 247).

A description of the method used to collect the data is a critical component of the method section. This information might be included in a subsection labeled *Instruments*, *Measures*, or *Data Collection*. In rare cases, this description may be accomplished in three or four sentences, such as when a standard physiologic measure has been used. More often, a detailed explanation of the study instruments or procedures, and a rationale for their use, are required to communicate how data were gathered. When it is not feasible to include actual instruments, their form and content should be described in as much detail as possible. If instruments were constructed specifically for the project, the report should describe their development, methods used for pretesting, revisions made as a result of pretesting, scoring procedures, and guidelines for interpretation. If special equipment was used (e.g., to gather biophysiologic or observational data), it should be described, including information about the manufacturer. The report should also indicate who collected the data (e.g., the authors, research assistants, graduate students, nurses) and what type of training they received.

TIP: Describe the measurement of all variables used in the analyses, together with information on the role the variable played (e.g., dependent variable), but provide most detail about key variables. A global statement usually suffices for background variables (e.g., "Background characteristics such as age, gender, and education were obtained from medical records").

 Example of a description of data collection:

Eller (2001), who studied quality of life among people living with HIV, described measurement of her dependent variable as follows:

> The Sickness Impact Profile (SIP) was used to measure quality of life. . . . The SIP consists of 136 items divided into 12 subscales that measure changes in behavior related to sickness. The subject checks off phrases that describe current health-related state in each category. . . . Scale values are assigned to each item, and the score is calculated as the sum total of checked items. Higher scores indicate poorer quality of life. A global QOL score is the sum of all 12 categories. . . . The SIP . . . requires 20 to 30 minutes for completion (p. 409).

The report must also convince readers that the data collection methods were sound. Any information relating to quality of the data or the analysis, and the procedures used to evaluate that quality, should be described. For psychosocial instruments, results from psychometric assessments should be provided.

Example of a description of data quality: McCrone, Lenz, Tarzian, and Perkins (2001), who studied depression in patients after coronary artery bypass graft surgery, described data quality from the Center for Epidemiological Studies Depression scale (CES-D) as follows:

> In Radloff's developmental studies, the scale revealed internal consistency reliability ranging from 0.85 to 0.94, and test-retest reliabilities of 0.45 to 0.70. Cronbach's alpha for *this* study ranged from 0.91 to 0.95. Construct, criterion-related, content, concurrent, and discriminant validity have also been shown (Radloff, 1977) (p. 158).

The method section (sometimes in a separate *Procedures* subsection) also provides information about steps used to collect the data and to protect human (or animal) subjects. In an interview study, where were interviews conducted, who conducted them, and how long did the average interview last?

In an observational study, what was the role of the observer in relation to subjects? When questionnaires are used, how were they delivered to respondents, and were follow-up procedures used to increase responses? Any unforeseen events occurring during data collection that could affect the findings should be described and assessed. It is also useful to indicate *when* data were collected because changes in economic, social, or medical trends may need to be taken into account in interpreting the results.

In experimental studies, the procedures subsection may include detailed information about the actual intervention (i.e., about the main independent variable). What exactly did the intervention entail? How and by whom was the treatment administered? What type of special training was required by those administering the treatment? What was done with subjects in the control group? How much time elapsed between the intervention and the measurement of the dependent variable?

Example of a description of procedures: Whitney and Parkman (2002) studied the effect of an intervention of early postoperative walking after total hip replacement. They described procedures as follows:

> Subjects enrolled into the study were randomly assigned after surgery to receive standard postoperative exercise (control, $n = 27$) or 4 days of augmented physical activity (experimental, $n = 31$) beginning the day of surgery and continuing for the next 3 days. Those randomized to the intervention group were taught isometric exercises for the gluteus and quadriceps muscles and began these on the day of surgery. On the first postoperative day, the intervention group began isotonic exercises for the biceps and triceps muscles. The intervention was designed to increase postoperative walking, and subjects followed a walking protocol in which distances increased daily (p. 21).

Analytic procedures are described either in the method or results section. It is usually sufficient to identify the statistical procedures used; computational formulas or references for commonly used statistics such as analysis of variance are not necessary. For unusual procedures, or unusual applications of a common procedure, a technical reference justifying the approach should be noted. If a statistical procedure was used to control extraneous variables, the specific variables controlled should be mentioned. The level of significance is typically set at .05 for two-tailed tests, which may or may not be explicitly stated; however, if a different significance level or one-tailed tests were used, this must be specified.

Example of a description of data analysis: Whitman, Davison, Sereika, and Rudy (2001) studied hospital staffing levels (e.g., worked hours per patient day, or WHPPD) in relation to the use of restraint. A subsection labeled *Data Analysis* stated:

Descriptive statistics (means, standard deviations, percentages) were tabulated for all variables. Chi-square test for goodness-of-fit was used to investigate the distribution of restraint episodes across the days of the week and shifts. Spearman rho correlations were used to describe and test the relationship between WHPPD and unit monthly mean restraint application duration rate (RADR). The level of significance was set at .05 (two-tailed) (p. 358).

The Results Section

Readers scrutinize the method section to know if the study was done with rigor, but it is the results section that is at the heart of the report. In a quantitative study, the results of the statistical analyses are summarized in a factual manner. If both descriptive and inferential statistics have been used, descriptive statistics ordinarily come first, to provide an overview of study variables. If key research questions involve comparing groups with regard to dependent variables (e.g., in an experimental or case–control study), the early part of the results section usually provides information about the groups' comparability with regard to extraneous variables, so readers can evaluate selection bias.

Example from a results section: Wang, Redeker, Moreyra, and Diamond (2001) used a quasi-experimental design to compare the effects of 4 hours versus 6 hours of bed rest after cardiac catheterization on patients' safety and comfort. Their results section began as follows:

Table 1 presents the demographic and clinical characteristics of the two sample groups. Groups were comparable on age, gender, weight, systolic and diastolic blood pressure, FBS (fasting blood sugar), PT (serum prothrombin time), aspirin dosage, and total amount of contrast media used (p. 34) [Table not shown].

Research results are then usually ordered in terms of their overall importance. If, however, research questions or hypotheses have been numbered in the introduction, the analyses addressing them should be ordered in the same sequence. The researcher must be careful to report all results as accurately and completely as possible, regardless of whether the hypotheses were supported.

Three pieces of information are normally included when reporting the results of statistical tests: the value of the calculated statistic, degrees of freedom, and significance level. For instance, it might be stated, "A chi-square test revealed that patients who were exposed to the experimental intervention were significantly less likely to develop decubitus ulcers than patients in the control group ($\chi^2 = 8.23$, $df = 1$, $p = .008$)." For some journals and conferences, especially ones with a medical audience, it has become standard to report confidence intervals as well as significance levels. If effect sizes have been computed, they should also be reported in the results section.

TIP: The inclusion of effect sizes in research reports can contribute to developing a strong base of evidence in a profession. Effect sizes help in interpreting results of individual studies, and are also useful for pooling information from multiple studies on a topic in meta-analyses. Beck (1999) has suggested further guidelines for reporting quantitative results to facilitate the work of meta-analysts, who are often plagued with problems in retrieving data from the primary studies. For example, if results are reported as being nonsignificant or significant below a standard probability level (e.g., $p < .01$), it may be difficult for meta-analysts to perform the necessary calculations. Whenever possible, exact p-levels (e.g., $p = .008$) should be reported, together with information on degrees of freedom and whether a one-tailed or two-tailed test was used. Beck also urged the reporting of group means and standard deviations even when group differences are not significant.

When results from several statistical analyses are reported, it is useful to summarize them in a **table**. Good tables, with precise headings and titles, are an important way to economize on space and to avoid dull, repetitive statements. When tables are used to present statistical information, the text should refer to the table by number (e.g., "As shown in Table 2, patients in the experimental group . . . "). Box 24-1 presents some suggestions regarding the construction of effective statistical tables.

 TIP: Do not repeat statistical information in both the text and in tables. Tables should be used to display information that would be monotonous to present in the text—and to display it in such a way that the numbers and patterns among the numbers are more comprehensible. The text can then be used to highlight the major thrust of the tables.

Figures may also be used to summarize results. Figures that display the results in graphic form are used less as an economy than as a means of dramatizing important findings and relationships. Figures are especially helpful for displaying information on some phenomenon over time, or for portraying conceptual or empirical models. Oermann (2001) and Browner (1998) offer guidelines on constructing figures and tables.

Example from results section:
Maloni, Kane, Suen, and Wang (2002) studied the trajectory of dysphoria (a combination of symptoms of negative affect) among high-risk pregnant hospitalized women on bed rest. A segment of their results section follows:

> Dysphoria significantly decreased across time from admission through the postpartum (F (5) = 23.58, $p < .001$, eta squared 0.276) [Figure 24-1] and was highest upon antepartum hospital admission. There was a significant decrease between hospital admission and the last antepartum measure ($p < .001$), and between the last antepartum measure and 2 days after delivery of the infant ($p = .005$) (p. 95).

BOX 24.1 Guidelines for Preparing Statistical Tables

1. Number tables so they can be referenced in the text.
2. Give tables a clear, brief explanatory title.
3. Avoid both overly simple tables with information more efficiently presented in the text, and overly complex tables that intimidate and confuse readers.
4. Arrange data in such a way that patterns are obvious at a glance; take care to organize information in an intelligible way.
5. Give each column and row of data a heading that is succinct but clear; table headings should establish the logic of the table structure.
6. Express data values to the number of decimal places justified by the precision of the measurement. In general, it is preferable to report numbers to one decimal place (or to two decimal places for correlation coefficients) because rounded values are easier to absorb than more precise ones. Report all values in a table to the same level of precision.
7. Make each table a "stand-alone" presentation, capable of being understood without reference to the text.
8. Clearly indicate probability levels, either by indicating the actual p values or by using asterisks and a probability level footnote. The usual convention is to use one asterisk when $p < 05$, two when $p < .01$, and three when $p < .001$.
9. Indicate units of measurement for numbers in the table whenever appropriate (e.g., pounds, milligrams, beats per minute).
10. Use footnotes to explain abbreviations or special symbols used in the table, except commonly understood abbreviations such as N.

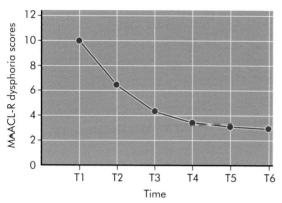

FIGURE 24.1 MAACL-R dysphoria from antepartum hospital through 6 weeks postpartum. (N = 63) T1 = antepartum admission; T2 = last antepartum; T3 = 2 days postpartum; T4 = 2 weeks postpartum; T5 = 4 weeks postpartum; T6 = 6 weeks postpartum. Used with permission from Maloni, J. A., et al., (2002) p. 97.

The write-up of statistical results is often a difficult task for beginning researchers because they are unsure about what to say and how to say it. Although we discuss style in a later section, it is difficult to avoid the mention of style here. By now, it should be clear that research evidence does not constitute *proof* of anything, but the point bears repeating. The report should never claim that the data proved, verified, confirmed, or demonstrated that hypotheses were correct or incorrect. Hypotheses are supported or unsupported, accepted or rejected.

Example from results section:
Lindgren (2001) studied the role of prenatal depression on pregnant women's health practices and fetal attachment. She stated some of the results of her hypothesis tests as follows:

> Hypothesis 1, that women who had higher levels of depressive symptoms would have lower levels of maternal-fetal attachment, was not supported by bivariate correlation results ($r = -.09$; $p > .05$). Hypothesis 2, that women who had higher levels of depressive symptoms would report fewer positive health practices, was supported ($r = -.41$; $p < .05$) (p. 210).

The Discussion Section

A report of the findings is never sufficient to convey their significance. The meaning that researchers give to the results plays a rightful and important role in the report. The discussion section is devoted to a thoughtful (and, it is hoped, insightful) analysis of the findings, leading to a discussion of their clinical and theoretical utility. A typical discussion section addresses the following questions:

What were the main findings?

What do the findings mean?

What evidence is there that the results and the interpretations are valid? What limitations might threaten validity?

How do the results compare with prior knowledge on the topic?

What can be concluded about the findings vis-à-vis their use in nursing practice, in nursing theory, and in future nursing research?

TIP: The discussion is typically the most challenging section to write. It deserves your most intense intellectual and creative effort—and careful review by peers. The peers should be asked to comment on how persuasive your arguments are, how well organized the section is, and whether it is too long, which is a common flaw.

Typically, the discussion section begins with a summary of the main findings, tied back to the introduction where the hypotheses, aims, or research questions were stated. The summary should be very brief, however, because the focus of the discussion is on making sense of (and not merely repeating) the results.

Example from discussion section:
Issel and Anderson (2001) studied community-based case managers' (CM) role in organizational decision making. They began their discussion as follows:

> Overall, the results supported the hypotheses and provided information on which activities and mechanisms are related to perceived CM influence. This is the first-known study in which CM PDM (participation in decision making) in a community-based setting was

examined, and the findings reveal that CMs did participate in organizational-level decision making and influence final choices (p. 368).

Interpretation of results is a global process, encompassing knowledge of the results, methods, sample characteristics, related research findings, clinical dimensions, and theoretical issues. Researchers should justify their interpretations, explicitly stating why alternative explanations have been ruled out. Unsupported conclusions are among the most common problems in discussion sections (Byrne, 1998). If the findings conflict with those of earlier studies, tentative explanations should be offered. A discussion of the generalizability of study findings should also be included.

Although readers should be told enough about the study's methods to identify its major weaknesses, report writers should point out limitations themselves. Researchers are in the best position to detect and assess the impact of sampling deficiencies, design constraints, data quality problems, and so forth, and it is a professional responsibility to alert readers to these difficulties. Moreover, if writers show their awareness of the study's limitations, readers will know that these limitations were considered in the interpretation.

Example from discussion section:
Melnyk and her colleagues (2001) undertook a pilot study to evaluate the effectiveness of a parent-focused intervention (COPE) on infants' cognitive development. They cited several study limitations, including the following:

> . . . a major limitation of this study was its small sample size, which resulted in large variances and limited power to detect statistically significant differences between groups, even when clinically meaningful differences existed (pp. 386–387.)

The implications derived from a study are often speculative and, therefore, should be couched in tentative terms. For instance, the kind of language appropriate for a discussion of the interpretation is illustrated by the following sentence: "The results *suggest* that it may be possible to improve nurse–physician interaction by modifying the

medical student's stereotype of the nurse as the physician's 'handmaiden.'" The interpretation is, in essence, a hypothesis that can presumably be tested in another research project. The discussion section, therefore, should include recommendations for studies that would help to test this hypothesis as well as suggestions for other studies to answer questions raised by the findings.

 Example from "Implications for clinical practice" subsection:
Gagnon, Waghorn, Jones, and Yang (2001), who studied the indicators nurses use in deciding to test healthy newborns for serum bilirubin, stated the following:

> Our data and the results of other studies suggest that newborns are being overtested for bilirubin levels. Our study shows that nurses use the presence of jaundice as the main reason for testing. Because the literature suggests that jaundice is common in newborns, exclusive use of the presence of jaundice may be inadequate information upon which to base the need for a test. Nurses may want to consider a more complete assessment before deciding to test for hyperbilirubinemia in the context of a newborn with physiologic jaundice (pp. 631–632.)

Other Aspects of the Report

The materials covered in the four major IMRAD sections are found in some form in virtually all quantitative research reports, although the organization might differ slightly. In addition to these major divisions, other aspects of the report deserve mention.

Title. Every research report should have a title indicating the nature of the study to prospective readers. The phrases "Research Report" or "Report of a Nursing Research Study" are inadequate. Insofar as possible, the dependent and independent variables (or central phenomenon under study) should be named in the title. It is also desirable to indicate the study population. However, the title should be brief (no more than about 15 words), so writers must balance clarity with brevity. The length of titles can often be reduced by omitting unnecessary terms such as "A Study of . . . ," "Report of . . ." or "An

Investigation To Examine the Effects of . . .," and so forth. The title should communicate concisely what was studied—and stimulate interest in the research.

Examples of research titles:
- "Self-reported reasons men decide not to participate in free prostate cancer screening" (Weinrich, Weinrich, Priest, & Fodi, 2003)
- "Effectiveness of home-based cardiac rehabilitation for special needs patients" (Warrington, Cholowski, & Peters, 2003).
- "The temperament profiles of school-aged children" (McClowry, 2002)

Abstract. Research reports usually include an abstract or, less often, a summary. Abstracts, it may be recalled, are brief descriptions of the problem, methods, and findings of the study, written so readers can decide whether to read the entire report. As noted in Chapter 5, abstracts for journals can either be in a traditional (unstructured) paragraph of 100 to 200 words, or in a structured form with subheadings. Examples of both types were presented in Box 5-2. Sometimes, a report concludes with a brief summary, and the summary may substitute for the abstract.

TIP: Take the time to write a compelling abstract. The abstract is your first main point of contact with reviewers and readers, so it deserves careful attention. It should demonstrate that your study is important clinically and that it was done with conceptual and methodologic rigor.

Key Words. It is often necessary to include key words that will be used in indexes to help others locate your study. Usually 5 to 10 key words suffice; indexing services may add other key words. Ideally, the key words identified conform to subject headings used in CINAHL or *Index Medicus*. Substantive, methodologic, and theoretical terms can be used as key words.

Example of key words:
Rockwell and Riegel (2001) studied predictors of self-care among people with heart failure. The key words used to index their study in CINAHL were:

Adult	*Heart Failure, Congestive	Scales
Age Factors	Inpatients	*Self-Care
Aged	Male	Self Report
Analysis of Variance	Middle Age	Severity of Illness
Comorbidity	*Models, Theoretical	Sex Factors
Conceptual Framework	Nonexperimental Studies	Socioeconomic Factors
Correlational Studies	Patient Compliance	Summated Rating Scaling
Education	Power Analysis	Support, Psychosocial
Female	Questionnaires	Surveys

Indicates main focus of paper

References. Each report concludes with a list of references cited in the text, using a reference style required by those reviewing the manuscript or report. References can be cumbersome to prepare, although there are some software programs to facilitate the preparation of reference lists (e.g., EndNote, ProCite, Reference Manager, Format Ease).

Acknowledgments. People who helped with the research but whose contribution does not qualify them for authorship are sometimes acknowledged at the end of the report. This might include statistical consultants, data collectors, and reviewers of the manuscript. The acknowledgments should also give credit to organizations that made the project possible, such as funding agencies or organizations that helped with subject recruitment.

Example of acknowledgments:
McDougall (2002) studied memory improvement in octogenarians. The following is excerpted from his acknowledgments:

This study was supported by the Claude D. Pepper Older Americans Independence Center at Case Western Reserve University Medical School. The author acknowledges the assistance of Jacquelyn Bayler, MSN . . .; the staff of Breckenridge Village in Willoughby, Ohio; and the significant contributions of Albert Bandura, PhD and Bert Hayslip, PhD for suggestions with research findings (p. 9).

Qualitative Research Reports

Qualitative research reports often follow the IMRAD format, or something akin to it. They can, however, be structured in a less standard fashion, offering more room for creativity—but also more challenges in determining how best to proceed. As Sandelowski (1998) has noted, there is no single style for reporting qualitative findings.

 Example of a nontraditional qualitative report organization:
Ritchie (2001) studied community health nurses' work in Australia with aboriginal clients, focusing on nurses' perceptions of empowering their clients. Her main headings were as follows:

> Empowerment Characteristics; Empowerment and Community Health Nursing; The Research Setting; The Research and Participants; Data Collection and Analysis; The Sociopolitical Context for Community Health Nursing Practice; Community Health Nursing Practice, Empowerment, and the Sociopolitical Context; and Discussion.

Even in this example, however, we can see that the author began by discussing the problem and its context, then described aspects of the study's methods, presented results, and discussed their implications. Thus, we present some issues of particular relevance for writing qualitative reports within the IMRAD structure.

Introduction

Qualitative reports usually begin with a statement of the problem, in a similar fashion to quantitative reports, but the focus is more squarely on the phenomenon under study. The way in which the problem is expressed and the types of questions the researchers sought to answer are usually tied to the research tradition underlying the study (e.g., grounded theory, ethnography), which is usually explicitly stated in the introduction. Prior research relating to the phenomenon under study may be summarized in the introduction, but sometimes this information is included in the discussion.

In many qualitative studies, but especially in ethnographic ones, it is critical to explain the cultural context of the study. In studies with an ideologic orientation (e.g., in critical theory or feminist research), it is also important to describe the sociopolitical context.

 Example from the introduction:
Choudry (2001) studied the resettlement experiences of South Asian women in Canada, and included an introductory section labeled "Cultural Context," which began as follows:

> There are significant differences between Canadian and South Asian culture. Although Indian culture encompasses several spoken languages and various religious traditions, people's behavior reflects the dominant Hindu cultural traditions and values. . . . The following description of South Asian culture will help the reader understand the participants' experiences in their cultural context (p. 378).

In other qualitative studies using phenomenological or grounded theory designs, the philosophy of phenomenology or symbolic interaction, respectively, may be discussed.

As another aspect of explaining the study's background, qualitative researchers sometimes provide information about their personal experiences or qualifications relevant to the conduct of the research. If a researcher who is studying decisions about long-term care placements is caring for two elderly parents and participates in a caregiver support group, this is relevant for readers' understanding of the study. In descriptive phenomenological studies, researchers may discuss their personal experiences in relation to the phenomenon being studied in order to share with the readers what they bracketed.

The concluding paragraph of the introduction usually offers a succinct summary of the purpose of the study or the research questions.

 Example from the introduction:
Norton and Bowers (2001) concluded their introduction with the following summary:

> The purpose of this study was to develop a grounded theory of how decisions were negotiated among providers and family members near the end of a patient's life. During the development of the theory . . ., identification was made of several strategies used to assist patients and families move

from curative to palliative treatment choices and goals. These strategies are the focus of this article (pp. 260–261).

Method

Although the research tradition of the study is often noted in the introduction, the method section usually elaborates on specific methods used in conjunction with that tradition. Design features such as whether the study was longitudinal should also be noted.

Example of a description of research design: Orshan, Furniss, Forst, and Santoro (2001) in their study of the lived experience of premature ovarian failure described their study design as follows:

Phenomenology focuses on the meaning of an experiential phenomenon of a human experience from the perspective of the individuals who experience it. . . . Within the phenomenological perspective, the perception of the individual who is describing her experience is accepted as the individual's reality. . . . The lived experience of a phenomenon does not evolve in a vacuum. Rather, the perception of the phenomenon emerges through the individuals' perceptions of their entire world—past, present, and future (p. 203).

The method section should provide a solid description of the research setting, so that readers can assess the transferability of findings. Study participants and methods by which they were selected should also be described. Even when samples are small, it may be useful to provide a table summarizing participants' main characteristics. If researchers have a personal connection to participants or to groups with which they are affiliated, this connection should be noted. At times, to disguise a group or institution, it may be necessary to omit potentially identifying information. Demographic characteristics of study participants that are not central to the story line may be changed to protect participants' confidentiality (Lipson, 1997).

Qualitative reports usually cannot provide specific information about data collection, inasmuch as formal instruments are not used, and questions and observations evolve in the field. Some researchers do, however, provide a sample of questions, especially if a topic guide was used. The description of

data collection methods should include how data were collected (e.g., interview or observation), how long data collection sessions lasted, who collected the data, how data collectors were trained, and methods used to record the data.

Example of a description of data collection: Kettunen, Poskiparta, Liimatainen, Sjögren, and Karhila (2001), who explored patients' taciturnity during counseling situations with a nurse, used the following methods to collect data:

This article is based on qualitative data gathered from a total of 38 nurse-patient health counseling sessions, which were videotaped in 7 different wards . . . of a Finnish hospital. Interviews with the nurses and patients after their sessions, during which they were encouraged to express their perceptions and evaluations of the counseling, were also collected. . . . All data were gathered by one member of the research group (pp. 401–402).

Information about data quality is particularly important in qualitative studies because the analysis depends so heavily on researchers' interpretation of the data. The more information included in the report about steps researchers took to ensure the trustworthiness of the data, the more confident readers can be that the findings are valid.

Example of a description of data quality: Kelly and Morgan-Kidd (2001), who studied social influences on at-risk girls' sexual behaviors, offered the following evidence about the quality of their focus group interview data:

Both authors . . . read the transcripts, labeled significant statements and key phrases, and independently assigned tentative codes. Areas of coding disagreement were discussed and resolved. . . . To verify the validity of the analysis, the investigators maintained an audit trail. . . . An anthropologist and a nurse-researcher who were not involved in the research but who were familiar with the study population reviewed the analysis and offered opinions . . . (that) were integrated into the final analysis (p. 484).

Quantitative reports typically have brief descriptions of data analysis techniques because standard statistical procedures are widely used and understood. By contrast, analytic procedures are often described in some detail in qualitative reports because readers need to understand how researchers organized, synthesized, and made sense of their data. If a computer program was used to manage and analyze data, the specific program should be mentioned.

 Example of a description of data analysis: Martell (2001), who conducted a grounded theory study of the postpartum experience, described her analysis as follows:

> Constant comparative analysis was used to derive a theoretical description from the interview data. The data were separated into categories derived inductively; labels for the categories were taken from the participants' own words. The categories were examined, compared, and recombined to uncover the underlying processes of the participants' experiences. As the study progressed, categories were changed, collapsed, or expanded. . . . Throughout these processes, the investigator took notes or memos about her interpretations (p. 498).

Results

In qualitative results sections, researchers summarize their thematic analysis and, in the case of grounded theory studies, the theory that emerged. This section can be organized in a number of ways. For example, if a process is being described, results may be presented chronologically, corresponding to the unfolding of the process. Key themes are often used as subheadings, organized in order of salience to participants or to a theory.

Example of thematic organization of results: Knobf (2002) did a grounded theory study of the experience of premature menopause among women with breast cancer. Her results section had the following subheadings, which corresponded to the stages uncovered in the research: *Being Focused*; *Facing Uncertainty*; *Becoming Menopausal*; and *Balancing*.

Metaphors are sometimes used to illuminate qualitative findings. Richardson (1994) referred to the metaphor as a literary device that is the spine or backbone of qualitative writing. She warned, however, that researchers must follow through on the details of the metaphors they have chosen.

Example of using metaphors in qualitative results:

Clemmens (2002) used the metaphor of a storm (specifically, a Nor'easter) to bring to life the results of her phenomenological study of adolescent mothers' experiences of feeling depressed. An example of her use of the storm metaphor can be seen in her second of six themes: "Being pulled and torn between two realities: like you've been swept up and pulled by the storm's strong opposing winds. It throws you off balance" (p. 557). Clemmens further explained this visual image: "Nor'easters are created by strong easterly flows of air to the north and opposing westerly flows from behind creating gusty winds that seem to pull in several directions. Adolescent mothers felt pulled and torn by the two realities of being both mothers and adolescents in school" (p. 557).

Sandelowski (1998) emphasizes the importance of developing a story line before beginning to write the findings. Because of the richness of qualitative data, researchers have to decide which story, or how much of it, they want to tell. They must also make a decision about how best to balance description and interpretation. The results section in a qualitative paper, unlike that in a quantitative one, intertwines data and interpretations of those data. It is important, however, that sufficient emphasis be given to the voices, actions, and experiences of participants themselves so that readers can gain an appreciation of their lives and their worlds. Most often, this occurs through the inclusion of direct quotes to illustrate important points. Because of space constraints in journals, quotes cannot be extensive, and great care must be exercised in selecting the best possible exemplars. Of course, quotes must be presented in a way that maintains participants' confidentiality (i.e., without divulging their names and identifying information). Using quotes is not only a skill but a complex process. When inserting quotes in the results section, researchers must pay attention to how the quote is introduced and how it is put in context. Quotes should not be used haphazardly or just inserted one right after the other in a string.

TIP: Although the analysis of qualitative data should be done with verbatim transcripts of interviews or dialogue, participant quotes should be edited for inclusion in a report. The quotes should maintain the integrity of the data, but should omit distracting or irrelevant materials (e.g., through the use of three ellipsis points, such as . . .).

Example of using quotes in results section: George (2002) studied women's menopausal experiences. One theme had to do with women's need to "sort things out" (i.e., to understand the context of the experience). Here is one excerpt from her transcripts:

> When I look back, it was just a very different kind of time for me. About a year before I started treatment for menopause, I really hit an extended period of time where I was clearly depressed. At the time I didn't know what it was. . . . I'm not sure whether it was menopause that played a part in the depression, or whether it was a time in my life for different changes (p. 82).

Figures, diagrams, and word tables that organize concepts are often extremely useful in qualitative studies in summarizing an overall conceptualization of the phenomena under study. Grounded theory studies are especially likely to benefit from a schematic presentation of the basic social process. Ethnographic and ethnoscience studies often present taxonomies in tabular form.

Discussion

In qualitative studies, the findings and the interpretation are typically presented together in the results section because the task of integrating qualitative materials is necessarily interpretive. The discussion section of a qualitative report, therefore, is not so much designed to give meaning to the results, but to summarize them, link them to other research, and suggest their implications for theory, practice, or future research. In some cases, researchers offer explicit recommendations about how their research can be corroborated (or how hypotheses can be tested) through quantitative studies. Sandelowski (1998) alerts qualitative researchers that they must pay attention not only to the content of the infor-

mation in their reports but to their form. Poor form can seriously impede the readers' understanding of the results and discussion sections. Van Manen (1997) warns qualitative researchers that they are not just writers who write up their research reports, but authors who write "from the midst of life experience where meanings resonate and reverberate with reflective being" (p. 368).

Example from discussion: Borrayo and Jenkins (2001) conducted a grounded theory study to understand how a cultural explanatory model (CEM) of breast cancer might influence breast cancer screening among Mexican-American women. Their discussion noted,

> . . . future research should quantitatively measure the elements of these women's cancer-relevant CEM in their sociocultural context. . . . (p. 822).

Other Aspects of a Qualitative Report

Qualitative reports, like quantitative ones, include abstracts, key words, references, and acknowledgments. Abstracts for journals that feature qualitative reports (e.g., *Western Journal of Nursing Research* and *Qualitative Health Research*) tend to be the traditional single-paragraph type—that is, not structured abstracts. The abstract frequently indicates the research tradition underlying the study.

The titles of qualitative reports usually state the central phenomenon under scrutiny. Phenomenological studies often have titles that include such words as "the lived experience of . . . " or "the meaning of. . . . " Grounded theory studies often indicate something about the *findings* in the title—for example, noting the core category or basic social process. Ethnographic titles usually indicate the culture being studied. Two-part titles are not uncommon, with substance and method, research tradition and findings, or theme and meaning, separated by a colon.

Examples of qualitative titles:
- Ethnography—"Characteristics of African American women caregivers of children with asthma" (Sterling & Peterson, 2003)
- Grounded theory—"Redefining parental identity: Caregiving and schizophrenia" (Milliken & Northcutt, 2003).

- Phenomenology—"The experience of women receiving brachytherapy for gynecologic cancer" (Velji & Fitch, 2001)
- Participatory action research—"Formerly incarcerated women create healthy lives through participatory action research" (Parson & Warner-Robbins, 2002)

Finally, qualitative reports may also include a brief biography of the researchers, summarizing aspects of their professional and personal lives that are relevant to the research.

THE STYLE OF RESEARCH REPORTS

Research reports—especially for quantitative studies—are usually written in a distinctive style. Some stylistic guidelines were discussed previously in this chapter and in Chapter 5, but additional points are elaborated on in this section.

A research report is not an essay. It is an account of how and why a problem was studied, and what was discovered as a result. The report should in general not include overtly subjective statements, emotionally laden statements, or exaggerations. This is not to say that the researchers' story should be told in a dreary manner. Indeed, in qualitative reports there are ample opportunities to enliven the narration with rich description, direct quotes, and insightful interpretation. Authors of quantitative reports, although somewhat constrained by structure and the need to include numeric information, should strive to keep the presentation lively.

In quantitative reports, personal pronouns such as "I," "my," and "we" are often avoided because the passive voice and impersonal pronouns suggest greater impartiality. Qualitative reports, by contrast, are often written in the first person and in an active voice. Some qualitative researchers (e.g., Webb, 1992) have argued that the use of the neutral, anonymous third person in quantitative research is actually deceptive because it suggests greater objectivity than may be warranted. It is likely that the report-writing styles of researchers working within different paradigms will continue to diverge. Even among quantitative researchers, however, there is a trend toward striking a greater balance between active and passive voice and first-person and third-person narration. If a direct presentation can be made without suggesting bias, a more readable and lively product usually results.

It is not easy to write simply and clearly, but these are important goals of scientific writing. The use of pretentious words or technical jargon does little to enhance the communicative value of the report. Avoiding jargon and highly technical terms is especially important in communicating research findings to practicing nurses. Also, complex sentence constructions are not necessarily the best way to convey ideas. The style should be concise and straightforward. If writers can add elegance to their reports without interfering with clarity and accuracy, so much the better, but the product is not expected to be a literary achievement. Needless to say, this does not imply that grammatical and spelling accuracy should be sacrificed. The research report should reflect scholarship, not pedantry.

With regard to references and specific technical aspects of the manuscript, various styles have been developed. The writer may be able to select a style, but often the style is imposed by journal editors and university regulations. Specialized manuals such as those of the University of Chicago Press (1993), the American Psychological Association (2001), and the American Medical Association (1997) are widely used for reference styles.

A common flaw in reports of beginning researchers is inadequate organization. The overall structure is fairly standard, but the organization within sections and subsections needs careful attention. Sequences should be in an orderly progression with appropriate transitions. Themes or ideas should not be introduced abruptly or abandoned suddenly. Continuity and logical thematic development are critical to good communication.

It may seem a trivial point, but methods and results should be described in the past tense. For example, it is inappropriate to say, "Nurses who receive special training perform triage functions significantly better than those without training." In this sentence, "receive" and "perform" should be changed to "received" and "performed." The present tense implies that the results apply to all nurses, when in fact the statement pertains only to a particular sample whose behavior was observed in the past.

TYPES OF RESEARCH REPORTS

Although the general form and structure of research reports are fairly consistent across different types of reports, certain requirements vary. This section describes features of four major kinds of research reports: theses and dissertations, traditional journal articles, on-line reports, and presentations at professional meetings. Reports for class projects are excluded—not because they are unimportant but rather because they so closely resemble theses on a smaller scale. Final reports to agencies that have sponsored research also are not described. Most funding agencies issue reporting guidelines that can be secured from project officers.

Theses and Dissertations

Most doctoral degrees are granted on the successful completion of an empirical research project. Empirical theses are sometimes required of master's degree candidates as well. Most universities have a preferred format for their dissertations. Until recently, most schools used a traditional IMRAD format. The following organization for a traditional dissertation is typical:

Preliminary Pages
  Title Page
  Acknowledgment Page
  Table of Contents
  List of Tables
  List of Figures
Main Body
  Chapter I. Introduction
  Chapter II. Review of the Literature
  Chapter III. Methods

Chapter IV. Results
Chapter V. Discussion and Summary
Supplementary Pages
  Bibliography
  Appendix

The preliminary pages or **front matter** for dissertations are much the same as those for a scholarly book. The title page indicates the title of the study, the author's name, the degree requirement being fulfilled, the name of the university awarding the degree, the date of submission of the report, and the signatures of the dissertation committee members. The acknowledgment page gives writers the opportunity to express appreciation to those who contributed to the project. The table of contents outlines the major sections and subsections of the report, indicating on which page the reader will find those sections of interest. The lists of tables and figures identify by number, title, and page the tables and figures that appear in the text.

The main body of a traditionally formatted dissertation incorporates the IMRAD sections described earlier. The literature review often is so extensive that a separate chapter may be devoted to it. When a short review is sufficient, the first two chapters may be combined. In some cases, a separate chapter may also be required to elaborate the study's conceptual framework.

The supplementary pages include a bibliography or list of references used to prepare the report and one or more appendixes. An appendix contains information and materials relevant to the study that are either too lengthy or too tangential to be incorporated into the body of the report. Data collection instruments, scoring instructions, codebooks, cover letters, permission letters, category schemes, and peripheral statistical tables are examples of the kinds of materials included in the appendix. Some universities also require the inclusion of a brief *curriculum vitae* of the author.

A new approach to formatting dissertations or theses is the **paper format thesis**. The front matter and material at the end are similar to those in a traditionally formatted thesis, but the main sections differ. In a typical paper format thesis, there is an introduction, one or two publishable papers, and then a conclusion (Morris & Tipples, 1998). Such a format obviously permits students to move directly from thesis to journal submission, but is somewhat more demanding than the traditional format. Morris and Tipples offered three possible scenarios for the papers to be included in the paper format thesis: (1) one paper focusing on a literature review followed by a second paper discussing the research results; (2) two or more papers focusing on different research findings for the single research project; and (3) one methodologic paper (e.g., describing the development of an instrument) and the second presenting research findings.

If an academic institution does not use the paper format thesis, a student will need to adapt the thesis or dissertation before submitting it for publication. This revision of the thesis/dissertation takes skill. Johnson (1996) interviewed 15 journal editors for advice on converting a thesis style to an acceptable manuscript format. Figure 24-2 summarizes suggested changes to facilitate acceptance of a manuscript for publication in a nursing journal. Boyle (1997) also has provided pointers to new recipients of doctoral degrees on how to publish their qualitative dissertations. This advice focuses on how to divide up or dissect the dissertation to generate two or more publications.

Journal Articles

Progress in nursing research depends on researchers' efforts to share their work. Dissertations and final reports to funders, which are too lengthy and inaccessible for widespread use, are read only by a handful of people. Publication in a professional journal ensures broad circulation of research findings. From a personal point of view, it is exciting and professionally advantageous to have journal publications. This section discusses issues relating to research reports in journals.

Selecting a Journal

Before writing begins, there should be a clear idea of the journal to which a manuscript will be submitted. Journals differ in their goals, types of manuscript sought, and readership; these factors need to be matched against personal interests and preferences. All journals issue goal statements, as well as guidelines for preparing and submitting a manuscript. This information is published in journals themselves and on their websites. Table 24-1

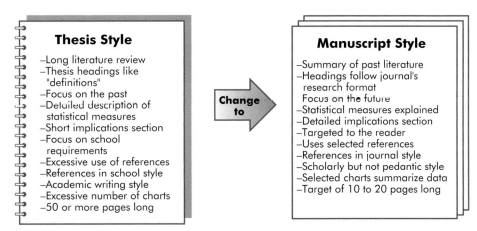

Thesis Style

–Long literature review
–Thesis headings like "definitions"
–Focus on the past
–Detailed description of statistical measures
–Short implications section
–Focus on school requirements
–Excessive use of references
–References in school style
–Academic writing style
–Excessive number of charts
–50 or more pages long

Change to

Manuscript Style

–Summary of past literature
–Headings follow journal's research format
–Focus on the future
–Statistical measures explained
–Detailed implications section
–Targeted to the reader
–Uses selected references
–References in journal style
–Scholarly but not pedantic style
–Selected charts summarize data
–Target of 10 to 20 pages long

FIGURE 24.2 Suggested changes to convert theses to manuscripts. Adapted with permission from Johnson, S. H. (1996) Adapting a thesis to publication style: Meeting editor's expectations. *Dimensions of Critical Care Nursing, 15,* 160–167.

TABLE 24.1 Peer-Reviewed Nursing Journals With High Concentration of Research Articles

NAME OF JOURNAL	WEBSITE	REFERENCE STYLE*		
		APA	Biomed	Other
American Journal of Critical Care	www.aacn.org		X	
American Journal of Infection Control	www.harcourthealth.com		X	
Applied Nursing Research	www.harcourthealth.com	X		
Archives of Psychiatric Nursing	www.harcourthealth.com	X		
Australian Journal of Advanced Nursing	www.anf.org.au			X
Canadian Journal of Nursing Research	www.nursing.mcgill.ca/cjnr/home/author/html	X		
Clinical Nursing Research	www.sagepub.com	X		
Heart & Lung	www.harcourthealth.com		X	
International Journal of Nursing Practice	www.blackwell-synergy.com		X	
International Journal of Nursing Studies	www.elsevier.com			X
Issues in Mental Health Nursing	www.taylorandfrancis.com	X		
Journal of Advanced Nursing	www.blackwell-synergy.com			X
Journal of Family Nursing	www.sagepub.com	X		
Journal of National Black Nurses Association	www.nbna.org	X		
Journal of Nursing Measurement	www.springerjournals.com	X		
Journal of Obstetric, Gynecologic, and Neonatal Nursing	www.sagepub.com	X		
Journal of Pediatric Nursing	www.harcourthealth.com	X		
Nursing History Review	www.springerjournals.com			X
Nursing Research	www.nursingcenter.com	X		
Public Health Nursing	www.blackwell-synergy.com	X		
Qualitative Health Research	www.sagepub.com	X		
Research in Nursing & Health	www.interscience.wiley.com	X		
Western Journal of Nursing Research	www.sagepub.com	X		

*APA, American Psychological Association (2001); Biomed, International Committee of Medical Journal Editors (1997).

presents a list of nursing journals that devote 50% or more of their space to research articles, together with their Internet addresses.

Example of statement of journal goal:

Qualitative Health Research is an international, interdisciplinary refereed journal for the enhancement of health care and to further the development and understanding of qualitative research methods in health care settings. We welcome manuscripts in the following areas: the description and analysis of the illness experience, health and health-seeking behaviors, the experience of caregivers, the sociocultural organization of health care, health care policy, and related topics. We also seek critical reviews and commentaries addressing conceptual, theoretical, methodological, and ethical issues pertaining to qualitative inquiry.

Journals also differ in prestige, acceptance rates, and circulation, and these may also need to be taken into account in selecting a journal. Northam, Trubenbach, and Bentov (2000), in their article on publishing opportunities for nurses, offered information on editorial style, number of issues annually, time for acceptance, time for publication, reasons for rejection, and acceptance rate for 83 U.S. journals in nursing and related health fields. Results of their survey show that some journals are far more competitive than others. For example, *Nursing Research* accepts only 20% of submitted manuscripts, whereas the acceptance rates for many specialty journals that accept research reports is greater than 50%. A supplementary resource for identifying potential journals is the Key Nursing Journals Chart (Allen, 2000), which can be accessed at the following website: http://nahrs.library.kent.edu/resource/reports/specr pts.htm. The chart indicates journal circulation, number of articles published each year, percentage of research articles published, and other valuable information for numerous nursing journals. Also, McConnell (2000) has compiled information about 82 non-U.S. nursing journals from 13 countries.

It is sometimes useful to send a **query letter** to a journal to ask the editor whether there is any interest in a proposed manuscript. The query letter should briefly describe the topic of the paper, the methods used, the researchers' qualifications, a preliminary title, and a tentative submission date. Query letters are not essential if researchers have done a lot of homework about the journal's goals and the type of articles it publishes. Query letters do, however, avoid problems that can arise if editors have recently accepted several papers on a similar topic and do not wish to consider another. Indeed, the top three reasons cited by the survey of 83 journal editors for rejecting manuscripts were the topic was not suitable for the journal's focus, the topic was not current, and similar articles recently had been published (Northam et al., 2000). Query letters can be submitted by traditional mail or, usually, by e-mail using contact information provided at the journal's website.

Query letters can be sent to multiple journals simultaneously, but ultimately the manuscript can be submitted only to one—or rather, only to one at a time. If several editors express interest in reviewing a manuscript, journals can be prioritized according to criteria previously described. The priority list should not be discarded because the manuscript can be resubmitted to the next journal on the list if the journal of first choice rejects it.

Preparing the Manuscript

Once a journal has been selected, the information included in the journal's **Instructions to Authors** should be carefully reviewed. These instructions typically tell prospective authors such information as maximum page length; what size paper, font, and margins are permissible; what type of abstract is desired; what reference style should be used; how many copies should be submitted; and whether an electronic file is required (and what software package is preferred). It is important to adhere to the journal's guidelines to avoid rejection for a nonsubstantive reason.

TIP: Don't begin to write until you have carefully examined a high-quality research report that you can use as a model. Select as a model a journal article on a topic similar to your own (or one that uses similar methods) in the journal you have selected as first choice.

TABLE 24.2 Example of a Manuscript Organization With Examples of Page Allocations

SECTION	NUMBER OF PAGES
Title page (title, authors, affiliations and credentials, contact information for corresponding author)	1
Abstract and key words	1
Text: Introduction	2
Methods	4
Results	4
Discussion	2
References	2
Tables/figures (plus legends and footnotes)	3
Acknowledgments, financial support for the study	1
Total number of pages:	18

Typically, a manuscript for journals must be no more than 15 to 20 double-spaced, typed pages (with 1-inch margins) in its entirety, including tables, references, the abstract, and so on. As an example, Table 24-2 shows what a complete manuscript might look like, in terms of contents and page numbers.

Care should be taken in using and preparing references. Some nursing journals suggest that references be limited to no more than 15 citations. In general, only published work can be included in the reference list (e.g., not papers at a conference or manuscripts submitted but not accepted for publication). As Table 24-1 shows, most journals use the reference style of the American Psychological Association (2001), which is the style we use throughout this book.

TIP: First (and even second) drafts of manuscripts are rarely ready for submission. You can often be more objective in critiquing your own paper if you put it aside for a few days and then reread it with a fresh outlook. A review of the draft by colleagues or advisers can be invaluable in improving its quality.

Submission of a Manuscript

When the manuscript is ready for journal submission, the required number of copies should be sent to the editor with a cover letter. The cover letter should include the following information: title of the paper, name and contact information of the **corresponding author** (the author with whom the journal communicates—usually, but not always, the lead author), and assurances that (1) the paper is original and has not been published or submitted elsewhere; (2) all authors have read and approved the manuscript; and (3) (in certain situations) there are no conflicts of interest. The cover letter should be signed by all authors. Some journals also require a signed copyright transfer form, which transfers all copyright ownership of the manuscript to the journal and warrants that all authors signing the form participated sufficiently in the research to justify authorship.

Manuscript Review

Most nursing journals that include research reports—including all those listed in Table 24-1—have a policy of independent, anonymous (sometimes referred to as **blind**) **peer reviews** by two or more experts in the field. By "anonymous," we mean that reviewers do not know the identity of the authors, and authors do not learn the identity of reviewers. Journals that have such a policy are **refereed journals**, and are in general more prestigious than nonrefereed journals.

TIP: When submitting a manuscript to a refereed journal, authors' names should not appear anywhere except on the title page.

Peer reviewers make recommendations to the editors about whether to accept the manuscript for publication, accept it contingent on revisions, or reject it. Relatively few papers are accepted outright—both substantive and editorial revisions are the norm.

Example of reviewer recommendation categories:
The journal *Research in Nursing & Health* asks reviewers to make one of six recommendations to the editorial staff: (1) Highly recommend; few revisions needed; (2) Publish if suggested revisions are satisfactorily completed; (3) Major revisions needed; revised version should be re-reviewed; (4) May have potential; encourage resubmission as a new manuscript; (5) Reject; do not encourage resubmission; and (6) Not appropriate for journal; send to another type of journal.

Authors are sent information about the editors' decision, together with reviewers' comments. When resubmitting a revised manuscript to the same journal, each reviewer recommendation should be addressed, either by making the requested change, or by explaining in the cover letter accompanying the resubmission the rationale for not revising. Defending some aspect of a paper against a reviewer's recommendation sometimes requires a citation or other supporting information. If the manuscript is rejected, the reviewers' comments should be taken into consideration before submitting it to another journal.

TIP: Try not be too disheartened by a rejection. A rejection by one journal should not discourage you from sending the manuscript to another

one. Competition for journal space is keen, and a rejection does not necessarily mean that a study is unworthy of publication. Manuscripts may need to be reviewed by several journals before final acceptance.

Typically, many months go by between submission of the original manuscript and the publication of a journal article, especially if there are revisions—as there usually are. For example, according to information provided in the Northam et al. (2000) survey, an average of 7 months elapses between submission and acceptance in *Western Journal of Nursing Research*, and an additional 18 months elapses before publication.

Example of journal timeline:
Beck (2002) completed a metasynthesis of qualitative studies on mothering multiples and submitted her paper to *MCN: The American Journal of Maternal/Child Nursing*. The timeline for acceptance and publication of this manuscript, which was relatively fast, is as follows:

January 23, 2001	Manuscript sent to *MCN* editor for review
March 28, 2001	Letter from editor informing of a revise and resubmit decision
April 27, 2001	Revised manuscript resubmitted
May 24, 2001	Revised manuscript accepted for publication
July/Aug., 2002	Publication in journal

Electronic Publication

Computers and the Internet have changed forever how information of all types is retrieved and disseminated. Many nurse researchers are exploring opportunities to share their research findings through electronic publication.

Most journals that publish in hard copy format (e.g., *Nursing Research*) now also have on-line capabilities. Such mechanisms, which serve as a document delivery system, expand a journal's circulation and make research findings accessible worldwide. There are few implications for authors, however.

Such electronic publication is just a method of distributing reports already available in hard copy and that are subject to the journal's standard page limitations, peer review process, and so on.

There are, however, many other ways to disseminate research findings on the Internet. For example, some researchers or research teams develop their own web page with information about their studies. When there are hyperlinks embedded in the websites, consumers can navigate between files and websites to retrieve relevant information on a topic of interest. At the other extreme are peer-reviewed electronic journals (**ejournals**) that are exclusively in on-line format. Examples include the *Online Journal of Knowledge Synthesis in Nursing* and the *Online Journal of Issues in Nursing*. In between are a variety of outlets of research communication, such as websites of nursing and health organizations and electronic magazines (**ezines**) in health fields.

Electronic publication offers numerous advantages. Dissemination can occur much more rapidly, cutting down dramatically on publication lag time. Electronic research reports are accessible to a broad, worldwide audience of potential consumers. Typically, there are no page limitations, enabling researchers to describe and discuss complex studies more fully. Qualitative researchers are able to use more extensive quotes from their raw data, for example. Research reports on the Internet can incorporate a wide variety of graphic material, including audio and video supplements not possible in hard copy journals. Raw data can also be appended to reports on the Internet for secondary analysis by other researchers.

Still, there are some potential drawbacks, including technological requirements. One issue concerns peer review. Although many on-line journals perform peer reviews, there are many opportunities to "publish" results on the Internet without a peer review process. Sparks (1999) points out that there are also non–peer-reviewed traditional journals, and so concludes that concern about peer review in electronic publishing is a red herring. However, nonrefereed journal articles are not as accessible to a worldwide market as nonreviewed information on the Internet. There is a much greater risk of

there being a glut of low-quality research available for consumption as a result of the Internet than there was previously. Responsible researchers who want their evidence to have an impact on nursing practice should seek publication in outlets that subject manuscripts to a review process.

TIP: The rapid expansion of on-line publishing opportunities makes in impossible to list them. There are, however, websites that maintain such listings, including:

http://www.nursefriendly.com
http://www.nursing-portal.com
http://www.healthweb.org

Presentations at Professional Conferences

Numerous professional organizations sponsor annual meetings at which nursing studies are presented, either through the reading of a research report or through visual display in a poster session. The American Nurses' Association is an example of an organization that holds meetings at which nurses have an opportunity to share their knowledge with others interested in their topic. Many local chapters of Sigma Theta Tau devote one or more of their annual activities to research reports. Examples of regional organizations that sponsor research conferences are the Western Society for Research in Nursing, the Southern Council on Collegiate Education for Nursing, the Eastern Nursing Research Society, and the Midwest Nursing Research Society.

Presentation of research results at a conference has two distinct advantages over journal publication. First, there is usually less time elapsed between the completion of a study and its communication to others when a presentation is made at a meeting. Second, there is an opportunity for dialogue between researchers and the audience at a conference. Listeners can request clarification on certain points or can make useful suggestions. For this reason, professional conferences are particularly good forums for presenting results to clinical audiences. Researchers also can take advantage of meeting and talking with others attending the conference who are working on similar problems in different parts of the country.

The mechanism for submitting a presentation to a conference is somewhat simpler than in the case of journal submission. The association sponsoring the conference ordinarily publishes an announcement or **Call for Abstracts** in its newsletter, journal, or website about 6 to 9 months before the meeting date. The notice indicates topics of interest, submission requirements, and deadlines for submitting a proposed paper or poster. Most universities and major health care agencies receive and post Call for Abstracts notices. The *Western Journal of Nursing Research* also publishes a calendar of national and international conferences at the beginning of each issue, and the Sigma Theta Tau International website (www.nursingsociety.org) maintains a listing of research conferences.

Oral Reports

Most conferences require prospective presenters to submit an abstract of 500 to 1000 words rather than a complete paper. Abstracts can usually be (and in some cases *must* be) submitted on-line. Each conference has its own guidelines for abstract content and form. In some cases, abstracts are submitted to the organizer of a particular session on a given topic; in other cases, conference sessions are organized after-the-fact, with related papers grouped together. Abstracts are evaluated on the basis of the quality and originality of the research, and the appropriateness of the paper for the conference audience. If abstracts are accepted, researchers are committed to appear at the conference to make a presentation.

Research reports presented at professional meetings usually follow a traditional IMRAD format. The time allotted for presentation usually is about 10 to 15 minutes, with up to 5 minutes for questions from the audience. Therefore, only the most important aspects of the study—with special emphasis on the results—can be included. It is especially challenging to condense a qualitative report to a brief oral summary without losing the rich, in-depth character of the data. A handy rule of thumb is that a page of double-spaced text requires $2\frac{1}{2}$ to 3 minutes to read aloud. Although most conference presenters do prepare a written paper or a script, presentations are most effective if they are delivered informally or conversationally, rather than if they are read verbatim. The presentation should be rehearsed to gain familiarity and comfort with the script, and to ensure that time limits are not exceeded.

TIP: Most conferences presentations can be greatly enhanced by including vivid visual materials (e.g., slides, transparencies, Power Point materials). The visual aids should be kept very simple for biggest impact. Tables are difficult to read on slides or transparencies; they can, however, be distributed to members of the audience in hard copy form. Make sure a sufficient number of copies is available.

The question-and-answer period can be a fruitful opportunity to expand on various aspects of the research and to get early feedback about the study. It is useful to make note of audience comments because these can be helpful in turning the conference presentation into a manuscript for journal submission.

Poster Presentations

Researchers sometimes elect to present their findings in poster sessions. (Abstracts, often similar to those required for oral presentations, must be submitted to conference organizers according to specific guidelines.) In poster sessions, several researchers simultaneously present visual displays summarizing the highlights of the study, and conference attendees circulate around the exhibit area perusing displays. In this fashion, those interested in a particular topic can devote time to discussing the study with the researcher and bypass posters dealing with topics of less interest. Poster sessions are thus efficient and encourage one-on-one discussions. Poster sessions are typically 1 to 2 hours in length; researchers should stand near their posters throughout the session to ensure effective communication.

It is challenging to design an effective poster. The poster must convey essential information about the background, design, and results of a study, in a format that can be perused in minutes. Bullet points, graphs, and photos are especially useful devices on a poster for communicating a lot of information quickly. Large, bold fonts are essential, because posters are often read from a distance of several feet. Another issue is that posters must be sturdily constructed for transport to the conference site. It is important to follow the conference guidelines in determining such matters as poster size (often 4 ft high × 6 or 8 ft wide), format, allowable display materials, and so on.

Wilson and Hutchinson (1997) recommend a three-phase process to presenting effective posters. In the prepresentation phase, researchers target the audience, obtain official guidelines, write an abstract/title, and design a poster based on principles of visual literacy. In the presentation phase, Wilson and Hutchinson suggest items to bring to the actual poster session, such as data collection instruments, bibliographic information, business cards, and pages of stick-on mailing labels so that those interested in additional information can write their names and addresses on the labels. In the postpresentation phase, presenters should evaluate the effectiveness of their poster. One approach is to ask viewers to complete a simple evaluation form regarding the poster. Bushy (1991) designed a 30-item Research-Poster Appraisal Tool (R-PAT) that researchers can use. Several authors have offered further advice on preparing for poster sessions (e.g., Lippman & Ponton, 1989; McDaniel, Bach, & Poole, 1993; and Moore, Augspurger, King, & Proffitt, 2001).

Russell, Gregory, and Gates (1996) alert qualitative researchers to the special challenges that await them in regard to designing a poster. Findings from quantitative research can be condensed and presented in numeric tables. The rich data from qualitative research, including participants' quotes, themes, and so forth, present more of a challenge in trying to summarize them concisely.

SUMMARY POINTS

- In developing a dissemination plan, researchers need to select a communication outlet (e.g., journal article versus conference presentation), identify the audience whom they wish to reach, and decide on the content that can be effectively communicated in a single outlet.
- In the planning stage, researchers need to decide authorship credits (if there are multiple authors), who the **lead author** and **corresponding author** will be, and in what order authors' names will be listed.
- Quantitative reports (and many qualitative reports) typically follow the **IMRAD format**, with the following sections: introduction, method, results, and discussion.
- The introduction acquaints readers with the research problem. It includes the problem statement, the phenomenon under study, research hypotheses or questions, importance of the research, a summary of relevant related literature, identification of a theoretical framework, and definitions of the concepts being studied. In qualitative reports, the introduction also indicates the research tradition and, if relevant, the researchers' connection to the problem.
- The method section describes what researchers did to solve the research problem. It normally includes a description of the study design (or an elaboration of the research tradition); the study participants and how they were selected; instruments and procedures used to collect and evaluate the data; and techniques used to analyze the data.
- In the results section, findings from the analyses are summarized. Quantitative reports summarize analyses in order of importance, or in the sequence in which hypotheses were presented. Qualitative reports summarize findings sequentially (if a process is being described) or in the order of salience of themes.
- Results sections in qualitative reports necessarily intertwine description and interpretation. Quotes from transcripts are essential for giving voice to study participants.
- Both qualitative and quantitative researchers include **figures** and **tables** that dramatize or succinctly summarize major findings or conceptual schema.

- The discussion section presents the interpretation of results, how the findings relate to earlier research, study limitations, and implications of the findings for nursing practice and future research.
- Additional items to be included with research reports include a title, abstract, key words, acknowledgments, and references.
- Research reports should be written simply and clearly, with a minimum of jargon or emotionally laden statements.
- The major types of research reports are theses and dissertations, journal articles, on-line publications, and presentations at professional meetings.
- Theses and dissertations normally follow a standard IMRAD format, but some schools are now accepting **paper format theses**, which include an introduction, one or more papers ready to submit for publication, and a conclusion.
- In selecting a journal for publication, the following factors should be kept in mind: the journal's goals and audience, its prestige and acceptance rates, how often it publishes, and its circulation.
- Before beginning to prepare a **manuscript** for submission to a journal, researchers need carefully to review the journal's **Instructions to Authors**. Most journals limit manuscripts to 15 to 20 typed, double-spaced pages, for example.
- Most nursing journals that publish research reports are **refereed journals** with a policy of basing publication decisions on **peer reviews** that are usually **blind reviews** (identities of authors and reviewers are not divulged).
- There are many new opportunities for electronic publishing that nurse researchers can explore, including publications in **ejournals** and **ezines**. Electronic publishing offers the advantage of speedy dissemination to a worldwide audience. Peer-reviewed electronic publications are preferred for building a strong evidence base for nursing practice.
- Nurse researchers can also present their research at professional conferences, either through a 10- to 15-minute oral report to a seated audience, or in a **poster session** in which the "audience" moves around a room perusing research summaries attached to posters. Sponsoring organizations usually issue a **Call for Abstracts** for the conference 6 to 9 months before it is held.

STUDY ACTIVITIES

Chapter 24 of the accompanying *Study Guide for Nursing Research: Principles and Methods, 7th ed.*, offers various exercises and study suggestions for reinforcing the concepts presented in this chapter. In addition, the following questions can be addressed:

1. Skim a qualitative and a quantitative research report. Make a bullet-point list of differences in style and organization between the two.
2. What are the similarities and differences of research reports that are written for journal publication and for presentation at a professional meeting?
3. Read a research report. Now write a two- to three-page summary of the report that communicates the major points of the report to a clinical audience with minimal research skills.

SUGGESTED READINGS

Methodologic/Stylistic References

Aaronson, L. S. (1994). Milking data or meeting commitments: How many papers from one study? *Nursing Research, 43*, 60–62.

American Medical Association. (1998). *American Medical Association manual of style: A guide for authors and editors* (9th ed.). Philadelphia: Lippincott Williams & Wilkins.

American Psychological Association. (2001). *Publication manual of the American Psychological Association* (5th ed.). Washington, DC: Author.

Beck, C. T. (1999). Facilitating the work of a meta-analyst. *Research in Nursing & Health, 22*, 523–530.

Bolker, J. (1998). *Writing your dissertation in 15 minutes a day: A guide to starting, revising, and finishing your doctoral dissertation*. New York: Henry Holt.

Boyle, J. S. (1997). Writing up: Dissecting the dissertation. In J. M. Morse (Ed.), *Completing a qualitative project: Details and dialogue* (pp. 9–37). Thousand Oaks, CA: Sage.

Browner, W. S. (1999). *Publishing and presenting clinical research*. Philadelphia: Lippincott Williams & Wilkins.

Bushy, A. (1991) . A rating scale to evaluate research posters. *Nurse Educator, 16*, 11–15.

Byrne, D. W. (1998). *Publishing your medical research paper: What they don't teach you in medical school*. Philadelphia: Lippincott Williams & Wilkins.

Davis, G. B., & Parker, C. (1997). *Writing the doctoral dissertation: A systematic approach* (2nd ed.). Hauppauge, NY: Barron's Educational Series.

Duncan, A. M. (1999). Authorship, dissemination of research findings, and related matters. *Applied Nursing Research, 12*, 101–106.

Erlen, J. A., Siminoff, L. A., Sereika, S. M., & Sutton, L. B. (1997). Multiple authorship: Issues and recommendations. *Journal of Professional Nursing, 13*, 262–270.

Gelfand, H., & Walker, C. (1990). *Mastering APA style: Students' workbook and training guide* (4th ed.). Washington, DC: American Psychological Association.

Hanson, S. M. H. (1988). Collaborative research and authorship credit: Beginning guidelines. *Nursing Research, 37*, 49–52.

Hayes, P. (1992). "De-jargonizing" research communication. *Clinical Nursing Research, 1*, 219–220.

Iles, R. (1997). *Guidebook to better medical writing*. Olathe, KA: Island Press.

International Committee of Medical Journal Editors. (1997). Uniform requirements for manuscripts submitted to biomedical journals. *Annals of Internal Medicine, 126*, 35–47 (available at www.icmje.org).

Jackle, M. (1989). Presenting research to nurses in clinical practice. *Applied Nursing Research, 2*, 191–193.

Johnson, S. H. (1996). Adapting a thesis to publication style: Meeting editor's expectations. *Dimensions of Critical Care Nursing, 15*, 160–167.

Lang, T. A., & Secic, M. (1997). *How to report statistics in medicine: Annotated guidelines for authors, editors, and reviewers*. New York: American College of Physicians.

Lippman, D. T., & Ponton, K. S. (1989). Designing a research poster with impact. *Western Journal of Nursing Research, 11*, 477–485.

Lipson, J. G. (1997). The politics of publishing: Protecting participants' confidentiality. In J. M. Morse (Ed.) *Completing a qualitative project: Details and dialogue* (pp. 39–58). Thousand Oaks, CA: Sage.

Madsen, D. (1991). *Successful dissertations and theses: A guide to graduate student research from proposal to completion*. New York: Jossey-Bass.

Markman, R. H., & Waddell, M. J. (1989). *Ten steps in writing the research paper* (4th ed.). Hauppauge, NY: Barron's Educational Series.

McConnell, E. A. (2000). Publishing opportunities outside the United States. *Journal of Nursing Scholarship, 32*, 87–92.

McDaniel, R. W., Bach, C. A., & Poole, M. J. (1993). Poster update: Getting their attention. *Nursing Research, 42*, 302–304.

McKinney, V., & Burns, N. (1993). The effective presentation of graphs. *Nursing Research, 42*, 250–252.

Meloy, J. M. (1994). *Writing the qualitative dissertation: Understanding by doing*. Mahwah, NJ: Lawrence Erlbaum.

Miracle, V. A., & King, K. C. (1994). Presenting research: Effective paper presentations and impressive poster presentations. *Applied Nursing Research, 7*, 147–151.

Moore, L. W., Augspurger, P., King, M. O., & Proffitt, C. (2001). Insights on the poster presentation and presentation process. *Applied Nursing Research, 14*, 100–104.

Morris, H. M., & Tipples, G. (1998). Choosing to write the paper format thesis. *Journal of Nursing Education, 37*, 173–175.

Northam, S., Trubenbach, M., & Bentov, L. (2000). Nursing journal survey: Information to help you publish. *Nurse Educator, 25*, 227–236.

Oermann, M. (2002). *Writing for publication in nursing*. Philadelphia: Lippincott Williams & Wilkins.

Richardson, L. (1994). Writing: A method of inquiry. In N. K. Denzin & Y. S. Lincoln (Eds.), *Handbook of qualitative research* (pp. 516–529). Thousand Oaks, CA: Sage.

Russell, C. K., Gregory, D. M., & Gates, M. F. (1996). Aesthetics and substance in qualitative research posters. *Qualitative Health Research, 6*, 542–553.

Sandelowski, M. (1998). Writing a good read: Strategies for re-presenting qualitative data. *Research in Nursing & Health, 21*, 375–382.

Sparks, S. (1999). Electronic publishing and nursing research. *Nursing Research, 48*, 50–54.

Strunk, W., Jr., White, E. B., & Angell, R. (2000). *The elements of style* (4th ed.). Boston: Allyn & Bacon.

Tornquist, E. M. (1999). *From proposal to publication: An informal guide to writing about nursing research* (2nd ed.). Menlo Park, CA: Addison-Wesley.

Tornquist, E. M., Funk, S. G., & Champagne, M. T. (1989). Writing research reports for clinical audiences. *Western Journal of Nursing Research, 11*, 576–582.

Turabian, K. L. (1996). *A manual for writers of term papers, theses, and dissertations* (6th ed.). Chicago: University of Chicago Press.

University of Chicago Press. (1993). *The Chicago manual of style* (14th ed.). Chicago: Author.

Van Manen, M. (1997). From meaning to method. *Qualitative Health Research, 7*, 345–369.

Webb, C. (1992). The use of the first person in academic writing. *Journal of Advanced Nursing, 17*, 747–752.

Wilson, H. S., & Hutchinson, S. A. (1997). Presenting qualitative research up close: Visual literacy in poster sessions. In J. M. Morse (Ed.), *Completing a qualitative project* (pp. 63–85). Thousand Oaks, CA: Sage.

Zeiger, M. (1999). *Essentials of writing biomedical research papers* (2nd ed.). New York: McGraw-Hill.

Zinsser, W. K. (1998). *On writing well: The classic guide to writing nonfiction* (6th ed.). New York: Harper.

Studies Cited in Chapter 24

Beck, C. T. (2002). Mothering multiples: A meta-synthesis of qualitative research. *MCN: The American Journal of Maternal/Child Nursing, 27*, 214–221.

Borrayo, E. A., & Jenkins, S. R. (2001). Feeling healthy: So why should Mexican-descent women screen for breast cancer? *Qualitative Health Research, 11*, 812–823.

Choudry, U. K. (2001). Uprooting and resettlement experiences of South Asian immigrant women. *Western Journal of Nursing Research, 23*, 376–393.

Clemmens, D. A. (2002). Adolescent mothers' depression after the birth of their babies: Breathing the storm. *Adolescence, 37*, 550–563.

Davies, B. L., & Hodnett, E. (2002). Labor support: Nurses' self-efficacy and views about factors influencing implementation. *Journal of Obstetric, Gynecologic, and Neonatal Nursing, 31*, 48–56.

Eller, L. S. (2001). Quality of life in persons living with HIV. *Clinical Nursing Research, 10*, 401–423.

Gagnon, A. J., Waghorn, K., Jones, M. A., & Yang, H. (2001). Indicators nurses employ in deciding to test for hyperbilirubinemia. *Journal of Obstetric, Gynecologic, and Neonatal Nursing, 30*, 626–633.

George, S. A. (2002). The menopause experience: A woman's perspective. *Journal of Obstetric, Gynecologic, and Neonatal Nursing, 31*, 77–85.

Issel, L. M., & Anderson, R. A. (2001). Intensity of case managers' participation in organizational decision making. *Research in Nursing & Health, 24*, 361–372.

Kang, D., & Fox, C. (2001). Th1 and Th2 cytokine responses to academic stress. *Research in Nursing & Health, 24*, 245–257.

Kelly, P. J., & Morgan-Kidd, J. (2001). Social influences on the sexual behaviors of adolescent girls in at-risk circumstances. *Journal of Obstetric, Gynecologic, and Neonatal Nursing, 30*, 481–489.

Kettunen, T., Poskiparta, M., Liimatainen, L., Sjögren, A., & Karhila, P. (2001). Taciturn patients in health counseling at a hospital: Passive recipients or active participators? *Qualitative Health Research, 11*, 399–422.

Knobf, M. T. (2002). The experience of premature menopause in women with early stage breast cancer. *Nursing Research, 51*, 9–17.

Lampic, C., Thurfjell, E., Bergh, J., Carolsson, M., & Sjödén, P. (2002). Life values before versus after a breast cancer diagnosis. *Research in Nursing & Health, 25*, 89–98.

Lindgren, K. (2001). Relationship among maternal-fetal attachment, prenatal depression, and health practices in pregnancy. *Research in Nursing & Health, 24*, 203–217.

Maloni, J. A. Kane, J. H., Suen, L. J., & Wang, K. K. (2002). Dysphoria among high-risk pregnant hospitalized women on bed rest. *Nursing Research, 51*, 92–99.

Martell, L. K. (2001). Heading toward the new normal: A contemporary postpartum experience. *Journal of Obstetric, Gynecologic, and Neonatal Nursing, 30*, 496–506.

McClowry, S. G. (2002). The temperament profiles of school-aged children. *Journal of Pediatric Nursing, 17*, 3–10.

McCrone, S., Lenz, E., Tarzian, A., & Perkins, S. (2001). Anxiety and depression: Incidence and patterns in patients after coronary artery bypass graft surgery. *Applied Nursing Research, 14*, 155–164.

McDougall, G. J. (2002). Memory improvement in octogenarians. *Applied Nursing Research, 15*, 2–10.

Melnyk, B. M., Alpert-Gillis, L., Feinstein, N. F., Fairbanks, E., Schutz-Czarniak, J., Hust, D., Sherman, L., LeMoine, C., Moldenhauser, Z., Small, L., Bender, N., & Sinkin, R. (2001). Improving cognitive development of low-birth-weight premature infants with the COPE program: A pilot study of the benefit of early NICU intervention with mothers. *Research in Nursing & Health, 24*, 373–389.

Milliken, P. J., & Northcutt, H. C. (2003). Redefining parental identity: Caregiving and schizophrenia. *Qualitative Health Research, 13*, 100–113.

Norton, S. A., & Bowers, B. J. (2001). Working toward consensus: Providers' strategies to shift patients from curative to palliative treatment choices. *Research in Nursing & Health, 24,* 258–269.

Orshan, S. A., Furniss, K. K., Forst, C., & Santoro, N. (2001). The lived experience of premature ovarian failure. *Journal of Obstetric, Gynecologic, and Neonatal Nursing, 30,* 202–208.

Parson, M. L., & Warner Robbins, C. (2002). Formerly incarcerated women create healthy lives through participatory action research. *Holistic Nursing Practice, 16,* 40–49.

Pridham, K. E., Brown, R., Sondel, S., Clark, R., & Green, C. (2001). Effects of biologic and experiential conditions on the pattern of growth in weight of premature and full-term infants. *Research in Nursing & Health, 24,* 283–297.

Ritchie, L. (2001). Empowerment and Australian community health nurses' work with Aboriginal clients. *Qualitative Health Research, 11,* 190–205.

Rockwell J. M., & Riegel, B. (2001). Predictors of self-care in persons with heart failure. *Heart & Lung, 30,* 18–25.

Sterling, Y. M., & Peterson, J. W. (2003). Characteristics of African American women caregivers of children with asthma. *MCN: The American Journal of Maternal/Child Nursing, 28,* 32–38.

Velji, K. & Fitch, M. (2001). The experience of women receiving brachytherapy for gynecologic cancer. *Oncology Nursing Forum, 28,* 743–751.

Wang, S., Redeker, N. S., Moreyra, A. E., & Diamond, M. R. (2001). Comparison of comfort and local complications after cardiac catheterization. *Clinical Nursing Research, 10,* 29–39.

Warrington, D., Cholowski, K., & Peters, D. (2003). Effectiveness of home-based cardiac rehabilitation for special needs patients. *Journal of Advanced Nursing, 41,* 121–9.

Weinrich, S. P., Weinrich, M. C., Priest, J., & Fodi, C. (2003). Self-reported reasons men decide not to participate in free prostate cancer screening. *Oncology Nursing Forum, 30,* E12–16.

Whitman, G. R., Davidson, L.J., Sereika, S. M., & Rudy, E. B. (2001). Staffing and pattern of mechanical restraint use across a multiple hospital system. *Nursing Research, 50,* 356–362.

Whitney, J., & Parkman, S. (2002). Preoperative physical activity, anesthesia, and analgesia: Effects on early postoperative walking after total hip replacement. *Applied Nursing Research, 15,* 19–27.

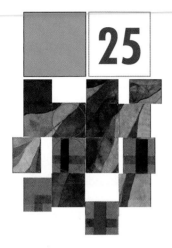

25

Writing a Research Proposal

OVERVIEW OF RESEARCH PROPOSALS

Research proposals are documents describing what researchers propose to study, prepared before a project has commenced. Proposals serve to communicate the research problem, its significance, and planned procedures for solving the problem to an interested party. Research proposals are written by both students seeking approval for empirical research projects and by seasoned researchers seeking financial or institutional support. In this section, we provide some general information regarding the content and preparation of research proposals.

Functions of a Proposal

Research proposals are an integral part of most studies, and are typically prepared after a researcher has identified a topic, developed research questions or hypotheses, and undertaken a literature review. Regardless of intended audience (e.g., faculty advisers, sponsors), proposals can serve several important functions.

Research proposals usually help researchers to clarify their own thinking. By committing ideas to writing, ambiguities about how to proceed can be identified and dealt with at an early stage. Proposals are intended to synthesize researchers'

critical thinking, and can serve to ensure that the research questions and proposed methods are sufficiently refined to warrant initiation of the study. Also, research proposals are reviewed by others who can offer suggestions for conceptual and methodologic improvements, and thus represent a mechanism for improving the study's contribution to knowledge.

Proposals represent the means for opening communication between researchers and parties interested in the conduct of research. Those parties are typically either funding agencies or faculty advisers, whose job it is to accept or reject the proposed plan, or to demand modifications. An accepted proposal is a two-way contract: those accepting the proposal are effectively saying, "We are willing to offer our (emotional or financial) support, as long as the investigation proceeds as proposed," and those writing the proposal are saying, "If you will offer support, then I will conduct the project as proposed."

Proposals often serve as the basis for negotiating with other parties as well. For example, a full or abridged proposal may be required to obtain institutional approval for the conduct of a study (e.g., for gaining access to study participants or for using facilities or equipment). Proposals are often incorporated into submissions to human subjects committees or Institutional Review Boards.

Finally, many studies are undertaken collaboratively. In such situations, proposals can help ensure that all researchers are "on the same page" about how the study is to proceed, and who is responsible for which tasks. Having a shared and agreed-upon document enhances communication among researchers and minimizes the possibility of friction.

Proposal Content

Reviewers of research proposals, whether they are faculty, funding sponsors, or peer reviewers, want a clear idea of what the researcher plans to study, what specific methods will be used to accomplish study goals, how and when various tasks are to be accomplished, and whether the researcher is capable of successfully completing the project. Proposals are usually evaluated on a number of criteria, including the importance of the research question, the contribution the study is likely to make to an evidence base, the adequacy of the research methods, the availability of appropriate personnel and facilities, and, if money is being requested, the reasonableness of the budget.

Proposal authors are usually given instructions indicating how the proposal should be structured. Funding agencies, for example, often supply an application kit that includes forms to be completed and specifies the format for organizing the contents of the proposal. Universities usually issue guidelines for their dissertation proposals. Despite the fact that formats and the amount of detail required may vary widely, there is some similarity in the type of information that is expected in research proposals. The content and organization are broadly similar to that for a research report, but proposals are written in the future tense (i.e., indicating what the researcher *will* do) and obviously do not include results and conclusions.

Front Matter
Proposals typically begin with what is referred to as **front matter**, which orients readers to the study and, in the case of proposals for funding, contains administrative information. The front matter typically includes, at a minimum, a cover page that indicates the title of the proposed study and the author's name and institution. For dissertations and theses, the cover page may also include the names of the advisory committee members.

The proposed title should be given careful thought. It is the first thing that reviewers will see, and should therefore be crafted to create a good impression. The title should be concise and informative, but should also be compelling and interesting. Like report titles, proposal titles should indicate the phenomena to be studied, and the population of interest.

Abstract
Proposals almost always begin with a brief synopsis of the proposed project. The abstract helps to establish a frame of reference for reviewers. The abstract should be brief (usually about 200 to 300 words) and should state succinctly the study objectives and methods to be used. Like the title, the abstract should be written with care to create a positive impression: It should persuade reviewers that the study has merit and would be undertaken with rigor. Although an abstract appears at the beginning of a proposal, it is often written last.

The Problem and Its Significance
The problem that the intended research will address is identified early in the proposal. The problem statement should clearly indicate the scope and importance of the problem, conveying any potential application to clinical practice. Care should be taken to be precise and to identify a problem of manageable proportions—a broad and complex problem is unlikely to be solvable. The proposal needs to describe clearly how the proposed research will contribute to knowledge and to the enhancement of evidence-based practice. The proposal should indicate the expected generalizability of the research, its contribution to theory, its potential for improving nursing practice, and possible applications or consequences of the knowledge to be gained.

Background of the Problem
A section of the proposal is usually devoted to a description of how the intended research builds on an

existing base of evidence, and how, if appropriate, it is linked to a conceptual model. The background material should strengthen arguments about the study's significance, orient readers to what is already known about the problem, and indicate how the proposed study will augment that knowledge; it should also serve as a demonstration of the researcher's command of current knowledge in a field. This section should, however, be tightly written to provide a strong foundation for the new study, and should not merely be a long catalogue of earlier work. An integrated and critical review of existing research and theory relevant to the project should provide a solid rationale for the new study.

 TIP: Beginning proposal writers sometimes forget that they are "selling" a product: themselves and their ideas. It is appropriate, therefore, to do a little marketing. If you do not sound convinced that the proposed study is important and will be executed with skill, then reviewers will not be persuaded either. The proposal should be written in a positive, confident tone. Instead of saying, "The study will *try* to . . . ," it is better to indicate more positively what the study *will* achieve. Similarly, it is more optimistic to specify what you *will* do, rather than what you *would* do, if approved. There is no need to brag or promise what cannot be accomplished, but you should put the proposed project in a positive light.

Objectives

Specific, achievable objectives provide the reader with clear criteria against which the proposed research methods can be assessed. Objectives stated as research hypotheses or specific models to be tested are often preferred. Whenever the theoretical background of the study, existing knowledge, or the researcher's experience permits an explicit prediction of outcomes, these predictions should be included in the proposal. In exploratory or descriptive research, which may not have hypotheses, the objectives may be most conveniently phrased as questions.

 TIP: Avoid using null hypotheses, which create an amateurish impression.

Method

The explanation of the research methods should be thorough enough that readers will have no question about how research objectives will be addressed. A thorough method section includes the following:

1. The research design, including a discussion of comparison group strategies, methods of controlling extraneous variables, number of data collection points, and so on; in a qualitative study, the research tradition should be described.
2. The experimental intervention (if applicable), including a description of both the treatment and the control group condition.
3. The sampling plan, including the specific sampling design, recruitment of study participants, definition of the population with exclusion or inclusion criteria, and number of participants expected.
4. Data collection methods and operational definitions of key variables (in proposals for funding, actual instruments are sometimes included in an appendix).
5. Procedures to be adopted, such as what equipment will be used to administer a treatment or collect data, how participants will be assigned to groups, and so on.
6. Strategies for coding, storing, reducing, and analyzing data, including any software to be used.
7. Methods of safeguarding human (or animal) subjects, including methods of maintaining confidentiality, securing informed consent, and minimizing risks.

The description of methods should also include a discussion of the rationale for the proposed methods, potential methodologic problems, and intended strategies for handling such problems.

The Work Plan

Researchers often describe their proposed plan for managing the flow of work on the project. Researchers indicate in the **work plan** the sequence of tasks to be performed, the anticipated length of time required for their completion, and the personnel required for their accomplishment. Work plans indicate how realistic and thorough researchers have been in designing their studies. In proposals for theses and dissertations, a detailed work plan is unnecessary, but a time table or tentative schedule is usually required.

Personnel

In proposals to funding agencies, the qualifications of key project personnel are described, and curricula vitae are usually appended. The research competencies of the project director and other team members are typically given major consideration in evaluating such proposals. Funders will scrutinize such factors as the researchers' training and education, experience, publications, and track record of doing research.

Facilities

Proposals should document what special facilities or equipment will be required by the project, and whether they will be available. Access to physiologic instrumentation, laboratories, clinical records, data processing equipment, special documents, and study participants should be described to reassure sponsors or advisers that the project can proceed as planned. The willingness of the institution with which the researcher is affiliated to allocate space, equipment, services, or data should also be indicated.

Budget

Budgets translate project activities into monetary terms, and are an extremely important part of research proposals requesting financial support; they are sometimes included in student proposals as well. Budgets are statements of how much money will be required to accomplish the various tasks. A well-conceived work plan greatly facilitates the preparation of the budget. An example of a budget is presented later in this chapter.

Proposals for Qualitative Studies

Preparing proposals for qualitative research entails special challenges. The main issue is that the nature of the inquiry and the standard demands of a proposal put researchers into what Morse and Field (1995) describe as a paradoxical situation: "Researchers have deliberately selected a qualitative method because little is known about the area—yet how can they write about, for instance, how they are going to analyze data when the nature of the data are not known?" (p. 43).

Decisions for qualitative studies evolve in the field, and therefore it is seldom possible to provide detailed or in-depth information about such matters as sample size, data collection strategies, data analysis, and so on. Enough detail needs to be provided on data analysis, however, that the reviewers will have confidence that the researcher will do justice to the data collected (Morse & Richards, 2002). For example, if a computer program will be used to help analyze the data, the specific software should be identified and also the rationale for choosing it. Even literature reviews for qualitative proposals are typically lean because there is not much prior research about the phenomenon of interest.

Qualitative researchers, therefore, must persuade reviewers that the topic is important and worth studying, that they are sufficiently knowledgeable about the challenges of field work and adequately skillful in eliciting rich data, and, in short, that the project would be a very good risk. Tripp-Reimer and Cohen (1991) warn researchers that poorly defined qualitative jargon used in a proposal is especially susceptible to criticism. Morse and Richards (2002) stress that there must be methodologic congruence throughout a qualitative proposal. Each qualitative tradition uses its own particular perspective and strategies to achieve its analytic goals, and the proposal must reflect in a systematic fashion the assumptions, questions, data collection strategies, and analytic methods of the chosen tradition. Sandelowski, Davis, and Harris (1989), Morse (1994), and Morse and Field (1995) offer advice about strategies of developing successful qualitative research proposals.

Tips on Proposal Preparation

Although it would be impossible to tell readers exactly what steps to follow to produce a successful proposal, we can offer some advice that might help to minimize the anxiety and trepidation that often accompany the proposal preparation. Some tips are especially relevant for researchers preparing proposals for funding.

Selection of an Important Problem

There is probably nothing more critical to the success of a proposal than selecting a problem that has clinical, theoretical, or social significance. The proposal must make a persuasive argument that the proposed research could make a notable contribution to an important topic.

Kuzel (2002), who shared some lessons about securing funding for a qualitative study, noted that qualitative researchers could profit by taking advantage of certain "hot topics" that have the special attention of the public and government officials. Proposals can sometimes be cast in such a way that they are linked to topics of national concern, and such a linkage can help to secure a favorable review. Kuzel used as an example his funded study of quality of care and medical errors in primary care practices, with emphasis on patient perspectives. The proposal was submitted at a time when the U.S. government was putting additional resources into research to enhance patient safety, and noted that there was little doubt that "the reframing of 'quality' under the name of 'patient safety' has captured the stage and is likely to have an enduring effect on what work receives funding" (p. 141). This advice about being sensitive to political realities is equally true for quantitative research.

Review of a Successful Proposal

Although there is no substitute for actually writing a proposal as a learning experience, novice proposal writers can often profit considerably by seeing the real thing. The information in this chapter provides some guidelines, but reviewing a successful proposal can do more to acquaint neophyte researchers with how the pieces fit together than all the textbooks in the world.

Chances are some of your colleagues or fellow students have written a proposal that has been accepted (either by a funding sponsor or by a dissertation committee), and many people are glad to share their successful efforts with others. Also, proposals funded by the federal government are usually in the public domain. That means that you can ask to see a copy of proposals that have obtained federal funding by writing to the sponsoring agency.

In recognition of the need of beginning researchers to become familiar with successful proposals, several journals have published proposals in their entirety (with the exception of administrative information such as budgets), together with the critique of the proposal prepared by a panel of expert reviewers. For example, the first such published proposal was a grant application funded by the Division of Nursing entitled, "Couvade: Patterns, Predictors, and Nursing Management" (Clinton, 1985). A more recent example is a proposal for a study of comprehensive discharge planning for the elderly (Naylor, 1990). Brown and her colleagues (1997) published a report about their resubmission of a grant application that was not originally funded, and how they responded to reviewers' critiques. Morse and Field's (1995) book includes in an appendix a full qualitative proposal that was funded by the National Institute of Nursing Research (NINR). Finally, some books that offer advice about writing dissertations include a full dissertation proposal (e.g., Madsen, 1991).

Input From Key People

Faculty advisers and staff at funding agencies are good sources to tap when preparing a proposal. Students should have a firm grasp of their adviser's expectations before they begin to write a proposal. Grey (2000), in her tips on **grantsmanship** (the set of skills involved in securing project funding) urges researchers to "talk it up" (p. 91), that is, to call program staff in agencies and foundations, or to send letters of inquiry about possible interest in a project. Grey also notes the importance of *listening* to what these people say and following their recommendations.

Kuzel (2002) also suggests seeking the advice of researchers who have had experience with the proposal development process. He noted that, "There is no substitute for people who can speak from experience" (p. 141). For students, peers who have gone through a proposal hearing (or who have already defended their dissertation) can offer important perspectives, especially if there is overlap among members of the dissertation committee. Researchers seeking funding can benefit from discussions with others who have been successful (or even those who have been unsuccessful) in getting research support from the agency in question.

Adherence to Instructions

Agencies or universities that evaluate proposals usually have written instructions on what is required. It is crucial to read these instructions carefully, and to follow them precisely. Proposals are sometimes rejected without review if they do not adhere to such guidelines as minimum font size or page limitations. For example, the instructions for grant applications to the National Institutes of Health (NIH) state the following about font size: "The height of the letters must not be smaller than 10 point; Helvetica or Arial 12-point is the NIH suggested font." It is wise to use the suggested font, and fatal to ignore the font limitations: "Deviations from the font size specifications . . . will be grounds for the Public Health Service to reject and return the entire application without peer review."

Justification of Decisions

Proposals often fail because they do not provide reviewers with confidence that key decisions have a justifiable rationale. Almost every aspect of a proposal involves a decision—the selected problem, the qualitative research tradition proposed, the population under study, the research site, the sample size, the data collection procedures, the comparison group to be used, the extraneous variables to be controlled, the analytic procedures to be used, the personnel who will work on the project, and so on. These decisions should be made carefully, keeping in mind the costs and benefits of alternative decisions. When you are satisfied that you have made the right decision, defend your decision by sharing the rationale with reviewers. In general, insufficient detail is more detrimental to the proposal than an overabundance of detail, although page constraints may make full elaboration impossible.

Attending to Evaluation Criteria

When funding is at stake, the funding agency often provides information about the criteria that reviewers use to make funding decisions. In some cases, the criteria are simply a list of factors that reviewers must take into consideration in making a global assessment of the proposal's quality. In other cases, however, the agency specifies exactly how many points will be assigned to different aspects of the proposal. As an example, in 2001 the National Institute of Child Health and Human Development (NICHD; an institute within NIH) requested proposals for studies about the behavioral and environmental risk factors for childhood drowning. The guidelines indicated that competing proposals would be evaluated in terms of four factors: technical approach, past performance, cost, and small disadvantaged business participation, with technical approach being of paramount importance. Technical evaluation criteria, together with the points to be allocated for each, included the following:

1. *Understanding of Project Requirements.* Offerors shall demonstrate a clear understanding of the nature of the problem, the purpose of the research, the realities of data collection and data management, and problems that may impede the research and possible solutions. (0 to 30 points)
2. *Previous Experience.* Offerors shall provide evidence that they have previous experience with epidemiologic studies that have used a case-control design, and with the tasks involved in the coordination and implementation of multi-site studies. (0 to 30 points)
3. *Qualifications of Personnel.* Key personnel shall have practical expertise and experience in the design and conduct of case-control studies and collection of population-based data. The offerors shall allocate sufficient professional and other staff effort to accomplish the study. (0 to 25 points)
4. *Facilities.* Offerors shall demonstrate that adequate facilities and software will be employed for data collection, data management, and analysis. (0 to 15 points)

In this example, a maximum of 100 points was awarded for the technical approach of each competing proposal. The proposals with the highest scores would ordinarily be most likely to obtain funding, unless other factors such as cost made the proposal noncompetitive. Therefore, researchers should pay particular attention to those aspects of the proposal that contribute most to an overall high score. In this example, it would have made little sense to put 85% of the proposal development effort into a description of the facilities, when a maximum of 15 points could be given for this aspect.

Different agencies establish different criteria for various types of research projects. Wise researchers learn what those criteria are and pay careful attention to them in developing their proposals.

The Research Team

For funded research, it is prudent to be judicious in putting together a research team: Reviewers often give considerable weight to the qualifications of the people who will conduct the research. In the example cited earlier, a full 25 of the 100 points were based on the expertise of the research personnel and their time allocations.

The person who is in the lead role on the project (the principal investigator, or PI) should carefully scrutinize the qualifications of the research team. It is not enough to have a team of competent people; it is necessary to have the right mix of competence. A project team of three brilliant theorists without statistical skills in a project that proposes sophisticated multivariate techniques may have difficulty convincing reviewers that the project would be successful. Gaps and weaknesses can often be compensated for by the judicious use of consultants.

Another shortcoming of some project teams is that there are too many researchers with small time commitments. It is usually unwise to load up a project staff with five or more top-level professionals who are able to contribute only 5% to 10% of their time to the project. Such projects often run into management difficulties because no one person is ever really in control of the flow of work. Although collaborative efforts are to be commended, you should be able to *justify* the inclusion of every staff person and to identify the unique contribution that each will make to the successful completion of the project.

Proposal Critique

Before formal submission of a proposal, a draft should be reviewed by at least one other person—but preferably by more than one. Reviewers should be selected to provide feedback regarding substantive issues, methodologic rigor, and style and flow of the writing. If the proposal is being submitted for funding, one reviewer ideally would be someone who is knowledgeable about the funding source and has received funding. If a consultant has been proposed because of specialized expertise that you believe will strengthen the study, then it would be advantageous to have that consultant participate in the proposal development by reviewing the draft and making recommendations for its improvement.

In universities, mock review panels are often held before submitting a proposal to the funding agency. Faculty and students are invited to these mock reviews and provide valuable feedback to the researchers on their proposals.

PROPOSALS FOR THESES AND DISSERTATIONS

Sternberg (1981), in his book on doing doctoral dissertations, argues that dissertation proposals are often a bigger hurdle than dissertations themselves, and that many doctoral candidates fail at the proposal development stage rather than at the stage of writing or defending the dissertation. Much of the advice we have offered thus far applies equally to proposals for theses and dissertations as for grant applications, but a few additional pieces of advice might prove helpful.

The Dissertation Committee

Choosing the right adviser (if an adviser is chosen rather than appointed) is almost as important as choosing the right topic to research. The ideal adviser is one who is a mentor, an expert with a strong reputation in the chosen field, a good teacher, a patient and supportive coach and critic, and an advocate. The ideal adviser is also a person who has sufficient time and interest to devote to your research and someone who is likely to stick with your project until its completion. This means that it might matter whether the prospective adviser has plans for a sabbatical leave, or is nearing retirement. Having consistent guidance throughout the project may be more helpful than having brilliant mentoring for only part of the project and then having to switch horses in midstream.

Dissertation committees often involve three or more members. If the adviser lacks certain of the "ideal" characteristics (e.g., he or she is a younger faculty member who has not yet firmly established a professional reputation), it is wise to balance those characteristics across committee members by seeking people with complementary talents and qualities. Putting together a group who will work well together and who have no personal antagonism toward each other can, however, be a tricky business. The adviser can usually make useful suggestions about other committee members.

Once a committee has been chosen, it is good to develop a working relationship with members and learn about their viewpoints before and during the proposal development stage. This means, at a minimum, becoming familiar with their research and the methodologic strategies they have favored. It also means meeting with them and sounding them out with ideas about topics and methods. If the suggestions from two or more members are at odds, it is prudent to seek your adviser's counsel on how to resolve this.

TIP: When meeting with your adviser and committee members, take notes about their suggestions, and write them out in more detail after the meeting while they are still fresh in your mind. The notes should be reviewed while developing the proposal.

Practices vary from one institution to another and from adviser to adviser, but some faculty require or prefer a written preproposal or prospectus before giving the go-ahead to prepare the full proposal. The prospectus is usually a three- to four-page paper outlining the research questions and the proposed methods.

Content of Dissertation Proposals

Most dissertation and thesis proposals follow a format roughly similar to the one described earlier in this chapter. Specific requirements regarding length and format vary in different settings, however, and it is important to know at the outset what is expected.

Dissertation proposals are typically 20 to 40 pages in length. In some cases, however, committees prefer what Sternberg (1981) describes as a "mini-dissertation," that is, a document with fully developed sections that can be inserted with minor adaptation into the dissertation itself. For example, the review of the literature, theoretical framework, hypothesis formulation, and the bibliography may be sufficiently refined at the proposal stage that they can be incorporated into the final product.

Sternberg argues that literature reviews are often the single most important section of a dissertation proposal (at least for quantitative studies) and thus merit special attention: "There is nothing better than a long, complete, thoughtful review of the literature in conveying to faculty the image (and reality) of a candidate who means business, is in the driver's seat . . . " (p. 93). Although not all committees want lengthy literature reviews, they certainly want to be assured that students are in command of knowledge in their field of inquiry.

Dissertation proposals sometimes include elements not normally found in proposals to funding agencies. One such element may be table shells (see Chapter 22), which are designed to show the committee that the student knows how to analyze data and present results effectively. Another element is a draft of the table of contents for the dissertation. The table of contents serves as an outline for the final product, and demonstrates to the committee that the student knows how to organize material.

FUNDING FOR RESEARCH PROPOSALS

Funding for research projects is becoming more and more difficult to obtain. The problem lies primarily in the extremely keen and growing competition among researchers. As increasing numbers of nurses become prepared to carry out significant research, so too will applications for research funds increase. Successful proposal writers need to have good research and proposal-writing skills, and they must also know how and from whom funding is available.

Federal Funding in the United States

In the United States, the federal government is the largest contributor to the support of research activities. The two major types of federal disbursements are grants and contracts. **Grants** are awarded for proposals in which researchers develop their own research ideas. Nurse researchers who identify an important research problem can seek federal funds through a grant program of one or more agencies of the government, such as NIH or the Agency for Healthcare Research and Quality (AHRQ; formerly the Agency for Health Care Policy and Research).

There are three basic mechanisms for funding federal grants, which can usually be awarded to researchers in both domestic and foreign institutions. One mechanism is for agencies and institutes to issue broad objectives relating to an overall mission. For example, as discussed in Chapter 1, NINR identified several areas of special interest for the years 2000 through 2002 (e.g., "chronic illnesses or conditions, such as management of chronic pain and care of children with asthma").

A second mechanism is for an agency to issue **program announcements** periodically, which describe new, continuing, or expanded program interests. For example, in December, 2001, NINR issued a joint program announcement with several other NIH institutes titled "Social and Cultural Dimensions of Health." The program announcement identified several specific objectives within this topic area and invited grant applications in five areas: (1) basic social and cultural constructs and processes used in health research; (2) etiology of health and illness; (3) consequences of poor health for individuals and social groups; (4) linking science to practice to improve prevention, treatment, health services, and dissemination; and (5) ethical issues in social and cultural research. Researchers apply for funding from this grant program through the process described in the next section. Program announcements are publicized by various government agencies on the Internet. Also, *The Catalogue of Federal Domestic Assistance* publishes information about all federal programs that provide any kind of aid. Information from this publication can be accessed through the Internet (http://www.cfda.gov).

The third grant-funding mechanism offers federal agencies a means of identifying a more specific topic area in which they are especially interested in receiving applications by a **Request for Applications (RFA)**. As an example, NINR issued an RFA titled "Informal Caregiving Research for Chronic Conditions" in November, 2001. Unlike a program announcement, an RFA usually specifies a deadline for the receipt of proposals (in this case, proposals were due February 26, 2002). General guidelines and goals for the competition are also specified, but researchers have considerable liberty to develop the specific research problem. Notices of such grant competitions are announced on the Internet on the websites specific to each funding agency and are also published in *The Federal Register*, which is a daily publication of the Government Printing Office (http://www.access.gpo.gov/su_docs).

Example of federal funding:
AHRQ awarded Marita Titler a grant of $1.46 million for a 3-year project titled "Evidence based practice: From book to bedside." The study, scheduled for completion in September, 2002, involved a randomized evaluation in 12 hospitals in 3 states to determine if a multidimensional organizational intervention alters nurse and physician behavior regarding the translation of research on acute pain management for the hospitalized elderly into clinical practice.

The second major type of government funding (and this may occur at both the federal and state level) is in the form of **contracts**. An agency that identifies the need for a specific study issues a **Request for Proposals (RFP)**, which details the *exact* work that the government wants done and the specific problem to be addressed. Proposals in response to RFPs describe the methods researchers would use in addressing the research problem, the project staff and facilities, and the cost of doing the study in the proposed way. Contracts are usually awarded to only one of the competitors. The contract method of securing research support severely constrains the kinds of work in which investigators can engage—researchers responding to an RFP usually have no latitude in developing the research objectives. For this reason, most nurse researchers probably will want to compete for grants rather than contracts. Nevertheless, many interesting RFPs have been issued by NIH and other agencies. For example, the previously mentioned NICHD-funded solicitation about the behavioral and environmental risk factors for childhood drowning was issued as an RFP; another NIH RFP requested proposals for a study of "Ethnic Differences in Life Style, Psychological Factors, and Medical Care During Pregnancy."

A summary of every federal RFP is printed in *Commerce Business Daily,* which is published every government workday; information can be accessed on the Internet (http://cbdnet.gpo.gov). Also, NIH publishes a weekly bulletin called the *NIH Guide for Grants and Contracts*; the contents of the bulletin are available on the Internet through the NIH website. This bulletin announces new NIH initiatives, including RFAs and RFPs issued by NIH.

In addition to grants and contracts, NIH (and other federal agencies) offers career development support for researchers, including support for doctoral research. For example, at NIH there are two types of mentored career development grant programs, the Mentored Research Scientist Development Award (K01) and the Mentored Patient-Oriented Research Career Development Award (K23). These grants provide sponsored research experience for doctorally prepared researchers who need a mentored research experience with an expert sponsor. The awards provide an opportunity for individuals to gain expertise in new research areas or in areas that would demonstrably enhance their research careers.

Government funding for research is, of course, also available to nurse researchers in countries other than the United States. In Canada, for example, various types of health research are sponsored by the Canadian Institutes of Health Research (CIHR). The objective of CIHR is "to excel, according to internationally accepted standards of scientific excellence, in the creation of new knowledge and its translation into improved health for Canadians, more effective health services and products and a strengthened health care system." Information about CIHR's program of grants, training awards, and other funding opportunities is available at its website (http://www.cihr.ca)

Private Funds

Health care research is supported by a number of philanthropic foundations, professional organizations, and corporations. Many researchers prefer private funding to government support because there is often less "red tape." Private organizations are typically less rigid in their proposal and reporting requirements, approval of instruments, and monitoring of progress. Not surprisingly, private organizations are besieged with proposed research projects.

Information about philanthropic foundations that support research is available through the Foundation Center (http://www.fdncenter.org). The Foundation Center offers a wide variety of resources on foundation funding and how to secure it. The most comprehensive resource for identifying funding opportunities is the Center's *The Foundation Directory*, now available on-line for a fee. The online service allows subscriptions at various levels, from the basic level (access to information about the 10,000 largest foundations) to the platinum level (access to information about a universe of over 65,000 grantmakers). The directory lists the purposes and activities of the foundations and information for contacting them. The Foundation Center also offers seminars and training on grant writing and funding opportunities in locations around the United States, and has published two additional resources of relevance: *Guide to Grantseeking on the Web* and the *National Guide to Funding in Health*. Another resource for information on funding is the Community of Science, which maintains a database on funding opportunities (http://www.cos.com).

Example of foundation funding:
The Patrick and Catherine Weldon Donaghue Medical Research Foundation (in West Hartford, Connecticut) is dedicated to the promotion of useful knowledge about human health through research. The second author of this book (Beck) has been awarded grants by this private foundation to develop and psychometrically test her Postpartum Depression Screening Scale.

Professional associations, such as the American Nurses' Foundation, Sigma Theta Tau, the American Association of University Women, and the Social Science Research Council, offer funds for conducting research. Health organizations, such as the American Heart Association and the American Cancer Society, also support research activities.

Finally, funds for research are sometimes donated by private corporations, particularly those dealing with health care products. The Foundation Center publishes a directory of corporate grant-makers and provides links through its website to a number of corporate philanthropic programs. Additional information concerning the requirements and interests of corporations should be obtained either from the organization directly or from personnel in research administration offices of universities, hospitals, or other agencies with which you are affiliated.

GRANT APPLICATIONS TO THE NATIONAL INSTITUTES OF HEALTH

NIH funds a considerable number of nursing studies through NINR and through other institutes and agencies in NIH. Because of the importance of NINR as a funding source for nurse researchers, this section describes the process of proposal submission and review at NIH. (It should be noted that AHRQ, which also funds nurse-initiated studies, uses the same application kit and similar application and review procedures.)

NIH Applications

Applications for grant funding through NIH are made by completing Public Health Service Grant Application Form PHS 398 (revised May, 2001), which is available through the office of sponsored research at most universities and hospitals. Copies of the application kit can also be downloaded from the NIH website at http://www.nih.gov under their "Grants and Opportunities" section, and are available in a "fillable" format.

New grant applications are usually processed in three cycles annually. The schedule for submission and review of new grant applications is shown in Table 25-1. Grant applications may be submitted on the proper forms at any time during the year, but proposals received after one receipt date will be held for another cycle. For example, if a proposal is received by NIH on February 2, it is considered with proposals received by June 1, not February 1.

Types of NIH Grants

NIH awards different types of grants, and each has its own objectives and review criteria. The basic grant program—and the primary funding mechanism for independent research—is the **Research Project Grant** (R01). The objective of the R01 grant is to support discrete, specific research projects in areas reflecting the interests and competencies of a PI. As of February, 2003, the five explicitly stated review criteria are as follows:

1. *Significance*. Does this study address an important problem? If the aims of the application are achieved, how will scientific knowledge be advanced? What will be the effect of the study on the concepts or methods that drive this field?

TABLE 25.1 Schedule for Processing New Research Grant Applications, National Institutes of Health

APPLICATION DEADLINE	SCIENTIFIC MERIT REVIEW DATES	ADVISORY COUNCIL REVIEW DATES	EARLIEST POSSIBLE START DATES
February 1	June/July	September/October	December
June 1	October/November	January/February	April
October 1	February/March	May/June	July

2. *Approach.* Are the conceptual framework, design, methods, and analyses adequately developed, and appropriate to the aims of the project? Does the applicant acknowledge potential problem areas and consider alternative tactics?

3. *Innovation.* Does the project employ novel concepts, approaches, or methods? Are the aims original and innovative? Does the project challenge existing paradigms or develop new methods or technologies?

4. *Investigator.* Is the investigator appropriately trained and well suited to carry out this work? Is the work proposed appropriate to the experience level of the principal investigator and other researchers?

5. *Environment.* Does the scientific environment in which the work will be done contribute to the probability of success? Do the proposed experiments take advantage of unique features of the scientific environment or employ useful collaborative arrangements? Is there evidence of institutional support?

In addition to these five explicit criteria, other factors are relevant in evaluating R01 proposals, including the reasonableness of the proposed budget, the adequacy of protections for human subjects or research animals, and the appropriateness of the sampling plan in terms of including women, minorities, and children as study participants.

Until 1998, there was a special funding mechanism at NIH for new investigators. The First Independent Research Support and Transition (FIRST or R29) program was designed to provide an initial period of support for newly independent researchers. Although this opportunity is no longer available, NIH does recognize the need to support and encourage new investigators. As of this writing, R01 applications from new investigators are identified as such to reviewers, who are instructed to use less stringent criteria. For example, in evaluating the qualifications of new investigators, more emphasis is to be placed on their training and research potential than on their track record and number of publications.

A special program (R15) has been established for researchers working in educational institutions that have not been major participants in NIH programs. These are the **Academic Research Enhancement Awards** (AREA), the objective of which is to stimulate research in institutions that provide baccalaureate training for many individuals who go on to do health-related research. AREA grants enable qualified researchers to obtain support for small-scale research projects. The NIH website lists institutions that are not eligible to receive AREA grants. The review criteria for AREA grants are basically the same as for R01 grants.

TIP: If you have an idea for a study and are not sure which type of grant program is best suited to your project—or you are not sure whether the project is one in which NINR or another institute in NIH might be interested—it is advisable to contact NINR directly. NINR's Division of Extramural Affairs has staff who can provide feedback about whether your proposed project will fit in the program interests of NINR. The telephone number is 301-594-6906; information about NINR's ongoing areas of research interests and specific areas of current opportunity are available on the Internet (http://www.nih.gov/ninr). A one- to two-page concept paper can also be faxed to NINR at 301-480-8260 or e-mailed to the address listed on the NINR website.

Preparing a Grant Application for NIH

As indicated earlier, proposals to NIH must be submitted according to procedures described in the Public Health Service application kit. Each kit specifies exactly how the grant application should be prepared and what forms are to be used for supplying critical pieces of information. It is important to follow these instructions precisely. In the sections that follow, we describe the various components of an application and provide some tips that should be helpful in completing certain sections.*

Front Matter

The front matter of grant applications consists of various forms that help in processing the application and provide administrative information. Proposal writers often fail to give the front matter the attention it merits, but careful attention to detail in this first section is very important. The forms included in Section 1 are as follows:

- *Face page.* On the face page form, researchers provide the title of the project (not to exceed 56 spaces), the name and institutional affiliation of the PI, the costs for the initial budget period and for the entire proposed period of support, the proposed period of support, and other administrative information.
- *Abstract of research plan.* Page 2 is a form that asks for a half-page abstract or description of

the proposed study, the designation of the performance sites, and a listing of the key professional personnel who would work on the study. The abstract must fit into the space allocated.

- *Table of contents.* Page 3 indicates on what pages various sections and subsections of the proposal are to be found.
- *Budget.* Until recently, applicants were required to itemize all costs that would be incurred by the project during the first 12 months. Detailed budgets are no longer necessary if annual direct project costs do not exceed $250,000. Instead, applicants complete a budget justification page for these new **modular research grant applications**, which are paid in modules of $25,000 of direct project costs. Figure 25-1 provides a sample of such a budget justification page. (Note that this budget requests funding over a 2-year period; the maximum project period for R01 grants is 5 years). Of course, researchers must still estimate their financial needs by preparing a more detailed budget for themselves. Figure 25-2 presents an example of how the estimate was made for the budget justification page shown in Figure 25-1. Note that the NIH budget forms should indicate **direct costs** (specific project-related costs) only; **indirect costs** (institutional **overhead**) are not shown. Beginning researchers are likely to need the assistance of a research administrator or an experienced, funded researcher in developing their first budget.
- *Biographic sketches.* Format pages are provided to summarize salient aspects of the education and experience of key project personnel. Sketches must be included for the PI and any other proposed staff considered to be key to the project's success. The sketch must list, in addition to education and training, a description of (a) positions and honors; (b) selected peer-reviewed publications or manuscripts in press; and (c) selected ongoing and completed research support. A maximum of four pages is permitted for each person.
- *Resources.* On this form, researchers must designate the availability of needed facilities and

---

*The application kit for NIH grants changes periodically. Therefore, the instructions in a current version of Form PHS 398 should be carefully reviewed and followed in preparing a grant application rather than relying exclusively on information in this chapter.

BUDGET JUSTIFICATION PAGE
MODULAR RESEARCH GRANT APPLICATION

Initial Budget Period	Second Year of Support	Third Year of Support	Fourth Year of Support	Fifth Year of Support
$ 150,000	$150,000		$	$

Total Direct Costs Requested for Entire Project Period	$300,000

Personnel

Stephanie Tacy, Ph.D., Principal Investigator (30% effort) will be responsible for overall project conceptualization and management, instrument development, data quality control, data analysis, and report preparation.

Linda McGann, Ph.D., Co-Investigator (25% effort) will contribute to conceptualization of the project, instrumentation, training of the interviewer, development of a coding scheme, analysis of the data, and report preparation.

Philomena Tucker, M.S.N., will serve as the interviewer on the project. She will work at 100% effort during the first 18 months of the project and will be responsible for all data collection.

To be Appointed, Research Assistant (25% effort) will be assigned such tasks as library research, instrument pretests, and data coding.

To be Appointed, Secretary (50% effort) will perform secretarial and clerical functions, including the scheduling of all interviews, maintenance of project records, preparation of forms, issuance of subject stipends, etc.

Norma Carlson, Ph.D., Statistical Consultant with expertise in LISREL, will provide guidance with regard to the statistical analysis of the data. Dr. Carlson is budgeted for 10 days in Year 1 and 15 days in Year 2 of the study.

Michelle Kerls, Ph.D. Measurement Consultant, will provide guidance with regard to instrument development and psychometric testing. She will devote 20 days of her time during Year 1 of the project.

Consortium

There are no consortium arrangements for this project.

FIGURE 25.1 Sample budget justification page.

Personnel

	Salary	Effort	Salary Requested	Fringe	Total	
S. Tacy	$90,000	30%	$30,000	$9,000	$39,000	
L. McGann	60,000	25%	15,000	4,500	19,500	
P. Tucker	35,000	100%	35,000	10,500	45,500	
TBA	20,000	25%	5,000	1,500	6,500	
TBA	25,000	50%	12,500	3,750	16,250	
						126,750

Consultants

N. Carlson	10 days @ $500	5,000	
M. Kerls	20 days @ $300	6,000	
			11,000

Other

Laptop computer	2,150	
Office supplies, publications ($75/mo)	900	
Photocopying/printing ($50/mo)	600	
Postage/courier ($75/mo)	900	
Telephone ($100/mo)	1,200	
Travel expenses (interviewer travel, professional conferences)	2,000	
Subject stipends (300 × $15)	4,500	
		12,250
		$150,000

FIGURE 25.2   Estimated budget for first year of project.

equipment in the following categories: laboratory; clinical; animal; computer; office; and other.

Research Plan Section

The main section of the NIH grant application is devoted to the research plan. This section consists of 10 parts (though not all 10 are relevant to every application). Parts a through d of the research plan, combined, must not exceed 25 single-spaced pages, including any figures, charts, or tables.

Applications that do not adhere to this page restriction are returned without review.

a. *Specific aims*. Researchers must provide a succinct summary of the research problem and the specific objectives to be undertaken, including any hypotheses to be tested. The application guidelines suggest that Part a be restricted to a single page.

b. *Background and significance*. In Part b, researchers must convince reviewers that the proposed study idea is sound and has important clinical or theoretical relevance. Researchers provide the context for the study in this section, usually through a brief analysis of existing knowledge and gaps on the topic and through a discussion of a conceptual framework. Within this context, investigators must demonstrate the significance of and need for the proposed project. NIH recommends restricting this section to two to three pages. This is often a challenging task, but we urge you not to be tempted to exceed the three-page guideline. Space should be conserved for a full elaboration of the proposed research methods.

c. *Preliminary studies.* This section is reserved for a description of the project team's previous work that is relevant to the proposed study. This section (although it is optional for new applications and is required only for continuation proposals) gives you an opportunity to persuade reviewers that you have the skills and background needed to do the research. The Preliminary Studies section provides a forum for the description of any relevant work key research staff have either completed or are in the process of doing. If the only relevant research you have completed is your dissertation, here is an opportunity to describe that research in full. If you have completed relevant research that has led to publications, you should reference them in this section and include copies of them as appendices. Other items that might be described include previous uses of an instrument or an experimental procedure that will be used in the new study, relevant clinical or teaching experience, membership on task forces or in organizations that have provided a perspective on the research problem, or the results of a pilot study that involved a similar research problem. The point is that this section allows you to demonstrate that the proposed work grew out of some ongoing commitment to, interest in, or experience with the topic. For new applications, no more than six to eight pages should be devoted to Part c, and fewer pages are often sufficient.

TIP: Many novice researchers mistakenly believe that the Preliminary Studies section is designed for a literature review. If you make this mistake, it will indicate that you are a novice and unable to follow instructions.

d. *Research design and methods.* It is in Part d that you must describe the methods you will use to conduct the study. This section should be succinct but with sufficient detail to persuade reviewers that you have a sound rationale for your methodologic decisions. Although there are no specific page limitations associated with this section of the application, keep in mind that you have up to 25 pages in total for Parts a through d combined.

The number of subsections in the methods section varies from one application to another. Each subsection should be labeled clearly to facilitate the review process. As is true in organizing any written material, it is often useful to begin with an outline. Here is an outline of the sections used in a successful grant application (by Polit) for a nonexperimental study of parenting behavior and family environments among low-income teenage mothers:

• Overview of the Research Design
• Sampling
• Research Variables and Measuring Instruments
• Data Collection Procedures
• Data Analysis
• Research Products
• Project Schedule

Morse prepared a grant application for a qualitative study entitled "Finding comfort for the improvement of nursing care" (Morse & Field, 1995). The outline of subsections for her "Part d" of the grant application was as follows:

• Study I: The Meaning of Comfort (a phenomenological study)
  ◦ Method
  ◦ Subject Selection
  ◦ Data Collection
  ◦ Data Analysis

- Study II: The Components of Comfort (an ethnoscience study)
  - ◦ Method
  - ◦ Subject Selection
  - ◦ Procedure
- Study III: Explication of the Process of Comfort (a grounded theory study)
  - ◦ Method
  - ◦ Sample Selection
  - ◦ Procedure
  - ◦ Data Analysis
- Reliability and Validity
- Summary of Research Methods
- Researcher

Section d, then, includes the plan for the conduct of the study, and should be as thorough and complete as possible regarding research design, interventions, sampling, data collection, and data analysis.

With regard to sampling, review panels increasingly expect to see a power analysis that justifies the adequacy of the specified sample size in quantitative projects. It is also advisable to document your access to the specified subject pool. For instance, if the proposal indicates that patients and personnel from Park Memorial Hospital will participate in the study, then you should include a letter of cooperation from an administrator of the hospital with the application. One further issue relating to the sample is that NIH policy requires that women and members of minority groups be included in all NIH-supported projects involving humans, unless a clear and compelling justification for their exclusion can be established. Guidelines for the inclusion of women and minorities should be reviewed before developing a sampling plan; the guidelines can be found on the NIH website in the *NIH Guide for Grants and Contracts*, Volume 23, March 11, 1994. NIH has also developed policies regarding the inclusion of children in research projects; the policy was issued in the *NIH Guide* on March 6, 1998.

Given page constraints, it is not normally possible to describe data collection techniques and procedures in much detail (although copies of instruments or topic guides can be included in an appendix). If a new instrument is to be developed as part of the project, however, the proposed procedures for its development *and* evaluation should be described. For qualitative studies, the data collection section should describe the procedures that will be implemented to enhance and assess the trustworthiness of the data.

Although the grant application kit does not specifically request a project schedule or work plan, it is often useful to develop and include one (unless the page limitation makes it impossible to do so). A work plan helps reviewers assess how realistic you have been in planning the project, and it should help you to develop an estimate of needed resources (i.e., your budget). Flow charts and other diagrams are often useful for highlighting the sequencing and interrelationships of project activities. (Figure 3.1 in Chapter 3 presents such a flow chart.)

e. *Human subjects*. Researchers who plan to collect data from human subjects have to complete a section on protection of subjects. Researchers can determine whether the proposed study meets human subjects requirements by consulting a decision tree available at the website of the Office of Human Research Protections (http://ohrp.osophs.dhhs.gov). In the Human Subjects section, applicants must either address the involvement of human subjects and describe protections from research risks or provide a justification for exemption with enough information that reviewers can determine the appropriateness of requests for exemption. If no exemption is sought, the section must address four issues, as outlined in the application kit. This section must also include various types of information regarding the inclusion of women, minorities, and children. If the project involves a clinical trial, the application must also include a "Data and Safety Monitoring Plan." This section of the proposal often serves as the cornerstone of the document submitted to Institutional Review Boards.

TIP: NIH now requires funded investigators to document that they have had specific training regarding protection of human study participants. Even researchers whose studies are exempt from an institutional review board review must demonstrate that they have had appropriate education.

    f. *Vertebrate animals.* If your proposed research involves the use of vertebrate animals, this section must contain a justification of their use and a description of the procedures used to safeguard their welfare.

    g. *Literature cited.* This subsection of the Research Plan consists of a list of references used in the text of the grant application. Any reference style is acceptable. Although there are no longer any page restrictions for this section, NIH encourages applicants to be concise and to select only the most pertinent and recent references.

    h. *Consortium or contractual arrangements.* If the proposed project will involve the collaboration of two or more different institutions (e.g., if a separate organization will be used to perform laboratory analyses, under a subcontract agreement), then details about the nature of the arrangements must be described in this section.

    i. *Consultants.* If you plan to include consultants to help with specific tasks on the proposed project, you must include a letter from each consultant, confirming his or her willingness to serve on the project. Letters are also needed from collaborators on the project, if they are affiliated with an institution different from your own.

Appendices

Grant applications often include appended materials. These materials might be, for example, instruments to be used in the project, detailed calculations on sample size estimates, scoring or coding instructions for instruments, letters of cooperation from institutions that will provide access to subjects, complex statistical models, and other supplementary materials in support of the application. Researchers can also submit copies of up to 10 published papers or papers accepted for publication (but *not* papers submitted for publication but not yet accepted). Appended materials are not made available to the entire review panel, so essential information should not be relegated to the appendix.

The Review Process

Grant applications submitted to NIH are received by the NIH Center for Scientific Review, where they are reviewed for completeness and relevance to NIH. Acceptable applications are assigned to an appropriate Institute or Center, and to a peer review group. Most applications by nurse researchers are assigned to NINR, unless the content of the proposal is better suited to another Institute. NIH encourages applicants to enclose a cover letter with their applications suggesting an assignment to a specific Institute, and outlining how the research is congruent with the mission of that Institute.

    As the schedule in Table 25-1 indicates, NIH uses a sequential, dual review system for making decisions about its grant applications. The first level involves a panel of peer reviewers (not employed by NIH), who evaluate the grant application for its scientific merit. These review panels are called **scientific review groups** (SRGs) or, more commonly, **study sections**. Each panel consists of about 15 to 20 researchers with backgrounds appropriate to the specific study section for which they have been selected. Appointments to the review panels are usually for 4-year terms and are staggered so that about one-fourth of each panel is new each year.

TIP: The Nursing Research Study Section has 18 members. The names of study section members are available at http://www.drg.nih.gov/Committees/rosterindex.asp#A. This information may be helpful in developing a grant application, *but* you should never contact a study section member directly.

    The second level of review is by an Advisory Council, which includes both scientific and lay representatives. The Advisory Council considers not only the scientific merit of an application but the relevance of the proposed study to the programs and priorities of the Center or Institute to which the application has been submitted, as well as budgetary considerations.

NIH has recently instituted a triage system for the first level of review. Study section members are sent applications and asked to evaluate whether they are in the upper half or lower half in terms of quality and likelihood for funding. Normally, each application is formally reviewed by at least two assigned reviewers, who prepare written critiques. If two reviewers agree that an application is not in the upper half, it is designated as "unscored" and is not discussed at the study section meeting or assigned a score.

Applications in the upper half are discussed in full at study section meetings and assigned a **priority score** that reflects each reviewer's opinion of the merit of the application.* The ratings range from 1.0 (the best possible score) to 5.0 (the least favorable score), in increments of 0.1. Before the streamlined review procedures were instituted, priority scores typically ran the full range from 1.0 to 5.0. However, the full range is no longer routinely used because the only applications assigned a score are those previously designated as being in the upper half. Thus, priority scores tend to be between 1.0 and 3.0, but reviewers are free to "vote their conscience" and may therefore assign any priority score they think appropriate.

The individual scores from all study section members are then combined, averaged, and multiplied by 100 to yield scores that (technically) range from 100 to 500, with 100 being the best possible score. Among all scored applications, only those with the best priority scores actually obtain funding. Cut-off scores for funding vary from agency to agency and year to year, but a score of 200 or lower is often needed to get funding.

Each grant applicant, regardless of the study section's decision, is sent a summary of the peer review panel's evaluation. These **pink sheets** (so called because they are printed on pink paper) summarize the reviewers' comments in seven areas: (1) an overall description of the project; (2) a critique of the strengths and weaknesses of the proposal, based on the five criteria described in the section on R01 grants; (3) an overall evaluation of the project; (4) an evaluation of gender and minority representation; (5) a review of procedures relating to human subjects and animal welfare; (6) an assessment of the reasonableness of the budget; and (7) a discussion of other considerations, with emphasis on the protection of the rights of human subjects or the welfare of animal subjects. For applications that have been scored, applicants are also advised of the average priority score and percentile rank.

TIP: It often pays to be persistent. Unless an unfunded proposal is criticized in some fundamental way (e.g., the problem area was not judged to be significant), applications should be resubmitted, with revisions that reflect the concerns of the peer review panel. When a proposal is resubmitted, the next review panel members are given a copy of the original application and the pink sheet so that they can evaluate the degree to which criticisms have been addressed. Applications can be resubmitted up to three times.

RESEARCH EXAMPLES

NIH makes available the abstracts of all funded projects through a database known as Computer Retrieval of Information on Scientific Projects (CRISP), which can be searched by subject or researcher name on the Internet. Abstracts for two projects funded through NINR in 2001 are presented next.

Example From a Funded Quantitative Project

Ann Horgas of the University of Florida prepared the following abstract for a project entitled "Pain Assessment in Nursing Home Residents," which received funding from NINR in September, 2001, (scheduled for completion in August, 2003).

---

*Study sections sometimes vote to defer an application. **Deferrals** usually involve applications that reviewers consider meritorious but missing some crucial information that would permit them to make a final determination.

More than 1.5 million Americans reside in nursing homes, a number that is expected to rise dramatically over the next 20 years as the Baby Boomer generation ages. Approximately 80 percent of nursing home residents have painful diseases and at least 50 percent have significant cognitive impairment. Evidence suggests, however, that pain among nursing home residents is poorly assessed and inadequately managed, especially among those with dementia. Prior research has revealed that cognitively impaired persons verbally report less pain than intact elders do. This may be due, in part, to the tendency of cognitively impaired persons to verbally report less pain. No evidence is available, however, to indicate that persons with dementia feel less pain. In addition, most prior research has relied solely on self-report measures of pain, which may be biased by dementia-related memory and language deficits. Thus, observational measures of pain are greatly needed to detect pain in this vulnerable population. Before health care providers can effectively manage pain among elderly adults, they must be able to accurately assess it, especially in those who are less able to verbally report its presence. This proposed research would investigate verbal and non-verbal expressions of pain in elderly adults, with and without dementia. The sample will consist of 200 nursing home residents aged 65 and older, sampled roughly proportional to their age, gender, and ethnic/racial distribution in the population. Using a quasi-experimental design, an activity-based protocol (Keefe & Block, 1982) will be used to exacerbate pain. A multidimensional battery of pain and cognitive assessments will be used to investigate the following specific aims: 1) to confirm that persons with impaired cognitive status report less pain; 2) to investigate whether behavioral assessments of pain might be less sensitive to cognitive status effects; and 3) to investigate relationships between self-reported pain intensity and observed pain behaviors, and whether such relationships vary across cognitive status groups.

Example From a Funded Qualitative Project

Mary Johnson of Rush University submitted a successful application for a grounded theory study that was funded by NINR in August, 2001 (scheduled to end in July, 2003). She prepared the following abstract for the study, which was entitled "De-escalation Strategies of Psychiatric Nursing Staff":

Violence toward health care workers is a significant occupational health concern. In one study of psychiatric staff, 73 percent reported having been assaulted at least once during their career and 28 percent reported being assaulted at least four times. Aside from the cost to the institution, injuries to staff cause significant emotional, social, biophysical and cognitive responses in the victim. And yet, despite the large body of research related to institutional violence in general, there is a notable lack of theoretical work needed to provide a scientific base for nursing interventions with potentially violent psychiatric patients. The purpose of this study is to investigate, using grounded theory methodology, the day-to-day strategies that nursing staff use to prevent psychiatric patients from escalating to violence. The specific aims are (1) to identify and describe nursing interventions that are used to de-escalate psychiatric patients who are escalating out of control; (2) to describe the context and conditions under which specific interventions are used to assist patients to regain control; and (3) to construct a mid-range theory of the de-escalation process. The interactions between the nursing staff and the patients will be observed and both nursing staff and patients will be formally and informally interviewed. The data will be analyzed and a theoretical model will be constructed using the constant comparative method of grounded theory. The long-term goal is to use this theory of de-escalation as the basis for developing and testing innovative nursing interventions for preventing violence and/or restraint use in psychiatric inpatient units and other settings that treat potentially aggressive patients. This outcome would not only make a unique contribution to psychiatric nursing practice but would effectively decrease the costs to the institution and the use of potentially harmful interventions with patients.

SUMMARY POINTS

- A **research proposal** is a written document specifying what a researcher intends to study; proposals are written both by students seeking approval for dissertations and theses and by seasoned researchers seeking financial or institutional support.
- Proposals can serve a number of purposes, one of which is to establish a two-way contract between researchers and those from whom support is sought.
- Major components of a research proposal include **front matter** such as a cover page, an

abstract, statement of the problem, background and significance of the problem, specific objectives, methods, and work plan or schedule; proposals written for funding usually also include sections on personnel and facilities and a budget.

- Preparing proposals for qualitative studies is especially challenging because methodologic decisions are made in the field; qualitative proposals need to persuade reviewers that the proposed study is important and a good risk.
- Some suggestions for writing a strong proposal include selecting an important topic; reviewing a successful proposal; soliciting input from key people; adhering to proposal instructions; attending to any evaluation criteria; and having the draft proposal critiqued by one or more reviewers.
- Students preparing a proposal for a dissertation or thesis need to work closely with a well-chosen committee and adviser. Dissertation proposals are often "mini-dissertations" that include sections that can be incorporated into the dissertation.
- The set of skills associated with learning about funding opportunities and developing proposals that can be funded is referred to as **grantsmanship.**
- The federal government is the largest source of research funds for health researchers in the United States. In addition to regular grants programs, agencies of the federal government announce special funding programs in the form of **program announcements** and **Requests for Applications** (**RFAs**) for **grants** and **Requests for Proposals** (**RFPs**) for **contracts.**
- A major source of funding for nurse researchers is the National Institutes of Health (NIH), within which is housed the National Institute of Nursing Research (NINR). Nurses can apply for a variety of grants from NIH, the most common being the **Research Project Grant** (R01 grant) and the **AREA Grant** (R15).
- Grant applications to NIH, which are submitted on special forms and which must follow strict formatting guidelines, are reviewed three times a year in a dual review process. The first phase involves a review by a peer review panel (or **study section**) that evaluates each proposal's scientific merit; the second phase is a review by an Advisory Council.
- In NIH's new streamlined review procedure, the study section assigns **priority scores** only to applications judged to be in the top half of proposals based on their quality. A score of 100 represents the most meritorious ranking, and a score of 500 is the lowest possible score.
- Applicants for NIH grants are sent a "**pink sheet**" or summary statement, which offers a detailed critique of the proposal, together with information on the priority score and percentile ranking.

STUDY ACTIVITIES

Chapter 25 of the accompanying *Study Guide for Nursing Research: Principles and Methods, 7th ed.*, offers various exercises and study suggestions for reinforcing the concepts taught in this chapter. In addition, the following study questions can be addressed:

1. Suppose that you were planning to study the self-care behaviors of aging AIDS patients.
   a. Outline the methods you would recommend adopting.
   b. Develop a work plan.
   c. Prepare a hypothetical budget.
2. Suppose that you were interested in studying separation anxiety in hospitalized children. Using the references cited in this chapter, identify potential funding sources for your project.

SUGGESTED READINGS

Bauer, D. G., & the American Association of Colleges of Nursing. (1988). *The complete grants source book for nursing and health.* New York: Macmillan.

Brown, L. P., Meier, P., Spatz, D. L., Spitzer, A., Finkler, S. A., Jacobsen, B. S., & Zukowsky, K. (1997). Resubmission of a grant application. *Nursing Research, 46,* 119–122.

Clinton, J. (1985). Couvade: Patterns, predictors and nursing management: A research proposal submitted to the Division of Nursing. *Western Journal of Nursing Research, 7*, 221–248.

Cohen, M. Z., Knafl, K., & Dzurec, L. C. (1993). Grant writing for qualitative research. *Image: The Journal of Nursing Scholarship, 25*, 151–156.

Crane, H. C., & Broome, M. E. (2000). Tool for planning the grant application process. *Nursing Outlook, 48*, 288–293.

Davis, G. B., & Parker, C. (1997). *Writing the doctoral dissertation: A systematic approach* (2nd ed.). New York: Barron's.

Fuller, E. O., Hasselmeyer, E. G., Hunter, J. C., Abdellah, F. G., & Hinshaw, A. S. (1991). Summary statements of the NIH nursing research grant applications. *Nursing Research, 40*, 346–351.

Grey, M. (2000). Top 10 tips for successful grantsmanship. *Research in Nursing & Health, 23*, 91–92.

Kim, M. J. (1993). The current generation of research proposals: Reviewers' viewpoints. *Nursing Research, 42*, 118–119.

Krathwohl, D. R. (1988). *How to prepare a research proposal: Guidelines for funding and dissertations in the social and behavioral sciences* (3rd ed.). Syracuse, NY: Syracuse University Press.

Kuzel, A. J. (2002). Some lessons from the story of a funded project. *Qualitative Health Research, 12*, 140–142.

Lindquist, R. D., Tracy, M. F., & Treat-Jacobson, D. (1995). Peer review of nursing research proposals. *American Journal of Critical Care, 4*, 59–65.

Locke, L., Spirduso, W., & Silverman, S. (2000). *Proposals that work: A guide for planning disserta-tions and grant proposals* (4th ed.). Thousand Oaks, CA: Sage.

Madsen, D. (1991). *Successful dissertations and theses: A guide to graduate student research from proposal to completion* (revised ed.). San Francisco: Jossey Bass.

Morse, J. M. (1994). Designing funded qualitative research. In N. K. Denzin & Y. S. Lincoln (Eds.), *Handbook of qualitative research*. Thousand Oaks, CA: Sage.

Morse, J. M., & Field, P. A. (1995). *Qualitative research methods for health professionals* (2nd ed.). Thousand Oaks, CA: Sage.

Morse, J. M., & Richards, L. (2002). *Read me first for a user's guide to qualitative methods*. Thousand Oaks, CA: Sage.

Naylor, M. D. (1990). An example of a research grant application: Comprehensive discharge planning for the elderly. *Research in Nursing & Health, 13*, 327–347.

Sandelowski, M., Davis, D., & Harris, B. (1989). Artful design: Writing the proposal for research in the naturalist paradigm. *Research in Nursing & Health, 12*, 77–84.

Sternberg, D. (1981). *How to complete and survive a doctoral dissertation*. New York: St. Martin's Press.

Tornquist, E. M. & Funk, S. G. (1990). How to write a research grant proposal. *Image: The Journal of Nursing Scholarship, 22*, 44–51.

Tripp-Reimer, T., & Cohen, M.Z. (1991). Funding strategies for qualitative research. In J. M. Morse (Ed.), *Qualitative nursing research: A contemporary dialogue* (pp. 243–256). Newbury Park, CA: Sage.

PART

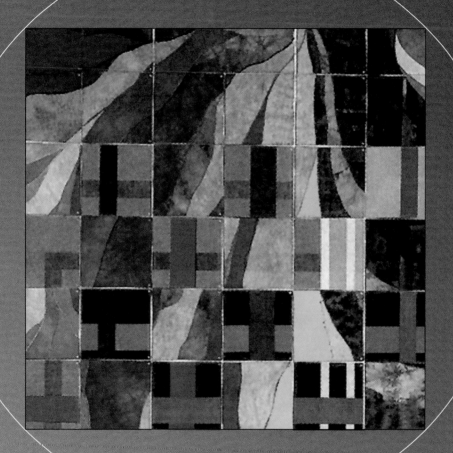

Using Research
Results

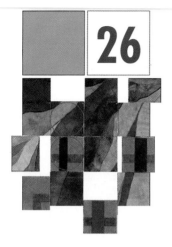

26

Evaluating Research Reports

esearch in a practicing profession such as nursing contributes not only scholarly knowledge but evidence to support and improve practice. Nursing research, then, has relevance for all nurses, not just the minority who actually do empirical studies. As professionals, nurses should possess skills to evaluate relevant research reports. We hope that this text has provided a foundation for the development of such skills. In this chapter, more specific guidelines for the critical appraisal of research reports are presented. The next chapter provides additional assistance regarding integrative reviews of a body of research.

THE RESEARCH CRITIQUE

Nursing practice can be based on solid evidence only if research reports are critically appraised. Consumers sometimes think that if a report was accepted for publication, the study must be sound. Unfortunately, this is not the case. Indeed, *most research has limitations and weaknesses.* Although disciplined research is the best possible means of answering many questions, no single study can provide conclusive evidence. Rather, evidence is accumulated through the conduct—and evaluation—of several studies addressing the same or a similar research question. Consumers who can do reflective and thorough **critiques** of research reports also play a role in advancing nursing knowledge.

Critiquing Research Decisions

Although no single study is infallible, there is a tremendous range in study quality—from nearly worthless to exemplary. Study quality is closely tied to the decisions researchers make in conceptualizing, designing, and executing studies and in interpreting and communicating results. Each study has its own particular flaws because each researcher, in addressing the same or a similar question, makes different decisions about how the study should be done. It is not uncommon for researchers who have made different decisions to arrive at different answers to the same question. It is precisely for this reason that consumers must be knowledgeable about the research process. As a consumer of research reports, you must be able to evaluate researchers' decisions so that you can determine how much faith to put in their conclusions. You must ask, What other approaches could have been adopted, and, if adopted, would the results have been more reliable, believable, or replicable? In other words, you must evaluate the impact of researchers' decisions on a study's ability to reveal the truth.

Purpose of Research Critiques

Research reports are evaluated for a variety of purposes. Students are often asked to prepare critiques to demonstrate their methodologic skills. Seasoned researchers are sometimes asked to write critiques of manuscripts to help journal editors make publication decisions or to accompany reports as published commentaries*; they may also be asked to present an oral critique if they are invited as discussants of a paper at a professional conference. Journal clubs in clinical settings may meet periodically to critique and discuss research studies. And, perhaps most important, critiquing individual studies plays a role in assembling evidence into integrative reviews of the literature on a topic. For all these purposes, the goal is to develop a balanced evaluation of a study's contribution to knowledge.

Research critiques are not just reviews or summaries of a study; rather, they are thoughtful critical appraisals of the strengths and limitations of a piece of research. A written critique should serve as a guide— to researchers, to editors, or to practitioners. Critiques should offer guidance about ways in which study results may have been compromised, and should provide guidance about alternative research strategies to address the research question. Critiques should thus help to advance a particular area of knowledge.

The function of critical evaluations of nursing studies is not to hunt for and expose mistakes. A good critique objectively and critically identifies adequacies and inadequacies, virtues as well as faults. Sometimes the need for such balance is obscured by the terms *critique* and *critical appraisal*, which connote unfavorable observations. The merits of a study are as important as its limitations in coming to conclusions about the worth of its findings. Therefore, research critiques should reflect a balanced consideration of a study's validity and significance.

Box 26-1 summarizes general guidelines to consider in preparing a written research critique. In the section that follows, we present some specific

BOX 26.1 Guidelines for the Conduct of a Written Research Critique

1. Be sure to comment on the study's strengths as well as weaknesses. The critique should be a balanced analysis of the study's worth. All reports have *some* positive features—be sure to find and note them.
2. Give specific examples of the study's strengths and limitations. Avoid vague generalizations of praise and fault finding.
3. Justify your criticisms. Offer a rationale for your concerns.
4. Be objective. Avoid being overly critical of a study because you are not interested in the topic or because your world view is inconsistent with the underlying paradigm.
5. Be sensitive in handling negative comments. Put yourself in the shoes of the researcher receiving the comments. Do not be condescending or sarcastic.
6. Don't just identify problems—suggest alternatives, indicating how a different approach would have solved a methodologic problem. Make sure the recommendations are practical.

guidelines for evaluating various aspects of research reports.

ELEMENTS OF A RESEARCH CRITIQUE

Research reports have several important dimensions that may need to be considered in a critical evaluation of a study's worth. These include the substantive/theoretical, methodologic, interpretive, ethical, and presentational/stylistic dimensions of a study. It should be noted, however, that some critiques—such as those prepared for journal editors—are likely to focus primarily on substantive and methodologic issues.

Substantive and Theoretical Dimensions

Readers of a research report need to determine whether a study was worthy in terms of the

---

*The *Western Journal of Nursing Research,* for example, often publishes research reports followed by one or two commentaries that include appraisals of the report.

significance of the problem, the soundness of the conceptualizations, and the appropriateness of the conceptual framework. The research problem should have clear relevance to some aspect of nursing. Thus, even before you learn *how* a study was done, you should evaluate whether the study should have been conducted. Of course, your own disciplinary orientation should not bear on an objective evaluation of the study's significance. A clinical nurse might not be intrigued by a study focusing on determinants of nursing turnover, but a nursing administrator trying to improve staffing decisions might find such a study useful. It is important, then, not to adopt a myopic view of a study's importance and relevance.

Many problems relevant to nursing are still not necessarily worthy of a new study. You must ask a question such as, Given what we know about this topic, is this research the right next step? Knowledge tends to be incremental. Researchers must consider how to advance knowledge on a topic in beneficial ways. They should avoid unnecessary replications of a study once a body of research clearly points to an answer, but they should also not leap several steps ahead when there is an insecure foundation. Sometimes, replication is exactly what is needed to enhance the credibility or generalizability of earlier findings.

An issue that has both substantive and methodologic implications is the congruence between the study question and the methods used to address it. There must be a good fit between the research problem on the one hand and the overall study design, the method of collecting research data, and the approach to analyzing those data on the other. Questions that deal with poorly understood phenomena, with processes, with the dynamics of a situation, or with in-depth description, for example, are usually best addressed with flexible designs, unstructured methods of data collection, and qualitative analysis. Questions that involve the measurement of well-defined variables, cause-and-effect relationships, or the effectiveness of a specific intervention, however, are usually better suited to more structured, quantitative approaches

using designs that offer control over the research situation.

Another issue is whether researchers have appropriately placed the research problem into a larger context, in terms of prior research and a conceptual framework. As we emphasized in Chapter 6, researchers do little to enhance the value of a study if the connection between the research problem and a conceptual framework is contrived. However, a specific research problem that is genuinely framed as a part of some larger intellectual issue can usually advance knowledge more than an inquiry that ignores its theoretical underpinnings. Even though qualitative studies are not viewed through the lens of a theoretical/conceptual framework, researchers should still address the philosophical or theoretical underpinnings of the chosen research tradition—for example, symbolic interaction should be addressed in a grounded theory study.

The substantive and theoretical dimensions of a study are normally communicated in a report's introduction. The manner in which introductory materials are presented is vital to the proper understanding and appreciation of what researchers have accomplished. Some guidelines for critiquing introductions to research reports are presented in Boxes 26-2 through 26-4.* Box 26-2 provides guidelines for critiquing the researcher's statement of the problem, research questions, and hypotheses. Boxes 26-3 and 26-4 suggest considerations relevant to a critique of the literature review and conceptual framework, respectively.

Methodologic Dimensions

Once a research problem has been identified, researchers make a number of important decisions about how to go about answering the research questions or testing the hypotheses. It is your job as a

---

*The questions included in the boxes in this chapter are not exhaustive. Many additional questions might need to be raised in dealing with a particular piece of research. Moreover, the boxes include many questions that do not apply to every piece of research. The questions are intended to represent a useful point of departure in undertaking a critique.

BOX 26.2 Guidelines for Critiquing Research Problems, Research Questions, and Hypotheses

1. Has the research problem been clearly identified? Has the researcher appropriately delimited its scope?
2. Does the problem have significance for nursing? How might the research contribute to nursing practice, administration, education, or policy?
3. Is there a good fit between the research problem and the paradigm within which the research was conducted?
4. Does the report formally present a statement of purpose, research questions, or hypotheses? Is this information communicated clearly and concisely, and is it placed in a logical and useful location?
5. Are purpose statements or questions worded appropriately (e.g., are key concepts/variables identified and the population of interest specified)?
6. If there are no formal hypotheses, is their absence justifiable? Are statistical tests used despite the absence of stated hypotheses?
7. Do hypotheses (if any) flow from a theory or previous research? Is there a justifiable basis for the predictions?
8. Are hypotheses (if any) properly worded—do they state a predicted relationship between two or more variables? Are they directional or nondirectional, and is there a rationale for how they were stated? Are they presented as research or as null hypotheses?

critiquer to evaluate those decisions and their conse-quences. In fact, the heart of a research critique lies in the analysis of the **methodologic decisions** adopted.

Although researchers make hundreds of deci-sions about the methods for conducting a study, there are some that are more critical than others. In a quan-titative study, the four major decision points on which you should focus critical attention are as follows:

• *Decision 1, Design*: What design will yield the most unambiguous and meaningful (internally valid) results about the relationship between the independent variable and dependent variable, or the most valid descriptions of concepts under

study? What extraneous variables need to be con-trolled, and how best can this be accomplished?
• *Decision 2, Sample*: Who should participate in the study? What are the characteristics of the popula-tion to which the findings should be generalized (external validity)? How large should the sample be, from where should participants be recruited, and what sampling approach should be used?
• *Decision 3, Data collection*: What method should be used to collect the data? How can the variables be operationalized and reliably and validly measured?
• *Decision 4, Data analysis*: What statistical analyses will provide the most appropriate tests

BOX 26.3 Guidelines for Critiquing Research Literature Reviews

1. Does the review seem thorough—does it include all or most of the major studies conducted on the topic? Does it include recent work?
2. Does the review cite primarily primary sources (the original studies)?
3. Is the review merely a summary of existing work, or does it critically appraise and compare key studies? Does the review identify important gaps in the literature?
4. Does the review use appropriate language, suggesting the tentativeness of prior findings? Is the review objective?
5. Is the review well organized? Is the development of ideas clear?
6. Does the review lay the foundation for undertaking the new study?

BOX 26.4 Guidelines for Critiquing Theoretical and Conceptual Frameworks

1. Does the research report describe a theoretical or conceptual framework for the study? If not, does the absence of a theoretical framework detract from the usefulness or significance of the research?
2. Does the report adequately describe the major features of the theory so that readers can understand the conceptual basis of the study?
3. Is the theory appropriate to the research problem? Would a different theoretical framework have been more appropriate?
4. Is the theoretical framework based on a conceptual model of nursing, or is it borrowed from another discipline? Is there adequate justification for the researcher's decision about the type of framework used?
5. Do the research problem and hypotheses flow naturally from the theoretical framework, or does the link between the problem and theory seem contrived?
6. Are the deductions from the theory or conceptual framework logical?
7. Are all the concepts adequately defined in a way that is consistent with the theory?
8. Does the researcher tie the findings of the study back to the framework at the end of the report? Do the findings support or undermine the framework?

of the research hypotheses or answers to the research questions?

In a quantitative study, these methodologic decisions are typically made up-front, and researchers then execute the prespecified plan. Qualitative researchers also make some up-front decisions, such as the research tradition that best matches the research question, (e.g., grounded theory versus phenomenology). Another up-front methodologic decision in qualitative research is the data analysis approach to be used. For example, in a phenomenological study, researchers usually prespecify whether the data will be analyzed by, say, Colaizzi's method or Giorgi's method. Ongoing methodologic decisions do occur while collecting and analyzing qualitative data, however. In qualitative studies, the major methodologic decisions you should consider in your critique are as follows:

• *Decision 1, Design*: Which research tradition best matches the research question?
• *Decision 2, Setting and study participants*: What setting will yield the richest information about the phenomenon under study? Who should participate, and how can participants be selected to enhance the study's theoretical

richness? How many participants are needed to achieve data saturation?
• *Decision 3, Data sources*: What should the sources of data be, and how should data be gathered? Should multiple sources of data (e.g., unstructured interviews and observations) be used to achieve method triangulation?
• *Decision 4, Data analysis*: What data analysis techniques are appropriate for the research tradition?
• *Decision 5, Quality enhancement*: What types of evidence can be obtained to support the credibility, transferability, dependability, and confirmability of the data, the analysis, and the interpretation?

Because of practical constraints, studies almost always entail compromises between what is ideal and what is feasible. For example, researchers might ideally want to collect data from 500 subjects, but, because of limited resources, they might have to be content with 200 subjects. Reviewers cannot realistically demand that researchers attain these methodologic ideals, but must evaluate how much damage has been done by failure to achieve them.

Various guidelines are presented in the following displays to help you in performing a critical

BOX 26.5 Guidelines for Critiquing Research Designs in Quantitative Studies

1. What would be the most rigorous research design for the research question? How does this correspond to the design actually used?
2. If there is an intervention, was a true experimental, quasi-experimental, or preexperimental design used, and how does this affect the believability of the findings?
3. If there is an intervention, was it described in sufficient detail? Was the intervention reliably implemented? Is there evidence of treatment "dilution" or contamination of treatments? Were participation levels in the treatment high?
4. If the design is nonexperimental, was the study *inherently* nonexperimental? If not, is there an adequate justification for failure to manipulate the independent variable?
5. What types of comparisons are specified in the design (e.g., before–after, between groups)? Do these comparisons adequately illuminate the relationship between independent and dependent variables? If there are no comparisons, does this pose difficulties for interpreting results?
6. Was the design longitudinal or cross-sectional—and was this appropriate? Was the number of data collection points reasonable?
7. What procedures were used to control external (situational) factors, and were they adequate and appropriate?
8. What procedures were used to control extraneous subject characteristics, and were they adequate and appropriate?
9. To what extent is the study internally valid? What alternative explanations must be considered (i.e., what are the threats to the study's internal validity)?
10. To what extent is the study externally valid? What are the threats to the study's external validity?
11. What are the major limitations of the design? Are these limitations acknowledged and taken into account in the interpretation of results?
12. Could the design have been strengthened by the inclusion of a qualitative component?

analysis of the research methods. Box 26-5 presents guidelines for critiquing the overall research design of quantitative studies, and Box 26-6 has guidelines for critiquing the design of qualitative and mixed-method studies. Sampling strategies can be evaluated using the questions included in Box 26-7 for quantitative studies or Box 26-8 for qualitative ones.

Six separate boxes are included here to assist with a critique of the researcher's data collection plan. Box 26-9 provides suggestions for critiquing the actual procedures used to collect the data. Explicit guidelines are provided for evaluating self-report approaches (Box 26-10), observational methods (Box 26-11), and biophysiologic measures (Box 26-12). Criteria are not provided for evaluating infrequently used data collection techniques (e.g., Q sorts), but other methods can be evaluated by considering one overarching ques-

tion: Was the data collection method the best possible approach to capturing key research variables? Boxes 25-13 and 25-14 suggest some guidelines for evaluating the overall quality of the data in quantitative and qualitative studies, respectively.

The analysis plan is the final methodologic area that requires a critical analysis. Box 26-15 lists a number of guiding questions of relevance for evaluating quantitative analyses, and Box 26-16 identifies questions for qualitative analyses. When a study has used both qualitative and quantitative analyses, questions from both boxes are likely to be applicable.

Ethical Dimensions

In performing a research critique, you may (depending on the purpose of the critique) need to

BOX 26.6 Guidelines for Critiquing Qualitative and Mixed-Method Designs

1. Is the research tradition for the qualitative study identified? If none was identified, can one be inferred? If more than one was identified, is this justifiable or does it suggest "method slurring?"
2. Is the research question congruent with the research tradition (i.e., is the domain of inquiry for the study congruent with the domain encompassed by the tradition)? Are the data sources, research methods, and analytic approach congruent with the research tradition?
3. How well is the design described? Is the design appropriate, given the research question? What design elements might have strengthened the study (e.g., a longitudinal perspective rather than a cross-sectional one)?
4. Is the study exclusively qualitative, or was the design mixed method, involving both qualitative and quantitative data? Could the design have been strengthened by the inclusion of a quantitative component?
5. If the study used a mixed-method design, how did the inclusion of both approaches contribute to enhanced theoretical insights, enhanced validity, or movement toward new frontiers?

consider whether the rights of human subjects were violated during the investigation. If there are any potential ethical concerns, you need to consider the impact of those problems on the scientific merit of the study on the one hand and on participants' well-being on the other. Guidelines for evaluating the ethical dimensions of a research report are presented in Box 26-17.

There are two main types of ethical transgressions in research studies. The first consists of inad-

vertent actions or activities that researchers did not interpret as creating an ethical dilemma. For example, in one study that examined married couples' experiences with sexually transmitted diseases, the researcher asked husbands and wives to complete, privately, self-administered questionnaires. The researcher offered to mail back copies of the questionnaires to couples who wanted an opportunity to discuss their responses. Although this offer was viewed as an opportunity to enhance couple

BOX 26.7 Guidelines for Critiquing Quantitative Sampling Designs

1. Is the target or accessible population identified and described? Are the eligibility criteria clearly specified? Would a more limited population specification have controlled for important sources of extraneous variation not covered by the research design?
2. What type of sampling plan was used? Does the report make clear whether probability or nonprobability sampling was used?
3. How were subjects recruited into the sample? Does the method suggest potential biases?
4. How adequate is the sampling plan in terms of yielding a representative sample?
5. If the sampling plan is weak (e.g., a convenience sample), are potential biases identified? Is the sampling plan justified, given the research problem?
6. Did some factor other than the sampling plan itself (e.g., a low response rate) affect the representativeness of the sample? Did the researcher take steps to produce a high response rate?
7. Are the size and key characteristics of the sample described?
8. Is the sample sufficiently large? Was the sample size justified on the basis of a power analysis?
9. To whom can the study results reasonably be generalized?

BOX 26.8 Guidelines for Critiquing
Qualitative Sampling Designs

1. Is the setting or study group adequately described? Is the setting appropriate for the research question?
2. Are the sample selection procedures described? What type of sampling strategy was used?
3. Given the information needs of the study, was the sampling approach appropriate? Were dimensions of the phenomenon under study adequately represented?
4. Is the sample size adequate? Did the researcher stipulate that information redundancy was achieved? Do the findings suggest a richly textured and comprehensive set of data without any apparent "holes" or thin areas?

communication, it is problematic. Some subjects may have felt compelled to say, under spousal pressure, that they wanted to share their responses, when, in fact, they wanted to keep their answers private. The use of the mail to return these sensitive completed questionnaires was also questionable. In this case, the ethical problem was inadvertent and could easily be resolved (e.g., the researcher could give out *blank* copies of the questionnaire for couples to go over together).

In other cases, researchers might be aware of having committed some violation of ethical principles, but made a conscious decision that the violation was modest in relation to the knowledge that could be gained by doing the study in a certain way. For example, a researcher may decide not to obtain informed consent from the parents of minor children attending a family planning clinic because to require such consent would probably dramatically reduce the number of minors willing to participate in the research and would lead to a biased sample of clinic users; it could also violate the minors' right to confidential treatment at the clinic. When researchers knowingly elect not to follow the ethical principles outlined in Chapter 7, you must evaluate the decision and the researcher's rationale.

Interpretive Dimensions

Research reports usually conclude with a Discussion, Conclusions, or Implications section. It is in the final section that researchers attempt to make sense of the analyses, to consider whether the findings support or fail to support hypotheses or theory, and to discuss what the findings imply for nursing. Inevitably, discussion sections are more subjective than other sections of a report, but they must also be based on a careful consideration of the evidence. In an appraisal of a report, unwarranted interpretations are fair game for criticism.

As a reviewer, you should be somewhat wary if a discussion section fails to point out any study limitations. Researchers are themselves in the best position to detect and assess the impact of sampling deficiencies, data quality problems, and so on, and it is a professional responsibility to alert readers to such issues. Moreover, when researchers note methodologic shortcomings, readers have some assurance that these limitations were considered in interpreting results.

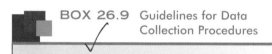

BOX 26.9 Guidelines for Data
Collection Procedures

1. How were data collected? Were multiple methods used and judiciously combined?
2. Who collected the data? Were data collectors judiciously chosen? Do they have traits (e.g., their professional role, their relationship with study participants) that could have undermined the collection of unbiased, high-quality data?
3. Was the training of data collectors adequate? Were steps taken to improve their ability to elicit or produce high-quality data or to monitor their performance?
4. Where and under what circumstances were data gathered? Was the setting for data collection appropriate?
5. Were other people present during data collection? Could the presence of others have resulted in any biases?
6. Did the collection of data place any burdens (in terms of time, stress, privacy issues) on participants? How might this have affected data quality?

BOX 26.10 Guidelines for Critiquing Self-Reports

INTERVIEWS AND QUESTIONNAIRES

1. Does the research question lend itself to self-report data? Would an alternative method have been more appropriate? Should another method have been used as a supplement?
2. How structured was the approach? Is the degree of structure consistent with the nature of the research question?
3. Do the questions asked adequately cover the complexities of the phenomenon under investigation?
4. Did the researcher use the best possible mode for collecting self-report data (i.e., personal interviews, telephone interviews, self-administered questionnaires), given the research question and respondent characteristics? Would an alternative method have improved data quality?
5. [If an instrument is available for review]: Was the instrument too long or too brief? Was there an appropriate blend of open-ended and closed-ended questions? Are questions clearly and sensitively worded? Is the ordering of questions appropriate? Are response alternatives comprehensive? Could questions lead to biased responses?
6. Were the instrument and data collection procedures adequately pretested?

SCALES

7. If a scale was used, is its use justified? Does it adequately capture the construct of interest?
8. If a new scale was developed for the study, is there adequate justification for not using an existing one? Was the new scale adequately tested and refined?
9. Does the report provide a rationale for using the selected scale (e.g., one particular scale to measure stress, as opposed to other available scales)?
10. Are procedures for eliminating or minimizing response-set biases described, and were they appropriate?

BOX 26.11 Guidelines for Critiquing Observational Methods

1. Does the research question lend itself to an observational approach? Would an alternative data collection method have been more appropriate? Should another method have been used as a supplement?
2. Is the degree of structure of the observational method consistent with the research question?
3. To what degree were observers concealed during data collection? What effect might their known presence have had on the behaviors and events under observation?
4. What was the unit of analysis of the observations? How much inference was required on the part of the observers, and to what extent might this have led to bias?
5. Where did observations take place? To what extent did the setting influence the "naturalness" of behaviors being observed?
6. How were data recorded (e.g., on field notes or checklists)? Did the recording procedures seem appropriate?
7. What steps were taken to minimize observer bias? How were observers trained, and how was their performance evaluated?
8. If a category scheme was developed, did it appear appropriate? Do the categories adequately cover the relevant behaviors? Was the scheme overly demanding of observers, leading to potential error? If the scheme was not exhaustive, did the omission of large realms of subject behavior result in an inadequate context for understanding the behaviors or interest?
9. How were events or behaviors sampled? Did this plan appear to yield an adequate or representative sample of relevant behaviors?

BOX 26.12 Guidelines for Critiquing
Biophysiologic Measures

1. Does the research question lend itself to the collection of biophysiologic data? Would an alternative data collection method have been more appropriate? Should another method have been used as a supplement?
2. Was the proper instrumentation used to obtain the biophysiologic measurements, or would an alternative have been more suitable?
3. Was care taken to obtain accurate data? For example, did the researcher's activities permit accurate recording?
4. Did the researcher have the skills necessary for proper use and interpretation of the biophysiologic measures?

 Example of researcher-noted limitations:
Lenz and Perkins (2000) conducted an experimental study of the effectiveness of a family-focused psychoeducational intervention for coronary artery bypass graft surgery patients and their family caregivers. The results failed to support hypotheses regarding improved physical and emotional outcomes for experimental group members. The researchers discussed several possible explanations for the results, including dilution of the treatment, small sample size, and limitations of the measures used.

Of course, researchers are unlikely to note *all* relevant shortcomings of their own work. The inclusion of comments about study limitations in the discussion section, although important, does not relieve you of the responsibility of appraising methodologic decisions. Your task as a reviewer is generally to contrast your own interpretation with that of the researcher and to challenge conclusions that do not appear to be supported by the results. If your objective reading of the research methods and study findings leads to an interpretation that is notably different from that of the researcher, then the study's interpretive dimension may be faulty.

It is often difficult to determine the validity of researchers' interpretations in qualitative studies.

BOX 26.13 Guidelines for Evaluating Data Quality in Quantitative Studies

1. Is there a congruence between the research variables as conceptualized (i.e., as discussed in the introduction) and as operationalized (i.e., as described in the methods section)?
2. If operational definitions (or scoring procedures) are specified, do they clearly indicate the rules of measurement? Do the rules seem sensible? Were data collected in such a way that measurement errors were minimized?
3. Does the report offer evidence of the reliability of measures? Does the evidence come from the research sample itself, or is it based on other studies? If the latter, is it reasonable to conclude that data quality for the research sample and the reliability sample would be similar (e.g., are sample characteristics similar)?
4. If reliability is reported, which estimation method was used? Was this method appropriate? Should an alternative or additional method of reliability appraisal have been used? Is the reliability sufficiently high?
5. Does the report offer evidence of the validity of the measures? Does the evidence come from the research sample itself, or is it based on other studies? If the latter, is it reasonable to believe that data quality for the research sample and the validity sample would be similar (e.g., are the sample characteristics similar)?
6. If validity information is reported, which validity approach was used? Was this method appropriate? Does the validity of the instrument appear to be adequate?
7. If there is no reliability or validity information, what conclusion can you reach about the quality of the data in the study?
8. Were the research hypotheses supported? If not, might data quality play a role in the failure to confirm the hypotheses?

BOX 26.14 Guidelines for Evaluating Data Quality in Qualitative Studies

1. Does there appear to be a strong relationship between the phenomena of interest as conceptualized (i.e., as described in the introduction) and as described in the discussion of the data collection approach?
2. Does the report discuss efforts to enhance or evaluate the trustworthiness of the data? If not, is there other information that allows you to conclude that data are of high quality?
3. Which techniques (if any) did the researcher use to enhance and appraise data quality? Was the investigator in the field an adequate amount of time? Was triangulation used, and, if so, of what type? Did the researcher search for disconfirming evidence? Were there peer debriefings or member checks? Do the researcher's qualifications enhance the credibility of the data? Did the report include information on the audit trial for data analysis?
4. Were the procedures used to enchance and document data quality adequate?
5. Given the efforts to enhance data quality, what can you conclude about the credibility, transferability, dependability, and confirmability of the data? In light of this assessment, how much faith can be placed in the results of the study?

BOX 26.15 Guidelines for Critiquing Quantitative Analyses

1. Does the report include any descriptive statistics? Do these statistics sufficiently describe the major characteristics of the researcher's data set?
2. Were indices of both central tendency and variability provided in the report? If not, how does the absence of this information affect the reader's understanding of the research variables?
3. Were the correct descriptive statistics used (e.g., was a median used when a mean would have been more appropriate)?
4. Does the report include any inferential statistics? Was a statistical test performed for each of the hypotheses or research questions? If inferential statistics were not used, should they have been?
5. Was the selected statistical test appropriate, given the level of measurement of the variables?
6. Was a parametric test used? Does it appear that the assumptions for the use of parametric tests were met? If a nonparametric test was used, should a more powerful parametric procedure have been used instead?
7. Were any multivariate procedures used? If so, does it appear that the researcher chose the appropriate test? If multivariate procedures were not used, should they have been? Would the use of a multivariate procedure have improved the researcher's ability to draw conclusions about the relationship between the dependent and independent variables?
8. In general, does the report provide a rationale for the use of the selected statistical tests? Does the report contain sufficient information for you to judge whether appropriate statistics were used?
9. Was there an appropriate amount of statistical information reported? Are the findings clearly and logically organized?
10. Were the results of any statistical tests significant? What do the tests tell you about the plausibility of the research hypotheses?
11. Were tables used judiciously to summarize large masses of statistical information? Are the tables clearly presented, with good titles and carefully labeled column headings? Is the information presented in the text consistent with the information presented in the tables? Is the information totally redundant?

BOX 26.16 Guidelines for Critiquing Qualitative Analyses

1. Given the nature of the data, were they best analyzed qualitatively? Were the data analysis techniques appropriate for the research design?
2. Is the initial categorization scheme described? If so, does the scheme appear logical and complete? Does there seem to be unnecessary overlap or redundancy in the categories?
3. Were manual methods used to index and organize the data, or was a computer program used?
4. Is the process by which a thematic analysis was performed described? What major themes emerged? If excerpts from the data are provided, do the themes appear to capture the meaning of the narratives—that is, does it appear that the researcher adequately interpreted the data and conceptualized the themes?
5. Is the analysis parsimonious—could two or more themes be collapsed into a broader and perhaps more useful conceptualization?
6. What evidence does the report provide that the researcher's analysis is accurate and replicable?
7. Were data displayed in a manner that allows you to verify the researcher's conclusions? Was a conceptual map, model, or diagram effectively displayed to communicate important processes?
8. Was the context of the phenomenon adequately described? Does the report give you a clear picture of the social or emotional world of study participants?
9. If the result of the study is an emergent theory or conceptualization, does it yield a meaningful and insightful picture of the phenomenon under study? Is the resulting theory or description trivial or obvious?

To help readers understand the lens through which they interpreted their data, qualitative researchers should make note of whether they (1) kept field notes or a journal of their actions and emotions during the investigation, (2) discussed their own behavior and experiences in relation to the participants' experiences, and (3) acknowledged any effects of their presence on the nature of the data collected. Reviewers should look for such information in critiquing qualitative reports.

BOX 26.17 Guidelines for Critiquing the Ethical Aspects of a Study

1. Were study participants subjected to any physical harm, discomfort, or psychological distress? Did the researchers take appropriate steps to remove or prevent harm or minimize discomfort?
2. Did benefits to participants outweigh any potential risks or actual discomfort they experienced? Did the benefits to society or nursing outweigh costs to participants?
3. Was any coercion or undue influence used in recruiting participants?
4. Were groups omitted from the inquiry (e.g., women, minorities) without a justifiable rationale?
5. Were vulnerable subjects used? Were special precautions instituted because of their vulnerable status?
6. Were participants deceived in any way? Were they fully aware of participating in a study and did they understand the purpose of the research?
7. Did participants have an opportunity to decline participation? Were appropriate consent procedures implemented? If not, were there valid and justifiable reasons?
8. Were participants told about any real or potential risks associated with participation in the study? Were study procedures fully described in advance?
9. Were appropriate steps taken to safeguard the privacy of participants?
10. Was the study approved and monitored by an Institutional Review Board or other similar ethics review committee? If not, did the researcher have any type of external review relating to ethical considerations?

In addition to contrasting your interpretation with that of the researcher (when this is possible), your critique should also draw conclusions about the stated implications of the study. Some researchers make rather grandiose claims or offer unfounded recommendations on the basis of modest results. Some guidelines for evaluating the researcher's interpretation and implications are offered in Box 26-18.

Presentational and Stylistic Dimensions

Although the worth of the study itself concerns primarily the dimensions we have reviewed thus far, the manner in which study information is communicated in the research report can also be critiqued in a comprehensive critical appraisal. Box 26-19 summarizes major points to consider in evaluating the presentation of a research report.

An important issue is whether the report provided sufficient information for a thoughtful critique of the other dimensions. For example, if the report does not describe how participants were selected, reviewers cannot comment on the adequacy of the sample, but they can criticize the absence of information on sampling. When vital pieces of information are missing, researchers leave readers little choice but to assume the worst because this would lead to the most cautious interpretation of the results.

The writing in a research report, as in any published document, should be clear, grammatical, concise, and well organized. Unnecessary jargon should be minimized, but colloquialisms usually should be avoided. Inadequate organization is

---

BOX 26.18 Guidelines for Critiquing the Interpretive Dimensions of a Research Report

INTERPRETATION OF THE FINDINGS

1. Are all important results discussed? If not, what is the likely explanation for omissions?
2. Are interpretations consistent with results? Do the interpretations take into account methodologic limitations?
3. What types of evidence are offered in support of the interpretation, and is that evidence persuasive? Are results interpreted in light of findings from other studies? Are results interpreted in terms of the original study hypotheses and the conceptual framework?
4. Are alternative explanations for the findings mentioned, and is the rationale for their rejection presented?
5. In quantitative studies, does the interpretation distinguish between practical and statistical significance?
6. Are any unwarranted interpretations of causality made?

IMPLICATIONS OF THE FINDINGS

7. Does the researcher offer implications of the research for nursing practice, nursing theory, or nursing research? Are implications of the study omitted, although a basis for them is apparent?
8. Are the stated implications appropriate, given the study's limitations?
9. Are generalizations made that are not warranted on the basis of the sample used?

RECOMMENDATIONS

10. Are specific recommendations made concerning how the study's methods could be improved? Are there recommendations for future research investigations?
11. Are recommendations for specific nursing actions presented?
12. Are recommendations consistent with the findings and with the existing body of knowledge?

BOX 26.19 Guidelines for Critiquing the Presentation of a Research Report

1. Does the report include a sufficient amount of detail to permit a thorough critique of the study's purpose, conceptual framework, design and methods, handling of critical ethical issues analysis of data, and interpretation?
2. Is the report well written and grammatical? Are pretentious words or jargon used when a simpler wording would have been possible?
3. Is the report well organized, or is the presentation confusing? Is there an orderly, logical presentation of ideas? Are transitions smooth, and is the report characterized by continuity of thought and expression?
4. Is the report sufficiently concise or does the author include a lot of irrelevant detail? Are important details omitted?
5. Does the report suggest overt biases?
6. Is the report written using tentative language as befits the nature of disciplined inquiry, or does the author talk about what the study did or did not "prove"?
7. Is sexist language avoided?
8. Does the title of the report adequately capture the key concepts and the population under investigation? Does the abstract (if any) adequately summarize the research problem, study methods, and important findings?

another presentation flaw in some research reports. Continuity and logical thematic development are critical to good communication of scientific information, but these qualities are often difficult to attain.

Styles of writing do differ for qualitative and quantitative reports, and it is unreasonable to apply the standards considered appropriate for one paradigm to the other. Quantitative research reports are typically written in a more formal, impersonal fashion, using either the third person or passive voice to connote objectivity. Qualitative studies are likely to be written in a more literary style, using the first or second person and active voice to connote proximity and intimacy with the data and the phenomenon under study. Regardless of style, however, you should, as a reviewer, be alert to indications of overt biases, unwarranted exaggerations, emotionally laden comments, or melodramatic language.

In summary, the research report is meant to be an account of how and why a problem was studied and what results were obtained. The report should be clearly written, cogent, and concise, and written in a manner that piques readers' interest and curiosity.

CONCLUSION

In concluding this chapter, several points about research critiques should be made. It should be apparent to those who have glanced through the questions in the boxes in this chapter that it will not always be possible to answer all questions satisfactorily. This is especially true for reports published as journal articles, in which the need for economy often translates into compressed methodologic descriptions. Furthermore, there are many questions listed that may have little or no relevance for particular studies. The inclusion of a question in the list does not necessarily imply that all reports should have all components mentioned. The questions are meant to suggest aspects of a study that often are deserving of consideration; they are not meant to lay traps for identifying omitted and perhaps unnecessary details.

It must be admitted that the answers to many questions will call on your judgment as much as, or even more than, your knowledge. An evaluation of whether the most appropriate data collection procedure was used for the research problem necessarily involves a degree of subjectivity. Issues concerning the appropriateness of various strategies and techniques are topics about which even experts disagree. You should strive to be as objective as possible and to indicate your reasoning for the judgments made.

One final note is that there is increasing interest in using quantitative methods to rate or score methodologic quality in individual studies, for the purposes of doing integrative reviews and meta-analyses. Such scoring systems are discussed in greater detail in the next chapter.

RESEARCH EXAMPLES

There are two complete research reports—one qualitative and the other quantitative—in the accompanying *Study Guide for Essentials of Nursing Research, 7th ed*. The guidelines in this chapter can be used to conduct a critical appraisal of these studies. In this section, we describe two studies by nurse researchers and present excerpts from published written commentaries. Note that the comments are not comprehensive—they do not cover all the dimensions of a research critique as described in this chapter. However, the excerpts provide a flavor for the kinds of things that are noted in a critique.

Example of a Quantitative Report and Critical Comments

Ross, Carswell, and Dalziel (2001) investigated family caregiving within institutional settings. Their published report was accompanied by a commentary by one reviewer.

Research Summary

Ross and her colleagues addressed several questions in their descriptive study of family caregiving to relatives within long-term care facilities, including the following: (1) How frequently do families visit after the admission of a relative? (2) What care-related activities do families carry out for their institutionalized relative? and (3) What are their care-related learning needs and resources?

Nineteen long-term care facilities in the Ottawa–Carleton region were identified, nine of

which were invited to participate in the study. Facilities were chosen to reflect diversity in size, urban/rural location, language, and type of ownership. Staff in these facilities identified family members who were personally involved with their relative, and 194 of those identified were randomly selected to be participants. Questionnaires that included both closed-ended and open-ended questions were mailed to selected family members, and a total of 122 completed questionnaires were returned.

Descriptive statistics (mostly percentages and means) were used to analyze the data. The findings indicated that families visited their institutionalized relatives frequently. While visiting, family members usually provided both direct care (e.g., grooming) and, especially, indirect care (e.g., communicating with staff). Most family members indicated an interest in learning to provide better emotional support. On the basis of their findings, the researchers made several recommendations for policy and practice, such as the development of mechanisms to facilitate the visiting experience and creating a comfortable environment.

Commentary

Penrod (2001) prepared a commentary that was published in the same issue as Ross and colleagues' study. Penrod had many favorable comments about the study and its purpose. For example, she noted the following:

> These authors cogently argue that we know little about what the visiting experience is like for family members. Observation of visible task performance provides a superficial glimpse of what is going on during these visits, but understanding these actions from the perspectives of the family members falls woefully short (p. 364).

Penrod did, however, express concerns about some methodologic aspects of the study. One concern focused on the sampling plan. Noting that the initial pool of eligibles had been identified by facility staff members, she commented that the researchers had not provided information about what selection criteria staff used. Moreover, by seeking residents whose family members were personally involved with their relative, there was a risk that results would be biased. Penrod concluded that "further clarification of sampling and selection would strengthen the study" (p. 365).

A more general concern related to the cross-sectional nature of the design. Penrod noted that caregivers' views and experiences are dynamic and change over time. This is of particular concern because the residents had lived in the facility for an average of 3.5 years, and presumably the range of time institutionalized varied widely. Penrod asked the following questions, which could best be answered by a longitudinal design, but which also could have been explored with the existing data, but were not:

> Did the caregivers' perceptions of frequency, duration, and reasons for visiting change over time? Did their views on task performance shift between direct and indirect care activities over this time? ... And was there any evidence of more dynamic learning needs as the caregivers lived through the initial admission and orientation processes followed by the deteriorating health status of their loved ones? (p. 365).

Penrod concluded by praising the contribution that the study made to an understanding of caregiving postplacement, but also commented that "the time has come to advance science beyond description of *what is* to begin exploring *what can be done* to maximize potential contributions of caregivers" (p. 367).

Example of a Qualitative Report and Critical Comments

Butler, Banfield, Sveinson, and Allen (1998) conducted a qualitative study to describe women's experiences with changes in sexual function after treatment for gynecologic cancer. Their research report, which appeared in *Western Journal of Nursing Research*, was followed by the commentaries of two reviewers.

Research Summary
Butler and her colleagues conducted a multimethod study that explored issues of sexual health for women with cervical and endometrial cancer. The qualitative portion of their study involved in-depth interviews with a sample of 17 women, using a semistructured interview guide. The questions were designed to stimulate discussion about how cancer and its treatment affected participants' views of themselves as women, as partners, and as mothers. The interviews, which were taped and transcribed, lasted approximately 90 minutes. Content analysis was used for data analysis. Three of the investigators independently coded the data; intercoder agreement was high.

Although the study's purpose was to pursue issues relating to sexual functioning, the women described a broader concept of sexual health in which functioning was only one aspect contributing to the view of self as a sexual being. The analysis revealed multiple components that need to be considered in developing a conceptual model of sexual health.

One of the central categories the women discussed was the effect of relationships—with health care personnel, family, friends, and partners—on their sexual well-being. The absence of discussions about sexual health by nurses and physicians suggested to the women that their sexuality was not really a medical concern. This interpretation was shared with their partners, resulting in couples making efforts to adjust with little information or support. The authors concluded that health care professionals should examine their own values and beliefs about sexuality and assess their knowledge and comfort level about these topics.

Commentary and Response
Downe-Wamboldt (1998) praised Butler and her colleagues for undertaking an interesting study on an important topic, and encouraged them to continue with research in this area: "The important topic of sexual health in the context of cancer care has received little attention from researchers, and this article makes a valuable contribution to the nursing literature" (p. 700).

Downe-Wamboldt did not offer any criticism of the actual study, except to note its limited generalizability, but made some suggestions about improving the report itself:

> To more meaningfully interpret the findings, it would have been helpful to have a description of the specific questions that were asked that provided the data for the study. Were there any questions that the women found too sensitive or were not comfortable to answer? The identified themes and relevant quotations generally provided a clear picture of how the themes emerged from the data. One notable exception is the theme of sexual health influenced by the environment. It is difficult to assess the validity of this theme based on the quality and quantity of quotations provided (pp. 700–701)

Alteneder (1998), who wrote a second commentary, also expressed a desire for more information than was provided in the report:

> The authors said that nurses rarely discussed sexual functioning; however, it would be of interest to the reader what the nurses did cover when they spoke on this topic .... Because 6 of the participants had no longer continued to be sexually active post-treatment, information about why they were no longer active would have added to the description of the women (p. 702).

This second commentator further suggested that the researchers could have improved the study by interviewing the women's partners; she also expressed some misgivings about the data collection:

> I have some concern about the use of the semistructured interview guide, which was reviewed for content and face validity by three oncology nurses and one physician. I feel that this type of study should be open to learn from the participants, and the restricting structure might inhibit the type of information received by the investigator (p. 702).

In their response, Butler and her colleagues (1998) provided the commentators with some of the information they were seeking (e.g., the six women's reasons for not being sexually active). They acknowledged the need for replication of the study, and also commented on data quality issues:

> The purpose statement may not have adequately reflected the depth of exploration provided by the semistructured interview guide .... The study participants did not appear to have any difficulty with questions asked during the interview and openly described how the cancer affected their well-being (p. 704).

SUMMARY POINTS

- A research **critique** is a careful, critical appraisal of the strengths and limitations of a study.
- In a comprehensive review of a research report, reviewers should consider five major dimensions of the study: the substantive and theoretical, methodologic, ethical, interpretive, and presentation and stylistic dimensions.
- In more targeted reviews, critiques focus primarily on the methodologic dimension.
- Researchers designing a study make a number of important **methodologic decisions** that affect the quality and integrity of the research. Consumers preparing a critique must evaluate the decisions the researchers made to determine how much faith can be placed in the results.

STUDY SUGGESTIONS

Chapter 26 of the accompanying *Study Guide for Nursing Research: Principles and Methods, 7th ed.*, offers various exercises and study suggestions for reinforcing the concepts presented in this chapter. Additionally, the following study questions can be addressed:

1. Read the article, "Self-care in adults with sickle-cell disease," by Jennifer Lenoci and colleagues (2002), *Western Journal of Nursing Research, 24,* 228–245. What limitations of the research methods did the authors identify? Do you agree? Do you have others to add?
2. Read an article from any issue of *Nursing Research* or any other nursing research journal and systematically assess the article according to the questions contained in this chapter. What are the merits and limitations of the report?
3. Read the article, "Narratives of family caregiving: Four story types," by Lioness Ayres (2000), *Research in Nursing & Health, 23,* 359–371. Develop some practice implications based on this research.

SUGGESTED READINGS

Methodologic References

Beck, C. T. (1993). Qualitative research: The evaluation of its credibility, fittingness, and auditability. *Western Journal of Nursing Research, 15,* 263–266.

Becker, P. H. (1993). Common pitfalls in published grounded theory research. *Qualitative Health Research, 3,* 254–260.

Cutcliffe, J. R., & McKenna, H. P. (1999). Establishing the credibility of qualitative research findings: The plot thickens. *Journal of Advanced Nursing, 30,* 374–380.

Evertz, J. (2001). Evaluating qualitative research. In P. L. Munhall (Ed.), *Nursing research: A qualitative perspective* (pp. 599–612). New York: NLN.

Gehlbach, S. H. (1992). *Interpreting the medical literature* (3rd ed.). Lexington, MA: The Collamore Press.

Giuffre, M. (1998). Critiquing a research article. *Journal of Perianesthesia Nursing, 13,* 104–108.

Horsley, J., & Crane, J. (1982). *Using research to improve nursing practice: A guide.* New York: Grune & Stratton.

Morse, J. M. (1991). Evaluating qualitative research. *Qualitative Health Research, 1,* 283–286.

Ryan-Wenger, N. M. (1992). Guidelines for critique of a research report. *Heart & Lung, 21,* 394–401.

Thorne, S. (1997). The art (and science) of critiquing qualitative research. In J. M. Morse (Ed.), *Completing a qualitative project* (pp. 117–132). Thousand Oaks, CA: Sage.

Topham, D. L., & DeSilva, P. (1988). Evaluating congruency between steps in the research process: A critique guide for use in clinical nursing practice. *Clinical Nurse Specialist, 2*, 97–102.

Wilson, H. S., & Hutchinson, S. A. (1996). Methodologic mistakes in grounded theory. *Nursing Research, 45*, 122–124.

Studies Cited in Chapter 26

Alteneder, R. A. (1998). Commentary. *Western Journal of Nursing Research, 20*, 701–703.

Butler, L., & Banfield, V. (1998). Response by Butler and Banfield, *Western Journal of Nursing Research, 20*, 703–705.

Butler, L., Banfield, V., Sveinson, T., & Allen, K. (1998). Conceptualizing sexual health in cancer care. *Western Journal of Nursing Research, 20*, 683–699.

Downe-Wamboldt, B. (1998). Commentary. *Western Journal of Nursing Research, 20*, 700–701.

Lenz, E. R., & Perkins, S. (2000). Coronary artery bypass graft surgery patients and their family member caregivers: Outcomes of a family-focused staged psychoeducational intervention, *Applied Nursing Research, 13*, 142–150.

Penrod, J. (2001). Commentary on "Family caregiving in long-term care facilities." *Clinical Nursing Research, 10*, 364–368.

Ross, M. M., Carswell, A., & Dalziel, W. B. (2001). Family caregiving in long-term care facilities. *Clinical Nursing Research, 10*, 347–363.

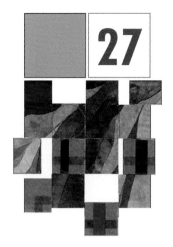

27

Utilizing Research: Putting Research Evidence Into Nursing Practice

Most nurse researchers want their findings to contribute to nursing practice, and there is growing interest among nurses in basing their practice on solid research evidence. In this chapter, we discuss various aspects of using nursing research to support an evidence-based practice (EBP).

RESEARCH UTILIZATION VERSUS EVIDENCE-BASED PRACTICE

The terms *research utilization* and *evidence-based practice* are sometimes used synonymously. Although there is overlap between the two concepts, they are, in fact, distinct. Research utilization (RU), the narrower of the two terms, is the use of the findings from a disciplined study or set of studies in a practical application that is unrelated to the original research. In projects that have had research utilization as a goal, the emphasis is on translating empirically derived knowledge into real-world applications. EBP involves making clinical decisions on the basis of the best possible evidence. Usually, the best evidence comes from rigorous research, but EBP also uses other sources of credible information.

Figure 27-1 provides a basic schema of how RU and EBP are interrelated. This section further explores and distinguishes the two concepts.

The Utilization of Nursing Research

During the 1980s and early 1990s, *research utilization* became an important buzz word, and several changes in nursing education and nursing research were prompted by the desire to develop a knowledge base for nursing practice. In education, nursing schools increasingly began to include courses on research methods so that students would become intelligent research consumers. In the research arena, there was a shift in focus toward clinical nursing problems. These changes, coupled with the completion of several large research utilization projects, played a role in sensitizing the nursing community to the desirability of using research as a basis for practice; they were not enough, however, to lead to widespread integration of research findings into the delivery of nursing care. Research utilization, as the nursing community has come to recognize, is a complex and nonlinear phenomenon that poses professional challenges.

The Research Utilization Continuum
As Figure 27-1 indicates, the start-point of research utilization is the emergence of new knowledge and new ideas. Research is conducted and, over time, knowledge on a topic accumulates. In turn, knowledge works its way into use—to varying degrees and at differing rates.

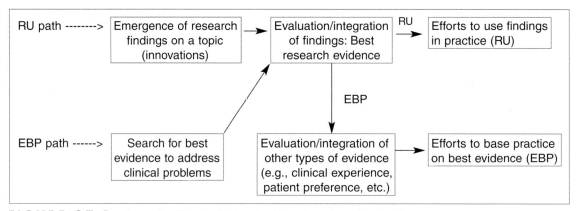

FIGURE 27.1 Research utilization (RU) and evidence-based practice (EBP).

Theorists who have studied the phenomenon of knowledge development and the diffusion of ideas typically recognize a continuum in terms of the specificity of the use to which research findings are put. At one end of the continuum are discrete, clearly identifiable attempts to base specific actions on research findings. For example, a series of studies in the 1960s and 1970s demonstrated that the optimal placement time of a glass thermometer for accurate oral temperature determination is 9 minutes (e.g., Nichols & Verhonick, 1968). When nurses specifically altered their behavior from shorter placement times to the empirically based recommendation of 9 minutes, this constituted an instance of research utilization at this end of the continuum. This type of utilization has been referred to as **instrumental utilization** (Caplan & Rich, 1975).

Research findings can, however, be used in a more diffuse manner—in a way that promotes cumulative awareness, understanding, or enlightenment. Caplan and Rich (1975) refer to this end of the utilization continuum as **conceptual utilization**. Thus, a practicing nurse may read a qualitative research report describing *courage* among individuals with long-term health problems as a dynamic process that includes efforts fully to accept reality and to develop problem-solving skills. The nurse may be reluctant to alter his or her own behavior or suggest an intervention based on the results, but the study may make the nurse more observant in working with patients with long-term illnesses; it

may also lead to informal efforts to promote problem-solving skills. Conceptual utilization, then, refers to situations in which users are influenced in their thinking about an issue based on their knowledge of studies but do not put this knowledge to any specific, documentable use.

The middle ground of this continuum involves the partial impact of research findings on nursing activities. This middle ground is frequently the result of a slow evolutionary process that does not reflect a conscious decision to use an innovative procedure but rather reflects what Weiss (1980) termed *knowledge creep* and *decision accretion*. **Knowledge creep** refers to an evolving "percolation" of research ideas and findings. **Decision accretion** refers to the manner in which momentum for a decision builds over time based on accumulated information gained through readings, informal discussions, meetings, and so on. Increasingly, however, nurses *are* making conscious decisions to use research in their clinical practice, and the EBP movement has contributed to this change.

Estabrooks (1999) recently studied research utilization by collecting survey data from 600 nurses in Canada. She found evidence to support three distinct types of research utilization: (1) **indirect research utilization**, involving changes in nurses' thinking and therefore analogous to conceptual utilization; (2) **direct research utilization**, involving the direct use of findings in giving patient care and therefore analogous to instrumental utilization; and (3)

persuasive utilization, involving the use of findings to persuade others (typically those in decision making positions) to make changes in policies or practices relevant to nursing care.

These varying ways of thinking about research utilization clearly suggest that both qualitative and quantitative research can play key roles in guiding and improving nursing practice. Indeed, Estabrooks (2001) argues that the process of implementing research findings into practice is essentially the same for both quantitative and qualitative research. What differentiates qualitative research, however, is its form. Because qualitative findings are presented in narrative form, Estabrooks claims that this type of research may have a privileged position in research utilization. Clinicians do not need a strong background in statistics to understand qualitative research, and thus one less step is required of readers of qualitative research. It is not necessary to translate the results into everyday language before the findings can be used conceptually.

The Research Utilization Process: Rogers' Diffusion of Innovations Theory

Several theorists have developed models of how knowledge gets disseminated and used. The most noteworthy is one that has influenced several research utilization projects in the nursing community, Rogers' (1995) Diffusion of Innovations Theory.

Rogers postulates that knowledge diffusion is an evolutionary process by which an innovation is communicated over time to members of a social system. The key elements in this process, all of which influence the rate and extent of innovation adoption, include the following:

1. The *innovation* is the new idea, practice, or procedure that, if adopted, will result in changes; the nature of the innovation strongly affects decisions about adoption.
2. *Communication channels* are the media through which information about the innovation is transmitted, and can include both mass media (e.g., journal articles, the Internet), or individual, face-to-face communication. Communication is most effective when there are shared beliefs, values,

and expectations on the part of the sender and receiver of information.
3. *Time* is a component of the theory in that the process of knowledge diffusion occurs over time; there are varying amounts of time that elapse between the creation of the knowledge and its dissemination, and between knowledge awareness and the decision to use or reject the innovation.
4. The *social system* is the set of interrelated units that solve problems and seek to accomplish a common goal; diffusion occurs within social systems that vary in their norms and receptivity to innovations.

Rogers characterized the innovation—adoption process as having five stages: knowledge, persuasion, decision, implementation, and confirmation. During the *knowledge stage*, individuals or groups become aware of the innovation, and during the *persuasion stage*, they form a positive attitude toward it. In the *decision stage*, a choice is made about whether to adopt or reject the innovation. The innovation is actually put into use during the *implementation stage*. Finally, the effectiveness of the innovation is evaluated during the *confirmation stage*, and decisions get made about continuation or discontinuation of the innovation.

Recent research on utilization has challenged the linear nature of the process, and Rogers himself acknowledges that stages can sometimes be skipped, but the general model has been a useful way to think about the research utilization process in nursing.

 Example of using Rogers' Diffusion of Innovations Theory:
Dooks (2001), using Rogers' model, explored possible reasons for the research—practice gap among oncology nurses relating to research on pain management.

Research Utilization in Nursing Practice
During the 1980s and 1990s, there was considerable concern that nurses had failed to use research findings as a basis for making decisions and for developing nursing interventions. This concern

was based on some studies suggesting that nurses were not always aware of research results or did not incorporate results into their practice. In one such study, Ketefian (1975) reported on the oral temperature determination practices of 87 registered nurses. The results of several studies in the late 1960s had clearly demonstrated that the optimal placement time for oral temperature determination using glass thermometers is 9 minutes. Ketefian's study was designed to learn what "happens to research findings relative to nursing practice after five or ten years of dissemination in the nursing literature" (p. 90). In Ketefian's study, only 1 of 87 nurses reported the correct placement time, suggesting that these practicing nurses were unaware of or ignored the research findings about optimal placement time. Other studies in the 1980s (e.g., Kirchhoff, 1982), were similarly discouraging.

Coyle and Sokop (1990) investigated practicing nurses' adoption of 14 nursing innovations that had been reported in the nursing research literature, replicating a study by Brett (1987). The 14 innovations were selected based on the following criteria: the scientific merit of the study, the significance of the findings for practice, and the findings' suitability for application to practice. A sample of 113 nurses practicing in 10 hospitals (randomly selected from the medium-sized hospitals in North Carolina) completed questionnaires that measured the nurses' awareness and use of the study findings. The results indicated much variation across the 14 innovations, with awareness of them ranging from 34% at one extreme to 94% at the other. Coyle and Sokop used a scheme to categorize each innovation according to its stage of adoption, based on Rogers' theory: awareness (indicating knowledge of the innovation); persuasion (indicating the nurses' belief that nurses should use the innovation in practice); occasional use in practice; and regular use in practice. Only 1 of the 14 studies was at the regular-use stage of adoption. Six studies were in the persuasion stage, indicating that the nurses knew of the innovation and thought it *should* be incorporated into nursing practice but were not

basing their own nursing decisions on it. Table 27-1 describes 4 of the 14 nursing innovations, 1 for each of the 4 stages of adoption.

More recently, Rutledge, Greene, Mooney, Nail, and Ropka (1996) studied the extent to which oncology staff nurses adopted eight research-based practices. The researchers found that awareness levels were high in their sample of over 1000 nurses, with between 53% and 96% of them reporting awareness of the eight practices. Moreover, almost 90% of aware nurses used seven of the practices at least some of the time. Similar results have been reported in a recent survey of nearly 1000 nurses in Scotland (Rodgers, 2000). The results of the recent studies are more encouraging than the studies by Ketefian and Kirchhoff because they suggest that, on average, practicing nurses are aware of many innovations based on research results, are persuaded that the innovations should be used, and are beginning to use them on occasion.

The need to reduce the gap between nursing research and nursing practice has been hotly discussed and has led to numerous formal attempts to bridge the gap. The best-known of several early nursing research utilization projects is the **Conduct and Utilization of Research in Nursing (CURN) Project**, a 5-year development project awarded to the Michigan Nurses' Association by the Division of Nursing in the 1970s. The major objective of the CURN project was to increase the use of research findings in the daily practice of registered nurses by disseminating current research findings, facilitating organizational changes needed to implement innovations, and encouraging collaborative clinical research. One CURN activity was to stimulate the conduct of research in clinical settings. The CURN project also focused on helping nurses to use research findings in their practice. The CURN project staff saw research utilization as primarily an organizational process, with the commitment of organizations that employ nurses as essential to the research utilization process (Horsley, Crane, & Bingle, 1978). The CURN project team concluded that research utilization by practicing nurses is feasible, but only if

TABLE 27.1 Extent of Adoption of Four Nursing Practices					
STAGE	**NURSING INNOVATION**	**AWARE (%)**	**PERSUADED (%)**	**USE SOMETIMES (%)**	**USE ALWAYS (%)**
Awareness	Elimination of lactose from the formulas of tube-feeding diets for adult patients minimizes diarrhea, distention, flatulence, and fullness and reduces patient rejection of feedings (Horsley, Crane, & Haller, 1981)	38	36	13	19
Persuasion	Accurate monitoring of oral temperatures can be achieved on patients receiving oxygen therapy by using an electronic thermometer placed in the sublingual pocket (Lim-Levy, 1982)	68	55	35	29
Occasional use	A formally planned and structured preoperative education program preceding elective surgery results in improved patient outcomes (King & Tarsitano, 1982)	83	81	48	23
Regular use	A closed sterile system of urinary drainage is effective in maintaining the sterility of urine in patients who are catheterized for less than 2 weeks; continuity of the closed drainage system should be maintained during irrigations, sampling procedures, and patient transport (Horsley, Crane, Haller, & Bingle, 1981)	94	91	84	6

Based on findings reported in Coyle, L. A., & Sokop, A. G. (1990). Innovation adoption behavior among nurses. *Nursing Research, 39,* 176–180. The sample consisted of 113 practicing nurses.

the research is relevant to practice and if the results are broadly disseminated.

During the 1980s and 1990s, utilization projects were undertaken by a growing number of hospitals and organizations, and descriptions of these projects began to appear regularly in the nursing research literature. These projects were generally institutional attempts to implement a change in nursing practice on the basis of research findings, and to evaluate the effects of the innovation. However,

during the 1990s, the call for research utilization began to be superceded by the push for EBP.

Evidence-Based Practice

The research utilization/innovation diffusion process begins with an empirically based innovation or new idea that gets scrutinized for possible adoption in practice settings. EBP, by contrast, begins with a search for information about how best to solve specific practice problems (see Fig. 27-1). Findings from rigorous research are considered the best possible source of information, but EBP also draws on other sources. A basic feature of EBP is that it deemphasizes decision making based on custom, authority opinion, or ritual. Rather, the emphasis is on identifying the best available research evidence and *integrating* it with clinical expertise, patient input, and existing resources.

The EBP movement has given rise to considerable debate, with both staunch, zealous advocates and skeptics who urge caution and a balanced approach to health care practice. Supporters argue that EBP offers a solution to sustaining high health care quality in our current cost-constrained environment. Their position is that a rational approach is needed to provide the best possible care to the most people, with the most cost-effective use of resources. Critics worry that the advantages of EBP are exaggerated and that individual clinical judgments and patient inputs are being devalued. Although there is a need for close scrutiny of how the EBP journey unfolds, it seems likely that the EBP path is the one that health care professions will follow in the early 21st century.

Overview of the Evidence-Based Practice Movement

One of the cornerstones of the EBP movement is the Cochrane Collaboration, which was founded in the United Kingdom based on the work of British epidemiologist Archie Cochrane. Cochrane published an influential book in the early 1970s that drew attention to the dearth of solid evidence about the effects of health care. He called for efforts to make research summaries (specifically, summaries of the results of clinical trials) available to health care decision-makers. This eventually led to the development of the Cochrane Center in Oxford in 1992, and an international collaboration called the Cochrane Collaboration, with centers now established in 15 locations throughout the world. The aim of the collaboration is to help people make good decisions about health care by preparing, maintaining, and disseminating systematic reviews of the effects of health care interventions. (For further information, see www.cochrane.org.)

At about the same time that the Cochrane Collaboration got under way, a group from McMaster Medical School in Canada developed a clinical learning strategy they called *evidence-based medicine*. Dr. David Sackett, a pioneer of evidence-based medicine at McMaster (who subsequently moved to Oxford, England to promote EBP), defined evidence-based medicine as "the conscientious, explicit, and judicious use of current best evidence in making decisions about the care of individual patients. The practice of evidence-based medicine means integrating individual clinical expertise with the best available external evidence from systematic research" (Sackett et al., 1996, p. 71). The evidence-based medicine movement has shifted over time to a broader conception of using best evidence by all health care practitioners (not just physicians) in a multidisciplinary team. EBP has been considered a major paradigm shift for health care education and practice.

Types of Evidence and Evidence Hierarchies

There is no consensus about what constitutes usable evidence for EBP, but there is general agreement that findings from rigorous studies are paramount. There is, however, some controversy about what constitutes "rigorous" research. In the initial phases of the EBP movement, there was a definite bias toward reliance on information from randomized clinical trials (RCTs), a bias stemming in part from the fact that the initial focus (e.g., at the Cochrane Collaboration) was on evidence about interventions rather than about other aspects of health care practice. This bias, in turn, led to some resistance to EBP by nurses who felt that evidence from qualitative and non-RCT studies would be ignored. As Closs and Cheater (1999) have noted, "Some antagonism towards EBN (evidence based nursing) seems to derive from viewing it as an unwelcome extension of the positivist tradition" (p. 13).

Positions about what constitutes useful evidence have loosened, but there have nevertheless been efforts to develop **evidence hierarchies** that rank studies according to the strength of evidence they provide. Several such hierarchies have been developed, many based on the one proposed by Archie

Cochrane. Most hierarchies put meta-analyses of RCT studies at the pinnacle and other types of nonresearch evidence (e.g., clinical expertise) at the base. As one example, Stetler, Brunell, Giuliano, Morse, Prince, and Newell-Stokes (1998) developed a six-level evidence hierarchy that also assigns grades on study quality (from A to D) within each of the six levels. The levels (from strongest to weakest) are as follows:

I. Meta-analyses of controlled studies
II. Individual experimental studies
III. Quasi-experimental studies (e.g., time series, nonequivalent control group) or matched case–control studies
IV. Nonexperimental studies (e.g., correlational, descriptive, qualitative studies)
V. Program evaluations, research utilization studies, quality improvement projects, case reports
VI. Opinions of respected authorities and of expert committees

To date, there have been relatively few published studies of RCTs (level II) in nursing, and even fewer published meta-analyses of RCT nursing studies (see, for example, Cullum, 1997). Therefore, evidence from other types of research will play an important role in evidence-based nursing practice. Moreover, the evidence hierarchies are sensibly applied only to certain types of questions, such as questions about the effectiveness of interventions. Many other clinical questions of importance to nurses can best be answered with rich descriptive and qualitative data from level IV and V studies.

Another issue is that there continue to be clinical practice questions for which there are relatively few research data. In such situations, an EBP will have to draw on other sources. Goode (2000) described an EBP model developed at the University of Colorado Hospital that includes nine nonresearch sources of evidence that can be used to supplement the core (i.e., findings from disciplined research). These nine alternative sources include the following: bench-marking data (e.g., national rates for cesarean deliveries); cost-effectiveness analyses; pathophysiologic data; retrospective or concurrent chart review; quality improvement and risk data; international, national, and local standards; institutional data collected for infection control purposes; patient preferences; and clinical expertise.

Thus, although EBP encompasses research utilization, both research and nonresearch sources of information play a role in EBP. Nurses and other health care professionals must be able to locate evidence, evaluate it, and integrate it with clinical judgment and patient preferences to determine the most clinically effective solutions to health problems. Note that an important feature of EBP is that it does not necessarily imply practice changes: The best evidence may confirm that existing practices are effective and cost-effective.

BARRIERS TO USING RESEARCH IN NURSING PRACTICE

The next section of this chapter describes approaches to undertaking a research utilization or EBP project. First, however, we review some of the barriers to research utilization and research-based EBP in nursing because it is useful to take these barriers into account in the planning and implementation of efforts to integrate research into practice. Several studies that have explored nurses' perceptions of barriers to research utilization have yielded remarkably similar results about constraints clinical nurses face (Funk, Tornquist, & Champagne, 1995).

Research-Related Barriers

For many nursing problems, the state of the art of research knowledge is fairly primitive. Results reported in the literature may not merit translation into practice if methodologic flaws are extensive. Thus, one impediment to using research in practice is that, for many nursing problems, a solid base of valid and trustworthy study results has not been developed.

As we have repeatedly stressed, most studies have flaws, and so if nurses were to wait for "perfect" studies before basing clinical decisions on research findings, they would have a very long wait indeed. It is precisely because of the limits of research methods that replication is essential. When repeated efforts to address a research question in different settings yield similar results, then there can be greater confidence in the findings. Single studies rarely provide an adequate basis for making changes in nursing practice. Therefore, another constraint to using research evidence is the dearth of published replications.

Finally, research is often reported in a way that makes findings inaccessible to practitioners. Complex statistical information and dense research jargon pose barriers to knowledge diffusion to most practicing nurses.

TIP: Given these issues, some tips for researchers interested in promoting the use of research findings in clinical practice are as follows:

- *Collaborate with clinicians.* Practicing nurses will be more willing to use research findings if researchers address pressing clinical questions.
- *Do high-quality research.* The quality of nursing studies has improved dramatically in the past two decades, but progress remains to be made to ensure valid and transferable findings.
- *Replicate.* Use of research results can rarely be justified based on a single study, so researchers must make a real commitment to replicating studies and publishing the results.
- *Communicate clearly.* A general aim should be to write research reports that are user-friendly, with a minimum of research jargon.
- *Present findings amenable to meta-analysis.* Integrative reviews of research findings are essential to EBP, and such reviews are increasingly using statistical methods of integration. Beck (1999) offers useful advice to researchers (and journal editors) about how to report results in a manner that facilitates meta-analysis.
- *Suggest clinical implications.* If an implications section with suggestions for clinical practice became a standard feature of research reports, then the burden of using research evidence would be lighter for nurse clinicians.
- *Disseminate aggressively.* If researchers fail to communicate the results of a study to other nurses, it is obvious that the results will never be used by practicing nurses.
- *Disseminate broadly.* It is especially important from a utilization standpoint for researchers to report their results in specialty journals, which are more likely to be read by practicing nurses than the nursing research journals. Researchers should also take steps to disseminate study findings at conferences, colloquia, and workshops attended by nurse clinicians.
- *Prepare integrative research reviews.* There is an urgent need for high-quality integrative reviews of research. Such reviews can play an invaluable role for practicing nurses, who usually do not have the time to do extensive literature reviews and who may have some difficulty in critically evaluating individual studies. Integrative reviews are a core feature of the EBP process.

Nurse-Related Barriers

Studies have found that many clinical nurses have characteristics that constrain the use of research evidence in practice. One issue concerns nurses' educational preparation and their research skills. Many have not received any formal instruction in research, and may lack the skills to judge the merits of a study. Courses on research methodology are now typically offered in baccalaureate nursing programs, but the ability to critique a research report is not necessarily sufficient for effectively incorporating research results into daily decision making.

Nurses' attitudes toward research and their motivation to engage in EBP have repeatedly been identified as potential barriers. Studies have found that the more positive the attitude, the more likely is the nurse to use research in practice. Some nurses see research utilization as little more than a "necessary evil" (Thompson, 2001), but there has been a trend toward more positive attitudes.

Another characteristic is one that is common to most humans: People are often resistant to change. Change requires effort, retraining, and restructuring of work habits. Change may also be perceived as threatening (e.g., changes may be perceived as affecting job security). Thus, there is likely to be some opposition to introducing innovations in the practice setting. However, there is evidence from a survey of more than 1200 nurses that nurses value nursing research and want to be involved in research-related activities (Rizzuto, Bostrom, Suter, & Chenitz, 1994).

 TIP: Every nurse can play a role in using research evidence. Here are some strategies:

- *Read widely and critically.* Professionally accountable nurses keep abreast of important developments and should read journals relating to their specialty, including research reports in them.
- *Attend professional conferences.* Many nursing conferences include presentations of studies that have clinical relevance. Conference attendees get opportunities to meet researchers and to explore practice implications.
- *Learn to expect evidence that a procedure is effective.* Every time nurses or nursing students are told about a standard nursing procedure, they have a right to ask the question: Why? Nurses need to develop expectations that the decisions they make in their clinical practice are based on sound rationales.
- *Become involved in a journal club.* Many organizations that employ nurses sponsor journal clubs that meet to review research articles that have potential relevance to practice.
- *Pursue and participate in RU/EBP projects.* Sometimes ideas for RU or EBP projects come from staff nurses (e.g., ideas may emerge within a journal club). Several studies have found that nurses who are involved in research-related activities (e.g., a utilization project or data collection activities) develop more positive attitudes toward research and better research skills.

Organizational Barriers

Many of the major impediments to using research in practice stem from the organizations that train and employ nurses. Organizations, perhaps to an even greater degree than individuals, resist change,

unless there is a strong organizational perception that there is something fundamentally wrong with the status quo. To challenge tradition and accepted practices, a spirit of intellectual curiosity and openness must prevail.

In many practice settings, administrators have established procedures to reward competence in nursing practice; however, few practice settings have established a system to reward nurses for critiquing nursing studies, for using research in practice, or for discussing research findings with clients. Thus, organizations have failed to motivate or reward nurses to seek ways to implement appropriate findings in their practice. Research review and use are often considered appropriate activities only when time is available, but available time is usually limited. In several studies of barriers to RU, one of the greatest reported barriers was "insufficient time on the job to implement new ideas."

Organizations also may be reluctant to expend resources for RU/EBP activities or for changing organizational policy. Resources may be required for the use of outside consultants, staff release time, library materials and Internet access, evaluating the effects of an innovation, and so on. With the push toward cost containment in health care settings, resource constraints may therefore pose a barrier to change—unless the project has cost containment as an explicit goal.

EBP will become part of organizational norms only if there is a commitment on the part of managers and administrators. Strong leadership in health care organizations is essential to making EBP happen.

 TIP: To promote the use of research evidence, administrators can adopt the following strategies:

- *Foster a climate of intellectual curiosity.* Open communication is important in persuading staff nurses that their experiences and problems are important and that the administration is willing to consider innovative solutions.
- *Offer emotional or moral support.* Administrators need to make their support visible by informing

staff and prospective staff of such support, by establishing RU or EBP committees, by helping to develop journal clubs, and by serving as role models for staff nurses.

- *Offer financial or resource support for utilization.* RU and EBP projects typically require some resources. If the administration expects nurses to engage in such activities on their own time and at their own expense, the message is that EBP is unimportant to those managing the organization.
- *Reward efforts for using research.* Administrators use various criteria to evaluate nursing performance. Research utilization should not be a primary criterion for evaluating nurses' performance, but its inclusion as one of several important criteria is likely to affect their behavior.
- *Seek opportunities for institutional RU or EBP projects.* Organizational efforts and commitment are essential for the type of RU/EBP projects we discuss in the next section.

Barriers Related to the Nursing Profession

Some impediments that contribute to the gap between research and practice are more global than those discussed previously and can be described as reflecting the state of the nursing profession or, even more broadly, the state of Western society.

It has sometimes been difficult to encourage clinicians and researchers to interact and collaborate. They are usually in different settings, have many different professional concerns, interact with different networks of nurses, and operate according to different philosophical systems. Relatively few systematic attempts have been made to form collaborative arrangements, and to date, even fewer of these arrangements have been formalized as permanent entities.

Phillips (1986) also noted two other noteworthy barriers to bridging the research—practice gap. One is the shortage of appropriate role models— nurses who can be emulated for their success in using or promoting the use of research in clinical practice. The other barrier is the historical "bag-

gage" that has defined nursing in such a way that practicing nurses may not typically perceive themselves as independent professionals capable of recommending changes based on research results. If practicing nurses believe that their role is to await direction from the medical community, and if they believe they have no power to be self-directed, then they will have difficulty in initiating innovations based on research findings. In the previously mentioned national survey, the barrier perceived by the largest percentage of nurses was the nurse's feeling that he or she did not have "enough authority to change patient care procedures" (Funk, Champagne, Wiese, & Tornquist, 1991). Fortunately, much progress has been made in our society and in the profession with regard to these two barriers. In particular, several professional nursing organizations have taken a strong stance to promote the use of research in practice.

Finally, some of the burden for changes in the profession must rest with nursing educators. As Funk and colleagues (1995) note, "The valuing of nursing research as the *sine qua non* on which practice is based must be conveyed throughout baccalaureate, associate degree, and diploma programs. This is not teaching of the conduct of research, but rather the valuing it as a way of knowing and as the foundation on which practice is based" (p. 400).

TIP: Educators could help to promote the use of research evidence through the following strategies:

- *Incorporate research findings into the curriculum.* Research findings should be integrated throughout the curriculum and, when possible, the efficacy of specific procedures should be documented by referring to relevant studies. When there is no relevant research, instructors should note the absence of empirical evidence supporting the technique.
- *Encourage research and research use.* Either by acting as role models to students (e.g., by discussing their own research) or by demonstrating positive attitudes toward research and its use in nursing, instructors can foster a spirit of

inquiry that is a precondition to effective research use.

• *Place demands on researchers.* Faculty reviewers of research proposals should demand that researchers demonstrate the proposed study's potential for clinical use; they can also demand that the researchers include a specific plan for dissemination or utilization.

THE PROCESS OF USING RESEARCH IN NURSING PRACTICE

In the years ahead, many of you are likely to be engaged in individual and institutional efforts to use research as a basis for clinical decisions. This section describes how that might be accomplished. We begin with an overview of two RU/EBP models developed by nurses.

Models for Evidence-Based Nursing Practice

During the 1980s and 1990s, a number of different models of research utilization were developed. These models offered guidelines for designing and implementing a utilization project in a practice setting. The most prominent of these models were the previously mentioned Diffusion of Innovations Theory, the Stetler model, and the Iowa model. The latter two models have been updated to incorporate EBP processes, rather than research utilization processes alone.

The Stetler Model

The **Stetler Model** of Research Utilization (Stetler, 1994) was designed with the assumption that research utilization could be undertaken not only by organizations, but by individual clinicians and managers. It was a model designed to promote and facilitate critical thinking about the application of research findings in practice. The updated and refined model is based on many of the same assumptions and strategies as the original, but provides "an enhanced approach to the overall application of research in the service setting" (Stetler, 2001,

p. 273). The current model, presented graphically in Figure 27-2, involves five sequential phases:

I. Preparation. In this phase, nurses define the underlying purpose and outcomes of the project; search, sort, and select sources of research evidence; consider external factors that can influence potential application and internal factors that can diminish objectivity; and affirm the priority of the perceived problem.

II. Validation. This phase involves a utilization-focused critique of each source of evidence, focusing in particular on whether it is sufficiently sound for *potential* application in practice. (The process stops at this point if the evidence sources are rejected.)

III. Comparative Evaluation and Decision-Making. This phase involves a synthesis of findings and the application of four criteria that, taken together, are used to determine the desirability and feasibility of applying findings from validated sources to nursing practice. These criteria (fit of setting, feasibility, current practice, and substantiating evidence) are summarized in Box 27-1. The end result of the comparative evaluation is to make a decision about using the study findings. If the decision is a rejection, no further steps are necessary.

IV. Translation/Application. This phase involves activities to (1) confirm how the findings will be used (e.g., formally or informally), and (2) spell out the operational details of the application, and implement them. The latter might involve the development of a guideline, detailed procedure, or plan of action, possibly including plans for formal organizational change.

V. Evaluation. In the final phase, the application is evaluated. Informal use of the innovation versus formal use would lead to different evaluative strategies.

Although the Stetler model originally was designed as a tool for individual practitioners, it has also been the basis of formal research utilization and EBP projects by groups of nurses.

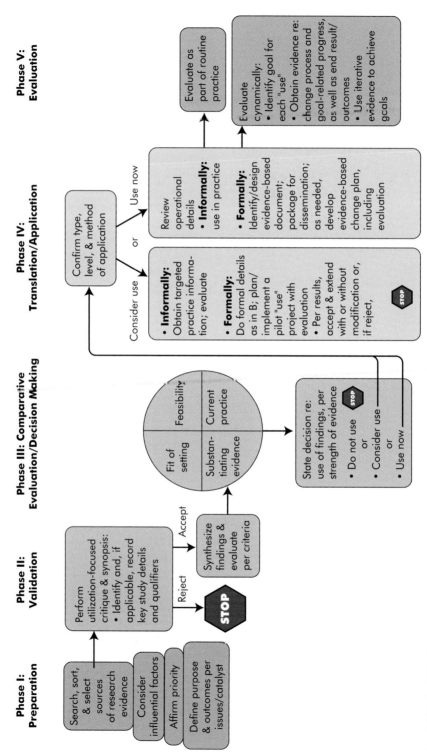

FIGURE 27.2 Stetler Model of Research Utilization to facilitate evidence-based practice. (Adapted from Stetler, C. B. (1994). Refinement of the Stetler/Marram model for application of research findings into practice. *Nursing Outlook, 42,* 15–25.)

BOX 27.1 Criteria for Comparative Evaluation Phase of Stetler's Model

1. FIT OF SETTING

Similarity of characteristics of sample to your client population
Similarity of study's environment to the one in which you work

2. FEASIBILITY

Potential risks of implementation to patients, staff, and the organization
Readiness for change among those who would be involved in a change in practice
Resource requirements and availability

3. CURRENT PRACTICE

Congruency of the study with your theoretical basis for current practice behavior

4. SUBSTANTIATING EVIDENCE

Availability of confirming evidence from other studies
Availability of confirming evidence from a meta-analysis or integrative review

Adapted from Stetler, C. B. (1994). Refinement of the Stetler/Marram model for application of research findings into practice. *Nursing Outlook, 42,* 15–25.

 Example of an application of the Stetler model:

Stetler, Corrigan, Sander-Buscemi, and Burns (1999) applied the Stetler model in a fall prevention project that was also designed to enhance evidence-based thinking.

The Iowa Model

Efforts to use research evidence to improve nursing practice are often addressed by groups of nurses interested in the same practice issue. Formal RU/EBP projects typically have followed systematic procedures using one of several models that have been developed, such as the Iowa Model of Research in Practice (Titler et al., 1994). This model, like the Stetler model, was revised recently, and renamed the **Iowa Model of Evidence-Based Practice to Promote Quality Care** (Titler et al., 2001). The current version of the Iowa model, shown in Figure 27-3, acknowledges that a formal RU/EBP project begins with a *trigger*—an impetus to explore possible changes to practice. The start-point can be either (1) a **knowledge-focused trigger** that emerges from awareness of innovative research findings (and thus follows a more traditional RU path, as in the top panel of Fig. 27-1); or (2) a **problem-focused trigger** that has its roots in a clinical or organizational problem (and thus follows a path that more closely resembles an EBP path). The model outlines a series of activities with three critical decision points:

1. Deciding whether the problem is a sufficient priority for the organization exploring possible changes; if yes, a team is formed to proceed with the project; if no, a new trigger would be sought;
2. Deciding whether there is a sufficient research base; if yes, the innovation is piloted in the practice setting; if no, the team would either search for other sources of evidence or conduct its own research; and

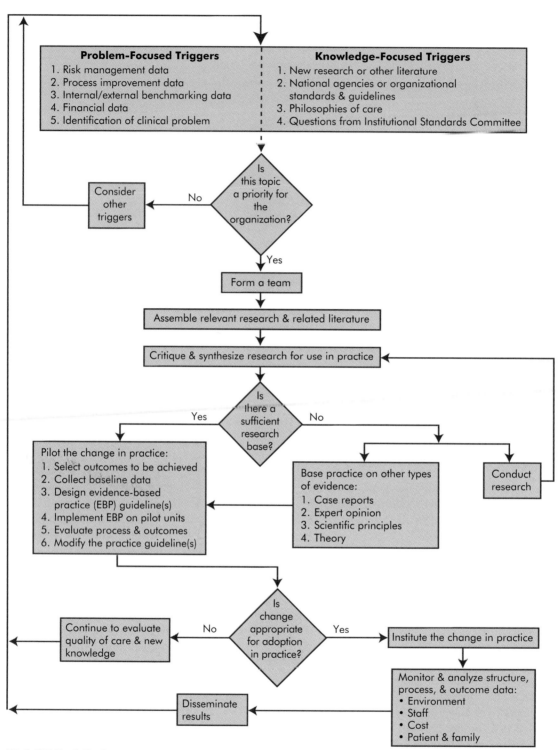

FIGURE 27.3 Iowa Model of Evidence-Based Practice to Promote Quality Care (Adapted from Titler, et al. (2001). The Iowa Model of Evidence-Based Practice to Promote Quality Care. *Critical Care Nursing Clinics of North America, 13,* 497–509.)

3. Deciding whether the change is appropriate for adoption in practice; if yes, a change would be instituted and monitored; if no, the team would continue to evaluate quality of care and search for new knowledge.

Example of an application of the Iowa model:

Montgomery, Hanrahan, Kottman, Otto, Barrett, and Hermiston (1999) used the Iowa model to develop a guideline for intravenous infiltration in pediatric patients.

Steps in Using Research in Nursing Practice

Using research to improve nursing practice involves a series of activities and decisions. The Stetler and Iowa models (as well as other models, such as the one proposed by Rosswurm and Larrabee [1999] and Soukup [2000]) are used as a basis for discussing major activities to support EBP.

Selecting a Topic or Problem

The Iowa model as well as the Center for Advanced Nursing Practice's model (Soukup, 2000) acknowledge that there are two types of stimulus for an EBP or RU endeavor—identification of a clinical practice problem in need of solution, or readings in the research literature. Problem-focused triggers may arise in the normal course of clinical practice or in the context of quality-assessment or quality-improvement efforts. This problem identification approach is likely to have staff support if the selected problem is one that numerous nurses have encountered, and is likely to have considerable clinical relevance because a specific clinical situation generated interest in the problem in the first place.

Gennaro (2001) advises nurses following this approach to begin by clarifying the practice problem that needs to be solved and framing it as a question. The goal can be finding the best way to anticipate a problem (how to *diagnose* it) or how best to solve a problem (how to *intervene*). Clinical practice questions may well take the form of "What is the best way to . . .?"—for example, "What is the

best way to encourage women to do breast self-examinations regularly?" Granger (2001) presents some useful suggestions about how to capture clinical questions.

TIP: Several websites may be helpful in framing a clinical practice question for EBP. For example, the University of Alberta offers an "Evidence-Based Medicine Tool Kit" that provides such assistance (www.med.ualberta.ca/ebm/ebm.htm). Another resource for framing an EBP question is the Health Web's website relating to evidence-based health care (www.uic.edu/depts/lib/ health/hw/ebhc).

A second catalyst for a utilization or EBP project begins with the research literature (i.e., the knowledge-focused trigger of the Iowa model). This approach could occur if, for example, a project emerged as a result of discussions in a journal club. In this approach, a preliminary assessment would need to be made of the clinical relevance of the research. The central issue here is whether a problem of significance to nurses will be solved by making some change or introducing a new intervention. Five questions relating to clinical relevance (shown in Box 27-2) can be applied to a research report or set of related reports. If the answer is "yes" to any of these questions, the process can move forward, but if it is determined that the research base is not clinically relevant, it would be necessary to start over.

With both types of triggers, it is important to ensure that there is a general consensus about the importance of the problem and the need for improving practice. Titler and colleagues (2001) include as the first decision point in their revised Iowa model the determination of whether the topic is a priority for the organization considering practice changes. They advise that the following issues be taken into account when finalizing a topic for EBP: the topic's fit with the organization's strategic plan; the magnitude of the problem; the number of people invested in the problem; support of nurse leaders and of those in other disciplines; costs; and possible barriers to change. Rosenfeld and colleagues (2000) present a model for examining and prioritizing practice problems as perceived by staff nurses.

BOX 27.2 Criteria for Evaluating the Clinical Relevance of a Body of Research

1. Does the research have the potential to help solve a problem that is currently being faced by practitioners?
2. Does the research have the potential to help with clinical decision making with respect to (a) making appropriate observations, (b) identifying client risks or complications, or (c) selecting an appropriate Intervention?
3. Are clinically relevant theoretical propositions tested by the research?
4. If the research involves an intervention, does the intervention have potential for implementation in clinical practice? Do nurses have control over the implementation of such interventions?
5. Can the measures used in the study be used in clinical practice?

Adapted from Tanner, C. A. (1987). Evaluating research for use in practice: Guidelines for the clinician. *Heart & Lung,* 16, 424–430.

TIP: The method of selecting a topic does not appear to have any bearing on the success of an RU/EBP project. What *is* important, however, is that the nursing staff who will implement an innovation are involved in topic selection and that key stakeholders are "on board."

Assembling and Evaluating Evidence

Once a clinical practice question has been selected and a team has been formed to work on the project, the next step is to search for and assemble research evidence (and other relevant evidence) on the topic. Chapter 5 provided information about locating research information, but some additional issues are relevant.

In doing a literature review as background for a new study, the central goal is to discover where the gaps are and how best to advance knowledge. For EBP or RU projects, which typically have as end products prescriptive practice protocols or guidelines, literature reviews are typically much more formalized. The emphasis is on amassing comprehensive information on the topic, weighing pieces of evidence, and integrating information to draw conclusions about the state of knowledge. Commentators have noted that **integrative reviews** have become a cornerstone of EBP (e.g., Jennings, 2000; Stevens, 2001).

High-quality integrative reviews represent a critical tool for EBP, and if the assembled RU/EBP team has the skills to complete one, this is clearly advantageous. It is, however, unlikely that every clinical organization will be able to marshal the skills needed to accomplish a high-quality critical review of the research literature on the chosen topic. Moreover, as Funk and her co-authors (1995) have noted, cost-efficiencies make this impractical: "With the shrinking health care dollar, we can no longer afford to have nurses in practice settings throughout the nation duplicating the work of searching for the most up-to-date literature, evaluating it, synthesizing it, and drawing practice conclusions" (p. 403).

Fortunately, many researchers and organizations have taken on the responsibility of preparing integrative reviews and making them available for EBP in professional journals and on the Internet. The previously mentioned Cochrane reviews are an especially important resource. These reports describe the background and objectives of the review, the methods used to search for, select, and evaluate studies, the main results, and the reviewers' conclusions. Cochrane reviews have been found to be more rigorous than those published in journals (Jadad et al., 1998), and have the advantage of being checked and updated regularly.

Example of Cochrane review conclusions: One Cochrane review that examined interventions for promoting smoking cessation during pregnancy came to the following conclusions: "Smoking cessation programs in pregnancy appear to reduce smoking, low birthweight and preterm birth, but no effect was detected for very low birthweight or perinatal mortality."

Another critical resource for those wishing to use available integrative reviews is the Agency for Healthcare Research and Quality (AHRQ). This agency awarded 12 5-year contracts in 1997 to establish Evidence-Based Practice Centers at institutions in the United States and Canada (e.g., at Johns Hopkins University, McMaster University); new 5-year contracts were awarded in 2002. Each center issues **evidence reports** that are based on rigorous integrative reviews of relevant scientific literature; dozens of these reports are now available to help "improve the quality, effectiveness, and appropriateness of clinical care" (AHRQ website, January, 2003, www.ahrq.gov).

Example of evidence reports from AHRQ EBP Centers: The titles of two evidence reports prepared by EBP Centers in 2001 are: *Preventing adolescent criminal and other health-risking behavior* and *Quality of life: Management of cancer-associated pain and related symptoms*.

Many other resources are available for locating integrative reviews. One particularly useful website at the University of Sheffield in the United Kingdom is referred to as "Netting the Web" (www.shef.ac.uk/uni/academic/R-Z/scharr/ir/netting.html). This site offers a comprehensive listing of other websites devoted to providing evidence for practice. Another useful website, also based in the United Kingdom, is the University of York's Centre for Evidence-Based Nursing (www.york.ac.uk/depts/hstd/centres/evidence/cebn.htm).

If an integrative review has been prepared by experts, it is possible that a formal evidence-based clinical guideline has been developed and can be used directly in an RU/EBP project. AHRQ, for example, has developed such guidelines on pain management, continence, and other problems of relevance to nurses. AHRQ no longer develops guidelines but helps to support the National Guideline Clearinghouse (www.guidelines.gov), which provides a comprehensive database of such guidelines. Nursing organizations (e.g., the Association of Women's Health, Obstetrics, and Neonatal Nurses [AWHONN]) have also developed clinical practice guidelines on several topics.

Of course, there are many clinical practice questions for which integrative reviews and clinical guidelines are not available. This may mean that an integrative review or synthesis of the research literature relating to the selected clinical question will need to be prepared. Some guidance on doing integrative reviews is provided later in this chapter.

TIP: If an integrative review already exists, it is wise to make sure that it is as up to date as possible and that new findings published after the review are taken into account. Moreover, even a published integrative review needs to be critiqued and the validity of its conclusions assessed. Stetler, Morsi, and colleagues (1998) offer a form for evaluating integrative reviews, and further advice is provided in a subsequent section of this chapter.

The review, evaluation, and synthesis of research evidence ideally would allow the RU/EBP team to draw conclusions about the sufficiency of the research base for guiding clinical practice. Adequacy of research evidence depends on such factors as the consistency of findings across studies, the quality and rigor of the studies, the strength of any observed effect, the transferability of the findings to clinical settings, and cost-effectiveness.

Coming to conclusions about the body of evidence can result in several possible outcomes and thus lead to different decisions for further action. First, if the research base is weak—or if there is a strong base with ambiguous conclusions—the team could opt to pursue one of three courses. The first is to go back to the beginning to pursue a new topic. A second option (preferable in the EBP environment) is to assemble other types of nonresearch evidence (e.g., through consultation with experts, surveys of clients, and so on) and assess whether that evidence suggests a practice change. Finally, another possibility is to pursue an original clinical study directly to address the practice question, thereby gathering new evidence and contributing to the base of practice knowledge. This last course of action may well be impractical for many, and would clearly result in years of delay before any further conclusions could be drawn.

If, on the other hand, there is a solid research base, the evidence could point in different directions. One possibility is that the evidence would support existing practices (which might lead to an analysis of why the clinical practice question emerged and what might make existing practices work more effectively). Another possibility is that there would be clearcut and compelling evidence that a clinical change is warranted, which would lead to the next set of activities.

Assessing Implementation Potential

Some models of RU/EBP move directly from the conclusion that evidence supports a change in practice to the pilot testing of the innovation. Others include steps first to evaluate the appropriateness of innovation within the specific organizational context; in some cases, such an assessment (or aspects of it) may be warranted even before embarking on efforts to assemble best evidence. Other models suggest evaluating issues of fit *after* the practice change has been implemented. We think a preliminary assessment of the implementation potential of an innovation is often sensible, although there may be situations with little need for such a formal assessment.

In determining the implementation potential of an innovation in a particular setting, several issues should be considered, particularly the transferability of the innovation, the feasibility of implementing it, and its cost–benefit ratio. Box 27-3 presents some relevant assessment questions for these three issues.

- *Transferability*. The main issue with regard to transferability is whether it makes good sense to implement an innovation in the new practice

setting. If there is some aspect of the practice setting that is fundamentally incongruent with the innovation—in terms of its philosophy, types of client served, personnel, or financial or administrative structure—then it might make little sense to try to adopt the innovation, even if it has been shown to be clinically effective in other contexts. One possibility, however, is that some organizational changes could be made to make the "fit" better.

- *Feasibility*. The feasibility questions in Box 27-3 address various practical concerns about the availability of staff and resources, the organizational climate, the need for and availability of external assistance, and the potential for clinical evaluation. An important issue here is whether nurses will have (or share) control over the innovation. When nurses do not have full control over the new procedure, it is important to recognize the interdependent nature of the project and to proceed as early as possible to establish the necessary cooperative arrangements.

- *Cost benefit ratio*. A critical part of any decision to proceed with an RU/EBP project is a careful assessment of the costs and benefits of the innovation. The cost–benefit assessment should encompass likely costs and benefits to various groups, including clients, staff, and the overall organization. Clearly, the most important factor is the client. If the degree of risk in introducing a new procedure is high, then the potential benefits must be great and the knowledge base must be extremely sound. A cost–benefit assessment should consider the opposite side of the coin as well: the costs and benefits of *not* instituting an innovation. It is sometimes easy to forget that the status quo bears its own risks and that failure to change—especially when such change is based on a firm knowledge base—is costly to clients, to organizations, and to the entire nursing community.

If the implementation assessment suggests that there might be problems in testing the innovation in that particular practice setting, then the team can either identify a new problem and begin the process

BOX 27.3 Criteria for Evaluating the Implementation Potential of an Innovation Under Scrutiny

TRANSFERABILITY OF THE FINDINGS

1. Will the innovation "fit" in the proposed setting?
2. How similar are the target population in the research and that in the new setting?
3. Is the philosophy of care underlying the innovation fundamentally different from the philosophy prevailing in the practice setting? How entrenched is the prevailing philosophy?
4. Is there a sufficiently large number of clients in the practice setting who could benefit from the innovation?
5. Will the innovation take too long to implement and evaluate?

FEASIBILITY

1. Will nurses have the freedom to carry out the innovation? Will they have the freedom to terminate the innovation if it is considered undesirable?
2. Will the implementation of the innovation interfere inordinately with current staff functions?
3. Does the administration support the innovation? Is the organizational climate conducive to research utilization?
4. Is there a fair degree of consensus among the staff and among the administrators that the innovation could be beneficial and should be tested? Are there major pockets of resistance or uncooperativeness that could undermine efforts to implement and evaluate the innovation?
5. To what extent will the implementation of the innovation cause friction within the organization? Does the utilization project have the support and cooperation of departments outside the nursing department?
6. Are the skills needed to carry out the utilization project (both the implementation and the clinical evaluation) available in the nursing staff? If not, how difficult will it be to collaborate with or to secure the assistance of others with the necessary skills?
7. Does the organization have the equipment and facilities necessary for the innovation? If not, is there a way to obtain the needed resources?
8. If nursing staff need to be released from other practice activities to learn about and implement the innovation, what is the likelihood that this will happen?
9. Are appropriate measuring tools available for a clinical evaluation of the innovation?

COST/BENEFIT RATIO OF THE INNOVATION

1. What are the risks to which clients would be exposed during the implementation of the innovation?
2. What are the potential benefits that could result from the implementation of the innovation?
3. What are the risks of maintaining current practices (i.e., the risks of *not* trying the innovation)?
4. What are the material costs of implementing the innovation? What are the costs in the short term during utilization, and what are the costs in the long run, if the change is to be institutionalized?
5. What are the material costs of *not* implementing the innovation (i.e., could the new procedure result in some efficiencies that could lower the cost of providing service)?
6. What are the potential nonmaterial costs of implementing the innovation to the organization (e.g., lower staff morale, staff turnover, absenteeism)?
7. What are the potential nonmaterial benefits of implementing the innovation (e.g., improved staff morale, improved staff recruitment)?

anew or consider adopting a plan to improve the implementation potential (e.g., seeking external resources if costs were the inhibiting factor).

TIP: Documentation of the implementation potential of an innovation is highly recommended. Committing ideas to writing is useful because it can help to resolve ambiguities, serve as a problem-solving tool if there are barriers to implementation, and be used to persuade others of the value of the project.

Developing, Implementing, and Evaluating the Innovation

If the implementation criteria are met, the team can design and pilot the innovation. Building on the Iowa model, this phase of the project likely would involve the following activities:

1. Developing an evaluation plan (e.g., identifying outcomes to be achieved, determining how many clients to involve in the pilot, deciding when and how often to take measurements);
2. Collecting baseline data relating to those outcomes, to develop a counterfactual against which the outcomes of the innovation would be assessed;
3. Developing a written EBP guideline based on the synthesis of evidence, preferably a guideline that is clear and user-friendly, and that uses such devices as flow charts and decision trees;
4. Training relevant staff in the use of the new guideline and, if necessary, "marketing" the innovation to users so that it is given a fair test;
5. Trying the guideline out on one or more units or with a sample of clients; and
6. Evaluating the pilot project, in terms of both process (e.g., how was the innovation received, to what extent were the guidelines actually followed, what implementation problems were encountered?) and outcomes (in terms of client outcomes and cost-effectiveness).

A variety of research designs can be used in the evaluation, of course, with the most rigorous being an experimental design. In most cases, however, a less formal evaluation will be more practical, comparing (for example) collected outcomes data or hospital records before and after the innovation, and gathering information about patient and staff satisfaction. Qualitative and mixed-method research designs can also contribute to evaluating an innovation (Sandelowski, 1996). A qualitative perspective can uncover subtleties about the innovation process and help explain research findings. Valuable information on the feasibility and participant burdens can be obtained.

Evaluation data should be gathered over a sufficiently long period (typically 6 to 12 months) to allow for a true test of a "mature" innovation. The end result of this process is a decision about whether to adopt the innovation, to modify it for ongoing use, or to revert to prior practices.

TIP: A final optional step, but one that is highly advisable, is the dissemination of the results of the project so that other practicing nurses can benefit.

RESEARCH INTEGRATION AND SYNTHESIS

Evidence-based practice relies on meticulous integration of research evidence on a topic. If practitioners are to glean best practices from research findings, they must take into account as much of the evidence as possible, organized and synthesized in a rigorous manner. This section provides some guidance in conducting integrative research reviews and evaluating reviews prepared by others.

An integrative review is not just a literature review—it is in itself a systematic inquiry that follows many of the same rules as those described in this book for primary studies. In other words, those doing an integrative review develop research questions or hypotheses; devise a sampling plan and data collection strategy; collect the relevant data; and analyze and interpret those data.

Integrative reviews can take various forms. Until recently, the most common type of integrative review was narrative (qualitative) integration that used various nonstatistical methods to merge and synthesize research findings. More recently, meta-analytic techniques that use a common metric for combining studies statistically have been increasingly used to integrate quantitative findings. (The reviews in the Cochrane Collaboration and the AHRQ EBP centers are meta-analyses.) Among qualitative researchers, the technique of metasynthesis has been developed to integrate and compare findings from qualitative studies. Many of the steps involved in these various approaches are similar, however; key differences are noted in the discussion that follows. The following activities assume that reviewers are developing an integrative review that will be in written form and shared with others.

Getting Started on an Integrative Review

An integrative review, like a primary study, begins with a problem statement and a research question or hypothesis. Care should be taken to develop a problem statement and questions that are clearly worded and sufficiently specific; key constructs should be conceptually defined. If there is an underlying theoretical model, it should be identified and its main features described.

 Example of a question from an integrative review:
Hill-Westmoreland, Soeken, and Spellbring (2002) conducted a meta-analysis that addressed the following question: "What are the effects of fall prevention programs on the proportion of falls in the elderly? Falls were conceptually defined as coming to rest on the ground, floor, or other lower level, unintentionally" (p. 2).

Integrative reviews are sometimes done by individuals, but it is preferable to have at least two reviewers. Multiple reviewers help not only in sharing the work load, but in minimizing subjectivity. Reviewers should have both substantive and clinical knowledge of the problem, and sufficiently strong methodologic skills to evaluate study quality.

Selecting a Sample

In an integrative review, the sample consists of the primary studies that have addressed a similar

research question. Reviewers must make a number of up-front decisions regarding the sample, which should be shared in the written review so that readers can evaluate how much confidence to place in the conclusions. The omission of information on sampling procedures results in a major threat to the validity of the review (Ganong, 1987). Sampling decisions include the following:

1. What are the exclusion or inclusion criteria for the search (e.g., Will foreign language reports be excluded? Will studies completed before a certain date be excluded?)
2. Will both published and unpublished reports be assembled?
3. What databases and other retrieval mechanisms will be used to locate the sample?
4. What key words or search terms will be used to identify relevant studies?

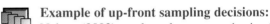 **Example of up-front sampling decisions:**
Nelson (2002) conducted a metasynthesis of qualitative studies related to mothering other-than-normal children. She explained that "I made a deliberate decision to include studies that used various qualitative methodologies and represented a wide variety of children because I was unable to locate a sufficient number of studies using the same qualitative methodology and focusing on one group of children. . . . I believed that the potential significance of synthesizing qualitative knowledge in the broad area of mothering other-than-normal children outweighed the limitations of the endeavor and was philosophically consistent with the qualitative paradigm" (p. 517).

In searching for a comprehensive sample of published and unpublished research reports, it is usually necessary to use techniques more exhaustive than simply doing a computerized literature search of a key database. Five search methods described in pathbreaking work by Cooper (1982, 1984) include the **ancestry approach** ("footnote chasing" of cited studies); the **descendancy approach** (searching forward in citation indexes for subsequent references to key studies), on-line searches (including Internet searches), informal contacts at research conferences, and the more traditional searches of bibliographic databases.

 Example of a search strategy from an integrative review:

Beck (2001), who updated an earlier meta-analysis on the predictors of postpartum depression, used all five of Cooper's search methods. She noted that, "The following on-line databases were searched for the 10-year period between 1990–2000: CINAHL, Medline, Psych Info, Eric, Popline, Social Work Abstracts, Dissertation Abstracts, and JRED. Examples of search terms included postpartum depression, postnatal depression, puerperal depression, predictors, and risk factors" (p. 276).

When a potential pool of studies has been identified, the next step is to screen them for appropriateness. Typically, many located studies are discarded because they turn out not to be relevant or do not, in fact, meet the sampling criteria. In some cases a second set of sampling criteria is used to screen out studies for methodologic rather than substantive reasons. For example, some reviewers exclude studies that did not use a true experimental design. Other reviewers assign quality ratings to all relevant studies, and then exclude studies from further analysis if the quality rating is too low (although, as we discuss later, there are alternatives for using data from low-quality studies). Yet another reason for excluding studies from the initial pool (particularly for meta-analyses) is that some provide insufficient information. All decisions relating to exclusions (normally made by at least two reviewers to ensure objectivity) should be well documented and justified.

Stetler and colleagues (1998) have noted that if the review involves an update to an existing integrative review, the earlier one should be thoroughly critiqued, using guidelines such as those provided in their article. They also recommend reading and critiquing a few of the primary studies in the initial review as a way of understanding the judgments that were made and the conclusions that were drawn.

 TIP: Full citations for the entire sample of studies should be included in the bibliography of the review. Often these are identified separately from other citations—for example, by noting them with asterisks.

Extracting and Recording Data

The next step in doing any type of integrative review is to extract relevant information about study characteristics, methodology, and findings. It is highly recommended that a written protocol or data collection form be used to record information—in numerically coded form for a meta-analysis. The goal of this task is to produce a data set, and procedures similar to those used in creating a data set with raw data from individual subjects also apply. Examples of the type of methodologic information to record include type of research design, extraneous variables controlled, length of follow-up (or timing of data collection vis-à-vis some event), sampling design, sample size, measurement information, and type of statistical analysis. Characteristics of the study participants are usually registered as well (e.g., age, gender, ethnicity, marital status, education). The data set should also include information about the data source (e.g., year of publication, type of publication, country where the study took place). If the inquiry involves multiple independent variables (e.g., multiple predictors of exercise behavior) or multiple dependent variables (e.g., different outcomes of an intervention), these also need to be recorded.

Finally, and most important, information about the results must be extracted and recorded. In a narrative review, results can be noted with a verbal summary and (or) with simple codes. Ganong (1987), for example, suggests a four-level code for the findings: positive, significant; positive, nonsignificant; negative, significant; negative, nonsignificant. In such a scheme, *positive* simply means that effects were in the hypothesized direction, and *negative* means they were in the opposite direction. In a metasynthesis, the results information to be recorded includes the key metaphors, for example, the themes, concepts, or phrases from each study. In a meta-analysis, as we subsequently discuss, the information to be recorded might include group means and standard deviations, confidence intervals, indices of relative risk, power estimates, and, most important, the effect size, that is, the index summarizing the magnitude of the relationship between the independent and dependent variables.

In narrative reviews (and sometimes in meta-analyses and metasyntheses as well), key information is often entered in summary tables that allow reviewers and readers to see at a glance the main characteristics of the knowledge base. Stetler, Morsi, and colleagues (1998) and Rosswurm and Larrabee (1999) provide templates for such tables.

 Example of a summary table in an integrative review:
Lanuza, Lefaiver, and Farcas (2000) conducted a narrative integrative review of research on quality of life among transplant candidates and recipients. Their summary table, based on a sample of 13 studies, incorporated information on the following: author, study site, study purpose, research design, sample size and characteristics, measurement instruments, and potential strengths and limitations.

Extraction and coding of information ideally should be completed by two or more people, at least for a portion of the studies in the sample. This allows for an assessment of interrater agreement, which should be sufficiently high to persuade readers of the review that the recorded information is accurate.

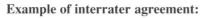 **Example of interrater agreement:**
In Beck's (2001) meta-analysis, one-fourth of the included studies (i.e., 20 of 84) were independently coded by Beck and a research assistant. Initial interrater agreement ranging from 85% to 100% was attained.

Evaluating Studies

In any integrative review, the evidence must be evaluated to determine how much confidence to place in

the findings. We have discussed the criteria for "scientific merit" throughout this book and, in Chapter 26, we presented guidelines for assessing whether the findings and conclusions of individual studies are accurate, believable, and generalizable or transferable. Strong studies clearly should be given more weight than weaker ones in coming to conclusions about "best practice" evidence.

In narrative reviews, evaluative information may be recorded as notes about key limitations and strengths of studies in the sample. For example, in the previously cited review on quality of life among lung transplant recipients, study limitations (e.g., "psychometrics of tools not addressed") and strengths (e.g., "two study sites") were noted in the summary table (Lanuza, Lefaiver, & Farcas, 2000, p. 185). For a metasynthesis, Paterson, Thorne, Canam, and Jillings (2001) have developed the Primary Research Appraisal Tool to use as a systematic means of reviewing and appraising each qualitative study.

In meta-analyses, the evaluation almost always involves a quantitative rating of each study in terms of the strength of evidence it yields. Some authors use the previously mentioned six-level graded evidence hierarchy for this purpose. Others, however, develop a formal assessment tool (or adapt one developed by others) because each review may require different criteria. For example, in Beck's (2001) study of the predictors of postpartum depression, most of the studies were in level IV of the evidence hierarchy (i.e., mostly nonexperimental studies), and therefore the hierarchy did not offer much possibility for discriminating studies of varying rigor. Examples of quality assessment instruments that have been used for rating the evidence quality of primary nursing studies include the ones proposed by Chalmers and co-workers (1981), and Sindhu, Carpenter, and Seers (1997). Moher, Jadad, Nichol, Penman, Tugwell, and Walsh (1995) provide an annotated bibliography of 25 scales and 9 checklists used to rate the quality of randomized clinical trials.

 Example of a quality assessment tool:
Beck (2001) developed a quality index, based on 11 criteria, that had scores ranging from

11 to 32. The criteria included first-author expertise; funding; type of sample; sample size; reliability and validity of instruments; type of measurement; type of diagnosis; research design; time dimensional design; and data analysis.

Quality assessments, to an even greater extent than the coding of study characteristics, require ratings by two or more qualified individuals. If there are disagreements between the two raters, there should be a discussion until a consensus has been reached or, if necessary, a third rater should be asked to help resolve the difference. Another issue concerns the "blinding" of raters with regard to the authorship and institutional affiliation of the primary study researchers. Although some rating scales use the credentials of the researchers as a criterion to be considered in the assessment, there is some evidence that blind assessments yield more consistent (and more conservative) scores than open assessments (Jadad et al., 1996).

What to *do* with the quality ratings has been the topic of some debate. As noted earlier, some reviewers (especially those doing narrative reviews) exclude studies deemed especially weak from the review altogether. The prevailing view appears to be to retain methodologically weak studies in the data set, but to "downweight" them (either qualitatively or quantitatively) in analyzing and synthesizing the findings. Lohr and Carey (1999), for example, argue that this approach "permits the users of scientific literature syntheses to understand the full range of evidence on a given topic and to choose, themselves, what weight to give to the poorer work" (p. 476). If studies with low quality ratings are retained in the data set for meta-analyses, the ratings can be used in a number of different ways. For example, weights proportional to the quality rating can be assigned so that the more rigorous studies "count" more in developing estimates of effects. Frequently, meta-analysts conduct what is referred to as **sensitivity analyses**. This means that they run their analyses including and excluding low-quality studies to see if including them changes the conclusions, or they compare the results for low-quality versus higher-quality stud-

ies. Several methodologic studies have found, at least in the case of clinical trials, that low-quality studies tend to lead to higher (and thus perhaps exaggerated) estimates of treatment benefits than high-quality ones (Khan, Daya, & Jadad, 1996; Moher et al., 1998).

Analyzing the Data

There are various methods of qualitatively analyzing the data for narrative reviews, although many reviewers appear to rely primarily on judgments without making clear the rules of inference that they used (Ganong, 1987). Inference is, of course, necessary only when the results of various studies are inconsistent (e.g., when some studies suggest a relationship between variables whereas others do not).

One approach to narrative integration uses what is referred to as the **voting method**. This procedure involves tallying the outcomes of studies in the data set to determine what outcome has received the greatest empirical support. This method, however, tends to ignore study quality, and it is not clear that it is preferable to a purely qualitative integration that relies on judgment. Ganong (1987) urges reviewers, even those using the voting method, to "search systematically across studies for explanations of varying results and should investigate all study characteristics possibly related to variations" (p. 9). Stetler, Morsi, and colleagues (1998) argue that the analysis and synthesis in narrative integrative reviews should be a group process and that the whole review team should meet to discuss their conclusions after reviewing a packet of synopsized studies and tables. In a narrative review, reviewers interpret the pattern of findings, draw conclusions about the evidence the findings yield, and derive implications for policy, practice, and further research.

In a metasynthesis, data analysis involves identifying the key metaphors in each qualitative study and then translating them into a synthesis that transforms these individual findings into a new conceptualization (Schreiber, Crooks, & Stern, 1997). Noblit and Hare (1988) provide one such data analytic approach for a metasynthesis. Their method consists of making a list of key metaphors from each study and determining their relation to each other. Are the metaphors, for example, directly comparable (reciprocal)? Are the metaphors in opposition to each other (refutational)? Next, the studies' metaphors are translated into each other. Noblit and Hare (p. 28) note that "translations are especially unique syntheses because they protect the particular, respect holism, and enable comparison. An adequate translation maintains the central metaphors and/or concepts of each account in their relation to other key metaphors or concepts in that account." This synthesis of qualitative studies creates a whole that is more than the sum of the parts of the individual studies. Sandelowski, Docherty, and Emden (1997, p. 370) warn that "Qualitative metasynthesis is not a trivial pursuit, but rather a complex exercise in interpretation; carefully peeling away the surface layers of studies to find their hearts and souls in a way that does the least damage to them."

 Example of data analysis in a metasynthesis:

Beck (2002) used Noblit and Hare's approach in her metasynthesis of 18 qualitative studies on postpartum depression. As part of the analysis, key metaphors were listed for each study and organized under four overarching themes, one being "spiraling downward." For instance, in Wood, Thomas, Droppelman, and Meighan's (1997) study, the key metaphors listed under this theme included "total isolation; façade of normalcy; obsessive thoughts; pervasive guilt; panic/overanxious/feels trapped; completely overwhelmed by infant demands; anger" (p. 459).

In meta-analysis, the data are analyzed quantitatively. An advantage of meta-analysis is that subjective judgment and interpretation play a much less crucial role than in the case of a narrative analysis. Readers of a meta-analysis can be confident that another analyst using the same data set would have come to exactly the same conclusions. The essence of a meta-analysis is that information from various studies is used to develop a common metric (an effect size); effect sizes are then combined across studies and averaged, yielding information about not only the *existence* of a relationship between variables, but about its *magnitude*. For example, meta-analysts can draw conclusions about how big an effect an intervention has (with a specified probability that the results are accurate), and this in turn can yield estimates of the intervention's cost-effectiveness. Also, in meta-analysis the relationship between methodologic quality and effect size can be examined directly. Finally, effect sizes can be computed separately for key subgroups (e.g., men versus women) to determine if effects differ for segments of the population.

Meta-analysis has its critics as well as advocates. One issue is the so-called "fruit problem," that is, the possibility of combining studies that conceptually do not belong with each other (apples and oranges). Another issue is that there is usually a bias in the studies appearing in published sources. Studies in which no group differences or no relationships between variables have been found are less likely to be published and, therefore, are less likely to be included in the meta-analysis. Narrative literature reviews are subject to the same two problems, however. Moreover, meta-analysis offers mechanisms to control for or examine these issues. For example, if there is concern that different methods of conceptualizing and measuring a dependent variable can lead to different conclusions (the fruit problem), separate analyses can be performed for the different measures to see if the results are similar. With regard to using only published studies in the data set, this problem can be partially addressed by making concerted efforts to identify relevant dissertations and conference papers. In addition, a **fail-safe number** can be calculated to estimate the number of studies reporting nonsignificant results that would be needed to reverse the conclusion of a significant effect in a meta-analysis (Wolf, 1986). The fail-safe number is compared to a tolerance level ($5k + 10$), where k is the number of studies included in the analysis (Rosenthal, 1991).

Example of calculating a fail-safe number:
Fetzer (2002) conducted a meta-analysis of the effect of a eutectic mixture of local anesthetics (EMLA) on reducing pain during venipuncture. All nine studies in the review reported a significant positive effect. The fail-safe number was calculated to be 374, which far exceeded the reasonable tolerance level of 55.

In a meta-analysis, a key analytic activity involves the calculation of an effect size for every study. The effect size, as noted earlier, represents the size of the impact of an intervention on an outcome, or the size of the association between two variables. The concept of effect size was explained in Chapter 20, which also indicated that formulas for effect size differ depending on the nature of the underlying statistical test. The simplest formula to understand is the effect size for the difference between two means (e.g., an experimental and control group). In this situation, the effect size is the mean for one group, minus the mean for the second group, divided by the common within-group standard deviation. Effect sizes for individual studies are then pooled and averaged to yield estimates of overall population effects. More sophisticated analyses are also possible, including a number of multivariate procedures. Further information on analytic procedures for meta-analysis is provided in Rosenthal (1991), Wolf (1986), and Lipsey and Wilson (2001).

The calculations for meta-analyses can be extremely laborious. Fortunately, there is meta-analytic software that can perform the statistical computations. One widely used software package is the Advanced BASIC Meta-Analysis program (Mullen, 1989), which has been described by Beck (1996).

Writing Up an Integrative Review

The report for an integrative review typically follows much the same format as for a research report for a primary study. That is, there is typically an introduction, method section, results section, and discussion. The method section should be thorough: Readers of the review need to be able to assess the validity of the findings by understanding and critiquing the procedures the reviewers used.

As Ganong (1987) has noted, "The purpose of integrative reviews—the summarization of accumulated evidence in primary research—is not achieved with reviews based on questionable or unclear methodology" (p. 10).

Guidelines for critiquing narrative integrative reviews and meta-analyses are available in Brown (1999) and Stetler, Morsi, and colleagues (1998). Those preparing integrative reviews would do well to consult such guidelines to ensure that they have prepared a maximally useful review that can make a contribution to nursing practice.

For a metasynthesis, alternatives to written reviews have been proposed. Noblit and Hare (1988) note, for example, that when the qualitative synthesis' purpose is to inform clinicians or practitioners, other forms of expressing the synthesis may be preferred, such as through music, artwork, plays, or videos.

RESEARCH EXAMPLE

Many EBP and research utilization projects are underway in practice settings, and some that have been described in the nursing literature offer rich information about planning and implementing such an endeavor. Projects have been undertaken by hospital—nursing school collaboratives (e.g., Flynn & Fink, 2001), by interdisciplinary teams within hospitals (e.g., Seemann, 2000), and by professional nursing organizations. Of particular note, AWHONN has conducted several major RU/EBP projects, one of which is described here.

An interdisciplinary team, under the leadership of neonatal clinical nurse specialist Carolyn H. Lund, undertook a 4-year project designed to develop and evaluate an evidence-based clinical practice guideline for assessment and routine care of neonatal skin (Lund, Kuller, Lane, Lott, Raines, & Thomas, 2001; Lund, Osborne, Kuller, Lane, Lott, & Raines, 2001). The project also sought to educate nurses about the scientific basis for the recommended skin care practices, and designed procedures to facilitate using the guideline in practice.

The project consisted of four 1-year phases. Phase 1 (Planning) involved forming the project team, synthesizing scientific and other evidence relating to neonatal skin care (Lund, Kuller, Lane, Lott, &

Raines, 1999), developing the evidence-based guideline, and developing data collection instruments. Ten areas of neonatal skin care were included in the practice guidelines: bathing, emollients, adhesives, skin disinfectants, control of transepidermal water loss, diaper dermatitis, cord and circumcision care, skin assessment, and prevention and treatment of skin breakdown. The quality of the scientific evidence in each of these areas determined the strength of each recommendation.

The second phase involved the implementation of the guidelines. Clinical sites (nurseries in the United States and Canada) were recruited through various means (e.g., bulletins published in *AWHONN Lifelines* and *JOGNN*) and invited to participate in an EBP project. More than 75 nurseries expressed an interest in participating, and ultimately 51 sites (representing 27 states) prepared preguideline and postguideline assessments. Each participating institution had a site coordinator who completed a variety of forms and underwent training in the use of the guidelines. Site coordinators provided information about their hospital's current skin care practices and took a knowledge test about neonatal skin care. The site coordinators also completed assessments of the skin condition of some 1371 infants (about 30 per site) before the implementation of the guidelines, and these assessments served as a baseline for evaluating the effectiveness of the new procedures. Skin assessments were done twice a week using an observational rating scale that evaluated dryness, erythema, and breakdown/excoriation.

Phase 3 of the project (Evaluation) involved an assessment of the outcomes. The evaluation addressed three broad questions: (1) Will nurses change clinical practices after receiving education and implementing a clinical practice guideline? (2) Will patient outcomes be positively affected by the use of the guideline in neonatal intensive care units (NICUs), special-care units (SCUs), and well-baby nursery settings? and (3) How does the caregiving environment influence skin integrity? Several specific hypotheses were tested (e.g., that the frequency of bathing would decrease, and that infant skin condition would improve). The results indicated that the guidelines were, in fact, integrated into care and that nurses changed their practices. For example, there was a significant and substantial decrease in the frequency of bathing in the NICU from preguideline to postguideline implementation, and a significant increase in emollient use. There was also

evidence that skin condition was improved, as reflected by less visible dryness, redness, and skin breakdown in all neonatal settings. Site coordinators reported a few problems during the course of the project (e.g., organizational barriers to changing products), but they mostly described the benefits of having an EBP guideline and of having participated in a national EBP project. All site coordinators except one reported that their units would continue using the guidelines after project completion, and the one exception indicated partial use of the guidelines.

Finally, in phase 4 of the project (Dissemination), the team made efforts to publish results, make presentations at conferences, and continue to advance evidence-based neonatal skin care through programmatic activities and educational products. The project team concluded that the results "support a wider dissemination of the project's practice guideline for neonatal skin care" (Lund, Osborne, et al., 2001, p. 41).

SUMMARY POINTS

- **Research utilization (RU)** and **evidence-based practice (EBP)** are overlapping concepts that concern efforts to use research as a basis for clinical decisions. RU starts with a research-based innovation that gets evaluated for possible use in practice. EBP starts with a search for the best possible evidence for a clinical problem, with emphasis on research-based evidence.

- Research utilization exists on a continuum, with direct utilization of some specific innovation at one end (**instrumental utilization**), and more diffuse situations in which users are influenced in their thinking about an issue based on research findings (**conceptual utilization**) at the other end.

- Rogers' **Diffusion of Innovations Theory** describes the innovation adoption process as occurring in five stages: the knowledge stage, persuasion stage, decision stage, implementation stage, and confirmation stage.

- Several major utilization projects have been implemented (e.g., the **Conduct and Utilization of Research in Nursing** or **CURN project**) that have demonstrated that research utilization can be increased, but have also shed light on barriers to utilization.

- EBP, which de-emphasizes clinical decision making based on custom or ritual, integrates the best available research evidence with other sources of data, including clinical expertise and patient preferences.

- Two of the cornerstones of the EBP movement are the Cochrane Collaboration (which is based on the work of British epidemiologist Archie Cochrane), and the clinical learning strategy called *evidence-based medicine* developed at the McMaster Medical School.

- EBP typically involves weighing various types of evidence, and often an **evidence hierarchy** is used to rank studies and other information according to the strength of evidence provided.

- In nursing, EBP and RU efforts often face a variety of barriers, including methodologically weak or unreplicated studies, nurses' limited training in research and EBP, resistance to change, lack of organizational support, resource constraints, and limited communication and collaboration between practitioners and researchers.

- Many models of RU and EBP have been developed, including models for individual clinicians (e.g., the **Stetler model**) and ones for organizations or groups of clinicians (e.g., the **Iowa Model of Evidence-Based Practice to Promote Quality Care**).

- Most models of utilization involve the following steps: selecting a topic or problem; assembling and evaluating evidence; assessing the implementation potential of an evidence-based innovation; developing or identifying EBP guidelines or protocols; implementing the innovation; evaluating outcomes; and deciding whether to adopt or modify the innovation or revert to prior practices.

- Assessing implementation potential includes the dimensions of transferability of findings, feasibility of using the findings in the new setting, and the cost–benefit ratio of a new practice.

- EBP relies on rigorous integration of research evidence on a topic through **integrative reviews**, which are rigorous, systematic inquiries with many similarities to original primary studies.

- Integrative reviews can involve either qualitative, narrative approaches to integration (including metasynthesis of qualitative studies), or quantitative (meta-analytic) methods.

- Integrative reviews typically involve the following activities: developing a question or hypothesis; assembling a review team; selecting a sample of studies to be included in the review; extracting and recording data from the sampled studies; doing quality assessments of the studies; analyzing the data; and writing up the review.

- Quality assessments (which may involve formal quantitative ratings) are sometimes used to exclude weak studies from integrative reviews, but can also be used in **sensitivity analyses** to determine if including or excluding weaker studies changes conclusions.

- Meta-analysis involves the computation of an effect size index (which quantifies the magnitude of relationship between the independent and dependent variables) for every study in the sample, and averaging across studies.

- In meta-analyses, a **fail-safe number** can be calculated to estimate the number of studies with nonsignificant results that would be needed to reverse the conclusion of a significant effect.

- In narrative reviews, integration might use a procedure known as the **voting method** (tallying outcomes to see which outcome had greatest empirical support if there are inconsistencies), or might be done in a strictly narrative fashion, with a qualitative analysis of patterns in the data.

STUDY ACTIVITIES

Chapter 27 of the accompanying *Study Guide for Nursing Research: Principles and Methods, 7th ed.*, offers various exercises and study suggestions for reinforcing the concepts taught in this chapter. In addition, the following study questions can be addressed:

1. Find an article in a recent issue of a nursing research journal that does not discuss the

implications of the study for nursing practice. Evaluate the study's relevance to nursing practice, and if appropriate, write one to two paragraphs summarizing the implications.

2. Consider your personal situation. What are the barriers that might inhibit your use of research findings? What steps might be taken to address those barriers?

SUGGESTED READINGS

Methodologic References

Beck, C. T. (1996). Use of a meta-analytic database management system. *Nursing Research, 45,* 181–184.

Beck, C. T. (1999). Facilitating the work of a meta-analyst. *Research in Nursing & Health, 22,* 523–530.

Brown, S. J. (1999). *Knowledge for health care practice: A guide to using research evidence.* Philadelphia: W. B. Saunders Company.

Caplan, N., & Rich, R. F. (1975). *The use of social science knowledge in policy decisions at the national level.* Ann Arbor, MI: Institute for Social Research, University of Michigan.

Chalmers, T. C., Smith, H., Blackburn, B., Silverman, B., Schroeder, B., Reitman, D., & Ambroz, A. (1981). A method for assessing the quality of a randomized control trial. *Controlled Clinical Trials, 2,* 31–49.

Closs, S. J., & Cheater, F. M. (1999). Evidence for nursing practice: A clarification of the issues. *Journal of Advanced Nursing, 30,* 10–17.

Cooper, H. (1982). Scientific guidelines for conducting integrative research reviews. *Review of Educational Research, 52,* 291–302.

Cooper, H. (1984). *The integrative research review: A social science approach.* Beverly Hills, CA: Sage.

Cullum, N. (1997). Identification and analysis of randomized controlled trials in nursing: A preliminary study. *Quality in Health Care, 6,* 2–6.

Dooks, P. (2001). Diffusion of pain management research into nursing practice. *Cancer Nursing, 24,* 99–103.

Estabrooks, C. A. (2001). Research utilization and qualitative research. In J. M. Morse, J. M. Swanson, & A. J. Kuzel (Eds.), *The nature of qualitative evidence* (pp. 275–298). Thousand Oaks, CA: Sage.

Funk, S. G., Champagne, M. T., Wiese, R. A., & Tornquist, E. M. (1991). Barriers to using research findings in practice: The clinician's perspective. *Applied Nursing Research, 4,* 90–95.

Funk, S. G., Tornquist, E. M., & Champagne, M. T. (1995). Barriers and facilitators of research utilization: An integrative review. *Nursing Clinics of North America, 30,* 395–407.

Ganong, L. H. (1987). Integrative reviews of nursing research. *Research in Nursing & Health, 10,* 1–11.

Gennaro, S. (2001). Making evidence-based practice a reality in your institution. *MCN: The American Journal of Maternal/Child Nursing, 26,* 236–244.

Goode, C. J. (2000). What constitutes "evidence" in evidence-based practice? *Applied Nursing Research, 13,* 222–225.

Granger, B. B. (2001). Research strategies for clinicians. *Critical Care Nursing Clinics of North America, 13,* 605–615.

Horsley, J. A., Crane, J., & Bingle, J. D. (1978). Research utilization as an organizational process. *Journal of Nursing Administration, 8,* 4–6.

Jadad, A. R., Cook, D. J., Jones, A., Klassen, T. P, Tugwell, P., Moher, M., & Moher, D. (1998). Methodology and reports of systematic reviews and meta-analyses: A comparison of Cochrane reviews with articles published in paper-based journals. *Journal of the American Medical Association, 280,* 278–280.

Jadad, A. R., Moore, R. A., Carroll, D., Jenkinson, C., Reynolds, D., Gavaghan, D., & McQuay, H. (1996). Assessing the quality of reports of randomized clinical trials: Is blinding necessary? *Controlled Clinical Trials, 17,* 1–12.

Jennings, B. M. (2000). Evidence-based practice: The road best traveled. *Research in Nursing & Health, 23,* 343–345.

Khan, K., Daya, S., & Jadad, A. (1996). The importance of quality of primary studies in producing unbiased systematic reviews. *Archives of Internal Medicine, 156,* 661–666.

Lipsey, M. W., & Wilson, D. B. (2001). *Practical meta-analysis.* Newbury Park, CA: Sage.

Lohr, K. N., & Carey, T. S. (1999). Assessing "best evidence": Issues in grading the quality of studies for systematic reviews. *The Joint Commission Journal on Quality Improvement, 25,* 470–479.

Moher, D., Jadad, A. R., Nichol, G., Penman, M., Tugwell, P., & Walsh, S. (1995). Assessing the quality of randomized clinical trials: An annotated bibliography of scales and checklists. *Controlled Clinical Trials, 16,* 62–73.

Moher, D., Pham, B., Jones, A., Cook, D. J., Jadad, A., Moher, M., Tugwell, P., & Klassen, T. (1998). Does quality of reports of randomised trials affect estimates of intervention efficacy reported in meta-analyses? *Lancet, 352,* 609–613.

Mullen, B. (1989). *Advanced BASIC: Meta-analysis.* Hillsdale, NJ: Erlbaum.

Noblit, G., & Hare, R. D. (1988). *Meta-ethnography: Synthesizing qualitative studies.* Newbury Park, CA: Sage

Paterson, B, I., Thorne, S. E., Canam, C., & Jillings, C. (2001). *Meta-study of qualitative health research.* Thousand Oaks, CA: Sage.

Phillips, L. R. F. (1986). *A clinician's guide to the critique and utilization of nursing research.* Norwalk, CT: Appleton-Century-Crofts.

Rogers, E. M. (1995). *Diffusion of innovations* (4th ed.). New York: Free Press.

Rosenfeld, P., Duthie, E., Bier, J., Bower-Ferres, S., Fulmer, T., Iervolino, L., McClure, M., McGivern, D., & Roncoli, M. (2000). Engaging staff nurses in evidence-based research to identify nursing practice problems and solutions. *Applied Nursing Research, 13,* 197–203.

Rosenthal, R. (1991). *Meta-analytic procedures for social research.* Newbury Park, CA: Sage.

Rosswurm, M. A., & Larrabee, J. H. (1999). A model for change to evidence-based practice. *Image: The Journal of Nursing Scholarship, 31,* 317–322.

Sackett, D. L., Rosenberg, W., Muir Gray, J. A., Haynes, R., & Richardson, W. (1996). Evidence based medicine: What it is and what it isn't. *British Medical Journal, 312,* 71–72.

Sandelowski, M. (1996). Using qualitative methods in intervention studies. *Research in Nursing & Health, 19,* 359–364.

Sandelowski, M., Docherty, S., & Emden, C. (1997). Qualitative metasynthesis: Issues and techniques. *Research in Nursing & Health, 20,* 365–371.

Schreiber, R., Crooks, D., & Stern, P. N. (1997). Qualitative meta-analysis. In J. M. Morse (Ed.), *Completing a qualitative project* (pp. 311–326). Thousand Oaks, CA: Sage.

Sindhu, F., Carpenter, L., & Seers, K. (1997). Development of a tool to rate the quality assessment of randomized clinical trials using a Delphi technique. *Journal of Advanced Nursing, 25,* 1262–1268.

Soukup, M., Sr. (2000). The Center for Advanced Nursing Practice evidence-based practice model: Promoting the scholarship of practice. *Nursing Clinics of North America, 35,* 301–309.

Stetler, C. B. (1994). Refinement of the Stetler/Marram model for application of research findings into practice. *Nursing Outlook, 42,* 15–25.

Stetler, C. B. (2001). Updating the Stetler model of research utilization to facilitate evidence-based practice. *Nursing Outlook, 49,* 272–279.

Stetler, C. B., Brunell, M., Giuliano, K. K., Morse, D., Prince, L., & Newell-Stokes, V. (1998). Evidence-based practice and the role of nursing leadership. *Journal of Nursing Administration, 28,* 45–53.

Stetler, C. B., Morsi, D., Rucki, S., Broughton, S., Corrigan, B., Fitzgerald, J., Giuliano, K., Havener, P., & Sheridan, E. A. (1998). Utilization-focused integrative reviews in a nursing service. *Applied Nursing Research, 11,* 195–206.

Stevens, K. R. (2001). Systematic reviews: The heart of evidence-based practice. *AACN Clinical Issues, 12,* 529–538.

Titler, M. G., Kleiber, C., Steelman, V., Goode, C., Rakel, B., Barry-Walker, J., Small, S., & Buckwalter, K. (1994). Infusing research into practice to promote quality care. *Nursing Research, 43,* 307–313.

Titler, M. G., Kleiber, C., Steelman, V., Rakel, B., Budreau, G., Everett, L., Buckwalter, K., Tripp-Reimer, T., & Goode, C. (2001). The Iowa model of evidence-based practice to promote quality care. *Critical Care Nursing Clinics of North America, 13,* 497–509.

Weiss, C, (1980) Knowledge creep and decision accretion. *Knowledge: Creation, Diffusion, Utilization, 1,* 381–404.

Wolf, F. M. (1986). *Meta-analysis: Quantitative methods for research synthesis.* Newbury Park, CA: Sage.

Studies Cited in Chapter 27

Beck, C. T. (2001). Predictors of postpartum depression: An update. *Nursing Research, 50,* 275–285.

Beck, C. T. (2002). Postpartum depression: A metasynthesis. *Qualitative Health Research, 12,* 453–472.

Brett, J. L. L. (1987). Use of nursing practice research findings. *Nursing Research, 36,* 344–349.

Coyle, L. A., & Sokop, A. G. (1990). Innovation adoption behavior among nurses. *Nursing Research, 39,* 176–180.

Estabrooks, C. A. (1999). The conceptual structure of research utilization. *Research in Nursing & Health, 22,* 203–216.

Fetzer, S. J. (2002). Reducing venipuncture and intravenous insertion pain with eutectic mixture of local anesthetic. *Nursing Research, 51,* 119–124.

Flynn, M. B., & Fink, R. (2001). Committing to evidence-based skin care practice. *Critical Care Nursing Clinics of North America, 13,* 555–567.

Hill-Westmoreland, E. E., Soeken, K., & Spellbring, A. M. (2002). A meta-analysis of fall prevention programs for the elderly: How effective are they? *Nursing Research, 51,* 1–8.

Ketefian, S. (1975). Application of selected nursing research findings into nursing practice. *Nursing Research, 24,* 89–92.

Kirchhoff, K. T. (1982). A diffusion survey of coronary precautions. *Nursing Research, 31,* 196–201.

Lanuza, D. M., Lefaiver, C. A., & Farcas, G. A. (2000). Research on the quality of life of lung transplant candidates and recipients: An integrative review. *Heart & Lung, 29,* 180–195.

Lund, C. H., Kuller, J., Lane, A. T., Lott, J. W., & Raines, D. A. (1999). Neonatal skin care: The scientific basis for practice. *Journal of Obstetric, Gynecologic, and Neonatal Nursing, 28,* 241–254.

Lund, C. H., Kuller, J., Lane, A. T., Lott, J. W., Raines, D. A., & Thomas, K. K. (2001). Neonatal skin care: Evaluation of the AWHONN/NANN research-based practice project on knowledge and skin care practices. *Journal of Obstetric, Gynecologic, and Neonatal Nursing, 30,* 30–40.

Lund, C. H., Osborne, J. W., Kuller, J., Lane, A.T., Lott, J. W., & Raines, D. A. (2001). Neonatal skin care: Clinical outcomes of the AWHONN/NANN evidence-based clinical practice guideline. *Journal of Obstetric, Gynecologic, and Neonatal Nursing, 30,* 41–51.

Montgomery, L., Hanrahan, K., Kottman, K., Otto, A., Barrett, T., & Hermiston, B. (1999). Guideline for i.v. infiltration in pediatric patients. *Pediatric Nursing, 25,* 167–169.

Nelson, A. M. (2002). A metasynthesis: Mothering other-than-normal children. *Qualitative Health Research, 12,* 515–530.

Nichols, G. A., & Verhonick, P. J. (1968). Placement times for oral temperatures: A nursing study replication. *Nursing Research, 17,* 159–161.

Rizzuto, C., Bostrom, J., Suter, W. N., & Chenitz, W. C. (1994). Predictors of nurses' involvement in research activities. *Western Journal of Nursing Research, 16,* 193–204.

Rodgers, S. E. (2000). The extent of nursing research utilization in general medical and surgical wards. *Journal of Advanced Nursing, 32,* 182–193.

Rutledge, D. N., Greene, P., Mooney, K., Nail, L. M., & Ropka, M. (1996). Use of research-based practices by oncology staff nurses. *Oncology Nursing Forum, 23,* 1235–1244.

Seemann, S. (2000). Interdisciplinary approach to a total knee replacement program. *Nursing Clinics of North America, 35,* 405–415.

Stetler, C. B., Corrigan, B., Sander-Buscemi, K., & Burns, M. (1999). Integration of evidence into practice and the change process: Fall prevention program as a model. *Outcomes Management for Nursing Practice, 3,* 102–111.

Thompson, C. J. (2001). The meaning of research utilization: A preliminary typology. *Critical Care Nursing Clinics of North America, 13,* 475–485.

Wood, A. F., Thomas, S. P., Droppleman, P. G., & Meighan, M. (1997). The downward spiral of postpartum depression. *MCN: The American Journal of Maternal/Child Nursing, 22,* 308–317.

APPENDIX

A *Statistical Tables*

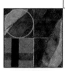

TABLE A-1 Distribution of *t* Probability

df	LEVEL OF SIGNIFICANCE FOR ONE-TAILED TEST					
	.10	.05	.025	.01	.005	.0005
	LEVEL OF SIGNIFICANCE FOR TWO-TAILED TEST					
df	.20	.10	.05	.02	.01	.001
1	3.078	6.314	12.706	31.821	63.657	636.619
2	1.886	2.920	4.303	6.965	9.925	31.598
3	1.638	2.353	3.182	4.541	5.841	12.941
4	1.533	2.132	2.776	3.747	4.604	8.610
5	1.476	2.015	2.571	3.376	4.032	6.859
6	1.440	1.953	2.447	3.143	3.707	5.959
7	1.415	1.895	2.365	2.998	3.449	5.405
8	1.397	1.860	2.306	2.896	3.355	5.041
9	1.383	1.833	2.262	2.821	3.250	4.781
10	1.372	1.812	2.228	2.765	3.169	4.587
11	1.363	1.796	2.201	2.718	3.106	4.437
12	1.356	1.782	2.179	2.681	3.055	4.318
13	1.350	1.771	2.160	2.650	3.012	4.221
14	1.345	1.761	2.145	2.624	2.977	4.140
15	1.341	1.753	2.131	2.602	2.947	4.073
16	1.337	1.746	2.120	2.583	2.921	4.015
17	1.333	1.740	2.110	2.567	2.898	3.965
18	1.330	1.734	2.101	2.552	2.878	3.922
19	1.328	1.729	2.093	2.539	2.861	3.883
20	1.325	1.725	2.086	2.528	2.845	3.850
21	1.323	1.721	2.080	2.518	2.831	3.819
22	1.321	1.717	2.074	2.508	2.819	3.792
23	1.319	1.714	2.069	2.500	2.807	3.767
24	1.318	1.711	2.064	2.492	2.797	3.745
25	1.316	1.708	2.060	2.485	2.787	3.725
26	1.315	1.706	2.056	2.479	2.779	3.707
27	1.314	1.703	2.052	2.473	2.771	3.690
28	1.313	1.701	2.048	2.467	2.763	3.674
29	1.311	1.699	2.045	2.462	2.756	3.659
30	1.310	1.697	2.042	2.457	2.750	3.646
40	1.303	1.684	2.021	2.423	2.704	3.551
60	1.296	1.671	2.000	2.390	2.660	3.460
120	1.289	1.658	1.980	2.358	2.617	3.373
∞	1.282	1.645	1.960	2.326	2.576	3.291

TABLE A-2 Significant Values of F
α = .05 (Two-Tailed)   α = .025 (one-tailed)

$\frac{df_B}{df_W}$	1	2	3	4	5	6	8	12	24	∞
1	161.4	199.5	215.7	224.6	230.2	234.0	238.9	243.9	249.0	254.3
2	18.51	19.00	19.16	19.25	19.30	19.33	19.37	19.41	19.45	19.50
3	10.13	9.55	9.28	9.12	9.01	8.94	8.84	8.74	8.64	8.53
4	7.71	6.94	6.59	6.39	6.26	6.16	6.04	5.91	5.77	5.63
5	6.61	5.79	5.41	5.19	5.05	4.95	4.82	4.68	4.53	4.36
6	5.99	5.14	4.76	4.53	4.39	4.28	4.15	4.00	3.84	3.67
7	5.59	4.74	4.35	4.12	3.97	3.87	3.73	3.57	3.41	3.23
8	5.32	4.46	4.07	3.84	3.69	3.58	3.44	3.28	3.12	2.93
9	5.12	4.26	3.86	3.63	3.48	3.37	3.23	3.07	2.90	2.71
10	4.96	4.10	3.71	3.48	3.33	3.22	3.07	2.91	2.74	2.54
11	4.84	3.98	3.59	3.36	3.20	3.09	2.95	2.79	2.61	2.40
12	4.75	3.88	3.49	3.26	3.11	3.00	2.85	2.69	2.50	2.30
13	4.67	3.80	3.41	3.18	3.02	2.92	2.77	2.60	2.42	2.21
14	4.60	3.74	3.34	3.11	2.96	2.85	2.70	2.53	2.35	2.13
15	4.54	3.68	3.29	3.06	2.90	2.79	2.64	2.48	2.29	2.07
16	4.49	3.63	3.24	3.01	2.85	2.74	2.59	2.42	2.24	2.01
17	4.45	3.59	3.20	2.96	2.81	2.70	2.55	2.38	2.19	1.96
18	4.41	3.55	3.16	2.93	2.77	2.66	2.51	2.34	2.15	1.92
19	4.38	3.52	3.13	2.90	2.74	2.63	2.48	2.31	2.11	1.88
20	4.35	3.49	3.10	2.87	2.71	2.60	2.45	2.28	2.08	1.84
21	4.32	3.47	3.07	2.84	2.68	2.57	2.42	2.25	2.05	1.81
22	4.30	3.44	3.05	2.82	2.66	2.55	2.40	2.23	2.03	1.78
23	4.28	3.42	3.03	2.80	2.64	2.53	2.38	2.20	2.00	1.76
24	4.26	3.40	3.01	2.78	2.62	2.51	2.36	2.18	1.98	1.73
25	4.24	3.38	2.99	2.76	2.60	2.49	2.34	2.16	1.96	1.71
26	4.22	3.37	2.98	2.74	2.59	2.47	2.32	2.15	1.95	1.69
27	4.21	3.35	2.96	2.73	2.57	2.46	2.30	2.13	1.93	1.67
28	4.20	3.34	2.95	2.71	2.56	2.44	2.29	2.12	1.91	1.65
29	4.18	3.33	2.93	2.70	2.54	2.43	2.28	2.10	1.90	1.64
30	4.17	3.32	2.92	2.69	2.53	2.42	2.27	2.09	1.89	1.62
40	4.08	3.23	2.84	2.61	2.45	2.34	2.18	2.00	1.79	1.51
60	4.00	3.15	2.76	2.52	2.37	2.25	2.10	1.92	1.70	1.39
120	3.92	3.07	2.68	2.45	2.29	2.17	2.02	1.83	1.61	1.25
∞	3.84	2.99	2.60	2.37	2.21	2.09	1.94	1.75	1.52	1.00

(continued)

TABLE A-2 Significant Values of *F* (continued)

$\alpha = .01$ (Two-Tailed) $\alpha = .005$(one-tailed)

$\dfrac{df_B}{df_W}$	1	2	3	4	5	6	8	12	24	∞
1	4052	4999	5403	5625	5764	5859	5981	6106	6234	6366
2	98.49	99.00	99.17	99.25	99.30	99.33	99.36	99.42	99.46	99.50
3	34.12	30.81	29.46	28.71	28.24	27.91	27.49	27.05	26.60	26.12
4	21.20	18.00	16.69	15.98	15.52	15.21	14.80	14.37	13.93	13.46
5	16.26	13.27	12.06	11.39	10.97	10.67	10.29	9.89	9.47	9.02
6	13.74	10.92	9.78	9.15	8.75	8.47	8.10	7.72	7.31	6.88
7	12.25	9.55	8.45	7.85	7.46	7.19	6.84	6.47	6.07	5.65
8	11.26	8.65	7.59	7.01	6.63	6.37	6.03	5.67	5.28	4.86
9	10.56	8.02	6.99	6.42	6.06	5.80	5.47	5.11	4.73	4.31
10	10.04	7.56	6.55	5.99	5.64	5.39	5.06	4.71	4.33	3.91
11	9.65	7.20	6.22	5.67	5.32	5.07	4.74	4.40	4.02	3.60
12	9.33	6.93	5.95	5.41	5.06	4.82	4.50	4.16	3.78	3.36
13	9.07	6.70	5.74	5.20	4.86	4.62	4.30	3.96	3.59	3.16
14	8.86	6.51	5.56	5.03	4.69	4.46	4.14	3.80	3.43	3.00
15	8.68	6.36	5.42	4.89	4.56	4.32	4.00	3.67	3.29	2.87
16	8.53	6.23	5.29	4.77	4.44	4.20	3.89	3.55	3.18	2.75
17	8.40	6.11	5.18	4.67	4.34	4.10	3.78	3.45	3.08	2.65
18	8.28	6.01	5.09	4.58	4.29	4.01	3.71	3.37	3.00	2.57
19	8.18	5.93	5.01	4.50	4.17	3.94	3.63	3.30	2.92	2.49
20	8.10	5.85	4.94	4.43	4.10	3.87	3.56	3.23	2.86	2.42
21	8.02	5.78	4.87	4.37	4.04	3.81	3.51	3.17	2.80	2.36
22	7.94	5.72	4.82	4.31	3.99	3.76	3.45	3.12	2.75	2.31
23	7.88	5.66	4.76	4.26	3.94	3.71	3.41	3.07	2.70	2.26
24	7.82	5.61	4.72	4.22	3.90	3.67	3.36	3.03	2.66	2.21
25	7.77	5.57	4.68	4.18	3.86	3.63	3.32	2.99	2.62	2.17
26	7.72	5.53	4.64	4.14	3.82	3.59	3.29	2.96	2.58	2.13
27	7.68	5.49	4.60	4.11	3.78	3.56	3.26	2.93	2.55	2.10
28	7.64	5.45	4.57	4.07	3.75	3.53	3.23	2.90	2.52	2.06
29	7.60	5.42	4.54	4.04	3.73	3.50	3.20	2.87	2.49	2.03
30	7.56	5.39	4.51	4.02	3.70	3.47	3.17	2.84	2.47	2.01
40	7.31	5.18	4.31	3.83	3.51	3.29	2.99	2.66	2.29	1.80
60	7.08	4.98	4.13	3.65	3.34	3.12	2.82	2.50	2.12	1.60
120	6.85	4.79	3.95	3.48	3.17	2.96	2.66	2.34	1.95	1.38
∞	6.64	4.60	3.78	3.32	3.02	2.80	2.51	2.18	1.79	1.00

(continued)

TABLE A-2 Significant Values of F (continued)

$\alpha = .001$ (Two-Tailed) $\alpha = .0005$ (one-tailed)

$\dfrac{df_B}{df_W}$	1	2	3	4	5	6	8	12	24	∞
1	405284	500000	540379	562500	576405	585937	598144	610667	623497	636619
2	998.5	999.0	999.2	999.2	999.3	999.3	999.4	999.4	999.5	999.5
3	167.5	148.5	141.1	137.1	134.6	132.8	130.6	128.3	125.9	123.5
4	74.14	61.25	56.18	53.44	51.71	50.53	49.00	47.41	45.77	44.05
5	47.04	36.61	33.20	31.09	29.75	28.84	27.64	26.42	25.14	23.78
6	35.51	27.00	23.70	21.90	20.81	20.03	19.03	17.99	16.89	15.75
7	29.22	21.69	18.77	17.19	16.21	15.52	14.63	13.71	12.73	11.69
8	25.42	18.49	15.83	14.39	13.49	12.86	17.04	11.19	10.30	9.34
9	22.86	16.39	13.90	12.56	11.71	11.13	10.37	9.57	8.72	7.81
10	21.04	14.91	12.55	11.28	10.48	9.92	9.20	8.45	7.64	6.76
11	19.69	13.81	11.56	10.35	9.58	9.05	8.35	7.63	6.85	6.00
12	18.64	12.97	10.80	9.63	8.89	8.38	7.71	7.00	6.25	5.42
13	17.81	12.31	10.21	9.07	8.35	7.86	7.21	6.52	5.78	4.97
14	17.14	11.78	9.73	8.62	7.92	7.43	6.80	6.13	5.41	4.60
15	16.59	11.34	9.34	8.25	7.57	7.09	6.47	5.81	5.10	4.31
16	16.12	10.97	9.00	7.94	7.27	6.81	6.19	5.55	4.85	4.06
17	15.72	10.66	8.73	7.68	7.02	6.56	5.96	5.32	4.63	3.85
18	15.38	10.39	8.49	7.46	6.81	6.35	5.76	5.13	4.45	3.67
19	15.08	10.16	8.28	7.26	6.61	6.18	5.59	4.97	4.29	3.52
20	14.82	9.95	8.10	7.10	6.46	6.02	5.44	4.82	4.15	3.38
21	14.59	9.77	7.94	6.95	6.32	5.88	5.31	4.70	4.03	3.26
22	14.38	9.61	7.80	6.81	6.19	5.76	5.19	4.58	3.92	3.15
23	14.19	9.47	7.67	6.69	6.08	5.65	5.09	4.48	3.82	3.05
24	14.03	9.34	7.55	6.59	5.98	5.55	4.99	4.39	3.74	2.97
25	13.88	9.22	7.45	6.49	5.88	5.46	4.91	4.31	3.66	2.89
26	13.74	9.12	7.36	6.41	5.80	5.38	4.83	4.24	3.59	2.82
27	13.61	9.02	7.27	6.33	5.73	5.31	4.76	4.17	3.52	2.75
28	13.50	8.93	7.19	6.25	5.66	5.24	4.69	4.11	3.46	2.70
29	13.39	8.85	7.12	6.19	5.59	5.18	4.64	4.05	3.41	2.64
30	13.29	8.77	7.05	6.12	5.53	5.12	4.58	4.00	3.36	2.59
40	12.61	8.25	6.60	5.70	5.13	4.73	4.21	3.64	3.01	2.23
60	11.97	7.76	6.17	5.31	4.76	4.37	3.87	3.31	2.69	1.90
120	11.38	7.31	5.79	4.95	4.42	4.04	3.55	3.02	2.40	1.56
∞	10.83	6.91	5.42	4.62	4.10	3.74	3.27	2.74	2.13	1.00

TABLE A-3 Distribution of χ^2 Probability

	LEVEL OF SIGNIFICANCE				
df	.10	.05	.02	.01	.001
1	2.71	3.84	5.41	6.63	10.83
2	4.61	5.99	7.82	9.21	13.82
3	6.25	7.82	9.84	11.34	16.27
4	7.78	9.49	11.67	13.28	18.46
5	9.24	11.07	13.39	15.09	20.52
6	10.64	12.59	15.03	16.81	22.46
7	12.02	14.07	16.62	18.48	24.32
8	13.36	15.51	18.17	20.09	26.12
9	14.68	16.92	19.68	21.67	27.88
10	15.99	18.31	21.16	23.21	29.59
11	17.28	19.68	22.62	24.72	31.26
12	18.55	21.03	24.05	26.22	32.91
13	19.81	22.36	25.47	27.69	34.53
14	21.06	23.68	26.87	29.14	36.12
15	22.31	25.00	28.26	30.58	37.70
16	23.54	26.30	29.63	32.00	39.25
17	24.77	27.59	31.00	33.41	40.79
18	25.99	28.87	32.35	34.81	42.31
19	27.20	30.14	33.69	36.19	43.82
20	28.41	31.41	35.02	37.57	45.32
21	29.62	32.67	36.34	38.93	46.80
22	30.81	33.92	37.66	40.29	48.27
23	32.01	35.17	38.97	41.64	49.73
24	33.20	36.42	40.27	42.98	51.18
25	34.38	37.65	41.57	44.31	52.62
26	35.56	38.89	42.86	45.64	54.05
27	36.74	40.11	44.14	46.96	55.48
28	37.92	41.34	45.42	48.28	56.89
29	39.09	42.56	46.69	49.59	58.30
30	40.26	43.77	47.96	50.89	59.70

TABLE A-4 Significant Values of the Correlation Coefficient

	LEVEL OF SIGNIFICANCE FOR ONE-TAILED TEST				
	.05	.025	.01	.005	.0005
	LEVEL OF SIGNIFICANCE FOR TWO-TAILED TEST				
df	.10	.05	.02	.01	.001
1	.98769	.99692	.999507	.999877	.9999988
2	.90000	.95000	.98000	.990000	.99900
3	.8054	.8783	.93433	.95873	.99116
4	.7293	.8114	.8822	.91720	.97406
5	.6694	.7545	.8329	.8745	.95074
6	.6215	.7067	.7887	.8343	.92493
7	.5822	.6664	.7498	.7977	.8982
8	.5494	.6319	.7155	.7646	.8721
9	.5214	.6021	.6851	.7348	.8471
10	.4973	.5760	.6581	.7079	.8233
11	.4762	.5529	.6339	.6835	.8010
12	.4575	.5324	.6120	.6614	.7800
13	.4409	.5139	.5923	.5411	.7603
14	.4259	.4973	.5742	.6226	.7420
15	.4124	.4821	.5577	.6055	.7246
16	.4000	.4683	.5425	.5897	.7084
17	.3887	.4555	.5285	.5751	.6932
18	.3783	.4438	.5155	.5614	.5687
19	.3687	.4329	.5034	.5487	.6652
20	.3598	.4227	.4921	.5368	.6524
25	.3233	.3809	.4451	.5869	.5974
30	.2960	.3494	.4093	.4487	.5541
35	.2746	.3246	.3810	.4182	.5189
40	.2573	.3044	.3578	.3932	.4896
45	.2428	.2875	.3384	.3721	.4648
50	.2306	.2732	.3218	.3541	.4433
60	.2108	.2500	.2948	.3248	.4078
70	.1954	.2319	.2737	.3017	.3799
80	.1829	.2172	.2565	.2830	.3568
90	.1726	.2050	.2422	.2673	.3375
100	.1638	.1946	.2301	.2540	.3211

GLOSSARY

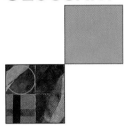

abstract   A brief description of a completed or proposed study, usually located at the beginning of a report or proposal.

accessible population   The population of people available for a particular study; often a nonrandom subset of the target population.

accidental sampling   Selection of the most readily available people as study participants; also called *convenience sampling*.

acquiescence response set   A bias in self-report instruments, especially in psychosocial scales, created when study participants characteristically agree with statements ("yea-say") independent of their content.

adjusted mean   The mean group value for the dependent variable, after statistically removing the effect of covariates.

after-only design   An experimental design in which data are collected from subjects only after an experimental intervention has been introduced.

alpha (α)   (1) In tests of statistical significance, the level designating the probability of committing a Type I error; (2) in estimates of internal consistency, a reliability coefficient, as in Cronbach's alpha.

alternative hypothesis   In hypothesis testing, a hypothesis different from the one being tested—usually, different from the null hypothesis.

analysis   The process of organizing and synthesizing data so as to answer research questions and test hypotheses.

analysis of covariance (ANCOVA)   A statistical procedure used to test mean differences among groups on a dependent variable, while controlling for one or more extraneous variables (covariates).

analysis of variance (ANOVA)   A statistical procedure for testing mean differences among three or more groups by comparing variability between groups to variability within groups.

analysis triangulation   The use of two or more analytic techniques to analyze the same set of data.

anonymity   Protection of participants in a study such that even the researcher cannot link individuals with the information provided.

applied research   Research designed to find a solution to an immediate practical problem.

assent   The affirmative agreement of a vulnerable subject (e.g., a child) to participate in a study.

associative relationship   An association between two variables that cannot be described as causal (i.e., one variable *causing* the other).

assumption   A basic principle that is accepted as being true based on logic or reason, but without proof or verification.

asymmetric distribution   A distribution of data values that is skewed, i.e., has two halves that are not mirror images of each other.

attribute variables   Preexisting characteristics of study participants, which the researcher simply observes or measures.

attrition   The loss of participants over the course of a study, which can create bias by changing the composition of the sample initially drawn—particularly if more participants are lost from one group than another, which can threaten the study's internal validity.

audio-CASI (computer assisted self-interview) An approach to collecting self-report data in which respondents listen to questions being read over headphones, and respond by entering information directly onto a computer.

audit trail   The systematic documentation of material that allows an independent auditor of a qualitative study to draw conclusions about the trustworthiness of the data.

auto-ethnography   Ethnographic studies in which researchers study their own culture or group.

axial coding   The second level of coding in a grounded theory study using the Strauss and Corbin approach, involving the process of categorizing, recategorizing, and condensing all first level codes by connecting a category and its subcategories.

back-translation   The translation of a translated text back into the original language, so that a comparison of the original and back-translated versions can be made.

baseline measure   A measure of the dependent variable prior to introducing an experimental intervention.

basic research   Research designed to extend the base of knowledge in a discipline for the sake of knowledge production or theory construction, rather than for solving an immediate problem.

basic social process (BSP)   The central social process emerging through an analysis of grounded theory data.

before-after design   An experimental design in which data are collected from research subjects both before and after the introduction of an experimental intervention.

behavioral objective   An intended outcome of a program or intervention, stated in terms of the behavior of those at whom the program is aimed.

beneficence   A fundamental ethical principle that seeks to prevent harm and exploitation of, and maximize benefits for, study participants.

beta (β)   (1) In multiple regression, the standardized coefficients indicating the relative weights of the independent variables in the regression equation; (2) in statistical testing, the probability of a Type II error.

between-subjects design   A research design in which there are separate groups of people being compared (e.g., smokers and nonsmokers).

bias   Any influence that produces a distortion in the results of a study.

bimodal distribution   A distribution of data values with two peaks (high frequencies).

bivariate statistics   Statistics derived from analyzing two variables simultaneously to assess the empirical relationship between them.

"blind" review   The review of a manuscript or proposal such that neither the author nor the reviewer is identified to the other party.

borrowed theory   A theory borrowed from another discipline to guide nursing practice or research.

bracketing   In phenomenological inquiries, the process of identifying and holding in abeyance any preconceived beliefs and opinions about the phenomena under study.

bricolage   The tendency in qualitative research to derive a complex array of data from a variety of sources, using a variety of methods.

calendar question   A question used to obtain retrospective information about the chronology of events and activities in people's lives.

canonical analysis   A statistical procedure for examining the relationship between two or more independent variables *and* two or more dependent variables.

carry-over effect   The influence that one treatment can have on subsequent treatments.

case-control design   A nonexperimental research design involving the comparison of a "case" (i.e., a person with the condition under scrutiny, such as lung cancer) and a matched control (a similar person without the condition).

case study   A research method involving a thorough, in-depth analysis of an individual, group, institution or other social unit.

categorical variable A variable with discrete values (e.g., gender) rather than values along a continuum (e.g., weight).

category system In observational studies, the prespecified plan for organizing and recording the behaviors and events under observation.

causal modeling The development and statistical testing of an explanatory model of hypothesized causal relationships among phenomena.

causal relationship A relationship between two variables such that the presence or absence of one variable (the "cause") determines the presence or absence, or value, of the other (the "effect").

cell (1) The intersection of a row and column in a table with two or more dimensions; (2) in an experimental design, the representation of an experimental condition in a schematic diagram.

census A survey covering an entire population.

central tendency A statistical index of the "typicalness" of a set of scores, derived from the center of the score distribution; indices of central tendency include the mode, median, and mean.

chi-square test A nonparametric test of statistical significance used to assess whether a relationship exists between two nominal-level variables; symbolized as χ^2.

clinical relevance The degree to which a study addresses a problem of significance to the practice of nursing.

clinical research Research designed to generate knowledge to guide nursing practice.

clinical trial A study designed to assess the safety and effectiveness of a new clinical treatment, sometimes involving several phases, one of which (Phase III) is a randomized clinical trial using an experimental design and, typically, a large and heterogeneous sample of subjects.

closed-ended question A question that offers respondents a set of mutually exclusive and jointly exhaustive alternative replies, from which the one most closely approximating the "right" answer must be chosen.

cluster analysis A multivariate statistical procedure used to cluster people or things based on patterns of association.

cluster randomization The random assignment of intact groups of subjects—rather than individual subjects—to treatment conditions.

cluster sampling A form of sampling in which large groupings ("clusters") are selected first (e.g., nursing schools), with successive subsampling of smaller units (e.g., nursing students).

code of ethics The fundamental ethical principles established by a discipline or institution to guide researchers' conduct in research with human (or animal) subjects.

codebook A record documenting categorization and coding decisions.

coding The process of transforming raw data into standardized form for data processing and analysis; in quantitative research, the process of attaching numbers to categories; in qualitative research, the process of identifying recurring words, themes, or concepts within the data.

coefficient alpha (Cronbach's alpha) A reliability index that estimates the internal consistency or homogeneity of a measure composed of several items or subparts.

coercion In a research context, the explicit or implicit use of threats (or excessive rewards) to gain people's cooperation in a study.

cognitive questioning A method sometimes used during a pretest of an instrument in which respondents are asked to talk about what comes to mind when they hear a question.

cognitive test An instrument designed to assess cognitive skills or cognitive functioning (e.g., an IQ test).

cohort comparison design A design that involves a comparison of two or more age cohorts.

cohort study A kind of trend study that focuses on a specific subpopulation (which is often an age-related subgroup) from which different samples are selected at different points in time (e.g., the cohort of nursing students who graduated between 1970 and 1974).

comparison group A group of subjects whose scores on a dependent variable are used to evaluate the outcomes of the group of primary interest (e.g., nonsmokers as a comparison group for smokers); term used in lieu of control group when the study design is not a true experiment.

component design   A study design for a mixed-method study in which qualitative and quantitative aspects are implemented as discrete components of the overall inquiry.

computer-assisted personal interviewing (CAPI)   In-person interviewing in which the interviewers read questions from, and enter responses onto, a laptop computer.

computer-assisted telephone interviewing (CATI)   Interviewing done over the telephone in which the interviewers read questions from, and enter responses onto, a computer.

concealment   A tactic involving the unobtrusive collection of research data without participants' knowledge or consent, used to obtain an accurate view of naturalistic behavior when the known presence of an observer would distort the behavior of interest.

concept   An abstraction based on observations of behaviors or characteristics (e.g., stress, pain).

conceptual definition   The abstract or theoretical meaning of the concepts being studied.

conceptual model   Interrelated concepts or abstractions assembled together in a rational scheme by virtue of their relevance to a common theme; sometimes called *conceptual framework.*

conceptual utilization   The use of research findings in a general, conceptual way to broaden one's thinking about an issue, without putting the knowledge to any specific, documentable use.

concurrent validity   The degree to which scores on an instrument are correlated with some external criterion, measured at the same time.

confirmatory factor analysis   A factor analysis, based on maximum likelihood estimation, designed to confirm a hypothesized measurement model.

confidence interval   The range of values within which a population parameter is estimated to lie.

confidence level   The estimated probability that a population parameter lies within a given confidence interval.

confidentiality   Protection of participants in a study such that individual identities are not linked to information provided and are never publicly divulged.

confirmability   A criterion for evaluating data quality with qualitative data, referring to the objectivity or neutrality of the data.

consent form   A written agreement signed by a study participant and a researcher concerning the terms and conditions of voluntary participation in a study.

consistency check   A procedure performed in cleaning a set of data to ensure that the data are internally consistent.

constant comparison   A procedure often used in a grounded theory analysis wherein newly collected data are compared in an ongoing fashion with data obtained earlier, to refine theoretically relevant categories.

construct   An abstraction or concept that is deliberately invented (constructed) by researchers for a scientific purpose (e.g., health locus of control).

construct validity   The degree to which an instrument measures the construct under investigation.

consumer   An individual who reads, reviews, and critiques research findings and who attempts to use and apply the findings in his or her practice.

contact information   Information obtained from study participants in longitudinal studies, to facilitate their relocation at a future date.

contamination   The inadvertent, undesirable influence of one experimental treatment condition on another treatment condition.

content analysis   The process of organizing and integrating narrative, qualitative information according to emerging themes and concepts.

content validity   The degree to which the items in an instrument adequately represent the universe of content for the concept being measured.

content validity index (CVI)   An indicator of the degree to which an instrument is content valid, based on average ratings of a panel of experts.

contingency table   A two-dimensional table that permits a crosstabulation of the frequencies of two categorical variables.

continuous variable   A variable that can take on an infinite range of values along a specified continuum (e.g., height).

control   The process of holding constant possible influences on the dependent variable under investigation.

control group   Subjects in an experiment who do not receive the experimental treatment and whose performance provides a baseline against which the effects of the treatment can be measured (see also *comparison group*).

convenience sampling   Selection of the most readily available persons as participants in a study; also called *accidental sampling.*

convergent validity   An approach to construct validation that involves assessing the degree to which two methods of measuring a construct are similar (i.e., converge).

core category   In a grounded theory study, the central phenomenon that is used to integrate all categories of the data.

correlation   An association or connection between variables, such that variation in one variable is related to variation in another.

correlation coefficient   An index summarizing the degree of relationship between variables, typically ranging from $+1.00$ (for a perfect positive relationship) through 0.0 (for no relationship) to -1.00 (for a perfect negative relationship).

correlation matrix   A two-dimensional display showing the correlation coefficients between all combinations of study variables.

correlational research   Research that explores the interrelationships among variables of interest without any active intervention by the researcher.

cost–benefit analysis   An evaluation of the monetary costs of a program or intervention relative to the monetary gains attributable to it.

counterbalancing   The process of systematically varying the order of presentation of stimuli or treatments to control for ordering effects, especially in a repeated measures design.

counterfactual   The condition or group used as a basis of comparison in a study.

covariate   A variable that is statistically controlled (held constant) in analysis of covariance. The covariate is typically an extraneous, confounding influence on the dependent variable or a preintervention measure of the dependent variable.

covert data collection   The collection of information in a study without participants' knowledge.

Cramér's *V*   An index describing the magnitude of relationship between nominal-level data, used when the contingency table to which it is applied is larger than 2×2.

credibility   A criterion for evaluating data quality in qualitative studies, referring to confidence in the truth of the data.

criterion variable   The criterion against which the effect of an independent variable is tested; sometimes used instead of *dependent variable.*

criterion-related validity   The degree to which scores on an instrument are correlated with some external criterion.

critical case sampling   A sampling approach used by qualitative researchers involving the purposeful selection of cases that are especially important or illustrative.

critical incident technique   A method of obtaining data from study participants by in-depth exploration of specific incidents and behaviors related to the topic under study.

critical region   The area in the sampling distribution representing values that are "improbable" if the null hypothesis is true.

critical theory   An approach to viewing the world that involves a critique of society, with the goal of envisioning new possibilities and effecting social change.

critique   An objective, critical, and balanced appraisal of a research report's various dimensions (e.g., conceptual, methodologic, ethical).

Cronbach's alpha   A widely used reliability index that estimates the internal consistency or homogeneity of a measure composed of several subparts; also called *coefficient alpha.*

crossover design   An experimental design in which one group of subjects is exposed to more than one condition or treatment in random order; sometimes called a *repeated measures design.*

cross-sectional design   A study design in which data are collected at one point in time; sometimes used to infer change over time when data are collected from different age or developmental groups.

crosstabulation   A determination of the number of cases occurring when two variables are considered simultaneously (e.g., gender—male/female—crosstabulated with smoking status—smoker/nonsmoker). The results are typically presented in a table with rows and columns divided according to the values of the variables.

data The pieces of information obtained in the course of a study (singular is *datum*).

data analysis The systematic organization and synthesis of research data, and the testing of research hypotheses using those data.

data cleaning The preparation of data for analysis by performing checks to ensure that the data are consistent and accurate.

data collection The gathering of information to address a research problem.

data collection protocols The formal procedures researchers develop to guide the collection of data in a standardized fashion in most quantitative studies.

data entry The process of entering data onto an input medium for computer analysis.

data saturation See *saturation*.

data set The total collection of data on all variables for all study participants.

data transformation A step often undertaken before data analysis, to put the data in a form that can be meaningfully analyzed (e.g., recoding of values).

data triangulation The use of multiple data sources for the purpose of validating conclusions.

debriefing Communication with study participants after participation is complete regarding various aspects of the study.

deception The deliberate withholding of information, or the provision of false information, to study participants, usually to reduce potential biases.

deductive reasoning The process of developing specific predictions from general principles (see also *inductive reasoning*).

degrees of freedom (*df*) A concept used in statistical testing, referring to the number of sample values free to vary (e.g., with a given sample mean, all but one value would be free to vary); degrees of freedom is often *N*-1, but different formulas are relevant for different tests.

Delphi technique A method of obtaining written judgments from a panel of experts about an issue of concern; experts are questioned individually in several rounds, with a summary of the panel's views circulated between rounds, to achieve some consensus.

demonstration A test of an innovative intervention, often on a large scale, to determine its effectiveness and the desirability of making practice or policy changes.

dependability A criterion for evaluating data quality in qualitative data, referring to the stability of data over time and over conditions.

dependent variable The variable hypothesized to depend on or be caused by another variable (the *independent variable*); the outcome variable of interest.

descriptive research Research studies that have as their main objective the accurate portrayal of the characteristics of persons, situations, or groups, and/or the frequency with which certain phenomena occur.

descriptive statistics Statistics used to describe and summarize data (e.g., mean, standard deviation).

descriptive theory A broad characterization that thoroughly accounts for a single phenomenon.

determinism The belief that phenomena are not haphazard or random, but rather have antecedent causes; an assumption in the positivist paradigm.

deviation score A score computed by subtracting an individual score value from the mean of all scores.

dichotomous variable A variable having only two values or categories (e.g., gender).

direct costs Specific project-related costs incurred in the course of a study (e.g., for salaries of research personnel, supplies, travel, and so on).

directional hypothesis A hypothesis that makes a specific prediction about the direction and nature of the relationship between two variables.

discrete variable A variable with a finite number of values between two points.

discriminant function analysis A statistical procedure used to predict group membership or status on a categorical (nominal level) variable on the basis of two or more independent variables.

discriminant validity An approach to construct validation that involves assessing the degree to which a single method of measuring two constructs yields different results (i.e., discriminates the two).

disproportionate sample   A sample in which the researcher samples differing proportions of study participants from different population strata to ensure adequate representation from smaller strata.

double-blind experiment   An experiment in which neither the subjects nor those who administer the treatment know who is in the experimental or control group.

dummy variable   Dichotomous variables created for use in many multivariate statistical analyses, typically using codes of 0 and 1 (e.g., female = 1, male = 0).

effect size   A statistical expression of the magnitude of the relationship between two variables, or the magnitude of the difference between groups with regard to some attribute of interest.

eigenvalue   In factor analysis, the value equal to the sum of the squared weights for each factor.

electronic database   Bibliographic files that can be accessed by computer for the purpose of conducting a literature review.

element   The most basic unit of a population from which a sample is drawn—typically humans in nursing research.

eligibility criteria   The criteria used to designate the specific attributes of the target population, and by which people are selected for participation in a study.

emergent design   A design that unfolds in the course of a qualitative study as the researcher makes ongoing design decisions reflecting what has already been learned.

emergent fit   A concept in grounded theory that involves comparing new data and new categories with previously existing conceptualizations.

emic perspective   A term used by ethnographers to refer to the way members of a culture themselves view their world; the "insider's view."

empirical evidence   Evidence rooted in objective reality and gathered using one's senses as the basis for generating knowledge.

endogenous variable   In path analysis, a variable whose variation is determined by other variables within the model.

equivalence   The degree of similarity between alternate forms of a measuring instrument.

error of measurement   The deviation between true scores and obtained scores of a measured characteristic.

error term   The mathematic expression (typically in a regression analysis) that represents all unknown or immeasurable attributes that can affect the dependent variable.

eta squared   In ANOVA, a statistic calculated to indicate the proportion of variance in the dependent variable explained by the independent variables, analogous to R^2 in multiple regression.

ethics   A system of moral values that is concerned with the degree to which research procedures adhere to professional, legal, and social obligations to the study participants.

ethnography   A branch of human inquiry, associated with the field of anthropology, that focuses on the culture of a group of people, with an effort to understand the world view of those under study.

ethnomethodology   A branch of human inquiry, associated with sociology, that focuses on the way in which people make sense of their everyday activities and come to behave in socially acceptable ways.

ethnonursing research   The study of human cultures, with a focus on a group's beliefs and practices relating to nursing care and related health behaviors.

etic perspective   A term used by ethnographers to refer to the "outsider's" view of the experiences of a cultural group.

evaluation research   Research that investigates how well a program, practice, or policy is working.

event sampling   In observational studies, a sampling plan that involves the selection of integral behaviors or events.

evidence-based practice   A practice that involves making clinical decisions on the best available evidence, with an emphasis on evidence from disciplined research.

evidence hierarchy   A ranked arrangement of the validity and dependability of evidence based on the rigor of the method that produced it.

ex post facto research   Nonexperimental research conducted after variations in the independent variable have occurred in the natural course of events and therefore any causal explanations are inferred "after the fact."

exclusion criteria   The criteria that specify characteristics that a population does *not* have.

exogenous variable   In path analysis, a variable whose determinants lie outside the model.

experiment   A study in which the researcher controls (manipulates) the independent variable and randomly assigns subjects to different conditions.

experimental group   The subjects who receive the experimental treatment or intervention.

experimental intervention   (experimental treatment) See *intervention; treatment.*

exploratory factor analysis   A factor analysis undertaken to determine the underlying dimensionality of a set of variables.

exploratory research   A study that explores the dimensions of a phenomenon or that develops or refines hypotheses about relationships between phenomena.

external criticism   In historical research, the systematic evaluation of the authenticity and genuineness of data.

external validity   The degree to which study results can be generalized to settings or samples other than the one studied.

extraneous variable   A variable that confounds the relationship between the independent and dependent variables and that needs to be controlled either in the research design or through statistical procedures.

extreme case sampling   A sampling approach used by qualitative researchers that involves the purposeful selection of the most extreme or unusual cases.

extreme response set   A bias in self-report instruments, especially in psychosocial scales, created when participants select extreme response alternatives (e.g., "strongly agree"), independent of the item's content.

F-ratio   The statistic obtained in several statistical tests (e.g., ANOVA) in which variation attributable to different sources (e.g., between groups and within groups) is compared.

face validity   The extent to which a measuring instrument looks as though it is measuring what it purports to measure.

factor analysis   A statistical procedure for reducing a large set of variables into a smaller set of variables with common characteristics or underlying dimensions.

factor extraction   The first phase of a factor analysis, which involves the extraction of as much variance as possible through the successive creation of linear combinations of the variables in the data set.

factor rotation   The second phase of factor analysis, during which the reference axes for the factors are moved such that variables more clearly align with a single factor.

factor score   A person's score on a latent variable (factor).

factor loading   In factor analysis, the weight associated with a variable on a given factor.

factorial design   An experimental design in which two or more independent variables are simultaneously manipulated, permitting a separate analysis of the main effects of the independent variables, plus the interaction effects of those variables.

feasibility study   A small-scale test to determine the feasibility of a larger study (*see also* pilot study).

feminist research   Research that seeks to understand, typically through qualitative approaches, how gender and a gendered social order shape women's lives and their consciousness.

field diary   A daily record of events and conversations in the field; also called a log.

field notes   The notes taken by researchers describing the unstructured observations they have made in the field, and their interpretation of those observations.

field research   Research in which the data are collected "in the field" from individuals in their normal roles, with the aim of understanding the practices, behaviors, and beliefs of individuals or groups as they normally function in real life.

findings   The results of the analysis of research data.

Fisher's exact test   A statistical procedure used to test the significance of the difference in proportions, used when the sample size is small or cells in the contingency table have no observations.

fit   In grounded theory analysis, the process of identifying characteristics of one piece of data and comparing them with the characteristics of another datum to determine similarity.

fixed alternative question   A question that offers respondents a set of prespecified responses, from which the respondent must choose the alternative that most closely approximates the correct response.

focus group interview   An interview with a group of individuals assembled to answer questions on a given topic.

focused interview   A loosely structured interview in which an interviewer guides the respondent through a set of questions using a topic guide.

follow-up study   A study undertaken to determine the outcomes of individuals with a specified condition or who have received a specified treatment.

forced-choice question   A question that requires respondents to choose between two statements that represent polar positions or characteristics.

formal grounded theory   A theory developed at a more abstract level of theory by compiling several substantive grounded theories.

formative evaluation   An ongoing assessment of a product or program as it is being developed, to optimize its quality and effectiveness.

framework   The conceptual underpinnings of a study; often called a *theoretical framework* in studies based on a theory, or *conceptual framework* in studies rooted in a specific conceptual model.

frequency distribution   A systematic array of numeric values from the lowest to the highest, together with a count of the number of times each value was obtained.

frequency polygon   Graphic display of a frequency distribution, in which dots connected by a straight line indicate the number of times score values occur in a data set.

Friedman test   A nonparametric analog of ANOVA, used with paired-groups or repeated measures situations.

full disclosure   The communication of complete information to potential study participants about the nature of the study, the right to refuse participation, and the likely risks and benefits that would be incurred.

functional relationship   A relationship between two variables in which it cannot be assumed that one variable caused the other, but it can be said that one variable changes values in relation to changes in the other variable.

gaining entrée   The process of gaining access to study participants in qualitative field studies through the cooperation of key actors in the selected community or site.

generalizability   The degree to which the research methods justify the inference that the findings are true for a broader group than study participants; in particular, the inference that the findings can be generalized from the sample to the population.

"going native"   A pitfall in ethnographic research wherein a researcher becomes too emotionally involved with participants and therefore loses the ability to observe objectively.

grand theory   A broad theory aimed at describing large segments of the physical, social, or behavioral world; also called a *macrotheory.*

grand tour question   A broad question asked in an unstructured interview to gain a general overview of a phenomenon, on the basis of which more focused questions are subsequently asked.

grant   A financial award made to a researcher or team of researchers to conduct a proposed project.

grantsmanship   The combined set of skills and knowledge needed to secure financial support for a research idea.

graphic rating scale   A scale in which respondents are asked to rate something (e.g., a concept or an issue) along an ordered bipolar continuum (e.g., "excellent" to "very poor").

grounded theory   An approach to collecting and analyzing qualitative data that aims to develop theories and theoretical propositions grounded in real-world observations.

Hawthorne effect   The effect on the dependent variable resulting from subjects' awareness that they are participants under study.

hermeneutics A qualitative research tradition, drawing on interpretive phenomenology, that focuses on the lived experiences of humans, and on how they interpret those experiences.

heterogeneity The degree to which objects are dissimilar (i.e., characterized by high variability) with respect to some attribute.

hierarchical multiple regression A multiple regression analysis in which predictor variables are entered into the equation in steps that are prespecified by the analyst.

histogram A graphic presentation of frequency distribution data.

historical research Systematic studies designed to discover facts and relationships about past events.

history threat The occurrence of events external to an intervention but concurrent with it, which can affect the dependent variable and threaten the study's internal validity.

homogeneity (1) In terms of the reliability of an instrument, the degree to which its subparts are internally consistent (i.e., are measuring the same critical attribute). (2) More generally, the degree to which objects are similar (i.e., characterized by low variability).

homegenous sampling A sampling approach used by qualitative researchers involving the deliberate selection of cases with limited variation.

hypothesis A statement of predicted relationships between variables.

identical (literal) replication An exact duplication of the original methods used in a prior study to determine if similar results are obtained.

impact analysis An evaluation of the effects of a program or intervention on outcomes of interest, net of other factors influencing those outcomes.

implementation analysis In an evaluation, a description of the process by which a program or intervention was implemented in practice.

implementation potential The extent to which an innovation is amenable to implementation in a new setting, an assessment of which is usually made in an evidence-based practice (or research utilization) project.

implied consent Consent to participate in a study that a researcher assumes has been given based on certain actions of the participant (such as returning a completed questionnaire).

IMRAD format The organization of a research report into four sections: the Introduction, Method, Research, and Discussion sections.

incidence rate The rate of new "cases" with a specified condition, determined by dividing the number of new cases over a given period of time by the number at risk of becoming a new case (i.e. free of the condition at the outset of the time period).

independent variable The variable that is believed to cause or influence the dependent variable; in experimental research, the manipulated (treatment) variable.

indirect costs The administrative costs included in a research budget, over and above the specific (direct) costs of conducting the study; also called *overhead*.

inductive reasoning The process of reasoning from specific observations to more general rules (see also *deductive reasoning*).

inferential statistics Statistics that permit inferences on whether relationships observed in a sample are likely to occur in the larger population.

informant A term used to refer to those individuals who provide information to researchers about a phenomenon under study (usually in qualitative studies).

informed consent An ethical principle that requires researchers to obtain the voluntary participation of subjects, after informing them of possible risks and benefits.

inquiry audit An independent scrutiny of qualitative data and relevant supporting documents by an external reviewer, to determine the dependability and confirmability of qualitative data.

Institutional Review Board (IRB) A group of individuals from an institution who convene to review proposed and ongoing studies with respect to ethical considerations.

instrument The device used to collect data (e.g., a questionnaire, test, observation schedule, etc.).

instrumental utilization Clearly identifiable attempts to base some specific action or intervention on the results of research findings.

instrumentation threat The threat to the internal validity of the study that can arise if the researcher changes the measuring instrument between two points of data collection.

integrated design A mixed method design in which there is integration of the method types during all phases of the project.

integrative review A review of research that amasses comprehensive information on a topic, weighs pieces of evidence, and integrates information to draw conclusions about the state of knowledge.

intensity sampling A sampling approach used by qualitative researchers involving the purposeful selection of intense (but not extreme) cases.

intention to treat A principle for analyzing data that involves the assumption that each person received the treatment to which he or she was assigned.

interaction effect The effect of two or more independent variables acting in combination (interactively) on a dependent variable rather than as unconnected factors.

intercoder reliability The degree to which two coders, operating independently, agree in their coding decisions.

internal consistency The degree to which the subparts of an instrument are all measuring the same attribute or dimension, as a measure of the instrument's reliability.

internal criticism In historical research, an evaluation of the worth of the historical evidence.

internal validity The degree to which it can be inferred that the experimental treatment (independent variable), rather than uncontrolled, extraneous factors, is responsible for observed effects.

interpretation The process of making sense of the results of a study and examining their implications.

interrater (interobserver) reliability The degree to which two raters or observers, operating independently, assign the same ratings or values for an attribute being measured or observed.

interrupted time series design. *See* time series design.

interval estimation A statistical estimation approach in which the researcher establishes a range of values that are likely, within a given level of confidence, to contain the true population parameter.

interval measure A level of measurement in which an attribute of a variable is rank ordered on a scale that has equal distances between points on that scale (e.g., Fahrenheit degrees).

intervention In experimental research, the experimental treatment or manipulation.

intervention protocol In experimental research, the specification of exactly what the treatment and the alternative condition (the counterfactual) will be, and how treatments are to be administered.

intervention research A systematic research approach distinguished not so much by a particular research methodology as by a distinctive *process* of planning, developing, implementing, testing, and disseminating interventions.

interview A method of data collection in which one person (an interviewer) asks questions of another person (a respondent); interviews are conducted either face-to-face or by telephone.

interview schedule The formal instrument, used in structured self-report studies, that specifies the wording of all questions to be asked of respondents.

intuiting The second step in descriptive phenomenology, which occurs when researchers remain open to the meaning attributed to the phenomenon by those who experienced it.

inverse relationship A relationship characterized by the tendency of high values on one variable to be associated with low values on the second variable; also called a *negative relationship.*

investigator triangulation The use of two or more researchers to analyze and interpret a data set, to enhance the validity of the findings.

item analysis A type of analysis used to assess whether items on a scale are tapping the same construct and are sufficiently discriminating.

isomorphism In measurement, the correspondence between the measures an instrument yields and reality.

item A single question on a test or questionnaire, or a single statement on an attitude or other scale (e.g., a final examination might consist of 100 items).

joint interview An interview where two or more people are interviewed simultaneously, typically using either a semi-structured or unstructured interview.

jottings Short notes jotted down quickly in the field so as to not distract researchers from their observations or their role as participating members of a group.

journal article A report appearing in professional journals such as *Nursing Research*.

journal club A group that meets regularly (often in clinical settings) to discuss and critique research reports appearing in journals, sometimes to assess the potential use of the findings in practice.

judgmental sampling A type of nonprobability sampling method in which the researcher selects study participants based on personal judgment about who will be most representative or informative; also called *purposive sampling*.

Kendall's tau A correlation coefficient used to indicate the magnitude of a relationship between ordinal-level variables.

key informant A person well-versed in the phenomenon of research interest and who is willing to share the information and insight with the researcher; key informants are often used in needs assessments and ethnographies.

known-groups technique A technique for estimating the construct validity of an instrument through an analysis of the degree to which the instrument separates groups predicted to differ based on known characteristics or theory.

Kruskal-Wallis test A nonparametric test used to test the difference between three or more independent groups, based on ranked scores.

Kuder-Richardson (KR-20) formula A method of calculating an internal consistency reliability coefficient for a scaled set of items when the items are dichotomous.

latent variable An unmeasured variable that represents an underlying, abstract construct (usually in the context of a LISREL analysis).

law A theory that has accrued such persuasive empirical support that it is accepted as true (e.g., Boyle's law of gases).

least-squares estimation A commonly used method of statistical estimation in which the solution minimizes the sums of squares of error terms; also called OLS (ordinary least squares).

level of measurement A system of classifying measurements according to the nature of the measurement and the type of mathematical operations to which they are amenable; the four levels are nominal, ordinal, interval, and ratio.

level of significance The risk of making a Type I error in a statistical analysis, established by the researcher beforehand (e.g., the .05 level).

life history A narrative self-report about a person's life experiences vis-à-vis a theme of interest.

life table analysis A statistical procedure used when the dependent variable represents a time interval between an initial event (e.g., onset of a disease) and an end event (e.g., death); also called *survival analysis*.

Likert scale A composite measure of attitudes involving the summation of scores on a set of items that respondents rate for their degree of agreement or disagreement.

linear regression An analysis for predicting the value of a dependent variable by determining a straight-line fit to the data that minimizes deviations from the line.

LISREL The widely used acronym for linear structural relation analysis, typically used for testing causal models.

listwise deletion A method of dealing with missing values in a data set that involves the elimination of cases with missing data.

literature review A critical summary of research on a topic of interest, often prepared to put a research problem in context.

log In participant observation studies, the observer's daily record of events and conversations that took place.

logical positivism The philosophy underlying the traditional scientific approach; see also *positivist paradigm*.

logistic regression A multivariate regression procedure that analyzes relationships between multiple independent variables and categorical dependent variables; also called *logit analysis*.

logit The natural log of the odds, used as the dependent variable in logistic regression; short for logistic probability unit.

longitudinal study   A study designed to collect data at more than one point in time, in contrast to a cross-sectional study.

macrotheory   A broad theory aimed at describing large segments of the physical, social, or behavioral world; also called a *grand theory.*

main effects   In a study with multiple independent variables, the effects of a single independent variable on the dependent variable.

manifest variable   An observed, measured variable that serves as an indicator of an underlying construct (i.e., a latent variable).

manipulation   An intervention or treatment introduced by the researcher in an experimental or quasi-experimental study to assess its impact on the dependent variable.

manipulation check   In experimental studies, a test to determine whether the manipulation was implemented as intended.

Mann-Whitney *U* test   A nonparametric statistic used to test the difference between two independent groups, based on ranked scores.

MANOVA   See *multivariate analysis of variance.*

marginals   The distribution of grouped data in a crosstabulation, so called because they are found in the margins of the table.

matching   The pairing of subjects in one group with those in another group based on their similarity on one or more dimension, to enhance the overall comparability of groups.

maturation threat   A threat to the internal validity of a study that results when changes to the outcome measure (dependent variable) result from the passage of time.

maximum likelihood estimation   An estimation approach (sometimes used in lieu of the least squares approach) in which the estimators are ones that estimate the parameters most likely to have generated the observed measurements.

maximum variation sampling   A sampling approach used by qualitative researchers involving the purposeful selection of cases with a wide range of variation.

McNemar test   A statistical test for comparing differences in proportions when values are derived from paired (nonindependent) groups.

mean   A descriptive statistic that is a measure of central tendency, computed by summing all scores and dividing by the number of subjects.

measurement   The assignment of numbers to objects according to specified rules to characterize quantities of some attribute.

measurement model   In LISREL, the model that stipulates the hypothesized relationships among the manifest and latent variables.

median   A descriptive statistic that is a measure of central tendency, representing the exact middle value in a score distribution; the value above and below which 50 percent of the scores lie.

median test   A nonparametric statistical test involving the comparison of median values of two independent groups to determine if the groups are from populations with different medians.

mediating variable   A variable that mediates or acts like a "go-between" in a chain linking two other variables (e.g., coping skills may be said to mediate the relationship between stressful events and anxiety).

member check   A method of validating the credibility of qualitative data through debriefings and discussions with informants.

meta-analysis   A technique for quantitatively combining and thus integrating the results of multiple studies on a given topic.

metamatrix   A device sometimes used in a mixed method study that permits researchers to recognize important patterns and themes across data sources and to develop hypotheses.

metasynthesis   The theories, grand narratives, generalizations, or interpretive translations produced from the integration or comparison of findings from qualitative studies.

method triangulation   The use of multiple methods of data collection about the same phenomenon, to enhance the validity of the findings.

methodologic notes   In observational field studies, the researcher's notes about the methods used in collecting data.

methodologic research   Research designed to develop or refine methods of obtaining, organizing, or analyzing data.

methods (research)   The steps, procedures, and strategies for gathering and analyzing data in a research investigation.

middle-range theory A theory that focuses on only a piece of reality or human experience, involving a selected number of concepts (e.g., theories of stress).

minimal risk Anticipated risks that are no greater than those ordinarily encountered in daily life or during the performance of routine tests or procedures.

missing values Values missing from a data set for some study participants, due, for example, to refusals, researcher error, or skip patterns.

mixed-mode strategy An approach to collecting survey data in which efforts are first made to conduct the interview by telephone, but then in-person interviewing is used if a telephone interview cannot be completed.

modality A characteristic of a frequency distribution describing the number of peaks; i.e., values with high frequencies.

moderator variable A variable that affects (moderates) the relationship between the independent and dependant variables.

mode A descriptive statistic that is a measure of central tendency; the score or value that occurs most frequently in a distribution of scores.

model A symbolic representation of concepts or variables, and interrelationships among them.

molar approach A way of making observations about behaviors that entails studying large units of behavior and treating them as a whole.

molecular approach A way of making observations about behavior that uses small and highly specific behaviors as units of observation.

mortality threat A threat to the internal validity of a study, referring to the differential loss of participants (attrition) from different groups.

multimethod research Generally, research in which multiple approaches are used to address a problem; often used to designate studies in which both qualitative and quantitative data are collected and analyzed.

multimodal distribution A distribution of values with more than one peak (high frequency).

multiple classification analysis A variant of multiple regression and ANCOVA that yields group means on the dependent variable adjusted for the effects of covariates.

multiple comparison procedures Statistical tests, normally applied after an ANOVA indicates statistically significant group differences, that compare different pairs of groups; also called *post hoc tests*.

multiple correlation coefficient An index (symbolized as R) that summarizes the degree of relationship between two or more independent variables and a dependent variable.

multiple regression analysis A statistical procedure for understanding the simultaneous effects of two or more independent (predictor) variables on a dependent variable.

multistage sampling A sampling strategy that proceeds through a set of stages from larger to smaller sampling units (e.g., from states, to nursing schools, to faculty members).

multitrait–multimethod matrix method A method of establishing the construct validity of an instrument that involves the use of multiple measures for a set of subjects; the target instrument is valid to the extent that there is a strong relationship between it and other measures purporting to measure the same attribute (convergence) and a weak relationship between it and other measures purporting to measure a different attribute (discriminability).

multivariate analysis of variance (MANOVA) A statistical procedure used to test the significance of differences between the means of two or more groups on two or more dependent variables, considered simultaneously.

multivariate statistics Statistical procedures designed to analyze the relationships among three or more variables; commonly used multivariate statistics include multiple regression, analysis of covariance, and factor analysis.

N The symbol designating the total number of subjects (e.g., "the total N was 500").

n The symbol designating the number of subjects in a subgroup or cell of a study (e.g., "each of the four groups had an n of 125, for a total N of 500").

narrative analysis A type of qualitative approach that focuses on the story as the object of the inquiry.

natural experiment   A nonexperimental study that takes advantage of some naturally occurring event or phenomenon (e.g., an earthquake) that is presumed to have implications for people's behavior or condition, typically by comparing people exposed to the event with those not exposed.

naturalistic paradigm   An alternative paradigm to the traditional positivist paradigm that holds that there are multiple interpretations of reality, and that the goal of research is to understand how individuals construct reality within their context; often associated with qualitative research.

naturalistic setting   A setting for the collection of research data that is natural to those being studied (e.g., homes, places of work, and so on).

needs assessment   A study designed to describe the needs of a group, community, or organization, usually as a guide to policy planning and resource allocation.

negative case analysis   A method of refining a hypothesis or theory in a qualitative study that involves the inclusion of cases that appear to disconfirm earlier hypotheses.

negative relationship   A relationship between two variables in which there is a tendency for higher values on one variable to be associated with lower values on the other (e.g., as temperature increases, people's productivity may decrease); also called an *inverse relationship*.

negative results   Research results that fail to support the researcher's hypotheses.

negatively skewed distribution   An asymmetric distribution of data values with a disproportionately high number of cases having high values—i.e., falling at the upper end of the distribution; when displayed graphically, the tail points to the left.

net effect   The effect of an independent variable on a dependent variable, after controlling for the effect of one or more covariates through multiple regression or ANCOVA.

network sampling   The sampling of participants based on referrals from others already in the sample; also called *snowball sampling*.

nocebo effect   Adverse side effect experienced by those receiving a placebo treatment.

nominal measure   The lowest level of measurement involving the assignment of characteristics into categories (e.g., males, category 1; females, category 2).

nominated sampling   A sampling method in which researchers ask early informants to make referrals to other potential participants.

nondirectional hypothesis   A research hypothesis that does not stipulate in advance the expected direction of the relationship between variables.

nonequivalent control group design   A quasi-experimental design involving a comparison group that was not developed on the basis of random assignment, but from whom preintervention data are obtained so that the initial equivalence of the groups can be assessed.

nonexperimental research   Studies in which the researcher collects data without introducing an intervention.

nonparametric statistical tests   A class of inferential statistical tests that do not involve rigorous assumptions about the distribution of critical variables; most often used with nominal or ordinal data.

nonprobability sampling   The selection of sampling units (e.g., participants) from a population using nonrandom procedures, as in convenience, judgmental, and quota sampling.

nonrecursive model   A causal model that predicts reciprocal effects (i.e., a variable can be both the cause of and an effect of another variable).

nonresponse bias   A bias that can result when a nonrandom subset of people invited to participate in a study fail to participate.

nonsignificant result   The result of a statistical test indicating that group differences or a relationship between variables could have occurred as a result of chance, at a given level of significance; sometimes abbreviated as NS.

normal distribution   A theoretical distribution that is bell-shaped and symmetrical; also called a *normal curve*.

norms   Test-performance standards, based on test score information from a large, representative sample.

null hypothesis   A hypothesis stating no relationship between the variables under study; used primarily in statistical testing as the hypothesis to be rejected.

nursing research Systematic inquiry designed to develop knowledge about issues of importance to the nursing profession.

objectivity The extent to which two independent researchers would arrive at similar judgments or conclusions (i.e., judgments not biased by personal values or beliefs).

oblique rotation In factor analysis, a rotation of factors such that the reference axes are allowed to move to acute or oblique angles and hence the factors are allowed to be correlated.

observational notes An observer's in-depth descriptions about events and conversations observed in naturalistic settings.

observational research Studies in which data are collected by observing and recording behaviors or activities relating to a phenomenon of interest.

observed (obtained) score The actual score or numerical value assigned to a person on a measure.

odds The ratio of two probabilities, namely, the probability of an event occurring to the probability that it will not occur.

odds ratio (OR) The ratio of one odds to another odds; used in logistic regression as a measure of association and as an estimate of relative risk.

on-protocol analysis A principle for analyzing data that includes data only from those members of a treatment group who actually received the treatment.

one-tailed test A test of statistical significance in which only values at one extreme (tail) of a distribution are considered in determining significance; used when the researcher can predict the direction of a relationship (see *directional hypothesis*).

open-ended question A question in an interview or questionnaire that does not restrict respondents' answers to preestablished alternatives.

open coding The first level of coding in a grounded theory study, referring to the basic descriptive coding of the content of narrative materials.

operational definition The definition of a concept or variable in terms of the procedures by which it is to be measured.

operationalization The process of translating research concepts into measurable phenomena.

oral history An unstructured self-report technique used to gather personal recollections of events and their perceived causes and consequences.

ordinal measure A level of measurement that rank orders phenomena along some dimension.

ordinary least squares (OLS) regression Regression analysis that uses the least-squares criterion for estimating the parameters in the regression equation.

orthogonal rotation In factor analysis, a rotation of factors such that the reference axes are kept at right angles, and hence the factors remain uncorrelated.

outcome analysis An evaluation of what happens with regard to outcomes of interest after implementing a program or intervention, without using an experimental design to assess net effects; see also *impact analysis*.

outcome measure A term sometimes used to refer to the dependent variable, i.e., the measure that captures the outcome of an intervention.

outcomes research Research designed to document the effectiveness of health care services and the end results of patient care.

outliers Values that lie outside the normal range of values for other cases in a data set.

p **value** In statistical testing, the probability that the obtained results are due to chance alone; the probability of committing a Type I error.

pair matching See *matching*.

pairwise deletion A method of dealing with missing values in a data set involving the deletion of cases with missing data on a selective basis (i.e., on a variable by variable basis).

panel study A type of longitudinal study in which data are collected from the same people (*a panel*) at two or more points in time, often in the context of a survey.

paradigm A way of looking at natural phenomena that encompasses a set of philosophical assumptions and that guides one's approach to inquiry.

parameter A characteristic of a population (e.g., the mean age of all U.S. citizens).

parametric statistical tests A class of inferential statistical tests that involve (a) assumptions about the distribution of the variables, (b) the estimation of a parameter, and (c) the use of interval or ratio measures.

participant See *study participant.*

participant observation A method of collecting data through the observation of a group or organization in which the researcher participates as a member.

participatory action research A research approach with an ideological perspective; based on the premise that the use and production of knowledge can be political and used to exert power.

path analysis A regression-based procedure for testing causal models, typically using nonexperimental data.

path coefficient The weight representing the impact of one variable on another in a path analytic causal model.

path diagram A graphic representation of the hypothesized linkages and causal flow among variables in a causal relationship.

Pearson's r A widely used correlation coefficient designating the magnitude of relationship between two variables measured on at least an interval scale; also called *the product-moment correlation.*

peer debriefing Sessions with peers to review and explore various aspects of a study—typically in a qualitative study.

peer reviewer A person who reviews and critiques a research report or proposal, who himself/-herself is a researcher (usually working on similar types of research problems as those under review), and who makes a recommendation about publishing or funding the research.

perfect relationship A correlation between two variables such that the values of one variable permit perfect prediction of the values of the other; designated as 1.00 or −1.00.

person triangulation The collection of data from different levels of persons, with the aim of validating data through multiple perspectives on the phenomenon.

personal notes In field studies, written comments about the observer's own feelings during the research process.

personal interview A face-to-face interview between an interviewer and a respondent.

phenomenon The abstract concept under study, most often used by qualitative researchers in lieu of the term "variable".

phenomenology A qualitative research tradition, with roots in philosophy and psychology, that focuses on the lived experience of humans.

phi coefficient A statistical index describing the magnitude of relationship between two dichotomous variables.

photo elicitation An interview stimulated and guided by photographic images.

pilot study A small scale version, or trial run, done in preparation for a major study.

pink sheet For grant applications submitted to the National Institutes of Health, the evaluation form containing the comments and priority score of the peer review panel.

placebo A sham or pseudo intervention, often used as a control condition.

placebo effect Changes in the dependant variable attributable to the placebo condition.

point estimation A statistical estimation procedure in which the researcher uses information from a sample to estimate the single value (statistic) that best represents the value of the population parameter.

point prevalence rate The number of people with a condition or disease divided by the total number at risk, multiplied by the number of people for whom the rate is being established (e.g., per 1000 population).

population The entire set of individuals (or objects) having some common characteristics (e.g., all RNs in the state of California); sometimes called *universe.*

positive relationship A relationship between two variables in which there is a tendency for high values on one variable to be associated with high values on the other (e.g., as physical activity increases, pulse rate also increases).

positive results Research results that are consistent with the researcher's hypotheses.

positively skewed distribution An asymmetric distribution of values with a disproportionately high number of cases having low values—i.e., falling at the lower end of the distribution; when displayed graphically, the tail points to the right.

positivist paradigm The traditional paradigm underlying the scientific approach, which assumes that there is a fixed, orderly reality that can be objectively studied; often associated with quantitative research.

post hoc test A test for comparing all possible pairs of groups following a significant test of overall group differences (e.g., in an ANOVA).

poster session A session at a professional conference in which several researchers simultaneously present visual displays summarizing their studies, while conference attendees circulate around the room perusing the displays.

posttest The collection of data after introducing an experimental intervention.

posttest-only design An experimental design in which data are collected from subjects only after the experimental intervention has been introduced; also called an *after-only design*.

power A research design's ability to detect relationships that exist among variables.

power analysis A procedure for estimating either the likelihood of committing a Type II error or sample size requirements.

prediction The use of empirical evidence to make forecasts about how variables will behave in a new setting and with different individuals.

predictive validity The degree to which an instrument can predict some criterion observed at a future time.

preexperimental design A research design that does not include mechanisms to compensate for the absence of either randomization or a control group.

pretest (1) The collection of data prior to the experimental intervention; sometimes called baseline data. (2) The trial administration of a newly developed instrument to identify flaws or assess time requirements.

pretest-posttest design An experimental design in which data are collected from research subjects both before and after introducing the experimental intervention; also called a *before-after design*.

prevalence study A study undertaken to determine the prevalence rate of some condition (e.g., a disease or a behavior, such as smoking) at a particular point in time.

primary source First-hand reports of facts, findings, or events; in research, the primary source is the original research report prepared by the investigator who conducted the study.

principal investigator (PI) The person who is the lead researcher and who will have primary responsibility for overseeing the project.

probability sampling The selection of sampling units (e.g., participants) from a population using random procedures, as in simple random sampling, cluster sampling, and systematic sampling.

probing Eliciting more useful or detailed information from a respondent in an interview than was volunteered in the first reply.

problem statement The statement of the research problem, often phrased in the form of a research question.

process analysis An evaluation focusing on the process by which a program or intervention gets implemented and used in practice.

process consent In a qualitative study, an ongoing, transactional process of negotiating consent with study participants, allowing them to play a collaborative role in the decision-making regarding their continued participation.

product moment correlation coefficient (r) A widely used correlation coefficient, designating the magnitude of relationship between two variables measured on at least an interval scale; also called *Pearson's r*.

projective technique A method of measuring psychological attributes (values, attitudes, personality) by providing respondents with unstructured stimuli to which to respond.

prolonged engagement In qualitative research, the investment of sufficient time during data collection to have an in-depth understanding of the group under study, thereby enhancing data credibility.

proportional hazards model A model applied in multivariate analyses in which independent variables are used to predict the risk (hazard) of experiencing an event at a given point in time.

proportionate sample A sample that results when the researcher samples from different strata of the population in proportion to their representation in the population.

proposal A document specifying what the researcher proposes to study; it communicates the research problem, its significance, planned procedures for solving the problem, and, when funding is sought, how much the study will cost.

prospective design A study design that begins with an examination of presumed causes (e.g., cigarette smoking) and then goes forward in time to observe presumed effects (e.g., lung cancer).

psychometric assessment An evalution of the quality of an instrument, based primarily on evidence of its reliability and validity.

psychometrics The theory underlying principles of measurement and the application of the theory in the development of measuring tools.

purposive (purposeful) sampling A nonprobability sampling method in which the researcher selects participants based on personal judgment about which ones will be most representative or informative; also called *judgmental sampling.*

Q sort A data collection method in which participants sort statements into a number of piles (usually 9 or 11) according to some bipolar dimension (e.g., most like me/least like me; most useful/least useful).

qualitative analysis The organization and interpretation of nonnumeric data for the purpose of discovering important underlying dimensions and patterns of relationships.

qualitative data Information collected in narrative (nonnumeric) form, such as the transcript of an unstructured interview.

qualitative outcome analysis (QOA). An approach to address the gap between qualitative research and clinical practice, involving the identification and evaluation of clinical interventions based on qualitative findings.

qualitative research The investigation of phenomena, typically in an in-depth and holistic fashion, through the collection of rich narrative materials using a flexible research design.

qualitizing The process of reading and interpreting quantitative data in a qualitative manner.

quantitative analysis The manipulation of numeric data through statistical procedures for the purpose of describing phenomena or assessing the magnitude and reliability of relationships among them.

quantitative data Information collected in a quantified (numeric) form.

quantitative research The investigation of phenomena that lend themselves to precise measurement and quantification, often involving a rigorous and controlled design.

quantitizing The process of coding and analyzing qualitative data quantitatively.

quasi-experiment An intervention study in which subjects are not randomly assigned to treatment conditions, but the researcher exercises certain controls to enhance the study's internal validity.

quasi-statistics An "accounting" system used to assess the validity of conclusions derived from qualitative analysis.

query letter A letter written to a journal editor to ask whether there is any interest in a proposed manuscript (or to a funding source to ask if there is interest in a proposed project).

questionnaire A method of gathering self-report information from respondents through self-administration of questions in a written format.

quota sampling The nonrandom selection of participants in which the researcher prespecifies characteristics of the sample to increase its representativeness.

r The symbol typically used to designate a bivariate correlation coefficient, summarizing the magnitude and direction of a relationship between two variables.

R The symbol used to designate the multiple correlation coefficient, indicating the magnitude (but not direction) of the relationship between the dependent variable and multiple independent variables, taken together.

R^2 The squared multiple correlation coefficient, indicating the proportion of variance in the dependent variable accounted for or explained by a group of independent variables.

random assignment The assignment of subjects to treatment conditions in a random manner (i.e., in a manner determined by chance alone); also called *randomization.*

random number table A table displaying hundreds of digits (from 0 to 9) in random order; each number is equally likely to follow any other.

random sampling The selection of a sample such that each member of a population has an equal probability of being included.

randomization The assignment of subjects to treatment conditions in a random manner (i.e., in a manner determined by chance alone); also called *random assignment.*

randomized block design An experimental design involving two or more factors (independent variables), only one of which in experimentally manipulated.

randomized clinical trial (RCT) A full experimental test of a new treatment, involving random assignment to treatment groups and, typically, a large and diverse sample (also known as a phase III clinical trial).

range A measure of variability, computed by subtracting the lowest value from the highest value in a distribution of scores.

ratio measure A level of measurement with equal distances between scores and a true meaningful zero point (e.g., weight).

raw data Data in the form in which they were collected, without being coded or analyzed.

reactivity A measurement distortion arising from the study participant's awareness of being observed, or, more generally, from the effect of the measurement procedure itself.

readability The ease with which research materials (e.g., a questionnaire) can be read by people with varying reading skills, often empirically determined through readability formulas.

receiver operating characteristic curve (ROC curve) A method used in developing and refining a screening instrument to determine the best cutoff point for "caseness."

rectangular matrix A matrix of data (variables × subjects) that contains no missing values for any variable.

recursive model A path model in which the causal flow is unidirectional, without any feedback loops; opposite of a nonrecursive model.

refereed journal A journal in which decisions about the acceptance of manuscripts are made based on recommendations from peer reviewers.

reflexive notes Notes that document a qualitative researcher's personal experiences, reflections, and progress in the field.

reflexivity In qualitative studies, critical self-reflection about one's own biases, preferences, and preconceptions.

regression analysis A statistical procedure for predicting values of a dependent variable based on the values of one or more independent variables.

relationship A bond or a connection between two or more variables.

relative risk An estimate of risk of "caseness" in one group compared to another, computed by dividing the rate for one group by the rate for another.

reliability The degree of consistency or dependability with which an instrument measures the attribute it is designed to measure.

reliability coefficient A quantitative index, usually ranging in value from .00 to 1.00, that provides an estimate of how reliable an instrument is; computed through such procedures as Cronbach's alpha technique, the split-half technique, test-retest approach, and interrater approaches.

repeated-measures design An experimental design in which one group of subjects is exposed to more than one condition or treatment in random order; also called a *crossover design.*

replication The deliberate repetition of research procedures in a second investigation for the purpose of determining if earlier results can be confirmed.

representative sample A sample whose characteristics are comparable to those of the population from which it is drawn.

research Systematic inquiry that uses orderly, disciplined methods to answer questions or solve problems.

research control See *control.*

research design The overall plan for addressing a research question, including specifications for enhancing the study's integrity.

research hypothesis The actual hypothesis a researcher wishes to test (as opposed to the *null* *hypothesis*), stating the anticipated relationship between two or more variables.

research methods   The techniques used to structure a study and to gather and analyze information in a systematic fashion.

research problem   A situation involving an enigmatic, perplexing, or conflictful condition that can be investigated through disciplined inquiry.

research proposal   See *proposal.*

research question   A statement of the specific query the researcher wants to answer to address a research problem.

research report   A document summarizing the main features of a study, including the research question, the methods used to address it, the findings, and the interpretation of the findings.

research utilization   The use of some aspect of a study in an application unrelated to the original research.

residuals   In multiple regression, the error term or unexplained variance.

respondent   In a self-report study, the study participant responding to questions posed by the researcher.

response rate   The rate of participation in a study, calculated by dividing the number of persons participating by the number of persons sampled.

response set bias   The measurement error introduced by the tendency of some individuals to respond to items in characteristic ways (e.g., always agreeing), independently of the items' content.

results   The answers to research questions, obtained through an analysis of the collected data; in a quantitative study, the information obtained through statistical tests.

retrospective design   A study design that begins with the manifestation of the dependent variable in the present (e.g., lung cancer) and then searches for the presumed cause occurring in the past (e.g., cigarette smoking).

risk–benefit ratio   The relative costs and benefits, to an individual subject and to society at large, of participation in a study; also, the relative costs and benefits of implementing an innovation.

rival hypothesis   An alternative explanation, competing with the researcher's hypothesis, for interpreting the results of a study.

sample   A subset of a population, selected to participate in a study.

sampling   The process of selecting a portion of the population to represent the entire population.

sampling bias   Distortions that arise when a sample is not representative of the population from which it was drawn.

sampling distribution   A theoretical distribution of a statistic, using the values of the statistic computed from an infinite number of samples as the data points in the distribution.

sampling error   The fluctuation of the value of a statistic from one sample to another drawn from the same population.

sampling frame   A list of all the elements in the population, from which the sample is drawn.

sampling plan   The formal plan specifying a sampling method, a sample size, and procedures for recruiting subjects.

saturation   The collection of data in a qualitative study to the point where a sense of closure is attained because new data yield redundant information.

scale   A composite measure of an attribute, involving the combination of several items that have a logical and empirical relationship to each other, resulting in the assignment of a score to place people on a continuum with respect to the attribute.

scatter plot   A graphic representation of the relationship between two variables.

scientific method   A set of orderly, systematic, controlled procedures for acquiring dependable, empirical—and typically quantitative—information; the methodologic approach associated with the positivist paradigm.

scientific merit   The degree to which a study is methodologically and conceptually sound.

screening instrument   An instrument used to determine whether potential subjects for a study meet eligibility criteria (or for determining whether a person has a specified condition).

secondary analysis   A form of research in which the data collected by one researcher are reanalyzed by another investigator to answer new research questions.

secondary source   Second-hand accounts of events or facts; in a research context, a description of a study or studies prepared by someone other than the original researcher.

selective coding A level of coding in a grounded theory study that involves selecting the core category, systematically integrating relationships between the core category and other categories, and validating those relationships.

selection threat (self-selection) A threat to the internal validity of the study resulting from preexisting differences between groups under study; the differences affect the dependent variable in ways extraneous to the effect of the independent variable.

self-determination A person's ability to voluntarily decide whether or not to participate in a study.

self-report A method of collecting data that involves a direct report of information by the person who is being studied (e.g., by interview or questionnaire).

semantic differential A technique used to measure attitudes that asks respondents to rate a concept of interest on a series of bipolar rating scales.

semi-structured interview An interview in which the researcher has listed topics to cover rather than specific questions to ask.

sensitivity The ability of screening instruments to correctly identify a "case," i.e., to correctly diagnose a condition.

sensitivity analysis In a meta-analysis, a method to determine whether conclusions are sensitive to the quality of the studies included.

sequential clinical trial A clinical trial in which data are continuously analyzed and "stop rules" are used to decide when the evidence about the intervention's efficacy is sufficiently strong that the experiment can be stopped.

setting The physical location and conditions in which data collection takes place in a study.

significance level The probability that an observed relationship could be caused by chance (i.e., as a result of sampling error); significance at the .05 level indicates the probability that a relationship of the observed magnitude would be found by chance only 5 times out of 100.

sign system In structured observational research, a system for listing behaviors of interest, when the observation focuses on behaviors that may or may not be manifested by study participants.

sign test A nonparametric test for comparing two paired groups based on the relative ranking of values between the pairs.

simple random sampling The most basic type of probability sampling, wherein a sampling frame is created by enumerating all members of a population, and then selecting a sample from the sampling frame through completely random procedures.

simultaneous multiple regression A multiple regression analysis in which all predictor variables are entered into the equation simultaneously; sometimes called *direct* or *standard* multiple regression.

single-subject experiment An intervention study that typically uses time series designs to test the effectiveness of an intervention with a single subject.

site The overall location where a study is undertaken.

skewed distribution The asymmetric distribution of a set of data values around a central point.

snowball sampling The selection of participants through referrals from earlier participants; also called *network sampling.*

social desirability response set A bias in self-report instruments created when participants have a tendency to misrepresent their opinions in the direction of answers consistent with prevailing social norms.

Solomon four-group design An experimental design that uses a before-after design for one pair of experimental and control groups, and an after-only design for a second pair.

space triangulation The collection of data on the same phenomenon in multiple sites, to enhance the validity of the findings.

Spearman-Brown prophecy formula An equation for making corrections to a reliability estimate calculated by the split-half technique.

Spearman's rank-order correlation (Spearman's rho) A correlation coefficient indicating the magnitude of a relationship between variables measured on the ordinal scale.

specificity   The ability of a screening instrument to correctly identify noncases.

split-half technique   A method for estimating internal consistency reliability by correlating scores on half of the instrument with scores on the other half.

standard deviation   The most frequently used statistic for measuring the degree of variability in a set of scores.

standard error   The standard deviation of a sampling distribution, such as the sampling distribution of the mean.

standard scores   Scores expressed in terms of standard deviations from the mean, with raw scores transformed to have a mean of zero and a standard deviation of one; also called z scores.

statement of purpose   A broad declarative statement of the overall goals of a study.

statistic   An estimate of a parameter, calculated from sample data.

statistical analysis   The organization and analysis of quantitative data using statistical procedures, including both descriptive and inferential statistics.

statistical conclusion validity   The degree to which conclusions about relationships and differences from a statistical analysis of the data are legitimate.

statistical control   The use of statistical procedures to control extraneous influences on the dependent variable.

statistical inference   The process of inferring attributes about the population based on information from a sample, using laws of probability.

statistical power   The ability of the research design to detect true relationships among variables.

statistical significance   A term indicating that the results from an analysis of sample data are unlikely to have been caused by chance, at some specified level of probability.

statistical test   An analytic tool that estimates the probability that obtained results from a sample reflect true population values.

stepwise multiple regression   A multiple regression analysis in which predictor variables are entered into the equation in steps, in the order in which the increment to R is greatest.

stipend   A monetary payment to individuals participating in a study to serve as an incentive for participation and/or to compensate for time and expenses.

strata   Subdivisions of the population according to some characteristic (e.g., males and females); singular is *stratum.*

stratified random sampling   The random selection of study participants from two or more strata of the population independently.

structural equations   Equations representing the magnitude and nature of hypothesized relations among sets of variables in a theory.

structured data collection   An approach to collecting information from participants, either through self-report or observations, in which the researcher determines response categories in advance.

study section   Within the National Institutes of Health, a group of peer reviewers that evaluates grant applications in the first phase of the review process.

study participant   An individual who participates and provides information in a study.

subgroup effect   The differential effect of the independent variable on the dependent variable for various subsets of the sample.

subject   An individual who participates and provides data in a study; term used primarily in quantitative research.

summated rating scale   See *Likert scale.*

survey research   Nonexperimental research that focusses on obtaining information regarding the activities, beliefs, preferences, and attitudes of people via direct questioning of a sample of respondents.

survival analysis   A statistical procedure used when the dependent variable represents a time interval between an initial event (e.g., onset of a disease) and an end event (e.g., death); also called life *table analysis.*

symmetric distribution   A distribution of values with two halves that are mirror images of the each other; a distribution that is not skewed.

systematic extension replication   A replication of an earlier study wherein methods are not duplicated, but deliberate attempts are made to test the implication of the original research.

systematic sampling   The selection of study participants such that every *kth* (e.g., every tenth) person (or element) in a sampling frame or list is chosen.

table of random numbers   See *random number table*.

table shells   A table without any numeric values, prepared in advance of data analysis as a guide to the analyses to be performed.

target population   The entire population in which the researcher is interested and to which he or she would like to generalize the results of a study.

test statistic   A statistic used to test for the statistical significance of relationships between variables; the sampling distributions of test statistics are known for circumstances in which the null hypothesis is true; examples include chi-square, *F*-ratio, *t*, and Pearson's *r*.

test–retest reliability   Assessment of the stability of an instrument by correlating the scores obtained on repeated administrations.

testing threat   A threat to a study's internal validity that occurs when the administration of a pretest or baseline measure of a dependent variable results in changes on the variable, apart from the effect of the independent variable.

theme   A recurring regularity emerging from an analysis of qualitative data.

theoretical notes   In field studies, notes detailing the researcher's interpretations of observed behavior.

theoretical sampling   In qualitative studies, the selection of sample members based on emerging findings as the study progresses, to ensure adequate representation of important themes.

theory   An abstract generalization that presents a systematic explanation about the relationships among phenomena.

theory triangulation   The use of competing theories or hypotheses in the analysis and interpretation of data.

thick description   A rich and thorough description of the research context in a qualitative study.

time sampling   In observational research, the selection of time periods during which observations will take place.

time series design   A quasi-experimental design involving the collection of data over an extended time period, with multiple data collection points both prior to and after an intervention.

time triangulation   The collection of data on the same phenomenon or about the same people at different points in time, to enhance the validity of the findings.

topic guide   A list of broad question areas to be covered in a semistructured interview or focus group interview.

tracing   Procedures used to relocate subjects to avoid attrition in a longitudinal study.

transferability   The extent to which findings can be transferred to other settings or groups—often used in qualitative studies and analogous to generalizability.

treatment   The experimental intervention under study; the condition being manipulated.

treatment group   The group receiving the intervention being tested; the experimental group.

trend study   A form of longitudinal study in which different samples from a population are studied over time with respect to some phenomenon (e.g., annual Gallup polls on abortion attitudes).

triangulation   The use of multiple methods to collect and interpret data about a phenomenon, so as to converge on an accurate representation of reality.

true score   A hypothetical score that would be obtained if a measure were infallible.

trustworthiness   The degree of confidence qualitative researchers have in their data, assessed using the criteria of credibility, transferability, dependability, and confirmability.

***t*-test**   A parametric statistical test for analyzing the difference between two means.

Type I error   An error created by rejecting the null hypothesis when it is true (i.e., the researcher concludes that a relationship exists when in fact it does not).

Type II error   An error created by accepting the null hypothesis when it is false (i.e., the researcher concludes that *no* relationship exists when in fact it does).

two-tailed tests Statistical tests in which both ends of the sampling distribution are used to determine improbable values.

unimodal distribution A distribution of values with one peak (high frequency).

unit of analysis The basic unit or focus of a researcher's analysis; in nursing research, the unit of analysis is typically the individual study participant.

univariate descriptive study A study that gathers information on the occurrence, frequency of occurrence, or average value of the variables of interest, one variable at a time, without focusing on interrelationships among variables.

univariate statistics Statistical procedures for analyzing a single variable for purposes of description.

unstructured interview An oral self-report in which the researcher asks a respondent questions without having a predetermined plan regarding the content or flow of information to be gathered.

unstructured observation The collection of descriptive information through direct observation that is not guided by a formal, prespecified plan for observing, enumerating, or recording the information.

utilization See *research utilization.*

validity The degree to which an instrument measures what it is intended to measure.

validity coefficient A quantitative index, usually ranging in value from .00 to 1.00, that provides an estimate of how valid an instrument is.

variability The degree to which values on a set of scores are dispersed.

variable An attribute of a person or object that varies, that is, takes on different values (e.g., body temperature, age, heart rate).

variance A measure of variability or dispersion, equal to the standard deviation squared.

vignette A brief description of an event, person, or situation about which respondents are asked to describe their reactions.

virtual (operational) replication A replication of an earlier study wherein the researcher approximates the methods used in the reference study.

visual analogue scale A scaling procedure used to measure certain clinical symptoms (e.g., pain, fatigue) by having people indicate on a straight line the intensity of the symptom.

vulnerable subjects Special groups of people whose rights in research studies need special protection because of their inability to provide meaningful informed consent or because their circumstances place them at higher-than-average-risk of adverse effects; examples include young children, the mentally retarded, and unconscious patients.

weighting A correction procedure used to arrive at population values when a disproportionate sampling design has been used.

Wilcoxon signed ranks test A nonparametric statistical test for comparing two paired groups, based on the relative ranking of values between the pairs.

wild code A coded value that is not legitimate within the coding scheme for that data set.

Wilk's lambda An index used in discriminant function analysis to indicate the proportion of variance in the dependent variable *un*accounted for by predictors; $(\lambda) = 1 - R^2$.

within-subjects design A research design in which a single group of subjects is compared under different conditions or at different points in time (e.g., before and after surgery).

z **score** A standard score, expressed in terms of standard deviations from the mean.

INDEX

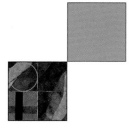

Page numbers in bold type indicate glossary entries.